Steve Goldstein

MAYO
INTERNAL MEDICINE
BOARD REVIEW
2000 - 01

MAYO
INTERNAL MEDICINE
BOARD REVIEW
2000 - 01

Udaya B. S. Prakash, M.D.
Editor-in-Chief

Thomas M. Habermann, M.D.
Associate Editor

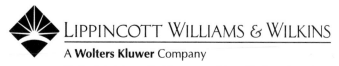

LIPPINCOTT WILLIAMS & WILKINS
A **Wolters Kluwer** Company
Philadelphia · Baltimore · New York · London
Buenos Aires · Hong Kong · Sydney · Tokyo

Acquisitions Editor: Richard Winters
Developmental Editor: Delois Patterson
Production Editor: Robert Pancotti
Manufacturing Manager: Tim Reynolds
Cover Designer: Jeffrey A. Satre
Printer: Courier Westford

Library of Congress Cataloging-in-Publication Data

Mayo internal medicine board review, 2000-01 / Udaya B.S. Prakash,
    editor-in-chief.
        p.   cm.
    Includes bibliographical references and index.
    ISBN 0-7817-2393-0
    1. Internal medicine—Outlines, syllabi, etc. 2. Internal medicine—
Examinations, questions, etc. I. Prakash, Udaya B.S. II. Mayo Foundation
for Medical Education and Research.
    [DNLM: 1. Internal Medicine—Examination Questions.
    2. Internal Medicine—Outlines. WB 18.2 M473 2000]
RC59.M392 2000
616'.0076—dc21
                                                            99-054284

Care has been taken to confirm the accuracy of the information presented and to describe generally accepted practices. However, the authors, editors, and publisher are not responsible for errors or omissions or for any consequences from application of the information in this book and make no warranty, express or implied, with respect to the contents of the publication. This book should not be relied on apart from the advice of a qualified health care provider.

The authors, editors, and publisher have exerted efforts to ensure that drug selection and dosage set forth in this text are in accordance with current recommendations and practice at the time of publication. However, in view of ongoing research, changes in government regulations, and the constant flow of information relating to drug therapy and drug reactions, the reader is urged to check the package insert for each drug for any change in indications and dosage and for added warnings and precautions. This is particularly important when the recommended agent is a new or infrequently employed drug.

Some drugs and medical devices presented in this publication have Food and Drug Administration (FDA) clearance for limited use in restricted research settings. It is the responsibility of the health care providers to ascertain the FDA status of each drug or device planned for use in their clinical practice.

DEDICATED TO

Residents and Fellows, past and present, of
Mayo Clinic and Mayo Foundation and
Mayo Graduate School of Medicine

FOREWORD

The fourth edition of *Mayo Internal Medicine Board Review 2000-01* is a manifestation of the continued commitment of the faculty members of the Department of Internal Medicine to the academic enterprise and to providing an up-to-date resource in clinical internal medicine. One of the key traditions in medicine is the passing of knowledge from physician to physician. Charles H. Mayo, M.D., once wrote, "There are two objects of medical education: to heal the sick and to advance the science." This edition provides information that will help to promote these two goals. In addition, it will aid in the study of medicine and care of patients.

Nicholas F. LaRusso, M.D.
Chair, Department of Internal Medicine
Mayo Clinic, Rochester, Minnesota

EDITORIAL AND PRODUCTION STAFF

Editor-in-Chief   Udaya B. S. Prakash, M.D.

Associate Editor   Thomas M. Habermann, M.D.

Editors   O. E. Millhouse, Ph.D.
                                             LeAnn M. Stee

Art Director   Jeffrey A. Satre

Editorial Assistant   Margery J. Lovejoy

Proofreader   Dorothy L. Tienter

Computer Scientific Illustrators   Marcia W. Blackburn
                                             Mark J. Curry
                                             Diane M. Knight

Digital Printing Coordinator   Thomas F. Flood

Production Advisers   Vicky L. Huebner
                                             Roberta J. Schwartz
                                             Ronald R. Ward

PREFACE

Among the greatest achievements of the 20th century are the astounding advances in the field of medicine. The new century and the millennium will undoubtedly bring forth further advances in medicine at a greater pace. These changes require physicians to remain abreast of the latest developments in their areas of expertise. To assist physicians in this endeavor, the Mayo Clinic remains committed to providing continuing medical education to physicians on a timely basis. This book, *Mayo Internal Medicine Board Review 2000-01*, is designed to meet the needs of physicians-in-training and practicing clinicians by not only updating their knowledge in internal medicine but also helping them prepare for the certifying and recertifying examinations in internal medicine.

The success of the earlier editions of the *Mayo Internal Medicine Board Review* is exemplified by use of the book as the course syllabus for several board review courses and by the publication of similar board review books by other authors. The authors of this edition are very gratified by the response of the readers to the earlier editions. The positive reaction and the success enjoyed by the earlier editions prompted the Department of Internal Medicine at Mayo Clinic to proceed with the publication of this, the fourth edition of *Mayo Internal Medicine Board Review 2000-01*. On behalf of the authors, the production staff, and the Department of Internal Medicine at Mayo, I am pleased and honored to present the latest edition to our readers.

Once again, the topics are divided into major subspecialty areas and are authored by physicians with special interest and clinical expertise in respective subjects. The other formats remain unchanged. The repetition of important points in the form of "pearls" after many of the paragraphs is aimed at stressing the clinical aspects of the topics. Many readers have informed us that this format helped them in their last-minute preparation for the boards. The multiple-choice questions with a single answer follow each chapter. As many clinical cases as possible are included in the questions. This edition has more than 500 multiple-choice questions. Answers with explanatory notes follow the questions. The material in the questions and answers is not included in the index.

Several points from the earlier editions need repetition. This book is not a comprehensive textbook of internal medicine. It should be used only as a guide containing selected topics considered important for physicians preparing for either the certifying or the recertifying examinations offered by the American Board of Internal Medicine or other examining institutions. This book is prepared under the assumption that readers have studied at length one of the standard textbooks of internal medicine before studying this review.

The authors and I thank readers who offered many important ideas for improvement. I am grateful to the authors of the previous editions who provided input into this edition and permitted the use of some of their material in this edition. I am indebted to all authors for their timely completion of the manuscripts. Once again, I thank the staff of the Section of Scientific Publications, Department of Internal Medicine, and Visual Information Services at Mayo Clinic for their help in bringing forth this edition. The support and cooperation by the publisher, Lippincott Williams & Wilkins, is gratefully acknowledged.

I trust that the fourth edition of the *Mayo Internal Medicine Board Review* will be granted the same accolades earned by the earlier editions.

Udaya B. S. Prakash, M.D.
Editor-in-Chief

MAYO
INTERNAL MEDICINE
BOARD REVIEW
2000 - 01

CHAPTER 1

THE BOARD EXAMINATION

Udaya B. S. Prakash, M.D.
Darryl S. Chutka, M.D.

A substantial number of physicians take the American Board of Internal Medicine (ABIM) certifying examination in internal medicine (IM) annually. The total number of candidates who took the ABIM certifying examination in 1998 was 10,603: 7,345 were first-time takers and 3,258 were repeaters. Of this group, 66% passed: 84% of those taking the examination for the first time and 27% of the repeaters. A greater importance is being placed on achieving board certification. Many managed-care organizations are now insisting on board certification before employment. The discussion in this chapter is aimed primarily at candidates preparing for the ABIM's certifying or recertifying examinations in IM. However, candidates preparing for non-ABIM examinations also may benefit from the discussion, which covers various aspects of preparation for an examination, strategies to answer the questions effectively, and avoidance of pitfalls.

AIM OF THE EXAMINATION

The ABIM has stated that the certifying examination tests the breadth and depth of a candidate's knowledge in IM to ensure that the candidate has attained the necessary proficiency required for the practice of IM. According to the ABIM, the examination has two goals: the first is to ensure competence in the diagnosis and treatment of common disorders that have important consequences for patients, and the second is to ensure excellence in the broad domain of IM.

EXAMINATION FORMAT

The examination for ABIM certification in IM requires 2 days to complete and is divided into four sections; morning sessions are 4 hours and afternoon sessions are 3.5 hours. The dates for the next two examinations are as follows: August 22-23, 2000, and August 21-22, 2001. More details regarding the examination, training requirements, eligibility requirements, application forms, and other related information can be obtained from the American Board of Internal Medicine,

510 Walnut Street, Suite 1700, Philadelphia, PA 19106-3699 (telephone numbers: 215-446-3500 or 800-441-2246; fax number: 215-446-3470). The Internet address of the ABIM is http://www.abim.org.

The examination consists of several hundred questions. Candidates should know that several questions known as field questions or pretest questions are included for experimental purposes only. These cannot be identified during the examination, and the answers to these are not scored. Because there is no penalty for guessing the answers, candidates should *answer every question*. Marking multiple answers for a single question is not allowed and will cause the question to be scored as incorrect. Most questions (75%) are based on the presentations of patients. Among these, 75% are in the setting of outpatient or emergency room encounters, and the remaining 25% are in the inpatient setting, including the critical care unit and nursing home. The ability to answer these questions requires integration of information provided from several sources (such as history, physical examination, laboratory test results, and consultations), prioritization of alternatives, or use of clinical judgment in reaching a correct conclusion. The overall ability to manage the patient in the most cost-effective fashion is stressed. Questions that require simple recall of medical facts are in the minority. The question format and examples are shown below.

- Candidates should answer every question; there is no penalty for guessing.
- Most questions (75%) are based on presentations of patients.
- Questions that require simple recall of medical facts are in the minority.

A list of normal laboratory values and illustrative materials (electrocardiograms, blood smears, Gram stains, urine sediments, chest radiographs, and photomicrographs) necessary to answer questions are provided in a separate atlas. Candidates should interpret the abnormal values on the basis of the normal values provided in the atlas and not on the basis of the normal values to which they are accustomed in their practice or training. Candidates for the certifying examination receive an information booklet several weeks before the examination. The booklet provides a detailed description of the examination, including the types of questions used. Although much of the information contained in this chapter is borrowed from the previous information booklets, candidates for ABIM examinations should read the booklet that is sent to them because the ABIM may change the format of the examination.

- A list of normal laboratory values and illustrative materials necessary to answer questions are provided.
- Read the information booklet sent several weeks before the examination by the ABIM.

SCORING

The passing scores reflect predetermined standards set by the ABIM. Passing scores are determined before the examination and therefore are not dependent on the performance of any group of candidates taking the examination.

- Passing scores are set before the examination.

THE CONTENT

The questions in the examination cover a broad area of IM, as listed below. They are divided into "primary" and "cross-content" groups. In the past few years, the subspecialties included in the primary content areas have included cardiovascular diseases, gastroenterology, pulmonary diseases, infectious diseases, rheumatology/orthopedics, endocrinology/metabolism, oncology, hematology, nephrology/urology, neurology, psychiatry, allergy and immunology, dermatology, obstetrics/gynecology, ophthalmology, otolaryngology, and miscellaneous. The specialties in the cross-content group have included adolescent medicine, critical care medicine, clinical epidemiology, ethics, geriatrics, nutrition, occupational medicine, preventive medicine, and substance abuse. Approximately 75% of the questions test knowledge in the following major specialties in IM: cardiology, endocrinology, gastroenterology, hematology, infectious diseases, nephrology, oncology, pulmonary diseases, and rheumatology. The remaining 25% of questions cover allergy/immunology, dermatology, gynecology, neurology, ophthalmology, and psychiatry. Independent of primary content, about 40% of the questions encompass the cross-content topics.

- About 75% of the questions test knowledge in the major specialties.
- About 25% of the questions cover allergy/immunology, dermatology, gynecology, neurology, ophthalmology, and psychiatry.
- About 40% of all questions encompass the cross-content topics: adolescent medicine, critical care medicine, clinical epidemiology, ethics, geriatrics, nutrition, occupational medicine, preventive medicine, and substance abuse.

Table 1-1 shows the distribution of the contents for a recent ABIM certifying examination in IM.

Table 1-1.—Contents of the 1999 Certification Examination of the American Board of Internal Medicine

Content	Percent
Primary content	
Cardiovascular	14
Gastroenterology	10
Pulmonary	10
Infectious disease	9
Rheumatology/orthopedics	8
Endocrinology/metabolism	7
Medical oncology	7
Hematology	6
Nephrology/urology	6
Allergy/immunology	5
Psychiatry	4
Neurology	4
Dermatology	3
Obstetrics/gynecology	2
Ophthalmology	2
Miscellaneous	3
Cross-content	
Geriatric medicine	10
Critical care medicine	10
Prevention	6
Women's health	6
Clinical epidemiology	3
Ethics	3
Nutrition	3
Adolescent medicine	2
Occupational/environmental medicine	2
Substance abuse	2

From ABIM News Update: 1999 Internal Medicine Certification Examination. American Board of Internal Medicine, Philadelphia, Spring 1999. By permission.

QUESTION FORMAT

All questions are multiple-choice, single-best–answer type. This format reflects a change that began with the 1995 examination. The question may include a case history, a brief statement, a radiograph, a graph, or a picture (such as a blood smear or Gram stain). Each question has five possible answers, and the candidates should identify the *single-best* answer. It is essential to realize that more than one answer may appear correct or partially correct for a question. It is also possible that the traditionally correct answer will not be listed as an option. In these situations, the one answer that is better than the others should be selected. As noted above, most questions are based on encounters with patients. Some questions are progressive; that is, more than one question is based on the same patient. The examples in this chapter, the questions at the end of each chapter in this book, and the examples included in the ABIM's information booklet should help candidates become familiar with the question format. Furthermore, the national in-training examination taken by the majority of all second-year residents in IM provides ample opportunity to become familiar with the question format.

- All questions are of the *single-best–answer* type.
- Become familiar with the question format by using various study guides.

EXAMPLES

Select *one best answer* for each of the following questions (answers are provided on page 5).

1. A 56-year-old woman is referred to you for an evaluation of dyspnea and chest pain of 6 weeks in duration. The chest pain is nonpleuritic, nonexertional, and located along the lower right lateral chest cage. She has no fever, cough, or chills. During the past few weeks, she has been experiencing constant low back pain. The patient underwent right mastectomy 4 years ago because of carcinoma of the breast with metastatic involvement of the right axillary lymph nodes. She received radiotherapy followed by chemotherapy for 24 months. Examination now reveals diminished breath sounds in the right lower lung field. The remainder of the examination is unremarkable. A chest radiograph suggests a moderate right pleural effusion. Which of the following is most likely to be helpful in confirming the suspected diagnosis?
   a. Bone scan with technetium 99m diphosphonate
   b. Bone marrow aspirate and biopsy
   c. Scalene fat pad biopsy
   d. Thoracentesis
   e. Mammography

2. A 20-year-old male military recruit returns home from several weeks of summer training in boot camp. He appears in your office the following day with a 12-day history of fever (38°C), coryza, pharyngitis, and cough. Physical examination discloses a bullous lesion over the right tympanic membrane and scattered crackles in both lung fields. Blood cell count reveals mild thrombocytopenia. A chest radiograph demonstrates patchy alveolar-interstitial infiltrates in both lungs. Which of the following is the best treatment for this patient?
   a. Erythromycin
   b. Penicillin
   c. Trimethoprim
   d. Clindamycin
   e. Ceftazidime

3. A 49-year-old male executive comes to your office with a 6-month history of cough, shortness of breath, and chest tightness soon after significant exertion. He notices these symptoms soon after he finishes a game of racquetball. He is a nonsmoker and has no risk factors for coronary artery disease. Results of physical examination in your office are normal. His weight is normal for his height. The chest radiograph is normal. A treadmill test for ischemic heart disease is negative. Which of the following diagnostic tests is indicated?
   a. Computed tomography of the chest
   b. Arterial blood gas studies at rest and after exercise
   c. Spirometry before and after exercise
   d. Ventilation-perfusion lung scan
   e. Cardiopulmonary exercise testing

4. Which of the following is *not* a clinical feature of infection caused by *Pneumocystis carinii* in adult patients with acquired immunodeficiency syndrome (AIDS) when compared with immunosuppressed patients without AIDS?
   a. Longer duration of symptoms
   b. Higher arterial oxygen tension
   c. Greater incidence of side effects from trimethoprim-sulfamethoxazole
   d. Recurrence or persistence of *P. carinii* infection
   e. The number of organisms seen microscopically is usually scanty

5. A hospitalized patient with AIDS dies of disseminated infection caused by *Mycobacterium avium* complex. Cough develops in the 28-year-old resident physician who cared for this patient. A chest radiograph reveals a nodular infiltrate in the right upper lobe. Tuberculin skin test (PPD) is positive (12 mm). Which of the following is the most appropriate next step?

a. Begin antituberculous therapy with at least four drugs because *M. avium* is resistant to two-drug therapy
b. Obtain sputum and gastric washings for stain and culture of tubercle bacilli
c. Order human immunodeficiency virus (HIV) serologic testing now and in 6 months
d. Begin prophylactic isoniazid therapy 300 mg/day for 12 months
e. Treat with isoniazid 300 mg/day and rifampin 600 mg/day for 9 months

6. A 37-year-old woman presents with a history of recurrent palpebral swelling, laryngospasm, and urticaria-like skin lesions. A similar history is present among three family members. Which one of the following is *not* true of this disease?
    a. It can be mediated by IgE and IgG
    b. The precise cause is not identifiable in most patients
    c. It may be precipitated by drugs, contrast dye, or surgical procedures
    d. It is associated with a high mortality
    e. C1-esterase inhibitor is always absent

7. Which of the following pulmonary diagnoses cannot be established by bronchoalveolar lavage?
    a. Pulmonary alveolar proteinosis
    b. *Pneumocystis carinii* infection
    c. Pulmonary tuberculosis
    d. Idiopathic pulmonary fibrosis
    e. Lymphangitic pulmonary metastasis

8. A 68-year-old woman, nonsmoker, presents with an 8-week history of low-grade fever, malaise, myalgias, sore throat, hoarseness, and cough. She also complains of headaches, cramps in the jaws, and intermittent visual blurring. The leukocyte count is normal, and the erythrocyte sedimentation rate is 86 mm in 1 hr. A chest radiograph is normal. Which of the following treatments is likely to resolve these symptoms?
    a. Cranial radiation and chemotherapy
    b. Itraconazole
    c. Corticosteroid
    d. Amantadine
    e. Antiplatelet therapy (aspirin)

9. A 34-year-old woman comes to your office with a 4-week history of hemoptysis, intermittent wheeze, and generalized weakness. Examination reveals that her blood pressure is 186/112 mm Hg. She appears cushingoid and has noted these changes taking place during the past 12 weeks. Auscultation discloses localized wheezing in the left mid-lung area. The chest radiograph indicates partial atelectasis of the left upper lobe. She is referred to you for further evaluations. Which of the following is least likely to provide useful information for diagnosis and treatment?
    a. Serum adrenocorticotropic hormone (ACTH) level
    b. 24-Hour urine test for 5-hydroxyindoleacetic acid (5-HIAA) level
    c. Bronchoscopy
    d. Computed tomography of the chest
    e. Serum potassium level

10. A lung biopsy in a middle-aged man with a diffuse lung process is interpreted as showing lymphocytic interstitial pneumonitis. This abnormality may be encountered in all of the following *except*:
    a. Diffuse alveolar cell carcinoma
    b. Chronic lymphocytic leukemia
    c. Sjögren syndrome
    d. Patients with acquired immunodeficiency syndrome (AIDS)
    e. Lymphomatoid granulomatosis

11. A 42-year-old man who is an office worker presents to the emergency room with acute dyspnea. He has smoked 1 1/2 packs per day for 25 years and had been relatively asymptomatic except for a smoker's cough and mild dyspnea on exertion. Physical examination findings are not remarkable except for slightly diminished intensity of breath sounds over the right lung and some prolonged expiratory slowing, consistent with obstructive lung disease. The chest radiograph is shown below. Which of the following entities is most likely responsible for this patient's symptoms?
    a. Pulmonary alveolar proteinosis
    b. Silicosis
    c. Pulmonary eosinophilic granuloma (histiocytosis X)
    d. Idiopathic pulmonary fibrosis
    e. Sarcoidosis

12. In a 34-year-old man with acute myelomonocytic leukemia, fever and progressive respiratory distress develop, and the chest radiograph shows diffuse alveolar infiltrates. The patient completed intensive chemotherapy 6 weeks earlier. The total leukocyte count has remained less than 900/mm^3 for more than 3 weeks. He is currently (for at least 10 days) receiving a cephalosporin (ceftazidime). Which of the following is the most appropriate therapy for this patient?
    a. Clindamycin
    b. Blood transfusion to increase the number of circulating leukocytes

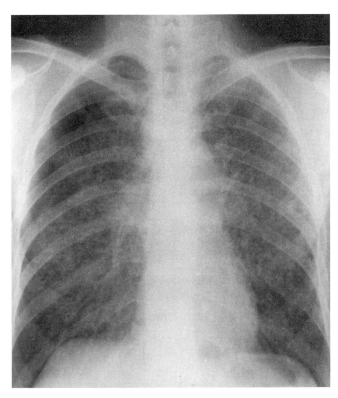

(Chest radiograph courtesy of Edward C. Rosenow III, M.D.)

    c. Antituberculous (triple-drug) therapy
    d. Amphotericin intravenously
    e. Pentamidine aerosol

The answers to the questions are as follows: 1, d (metastatic pleural effusion); 2, a (*Mycoplasma* infection); 3, c (exercise-induced asthma); 4, e; 5, b; 6, e (hereditary angioneurotic edema); 7, d; 8, c (giant cell arteritis); 9, b (bronchial carcinoid); 10, a; 11, c (pulmonary eosinophilic granuloma with spontaneous pneumothorax); 12, d (disseminated aspergillosis in a leukopenic patient).

Questions 1 through 3 are examples of questions that are aimed at evaluating knowledge and judgment about problems that are encountered frequently in practice and for which physician intervention makes a significant difference. These questions judge the candidate's minimal level of clinical competence. Questions 1 through 3 include descriptions of typical clinical features of metastatic breast carcinoma, *Mycoplasma* pneumonia, and exercise-induced asthma, respectively. Therefore, the decision making is relatively easy and straightforward. Questions 4 through 12 are more difficult to answer because they are structured to reflect excellence in clinical competence rather than just minimal competence. In other words, they require more extensive knowledge (that is, knowledge beyond that required for minimal competence) in IM and its subspecialties. Although most of the questions in this chapter are based on encounters with patients, some (questions 4, 7, and 10) require recall of well-known medical facts. A minority of questions in the ABIM examination are in this category.

PREPARATION FOR THE TEST

Training during medical school forms the foundation on which advanced clinical knowledge is accumulated during residency training. However, the serious preparation for the examination actually starts at the beginning of the residency training in IM. Most candidates will require a minimum of 6 to 8 months of intense preparation for the examination. Cramming just before the examination is counterproductive. Some of the methods for preparation for the board examination are described below. Additionally, each candidate may develop her or his own system.

- Preparation for the ABIM examination starts at the beginning of the residency training in IM.

It is essential that each candidate study a standard textbook of medicine from beginning to end. Any of the standard textbooks on IM should provide a good basic knowledge base in all areas of IM. Ideally, the candidate should read one good textbook and not jump from one to another, except for reading certain chapters that are outstanding in a particular textbook (see below). This book and similar board review syllabi are excellent tools for brushing up on important board-relevant information several weeks to months before the examination. They, however, cannot take the place of comprehensive textbooks of internal medicine. This book is designed as a study guide rather than a comprehensive textbook of medicine. Therefore, it should not be used as the sole source of medical information for the examination.

- Candidates should thoroughly study a standard textbook of medicine.
- This book is designed as only a study guide.

The Medical Knowledge Self-Assessment Program (MKSAP) prepared by the American College of Physicians is extremely valuable for obtaining practice in answering multiple-choice questions. The text contents, however, are uneven in the coverage of topics. By design, the MKSAP is prepared for the continuing medical education of practicing (presumably ABIM-certified) internists rather than for those preparing for initial certification by the ABIM. For recertification purposes, MKSAP is a reasonable aid.

Formation of study groups, three to five candidates per group, permits study of different textbooks and review articles in journals. It is important that the group meet regularly and that each candidate be assigned reading materials. Selected review papers and state-of-the-art articles on common and important topics in IM should be included in the study materials. Indiscriminate reading of articles from many journals should be avoided. In any case, most candidates who begin preparation 6 to 8 months before the examination will not find time for extensive study of journal materials. The newer information in the recent (within 6 to 9 months of the examination) medical journals is unlikely to be included in the examination. Notes and other materials the candidates have gathered during their residency training are also good sources of information. These clinical "pearls" gathered from mentors will be of help in remembering certain important points.

- Study groups may help cover large amounts of information.
- Avoid indiscriminate reading of articles from many journals.
- Information in the recent (within 6 to 9 months of the examination) medical journals is unlikely to be included in the examination.

Certain diseases are more important because they are topical (for example, AIDS, tuberculosis, lipid disorders, and recent increase in morbidity and mortality due to asthma). Try to remember some of the uncommon manifestations of the most common diseases (such as polycythemia in common obstructive pulmonary disease) and common manifestations of uncommon diseases (such as pneumothorax in eosinophilic granuloma). Certain diseases, many peculiar and uncommon, are eminently "board-eligible," meaning that they may appear in the board examinations more frequently than in clinical practice. Most of these are covered in this book. Several formulas and points should be memorized (such as the alveolar gas equation). Most significantly, the clinical training obtained and the regular study habits formed during residency training are the most important aspects of preparation for the examination.

- Study as much as possible about board-eligible topics.
- Learn about the uncommon manifestations of common diseases and the common manifestations of uncommon diseases.

DAY OF THE EXAMINATION

Adequate time is allowed to read and answer all the questions; therefore, there is no need to rush or become anxious. You should watch the time to ensure that you are at least halfway through the examination when half of the time has elapsed. Start by answering the first question and continue sequentially (do not skip too many—see below). Several questions often follow a case presentation. At times, subsequent questions will give you information which may help you answer a previous question. Do not be alarmed by lengthy questions; look for the question's salient points. When faced with a confusing question, do not become distracted by that question. Mark it so you can find it later, then go to the next question and come back to the unanswered ones at the end. Extremely lengthy stem statements or case presentations are apparently intended to test the candidate's ability to separate the essential from the unnecessary or unimportant information. Carry a simple ruler (make sure it is allowed) to the examination. It can be used, for instance, to estimate the P50 point on the oxyhemoglobin dissociation curve or for drawing nomograms from memory.

- Look for the salient points in each question.
- Do not skip questions.

Some candidates may fail the examination despite the possession of an immense amount of knowledge and the clinical competence necessary to pass the examination. Their failure to pass the examination may be caused by the lack of ability to understand or interpret the questions properly. The ability to understand the nuances of the question format is sometimes referred to as "boardsmanship." Intelligent interpretation of the questions is very important for candidates who are not well versed in the format of multiple-choice questions. It is very important to read the final sentence (that appears just before the multiple answers) several times to understand how an answer should be selected. For example, the question may ask you to select the *correct* or *incorrect* answer. It is advisable to recheck the question format before selecting the correct answer. It is also important to read each answer option thoroughly through to the end. Occasionally a response may be only partially correct. Watch for qualifiers such as "next," "immediately," or "initially." Another hint for selecting the correct answers is to avoid answers that contain absolute or very restrictive words such as "always," "never," or "must." For example, if an answer states that "pneumonia vaccine must (or always, or never) be given to all patients with chronic obstructive pulmonary disease," it is likely an incorrect response. Another means to ensure that you know the correct answer is to cover the answers before tackling the question; read the question and then try to think of the answer before looking at the list of potential answers. Assume you have been given all the necessary information to answer the question. If the answer you had formulated is not among the list of answers provided, you may have interpreted the question incorrectly. When a patient's case is presented, write down the diagnosis before looking at the list of answers. It will be reassuring to realize (particularly if your diagnosis is supported by the answers) that you are on the "right track." If you do not know the answer to the question, very often you are able to rule out one or several answer options and improve your odds at guessing.

- Develop "boardsmanship."
- Do not select answers with absolute or very restrictive words such as "always," "never," or "must."
- Try to formulate your own answer before looking at the answers provided.

Candidates are well advised to use the basic fund of knowledge accumulated from clinical experience and reading to solve the questions. Approaching the questions as "real-life" encounters with patients is far better than trying to second-guess the examiners or trying to analyze whether the question is "tricky." As indicated above, the questions are never "tricky," and there is no reason for the ABIM to trick the candidates into choosing wrong answers.

- Approach questions as "real-life" encounters with patient.
- There are no "trick" questions.

It is better not to discuss the questions or answers (after the examination) with other candidates. Such discussions usually cause more consternation, although some candidates may derive a false sense of having performed well in the examination. In any case, the candidates are bound by their oath to the ABIM not to discuss or disseminate the questions.

CONNECTIONS

Associations, causes, complications, and other relationships between a phenomenon or disease and clinical features are important to remember and recognize. I call these "connections." For example, Table 1-2 lists some of the "connections" in infectious and occupational entities in pulmonary medicine. Each subspecialty has many similar connections, and candidates for the ABIM and other examinations may want to prepare lists like this for different areas.

RECERTIFICATION

The diplomate certificates issued to successful candidates who have passed the ABIM examination in IM in 1990 and thereafter are valid for 10 years. The first recertification examination under the new guidelines was administered in 1996 (see details below). The ABIM has stated that the recertification program is dedicated to promoting clinical excellence within the specialty of IM. The goals of the recertification program are to 1) improve the quality of patient care, 2) set high standards of clinical competence, and 3) foster the continuing scholarship required for professional excellence over a lifetime of practice. For the first recertification examination in 1996, 256 candidates took the examination. The overall pass rate for 1996 was 93%. In 1997, 153 candidates took the

examination, and the pass rate was 91%. In 1998, 297 candidates took the examination, and the pass rate was 87%.

- Certificates issued to successful candidates who have passed the ABIM examination in IM in 1990 and thereafter are valid for 10 years.
- The first recertification examination under the new guidelines was administered in 1996.

The recertification program consists of three steps:

1. Each applicant is expected to demonstrate evidence of competence, as determined by a valid license to practice medicine, and evidence from the chief-of-staff or the credentials committee indicating good standing and satisfactory clinical competence in one's clinic or hospital.
2. Completion of the Self-Evaluation Process (SEP), an at-home, open-book examination. A total of five SEP modules must be completed successfully. Three modules must be in general internal medicine, and the fourth and fifth modules may be either in general internal medicine or in any of the other modules available. Each SEP module consists of 60 questions that test the candidate on recent clinical advances in internal medicine and in more established principles of internal medicine. The modules may be completed at the pace set by each applicant. Each SEP module obtained should be returned for scoring within 90 days. A minimal passing score must be attained for each module. The modules are returned to the applicant with the incorrect responses identified; if the applicant does not meet the minimal standard of correct responses, the module is to be sent back with appropriate corrections made. All five modules must be passed before the applicant is allowed to take the final examination.
3. A proctored, written final examination is offered annually at multiple testing centers. The format of the final examination is somewhat similar to that of the internal medicine certifying examination (three modules, with each module consisting of 60 single-best–answer, multiple-choice questions). The questions on the final examination address well-established knowledge and clinical judgment in internal medicine. Candidates must correctly answer a predetermined percentage of questions. If the candidate is unsuccessful in passing the final examination, the candidate must start the recertification process over with the SEP modules.

- Applicant must pass five SEP modules.
- Applicant must pass a final examination (a written, proctored examination).

Details of the recertification program can be obtained by writing to the ABIM offices at the American Board of Internal Medicine, 510 Walnut Street, Suite 1700, Philadelphia, PA 19106-3699 (telephone numbers: 215-446-3500 or 800-441-2246; fax number: 215-446-3470). The Internet address of the ABIM is http://www.abim.org.

Table 1-2.—Example of "Connections" Between Etiologic Factors and Diseases

Etiologic factor	Agent, disease
Cattle, swine, horses, wool, hide	Anthrax
Abattoir worker, veterinarian	Brucellosis
Travel to Southeast Asia, South America	Melioidosis
Squirrels, chipmunks, rabbits, rats	Plague
Rabbits, squirrels, infected flies, or ticks	Tularemia
Birds	Psittacosis, histoplasmosis
Rats, dogs, cats, cattle, swine	Leptospirosis
Goats, cattle, swine	Q-fever
Soil, water-cooling tower	Legionellosis
Military camps	Mycoplasmosis
Chicken coop, starling roosts, caves	Histoplasmosis
Soil	Blastomycosis
Travel in Southwestern United States	Coccidioidomycosis
Ohio and Mississippi river valleys	Histoplasmosis
Decaying wood	Histoplasmosis
Gardeners, florists, straw, plants	Sporotrichosis
Progressive, massive fibrosis	Silicosis, coal, hematite, kaolin, graphite, asbestosis
Autoimmune mechanism	Silicosis, asbestosis, berylliosis
Monday morning sickness	Byssinosis, bagassosis, metal fume fever
Metals and fumes producing asthma	Baker's asthma, meat wrapper's asthma, printer's asthma, nickel, platinum, toluene diisocyanate (TDI), cigarette cutter's asthma
Increased incidence of tuberculosis	Silicosis, hematite lung
Increased incidence of carcinoma	Asbestos, hematite, arsenic, nickel, uranium, chromate
Welder prone to develop	Siderosis, pulmonary edema, bronchitis, emphysema
Centrilobar emphysema	Coal, hematite
Generalized emphysema	Cadmium, bauxite
Silo filler's lung produced by	Nitrogen dioxide
Farmer's lung produced by	*Thermoactinomyces, Micropolyspora*
Asbestos exposure	Mesothelioma, bronchogenic carcinoma, gastrointestinal cancer
Eggshell calcification	Silicosis, sarcoid
Sarcoid-like disease	Berylliosis
Diaphragmatic calcification	Asbestosis (also ankylosing spondylitis)
Nonfibrogenic pneumoconioses	Tin, emery, antimony, titanium, barium
Minimal pathology in lungs	Siderosis, baritosis, stannosis
Bullous emphysema	Bauxite lung

CHAPTER 2
ALLERGY

James T.-C. Li, M.D., Ph.D.

ALLERGY TESTING

Standard allergy testing relies on identifying the allergen-specific IgE antibody. Two classic means of doing this are the immediate wheal-and-flare skin test (a small amount of antigen is introduced into the skin and evaluated at 15 minutes for the presence of an immediate wheal-and-flare reaction) and in vitro testing.

Allergy practices without a clear scientific basis include cytotoxic testing, provocation-neutralization testing or treatment, "yeast allergy," and sublingual immunotherapy.

Patch Tests and Prick (Cutaneous) Tests

Many people seem confused about the concept of patch testing of skin as opposed to immediate wheal-and-flare skin testing. Patch testing is used to investigate contact dermatitis, a type IV hypersensitivity reaction. Patch tests require about 96 hours for complete evaluation (similar to tuberculin skin reactivity that requires 72 hours). Patch testing is useful only for investigating type IV hypersensitivity reactions leading to contact dermatitis. Most substances that cause contact dermatitis are small organic molecules that can penetrate various barriers inherent in the skin surface. The mechanisms of hypersensitivity postulated to explain these reactions usually involve haptenation of endogenous dermal proteins.

Inhalant allergens generally are sizable intact proteins in which each molecule can be multivalent with respect to IgE binding. Such molecules penetrate skin poorly and are seldom involved in cutaneous type IV hypersensitivity reactions.

- Patch testing is used to investigate contact dermatitis.
- Prick (immediate) skin testing is used to investigate respiratory allergy to pollens and molds.

Prick, scratch, and intradermal testing involve introducing allergen to the skin layers below the external keratin layer. Each of these techniques is increasingly sensitive (but less specific)

as allergen is introduced more closely to responding cells and at higher doses. We perform allergen skin tests by the prick technique because it adequately identifies patients with significant clinical sensitivities without identifying a large number of those with minimal levels of IgE antibody and no clinical sensitivity. We use scratch or intradermal testing in selective cases, including the protocol for evaluating stinging insect venoms and for penicillin. Drugs with antihistamine properties, such as H_1 receptor antagonists, and many anticholinergic and tricyclic antidepressant drugs can suppress immediate allergy skin tests. H_2 receptor antagonists have a small suppressive effect. Corticosteroids can suppress the delayed type hypersensitivity response but not the immediate response.

- Intradermal skin tests are more sensitive but less specific than prick skin tests.
- Intradermal skin testing is used to investigate allergy to insect venoms and penicillin.

In Vitro Allergy Testing

In vitro allergy testing involves chemically coupling allergen protein molecules to a solid-phase substance. The test is conducted by incubating a serum (from patient) that may contain IgE antibody specific for the allergen that has been immobilized to the membrane for a standard period of time. The solid phase is then washed free of nonbinding materials from the serum and incubated in a second solution containing a signal reagent (e.g., radiolabeled anti-IgE antibody). The various wells are counted, and the radioactivity is correlated directly with the preparation of a standard curve in which known amounts of allergen-specific IgE antibody were incubated with a set of standard preparations of a solid phase. In vitro allergy testing uses the principles of radioimmunoassay or chromogen activation.

It is important to understand that this test only identifies the presence of allergen-specific IgE antibody in the same way that the allergen skin test does. Generally, in vitro allergy testing is not as sensitive as any form of skin testing and has some limitations because of the potential for chemical modification of the protein while coupling it to the solid phase by means of covalent reaction. It generally is more expensive than allergen skin tests and has no advantage in routine clinical work. In vitro allergy testing may be useful clinically for patients 1) who have been taking antihistamines and in whom no positive histamine responsiveness can be induced in the skin and 2) who have primary cutaneous diseases that make allergen skin testing impractical or inaccurate (e.g., severe atopic eczema with most of the skin involved in a flare).

- Skin testing is more sensitive and less expensive than in vitro allergy testing.

ASTHMA

Pathology

The pathologic features of asthma have been studied chiefly in fatal cases; some bronchoscopic data are available about mild and moderate asthma.

The histologic hallmarks of asthma are listed in Table 2-1.

- Histologic hallmarks of asthma: mucus gland hypertrophy, mucus hypersecretion, epithelial desquamation, widening of basement membrane, infiltration of eosinophils.

Pathophysiology

Bronchial hyperresponsiveness is common to all forms of asthma. Bronchial hyperresponsiveness is measured by assessing pulmonary function before and after exposure to methacholine, histamine, cold air, or exercise. Prolonged aerosol corticosteroid therapy reduces bronchial hyperre-

Table 2-1.—Histologic Hallmarks of Asthma

Mucus gland hypertrophy
Mucus hypersecretion
Alteration of tinctorial and viscoelastic properties of mucus
Widening of basement membrane zone of bronchial epithelial
  membrane
Increased number of intraepithelial leukocytes and mast cells
Round cell infiltration of bronchial submucosa
Intense eosinophilic infiltration of submucosa
Widespread damage to bronchial epithelium
    Large areas of complete desquamation of epithelium into
      airway lumen
    Mucus plugs filled with eosinophils and their products

---

sponsiveness. Prolonged therapy with certain other anti-inflammatory drugs, for example, sodium cromolyn or nedocromil, also reduces bronchial hyperresponsiveness. Note that although cromolyn and nedocromil both were originally touted as "anti-allergic" (they inhibit mast cell activation), they affect most cells involved in inflammation; also, the effects on these cells occur at lower doses than those that inhibit mast cell activation.

- Bronchial hyperresponsiveness generally is present in all forms of asthma.
- Prolonged aerosol corticosteroid therapy reduces bronchial responsiveness.

Persons who have allergic asthma generate mast cell and basophil mediators that have significant roles in the development of the endobronchial inflammation and smooth muscle changes that occur after acute exposure to allergen. Mast cells and basophils are prominent during the immediate reaction.

- In the immediate-phase reaction, mast cells and basophils are important.

In the so-called late-phase reaction to allergen exposure, the bronchi have histologic features of chronic inflammation, and eosinophils become prominent in the reaction.

- In the late-phase reaction, eosinophils become prominent.

Patients with negative allergy skin test results and chronic asthma seem to have an inflammatory infiltrate in the bronchi and a histologic picture dominated by eosinophils when asthma is active. Patients with sudden asphyxic asthma may have a neutrophilic rather than an eosinophilic infiltration of the airway.

Various hypotheses explain the development of nonallergic asthma. One proposal is that the initial inflammation represents an autoimmune reaction arising from a viral or other microbial infection in the lung and, for reasons unknown, inflammation becomes chronic and characterized by a lymphocyte cytokine profile in which interleukin-5 (IL-5) is prominent. The intense eosinophilic inflammation is thought to come from the IL-5 influence of T cells in the chronic inflammatory infiltrate. Airway macrophages and platelets have low-affinity IgE receptors on their membranes and are activated by cross-linking of these receptors by allergen, suggesting that some phases of lung inflammation in allergy may involve the macrophage as a primary responder cell.

- IL-5 stimulates eosinophils.
- Airway macrophages and platelets have low-affinity IgE receptors.

The two types of helper T cells are TH1 and TH2. In general, TH1 cells produce interferon-γ (IFN-γ) and IL-2, and TH2 cells produce IL-4 and IL-5. IL-4 stimulates IgE synthesis. Hence, many clinical scientists believe that atopic asthma is caused by a preferential activation of TH2 lymphocytes.

- IL-4 stimulates IgE synthesis.
- TH2 lymphocytes produce IL-4 and IL-5.

Important characteristics of cytokines are summarized in Table 2-2.

Genetics of Asthma

The genetics of asthma is complex and confounded by environmental factors. No "asthma gene" has been discovered.

The gene encoding the beta subunit of the high-affinity IgE receptor is located on chromosome 11q13 and is linked to total IgE, atopy, and bronchial hyperreactivity. Polymorphic variants of the β_2-adrenergic receptor are linked to bronchial hyperreactivity. The gene for IL-4 is located on chromosome 5q31 and is linked to total IgE.

Occupational Asthma

Every patient interviewed about a history of allergy or asthma must provide an adequate occupational history. A large fraction of occupational asthma escapes diagnosis because physicians obtain an inadequate occupational history. An enormous range of possible industrial circumstances may lead to exposure and resultant disease. The most widely recognized types of occupational asthma are listed in Table 2-3.

- Inquiry into a possible occupational cause of asthma is important in all patients with asthma.

As new industrial processes and products evolve, occupational asthma may become more common. An example of

Table 2-2.—Characteristics of Cytokines

Cytokine	Major actions	Primary sources
IL-1	Lymphocyte activation	Macrophages
	Fibroblast activation	Endothelial cells
	Fever	Lymphocytes
IL-2	T- and B-cell activation	T cells (TH1)
IL-3	Mast cell proliferation	T cells
	Neutrophil, macrophage maturation	Mast cells
IL-4	IgE synthesis	T cells (TH2)
IL-5	Eosinophil proliferation and differentiation	T cells (TH2)
IL-6	IgG synthesis	Fibroblasts
	Lymphocyte activation	T cells
IL-8	Neutrophil chemotaxis	Fibroblasts
		Endothelial cells
		Monocytes
IL-10	Inhibits IFN-γ, IL-1 production	T cells
		Macrophages
IL-13	Promotes IgE synthesis	T cells
IFN-α	Antiviral activity	Leukocytes
IFN-γ	Activates macrophages	T cells (TH1)
	Stimulates MHC expression	
	Inhibits TH2 activity	
TNF-γ	Antitumor cell activity	Lymphocytes
		Macrophages
TNF-β	Antitumor cell activity	T cells
GM-CSF	Stimulates mast cells, granulocytes, macrophages	Lymphocytes
		Mast cells
		Macrophages

GM-CSF, granulocyte-macrophage colony-stimulating factor; IFN, interferon; IL, interleukin; MHC, major histocompatibility complex; TH, helper T cell; TNF, tumor necrosis factor.

Table 2-3.—Industrial Agents That Can Cause Asthma

Metals
   Salts of platinum, nickel, chrome
Wood dusts
   Mahogany
   Oak
   Redwood
   Western red cedar (plicatic acid)
Vegetable dusts
   Castor bean
   Cotton dust
   Cottonseed
   Flour
   Grain (mite, weevil antigens)
   Green coffee
   Gums
Industrial chemicals and plastics
   Ethylenediamine
   Phthalic and trimellitic anhydrides
   Polyvinyl chloride
   Toluene diisocyanate
Pharmaceutical agents
   Phenylglycine acid chloride
   Penicillins
   Spiramycin
Food industry agents
   Egg protein
   Polyvinylchloride
Biologic enzymes
   Bacillus subtilis (laundry detergent workers)
   Pancreatic enzymes
Animal emanations
   Canine or feline saliva
   Horse dander (racing workers)
   Rodent urine (laboratory animal workers)

a potentially huge problem is latex-induced asthma among medical workers with the widespread use of latex gloves for medical workers. The incidence of occupational asthma is estimated to be 6% to 15% of all adult-onset asthmatics.

● Allergy to latex is an important cause of occupational asthma.

Gastroesophageal Reflux and Asthma

The role of gastroesophageal reflux in asthma is not known. Two mechanistic hypotheses are 1) reflux bronchospasm from acid in the distal esophagus and 2) recurrent aspiration of gastric contents. Although a well-documented reflex in dogs links acid in the distal esophagus to vagally mediated bronchospasm, this reflex had not been demonstrated consistently in humans. The other hypothesis is that gastric contents reach the tracheobronchial tree by ascending to the hypopharynx.

Asthma-Provoking Drugs

It is important to recognize the potentially severe adverse response that patients with asthma may show to β-blocking drugs. Asthmatics with glaucoma treated with ophthalmic preparations of timolol and betaxolol (betaxolol is less likely to cause problems) may experience bronchospasm.

● β-Blocking drugs, including eyedrops, can cause severe adverse responses.
● Note that so-called β_1 selective agents such as atenolol may also provoke asthma.

Persons taking angiotensin-converting enzyme (ACE) inhibitor drugs may develop a chronic cough that can mimic asthma. This cough may not be accompanied by additional bronchospasm.

● ACE inhibitors can cause coughing.

Aspirin ingestion can cause acute, severe, and fatal asthma in a small subset of patients with asthma. The cause of the reaction is unknown but probably involves the generation of leukotrienes. Most of the affected patients have nasal polyposis and hyperplastic pansinus mucosal disease and are steroid-dependent for control of asthma. However, not all asthmatics with this reaction to aspirin fit the profile. Many nonsteroidal anti-inflammatory drugs can trigger the reaction to aspirin; the likelihood of a drug causing the reaction correlates with its potency of inhibiting cyclooxygenase enzyme. Structural aspects of the drug seem unrelated to its tendency to provoke the reaction. Only nonacetylated salicylates such as choline salicylate (a weak cyclooxygenase inhibitor) seem not to provoke the reaction. Leukotriene-modifying drugs may be particularly helpful in aspirin-sensitive asthma.

● Aspirin and other nonsteroidal anti-inflammatory agents can cause acute, severe asthma.
● Asthma, nasal polyposis, and aspirin sensitivity form the aspirin triad.
● Leukotriene modifiers may be helpful in aspirin-sensitive asthma.

Traditionally, asthmatic patients have been warned not to use antihistamines, because anticholinergic activity of some antihistamines was thought to cause drying of lower respiratory tract secretions, further worsening the asthma. However, antihistamines do not worsen asthma, and in fact, some studies have shown a beneficial effect. Thus, on occasion, we specifically prescribe antihistamine for asthma, because the drug may have some beneficial effect on asthmatic inflammation.

● Antihistamines are not contraindicated in asthma.

Cigarette Smoking and Asthma

A combination of asthma and cigarette smoking leads to accelerated chronic obstructive pulmonary disease. Because of accelerated decline in irreversible obstruction, all asthmatic patients who smoke should be told to stop smoking.

Environmental tobacco smoke is an important asthma trigger. In particular, asthmatic children exposed to environmental smoke have more respiratory infections and asthma attacks.

Medical History

A medical history for asthma includes careful inquiry about symptoms, provoking factors, alleviating factors, and severity. Patients with significant respiratory allergy have symptoms when exposed to aeroallergens and often have seasonal variation of symptoms. You can be reasonably certain someone does not have allergic asthma if allergy skin test results are negative.

● In allergic asthma, symptoms are sporadic and they are consistently related to exposure or are seasonal.

Respiratory infections (particularly viral), cold air, exercise, and respiratory irritants can trigger allergic and nonallergic asthma.

● Allergic patients are likely to respond to many nonimmunologic triggers.
● Cold dry air can trigger asthma.

Assessment of Severity

Asthma is mild-intermittent if the symptoms are intermittent, continuous treatment is not needed, and the flow-volume curve during formal pulmonary function testing is normal between episodes of symptoms. Even in patients fitting this description, inflammation (albeit patchy) in airways is significant, and corticosteroid inhaled on a regular basis diminishes bronchial hyperresponsiveness.

● Corticosteroid inhaled on a regular basis diminishes bronchial hyperresponsiveness.

Asthma is mild-persistent or moderate when 1) the symptoms occur with some regularity or daily, 2) there is some nocturnal occurrence of symptoms, or 3) asthma exacerbations are troublesome. For many of these patients, the flow-volume curve is rarely normal, and complete pulmonary function testing may show evidence of hyperinflation, as indicated by increased residual volume or an increase above expected levels for the diffusing capacity of the lung for CO_2. Patients with mild, moderate, or severe asthma should receive treatment with anti-inflammatory medications, often with inhaled corticosteroids.

Asthma is severe when symptoms are present almost continuously and when the upper end of the dose range of the usual medications is needed to control the asthma. Most patients with severe asthma require either large doses of inhaled corticosteroid or oral prednisone daily for adequate control. Most of them have been hospitalized more than once and for more than overnight observation. The severity of asthma can change over time. Note that one of the first signs that asthma is not well-controlled is the emergence of the nocturnal symptoms.

● Nocturnal symptoms suggest that asthma is worsening.

Methacholine Bronchial Challenge

A patient with a history suggestive of episodic asthma but who on the day of the examination has normal pulmonary function test results is a reasonable candidate for methacholine bronchial challenge. The methacholine bronchial challenge is useful in evaluating patients for cough in whom baseline pulmonary function appears normal. Positive results indicate that bronchial hyperresponsiveness is present (Table 2-4). Some consider isocapneic hyperventilation with subfreezing dry air (by either exercise or breathing CO_2/air mixture) or exercise as alternatives to methacholine challenge.

Do not perform a methacholine challenge in patients with severe airway obstruction. Usually, a 20% decrease in forced expiratory volume in 1 second (FEV_1) is considered a positive result.

● Patients with suspected asthma and normal results on pulmonary function tests can benefit from methacholine testing.

Table 2-4.—Medical Conditions Associated With Positive Findings on Methacholine Challenge

Current asthma
Past history of asthma
Chronic obstructive pulmonary disease
Smoking
Recent respiratory infection
Chronic cough
Allergic rhinitis

Differential Diagnosis

The differential diagnosis of wheezing is given in Table 2-5.

Medications for Asthma

Medications for asthma are listed in Table 2-6. Currently, the only anticholinergic drug available in the U.S. for treating asthma is ipratropium bromide, although it is approved for only chronic obstructive pulmonary disease. Several short-acting β-adrenergic compounds are available, but albuterol or pirbuterol is probably prescribed most. More side effects occur when they are given orally rather than by inhalation. Nebulized β-agonists are infrequently used chronically in adult asthma, although they may be life-saving in acute attacks. For home use, the metered-dose inhaler is the preferred delivery system. Salmeterol and formoterol are two long-acting inhaled β-agonists. Both are used in combination with inhaled corticosteroids. Theophylline is effective for asthma but has a narrow therapeutic index. Note that drug interactions (cimetidine, erythromycin, and quinolone antibiotics) can increase the serum level of theophylline.

- Theophylline has a narrow therapeutic index.
- β-Agonists are best delivered by the inhaler route.

Cromolyn and nedocromil are inhaled anti-inflammatory medications that are appropriate for treatment of mild or moderate asthma. The 5-lipoxygenase inhibitor zileuton and the leukotriene antagonists zafirlukast and montelukast are approved for treatment in mild-persistent asthma. These agents work by decreasing the inflammatory effects of leukotrienes. Zileuton can cause increased values on liver function tests. Cases of Churg-Strauss vasculitis have been linked to zafirlukast.

Corticosteroid Therapy

Because of the potential long-term benefits of reduced bronchial hyperresponsiveness and reduced airway remodeling (fibrosis), many experts recommend inhaled glucocorticoids for mild asthma. Long-term use of β-agonist bronchodilators may adversely affect asthma; this also argues for earlier use of inhaled glucocorticoids. Asthma mortality has been linked to the heavy use of β-agonist inhalers. This association may simply reflect that patients with more severe asthma (who are more likely to die of an asthma attack) use more β-agonist inhalers. However, prolonged and heavy use of inhaled β-agonists may have a direct, deleterious effect on asthma, but this has not been proved. Certainly, asthmatic patients with regularly recurring symptoms probably should have inhaled corticosteroids (or cromolyn or nedocromil) as part of the treatment.

- Prescribe inhaled glucocorticoids for moderate and severe asthma.

Table 2-5.—Differential Diagnosis of Wheezing

Pulmonary embolism
Cardiac failure
Foreign body
Central airway tumors
Aspiration
Carcinoid syndrome
Chondromalacia/polychondritis
Löffler syndrome
Bronchiectasis
Tropical eosinophilia
Hyperventilation syndrome
Laryngeal edema
Vascular ring affecting trachea
Factitious (including psychophysiologic vocal cord adduction)
α_1-Antiprotease deficiency
Immotile cilia syndrome
Bronchopulmonary dysplasia
Bronchiolitis (including bronchiolitis obliterans), croup
Cystic fibrosis

Table 2-6.—Medications for Asthma

Bronchodilator compounds
    Anticholinergic drugs (ipratropium bromide)
    β_2-Agonist drugs
        Short acting (albuterol, pirbuterol)
        Long acting (salmeterol, formoterol)
    Methylxanthines (theophylline)
"Anti-allergic" compounds
    Cromolyn
    Nedocromil
Glucocorticoids
    Systemic
        Prednisone
        Methylprednisolone
    Topical
        Triamcinolone acetonide
        Beclomethasone
        Flunisolide, budesonide
Antileukotrienes
    Leukotriene receptor antagonists
    Lipoxygenase inhibitors

- Long-term use of β-agonist bronchodilators may worsen asthma.

The inflammatory infiltrate in the bronchial submucosa likely depends on lymphokine secretory patterns. Corticosteroids may interfere at several levels in the lymphokine cascade.

Bronchoalveolar lavage and biopsy studies show that corticosteroids inhibit IL-4, IL-5, and granulocyte-macrophage colony-stimulating factor (GM-CSF) in asthma.

- Corticosteroids reduce airway inflammation by modulating cytokines.

Monocytes or platelets may be important in the asthmatic process. Corticosteroids modify activation pathways for monocytes and platelets.

- Corticosteroids can inhibit the inflammatory properties of monocytes and platelets.

Furthermore, corticosteroids have vasoconstrictive properties, which reduce vascular congestive changes in the mucosa, and they tend to reduce mucus gland secretion.

- Corticosteroids have vasoconstrictive properties.
- Corticosteroids reduce mucus gland secretion.

The most common adverse effects of inhaled corticosteroids are dysphonia and thrush. These unwanted effects occur in about 10% of patients and can be reduced by using a spacer device and rinsing the mouth after administration. Usually, oral thrush can be treated successfully with oral antifungal agents. Dysphonia, when persistent, should be treated by reducing or discontinuing the use of inhaled corticosteroids.

Detailed study of the systemic effects of inhaled corticosteroids shows that these agents are much safer than oral corticosteroids. Nevertheless, there is evidence that inhaled corticosteroids can affect the hypothalamic-pituitary-adrenal axis and bone metabolism. Inhaled corticosteroids may increase the risk of future development of glaucoma, cataracts, and osteoporosis. Inhaled corticosteroids can also decrease growth velocity in children and adolescents. The effect of inhaled corticosteroids on adult height is not known, but it may be small or minimal.

Poor inhaler technique and poor compliance can result in poor control of asthma. Therefore, all patients using a metered-dose inhaler should be taught the proper technique of using these devices. Most patients using inhaled corticosteroids should be using a spacer device with the inhaler.

- The most common cause of poor results is poor inhaler technique.

- Patients should use a spacer device with inhaled corticosteroids.

Goals of Asthma Management

The goals of asthma management are listed in Table 2-7.

Management of Chronic Asthma

Baseline spirometry is recommended for all patients with asthma, and home peak flow monitoring is recommended for patients with moderate and severe asthma (Fig. 2-1).

- Spirometry is recommended for all asthma patients.
- Home peak flow monitoring is recommended for those with moderate and severe asthma.

Environmental triggers should be discussed with all asthmatic patients, and allergy testing should be offered to patients with suspected allergic asthma or to those whose asthma is not well controlled. Although allergy immunotherapy is effective, it is recommended only for patients with allergic asthma who have undergone a careful evaluation by an allergist.

Management of Acute Asthma

Inhaled β-agonists, measurements of lung function, and systemic corticosteroids (for most patients) are the cornerstones of managing acute asthma (Fig. 2-2). Generally, nebulized albuterol, administered repeatedly if necessary, is the first line of treatment. Delivery of β-agonist by metered-dose inhaler can be substituted in less severe asthma attacks. Inhaled β-agonist delivered by continuous nebulization may be appropriate for more severe patients.

- Inhaled β-agonist can be delivered by intermittent nebulization, continuous nebulization, or metered-dose inhaler.

It is important to measure lung function (usually peak expiratory flow rate [PEFR] but also FEV whenever possible) at presentation and after administration of bronchodilators. These measurements provide invaluable information that allows

Table 2-7.—Goals of Asthma Management

No asthma symptoms
No asthma attacks
Normal activity level
Normal lung function
Use of safest and least amount of medication necessary
Establish therapeutic relationship between patient and provider

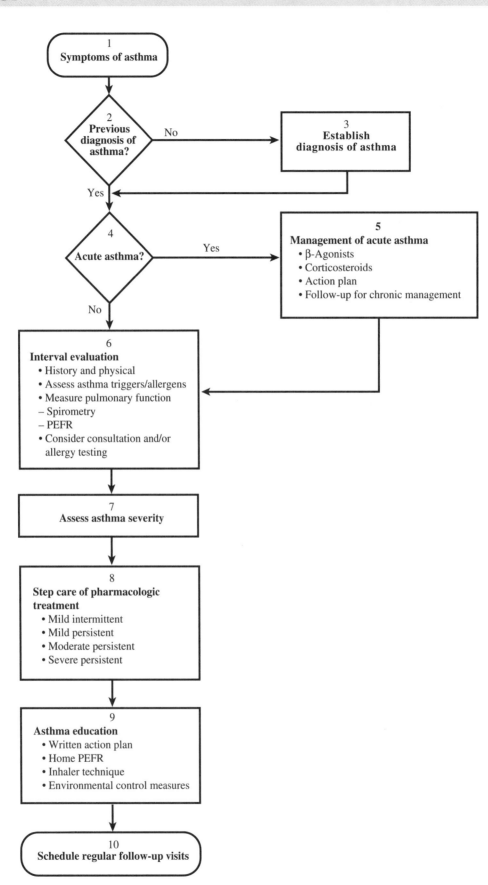

Fig. 2-1. Diagnosis and management of asthma. PEFR, peak expiratory flow rate.

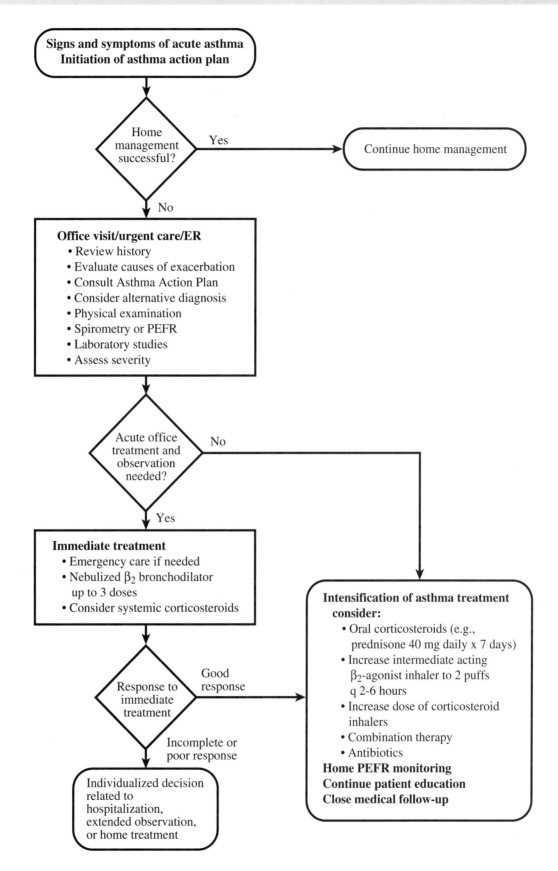

Fig. 2-2. Management of acute asthma in adults. ER, emergency room; PEFR, peak expiratory flow rate. (By permission of Institute of Clinical Systems Integration.)

the physician to assess the severity of the asthma attack and the response (if any) to treatment.

Patients who do not have a prompt and full response to inhaled β-agonists should receive a course of systemic corticosteroids. The most severe and poorly responsive patients should be treated in the hospital or intensive care unit.

- Measure pulmonary function at presentation and after giving bronchodilators.
- Most patients with acute asthma need a course of systemic corticosteroids.

Allergic Bronchopulmonary Aspergillosis

Allergic bronchopulmonary aspergillosis is an obstructive lung disease caused by an allergic reaction to *Aspergillus* in the lower airway. The typical clinical presentation is severe steroid-dependent asthma. Most of the patients with this condition have coexisting asthma or cystic fibrosis.

- Allergic bronchopulmonary aspergillosis develops in patients with asthma or chronic obstructive pulmonary disease.

The diagnostic features of allergic bronchopulmonary aspergillosis are summarized in Table 2-8. Fungi other than *Aspergillus fumigatus* can cause an allergic bronchopulmonary mycosis similar to allergic bronchopulmonary aspergillosis.

Chest radiography can show transient or permanent infiltrates and central bronchiectasis, usually affecting the upper lobes (Fig. 2-3). Advanced cases show extensive pulmonary fibrosis.

Allergic bronchopulmonary aspergillosis is treated with systemic corticosteroids. Total serum IgE may be helpful in following the course of the disease. Antifungal therapy has not been effective.

CHRONIC RHINITIS

Medical History

Vasomotor rhinitis is defined as nasal symptoms occurring in response to nonspecific stimuli. Common triggers of vasomotor rhinitis are strong odors, respiratory irritants such as dust or smoke, changes in temperature, changes in body position, and ingestants such as spicy food or alcohol.

- Vasomotor rhinitis is nasal symptoms in response to nonspecific stimuli.

Historical factors favoring a diagnosis of allergic rhinitis include a history of nasal symptoms that have a recurrent seasonal pattern (e.g., every August and September) or seem to be

Table 2-8.—Diagnostic Features of Allergic Bronchopulmonary Aspergillosis

Clinical asthma
Bronchiectasis (usually proximal)
Increased total serum IgE
IgE antibody to *Aspergillus* (by skin test or in vitro assay)
Precipitins or IgG antibody to *Aspergillus*
Radiographic infiltrates (often upper lobes)
Peripheral blood eosinophilia

provoked by the person being near animals. Factors favoring vasomotor rhinitis include strong odors and humidity and temperature changes.

- Allergic rhinitis has a recurrent seasonal pattern and may be provoked by being near animals.
- Triggers of vasomotor rhinitis include humidity and temperature changes and strong odors.

Factors favoring both allergic rhinitis and vasomotor rhinitis (thus, without differential diagnostic value) include perennial symptoms, intolerance of cigarette smoke, and history of "dust" sensitivity. Factors that suggest fixed nasal obstruction (which

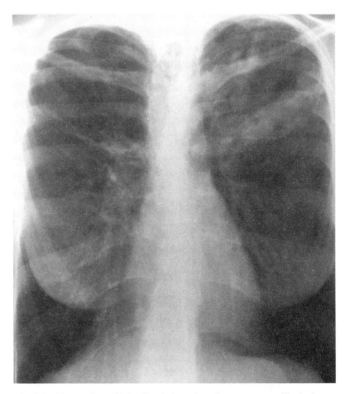

Fig. 2-3. Chest radiograph in allergic bronchopulmonary aspergillosis shows cylindrical infiltrates involving the upper lobes.

should prompt physicians to consider other diagnoses) include unilateral nasal obstruction, unilateral facial pain, unilateral nasal purulence, nasal voice but no nasal symptoms, disturbances of olfaction without any nasal symptoms, and unilateral nasal bleeding (Table 2-9).

- Perennial symptoms, intolerance of cigarette smoke, and history of "dust" sensitivity are common to allergic and vasomotor rhinitis.
- Dust mite sensitivity is a common cause of perennial allergic rhinitis.

Allergy Skin Tests in Allergic Rhinitis

The interpretation of allergy skin test results must be tailored to the unique features of each patient.

1. For patients with perennial symptoms and negative results on allergy skin tests, the diagnosis is vasomotor rhinitis.
2. For patients with seasonal symptoms and appropriately positive allergy skin tests, the diagnosis is seasonal allergic rhinitis.
3. For patients with perennial symptoms, allergy skin tests positive for house dust mite suggest house dust mite allergic rhinitis. These patients should proceed with dust mite allergen avoidance, that is, have the patient encase bedding with allergy-proof encasements, remove carpeting from the bedroom, and lower the relative humidity in the house to 40% to 50% or less.

Corticosteroid Therapy for Rhinitis

The need for systemic corticosteroid treatment for rhinitis is limited. Occasionally, patients with severe symptoms of hay fever may benefit greatly from 5 days of 10-mg prednisone (10 mg four times daily by mouth for 5 days). This may induce sufficient improvement so that topical corticosteroids can penetrate the nose and satisfactory levels of antihistamine can be established in the blood. Patients with severe nasal polyposis may warrant a longer course of oral corticosteroids. Sometimes, recurrence of nasal polyps can be prevented by continued use of topical corticosteroids. Polypectomy may be required if

Table 2-9.—Differential Diagnosis of Chronic Rhinitis

Allergic rhinitis
Vasomotor rhinitis
Rhinitis medicamentosus
Sinusitis
Nasal polyposis
Nasal septal deviation
Foreign body
Tumor

nasal polyps fail to respond to treatment with systemic and intranasal corticosteroids.

- Treatment of nasal polyposis can include oral prednisone followed by topical corticosteroids.

In contrast with systemic corticosteroid therapy, topical corticosteroid agents for the nose are easy to use and have few adverse systemic effects. Intranasal corticosteroids may reduce growth velocity in children.

- Intranasal corticosteroids may reduce growth velocity in children.

Most people are aware that treatment with decongestant nasal sprays is a bad idea because of the "addictive" potential (a vicious cycle of rhinitis medicamentosa caused by topical vasoconstrictors is common knowledge). Reassure patients that topical corticosteroid does not induce any dependence.

- Unlike decongestant nasal sprays, topical intranasal corticosteroid does not induce tachyphylaxis and rebound congestion.

A significant number of patients with vasomotor rhinitis also have a good response to intranasal corticosteroid therapy, especially if the patient has the nasal eosinophilia and/or nasal polyposis form of vasomotor rhinitis.

- Many patients with vasomotor rhinitis have a good response to topical aerosol corticosteroid therapy.

If a hay fever patient does not receive adequate relief with topical steroid plus antihistamine therapy, it may indicate the need for systemic corticosteroid and for initiating immunotherapy.

- If pharmacologic management fails, allergy immunotherapy should be considered for patients with allergic rhinitis.

An unusual side effect of intranasal corticosteroids is nasal septal perforation. Dry powder spray cannisters deliver a powerful jet of particulates, and a few patients have misdirected the jet to the nasal septum.

- Nasal topical corticosteroid sprays rarely can cause nasal septal perforation.

Antihistamines and Decongestants

Antihistamines antagonize the interaction of histamine with its receptors. Histamine may be more effective than other mediators for nasal itch and sneezing. These are symptoms most often responsive to antihistamine therapy.

Two decongestants, pseudoephedrine and phenylpropanolamine, are the most common agents in nonprescription drugs for treating cold symptoms/rhinitis and usually are the active agents in widely used proprietary prescription agents. A large number of prescription and nonprescription combination agents combine antihistamine and decongestant. Decongestant preparations are often the only therapeutic option for patients with vasomotor rhinitis unresponsive to topical glucocorticoids.

● Pseudoephedrine and phenylpropanolamine are the most common decongestant agents in nonprescription preparations.

Note that middle-aged and older men may have urinary retention caused by antihistamines (principally the older drugs that have anticholinergic effects) and decongestants; these patients should be alerted to this. Although there has been concern for years that decongestants may exacerbate hypertension because they are α-adrenergic agonists, no clinically significant hypertensive response has been seen in stable medicated patients with hypertension.

● Antihistamines and decongestants may cause urinary retention in men.

For antihistamines with anticholinergic activity, patients, especially older ones, should be warned about possible dizziness, dry mouth, blurred vision, and drowsiness.

● The elderly are more sensitive to the anticholinergic effects of antihistamines.

Immunotherapy for Allergic Rhinitis

Until topical nasal glucocorticoid sprays were introduced, allergen immunotherapy was considered "first-line" therapy for allergic rhinitis when the relevant allergen was seasonal pollen of grass, trees, or weeds. Immunotherapy became "second-line" therapy after topical corticosteroids were introduced because 1) immunotherapy has no greater efficacy than glucocorticoids and 2) immunotherapy carries a small risk of anaphylaxis to the immunotherapy injection itself. However, immunotherapy for allergic rhinitis can be appropriate first-line therapy in selected patients.

● Controlled trials have shown that immunotherapy is effective for allergic rhinitis.
● Anaphylaxis is a risk of immunotherapy.
● Immunotherapy for allergic rhinitis is first-line therapy in selected patients.

Immunotherapy is usually reserved for patients who get no satisfactory relief with topical steroids or who cannot tolerate nasal sprays or antihistamines. Controlled trials have shown a benefit for pollen, dust mite, and cat allergy and a variable benefit for mold allergy. Immunotherapy is not given for food allergy or for nonallergic rhinitis. The practice is less uniform with respect to mold allergens, with endorsement divided in the subspecialty.

● Immunotherapy is usually reserved for patients who get no relief with intranasal glucocorticoids or who cannot tolerate allergy medications.

Environmental Modification

House Dust Mite

House dust mites are so small they cannot maintain their own internal water unless ambient conditions are high humidity. They eat all kinds of organic matter but seem to favor mold and epidermal scale shed by humans. They occur in all human habitations, although the population size varies with local conditions. The only geographic areas free of house dust mites are those at great elevations with extreme dryness.

● House dust mites require high humidity.
● They are found in nearly all human habitations.

Areas in the home harboring the most significant mite populations are bedding and fabric-upholstered furniture (heavily used) and any area where carpeting is on concrete (when concrete is in contact with grade). Although carpeting is often cited as a significant mite-related problem, carpet on wooden floors in a dry, well-ventilated house usually harbors small numbers of dust mites. Aerosal dispersion of allergen from this source is not great compared with that from bedding and furniture. To prevent egress of allergen when the mattress and pillows are compressed by occupancy of the bed, encase the bedding (and sometimes, when practical, furniture cushions) in plastic dust-proof encasements. To some degree, this also prevents infusion of water vapor into the bedding matrix. These two factors combine to significantly reduce the amount of airborne allergen. Measures for controlling dust mites are listed in Table 2-10.

● Dust mite is an important respiratory allergen.
● The most significant mite population is in bedding and fabric-upholstered furniture.
● Plastic encasements prevent egress of allergen.

Recently, chemical sprays (acaricides) capable of either killing mites or denaturing the protein allergens from them have been marketed. Despite immunochemical evidence that the allergen is denatured by denaturant and mites are killed by acaricides, neither agent is substantially helpful when applied in the home.

Pollens

Air conditioning, which enables the warm-season home to remain tightly closed, is the principal defense against pollinosis. Most masks purchased at local pharmacies are **not** capable of excluding pollen particles and, thus, are not worth the expense. Some masks can protect the wearer from allergen exposure, such as industrial-quality respirators designed specifically to pass rigorous testing by the Occupational Safety and Health Administration (OSHA) and National Institute for Occupational Safety and Health (NIOSH) that qualify them capable of excluding a wide spectrum of particulates, including pollen and mold. These masks allow allergic patients to mow the lawn and do yard work otherwise intolerable because of exposure to pollen allergen.

- Only industrial-quality masks are capable of excluding pollen particles.

Animal Danders

No measure can compare with getting the animal completely out of the house. No air filtration scheme that is feasible for average homeowners to install can eliminate allergen from an actively elaborating animal. If complete removal is not tenable, some partial measure must be considered.

If the house is heated or cooled by a forced-air system with ductwork, confining the pet to a single room in the house is only partially effective in reducing overall exposure, because air from every room is collected through the air-return ductwork and redistributed through a central plenum. If air-return ducts are sealed in the room where the animal is kept and air can escape from the room only by infiltration, exposure may be reduced. The room selected for this measure should be as far as possible from the bedroom of the allergic patient. Naturally, the allergic patient should avoid close contact with the animal

Table 2-10.—Dust Mite Control

Encase bedding and pillows in airtight encasements
Remove carpeting in bedroom
Remove upholstered furniture from bedroom
Remove all carpeting laid on concrete
Discontinue use of humidifier
Wash bedding in hot water
Run dehumidifier

---

and should consider using a mask if animal handling or entry into the room where the animal is kept is necessary. Most animal danders have little or nothing to do with animal hair, so its shedding status is irrelevant. Bathing cats about once every other week may reduce the allergen load in the environment.

- Complete avoidance is the only entirely effective way to manage allergy to household pets.

Sinusitis

Sinusitis is closely associated with edematous obstruction of the sinus ostia (the osteomeatal complex). Poor drainage of the sinus cavities predisposes to infection, particularly by microorganisms that thrive in low oxygen environments (e.g., anaerobes). In adults, *Streptococcus pneumoniae*, *Haemophilus influenzae*, anaerobes, and viruses are common pathogens. In addition, *Branhamella catarrhalis* is an important pathogen in children.

Important clinical features of acute sinusitis are nasal discharge, tooth pain, cough, and poor response to decongestants. Findings on paranasal sinus transillumination may be abnormal.

- Purulent nasal discharge, tooth pain, and abnormal transillumination are important clinical features of sinusitis.

Physicians should be aware of the complications of sinusitis, which can be life-threatening (Table 2-11). Mucormycosis can cause recurrent or persistent sinusitis refractory to antibiotics. Allergic fungal sinusitis is characterized by persistent sinusitis, eosinophilia, increased total IgE, antifungal (usually *Aspergillus*) IgE antibodies, and fungal colonization of the sinuses. Wegener granulomatosis, ciliary dysmotility, and hypogammaglobulinemia are medical conditions that can cause refractory sinusitis (Table 2-12).

Untreated sinusitis can cause osteomyelitis, orbital and periorbital cellulitis, meningitis, and brain abscess. Cavernous sinus thrombosis, an especially serious complication, can lead to retrobulbar pain, extraocular muscle paralysis, and blindness.

Persistent, refractory, and complicated sinusitis should be evaluated by a specialist. Sinus computed tomography (CT) is the preferred imaging study for these patients (Fig. 2-4).

Amoxicillin, 500 mg three times daily, or trimethoprim-sulfamethoxazole (one double-strength capsule twice daily) for 10 to14 days is the treatment of choice for uncomplicated maxillary sinusitis.

The sensitivity of plain film radiographs of the sinuses is not as good as CT scanning (using coronal sectioning technique). Good-quality coronal CT scans reveal greater detail about sinus mucosal surfaces, but CT usually is not necessary in acute uncomplicated sinusitis. However, CT scanning is indicated for patients being considered for a sinus operation and for those in whom standard treatment for sinusitis fails. Be aware that patients with extensive dental restorations that contain metal may generate too much artifact for CT to be useful. For these patients, magnetic resonance imaging (MRI) techniques are better.

- Sinus imaging is indicated for recurrent sinusitis.
- Sinus CT is preferred to sinus radiography for complicated sinusitis.

URTICARIA AND ANGIOEDEMA

The distinction between acute and chronic urticaria is arbitrary and based on the duration of the urticaria. If it has been present for 6 weeks or longer, it is called chronic urticaria.

Secondary Urticaria

Most patients simply have urticaria as a skin disease (chronic idiopathic urticaria). Urticaria is occasionally the presenting sign of more serious internal disease. It can be a sign of lupus erythematosus and other connective tissue diseases, particularly of the more difficult to categorize "overlap" syndromes. Malignancy, mainly of the gastrointestinal tract, and lymphoproliferative diseases are associated with urticaria, as occult infection may be, particularly of the gallbladder and dentition. Immune-complex disease has been associated with urticaria, usually with urticarial vasculitis, and hepatitis B virus has been identified as an antigen in the cases of urticaria and immune-complex disease.

- Urticaria can be associated with lupus erythematosus and other connective tissue diseases, malignancy, infection, and immune-complex disease.

A common cause of acute urticaria and angioedema (other than the idiopathic variety) is drug or food allergy. However, drug or food allergy usually does not cause chronic urticaria.

- Chronic urticaria and angioedema are often idiopathic.
- A common secondary cause of acute urticaria and angioedema is drug or food allergy.

Relationship Between Urticaria and Angioedema

In common idiopathic urticaria, the lesions itch intensely because histamine is one of the causes of wheal formation.

- Typical urticarial lesions last 2-18 hours and are pruritic.

The pathophysiology is similar for urticaria and angioedema. The critical factor is the type of tissue in which the capillary leak and mediator release occur. Urticaria occurs when the capillary events are in the tightly welded tissue wall of

Table 2-11. —Complications of Sinusitis

Osteomyelitis
Meningitis
Subdural abscess
Extradural abscess
Orbital infection
Cellulitis
Cavernous sinus thrombosis

Table 2-12.—Causes of Persistent or Recurrent Sinusitis

Nasal polyposis
Mucormycosis
Allergic fungal sinusitis
Ciliary dyskinesia
Wegener granulomatosis
Hypogammaglobulinemia
Tumor

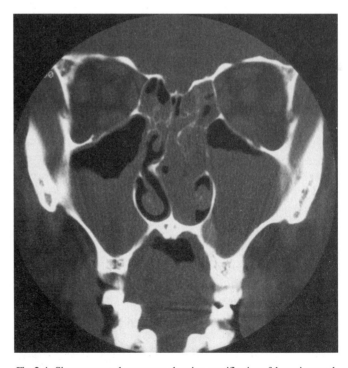

Fig. 2-4. Sinus computed tomogram showing opacification of the ostiomeatal complex on the left, subtotal opacification of the right maxillary sinus, and an air-fluid level in the left maxillary antrum.

the skin—the epidermis. Angioedema occurs when capillary events affect vessels in loose connective tissue of the deeper layers—the dermis. Virtually all patients with the common idiopathic type of urticaria also have angioedema from time to time. When urticaria is caused by allergic reactions, angioedema may also occur. The only exception is with the hereditary angioneurotic edema type of disease (HANE), which is not related to mast cell mediator release but is a complement disorder. Patients with this form of angioedema rarely have urticaria.

C1 Esterase Inhibitor Deficiency

If HANE is strongly suspected, the diagnosis can be proved by the appropriate measurement of complement factors (C1 esterase inhibitor, quantitative and functional, and C4 [also, C2, if seen during an episode of swelling]).

- C1 esterase inhibitor levels and C4 are decreased in hereditary angioedema.

The duration of individual swellings varies. Many HANE patients have had at least one hospitalization for what appeared to be intestinal obstruction. If they avoid laparotomy on these occasions, the obstruction usually resolves in 3 to 5 days. Cramps and diarrhea may occur.

Lesions in the HANE type do not itch. The response to epinephrine is a useful differential point: HANE lesions do not respond well to epinephrine, but common angioedema usually melts away in 15 minutes or less. Laryngeal edema almost never occurs in the common idiopathic type of disease (although it may occur in allergic reactions, most often in insect-sting anaphylaxis cases); however, it is relatively common in HANE (earlier papers quoted a 30% mortality rate in HANE, with all deaths due to laryngeal edema). Finally, HANE episodes may be related to local tissue trauma in a high percentage of cases, with dental work often regarded as the classic precipitating factor.

- Most HANE patients have been hospitalized for "intestinal obstruction."
- HANE lesions do not respond well to epinephrine.
- In HANE, laryngeal edema is relatively common.
- Dental work is the classic precipitating factor for HANE.

The common idiopathic form of urticaria and angioedema is usually unrelated to antecedent trauma except in special cases of delayed-pressure urticaria, in which hives and angioedema follow minor trauma or pressure (e.g., to the hands while playing golf) of soft tissues. The response to pressure distinguishes this special form of physical urticaria from HANE.

It is reasonable to perform C4, C1 esterase inhibitor assays (functional and quantitative) for all patients with unexplained recurrent angioedema, especially if urticaria is not present.

The five types of HANE-like disorders are as follows:

1. Classic HANE is a genetic dysregulation of gene function for C1 inhibitor that is inherited in an autosomal-dominant pattern. Therapy with androgens (testosterone, stanozolol, danazol) reverses the dysregulation and allows expression of the otherwise normal gene, resulting in half-normal plasma levels of C1, which is sufficient to eliminate the clinical manifestations of the disease.

- Classic HANE is a genetic dysregulation (autosomal dominant).
- Testosterone, stanozolol, and danazol reverse the dysregulation.

2. In some cases of HANE, the gene for the C1 inhibitor mutates, rendering the molecule functionally ineffective but quantifiable in the blood. Thus, plasma levels of the C1 inhibitor molecule may be normal in these cases. This is the basis for requesting immunochemical and functional measures of serum C1 inhibitor (with immunochemical measures only, the diagnosis is missed in cases of normal levels of an inactive molecule). Both classic HANE (low levels of C1 esterase inhibitor) and classic HANE with mutated gene for C1 inhibitor (nonfunctional C1 esterase inhibitor) are inherited forms of the disease. However, both forms may be seen in which the proband starts the mutational line, so the family history is not positive in all cases.

- Hereditary angioedema with normal levels of C1 esterase inhibitor but nonfunctional (by esterase assay) indicates a gene mutation.

3. C1 esterase inhibitor deficiency may be an acquired disorder with malignancy or lymphoproliferative disease. Plasma levels for C1, C4, and C1 esterase inhibitor are low in acquired C1 esterase inhibitor deficiency. The hypothesis for the pathogenesis of this form of angioedema is that the tumor has or releases determinants that fix complement, and with constant *consumption* of complement components, a point is reached at which the biosynthesis of C1 inhibitor cannot keep up with the consumption rate, and the relative deficiency of C1 inhibitor allows episodes of swelling.

- C1 esterase inhibitor deficiency can be an acquired disorder in malignancy or lymphoproliferative disease.
- C1 levels are low in acquired C1 esterase inhibitor deficiency.

4. and 5. Basically, these two types are autoimmune disorders in which antibody to the catalytic site on C1 inhibitor or

to the binding site for C1 inhibitor on C1q interferes with the function of C1 inhibitor, hastening its destruction.

Physical Urticaria

Heat, light, cold, vibration, and trauma/pressure have been reported to cause hives in susceptible persons. Getting the history is the only way to suspect the diagnosis, which can be confirmed by applying each of the stimuli to the patient's skin in the laboratory. Heat can be applied by placing coins (soaked in hot water for a few minutes) on the patient's forearm. Cold can be applied with coins kept in a freezer or with ice cubes. For vibration, use a laboratory vortex mixer or any common vibrator. A pair of sandbags connected by a strap can be draped over the patient to create enough pressure to cause symptoms in the patients with delayed pressure urticaria. Note that unlike most cases of common idiopathic urticaria (in which the lesions affect essentially all skin surfaces), many cases of physical urticarias seem to involve only certain areas of skin. Thus, challenges will be positive only in the areas usually involved and negative in other areas. Directing challenges to the appropriate area depends on the history.

● For physical urticaria, the history is the only way to suspect the diagnosis, which can be confirmed by applying stimuli to the patient's skin.

Food Allergy in Chronic Urticaria

Food allergy almost never causes chronic urticaria. However, urticaria can be an acute manifestation of true food allergy.

● Food allergy almost never causes *chronic* urticaria.
● Food allergy may cause *acute* urticaria, angioedema, or anaphylaxis.

Histopathology of Chronic Urticaria

Chronic urticaria is characterized by mononuclear cell perivascular cuffing around dermal capillaries, particularly involving the capillary loops that interdigitate with the rete pegs of the epidermis. This mononuclear cell cuff is mostly helper T cells, with some monocytes, macrophages, B cells, and mast cells. This is the usual histologic location for most skin mast cells. It appears there is about a tenfold increase in the number of mast cells in the cuff compared with the normal value. However, the number of mast cells is still small compared with that of other round cells in the cuff. This histologic picture is consistent throughout the skin, regardless of recent active urtication. Most pathologists consider "vasculitis" to indicate actual necrosis of the structural elements of blood vessels; thus, the typical features of chronic urticaria do not meet the criteria for vasculitis. Immunofluorescence studies on chronic urticaria biopsy samples for fibrin, complement, and immunoglobulin deposition in blood vessels are negative.

Urticarial vasculitis shows the usual histologic features of leukocytoclastic vasculitis.

● Characteristic of chronic urticaria: a mononuclear cell perivascular cuff around capillaries.

Management of Urticaria

The history is of utmost importance if the 2% to 4% of cases of chronic urticaria actually due to allergic causes are to be discovered. A complete physical examination is needed, with particular attention to the skin (including some test for dermatographism), to evaluate for the vasculitic nature of the lesions, and to the liver, lymph nodes, and mucous membranes. Laboratory testing need not be exhaustive: chest radiography, a complete blood count with differential to discover eosinophilia, liver enzymes, erythrocyte sedimentation rate, serum protein electrophoresis, total hemolytic complement, antinuclear antibody, urinalysis, and stool examination for parasites. Only if the patient seems to have a strong allergic diathesis and some element in the history suggests an allergic cause is allergy skin testing indicated. However, patients with idiopathic urticaria often have fixed ideas about an allergy causing their problem, and skin testing often helps to dissuade them of this idea.

● The history is of utmost importance in diagnosing allergic urticaria.
● Laboratory testing may include chest radiography, eosinophil count, liver enzymes, erythrocyte sedimentation rate, serum protein electrophoresis, total hemolytic complement, and stool examination for parasites.

Management of urticaria and angioedema is usually with H_1 antagonists; the addition of H_2 antagonists may be helpful. Tricyclic antidepressants, such as doxepin, have potent antihistamine effects and are useful. Systemic corticosteroids can be used for acute urticaria and angioedema or for very severe chronic idiopathic urticaria and angioedema.

● Urticaria and angioedema: usual management is with H_1 antagonists.
● Urticaria and angioedema: systemic corticosteroids for severe cases.

FOOD ALLERGY

Clinical History

The clinical syndrome of food allergy should prompt patients to provide a history containing some or all the following: for very sensitive persons, some tingling, itching, and a metallic taste in the mouth occur while the food is still in the mouth. Within 15 minutes after swallowing the food, some epigastric distress may occur. There may be nausea and, occasionally with marked sensitivity, vomiting. Abdominal cramping is felt chiefly in the periumbilical area (small bowel phase), and lower abdominal cramping and watery diarrhea may occur. Urticaria or angioedema may occur in any distribution or there may be only itching of the palms and soles. With increasing clinical sensitivity to the offending allergen, anaphylactic symptoms may emerge, including tachycardia, hypotension, generalized flushing, and alterations of consciousness.

In extremely sensitive persons, generalized flushing, hypotension, and tachycardia may occur before the other symptoms. Most patients with a food allergy can identify the offending foods. The diagnosis should be confirmed by skin testing or in vitro measurement of allergen-specific IgE antibody.

- Allergic reactions to food usually include pruritus, urticaria, or angioedema.

Common Causes of Food Allergy

Table 2-13 lists items considered the most common allergens.

Food-Related Anaphylaxis

Food-induced anaphylaxis is the same process involved in acute urticaria or angioedema to food allergens except the severity of the reaction is greater in anaphylaxis. Relatively few foods are involved in food-induced anaphylaxis; the main ones are peanuts, shellfish, and nuts. Patients with latex allergy can develop food allergy to banana, avocado, kiwifruit, and other fruits.

- Anaphylaxis to food can be life-threatening.
- There is cross-sensitivity between latex and banana, avocado, and kiwifruit.

Allergy Skin Testing in Food Allergy

Patients presenting with food-related symptoms may have food allergy, food intolerance, irritable bowel syndrome, nonspecific dyspepsia, or one of a large number of nonallergic

Table 2-13.—Common Causes of Food Allergy

Eggs	Shellfish
Milk	Soybean
Nuts	Wheat
Peanuts	

conditions. A careful and detailed history on the nature of the "reaction," the reproducibility of the association of food and symptoms, and the timing of symptoms in relation to the ingestion of food can help the clinician form a clinical impression.

In many cases, allergy skin tests to foods can be helpful. If the allergy skin tests are negative (and the clinical suspicion for food allergy is low), the patient can be reassured that food allergy is not the cause of the symptoms. If the allergy skin tests are positive (and the clinical suspicion for food allergy is high), then the patient should be counseled on the management of the food allergy. For highly sensitive persons, this includes strict and rigorous avoidance of the offending foods. These patients should also be given epinephrine for self-administration in case of emergency.

When the diagnosis of food allergy is uncertain or if the symptoms are mild and nonspecific, sometimes oral food challenges can be helpful. An open challenge is usually performed first. If negative, the diagnosis of food allergy is excluded. If positive, a blinded placebo-controlled challenge can be performed.

- Positive results on skin tests and double-blind food challenges can confirm the diagnosis of food allergy.
- If results of food skin tests are negative, food allergy is unlikely.
- Patients with anaphylaxis to food should strictly avoid the offending food and carry an epinephrine kit.

STINGING INSECT ALLERGY

In patients clinically sensitive to Hymenoptera, reactions to a sting can be either large local reactions or the systemic, anaphylactic reactions. In the large local sting reaction, swelling at the sting site may be dramatic but there are no symptoms distant from that site. Stings of the head, neck, and dorsum of the hands are particularly prone to large local reactions.

Anaphylaxis caused by allergy to stinging insects is similar to all other forms of anaphylaxis. Thus, the onset of anaphylaxis may be very rapid, often within 1 or 2 minutes. Pruritus of the palms and soles is the most common initial manifestation and frequently is followed by generalized flushing, urticaria, angioedema, or hypotension (or a combination of these). The reason for attaching importance to whether a stinging insect reaction is a large local or a generalized one is that allergy skin testing and allergen immunotherapy are recommended only for generalized reactions. Patients who experience a large local reaction are not at increased risk for future anaphylaxis.

- Two varieties of reaction to sting: large local and anaphylactic.

Bee and Vespid Allergy

Yellow jackets, wasps, and hornets are vespids, and their venoms cross-react to a substantial degree. The venom of honeybees (order Apidaea) does **not** cross-react with that of vespids. Unless the patient actually captures the insect delivering the sting, uncertainty will likely attend many cases of insect-stinging anaphylaxis. Thus, we usually conduct skin testing to honeybee and each of the vespids. To interpret skin tests accurately, it is helpful to know which insect caused the sting producing the generalized reaction. Often, the circumstances of the sting can help determine the type of insect responsible. Multiple stings received while mowing the grass or doing other landscape jobs that may disturb yellow-jacket burrows in the ground are likely causes of yellow-jacket stings. A single sting received while near picnic tables or refuse containers at picnic areas is likely from a yellow jacket or possibly a hornet. Stings received while working around the house exterior (painting, cleaning eaves and gutters, attic work) are most likely from wasps.

- Yellow jackets, wasps, and hornets are vespids and their venoms cross-react.
- Venom of bees does not cross-react with that of vespids.
- It is helpful to know which insect caused the sting.

Allergy Testing

Patients who have had a generalized reaction warrant allergen skin testing. Patients who have had a large local reaction to one of the Hymenoptera stings do **not** warrant allergen skin testing because they are not at increased risk for future anaphylaxis.

- Generalized reaction warrants allergen skin testing.
- Large local reaction does not warrant allergen skin testing.

In many cases, skin testing should be delayed for at least 1 month after a sting-induced general reaction, because tests conducted closer to the time of the sting have a substantial risk of being falsely negative. Positive results on skin testing that correlate with the clinical history are sufficient evidence for considering Hymenoptera venom immunotherapy.

- Skin testing should be delayed for at least 1 month after a sting-induced general reaction.
- Patients with clinical anaphylaxis and positive results on venom skin tests may benefit from venom immunotherapy.

Venom Immunotherapy

The decision to undertake venom immunotherapy can be reached only after a discussion between the patient and physician. General indications for venom immunotherapy are listed in Table 2-14. Patients must understand that once initiated

Table 2-14.—Indications for Venom Immunotherapy

History of anaphylaxis to a sting
Positive results on skin tests to venom implicated historically in the anaphylactic reaction
Patient's level of anxiety disrupts usual habits and activities in warm months
Occupational—higher than usual risk of sting
House painters
Outdoor construction workers
Forestry workers

the immunotherapy injection schedule has to be maintained and that there is a small risk of the immunotherapy inducing anaphylaxis. It is important that patients understand that despite receiving allergy immunotherapy, they must carry epinephrine when outdoors, because of the 2% to 10% possibility that immunotherapy will not provide suitable protection. Most, but not all, patients can safely discontinue venom immunotherapy after 3 to 5 years of treatment.

- There is a small risk that immunotherapy will induce anaphylaxis.
- There is a 2%-10% chance that immunotherapy will not provide protection.

Avoidance

Table 2-15 lists the warnings that every patient with stinging-insect hypersensitivity should receive.

The circumstances of each patient may provide additional entries to the list in Table 2-15. Also, patients need to know how to use self-injectable epinephrine in its several forms. Many patients wear an anaphylaxis identification bracelet.

- All patients with stinging-insect sensitivity should carry an epinephrine kit.

Anaphylaxis

Anaphylaxis is a generalized reaction characterized by flushing, hypotension, and tachycardia. Urticaria and angioedema may occur in many cases, and in patients with moderate-to-severe asthma or rhinitis as a preexisting condition, the asthma and rhinitis can be made worse. This definition of anaphylaxis is based on clinical manifestations. A cellular and molecular definition of anaphylaxis is "a generalized allergic reaction in which large quantities of both preformed and newly synthesized mediators are released from activated basophils and mast cells." The dominant mediators of acute anaphylaxis are histamine and prostaglandin D_2. The serum levels of tryptase may be increased for a few hours after clinical anaphylaxis. Physiologically, the hypotension of anaphylaxis is caused by peripheral vasodilatation and not by impaired cardiac contractility. Anaphylaxis is characterized by a hyperdynamic state. For these reasons, anaphylaxis can be fatal in patients with preexisting fixed vascular obstructive disease in whom a decrease in perfusion pressure leads to a critical reduction in flow (stroke) or in patients in whom laryngeal edema develops and completely occludes the airway.

- The clinical hallmarks of anaphylaxis are flushing, hypotension, and tachycardia.
- Urticaria and angioedema may be present.
- Histamine and prostaglandin D_2 are the dominant mediators of acute anaphylaxis.
- Peripheral vasodilatation causes hypotension of anaphylaxis.

Latex allergy is an important cause of intraoperative anaphylaxis. Patients with intraoperative anaphylaxis should be evaluated for possible latex allergy, usually by a skin test or in vitro assay. When persons with known latex allergy undergo invasive procedures, a latex-free environment is necessary. Patients with spina bifida or those with dermatitis, rhinitis, or asthma caused by latex allergy are at increased risk for anaphylaxis to latex.

- Latex allergy is an important cause of intraoperative anaphylaxis.

Table 2-15.—Do's and Don'ts for Patients With Hypersensitivity to Insect Stings

---

Avoid looking or smelling like a flower
    Avoid flowered prints for clothes
    Avoid cosmetics and fragrances, especially ones derived from flowering plants
Never drink from a soft-drink can out-of-doors during the warm months--a yellow jacket can land **on** or **in** the can while you are not watching and go inside the can and sting the inside of your mouth (one of the most dangerous places for a sensitive patient to be stung) when you take a drink
Avoid doing outdoor maintenance and yard work
Never reach into a mailbox without first looking in it
Never go barefoot
Always look at the underside of picnic table benches and park benches before sitting down
Never attempt physically to eject a stinging insect from the interior of an automobile but pull over, get out, and let someone else remove the insect

---

DRUG ALLERGY

Classes of Drug Allergy

Drug Allergy Not Involving IgE or Immediate-Type Reactions

Stevens-Johnson Syndrome

Stevens-Johnson syndrome is a bullous skin and mucosal reaction; very large blisters appear over much of the skin surface, in the mouth, and along the gastrointestinal tract. Because of the propensity of the blisters to break down and become infected, the reaction often is life-threatening. Treatment consists of stopping the drug causing the reaction, giving systemic steroids, and providing supportive care. The patients are often treated in burn units. Penicillin, sulfonamides, barbiturates, diphenylhydantoin, warfarin, and phenothiazines are well-known causes. A drug-induced Stevens-Johnson reaction is an absolute contraindication to giving a causative drug to the patient.

- Stevens-Johnson syndrome is life-threatening and is an absolute contraindication for rechallenge with the drug.

Toxic Epidermal Necrolysis Syndrome

Clinically, toxic epidermal necrolysis syndrome is almost indistinguishable from Stevens-Johnson syndrome. Histologically, the cleavage plane for the blisters is deeper than in Stevens-Johnson syndrome. The cleavage plane is *at* the basement membrane of the epidermis, so even the basal cell layer is lost. This makes toxic epidermal necrolysis syndrome even more devastating than Stevens-Johnson syndrome, because healing occurs with much scarring. Often, healing cannot be accomplished without skin grafting, so the mortality rate is even higher than in Stevens-Johnson syndrome. Patients with toxic epidermal necrolysis are always cared for in a burn unit because of full-thickness burns over 80% to 90% of the skin. The mortality rate is very high, as in burn patients with damage of this extent.

- Toxic epidermal necrolysis syndrome is a life-threatening exfoliative dermatitis.

Macular "Drug Red" Syndrome

Macular "drug red" syndrome is a generalized skin rash that is fairly characteristic because it is intensely bright red. It is nonpruritic, flat (macular), and usually causes no significant discomfort. It cannot be predicted, and because it is potentially related to the serious syndromes above, most physicians regard this type of rash as a strong contraindication to giving the drug anytime in the future.

- Macular "drug red" rash is intensely bright red, nonpruritic, and flat (macular).

Ampicillin-Mononucleosis Rash

Ampicillin-mononucleosis rash is a unique drug rash occurring when ampicillin is given to an acutely ill febrile patient who has mononucleosis. The rash is papular, nonpruritic, rose-colored, usually on the abdomen, and has a granular feel when the fingers brush lightly over the surface of the involved skin. It is not known why the rash is specific for ampicillin and mononucleosis.

- Ampicillin-mononucleosis rash is papular, nonpruritic, rose-colored, and on the abdomen.

Fixed Drug Eruptions

Fixed drug eruptions are red to red-brown macules that appear on a certain area of the patient's skin; any part of the body can be affected. The macules do not itch or have other signs of inflammation, although fever is associated with their appearance in a few patients. The unique aspect of this allergic phenomenon is that if a patient is given the drug of cause in the future, exactly the same skin areas have the rash. Resolution of the macules often includes postinflammatory hyperpigmentation. Except for cosmetic problems due to skin discolorations, the phenomenon does not seem serious. Antibiotics and sulfonamides are the most frequently recognized causes.

- In fixed drug eruptions, the same area of skin is affected.

Erythema Nodosum

Erythema nodosum is a characteristic rash of red nodules about the size of a quarter, usually nonpruritic and appearing only over the anterior aspects of the lower legs. Histopathologically, the nodules are plaques of infiltrating mononuclear cells. Erythema nodosum is associated with several connective tissue diseases, viral infections, and drug allergy.

- Erythema nodosum rash is usually nonpruritic, appearing only over the anterior aspect of the lower legs.
- It is associated with several connective tissue diseases, viral infections, and drug allergy.

Contact Dermatitis

Contact dermatitis can occur with various drugs. Commonly, it is a form of drug allergy that is an occupational disease in medical or healthcare workers. In some patients receiving topical drugs on the skin, allergy develops to the drug or various elements in its pharmaceutical formulation, for example, fillers, stabilizers, antibacterials, and emulsifiers. Contact dermatitis is a manifestation of type IV hypersensitivity and clinically appears as an area of reddening on the skin which progresses to a granular weeping eczematous eruption of the skin, with some dermal thickening and a plaque-like quality of the surrounding skin. Histopathologically, the affected area is infiltrated by mononuclear cells. When patients receiving treatment for some kind of dermatitis develop contact hypersensitivity to corticosteroids or other drugs used in treatment, a particularly difficult diagnostic problem arises, unless the physician is alert to this possibility. When contact hypersensitivity to a drug occurs, it does not increase the probability of acute type I hypersensitivity and is not associated with serious exfoliative syndromes. However, patients can develop exquisite cutaneous sensitivity of this type so that almost no avoidance technique in the workplace completely eliminates dermatitis; even protective gloves are only partly helpful. Thus, it can be occupationally disabling.

- Contact dermatitis is a form of drug allergy.
- It is a manifestation of type IV hypersensitivity.

Penicillin Allergy

Penicillin can cause anaphylaxis in sensitive persons. It is an IgE-mediated process that can be evaluated by skin testing to penicillin major and minor determinants. Patients with positive results on skin testing and a clinical history of penicillin allergy can be desensitized to penicillin, but the procedure may be hazardous.

- Penicillin can cause anaphylaxis.
- It is an IgE-mediated process diagnosed by penicillin skin testing.
- Patients can be desensitized, but the procedure may be hazardous.

Penicillin skin tests can be helpful in determining whether it is safe to administer penicillin to a patient with suspected penicillin allergy. About 85% of patients with a history of penicillin allergy have negative skin tests to the major and minor determinants of penicillin. These patients generally are not at increased risk for anaphylaxis, and most can receive penicillin safely. If penicillin skin tests are positive, there is a 40% to 60% chance that an allergic reaction will develop if the patient is challenged with penicillin. Most of these patients should avoid penicillin and related drugs. However, if there is a strong indication for penicillin treatment, desensitization can be considered. The desensitization procedure involves the administration of progressively increasing doses of penicillin. Desensitization can be accomplished by the oral or intravenous route and is usually performed in a hospital setting.

Ampicillin, amoxicillin, nafcillin, and other β-lactam antibiotics cross-react strongly with penicillin. Early studies suggested that up to 20% to 30% of patients with penicillin allergy were also allergic to cephalosporins. More recent studies have suggested that the cross-sensitivity of penicillin with cephalosporins is much less, about 5%. Most studies have suggested that aztreonam does not cross-react with penicillin.

Radiographic Contrast Media Reactions

Radiographic contrast media can cause reactions that have the clinical appearance of anaphylaxis. Estimates of the frequency of these reactions are 2% to 6% of procedures involving intravenous contrast media. The incidence of intra-arterial contrast-induced reactions is lower. The anaphylactoid reactions **do not** involve IgE antibody (thus, the reason for the term "anaphylact**oid**" reactions). Radiocontrast media appear to induce mediator release on the basis of some other property intrinsic to the contrast agent. The tonicity or ionic strength of the media seems particularly related to anaphylactoid reactions. With availability of low ionic strength media, the incidence of reactions has been lower.

- The frequency of contrast media reactions is 2%-6% of procedures.
- The reaction does not involve IgE antibody.
- Nonionic or low osmolar contrast media cause fewer anaphylactoid reactions than standard contrast media.

The frequency of radiocontrast media reactions can be reduced with the use of low ionic strength media in patients with a history of asthma or atopy. Patients with a history of reaction to radiocontrast media who subsequently need radiographic contrast media procedures can be pretreated with a protocol of 50 mg oral prednisone every 6 hours for three doses, with the last dose 1 hour before the procedure. At the time of the last dose, also give 50 mg of diphenhydramine or equivalent. Some studies show that the addition of oral ephedrine can be beneficial. However, most studies show that the addition of an H_2 antagonist is unnecessary.

- Patients with a history of systemic reactions to radiocontrast media 1) should be pretreated with systemic corticosteroids and an H_1 antagonist and 2) should be offered nonionic contrast agents.

Mastocytosis

Systemic mastocytosis is a disorder of abnormal proliferation of mast cells. The skin, bone marrow, liver, spleen, lymph nodes, and gastrointestinal tract can be affected.

The clinical manifestations vary but can include flushing, pruritus, urticaria, unexplained syncope, fatigue, and dyspepsia. Bone marrow biopsy with special stains for mast cells (toluidine blue, Giemsa, chloral acetate esterase, and immunochemical stains for tryptase) is the most direct diagnostic study. Serum levels of tryptase and urinary concentrations of histamine and histamine metabolites may be increased.

Treatment initially consists of antihistamines. Cromolyn given orally can be beneficial, especially in patients with gastrointestinal symptoms. Corticosteroids should be considered in severe cases, and interferon is a promising investigational treatment.

Eosinophilia

The differential diagnosis of eosinophilia is given in Table 2-16. The eosinophil myalgia syndrome is a systemic illness associated with a contaminant in specific batches of L-tryptophan preparations (these contaminated products are no longer available).

The clinical manifestations include weight loss, muscle weakness, and cutaneous induration. The laboratory hallmark is peripheral and tissue eosinophilia. Follow-up studies show that many affected patients continue to have significant disability months and years after the acute illness. Although corticosteroids are used in the treatment of this disorder, there is no evidence that corticosteroid therapy alters long-term disability or mortality.

Hypereosinophilia syndrome is an idiopathic disorder

Table 2-16.—Common Causes of Eosinophilia

Atopic
Allergic rhinitis
Allergic bronchopulmonary aspergillosis
Asthma
Atopic dermatitis
Drug hypersensitivity
Pulmonary
Eosinophilic pneumonia
Löffler syndrome
Proliferative/neoplastic
Idiopathic hypereosinophilic syndrome
Eosinophilic leukemia
Vasculitis/connective tissue
Churg-Strauss vasculitis
Eosinophilic fasciitis
Eosinophilic gastroenteritis
Infectious
Visceral larva migrans
Helminth
Toxic
Eosinophil myalgia syndrome
Toxic oil syndrome

characterized by 1) a total eosinophil count greater than 1,500/μL for 6 months or longer, 2) signs or symptoms of organ involvement, and 3) no other known cause of eosinophilia. The syndrome typically affects persons in the third through sixth decades of life; women are affected more often than men. It usually is a multisystem disorder affecting the heart, lungs, nervous system, or skin. Symptoms include fatigue, cough, shortness of breath, or rash. Cardiac involvement in hypereosinophilia syndrome is especially important: endomyocardial fibrosis, murothrombi, and mitral and tricuspid incompetence can occur. The clinical syndrome is one of a restrictive cardiomyopathy with congestive heart failure. Echocardiography and endomyocardial biopsy are two important diagnostic tests.

Treatment of hypereosinophila syndrome usually includes systemic corticosteroids. Hydroxyurea or vincristine can be useful in refractory cases.

Common Variable Immunodeficiency

Common variable immunodeficiency can affect persons of all ages, both males and females. It is not a hereditary disorder. Patients have recurrent infections and hypogammaglobulinemia. Recurrent pyogenic infections include chronic otitis media, chronic or recurrent sinusitis, pneumonia, and bronchiectasis.

Patients with common variable immunodeficiency often have autoimmune or gastrointestinal disturbances. About one-half of patients have chronic diarrhea and malabsorption. There may be steatorrhea, protein-losing enteropathy, ulcerative colitis, or Crohn disease. Other gastrointestinal problems associated with the disease are atrophic gastritis, pernicious anemia, giardiasis, and chronic active hepatitis. Pathologic changes in the gastrointestinal tract mucosa include loss of villi, nodular lymphoid hyperplasia, and diffuse lymphoid infiltration.

Autoimmune anemia, thrombocytopenia, or neutropenia is present in 10% to 50% of patients. Inflammatory arthritis and lymphoid interstitial pneumonia are other associated conditions. Also, patients have an increased risk of developing malignancy, particularly a lymphoid malignancy such as non-Hodgkin lymphoma.

The diagnosis of common variable immunodeficiency should be considered in patients with recurrent pyogenic infections and hypogammaglobulinemia. Associated gastrointestinal or autoimmune disease and the exclusion of hereditary primary immunodeficiencies support the diagnosis. Treatment is with intravenous gamma globulin.

Terminal Complement Component Deficiencies

Patients with deficiency of the terminal complement component C5, C6, C7, or C8 have increased susceptibility to meningococcal infections. The terminal complement components form the membrane attack complex that causes cell lysis; hence, deficiency of one of these components results in defective microbial killing. The terminal component C9 participates in membrane pore formation but is not essential for complement-mediated cell lysis. Thus, the rare patients with a C9 deficiency have limited increased susceptibility to infections.

Terminal complement component deficiency should be suspected in patients with recurrent meningococcal disease, a family history of meningococcal disease, systemic meningococcal infection, or those infected with an unusual serotype of meningococcus. Diagnosis is confirmed with assay of total hemolytic complement and measurement of individual complement components.

QUESTIONS

Multiple Choice (choose the one best answer)

1. A 13-year-old child presents with a 3-day history of left ear pain. There is a past history of hives following treatment with amoxicillin and sulfamethoxazole at ages 2 and 3, respectively. Allergy skin tests are performed to guide antibiotic treatment. The skin tests should be performed by which technique?
   a. Scratch
   b. Prick
   c. Patch
   d. Intradermal
   e. Punch

2. A 35-year-old farmer presents with a history of anaphylaxis to yellow jacket sting. Two months earlier she was stung on the left wrist by a (presumed) yellow jacket and 15 minutes later developed hives, periorbital edema, wheezing, and lightheadedness. Treatment with epinephrine, antihistamines, and systemic steroids was successful. The patient has stable, steroid-dependent asthma, and treated depression. Current medications include:

    Beclomethasone inhaler, 84 µg/puff, 4 puffs bid
    Loratidine, 10 mg qd
    Doxepin, 50 mg qd
    Prednisone, 10 mg qd

    Before allergy testing for evaluation of anaphylaxis, the patient should discontinue taking:
    a. Prednisone
    b. Loratadine
    c. Doxepin
    d. Loratadine and doxepin
    e. Loratadine, doxepin, and prednisone

3. A 44-year-old long-distance truck driver presents with a 10-year history of seasonal rhinitis. Symptoms include itchy watery eyes, sneezing, and rhinorrhea. Symptoms are present May through August each year and are completely absent in the winter. Current medications include:

    Ketoconazole, 200 mg once daily
    Digoxin, 0.25 mg once daily
    Acetaminophen, 500 mg as needed

    You prescribe:
    a. Astemizole
    b. Cetirizine
    c. Chlorpheniramine
    d. Diphenhydramine
    e. Fexofenadine

4. A 25-year-old woman presents with symptomatic asthma. She has searched Internet sites and asks about starting a 5-lipoxygenase inhibitor. She is referring to:
   a. Zileuton
   b. Zafirlukast
   c. Montelukast
   d. Pranlukast
   e. MK-886

5. A 32-year-old nurse has nasal congestion and rhinorrhea. She is fairly certain that the symptoms are worse at work and are aggravated when she dons protective latex gloves. This patient should also avoid:
   a. Vinyl gloves
   b. Toy balloons
   c. Plastic jewelry
   d. Automobile tires
   e. Latex paint

6. A 19-year-old college student has peanut allergy. In previous years, the ingestion of peanuts or peanut butter resulted in the development of hives and angioedema of the hands and face within 10 to 15 minutes. Most of these past episodes resolved spontaneously or with home treatment. Two weeks ago, the ingestion of a cookie containing peanuts resulted in generalized pruritus, scattered hives, angioedema of the tongue and lips, and lightheadedness. This spell was treated successfully in the emergency department with epinephrine, antihistamines, and corticosteroids. Your advice should include:
   a. Double-blind challenge with peanut
   b. Cetirizine, 10 mg daily
   c. Prednisone, 10 mg daily
   d. Rigorous avoidance of all peanut-containing food
   e. In vitro antibody test to peanut

7. A 48-year-old presents with a respiratory infection and a 4-day history of malaise, nasal congestion, and rhinorrhea. There is a nasal discharge of yellow-green secretions, more pronounced on the left. In addition, there is a sense of facial fullness, also more pronounced on the left, and some tooth pain in the upper left molar region. Your next step is:
   a. Sinus radiography
   b. Sinus computed tomography
   c. Treatment with trimethoprim-sulfamethoxazole
   d. Treatment with metronidazole
   e. Treatment with clindamycin

8. A 40-year-old man presents with continued asthma. Symptoms of wheeze and chest tightness occur several times daily, especially with exercise. He may awaken with wheezing about twice a week. He experiences asthma exacerbations requiring emergency treatment 4 or 5 times a year. The most recent FEV_1 was 54% of predicted, with 22% improvement after bronchodilator treatment. Compliance with his existing asthma program appears good and includes:

   Fluticasone inhaler (220 μg/puff), 4 puffs bid
   Salmeterol inhaler (21 μg/puff), 2 puffs bid
   Albuterol inhaler, 2 puffs tid

   Your advice is to add:
   a. Troleandomycin, 250 mg qid
   b. Prednisone, 20 mg qd
   c. Albuterol by nebulization qid
   d. Inhaled cromolyn, 2 puffs qid
   e. Cyclosporine, 25 mg bid

9. A 38-year-old patient presents with unexplained flushing. These spells are characterized by a feeling of warmth and pink color to the face and chest, and they may occur several times a week and are unprovoked. There also have been episodes of lightheadedness and two syncopal spells. Cardiac and neurologic work-up was negative. Laboratory studies were notable only for a hemoglobin of 10.8. You order:
   a. Serum C1 esterase inhibitor
   b. C4
   c. Urinary catecholamines
   d. Serum vasoactive intestinal polypeptide
   e. Serum tryptase

10. A 49-year-old asks about his allergy shots to honeybee venom. At age 44, he was stung on the neck by a honeybee, and 5 minutes later scattered hives developed. The hives resolved without treatment. He started immunotherapy to honeybee venom at that time. Although he carries epinephrine for self-administration, he has not been stung since the initial sting 5 years ago. The patient would like to discontinue the shots but asks for your advice. You recommend:
   a. Repeat the allergy skin test to bee venom
   b. Assay protective IgG antibody levels to bee venom
   c. Continue the shots indefinitely
   d. Continue the shots for another 3 to 5 years
   e. Discontinue the shots

ANSWERS

1. Answer d.
This patient should undergo penicillin allergy testing using the intradermal technique. Penicillin allergy intradermal skin tests have been well studied and have excellent predictive value. Prick skin tests for penicillin allergy have low sensitivity. Patch testing is reserved for evaluation of contact dermatitis.

2. Answer d.
Antihistamines should be discontinued before allergy skin tests to venoms. Also, medications with antihistamine properties should be discontinued, including tricyclic antidepressants, anticholinergic agents, and phenothiazines. Therefore, the antihistamine loratadine and the tricyclic antidepressant doxepin both should be discontinued before allergy testing. Corticosteroids generally do not interfere with immediate-type skin testing such as allergy testing.

3. Answer e.
This patient should be treated with an oral antihistamine. Antihistamines with sedating properties should be avoided in treating a truck driver, and chlorpheniramine and diphenhydramine are both potentially sedating. The antihistamine cetirizine also can be sedating but is not as likely to cause sedation as chlorpheniramine and diphenhydramine. Astemizole is a nonsedating antihistamine but has potential drug interactions with ketoconazole. Fexofenadine and loratadine are

nonsedating and do not have drug interactions with keto-conazole or macrolide antibiotics.

4. Answer a.

Zileuton is a 5-lipoxygenase inhibitor. Zafirlukast, mon-telukast, and pranlukast are leukotriene receptor antagonists. The product MK-886 is a member of a completely separate class of leukotriene-modifying agents called FLAP inhibitors.

5. Answer b.

This patient has presumed latex allergy. Toy balloons are generally made of latex and can precipitate local angioede-ma or even anaphylaxis. Vinyl gloves and plastic jewelry generally do not contain latex. Automobile tires are made of volcanized rubber and do not cause latex allergy. Latex paint contains polymers that, in fact, are not of latex origin.

6. Answer d.

This patient has a strong history of allergy to peanut. A double-blind challenge with peanut is potentially hazardous and should not be performed. Daily treatment with antihis-tamine or oral corticosteroid is generally not an effective pro-phylaxis for food allergy. An in vitro antibody test to peanut certainly is reasonable but response (d) is the better answer. In this patient, instructions should be given to strictly avoid even inadvertent peanut ingestion. This advice should be given even if the in vitro antibody test to peanut is negative or equivocal.

7. Answer c.

This patient presents with an acute uncomplicated sinusitis. Empiric treatment with an antibiotic such as trimethoprim-sulfamethoxazole is generally the recommended treatment. For uncomplicated sinusitis, sinus imaging with radiography or computed tomography is not necessary. Metronidazole and clin-damycin may be appropriate for chronic or persistent sinusitis.

8. Answer b.

This patient has severe asthma that is steroid-dependent or nearly steroid-dependent. Because of the suboptimal control of asthma, this patient should begin a trial of continuous oral prednisone. Albuterol by nebulization would not be expected to achieve significantly superior bronchodilatation to the exist-ing program of salmeterol and albuterol. Inhaled cromolyn has not been shown to have any steroid-sparing effect. Troleandomycin and cyclosporine are not accepted treatments for asthma.

9. Answer e.

This patient has suspected systemic mastocytosis. Serum tryptase is a diagnostic test that measures the level of mast cell tryptase in the serum. The fourth component of complement and the C1 esterase inhibitor assay are appropriate tests for suspected hereditary angioedema. Urinary catecholamines can be helpful for the diagnosis of pheochromocytoma, which is not characterized by flushing. Vasoactive intestinal polypep-tide would be a study appropriate in unexplained diarrhea.

10. Answer e.

This patient appropriately started immunotherapy to bee venom 5 years previously. Current evidence suggests that for most cases of stinging insect hypersensitivity, especially for milder reactions, immunotherapy can be discontinued after a total of 3 to 5 years of treatment. However, allergy skin tests usually remain positive, even during and after immunothera-py. Specific IgG antibody levels to bee venom increase with venom immunotherapy, but these are not predictive of whether a patient can safely discontinue immunotherapy.

NOTES

CHAPTER 3
CARDIOLOGY

Thomas Behrenbeck, M.D., Ph.D.
Kyle W. Klarich, M.D.
Carole A. Warnes, M.D.
Win-Kuang Shen, M.D.
Paul A. Friedman, M.D.
Rick A. Nishimura, M.D.
Barry L. Karon, M.D.

PART I
Thomas Behrenbeck, M.D., Ph.D.
Kyle W. Klarich, M.D.
Carole A. Warnes, M.D.

PHYSICAL EXAMINATION

Jugular Venous Pressure

This pressure is normally 6 to 8 cm H_2O and best evaluated with the patient at 45°. When the pressure is increased, consider not only biventricular failure but also constrictive pericarditis, pericardial tamponade, cor pulmonale (especially pulmonary embolus), and superior vena cava syndrome. The normal waves are *a*, which reflects atrial contraction; *c*, closure of tricuspid valve followed by the *x* descent; and *v*, ventricular filling followed by *y* descent.

- Normal jugular venous pressure is 6 to 8 cm H_2O.
- Normal waves are *a*, atrial contraction; *c*, closure of tricuspid valve; *v*, ventricular filling.
- *x* descent, downward motion of right ventricle.
- *y* descent, early right ventricular filling phase.

Abnormalities of the waves indicate various conditions, as follows:
1) Large "a" wave: tricuspid stenosis, right ventricular hypertrophy, pulmonary hypertension (that is, increased right ventricular end-diastolic pressure)
2) Cannon "a" wave: atria contracting intermittently against a closed atrioventricular valve (atrioventricular dissociation)
3) Large, fused cv wave: tricuspid regurgitation
4) Rapid x + y descent: constrictive pericarditis

5) Kussmaul sign: venous filling with inspiration, pericardial tamponade, or constriction

- Abnormalities of waves:
    large "a" wave: tricuspid stenosis; right ventricular hypertrophy, pulmonary hypertension.
    cannon "a" wave: atria contracting against closed atrioventricular valve (atrioventricular dissociation).
    rapid x + y descent: constrictive pericarditis.

Arterial Pulse

Palpation of the radial pulse is useful only for rate; check the brachial or carotid pulse for contour. "Tardus" describes the timing and rate of rise of upstroke, and "parvus" describes the volume. In hypertension, radiofemoral delay (check radial and femoral pulses simultaneously) may reveal accompanying aortic coarctation.

Abnormalities of the arterial pulse and their indicated conditions are as follows:
1) parvus and tardus: aortic stenosis
2) parvus only: low output, cardiomyopathy
3) bounding: aortic regurgitation or atrioventricular fistulae
4) bifid: hypertrophic obstructive cardiomyopathy (from midsystolic obstruction)
5) bisferiens: aortic stenosis and regurgitation

6) dicrotic: left ventricular failure with hypotension, low output, and increased peripheral resistance

- Abnormalities of arterial pulse:
  parvus and tardus: aortic stenosis.
  parvus only: low output, cardiomyopathy.
  bisferiens: aortic stenosis and regurgitation.

Apical Impulse

This is normally a discrete area of localized contraction. It is usually maximal at the fifth intercostal space, midclavicular line.

Abnormalities of the apical impulse and their indicated conditions are as follows:
1) apex displaced, impulse poor and diffuse: cardiomyopathy
2) sustained but not necessarily displaced: left ventricular hypertrophy, aortic stenosis, often with large "a" wave
3) trifid: hypertrophic cardiomyopathy
4) hyperdynamic, descended, and diffuse with rapid filling wave: mitral regurgitation, aortic regurgitation
5) tapping quality, localized: mitral stenosis

- Abnormalities of apical impulse:
  apex displaced, impulse poor and diffuse: cardiomyopathy.
  trifid: hypertrophic cardiomyopathy.
  tapping quality, localized: mitral stenosis.

Additional Cardiac Palpation

A palpable aortic (A_2) component at the right upper sternum suggests a dilated aorta (aneurysm, dissection, severe aortic regurgitation, poststenotic dilatation in aortic stenosis, hypertension).

Severe tricuspid regurgitation may result in a pulsatile liver palpable in the right epigastrium. Look for accompanying hepatojugular reflux. In patients with severe emphysema, the apical impulse rotates medially and may be appreciated in the epigastrium.

Right ventricular hypertrophy results in sustained lift, best appreciated in the fourth intercostal space 2 to 3 cm left parasternally. Diastolic overload (atrial septal defect, anomalous pulmonary venous return) results in a vigorous untoward motion but may not be sustained. In significant pulmonary hypertension, the pulmonic (P_2) component may be palpable (this may be physiologic in slender people with small anteroposterior diameter).

- Pressure overload usually results in sustained, lateralized impulses (left > right ventricle).
- Volume overload (regurgitant lesions, atrial septal defect) usually is appreciated as dynamic and forceful but not sustained impulses.

- Palpable A_2/P_2 components are pathologic in adults with average body habitus.

Thrills

These indicate turbulent flow (such as aortic stenosis, ventricular septal defect).

Heart Sounds

First

This consists of audible mitral valve closure followed shortly by tricuspid valve closure and normally silent aortic/pulmonic opening. A *loud* first heart sound occurs with a short P-R interval and mitral stenosis because the mitral valve is wide open when the left ventricle begins to contract and then slaps shut. The first heart sound is also augmented in hypercontractile states (fever, exercise, thyrotoxicosis, pheochromocytomas, anemia). The intensity of the first sound is *decreased* if the mitral valve is heavily calcified (severe mitral stenosis) and also if the P-R interval is long (occurs classically with acute rheumatic fever).

- Loud first heart sound: short P-R interval, mitral stenosis, hypercontractile states.
- Decreased intensity of first heart sound: mitral valve heavily calcified, long P-R interval.

Second

This consists of aortic closure followed by pulmonary closure. Intensity of both is increased by hypertension (loud P_2 with pulmonary hypertension, P_2 then audible at apex). Intensity is decreased with heavily calcified valves (severe aortic stenosis). Normally, the second sound widens on inspiration.

- The intensity of the second heart sound is increased by hypertension.
- The intensity is decreased with heavily calcified valves.

Abnormalities of splitting of the second heart sound and their indicated conditions are as follows:
1) fixed split, particularly during expiration: atrial septal defect, widest split occurs with a combination atrial septal defect and pulmonary stenosis
2) paradoxic split (caused by delay in aortic closure so it closes after pulmonary valve): left bundle branch block, left ventricular hypertrophy

- Abnormalities of splitting of second heart sound:
  fixed split: atrial septal defect.
  paradoxic split: left bundle branch block, left ventricular hypertrophy.

- Mnemonic for S_1-S_2: *Many Things Are Possible*

Third

This is probably caused by tensing of the chordae as the blood distends the left ventricle during diastole. It is heard normally in young people (younger than 30 years) and in older adults and is associated with volume load on the left ventricle such as aortic regurgitation, mitral regurgitation, and cardiomyopathy.

- Third heart sound is heard in young people (where it is normal) and older adults in association with volume load on left ventricle (e.g., aortic regurgitation, mitral regurgitation, cardiomyopathy).

Fourth

This occurs with the atrial kick as blood is forced into the left ventricle by atrial contraction. It occurs when the left ventricle is stiff and noncompliant but usually not failing, such as in aortic stenosis, systemic hypertension, hypertrophic cardiomyopathy, and ischemia.

- Fourth heart sound occurs in aortic stenosis, systemic hypertension, hypertrophic cardiomyopathy, and ischemia.

Opening Snap

This is virtually always caused by mitral stenosis, and the interval from the second heart sound to the opening snap helps determine the severity. With severe mitral stenosis, the left atrial pressure is very high and thus the valve opens earlier, and the interval is less than 60 m/s.

- Opening snap is virtually always caused by mitral stenosis.

Murmurs

The specific murmurs are discussed with the individual valvular lesions described later in this chapter, but some broad guidelines follow here.

A systolic ejection murmur begins after the first heart sound and ends before the second sound. It may have a diamond-shaped quality with crescendo and decrescendo components, but in general the more severe the obstruction (the narrower the orifice), the louder the murmur and the later the peak of the murmur. It may be preceded by an ejection click, if the pliability of the valve is preserved.

- Systolic ejection murmur: the more severe the obstruction, the louder the murmur and the later the peak.

A holosystolic murmur occurs when blood goes from a high-pressure to a low-pressure system (mitral regurgitation, ventricular septal defect). It engulfs the first and second heart sounds.

- Holosystolic murmur occurs with mitral regurgitation and ventricular septal defect.

MANEUVERS THAT ALTER CARDIAC MURMURS

- *Inspiration* increases venous return and so increases right-sided murmurs, pulmonary stenosis, pulmonary regurgitation.
- *Valsalva* increases intrathoracic pressure, inhibiting venous return to the right side of the heart.
- Most cardiac murmurs and sounds diminish in intensity during Valsalva maneuver because of decreased ventricular filling and decreased cardiac output (except hypertrophic obstructive cardiomyopathy and mitral valve prolapse).
- *Handgrip* increases cardiac output and systemic arterial pressure.
- A change in *posture* from supine to upright causes decrease in venous return; therefore, stroke volume decreases, and this decrease causes a reflex increase in heart rate and peripheral resistance.
- *Squatting* and the *Valsalva maneuver* have opposite hemodynamic effects. Squatting increases peripheral resistance and increases venous return.

The effects of maneuvers are shown in Table 3-1.

VALVULAR HEART DISEASE

Aortic Stenosis

Supravalvular

The two major types of supravalvular aortic stenosis are diaphragmatic and localized hourglass-shaped narrowing immediately above the aortic sinuses, often associated with hypoplasia of the ascending aorta.

Supravalvular aortic stenosis is associated with Williams syndrome, which is characterized by so-called elfin facies, mental retardation, and hypercalcemia. Systemic hypertension is a common association. An important feature is large, dilated, thick-walled coronary arteries because the coronary ostia are proximal to the obstruction, causing premature atherosclerosis.

Physical Examination

Findings include a prominent left ventricle, a thrill in the suprasternal notch and over the carotid artery (thrill is often more marked in right carotid artery and the pulse upstroke is often brisker on right side than left side), systolic murmur without

Table 3-1.—Effects of Physical Maneuvers and Other Factors on Valvular Diseases

		Effect on murmur			
Maneuver	Result	Mitral regurgitation	MVP	Aortic stenosis	HOCM
Amyl nitrite	↓ afterload	↓	↑/0	↑	↑
Valsalva	↓ preload	↓	↑	↓	↑
Handgrip	↑ afterload	↑	↓/0	↓	↓
Post-PVC	↑ contractility ↓ afterload	=	↓	↑	↑*

*Although the murmur ↑, the peripheral pulse ↓ because of the increase in outflow obstruction.
HOCM, hypertrophic obstructive cardiomyopathy; MVP, mitral valve prolapse; PVC, premature ventricular complex.

click, and a loud A$_2$, because the valve is intact and the stenosis is downstream.

- Features of supravalvular aortic stenosis: thrill in suprasternal notch and over carotid artery, systolic murmur without click, loud A$_2$.

Subvalvular

The types of subvalvular stenosis are discrete ("membranous") and fibromuscular (fixed or dynamic). These two types can coexist.

Physical Examination

Findings include a prominent left ventricle, reduced pulse pressure, no click, and arterial thrill when the stenosis is severe. Subvalvular aortic stenosis is commonly associated with aortic regurgitation because there is a jet lesion on the aortic valve cusps.

- Features of subvalvular aortic stenosis: prominent left ventricle, reduced pulse pressure, no click, arterial thrill when the stenosis is severe.
- Commonly associated with aortic regurgitation.

Diagnosis

The diagnosis can usually be made with two-dimensional and Doppler echocardiography, often without the need for cardiac catheterization. Two-dimensional echocardiography can determine the severity of the stenosis and the site and presence or absence of additional valvular abnormality. In addition, it can assess the presence or absence of left ventricular hypertrophy. If cardiac catheterization is performed, when the catheter is pulled back from the left ventricle toward the aorta there is a low subvalvular left ventricular pressure tracing before the aortic valve is crossed.

- The diagnosis of subvalvular aortic stenosis is made with two-dimensional and Doppler echocardiography.
- Echocardiography can assess the presence or absence of left ventricular hypertrophy.

Valvular

Types

The *congenital bicuspid* type occurs in 1% of the population. It may be associated with obstruction in infancy through early adulthood. It is the most common cause of aortic stenosis in adults younger than 55 years. Frequently, the valve is still pliable and auscultation is thus different from that of degenerative aortic valve disease. An ejection click often precedes the systolic murmur. The earlier the click (that is, the closer to the first sound), the more severe the stenosis. A$_2$ is delayed with progressive stenosis, and when severe there may be paradoxic splitting of the second sound. The lesion may be associated with coarctation (10%). The diagnosis can usually be made successfully with two-dimensional and Doppler echocardiography without the need for cardiac catheterization in young people.

- Congenital bicuspid valvular aortic stenosis occurs in 1% of population.
- It is the most common cause of aortic stenosis in adults younger than 55 years.
- An ejection click often precedes the systolic murmur.
- The earlier the click (closer to first heart sound), the more severe the stenosis.
- A$_2$ is delayed with progressive stenosis; when severe, there may be paradoxic splitting of second sound.

Degenerative aortic valve disease is the most common cause of aortic stenosis in adults older than 55 years. The valve is tricuspid and calcified. When calcification is extensive, A_2 becomes inaudible.

- Degenerative aortic valve disease is most common cause of aortic stenosis in adults older than 55 years.
- With extensive calcification, A_2 becomes inaudible.

The *rheumatic* type is less common. It is associated with thickening and fusion of the aortic cusps at the commissures. It always occurs with a rheumatic mitral valve, although important mitral stenosis or regurgitation may not always be evident. It usually occurs in early adulthood (age 40 to 60 years), usually 15 ± 5 years after acute rheumatic fever.

- Rheumatic type is less common cause of valvular aortic stenosis.
- Usually occurs at 40 to 60 years of age.

Symptoms

The classic symptoms include exertional dyspnea, syncope, angina, and sudden cardiac death. Most patients are symptom-free; the onset of symptoms is an ominous sign. The presence of angina does not necessarily indicate coexisting coronary disease.

- Symptoms of valvular type of aortic stenosis: exertional dyspnea, syncope, angina, sudden cardiac death.
- Angina does not necessarily indicate coexisting coronary disease.

Physical Examination

The pulse is parvus and tardus. The left ventricular impulse is localized, lateralized, and sustained. Arterial thrills may be palpable in the carotid, suprasternal notch, second intercostal space, or left and right sternal borders. A fourth heart sound may be present, both palpable and audible. A_2 is diminished or absent. The ejection systolic murmur becomes louder and peaks later with increasing severity, radiating to the carotid arteries and the apex.

- Pulse is parvus and tardus.
- Ejection systolic murmur becomes louder with increasing severity.

Diagnosis

Electrocardiography may show left ventricular hypertrophy (not a sensitive index, and echocardiography is better), but the results often are normal in young patients. Left bundle branch block is common, and in later stages of the condition conduction abnormalities may develop (e.g., complete heart block) if the calcium impinges on the conducting system. On chest radiography, the heart size is normal, until left ventricular

remodeling occurs in the late stages, even when the stenosis is severe. The aortic root may show post-stenotic dilatation. In degenerative aortic valve disease, calcium in the valve leaflets may be seen, especially on a penetrated lateral view.

- Electrocardiography is often normal in young patients.
- Left bundle branch block is common on electrocardiogram.
- Aortic root may show post-stenotic dilatation on chest radiograph.

Differential diagnoses include 1) hypertrophic cardiomyopathy (note different carotid upstroke and change in murmur with maneuvers) and 2) mitral regurgitation (murmur may radiate anteriorly and upward, particularly if there is rupture of a posterior mitral valve leaflet; there is *no* radiation to the carotid arteries).

Aortic stenosis can be diagnosed with bedside physical examination. The most important physical finding is the parvus and tardus pulse. However, the degree of aortic stenosis can be difficult to determine, particularly in older patients. Doppler echocardiography is useful for assessing gradients and correlates well with cardiac catheterization. Severe aortic stenosis is present when the mean Doppler gradient is more than 50 mm Hg and the valve area is less than 0.75 cm^2. Patients being considered for surgery should also have coronary angiography if they are older than 50 years.

- Aortic stenosis can be diagnosed with bedside physical examination.
- Most important physical finding: parvus and tardus pulse.
- Doppler echocardiography is useful for diagnosis.
- Severe aortic stenosis: gradient is more than 50 mm Hg, valve area is less than 0.75 cm^2.

Aortic Regurgitation

Etiology

Valvular

Causes of valvular aortic regurgitation include 1) congenital bicuspid valve, 2) rheumatic fever, 3) endocarditis, 4) degenerative aortic valve disease, 5) seronegative arthritis, 6) ankylosing spondylitis, and 7) rheumatoid arthritis.

Aortic Root Dilatation

Various conditions have been associated with aortic root dilatation. Marfan syndrome can be associated with progressive dilatation of the aortic root and sinuses (so-called cystic medial necrosis). Prophylactic β-adrenergic blocker therapy is effective in slowing the rate of aortic dilatation and reducing the development of aortic complications in some patients with Marfan syndrome. When the aortic root reaches 5.5 cm or more in diameter, it should be replaced. Syphilis is an uncommon cause of aortic regurgitation and usually causes aortic root dilatation above the sinuses (syphilis spares the sinuses). Remember that syphilis is associated with calcium in the aortic root on chest radiography. Age is also a related factor. With advancing age, the aorta dilates, and hypertension also tends to accelerate this process. Acute aortic regurgitation may be associated with an aortic dissection.

- Marfan syndrome can be associated with aortic root dilatation.
- Hypertension is a common cause of (usually mild) aortic regurgitation.
- Syphilis is uncommon cause of aortic regurgitation.

Symptoms

The symptoms of aortic regurgitation include fatigue, dyspnea, palpitations, and exertional angina.

Physical Examination

A bounding, collapsing Corrigan pulse resulting from wide pulse pressure is found. Other findings are de Musset head nodding, Durozier sign over the femoral artery, and Quincke sign (pulsatile capillary nail bed). The left ventricular impulse is diffuse and hyperdynamic, and the apex beat is often displaced downward. A diastolic decrescendo murmur is heard at either the left or the right sternal border, and the second heart sound may be paradoxically split because of increased left ventricular volume.

The duration of the murmur is related to the rate of pressure equilibration between the aorta and the left ventricle. Mild aortic regurgitation with physiologic diastolic pressures results in a holosystolic murmur. The shorter the murmur, the faster the pressure equilibration, the more severe the aortic regurgitation, or the higher the left ventricular end-diastolic pressure. The loudness of the murmur does not correlate with the severity of aortic regurgitation, particularly in acute aortic regurgitation (such as with dissection). A systolic flow murmur is common, because of the increased "shuttle" volume. It does not necessarily indicate coexistent aortic stenosis, and so the pulse upstroke should be checked.

- Findings indicative of aortic regurgitation: bounding, collapsing Corrigan pulse, diastolic decrescendo murmur, second heart sound may be paradoxically split.
- The duration, but not the loudness of the murmur, is related to the severity of the aortic regurgitation.

Diagnosis

On electrocardiography, features of left ventricular hypertrophy may be found. Ruptured sinus of Valsalva should be considered in the differential diagnosis. The diagnosis can be made at bedside clinical examination, but it can be missed if a patient with acute aortic regurgitation presents with little or no murmur. Doppler echocardiography is useful and also helps evaluate left ventricular size and function. If dissection is suspected, transthoracic echocardiography may be insufficient, and electron beam computed tomography, transesophageal echocardiography, magnetic resonance imaging, or even aortography may be needed.

- Electrocardiography may show left ventricular hypertrophy.
- Differential diagnosis: ruptured sinus of Valsalva.
- Doppler echocardiography is useful.

Timing of Surgery

The timing of surgical management is still controversial. Despite a large volume load on the left ventricle and compensatory left ventricular enlargement, patients with aortic regurgitation may remain asymptomatic for several years. The development of symptoms, however, usually reflects left ventricular dysfunction, and survival is limited unless surgical intervention is prompt. Once left ventricular dysfunction is established, patients are less likely to have a return of normal function after aortic valve replacement. There is still debate, however, regarding the timing of operation for patients who are asymptomatic or who have very mild symptoms. Other factors that have been used include echocardiographic data: a systolic dimension more than 55 mm or a diastolic dimension more than 80 mm. Asymptomatic patients with dilated left ventricles need to be followed carefully; if there is evidence of resting left ventricular systolic dysfunction, progressive diastolic dysfunction, or rapidly progressive left ventricular dilatation, surgery should be performed. Angiotensin-converting enzyme inhibitors help slow ventricular dilation in patients with severe aortic regurgitation and may help to delay surgery.

- Patients can be asymptomatic for several years.
- If symptoms develop, survival is limited unless surgical intervention is prompt.
- If ejection fraction decreases below normal, operation is needed.

When the cause of aortic regurgitation is acute infective endocarditis, antibiotic therapy should always be instituted first. Surgery is indicated for uncontrolled infection, development of left ventricular dysfunction, or pulmonary congestion. Conduction abnormalities suggest an aortic root abscess and are an urgent indication for operation.

- If cause of aortic regurgitation is acute infective endocarditis, antibiotic therapy should be given first.

- Indications for operation: uncontrolled infection, left ventricular dysfunction, pulmonary congestion.
- Conduction abnormalities suggest aortic root abscess.

Mitral Stenosis

Mitral stenosis is almost always due to rheumatic heart disease causing leaflet thickening with fusion of the commissures and later calcification. Symptoms do not usually develop for several years after mitral stenosis is apparent on physical examination. These symptoms are usually dyspnea and later orthopnea with paroxysmal nocturnal dyspnea. Atrial fibrillation usually causes significant deterioration of symptoms. Hemoptysis and pulmonary hypertension with signs of right-sided failure (i.e., ascites and peripheral edema) are late manifestations. Systemic emboli may also result from atrial fibrillation (about 20% without anticoagulation).

- Mitral stenosis is almost always due to rheumatic heart disease.
- Symptoms do not develop for several years after mitral stenosis is found on physical examination.
- Symptoms: dyspnea, orthopnea with paroxysmal nocturnal dyspnea.
- Atrial fibrillation causes significant deterioration of symptoms.

Physical Examination

The first heart sound is loud. The shorter the interval from the second heart sound (A_2) to the opening snap, the more severe the mitral stenosis. An opening snap occurs only with a pliable valve, and it disappears when the valve calcifies. The stenosis is mild if this interval is >90 ms, moderate if it is 80 ms, and severe if it is <60 ms. The diastolic murmur is a low-pitched apical rumble, and the longer it is, the more severe the stenosis. The murmur has presystolic accentuation if sinus rhythm is present. Right ventricular lift and increased P_2 are associated with pulmonary hypertension.

- Physical examination in mitral stenosis:
  loud first heart sound.
  the shorter the interval from A_2 to the opening snap, the more severe the stenosis.
  diastolic murmur is low-pitched apical rumble.
  the longer the murmur, the more severe the stenosis.

Diagnosis

Electrocardiography shows P mitrale and later right ventricular hypertrophy. Chest radiography (Fig. 3-1) shows straightening of the left heart border with a large left atrial shadow and dilated upper lobe pulmonary veins. With pulmonary hypertension, the central pulmonary arteries become prominent. In severe stenosis, Kerley B lines may

be present, indicating a pulmonary wedge pressure of more than 20 mm Hg.

- Electrocardiography shows P mitrale and later right ventricular hypertrophy.
- Chest radiography shows straightening of the left heart border, a large left atrial shadow, and dilated upper lobe pulmonary veins.
- In severe stenosis, Kerley B lines may be present.

Two-dimensional and Doppler echocardiography is the tool of choice to diagnose mitral stenosis and determine its severity. Information is gained about valve gradient and valve area (Table 3-2), and pulmonary artery pressures can be noninvasively assessed. Cardiac catheterization is usually unnecessary unless the coronary arteries need to be studied or the echocardiographic findings do not concur with the clinical situation. Severe stenosis usually correlates with a mean gradient of 12 or more mm Hg.

- Two-dimensional and Doppler echocardiography is used to diagnose mitral stenosis and determine severity.
- For diagnosis of mitral stenosis, cardiac catheterization is usually unnecessary.
- Severe stenosis correlates with a mean gradient of 12 or more mm Hg.

Indications for Surgery

Because there is no concern about left ventricular dysfunction (left ventricle is small and underfilled) in mitral stenosis, operation is not needed until there are symptoms

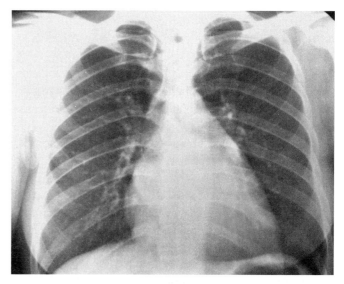

Fig. 3-1. Chest radiograph from a patient with severe mitral stenosis, showing a typical straight left heart border, prominent pulmonary artery, large left atrium, right ventricular contour, and pulmonary venous hypertension.

Table 3-2.—Severity of Mitral Stenosis, by Valve Area

Severity	Valve area, cm^2	Mean gradient, mm Hg	Systolic PAP, mm Hg
Mild	1.5-2	<6	Normal
Moderate	1-1.5	6-11	≤50
Severe	<1	≥12	>50

PAP, systolic pulmonary artery pressure.

of exertional dyspnea, pulmonary edema, or pulmonary hypertension with the risk of irreversible pulmonary vascular changes. Atrial fibrillation does not necessarily indicate the need for operation because it can often be controlled medically. Because atrial fibrillation is frequent and intermittent in the early stages, anticoagulation should be considered early. With a pliable valve that is noncalcified and has no regurgitation, a commissurotomy can be performed without valve replacement, and this may preclude the need for valve replacement for at least 10 years. Another consideration is a percutaneous balloon valvuloplasty if the valve is pliable and there is no regurgitation. This is probably the procedure of choice; results compare favorably with those of surgical commissurotomy.

- Operation for mitral stenosis is indicated with exertional dyspnea, pulmonary edema, or significant pulmonary hypertension.
- Atrial fibrillation is not necessarily indicative of operation (if it can be controlled medically). Consider anticoagulation.
- Percutaneous balloon valvuloplasty is probably procedure of choice if valve leaflets are pliable.

Mitral Regurgitation

Etiology

Causes of mitral regurgitation include the following: 1) rheumatic; 2) mitral valve prolapse (with or without ruptured chordae); 3) infective endocarditis; 4) papillary muscle dysfunction—as a result of ischemia, fibrosis, or rupture (note that the posteromedial papillary muscle with its single blood supply from the right coronary artery becomes infarcted more frequently than the anterior papillary muscle); 5) dilated left ventricle; 6) hypertrophic cardiomyopathy; 7) cleft mitral valve associated with primum atrial septal defect; 8) trauma; and 9) systemic lupus erythematosus. Mitral annular calcification, when severe, can also cause mitral regurgitation. This may be accelerated by systemic hypertension, diabetes, and hypercalcemic states (such as resulting from chronic renal failure).

- In mitral regurgitation, the posteromedial papillary muscle becomes infarcted more often than the anterior papillary muscle.
- Mitral annular calcification may be accelerated by systemic hypertension, diabetes, hypercalcemic states.

Symptoms

Fatigue, dyspnea (due to increased left atrial pressure), and pulmonary edema can be present. Symptoms worsen with atrial fibrillation.

Physical Examination

The findings include a diffuse and hyperdynamic left ventricular impulse, which may be visible, and a palpable rapid filling wave. The first heart sound is usually obliterated, and there is a holosystolic murmur. The second heart sound is widely split (early A$_2$), and there is a third heart sound. A low-pitched early diastolic rumble is significant for severe regurgitation, represents a volume murmur, and usually not coexisting mitral stenosis.

In acute mitral regurgitation, the murmur may be short because of increased left atrial pressure. In severe mitral regurgitation, the carotid upstroke may appear parvus, because of the low forward stroke volume, but not tardus. The left atrium may be palpable with systole, and the left ventricle with diastole; there may be both third and fourth heart sounds. If the cause is ruptured chordae, an anterior leaflet murmur radiates to the axilla and back, and a posterior leaflet murmur radiates to the base and carotids. Consider acute mitral regurgitation with a normal-sized heart, pulmonary edema, and acute onset of symptoms.

- Physical examination in mitral regurgitation:
    first heart sound is usually obliterated.
    holosystolic murmur is present.
    second heart sound is widely split (early A$_2$).
    low-pitched early diastolic rumble indicates severe regurgitation.

Diagnosis

Chest radiography may first show a dilated left atrium and then, as mitral regurgitation increases, dilatation of the left ventricle.

Pathophysiology

Mitral regurgitation "offloads" the left ventricle, so filling volume must increase to maintain adequate forward output. This results in a hyperdynamic ventricle, and thus many patients with significant mitral regurgitation remain asymptomatic for many years. A low or low-normal ejection fraction therefore suggests significant ventricular dysfunction.

- Many patients with mitral regurgitation remain asymptomatic for many years.
- Low or low-normal ejection fraction suggests significant ventricular dysfunction.

Timing of Surgery

Asymptomatic patients with a normal or hyperdynamic ejection fraction can continue to undergo regular observation. Operation should be considered for symptomatic patients (note that ventricular function significantly influences the postoperative outcome), and because "afterload is removed" when the mitral valve is replaced, left ventricular function may actually deteriorate temporarily. Mildly symptomatic patients may be considered for operation, particularly if serial examinations reveal progressive cardiac enlargement. Earlier operation may be indicated in those who are suitable for mitral valve repair rather than replacement.

- Symptomatic patients with mitral regurgitation should be considered for operation.
- Mildly symptomatic patients, particularly with progressive cardiac enlargement, may be considered for surgery to increase the chance for repair rather than replacement.

Tricuspid Stenosis

The cause of tricuspid stenosis is almost always rheumatic, and it is never an isolated lesion. Carcinoid syndrome may cause tricuspid stenosis, and in rare cases atrial tumors may be the cause.

- Cause of tricuspid stenosis is almost always rheumatic; rarely, carcinoid syndrome and atrial tumors may be the cause.

Tricuspid Regurgitation

This is usually caused by dilatation of the right ventricle. When there is right ventricular hypertension, tricuspid regurgitation is also common. It often accompanies mitral valve disease, but it may be related to 1) biventricular infarction, 2) primary pulmonary hypertension, 3) congenital heart disease (such as Ebstein anomaly), or 4) carcinoid syndrome—more commonly associated with tricuspid regurgitation than tricuspid stenosis.

- Tricuspid regurgitation is usually caused by dilatation of the right ventricle.
- It often accompanies mitral valve disease.

Tricuspid Valve Prolapse

This may occur as an isolated entity or in association with other connective tissue abnormalities. The tricuspid valve may prolapse or become flail as a result of trauma or endocarditis (commonly fungal or staphylococcal in drug addicts).

Physical Examination

Findings on physical examination include jugular venous distention with a prominent v wave, a prominent right ventricular impulse, a pansystolic murmur at the left sternal edge, possibly a right-sided third heart sound, and peripheral edema, ascites, and hepatomegaly.

Surgical Therapy

Tricuspid annuloplasty may be helpful if regurgitation is a result of right ventricular dilatation. However, if there is significant pulmonary hypertension, tricuspid valve replacement is usually required with either a biologic or a mechanical valve. Biologic prostheses in the tricuspid position do not degenerate as quickly as prostheses in the left side of the heart. In patients with endocarditis, the tricuspid valve can be removed completely, and patients may tolerate this well for several years.

CONGENITAL HEART DISEASE

Atrial Septal Defect

Secundum

Patients with secundum atrial septal defect often survive to adulthood and may be asymptomatic. The condition is often detected on routine examination with the finding of a murmur. If the defect has gone undetected, atrial fibrillation frequently develops in patients in their 50s with onset of symptoms, usually dyspnea with subsequent tricuspid regurgitation and right-sided heart failure. The condition may present with a neurologic event.

- Patients with secundum atrial septal defect often survive to adulthood and may be asymptomatic.
- Condition is found on routine examination with finding of murmur.
- Atrial fibrillation often develops in patients in their 50s with onset of symptoms.
- Condition may present with a neurologic event.

Physical Examination

Findings include a normal or slightly prominent jugular venous pressure, a right ventricular heave, an ejection systolic murmur in the pulmonary artery (never more than grade 3/6), a fixed splitting of the second sound, and a tricuspid diastolic flow rumble if the shunt is large.

- Findings of secundum atrial septal defect:
    ejection systolic murmur in pulmonary artery (never more than grade 3/6).
    fixed splitting of second sound.
    tricuspid diastolic flow rumble if shunt is large.

Diagnosis

Electrocardiography usually shows right bundle branch block. Chest radiography shows pulmonary plethora, a prominent pulmonary artery, and right ventricular enlargement (Fig. 3-2). Young patients (younger than 40 years) with secundum atrial septal defect and sinus rhythm do not have left atrial enlargement. If the chest radiograph shows left atrial enlargement, consider another lesion, particularly primum atrial septal defect with mitral regurgitation.

● If chest radiograph shows left atrial enlargement, consider primum atrial septal defect with mitral regurgitation.

Two-dimensional and color Doppler echocardiography can usually demonstrate the defect and right ventricular enlargement with volume overload. If visualization is poor, transesophageal echocardiography can be performed. Cardiac catheterization is usually unnecessary, unless coexisting coronary disease is suspected.

Sinus Venosus

An uncommon condition, this occurs in the superior portion of the atrial septum. It is often associated with anomalous pulmonary veins, usually the right upper. If echocardiography shows right ventricular volume overload and no secundum defect, consider sinus venosus atrial septal defect or anomalous pulmonary veins.

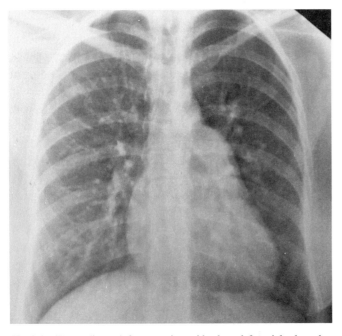

Fig. 3-2. Chest radiograph from a patient with a large left-to-right shunt due to a secundum atrial septal defect. Notice cardiac enlargement with right ventricular contour, very prominent pulmonary artery, and pulmonary plethora.

Primum (Partial Atrioventricular Canal)

This is a defect in the lower portion of the septum. The mitral valve is usually cleft and produces various degrees of regurgitation.

Diagnosis

On electrocardiography, findings are different from those of secundum type with left-axis deviation and right bundle branch block. More than 75% of patients have first-degree atrioventricular block. The chest radiographic findings are the same as those for secundum atrial septal defect, although there may be left atrial enlargement because of mitral regurgitation. Atrioventricular defects are the most common cardiac anomaly associated with Down syndrome.

● Electrocardiography shows left-axis deviation with right bundle branch block and, commonly, first-degree atrioventricular block.
● Atrioventricular defects are most common cardiac anomaly of Down syndrome.

Ventricular Septal Defect

Ventricular septal defect occurs in different parts of the ventricular septum, most commonly either in the membranous septum or in the muscular septum. Small defects produce a loud noise, and patients are often asymptomatic. The size of the hole determines the degree of left-to-right shunting. Small defects may have a long holosystolic murmur, often with a thrill at the left sternal edge, usually around the fourth interspace. Large defects may produce a mitral diastolic flow rumble at the apex, especially when the shunt is more than 2.5:1.

● Ventricular septal defects are most common in membranous septum or muscular septum.
● Small defects produce loud noise.
● Size of hole determines the degree of left-to-right shunting.

Patent Ductus Arteriosus

This condition is associated with maternal rubella. It produces essentially an "arteriovenous fistula." A small ductus is compatible with a normal lifespan. The ductus may calcify in adult life. A continuous "machinery" murmur envelops the second heart sound around the second interspace beneath the left clavicle. A large patent ductus arteriosus may produce ventricular failure. Surgical ligation is curative. Patients then do not need endocarditis prophylaxis.

All of the above-described shunt lesions, when large, may produce elevated pulmonary pressures and subsequently pulmonary vascular disease.

- Patent ductus arteriosus is associated with maternal rubella.
- Small ductus is compatible with normal lifespan.
- Continuous "machinery" murmur is present.
- Surgical ligation is curative, and endocarditis prophylaxis then is not needed.
- All described shunt lesions, when large, may produce elevated pulmonary pressures and subsequently pulmonary vascular disease.

Eisenmenger Syndrome

This syndrome develops in the first few years of life when a large shunt (usually a ventricular septal defect or patent ductus arteriosus) produces pulmonary hypertension and irreversible pulmonary vascular disease. This condition causes the shunt to reverse so that blood flows from the right to the left, and subsequent cyanosis occurs. Patients are then inoperable. Death commonly occurs in the third or fourth decade of life as a result of exercise-induced syncope, arrhythmia, hemoptysis, and stroke. The cyanosis produces significant erythrocytosis, often with hemoglobin values in the teens or 20s. There is no need to phlebotomize patients with a hemoglobin value less than 20 g/dL or a hematocrit value less than 65%. Also, repeated phlebotomies frequently lead to iron deficiency, and iron-deficient erythrocytes are more rigid than ordinary ones, and the risk of stroke is thereby increased. Phlebotomy may be necessary in symptomatic patients with a hemoglobin value more than 20 g/dL. Always remember to replace fluid concomitantly in patients with Eisenmenger syndrome because hypotension and syncope may be fatal.

- Eisenmenger syndrome develops in first few years of life.
- Syndrome produces pulmonary hypertension and irreversible pulmonary vascular disease.
- Death is common in the third or fourth decade of life.
- Associated conditions: exercise-induced syncope, arrhythmia, hemoptysis, stroke.
- Cyanosis produces significant erythrocytosis.

Pulmonary Stenosis

This may occur as an isolated lesion or in association with a ventricular septal defect. Valvular pulmonary stenosis often causes few or no symptoms. The valve is frequently pliable, and it may be bicuspid. Thickened dysplastic valves, often stenotic, occur in association with the Noonan syndrome.

- Thickened dysplastic valves, often stenotic, occur with the Noonan syndrome.

Physical Examination

Findings include a prominent "a" wave in the jugular venous pulse; right ventricular heave; ejection click—the earlier the click, the more severe the stenosis (the click indicates that the valve is pliable and noncalcified); ejection systolic murmur—the longer the murmur and the later peaking, the more severe the stenosis; and soft and late P_2 (with severe stenosis P_2 becomes inaudible).

- Findings of pulmonary stenosis:
    prominent "a" wave in the jugular venous pulse.
    ejection click (the earlier the click, the more severe the stenosis).
    soft and late P_2.

Diagnosis

Electrocardiography shows right ventricular hypertrophy. On chest radiography, pulmonary oligemia is found only with *very severe* pulmonary stenosis. There is poststenotic pulmonary dilatation, especially of the left pulmonary artery (Fig. 3-3).

The diagnosis can be reliably made with two-dimensional echocardiography, and Doppler reliably predicts the gradient and estimates right ventricular pressure. In asymptomatic patients, no treatment is indicated unless the right ventricular pressure approaches two-thirds that of the systemic pressure. Later in life, the valve may become calcified when the ejection click disappears. The treatment of choice for a pliable valve is percutaneous balloon valvuloplasty. This has essentially replaced surgical valvotomy.

- Diagnosis of pulmonary stenosis is made with two-dimensional and Doppler echocardiography.
- Treatment for pliable valve is percutaneous balloon valvuloplasty.

Coarctation of the Aorta

This is usually either a discrete or a long segment of narrowing adjacent to the left subclavian artery. It is more common in males and frequently is associated with a bicuspid aortic valve. Most cases of coarctation are diagnosed in childhood; only about 20% are diagnosed in adulthood. This is the most common cardiac anomaly associated with Turner syndrome. Other associations include aneurysms of the circle of Willis and aortic dissection or rupture. There is an increased incidence of aortic dissection or rupture in Turner syndrome even in the absence of coarctation. As a result of the coarctation, systemic collaterals develop from the subclavian and axillary arteries through the internal mammary, scapular, and intercostal arteries.

- Coarctation of aorta is more common in males.
- Condition is frequently associated with a bicuspid aortic valve.

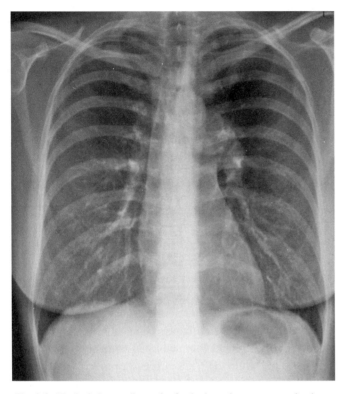

Fig. 3-3. Typical chest radiograph of valvular pulmonary stenosis, showing normal cardiac size and marked prominence of main and left pulmonary arteries, representing poststenotic dilatation. This does not occur with infundibular pulmonary stenosis. Lung fields appear mildly oligemic.

- Only 20% of cases are diagnosed in adulthood.
- It is the most common cardiac anomaly associated with Turner syndrome.
- Incidence of aortic dissection or rupture is increased in Turner syndrome even in the absence of coarctation.

There are five major complications of coarctation of the aorta: 1) cardiac failure, 2) aortic valve disease, 3) rupture or dissection, 4) endarteritis, and 5) rupture of an aneurysm of the circle of Willis—this is exacerbated by the presence of hypertension, which occurs in the upper limbs. Systemic hypertension may be the presenting feature in adults. Some patients complain of pain in the legs on exercise.

Physical Examination

Findings include an easily palpable brachial pulse; the femoral pulse is weak and delayed. There are differences in systolic pressure between the upper and lower extremities. Exercise may exaggerate the systemic hypertension. An ejection click is present when there is an associated bicuspid valve. A_2 may be loud as a result of hypertension. A fourth heart sound may be present with associated left ventricular hypertrophy and hypertension. Murmurs may originate from 1) the coarctation, which can produce a systolic murmur over

the left sternal edge and over the spine in the mid-thoracic region, and it sometimes extends into diastole in the form of a continuous murmur; 2) arterial collaterals, which are spread widely over the thorax; and 3) the bicuspid aortic valve, which may generate a systolic murmur.

- Findings of coarctation of aorta: easily palpable brachial pulse, weak and delayed femoral pulse, differences in systolic pressure between upper and lower extremities.
- Coarctation can produce a systolic murmur over the left sternal edge and over the spine in mid-thorax.
- Arterial collaterals are spread widely over thorax.

Diagnosis

Electrocardiography may be normal. With more severe coarctation or hypertension, left ventricular hypertrophy with or without repolarization changes is found. Chest radiography may show rib notching from the dilated and pulsatile intercostal arteries and a "3" configuration of the aortic knob, which represents the coarctation site with proximal and distal dilatations.

- Chest radiographic findings in coarctation of aorta are rib notching and a "3" configuration of the aortic knob.

The condition may be demonstrated by echocardiography and Doppler, although imaging may be difficult in this area, and additional visualization may be necessary with digital subtraction angiography, magnetic resonance imaging, or computed tomography. Angiography can also be performed.

Treatment

Balloon angioplasty has been performed in some patients, although it is associated with aneurysm formation and re-coarctation. Surgical treatment has been an accepted approach since 1945. However, there is a significant rate of hypertension after coarctation repair. As many as 75% of patients are hypertensive at 30-year follow-up. Surgically treated patients still often die prematurely of coronary disease, heart failure, stroke, or ruptured aorta. Age at operation is important. The 20-year survival rate is 91% in patients who have operation when they are less than 14 years old and 79% in patients who have operation when they are more than 14 years old.

- Surgical repair of coarctation of aorta is associated with significant rate of hypertension; 75% of patients are hypertensive at 30-year follow-up.
- Surgically treated patients often die prematurely of coronary disease, heart failure, stroke, or ruptured aorta.

Ebstein Anomaly

This unusual congenital lesion is thought to be associated with maternal lithium ingestion during pregnancy. It has a variable spectrum. It involves an inferior displacement of the tricuspid valve ring into the right ventricular cavity. The degree of displacement is variable, as is the degree of abnormality of the tricuspid valve. The inferior displacement results in "atrialization" of the right ventricle, the small contractile chamber beneath.

- Ebstein anomaly is thought to be associated with maternal lithium ingestion during pregnancy.
- Anomaly involves inferior displacement of the tricuspid valve ring into the right ventricular cavity.

Physical Examination

The extremities are usually cool, often with peripheral cyanosis (a reflection of low cardiac output). There may be an "a" wave in the jugular venous pressure (although this is variable because the large right atrium may accommodate a large tricuspid regurgitant volume). A subtle right ventricular lift is noted. The first heart sound has a loud tricuspid (T_1) component. A holosystolic murmur increases on inspiration at the left sternal edge from tricuspid regurgitation. One or more systolic clicks are noted (may be multiple). Common associated conditions are secundum atrial septal defect and preexcitation syndrome. Patients with secundum atrial septal defects are often very cyanotic because of the right-to-left shunting. They may present with neurologic events.

- Findings of Ebstein anomaly include cool extremities, often with peripheral cyanosis, and a holosystolic murmur that increases on inspiration.
- One or more systolic clicks are noted (may be multiple).
- Associated conditions: secundum atrial septal defect, and preexcitation syndrome.
- Patients with secundum atrial septal defects are often very cyanotic.
- They may present with neurologic events.

Diagnosis

Chest radiography shows a narrow pedicle with enlarged globular silhouette and right atrial enlargement. The lung fields are normal or oligemic. On electrocardiography, a tall P wave (Himalayan P waves) and right bundle branch block are found.

Two-dimensional and Doppler echocardiography delineates the anatomy precisely, and cardiac catheterization is unnecessary. Electrophysiology study may be necessary to delineate the bypass tract, if present.

PREGNANCY AND CARDIAC DISEASE

Physiologic Changes of Pregnancy

Plasma volume starts to increase in the first trimester, peaking around the second trimester to almost 50% above normal. An increase in red cell mass also begins early and peaks in the second trimester, but not to the same degree as the plasma volume; thus, there is a relative anemia. The cardiac output increases, and peripheral resistance decreases. Increased venous pressure in the lower extremities leads to pedal edema in 80% of healthy pregnant women.

- Physiologic changes of pregnancy include increased plasma volume, red cell mass, and cardiac output.
- Peripheral resistance decreases.

Because of these changes, the physical examination may suggest cardiac abnormalities to the unwary. Normal results of physical examination in a healthy pregnant woman include elevation of the jugular venous pressure, bounding carotid pulses, and an ejection systolic murmur in the pulmonary area (never more than grade 3/6). The second heart sound is loud, and there is a third heart sound or diastolic filling sound. A fourth heart sound occasionally may be heard.

- Ejection systolic murmur in the pulmonary area (never more than grade 3/6) is a normal finding in pregnancy.

Although a third heart sound or diastolic filling sound is common, a long rumble should raise the possibility of mitral stenosis. Because of the decrease in peripheral resistance and increased output changes, stenotic lesions are less well tolerated than regurgitant ones; for example, a patient with aortic stenosis has exaggeration of the aortic valve gradient, whereas a patient with mitral regurgitation experiences "afterload reduction" with peripheral vasodilatation and so tolerates pregnancy better. Functional class of the patient is a consideration in terms of whether pregnancy is possible. Patients who are in functional class III or IV have a maternal mortality rate approaching 7%.

- Third heart sound or diastolic filling sound is common in pregnancy, but a long rumble should raise the possibility of mitral stenosis.
- In patients in functional class III or IV, maternal mortality rate approaches 7%.

Pregnancy is *absolutely contraindicated* in patients with the following conditions: 1) Marfan syndrome with a dilated aortic root—increased risk of dissection and rupture because hormonal changes soften the connective tissue (unpredictable risk of dissection and rupture in Marfan syndrome and pregnancy even when aortic root has normal size), 2) Eisenmenger syndrome (maternal mortality rate is 50%), 3) primary pulmonary hypertension, 4) symptomatic severe aortic stenosis, 5) symptomatic severe mitral stenosis, and 6) symptomatic dilated cardiomyopathy.

Although not absolute contraindications, the following conditions are also of concern in pregnancy: 1) atrial septal defect (deep venous thrombosis may lead to paradoxical embolus) and 2) coarctation (increased risk of dissection and rupture).

Patients at risk during pregnancy should minimize activity (decreases cardiac output), reduce sodium in the diet, and minimize anemia with iron and vitamin supplements.

If symptoms deteriorate and congestive heart failure supervenes, bed rest may need to be instituted. Arrhythmias such as atrial fibrillation need to be treated promptly in these situations. If necessary, cardioversion can be performed with apparently low risk to the fetus. Fetal cardiac monitoring should be performed at the same time. Occasionally patients need operative intervention. Operation during the first trimester is associated with a significantly increased rate of fetal loss. Percutaneous aortic, mitral, and pulmonary balloon valvuloplasty have been performed during pregnancy and may obviate bypass. Careful lead shielding of the fetus is needed during these procedures.

Drugs

Many cardiac drugs cross the placenta into the fetus but yet can be used safely when necessary and are not absolutely contraindicated in pregnancy. These include digoxin, quinidine, procainamide, β-adrenergic blockers, and verapamil. The β-adrenergic blockers can be associated with growth retardation of the fetus, neonatal bradycardia, and hypoglycemia. They may need to be used, however, in large doses in patients with hypertrophic cardiomyopathy, and fetal growth must be monitored.

Drugs that should be avoided are captopril, which causes fetal renal dysgenesis; phenytoin, which causes hydantoin syndrome and teratogenicity; and warfarin, which causes teratogenicity and abortion. One noncardiac drug to avoid is tetracycline, which stains fetal teeth.

- Drugs to avoid in pregnancy: captopril, phenytoin, warfarin, and tetracycline.

Delivery

Delivery is a time of rapid hemodynamic swings. With each uterine contraction, about 500 mL of blood is released into the circulation. Cardiac output goes up with advancing labor. High-risk patients need careful monitoring with Swan-Ganz catheterization to maintain preload at an optimal level, maternal and fetal electrocardiography monitoring, careful analgesia and anesthesia to avoid hypotension, delivery in the left lateral position so the fetus is not lying on the inferior vena cava (this position

maintains venous return), and a short second stage (delivery may need to be facilitated if labor progresses slowly).

Vaginal delivery is safer for most women because the average blood loss is 500 to 800 mL; with cesarean section it is 800 mL. Usually, cesarean section is performed only for obstetric indications. The new guidelines of the American Heart Association state there is no need for antibiotic prophylaxis in an uncomplicated vaginal delivery.

- With each uterine contraction, 500 mL of blood is released into circulation.
- No need for antibiotic prophylaxis in uncomplicated vaginal delivery.

Prosthetic Valves and Pregnancy

Most women of childbearing age who need a valve replacement will receive a biologic valve, and if they are in sinus rhythm they will usually not be receiving anticoagulants. Women with mechanical valves will be taking warfarin, and this poses a problem with teratogenicity and increased risk of abortion. In general, diagnose pregnancy as soon as possible and switch the therapy to subcutaneous heparin, monitoring the activated partial thromboplastin time, and continue this approach throughout pregnancy. This agent is also associated with increased fetal loss, however, and an increased risk of maternal valve thrombosis.

- In pregnant patients with mechanical valves, switch therapy from warfarin to subcutaneous heparin.
- Heparin is associated with increased fetal loss.

PERICARDIAL DISEASE

The pericardium has an inner layer, the visceral pericardium, and an outer layer, the parietal pericardium. Space between the two layers contains approximately 15 to 25 mL of clear fluid. The pericardium has three main functions: prevent cardiac distention, limit cardiac displacement because of its attachment to neighboring structures, and protect the heart from nearby inflammation.

Acute or Subacute Inflammatory Pericarditis

Presenting Symptoms

The chest pain of pericarditis is often aggravated by movement of the trunk, by inspiration, and by coughing. The pain is often relieved by sitting up. *Low-grade fever* and malaise are other findings.

Diagnosis

Pericardial friction rub may be variable. Chest radiography

is usually normal. It may show globular enlargement if pericardial effusion is significant (at least 250 mL). Occasionally, pulmonary infiltrate or small pleural effusion is noted. Left pleural effusion predominates, and the cause is unknown. Electrocardiography shows acute concave ST elevation in all ventricular leads. The PR segment is also depressed in the early stages. Echocardiography allows easy diagnosis of pericardial effusion and determination of whether the pericardial effusion is hemodynamically significant.

- Chest pain is the presenting symptom of pericarditis.
- Electrocardiography shows concave ST elevation and depressed PR segment.

Causes

The causes of pericarditis include viral pericarditis, idiopathic pericarditis, autoimmune and collagen diseases (systemic lupus erythematosus, rheumatoid arthritis, scleroderma), and postmyocardial infarction. The postcardiotomy syndrome follows open heart procedures. It presents with pyrexia, increased sedimentation rate, and pleural or pericardial chest pain. It occurs weeks to months after operation. Its incidence decreases with age, and it usually responds to anti-inflammatory agents. Pericarditis is also associated with radiation and neoplasm, namely, Hodgkin disease, leukemia, and lymphoma. Breast, thyroid, and lung tumors can metastasize to the pericardium and cause pericarditis or pericardial effusion. Melanoma also metastasizes to the heart. Uremia and tuberculosis can also cause pericarditis. If no cause can be documented, idiopathic viral pericarditis is the most likely diagnosis, and treatment with nonsteroidal anti-inflammatory agents or high-dose aspirin usually resolves the condition.

- Causes of pericarditis: autoimmune and collagen diseases; postmyocardial infarction; radiation; neoplasm; breast, thyroid, and lung tumors; uremia; tuberculosis.

Pericardial Effusion

The response of the pericardium to inflammation is to exude fluid, fibrin, and blood cells, causing a pericardial effusion. The amount of effusion needed before it shows on the chest radiograph is 250 mL. If fluid accumulates slowly, the pericardial sac distends slowly with no cardiac compression. If fluid accumulates rapidly, such as with bleeding, tamponade can occur with relatively small amounts of fluid. Tamponade restricts the blood entering the ventricles and causes a decrease in ventricular volume. The raised intrapericardial pressure increases the ventricular end-diastolic pressure and mean atrial pressure, and the increased atrial pressure increases the venous pressure. The decreased ventricular volume and filling diminish cardiac output. Any of the previously listed causes of pericarditis can cause tamponade, but other acute causes of hemopericardium should be considered, such as ruptured myocardium after infarction, aortic dissection, ruptured aortic aneurysm, and sequelae of cardiac operation.

- Amount of pericardial effusion needed before it can be seen on chest radiograph is 250 mL.
- Tamponade can occur with small amounts of fluid.
- Tamponade restricts the blood entering the ventricles and decreases ventricular volume.

Clinical Features

Tamponade produces a continuum of features, depending on its severity. The blood pressure is low, the heart is small and quiet, tachycardia may be present, jugular venous pressure is increased, and pulsus paradoxus develops (increased flow of blood into the right heart during inspiration, decreased flow into the left heart). An increase in inspiratory distention of the neck veins (Kussmaul sign) is infrequent unless there is underlying constriction.

Treatment

Emergency pericardiocentesis is performed with echocardiography-directed guidance.

Constrictive Pericarditis

Diastolic filling of both ventricles is prevented by the pericardium. The smaller the ventricular volume, the higher the end-diastolic pressure. The most common causes are recurrent viral pericarditis, irradiation, previous open heart operation, tuberculosis, and neoplastic disease.

Symptoms

Dominantly right-sided failure, peripheral edema, ascites, and often dyspnea and fatigue are present.

- Symptoms of constrictive pericarditis: peripheral edema, ascites, dyspnea, and fatigue.

Physical Examination

The jugular venous pressure is elevated (remember to look at the patient when he or she is sitting or standing), and inspiratory distention of neck veins (Kussmaul sign) is present. The jugular venous pressure may show rapid descents, and pericardial knock is present in fewer than 50% of cases (sound is probably due to sudden cessation of ventricular filling). Ascites and peripheral edema may be present. Chest radiography may show pericardial calcification, but no specific changes are found on electrocardiography.

- Signs of constrictive pericarditis: elevated jugular venous pressure, inspiratory distention of neck veins, rapid descents of jugular venous pressure, and pericardial knock in less than 50%.

- Chest radiograph may show pericardial calcification.
- No specific changes are found on electrocardiography.

Diagnosis

Echocardiography and Doppler may be helpful, particularly Doppler, which shows respiratory changes in mitral and tricuspid inflow velocities. Other methods such as computed tomography and magnetic resonance imaging help to delineate the thickness of the pericardium. The major confounding diagnosis is restrictive cardiomyopathy, and the distinction can be very difficult. Diastolic expansion of both ventricles is affected equally; therefore, diastolic pressure is elevated and equal in all four chambers. Ventricular pressure curve shows characteristic "√⁻" from rapid ventricular filling and equalization of pressures (also may be seen in restrictive cardiomyopathy). The "a" and v waves are usually equal and x and y descents are rapid. If pulmonary artery systolic pressure is more than 50 mm Hg, myocardial disease is likely. If the end-diastolic pulmonary artery pressure is more than 30% of systolic pressure, myocardial disease is likely. Both of these findings are nonspecific, however. The treatment of choice for constrictive pericarditis is exploratory operation to remove the pericardium.

- Constrictive pericarditis is diagnosed from respiratory changes in mitral and tricuspid inflow velocities.
- Major confounding diagnosis is restrictive cardiomyopathy.
- Diastolic pressure is elevated and equal in all four chambers.

EVALUATION OF THE PATIENT WITH CARDIAC DISEASE BEFORE NONCARDIAC OPERATION

Risks

The major risk for most patients with cardiac disease who undergo noncardiac operations arises from the presence of coronary artery disease. In patients without previous evidence of heart disease, the risk of perioperative myocardial infarction during a noncardiac procedure is 0.15%. In patients with previous myocardial infarction, the frequency of reinfarction during a major noncardiac operation is about 6%. The risk of perioperative reinfarction is inversely related to the interval between preoperative infarction and noncardiac operation (Table 3-3). Aggressive perioperative management and invasive hemodynamic monitoring reduce these rates. The mortality rate from a perioperative myocardial infarction is approximately 50%.

- In patients without previous heart disease, the risk of perioperative myocardial infarction during a noncardiac operation is 0.15%.
- In patients with previous myocardial infarction, the risk of reinfarction during a major noncardiac operation is 6%.
- The risk of perioperative infarction is inversely related to the time from previous infarction to noncardiac operation.
- The mortality rate from perioperative myocardial infarction is 50%.

Certain surgical procedures are associated with a threefold greater chance of myocardial infarction: major intrathoracic, upper abdominal, and great vessel surgical procedures. Other preoperative cardiac risks include age more than 70 years, gallop of the third heart sound, jugular venous pressure more than 12 cm H_2O, and significant aortic stenosis. Electrocardiographic risk factors are a rhythm other than sinus, atrial ectopy, or more than 5 premature ventricular contractions per minute. Other factors to consider are general medical status (PaO_2 less than 60 or $PaCO_2$ more than 50 mm Hg, potassium less than 3 mEq/L, bicarbonate less than 20 mEq/L), blood urea nitrogen value more than 50 or creatinine value more than 3 mg/dL, chronic liver disease, general debilitation, and type of operation (such as emergency procedure or intraperitoneal, thoracic, or aortic procedure).

- Risk of myocardial infarction is threefold more with major intrathoracic, upper abdominal, and great vessel operations.

Because of a strong association between coronary disease and peripheral vascular disease, patients who are to undergo a peripheral vascular operation are at high risk of having important coronary disease. In patients having routine coronary angiography before a vascular operation, approximately 60% with clinically suspected ischemic heart disease have severe multivessel or even inoperable coronary artery disease. Approximately 20% of patients with no prior history to suggest coronary artery disease have diffuse, severe coronary artery disease.

Table 3-3.—Risk of Perioperative Reinfarction, by Time From Initial Infarction

Time from MI to noncardiac operation, mo	Risk of perioperative MI, %
<3	27-37
3-6	11-16
>6	4-5

MI, myocardial infarction.

- There is a strong association between coronary disease and peripheral vascular disease.
- At routine angiography before a vascular operation, 60% of patients with clinically suspected ischemic heart disease have severe multivessel or inoperable coronary artery disease.
- Of patients without a history of coronary artery disease, 20% have diffuse, severe coronary artery disease.

Use of a cardiac risk index (such as Goldman) has limitations because the risks are much higher in patients undergoing vascular operation. Risk indices depend on referral patient population, nature of the operation, expertise of the surgeon and anesthesiologist, and uncommon problems or events (such as emergency procedure).

A low risk score index does not exclude a patient from having a perioperative event but rather indicates a low probability of a cardiac event. Preoperative cardiovascular assessment with a thorough cardiac history is important, corroborated by examination, chest radiography, and electrocardiography. The absence or presence and severity of angina pectoris and the efficacy of current medical therapy need to be considered. The history and time of the previous myocardial infarction are important. If operation is not urgent, waiting more than 6 months after myocardial infarction is probably appropriate.

- Low risk score index does not exclude a perioperative event but does indicate low probability of cardiac event.
- Preoperative cardiovascular assessment is important.
- History and time of previous infarction are important.

Mild Angina

Most patients who can perform vigorous activity of daily living and are functional class I or II tolerate the stress of most noncardiac operations. However, if they are to undergo one of the more risky procedures (intrathoracic, upper abdominal, or vascular), preoperative stress testing should be considered. If functional limitation is not clear from the history, stress testing should be performed, if possible.

Class III or IV Angina

Significant limitation because of symptoms suggests the need for direct coronary angiography.

- Mild angina in most patients having noncardiac surgery does not require additional workup.
- Patients limited by class III or IV angina need direct coronary angiography.

Resting Electrocardiogram

The presence of a normal resting electrocardiogram infers a low probability of a perioperative cardiac event, as does the presence of nonspecific ST T-wave changes. Q waves suggestive of previous myocardial infarction increase the risk to 5%.

- A normal resting electrocardiogram infers a low probability for a perioperative cardiac event.
- Q waves on the resting electrocardiogram increase the risk up to 5%.

Exercise Testing

Different end points have been used in stress testing. This should be reserved for patients in whom coronary artery disease is highly suspected or for patients with known significant peripheral arteriopathy, which may prevent the occurrence of anginal symptoms. The absence of ischemia in an adequate exercise test (75% or more of predicted maximal heart rate, absolute peak heart rate 125 beats per minute, more than 5 METs workload) indicates a low probability of a perioperative event. If noncardiac causes prevent appropriate exercise (orthopedic problems, claudication), pharmacologic stress may be helpful (dobutamine echocardiography, adenosine, dipyridamole, dobutamine, thallium, sestamibi, radionuclide angiography). The negative predictive value is excellent, and the positive predictive value is high (about 30%) but not very specific.

The risk of delaying the planned procedure and the risk of a bypass procedure need to be weighed carefully (bypass, 2.3%; with left ventricular ejection fraction less than 50%, increase to 2.9%; in patients older than 70 years, 7.9%). Antianginal medication (β-adrenergic, nitrates) should be used liberally, and hemodynamic monitoring with right heart catheterization (Swan-Ganz) should be considered to avoid significant volume shifts.

- A negative exercise test with adequate workload indicates an excellent prognosis.
- A negative pharmacologic test is very helpful; however, a positive test does not necessarily identify the specific patient (30/70).
- Risk of planned operation (and its delay) need to be weighed carefully against the risk of a possible bypass procedure.
- Optimize (maximize) perioperative antianginal therapy.

Aortic or Mitral Stenosis

Assess stenosis with two-dimensional and Doppler echocardiography. If it is severe, patients should have cardiac operation before a noncardiac procedure. Percutaneous balloon valvuloplasty can occasionally be used to "get patients through" the operation. Asymptomatic patients with significant aortic stenosis can often tolerate a noncardiac operation safely with careful anesthesia and hemodynamic monitoring.

- If aortic or mitral stenosis is severe, cardiac operation should be done before noncardiac procedure.
- Asymptomatic patients with significant aortic stenosis can often tolerate a noncardiac operation safely.

Mechanical Valvular Prostheses

Management depends on the degree of operation being undertaken. Depending on the risk and degree of the procedure, anticoagulant therapy can be discontinued 1 to 3 days preoperatively and restarted 2 to 5 days postoperatively with a low risk of a thromboembolic event. The risk of bleeding complications may be higher, depending on the extent of the operation. For patients needing more extensive procedures, oral anticoagulation may be changed to heparin, discontinued 6 hours before operation with resumption 24 hours postoperatively, or days later if, surgically necessary.

THE HEART AND SYSTEMIC DISEASE

Many systemic diseases may have manifestations in the heart. This chapter describes those that are most likely to be included on the examination.

Common disease processes with cardiac involvement include deposition disorders, neurologic diseases, acquired diseases, malignancies, endocrine disorders, collagen and vascular diseases, autoimmune diseases, and infectious diseases.

Hyperthyroidism

Effects

The cardiovascular manifestations of hyperthyroidism include an increase in heart rate, stroke volume, and cardiac output. Peripheral vascular resistance is decreased, and thus there is a widened pulse pressure. All of these lead to an increase in myocardial oxygen consumption and therefore may precipitate angina. Other symptoms include palpitations, tachycardia, and shortness of breath on exertion.

- Cardiovascular effects of hyperthyroidism: increased heart rate, stroke volume, and cardiac output and decreased peripheral resistance with wide impulse pressure.
- Effects lead to increased myocardial work and oxygen consumption and perhaps angina.

Physical Examination

Common physical findings are tachycardia and a bounding pulse with forceful apical pulse and a systolic ejection murmur. Cardiac arrhythmias are common, particularly supraventricular tachycardia and atrial fibrillation. Atrial fibrillation occurs in 10% to 20% of patients with hyperthyroidism. Therefore, always suspect thyrotoxicosis in patients with atrial fibrillation and check the results of thyroid function studies.

- Findings of hyperthyroidism: tachycardia, bounding pulse, forceful apical impulse, and systolic ejection murmur.
- Cardiac arrhythmias are common, especially atrial fibrillation.
- Suspect thyrotoxicosis in patients with atrial fibrillation.

Hypothyroidism

Effects

Hypothyroidism leads to cardiac enlargement and infiltration of the myocardium with mucoprotein. This disorder decreases the metabolic rate and circulatory demand and causes bradycardia, decreased myocardial contractility and stroke volume, and an increase in peripheral resistance. The cardiomyopathy of hypothyroidism is reversible if detected early. It also can increase cholesterol levels and accelerate atherosclerosis.

Physical Examination

There may be cardiac enlargement due to the myocardial disease or to a commonly found pericardial effusion. Pericardial effusion is common in approximately a third of patients. The volume of pulses is decreased because of a decrease in myocardial contractility.

- Physical findings in hypothyroidism: cardiac enlargement, reduced myocardial contractility, and pericardial effusion (this occurs in a third of patients).
- Heart failure is rare, but reversible if found early.
- Atherosclerosis is accelerated.

Diabetes Mellitus

This condition frequently is associated with premature development of atherosclerosis. The prevalence is two times as common in diabetic men and three times as common in diabetic women than in a nondiabetic population. Patients with diabetes have an increased prevalence of hypertension and hyperlipidemia. Angina and myocardial infarction may often manifest as either atypical symptoms or silent ischemia. In fact, congestive heart failure may be the first manifestation of coronary artery disease among the diabetic population. There is also some possible evidence that cardiomyopathy unassociated with epicardial coronary atherosclerosis exists. This is speculated to be on the basis of small vessel disease.

- Key points: fatal myocardial infarction is more common in diabetics than in nondiabetics.
- Prevalence of hypertension is increased in diabetes.
- Incidence of silent myocardial ischemia is high.

Amyloidosis

Amyloidosis is the result of multiple diseases leading to the extracellular deposition of insoluble proteins in organs. Organs involved typically are the liver, kidney, heart, gastrointestinal tract, and nervous tissue. In primary amyloidosis, nearly 90% of patients have clinical manifestations of cardiac dysfunction. The heart is enlarged, most often a result of thickened ventricular myocardium from the protein infiltration. Abnormalities of diastolic function, conduction, and ultimately systolic dysfunction can occur. Amyloid deposition in the cardiac valve leads to atrioventricular valvular regurgitation, which is usually not severe. Secondary amyloidosis occurs in association with chronic disease such as rheumatoid arthritis, tuberculosis, chronic infection, neoplasia, and chronic renal failure. Cardiac involvement occurs in secondary amyloidosis, but it is usually not a prominent feature. The entity of senile amyloidosis does exist, and the heart is the organ most commonly involved. The prevalence of this disorder increases from age 60 on. Familial amyloidosis is autosomal dominant. The characteristic amyloid protein is pre-albumin and it can involve the heart.

Clinical Features

The following can occur in cardiac amyloid involvement: congestive heart failure, arrhythmias, sudden death, angina, light chest pain, pericardial effusion (usually not hemodynamically significant), and murmurs. The natural history of the disease is usually intractable because of ventricular cardiac failure. Diastolic abnormalities are early common manifestation and are classic for "restrictive cardiomyopathy." The restrictive classification indicates a poor prognosis.

Diagnosis

The diagnosis of cardiac involvement is made on the basis of electrocardiography, which shows a classic low-voltage QRS complex, which is nonspecific. In addition, echocardiography is particularly useful. It classically demonstrates an increase in left ventricular wall thickness, in contradistinction to the small voltage on electrocardiography. Tissue characteristics on ultrasonography are often described as granular. The atria are generally dilated. The cardiac valves may show some thickening and regurgitation. There may be a small pericardial effusion. Diastolic function is generally abnormal; in the early stages of the disease it shows a prolongation of the relaxation, and in the later stages it shows restrictive filling (consistent with high left ventricular filling pressures).

- In primary amyloidosis, 90% of patients have cardiac dysfunction.
- Echocardiographic features: thickened ventricular walls, granular myocardial appearance, dilated atria.
- Abnormal diastolic function: consistent with delay and relaxation in the early stages, and with restrictive (increased ventricular filling pressure) patterns in the later stages.
- Normal to reduced voltage on electrocardiography, in the face of "thick" walls on echocardiography.

Hemochromatosis

Hemochromatosis is an iron-storage disease. There is a primary or a secondary form related to exogenous iron (usually from repeated blood transfusions) deposits within the cardiac cells. Cardiac hemochromatosis generally does not occur alone and is accompanied by involvement of other organ systems, primarily the tetrad of diabetes, liver disease, brown skin pigmentation, and congestive heart disease. The condition may present with cardiomegaly, congestive heart failure, and arrhythmias. This disease has features of poor systolic and diastolic function. Once clinical cardiac symptoms appear, the prognosis is very poor unless treatment is initiated with a combination of phlebotomy and iron chelation.

- Hemochromatosis is related to iron deposits within cardiac cells.
- Cardiac hemochromatosis does not occur alone.
- Key to diagnosis is a tetrad of diabetes, liver disease, skin hyperpigmentation, and congestive heart failure.

Carcinoid Heart Disease

Metastatic (to liver or lungs) malignant carcinoid tumors produce serotonin-like substances that cause systemic flushing and diarrhea. These substances are also toxic to valvular tissues. They are metabolized in the liver and lungs. Cardiac involvement occurs after hepatic metastasis. Therefore, toxic effects generally affect right-sided cardiac valves unless there is a shunt (generally a patent foramen ovale) that allows right-to-left movement of blood substances. The leaflets become thickened, relatively immobile, and retracted. The result is regurgitation with an element of stenosis of both the tricuspid and the pulmonary valves. Surgical therapies include tricuspid valve replacement and pulmonary valve resection.

- Carcinoid tumors produce serotonin-like substances that cause flushing and diarrhea.
- Changes occur in the tricuspid and pulmonary valves. Dominant lesions are tricuspid regurgitation, pulmonary regurgitation, and stenosis.

Hypereosinophilic Syndrome

Effects

This syndrome affects young patients, generally male, who have a persistent eosinophil concentration of more than 1,500 per mm^2. The causes are several, including idiopathic hypereosinophilia, Löffler endocarditis, reactive or allergic eosinophilia, leukemic or neoplastic eosinophilia, or Churg-Strauss syndrome. All of these may have cardiac manifestations.

Clinical Features

Patients present with weight loss, fatigue, dyspnea, syncope, and systemic embolization. Cardiac manifestations include arrhythmias, myocarditis, conduction abnormalities, and thrombosis. Eosinophilic deposition occurs in the heart, where a clot forms in the apices of the ventricles and in the inflow portions under the mitral and tricuspid valves. This ultimately leads to matting down of the atrioventricular valve and causes significant regurgitation. The clot ultimately scars, leading to endomyocardial fibrosis and restrictive cardiomyopathy.

- Hypereosinophilic syndrome may be present in patients with a persistent eosinophil value of more than 1,500 per mm^2.
- Hypereosinophilic syndrome presents with restrictive cardiomyopathy and atrioventricular valve regurgitation.

Systemic Lupus Erythematosus

Effects

Systemic lupus erythematosus may involve any of the cardiac structures. Special features of involvement include the antiphospholipid syndrome, Libman-Sacks endocarditis, and congenital heart block in the offspring of mothers with lupus.

Offspring of mothers with anti-La and anti-Ro antibodies are at risk for development of both myocarditis and inflammation and fibrosis of the conduction system, which may lead to congenital heart block.

Cardiac involvement in patients with systemic lupus erythematosus may include pericarditis, which is characterized by a positive antinuclear antibody in the pericardial fluid, myocarditis (more common in patients with anti-Ro antibody), a valvulopathy, coronary arteritis, and Libman-Sacks endocarditis.

Libman-Sacks endocarditis is a noninfective vegetation that may be present in up to 50% of patients with systemic lupus erythematosus. It does not generally embolize or interfere with valvular function.

- The offspring of mothers with anti-La and anti-Ro antibodies are at risk for congenital heart block.

- Approximately a third of patients with systemic lupus erythematosus may have clinical evidence of cardiac involvement, including pericarditis, endocarditis, myocarditis, and coronary arteritis.

Scleroderma

Effects

Scleroderma affects the skin with sclerotic changes, the esophagus with dysphagia, and small vessels with manifestations such as Raynaud phenomenon. Cardiac involvement is manifested by intramural coronary involvement and immune-mediated endothelial injury, which is often associated with the Raynaud phenomenon clinically. Conduction defects occur in up to 20% of patients, and a pericardial effusion is found in a third of patients, but it is often asymptomatic. Indirect cardiac involvement due to pulmonary hypertension and cor pulmonale is frequent.

- Cardiac involvement is the third most common cause of mortality in patients with scleroderma.
- Coronary vasculitis is associated with clinical Raynaud phenomenon.
- Conduction defects may occur in up to 20% of patients.

Rheumatoid Arthritis

Effects

Rheumatoid arthritis may be associated with involvement of nearly all cardiac components, including pericardium, myocardium, valves, coronary arteries, and aorta. Rheumatoid arthritis may cause both granulomatous and nongranulomatous inflammation of valve leaflets, which rarely leads to severe valvular incompetence. Pericarditis of rheumatoid arthritis is usually associated with a low glucose level and complement depletion in the pericardial fluid. Rheumatoid nodules may be deposited in the conduction system, leading to degrees of heart block. Aortitis and pulmonary hypertension due to pulmonary vasculitis are very rare complications of rheumatoid arthritis.

- Pericardial fluid in patients with rheumatoid pericarditis will be low in glucose and complement and is associated with nodular rheumatoid arthritis.
- Granulomatous involvement in the conduction system may lead to heart block.
- Nongranulomatous and granulomatous involvement of valvular tissue may lead to incompetence of cardiac valve structures.

Ankylosing Spondylitis

Aortic dilatation and aortic regurgitation may be present in approximately 10% of patients. Aortic valve cusps become distorted and retracted, leading to significant aortic regurgitation. The conduction system may become involved as a result of both fibrosis and inflammation.

Marfan Syndrome

Marfan syndrome is an autosomal dominant condition associated with degenerative elastic tissues, leading to arachnodactyly, tall stature, pectus excavatum, kyphoscoliosis, and lenticular dislocation.

Common cardiac manifestations include mitral valve prolapse, aortic dilatation, and increased risks of aortic dissection, which may respond to long-term β-adrenergic blockade.

Friedreich Ataxia

This is autosomal recessive neurologic disorder that involves the heart in up to 90% of cases. It usually manifests as a symmetric hypertrophy, and less commonly a dilated cardiomyopathy.

Osteogenesis Imperfecta

Brittle bones, blue sclera, and deafness are the hallmarks of this condition, which leads to a lack of collagen-supporting matrix. Ultimately, there is a degeneration of elastic tissues, including aortic root dilatation, aortic regurgitation, annular dilatation, and chordal stretch leading to significant atrioventricular regurgitation.

Lyme Disease

Lyme disease is a spirochete infection by *Borrelia burgdorferi* organisms. Up to 10% of cases have clinical cardiac involvement. Cardiac manifestations include atrioventricular block and Lyme carditis. The diagnosis is generally made by biopsy of the right ventricular myocardium or gallium scanning.

Acquired Immunodeficiency Syndrome (AIDS)

Clinically apparent cardiac involvement may occur in up to 10% of patients with AIDS. Cardiac involvement has been reported as a myocarditis in up to 50% of patients at autopsy. This may be associated with ventricular arrhythmias, dilated cardiomyopathy, a pericarditis, or infectious or malignant invasion of the cardiac structures.

Cardiac Trauma

Contusion, in the acute stage, may lead to arrhythmia, increased cardiac enzyme values, transient regional wall motion abnormalities, and pericardial effusion or tamponade. It also has been reported to cause disruption of the aorta, valves (tricuspid valve most often), or right ventricular rupture.

Commotio cordis is characterized by mild trauma to the chest wall, which is generally a nonpenetrating blow such as that delivered by a baseball or softball. This can occur in the absence of underlying cardiac disease and leads to instantaneous cardiac arrest. Research indicates that the trauma must be delivered during the vulnerable phase of the cardiac cycle, which is described as 15 to 30 milliseconds before and after the T wave.

PROSTHETIC VALVES

Bioprostheses

These are made of animal or human tissue, which may be unmounted or mounted in a frame. Different types include 1) homograft (human tissue), either aortic or pulmonary; 2) heterograft (porcine valve), for example, Hancock or Carpentier-Edwards; and 3) pericardial (bovine valve), for example, Ionescu-Shiley. Tissue valves have the advantage that they are not as thrombogenic as mechanical valves; thus, most patients in sinus rhythm do not require anticoagulation. There is a risk of systemic embolism, however, with biologic prostheses in patients with atrial fibrillation, particularly with a mitral prosthesis. The disadvantage is that tissue valves degenerate and calcify and thus patients will need reoperation. Approximately 50% of patients will need valve replacement at 10 years. In young patients (20 years or younger), these valves may calcify very rapidly. Tissue valves last a little longer in the tricuspid position than in positions on the left side of the heart. Aortic valves have a slightly better durability than mitral valves. Prosthesis failure can be detected by clinical evaluation and two-dimensional and Doppler echocardiography.

- Tissue valves are not as thrombogenic as mechanical valves.
- Most patients with tissue valves who are in sinus rhythm do not require anticoagulation.
- There is a risk of systemic embolism with biologic prostheses in patients with atrial fibrillation, particularly with a mitral prosthesis.
- Tissue valves degenerate and calcify.
- About 50% of patients will need valve replacement.

Mechanical Valves

An example of a *ball valve* is the Starr-Edwards. It has excellent longevity and is a so-called high-profile valve. A small size may be associated with a higher transvalvular pressure gradient. Types of *tilting disc valves* are the Björk-Shiley and St. Jude. All mechanical valves have a risk of thromboembolism. Reported rates vary. For example, in a Mayo Clinic series of patients with a Starr-Edwards prosthesis, 81% were free of embolism at 5 years when the valve was in the aortic position, and 93% were free of embolism when it was in the mitral position. Hemolysis often occurs with mechanical prostheses, especially with perivalvular leak. Anticoagulation can also be associated with hemorrhage and thrombosis. The rate of minor hemorrhages is approximately 2% to 4% per year, and that of major hemorrhages is 1% to 2% per year.

- All mechanical valves have a risk of thromboembolism.
- Hemolysis often occurs with mechanical prostheses, especially with perivalvular leak.
- Anticoagulation can be associated with hemorrhage and thrombosis.

TUMORS OF THE HEART

Most cardiac tumors are metastatic. The most common primary cardiac tumor is myxoma.

Cardiac Myxoma

Most cardiac myxomas are sporadic, but there have been some reports of familial occurrence. A syndrome of cardiac myxomas with lentiginosis (spotty pigmentation) and recurrent myxomas has been recognized. About 75% are in the left atrium, 18% are in the right atrium, and the rest are in the ventricles. Most of the atrial tumors arise from the atrial septum, usually adjacent to the fossa ovalis. About 95% are single. Most myxomas have a short stalk, are gelatinous and friable, and tend to embolize. They occasionally calcify, so they may be visible on a chest radiograph.

The main clinical features are obstruction to blood flow, embolization, and systemic effects. Left atrial tumors prolapse into the mitral valve orifice and produce mitral stenosis. They mimic mitral valvular stenosis with symptoms of dyspnea, orthopnea, cough, pulmonary edema, and hemoptysis. Classically, symptoms occur with a change in body position. Physical findings suggest mitral stenosis. Pulmonary hypertension may also occur. An early diastolic sound, the tumor "plop," may be heard. This has a lower frequency than an opening snap.

- Most cardiac tumors are metastatic.
- Most common primary cardiac tumor is myxoma.
- 75% of cardiac myxomas are in the left atrium and 18% are in the right atrium; rest are in the ventricles.
- Clinical features are obstruction to blood flow, embolization, and systemic effects.
- Symptoms occur with a change in body position.
- An early diastolic sound, tumor "plop," may be heard.

Embolization

Systemic emboli may occur in 30% to 60% of patients with left-sided myxoma, frequently to the brain and lower extremities. Histologic examination of embolized material is important. Coronary embolization is rare, but it should be considered in a young patient with no known previous cardiac disease. Systemic effects are fatigue, fever, weight loss, and arthralgia. Systemic effects may be associated with an elevated sedimentation rate, leukocytosis, hypergammaglobulinemia, and anemia. Increased immunoglobulins are usually of IgG class.

Echocardiography is the preferred approach to diagnosis. Transesophageal echocardiography helps delineate the precise site of origin and accurately assesses tumor size and degree of mobility. Operation is indicated when the diagnosis is made.

- Systemic emboli occur in 30% to 60% of cases of left-sided myxoma, frequently to the brain and lower extremities.
- Coronary embolization is rare.
- Systemic effects: fatigue, fever, weight loss, and arthralgia.
- Systemic effects may be associated with elevated sedimentation rate, leukocytosis, hypergammaglobulinemia, and anemia.
- Increased immunoglobulins are usually IgG class.
- Echocardiography is the preferred approach for diagnosis.
- Operation is indicated.

Primary Cardiac Neoplasm

Rhabdomyoma is most common in women and children. It can produce obstruction of cardiac valves simulating other abnormalities and can cause cardiac arrhythmias. Other tumors, such as Kaposi sarcoma associated with acquired immunodeficiency syndrome (AIDS), do not usually cause cardiac symptoms.

Secondary tumors most often originate from bone, breast, lymphoma, leukemia, and thyroid. More than half of patients with malignant melanoma have metastases to the heart.

- Rhabdomyoma is most common in women and children.
- More than half of patients with malignant melanoma have metastases to heart.

IMAGING IN CARDIOLOGY

An important part of cardiology is the appropriate choice of an imaging method to aid in the diagnosis, quantification, and prognosis of various diseases. The most commonly ordered test is the assessment of left ventricular function. Various techniques are available, as outlined in Table 3-4. It is important for the clinician to focus the question and subsequently choose the most appropriate technique to answer the clinical question.

Contrast Angiography

This imaging method was the first to visualize the cardiac chambers and directly assess left ventricular size and function by injecting radiopaque material (iodine dye) into the cardiac chambers, which can be visualized with x-rays. Intracardiac access is usually required, and thus it is an invasive procedure, although new techniques (intravenous digital subtraction angiography) may allow a more noninvasive approach. With use of a 30° right ventricular oblique and an orthogonal (60°) left anterior oblique view (sometimes with a 20°- to 30°-cranial tilt to avoid foreshortening of the left ventricle), biplane views are obtained over several cycles to assess left ventricular volumes and regional wall motion abnormalities. Several algorithms have been developed to extrapolate the information of these two views to the entire heart. This requires certain assumptions about the ventricular shape (regularity) and contraction pattern (concentric), which may not hold true in ischemia with resting wall motion abnormalities and previous myocardial infarction. Another drawback is the need for ionizing radiation and possible allergies to iodine. These are usually overcome with appropriate preparation (steroids, antihistamine). Because coronary angiography, that is, the selective visualization of the coronary arteries, is the reference technique to assess the location (not necessarily the hemodynamic significance) of coronary artery stenosis, assessment of left ventricular function by contrast ventriculography should be performed only during accompanying coronary angiography. If the dye load needs to be minimized (renal failure), an alternative technique should be considered to save approximately 20 to 50 mL of contrast.

Echocardiography

Echocardiography uses a high-frequency (2 to 10 MHz) ultrasonic beam produced by a piezoelectric crystal from a transducer to generate images acquiring and processing the various acoustic echoes. Currently, three methods are readily available: M-mode, two-dimensional, and Doppler/color Doppler.

M-Mode

A single cursor (beam) traverses the object of interest and trades its motion through time. Identification of characteristic borders (endocardium, epicardium, aorta, atria, valve leaflets) allows measurements of function (motion). M-mode echocardiography, because of its ease of application, is still the most commonly used method to assess function despite several shortcomings.

M-mode echocardiography provides only limited information about the structure of interest. Because of its dependence on the transducer position, appropriate placement of the M-mode cursor may not be possible. Because it represents a single-dimensional measurement (centimeters), extrapolations (cubing the measurements) need to be made, which can compound measurement errors.

Two-Dimensional Echocardiography

Two-dimensional imaging provides a beat-to-beat tomogram of the heart. Outlining the endocardial and epicardial borders allows determination of left ventricular volumes in end-diastole and end-systole and subsequently stroke volume, ejection fraction, and muscle mass. The algorithms used are similar to those used in contrast ventriculography, requiring certain assumptions about ventricular shape and contraction. The technique is, however, completely noninvasive and thus lends itself to serial image acquisition. Its easy availability (mobile equipment, "uncomplicated" technology, additional information) has made it the most widely used imaging

Table 3-4.--Cardiac Imaging Methods

Method	LVEF	RV function	LV mass	RWMA	Cost effective*
Contrast angiography	Yes	No	No	Yes	++++†
Two-dimensional echocardiography	Yes	Yes	Yes	Yes	++
First-pass RNA	Yes	Yes, quantitative‡	No	No	+
Blood pool RNA	Yes	No	No	Yes	+
Magnetic resonance imaging	Yes	Yes, quantitative‡	Yes	Yes	+++/+
Electron beam computed tomography	Yes	Yes, quantitative‡	Yes	Yes	+++

*+, Least expensive; ++++, most expensive.

†If performed without coronary angiography.

‡Quantitative, absolute measurements of global ventricular volumes possible to facilitate measure of RV ejection fraction.

LV, left ventricular; LVEF, left ventricular ejection fraction; RNA, radionuclide angiography; RV, right ventricular; RWMA, regional wall motion abnormalities.

technology in cardiology. By assessing endocardial motion and wall thickening from various transducer positions, regional wall motion abnormalities also can be assessed. The morphology of valves (pliability, degree of calcification, morphologic abnormalities, that is, flail segments) and intracardial and pericardial structures also can be analyzed. With exercise or pharmacologic (usually dobutamine) stress, regional wall motion can be assessed both at rest and at stress for the diagnosis of coronary artery disease. Regional wall motion analysis requires a highly skilled interpreter, particularly in the presence of preexisting regional wall motion abnormalities.

Doppler/Color Doppler Echocardiography

Doppler/color Doppler echocardiography allows direct measurements of blood velocities across valves and along conduits (left ventricular outflow tract, vessels), which permit calculation of stroke volume, cardiac output, valve gradients, and severity of regurgitant lesions and semiquantitation of intracardiac and extracardiac shunts.

The crucial element for optimal echocardiographic image acquisition is the availability of appropriate acoustic "windows" to properly direct the ultrasound beam to the structure of interest. Obese patients, very cachectic patients, patients with significant lung disease (smokers, chronic obstructive pulmonary disease, restrictive lung disease) may pose insurmountable problems for transthoracic echocardiography (10% to 20%). Transesophageal echocardiography may overcome this problem, but it is an invasive approach. Echocardiography also requires the most operator experience and dependence for both image acquisition and interpretation.

Radionuclide Imaging

Radionuclide imaging principally uses two techniques: labeling erythrocytes with an isotope to assess endocardial motion or using perfusion tracers (thallium, sestamibi) to assess differences between resting and stress blood flow.

Radionuclide Angiography

Erythrocytes are labeled with technetium, which can be imaged by a gamma camera, which is placed usually in the anteroposterior, left anterior oblique, and lateral positions. To ensure sufficient photon capture, images are acquired over multiple cardiac cycles. This procedure requires electrocardiographic gating, which opens the aperture of the camera for fractions during the cardiac cycle. Patients with atrial fibrillation and markedly variable RR intervals are not suited for this approach. Quantification of left ventricular function is based on the number of photons in the ventricle at end-diastole and end-systole. This count-based method obviates any geometric assumptions and thus provides a very accurate assessment of left ventricular function, especially in patients with poor

function. Because radionuclide angiography is dependent on the number of photons available at end-diastole and end-systole, there is a very good signal with little noise in large, poorly contractile ventricles, allowing excellent discrimination between low ejection fractions, particularly during serial assessment. In contrast, echocardiography relies on the endocardial inward motion, which is poor in severely dysfunctional ventricles, introducing a higher signal-to-noise ratio which makes discrimination between low ejection fractions difficult.

First-Pass Radionuclide Angiography

Recently, techniques have been developed to follow the passage of a radioisotope bolus through the right and left cardiac system, allowing assessment of left ventricular function. Subsequently, the tracer distributes according to coronary blood flow, and perfusion images are obtained. This technique, based on dye-dilution and videodensitometric principles, allows easy, economical assessment of both right and left ventricular function. Drawbacks are difficulties in administering the bolus (poor intravenous access), which lead to early diffusion of the bolus with poor discrimination of the dextro and levo phases. Similar to radionuclide angiography, first-pass radionuclide angiography is extremely sensitive to dysrhythmias, particularly when they occur during the calculation phase of the first-pass acquisition.

Myocardial Perfusion Imaging

The two most commonly applied isotopes are thallium and sestamibi, which distribute to the myocardium according to blood flow. They are avidly taken up by the myocytes. These isotopes can subsequently be imaged at rest and after exercise (Fig. 3-4). Images are acquired by a planar technique in which the camera is positioned similar to that in radionuclide angiography in three positions. More accurate is a single photon emission computed tomography approach in which a camera rotates around the patient and takes images at certain, narrow-angle intervals to compose a complete three-dimensional image of the entire heart without super positrons. The views are then commonly displayed as short-axis tomograms spanning the entire heart (Fig. 3-4, upper left at stress; upper right at rest). The images are then compared with each other. During stress (exercise or pharmacologic), there is usually reduced uptake in the affected myocardium. Subsequently, at rest, there is redistribution of the isotope (thallium) where a preferential washout of the previously normal and a preferential uptake of the previously hypoperfused myocardium take place. With sestamibi, because the isotope is taken up irreversibly into the myocardium, a repeat resting injection is mandatory to reflect the resting flow conditions. The extent and the severity of the perfusion defect provide additional, important information in regard to the prognosis of the disease which goes beyond the mere diagnosis of the presence or absence of coronary artery disease. It is also helpful to assess residual ischemia in patients with previous myocardial infarction and to assess therapeutic efficacy in patients treated medically or by intervention. The result of the imaging studies should always be viewed in conjunction with the data available from the exercise or stress electrocardiogram.

Magnetic Resonance Imaging

Magnetic resonance imaging is a noninvasive, three-dimensional imaging technique that allows noninvasive assessment of left ventricular size, function, and muscle mass. The technique is extremely precise; however, its major drawback is its cumbersome application, duration of the study, and the complex post-processing.

Electron Beam Computed Tomography

Electron beam computed tomography is a scanner without any movable parts in which an electron beam is deflected via magnetic fields rapidly on several rings around the patient, allowing high-fidelity, high-resolution, three-dimensional images of the entire heart in rapid succession. Like all complex imaging techniques it is dependent on electrocardiographic gating; however, it requires only one beat to complete a cycle. Because the entire heart is encompassed in the scan, no geometric assumptions need to be made. It is ideally suited for serial studies in left ventricular remodeling because of its high precision and accuracy. Drawbacks are the requirements for a contrast agent to be administered into a peripheral vein and ionizing radiation.

Positron Emission Tomography

Positron emission tomography depends on the detection of a simultaneous pair of photons radiating into exact opposite directions. This principle, not unlike radionuclide angiography, allows high-spatial and temporal resolution imaging. Positron emission tomography currently is the reference standard for the assessment of myocardial viability. However, the complexity of the technology and the cost currently limit its use to tertiary academic centers.

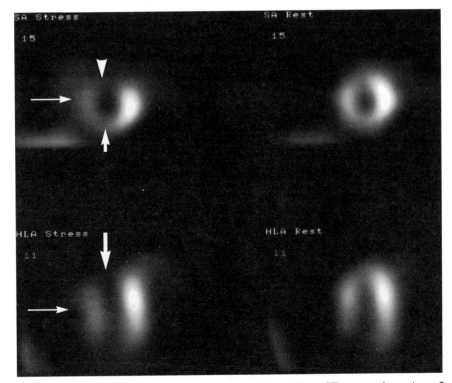

Fig. 3-4. Patient with exertional angina (class III) of recent onset. Low-level exercise with 1-mm ST-segment depression at 2 minutes into exercise. The left column depicts the stress images with a representative short-axis tomogram (upper left panel) and the horizontal long axis (lower left panel). In the right column are the rest images, with corresponding short-axis tomogram in the right upper panel and the corresponding horizontal long-axis tomogram in the right lower panel. Note the severely reduced uptake in the apical (*thick arrow*), septum (*thin arrows*), anterior (*arrowhead*), and inferior (*short arrow*) segments. At rest there is nearly complete normalization in all segments. Subsequent angiography indicated complete occlusion of the right coronary artery and 80% stenosis in the proximal left anterior descending coronary artery. The circumflex coronary artery did not show a critical lesion.

PART II
Win-K. Shen M.D.

MYOCARDIAL CELLULAR CONDUCTION

Cells in the sinus and atrioventricular (AV) nodes are slow-conducting and activated by the opening of calcium channels and blocked by calcium channel blockers such as verapamil. Cells in the atrium, His-Purkinje system, and ventricle are fast-conducting and activated by the opening of sodium channels and blocked by sodium channel blockers such as class I antiarrhythmic drugs (e.g., quinidine, lidocaine, and propafenone).

MECHANISMS OF ARRHYTHMIAS

Reentry

Three conditions are required for reentry to occur (Fig. 3-5 and 3-6): 1) two or more anatomically or functionally distinct pathways connected proximally and distally to form a closed circuit, 2) unidirectional block in one pathway, and 3) slowed conduction in the other pathway.

Reentry is the most common mechanism responsible for cardiac arrhythmias and can occur in a microreentrant circuit within the sinus node, AV node, or small area of injured myocardium bordering a myocardial infarction. Large reentrant circuits involve the atrium (as in atrial flutter) or the atrium, AV conduction system, ventricle, and accessory pathway (as in patients with Wolff-Parkinson-White syndrome).

- Reentry is the most common mechanism for cardiac arrhythmias.

Automaticity

Automatic rhythms occur when accelerated phase IV depolarization results in enhanced automaticity (Fig. 3-7). The sinus node demonstrates normal physiologic automaticity. When other cells in the heart have increased automaticity, they may exceed the rate of sinus node automaticity and replace the sinus node as the cardiac pacemaker. The factors that enhance automaticity are listed in Table 3-5.

Automaticity may be the mechanism responsible for multifocal atrial tachycardia in patients with decompensated lung disease and those with ventricular ectopy early after myocardial infarction. In both cases, automaticity is enhanced by increased sympathetic tone, hypoxia, acid-base and electrolyte disturbances, and atrial or ventricular stretch. Accelerated idioventricular rhythm may also be due to abnormal automaticity.

- Automaticity is enhanced by increased sympathetic tone, hypoxia, acid-base and electrolyte disturbances, and atrial or ventricular stretch.

Parasystole

Parasystole is a type of abnormal automaticity. It occurs when an ectopic focus in the atrium or ventricle is isolated from the dominant rhythm because of conduction block into the focus. Cells within this area undergo automatic depolarization and, because of entrance block, are not constantly reset

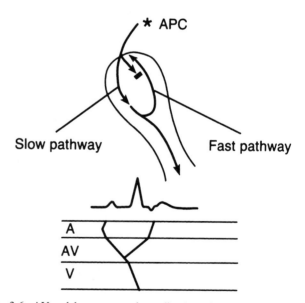

Fig. 3-6. AV nodal reentrant tachycardia. An atrial premature complex (APC) blocks in fast pathway but conducts over slow pathways to ventricle. Impulse then returns to atria over recovered fast pathway and can reenter slow pathway and initiate tachycardia. A, atrium; AV, atrioventricular node; V, ventricle.

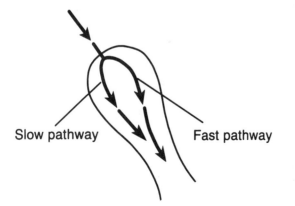

Fig. 3-5. Reentry within the atrioventricular (AV) node demonstrates the two limbs of reentrant circuit. Recent evidence suggests that a portion of the reentrant pathway is separate from the AV node.

Table 3-5.—Factors That Enhance Automaticity

Autonomic changes
    Increased sympathetic tone
    Decreased parasympathetic tone
Metabolic/ischemic changes
    Increased carbon dioxide
    Decreased oxygen
    Increased acidity
Mechanical factors
    Increased stretch
Drugs
    Isoproterenol
Electrolyte alterations
    Decreased potassium
    Increased calcium

by the dominant rhythm. These cells capture the regional myocardium unless the myocardium is refractory from a previously conducted beat. This mechanism causes 3% of premature ventricular complexes (PVCs) noted during routine monitoring and, in general, is benign.

- Parasystole is caused by an ectopic focus in the atrium or ventricle.
- Parasystole causes 3% of PVCs during routine monitoring.
- Parasystole is benign.

Triggered Activity

This mechanism for arrhythmias is so-named because each complex in the rhythm is generated (triggered) by the preceding one. The arrhythmia cannot begin without an initiating beat. Two types of triggered activity exist: delayed afterdepolarizations and early afterdepolarizations. *Delayed afterdepolarizations* arise during the resting phase of the action potential (phase 4) and may be the mechanism for digitalis-induced arrhythmias. *Early afterdepolarizations* arise during the plateau (phase 2) or repolarization (phase 3) of the action potential and may be responsible for the polymorphic ventricular tachycardia (torsades de pointes) caused by antiarrhythmic drugs such as quinidine.

DIAGNOSTIC TECHNIQUES

Ambulatory Electrocardiographic Monitoring and Transtelephonic Event Recording

Ambulatory (Holter) monitoring is used to document symptomatic and asymptomatic rhythm disturbances if they occur frequently enough to be recorded during the 24- or 48-hour recording period. It is also used to determine the effect of treatment, such as control of the ventricular response during atrial fibrillation. Patients may have adequate control of heart rate in response to atrial fibrillation at rest in the physician's office but inappropriately rapid heart rates in response to mild exercise. Such inappropriate rates can be shown by 24-hour monitoring or exercise testing.

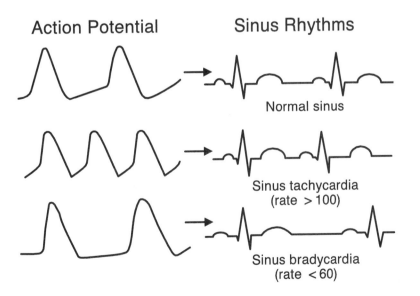

Fig. 3-7. Action potential corresponding to electrocardiographic manifestation of sinus node activity. Under physiologic conditions, sinus rate is a function of the slope of spontaneous depolarization during phase 4 of the action potential. A steep slope of the spontaneous depolarization corresponds to a faster sinus rate (sinus tachycardia). A flat slope of phase 4 depolarization corresponds to a slower sinus rate (sinus bradycardia).

Ambulatory monitoring can assess pacemaker function and determine the relationship of arrhythmia to daily activity (e.g., exercise). Also, ambulatory monitoring may be used to confirm episodes of myocardial ischemia, most of which are not usually associated with the typical symptoms of angina.

- Ambulatory monitoring assesses pacemaker function, documents the relationship of arrhythmia to daily activity, and confirms episodes of myocardial ischemia.

Transtelephonic event recording documents heart rate and rhythm during symptoms that occur infrequently. Patients either wear a device continuously for several days or weeks or briefly attach it to themselves during symptoms. The device permanently stores the electrocardiogram (ECG) in memory when the activation button is depressed, and this ECG is later transmitted over the telephone for evaluation. This device documents the rhythm when a patient experiences typical symptoms. About 20% of transmissions document abnormal heart rhythm, although often the transmissions are helpful for patient management even if a normal rhythm is identified. Continuous loop event recorders store the ECG that occurs 30 seconds to 4 minutes before the activation button is depressed and are very useful for patients whose symptoms are brief or of sudden onset. Implantable loop event recorders have been approved for clinical use; however, the guidelines for implantation have not been established.

- Transtelephonic event recording documents heart rate during symptoms that occur infrequently.
- About 20% of transmissions document abnormal heart rhythm.
- Transtelephonic event recording is often helpful for patient management even if normal rhythm is identified.

Exercise Testing

Exercise testing is helpful when patients describe symptoms consistent with cardiac arrhythmia which occur during exercise. This allows for evaluation in a controlled setting with ECG monitoring to determine whether a cardiac arrhythmia is causing the exercise-related symptoms. Exercise testing is also useful to determine whether the beneficial effect of a drug at rest is reversed with exercise. Patients with atrial fibrillation may have adequate control of heart rate at rest but poor control with moderate exercise. Those with ventricular tachycardia or complex ventricular ectopy may have adequate suppression of the arrhythmia at rest in response to medical therapy, only to have ventricular tachycardia with exercise. Sometimes, proarrhythmic effects of antiarrhythmic drugs can be provoked by exercise testing. This is particularly true of class IC drugs (flecainide and propafenone),

probably because of use-dependence and their long unbinding times from the sodium channel.

- Exercise testing evaluates cardiac arrhythmia during exercise.
- Exercise testing determines whether the effect of a drug is reversed with exercise.

PVCs occur during exercise testing in 10% of patients without and in 60% of those with coronary artery disease. The response of PVCs during exercise does not predict the severity of coronary artery disease. Elimination of PVCs with exercise is not an indication that coronary artery disease is less severe.

- PVCs occur during exercise in 10% of patients without and in 60% of those with coronary artery disease.
- Response of PVCs during exercise does not predict the severity of coronary artery disease.
- Elimination of PVCs with exercise does not indicate less severe coronary artery disease.

Exercise testing is useful for assessing sinus node function to determine whether there is chronotropic incompetence in a patient who complains of dyspnea on exertion or fatigue. It is also used to assess AV block. AV block at the AV node is usually benign and does not require pacing. This type of block (Wenckebach [Mobitz I]) improves with exercise when increased catecholamines enhance AV node conduction. AV block due to failure of conduction in the His-Purkinje system (Mobitz II) has a worse prognosis; it has a high incidence of complete heart block and requires pacing. This type of block often worsens with exercise because the increase in catecholamines enhances AV node conduction and results in increased frequency of activation of the diseased His-Purkinje system with progressive block.

- Exercise testing assesses sinus node function in patients with dyspnea on exertion.
- Mobitz I block may improve with exercise.
- Mobitz II block may worsen with exercise.
- Mobitz II block has a worse prognosis and requires pacing.

Signal-Averaged ECG

Signal-averaged ECG is a noninvasive test used to detect low-level signals, termed "late potentials," that result from delayed conduction through diseased myocardium. These signals usually arise in the border zone adjacent to a myocardial infarction, where conducting myocardial cells are mixed in among scar tissue. This disrupted architecture results in delayed conduction and is the substrate for myocardial reentry. Signal-averaged ECG amplifies this low-level signal by several thousandfold and averages multiple QRS complexes to eliminate random noise. The low-level activity is then measured to determine whether a late potential is present. Late potentials have independent prognostic value for identifying patients at risk for ventricular tachycardia after myocardial infarction and inducible ventricular tachycardia at the time of electrophysiologic testing. Signal-averaged ECG has a positive predictive accuracy of 25% to 50% and a negative predictive accuracy of 90% to 95% for identifying patients at risk for ventricular tachycardia. The test is used primarily to stratify patients at risk for ventricular tachycardia or ventricular fibrillation. It is not useful in the setting of right bundle branch block or in patients without coronary artery disease.

- Signal-averaged ECG is noninvasive.
- Signal-averaged ECG identifies patients at risk for ventricular tachycardia.

Heart Rate Variability

More recently, research has increased in assessing how much the heart rate varies as a predictor of future arrhythmic events. It has been shown that heart rate variability decreases when there is relatively more sympathetic versus parasympathetic tone; the converse is also true. Decreased heart rate variability after myocardial infarction identifies a group with increased risk of ventricular arrhythmias. Currently, this should be considered a research tool in most instances; it does not have widespread clinical applicability.

Electrophysiologic Testing

Electrophysiologic testing involves the placement of electrode catheters in the heart to record and to stimulate heart rhythm. In general, catheters are placed in the high right atrium, across the tricuspid valve in the region of the AV node and His bundle, in the right ventricular apex, and, in selected patients, in the coronary sinus to record from the left atrium and ventricle. This testing is indicated in patients with cardiogenic syncope of undetermined origin, for evaluation of the mechanism of supraventricular tachycardia, for assessing symptomatic patients with Wolff-Parkinson-White syndrome, and for evaluating patients with sustained ventricular tachycardia and survivors of out-of-hospital cardiac arrest. Ablative therapy can be curative for almost all patients with AV node reentry or Wolff-Parkinson-White syndrome, most patients with atrial tachycardia or typical atrial flutter, and selected patients with ventricular tachycardia. The complication rate of the test is 0.5% to 1%.

- Electrophysiologic testing is invasive.
- Electrophysiologic testing is indicated for cardiogenic syncope of undetermined origin.
- The complication rate is 0.5%-1%.

THERAPY

Pacing

Pacing uses a four-letter classification system (Table 3-6). The first letter is the chamber paced; the second letter, the chamber sensed; and the third letter, the mode of response. In practice, the fourth letter is used to designate whether the pacemaker will automatically increase its rate in response to activity detected by a sensor within the pacemaker pulse generator. Common pacing modes are VVI, which is ventricular paced, ventricular sensed, and inhibited in response to a ventricular event; VVIR, in which rate responsiveness (R) is added; DDD, which is atrial and ventricular paced and sensed and also triggered and inhibited in response to a sensed atrial or ventricular event; and DDDR, which adds rate response to the DDD mode.

Physiologic pacing attempts to maintain heart rate with normal AV synchrony and to increase heart rate in response to physical activity. DDD pacing is used to track atrial activation in patients with normal sinus node activity but some type of AV block. As sinus activity increases in response to

Table 3-6.—Code of Permanent Pacing

Chamber(s) paced	Chamber(s) sensed	Mode(s) of response	Programmable capabilities
V = Ventricle	V = Ventricle	T = Triggered	R = Rate modulated
A = Atrium	A = Atrium	I = Inhibited	
D = Dual (atrium and ventricle)	D = Dual (atrium and ventricle)	D = Dual (triggered and inhibited)	
	O = None	O = None	

exercise or some other stress, the pacemaker tracks this response and paces the ventricle with normal AV conduction delay (P-R interval) at a rate following the sinus rate. In patients who have chronic atrial fibrillation, rate-modulated pacing (the "R" in VVIR) is used to increase heart rate in response to physical demand. An external sensor that senses body motion, respiratory rate, and blood temperature, or some other sensor, is used to drive the pacemaker to keep up with increased metabolic demands. This type of pacemaker increases exercise endurance during treadmill testing. A patient with sinus node dysfunction and AV conduction system disease would benefit from DDDR pacing.

- Physiologic pacing maintains heart rate with normal AV synchrony and increases the rate during physical activity.
- Rate-modulated pacing increases exercise endurance during treadmill testing.

Pacemaker syndrome is a complication that occurs during ventricular pacing in patients who have intact retrograde conduction between the ventricle and the atrium (Fig. 3-8). When the ventricle is paced, the impulse conducts retrogradely to the atrium and simultaneous atrial and ventricular contractions result. Because the atria are contracting against closed tricuspid and mitral valves, the atrial contribution to ventricular filling is prevented and the atria are distended. The increased atrial pressure distends the neck veins and can result in hypotension; symptoms include a full sensation in the neck, light-headedness, and fatigue. These are eliminated with dual-chamber pacing.

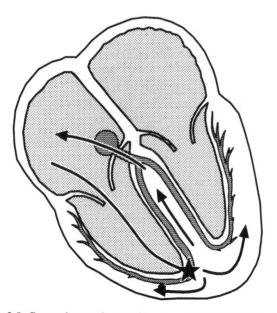

Fig. 3-8. Pacemaker syndrome with retrograde atrial activation during ventricular pacing (*star*), resulting in simultaneous atrial and ventricular contractions.

- Pacemaker syndrome is a complication of pacemakers.
- Atria contract against closed tricuspid and mitral valves.
- Increased atrial pressure distends neck veins and results in hypotension.
- Symptoms: full sensation in neck, light-headedness, and fatigue.
- Dual-chamber pacing eliminates symptoms.

Pacemaker-mediated tachycardia occurs with DDD pacing when there is intact retrograde conduction between the ventricle and atrium. In this type of tachycardia, the pacemaker generator acts as one limb of the reentrant circuit. Typically, a PVC occurs that conducts retrogradely to the atrium. The retrograde atrial activity is sensed by the pacemaker, which awaits the normal AV delay and then paces the ventricle. The ventricular activity conducts retrogradely to the atrium, and the reentrant circuit is completed. This abnormality is corrected through programming changes of the pacemaker generator.

- Pacemaker-mediated tachycardia occurs with DDD pacing when there is intact retrograde conduction between the ventricle and atrium.
- The abnormality is corrected by programming changes of the pacemaker generator.

Indications for Permanent Pacemaker Implantation

The guidelines for permanent pacemaker implantation are well established. Indications for specific conduction system disease are discussed below (Table 3-7). Indications for permanent pacemaker implantation generally have been grouped according to the following classification. 1) Class I indication: conditions for which there is general agreement that permanent pacemakers should be implanted. 2) Class II: conditions for which permanent pacemakers are frequently used but opinions differ about the necessity of implantation. 3) Class III: conditions for which there is general agreement that pacemakers are not necessary. It is important to bear in mind that if clinical symptoms such as syncope, presyncope, or exercise intolerance can be correlated with and attributed to a bradycardia disorder, this usually constitutes a class I indication for permanent pacemaker implantation. If symptoms cannot be correlated with bradycardia, it is less certain that permanent pacemaker implantation is indicated.

Antiarrhythmic Drugs

Therapeutic range, half-life, and routes of metabolism of antiarrhythmic drugs are listed in Table 3-8. The relative effectiveness of these drugs for treating PVCs, ventricular tachycardia, paroxysmal tachycardia using the AV node as part of the reentrant circuit, and atrial fibrillation are listed in

Table 3-9. The predominant target of the antiarrhythmic drugs is shown in Figure 3-9.

Half-life is an important concept in the use of antiarrhythmic drugs. It is the time required for 50% of the drug within the body to be eliminated. It takes five half-lives for a drug to reach steady state or to be eliminated. If a drug has a half-life of 90 minutes (e.g., lidocaine), a steady state will be reached in 6 hours; therefore, a loading dose is given to achieve a therapeutic level more promptly.

- Half-life is an important concept in the use of antiarrhythmic drugs.
- Half-life is the time required for 50% of the drug within the body to be eliminated.

Proarrhythmic effect (Table 3-10), a common problem of all antiarrhythmic drugs, occurs when the drug creates an adverse rhythm disturbance (Fig. 3-10), including sinus node suppression and sinus bradycardia, AV block, or increased frequency of or new-onset atrial or ventricular arrhythmias. It was first described in association with quinidine and causes quinidine syncope, which occurs in an estimated 3% of patients who take this drug. In such patients, a rapid ventricular tachycardia with polymorphic morphology, termed "torsades de pointes," develops. The frequency of proarrhythmia is higher in patients who have decreased ventricular function and a history of sustained ventricular tachycardia or ventricular fibrillation. Unfortunately,

Table 3-7.—Indications for Packemaker Implantation

Sinus node dysfunction
    Class I
        Documented symptomatic bradycardia
    Class II
        HR <40 beats/min, symptoms present but not clearly
            correlated with bradycardia
    Class III
        Asymptomatic bradycardia (<40 beats/min)
AV block
    Class I
        Symptomatic 2° or 3° AV block, permanent or
            intermittent
        Congenital 3° AV block with wide QRS
        Advanced AV block 14 days after cardiac surgery
    Class II
        Asymptomatic type II 2° or 3° AV block with
            ventricular rate >40 beats/min
    Class III
        Asymptomatic 1° and type I 2° AV block
Myocardial infarction
    Class I
        Recurrent type II 2° AV block and 3° AV block with
            wide QRS
        Transient advanced AV block in presence of BBB
    Class II
        Persistent advanced AV block with narrow QRS
        Acquired BBB in absence of AV block
    Class III
        Transient AV block in absence of BBB

AV, atrioventricular; BBB, bundle branch block.

Table 3-8.—Properties of Antiarrhythmic Drugs

Drug	Therapeutic range, µg/mL	Half-life, hr	Route of metabolism	
			Hepatic, %	Renal, %
Class IA				
Quinidine	2-5	6-8	80	20
Procainamide	4-10	3-6	50	50
Disopyramide	2-5	4-8	50	50
Class IB				
Lidocaine	1.5-5	1-4	100	...
Mexiletine	1-2	8-16	100	...
Tocainide	5-12	9-20	60	40
Phenytoin	10-20	24	~100	...
Class IC				
Flecainide	0.2-1	12-27	75	25
Propafenone	Not helpful[*]	2-10	100	...
Class I				
Moricizine	0.8-2.0	2-6[†]	60	40
Class III				
Amiodarone	1-2.5	25-110 days	100	...
Sotalol	~2.5	7-18	...	100

[*]Therapeutic effects for propafenone are generally associated with a QRS width increase of 10% above baseline.
[†]Effects of moricizine persist for 14-24 hours; thus, an unmeasured metabolite is suggested.
From MKSAP IX: Part C Book 1, 1992. American College of Physicians. By permission.

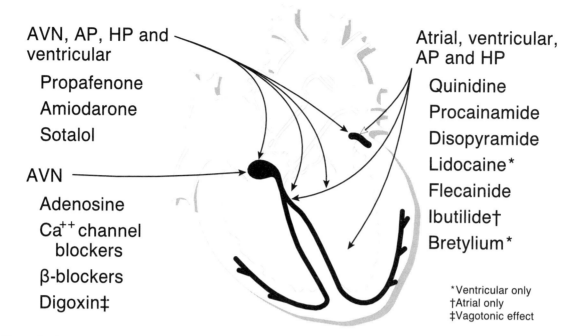

AVN, AP, HP and
ventricular

  Propafenone

  Amiodarone

  Sotalol

AVN

  Adenosine

  Ca^{++} channel
  blockers

  β-blockers

  Digoxin‡

Atrial, ventricular,
AP and HP

  Quinidine

  Procainamide

  Disopyramide

  Lidocaine*

  Flecainide

  Ibutilide†

  Bretylium*

*Ventricular only
†Atrial only
‡Vagotonic effect

Fig. 3-9. The predominant target of frequently used antiarrhythmic agents. AP, accessory pathway; AVN, atrioventricular node; HP, His-Purkinje system.

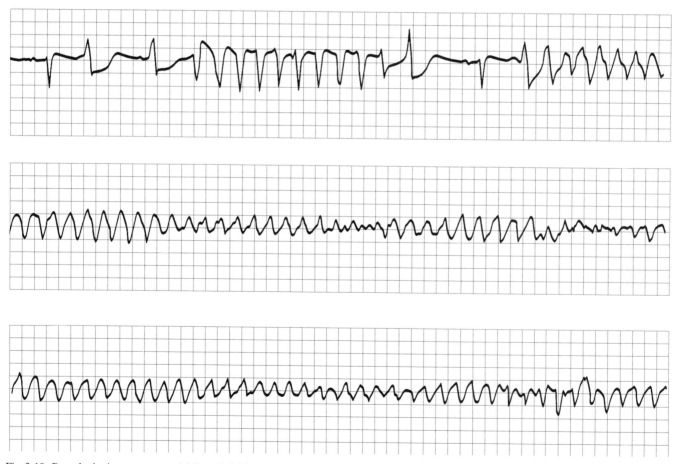

Fig. 3-10. Proarrhythmic response to quinidine. Quinidine resulted in prolongation of QT interval, and late-coupled premature ventricular complex initiated polymorphic ventricular tachycardia, termed "torsades de pointes."

Table 3-9.—Relative Effectiveness of Antiarrhythmic Drugs

Drug	Effectiveness*			
	PVCs	VT	PSVT	AF
Quinidine	2+	2+	2+	2+
Procainamide	2+	2+	2+	2+
Disopyramide	2+	2+	2+	2+
Lidocaine	2+	2+	0	0
Mexiletine	2+	2+	0	0
Tocainide	2+	1+	0	0
Flecainide	4+	2+	3+	2+
Propafenone	4+	2+	3+	2+
Moricizine	2+	2+	0-1+	0-1+
Amiodarone	4+	3+	3+	3+
Sotalol	3+	2-3+	3+	2+

*0, not effective; 1+, least effective; 4+, most effective.

AF, atrial fibrillation (prevention of paroxysmal AF); PSVT, paroxysmal tachycardia utilizing AV node as part of reentrant circuit; PVCs, premature ventricular complexes; VT, ventricular tachycardia.

it is these patients in whom antiarrhythmic drugs are most often required. Also, proarrhythmia can occur in structurally normal hearts.

- Proarrhythmic effect is a common problem of all antiarrhythmic drugs.
- Proarrhythmic effect occurs when a drug creates rhythm disturbance.
- Proarrhythmic effect causes quinidine syncope: a rapid ventricular tachycardia with polymorphic morphology (torsades de pointes).

The results of recent pharmacologic trials for the prevention of sudden cardiac death are summarized in Table 3-11.

The Cardiac Arrhythmia Suppression Trial (CAST) study indicated that patients with asymptomatic or mildly symptomatic ventricular ectopy after myocardial infarction had decreased survival rates with drug therapy, even though the drugs suppressed the spontaneous ectopy. These patients had approximately a threefold increase in death rate compared with the rate in patients taking placebo. The CAST study evaluated flecainide, encainide, and moricizine; however, similar results have been demonstrated for class IA drugs (quinidine, procainamide, and disopyramide) and the class IB drug mexiletine.

- The CAST study indicated decreased survival rate with drug therapy in patients with asymptomatic ventricular ectopy after infarction.

The final results on amiodarone therapy for long-term survival have been published recently. Results from two randomized trials on amiodarone after myocardial infarction (European Myocardial Infarction Amiodarone Trial [EMIAT], and Canadian Amiodarone Myocardial Infarction Arrhythmia Trial [CAMIAT]) suggest that amiodarone may improve arrhythmia-related death; however, overall mortality was not improved. Results from amiodarone trials in patients with congestive heart failure are also mixed. The Survival Trial of Antiarrhythmic Therapy in Patients With Congestive Heart Failure Arrhythmia (STAT-CHF) study showed that overall mortality was not significantly different between patients treated with amiodarone and those receiving placebo. The Gruppo de Estudio de la Sobrevida en la Insuficiencia Cardiaca en Argentia (GESICA) study (randomized trial of low-dose amiodarone in severe congestive heart failure) showed that low-dose amiodarone therapy reduced total mortality in comparison with placebo therapy in patients with congestive heart failure. The differences in outcome may be explained on the basis of differences in patient population. In the STAT-CHF study, approximately 70% of the study population had coronary artery disease, as compared with 30% in the GESICA study. Currently, the routine use of amiodarone in the post-myocardial infarction population or in patients with congestive heart failure is not recommended. However, if patients should have frequent and complex premature ventricular contractions associated with documented symptoms in the setting of compromised left ventricular dysfunction, it is not unreasonable to consider a trial of amiodarone therapy.

Adenosine slows conduction in the AV node and is eliminated by uptake in endothelial cells and erythrocytes. Its half-life is 10 seconds. Adenosine is indicated in supraventricular reentrant tachycardia that uses the AV node as part of the reentrant circuit (i.e., AV nodal reentry or reentry using an accessory pathway). The drug does not terminate atrial fibrillation, flutter, or tachycardia, and it slows the ventricular rate for only a few seconds because of its short half-life. Both adenosine and verapamil have equal efficacy at the highest recommended doses (adenosine, 12 mg; verapamil, 10 mg). Because of the short half-life of adenosine, approximately 10% of patients have recurrent supraventricular tachycardia after its administration, whereas recurrent supraventricular tachycardia is rare after termination by verapamil. In patients with a wide QRS tachycardia (ventricular tachycardia) or atrial fibrillation and associated Wolff-Parkinson-White syndrome, hemodynamic collapse is common when they are given verapamil. This problem is not associated with adenosine. The cost of adenosine is approximately twice that of verapamil.

- Adenosine slows conduction in the AV node.
- Adenosine is used for supraventricular reentrant tachycardia.

Table 3-10.—Toxicity and Side Effects of Antiarrhythmic Drugs

Drug	Frequency of side effects, %	Organ toxicity	% proarrhythmia during treatment for VT	Risk of congestive heart failure[*]		Side effects
				EF ≥ 30%	EF ≤ 30%	
Quinidine	30	Moderate	3	0	0	Nausea, abdominal pain, diarrhea, thrombocytopenia, hypotension, ↓ warfarin
Procainamide	30	High	2	0	1+	Lupus-like syndrome, rash, fever, headache, nausea, hallucinations, diarrhea
Disopyramide	30	Low	2	1+	4+	Dry mouth, urinary hesitancy, blurred vision, constipation, urinary retention
Lidocaine	40	Moderate	2	0	0	L-H, seizure, tremor, confusion, memory loss, nausea
Mexiletine	40	Low	2	0	0	L-H, tremor, ataxia, confusion, memory loss, altered liver function
Tocainide	40	High	2	0	0	L-H, tremor, ataxia, confusion, memory loss, blood dyscrasia, pulmonary fibrosis
Flecainide	30	Low	5	1+	3+	L-H, visual disturbance, headache, nausea
Propafenone	30	Low	5	0-1+	2+	L-H, headache, nausea, constipation, metallic taste, ↓ warfarin
Moricizine	30	Low	5	0	1+	L-H, nausea, headache, fatigue, dyspnea
Amiodarone	65	High	4	0	1+	Corneal deposits, photosensitivity, sleep disturbance, nausea, anorexia, tremor, ataxia, neuropathy, pulmonary fibrosis, thyroid disorders, hepatotoxicity, ↓ warfarin
Sotalol	30	Low	5	1+	3+	L-H, fatigue, dyspnea, nausea

[*]Congestive heart failure risk: 0, no risk; 4+, high risk.
EF, ejection fraction; L-H, light-headedness; PVC, premature ventricular complex; VT, sustained ventricular tachycardia.
Modified from MKSAP IX: Part C Book 1, 1992. American College of Physicians. By permission.

Table 3-11.—Results of Trials on Pharmacologic Prevention of Primary Sudden Cardiac Death

Trial	Patients	No.	Drug	Follow-up, mo	Total mortality, %		Significance
					Placebo	Drug	
Julian et al., 1982	MI < 2 wk	1,456	*d, l*-Sotalol	12	8.9	7.3	No
CAST, 1989	MI, EF < 0.55, > 6 PVCs/hr	1,455	Flecainide Encainide	10	3.0	7.7	Yes
CAST II, 1992	MI, EF ≤ 0.40, > 6 PVCs/hr	1,155	Moricizine	18	12.4	15.0	No
SWORT, 1996	MI, EF ≤ 0.40	3,121	*d*-Sotalol	5	3.1	5.0	Yes
Diamond-MI, 1997	MI	1,510	Dofetilide	≥ 12	32.0	31.0	No
GESICA, 1994	CHF	516	Amiodarone	24	41.4	33.5	Yes
STAT-CHF, 1995	CHF, EF < 0.4	674	Amiodarone	45	29.2 (2 yr)	30.6 (2 yr)	No
CAMIAT, 1997	MI, ≥ 10 PVCs/hr or ± NSVT	1,202	Amiodarone	22	11.4	9.4	No
EMIAT, 1997	MI, EF ≤ 0.4	1,486	Amiodarone	21	13.7	13.9	No

CHF, congestive heart failure; EF, ejection fraction; MI, myocardial infarction; NSVT, nonsustained ventricular tachycardia ; PVCs, premature ventricular complexes.

- Adenosine does not terminate atrial fibrillation, flutter, or tachycardia.
- The efficacy of 12 mg of adenosine is equal to that of 10 mg of verapamil.
- The cost of adenosine is twice that of verapamil.

Electrophysiology-Guided Serial Drug Testing

This technique is used to identify an effective drug for patients (before dismissal from the hospital) who have life-threatening arrhythmias and for whom outpatient management is unsafe. Arrhythmia is induced in the baseline state, an antiar-rhythmic drug is then administered orally, and the electro-physiologic study is repeated. A drug that prevents induction of tachycardia is termed effective. In patients who have ventricular tachycardia occurring spontaneously, the chance of that tachycardia being induced in the laboratory is 95% if the patients have underlying coronary artery disease and 75% if they have dilated cardiomyopathy or valvular heart disease. In patients who present with out-of-hospital cardiac arrest and ventricular fibrillation, the chance of life-threatening ventric-ular arrhythmia being induced at testing is 70%. For patients with ventricular tachycardia, an effective drug is identified for approximately 40%, and each drug has a 25% chance of being effective with electrophysiology-guided serial drug testing. For patients who survive cardiac arrest and have inducible ventricular tachycardia, the survival rate at 1 year is 95% if an effective drug is identified. Alternatively, the 1-year survival rate is 65% if an effective drug cannot be identified and 85% if ventricular tachycardia is not inducible during baseline study and no therapy is given.

- Electrophysiology-guided serial drug testing, performed before hospital dismissal, identifies an effective drug for patients with life-threatening arrhythmias.
- With out-of-hospital cardiac arrest and ventricular fibrilla-tion, the chance of inducing life-threatening arrhythmia during testing is 70%.
- Serial drug testing identifies an effective drug for 40% of patients with ventricular tachycardia.

Implantable Defibrillators

Because serial drug testing identifies only 40% of patients with life-threatening ventricular arrhythmias, an alternative therapy has been developed to treat recurrences of tachycardia. The most effective therapy has been the implantable cardioverter defibrillator. This device monitors the rhythm and treats a ventricular arrhythmia with up to 34-J shock or antitachycardia pacing as the initial therapy, followed by low-energy cardioversion and high-energy defibrillation if needed. Current limitations of the device are a battery life of 3 to 5 years, large and cumbersome size, and the presence of uncomfortable and potentially dangerous shocks during sinus rhythm or atrial fibrillation.

Implantable cardioverter defibrillators have improved mortality in patients surviving sudden cardiac death when compared with historical controls. Historically, such patients had a 70% survival rate at 1 year with either no treatment or empiric antiarrhythmic drug therapy. The use of the device has improved the overall 1-year survival rate to 90%; recurrent sudden cardiac death occurs in 2% of patients at 1 year and in 4% of patients at 4 years. The recent Antiarrhythmic Versus Implantable Defibrillator (AVID) trial reported, for the first time, that an implantable cardioverter defibrillator is superior in reducing overall mortality in comparison with empiric amiodarone therapy in patients with a history of out-of-hospital cardiac arrest or symptomatic sustained ventricular tachycardia.

Several ongoing trials are assessing the optimal therapy of implantable cardioverter defibrillator versus conventional pharmacologic therapy in preventing primary sudden cardiac death. A recent study (Multicenter Automatic Defibrillator Implantation Trial [MADIT]) has shown that implantable cardioverter defibrillators may improve survival in a highly selected patient population at high risk for sudden death (patients who have had a myocardial infarction, an ejection fraction <35% in the presence of nonsustained ventricular tachycardia, and electrophysiologically inducible sustained monomorphic ventricular tachycardia not suppressible with procainamide). The results of this study have not been confirmed by other ongoing trials. Currently, routine implantation as prophylaxis for sudden cardiac death in asymptomatic patients (without a history of sudden cardiac death or documented sustained ventricular arrhythmia) is not recommended.

Advances in technology have now made it possible to implant defibrillators in virtually all patients by using a nonthoracotomy approach. Also, the devices have been reduced in size so that most patients can have them implanted in the pectoral region, similar to a pacemaker.

- Limitations of implantable cardioverter defibrillator: battery life of 3-5 years, large size, uncomfortable and potentially dangerous shocks during sinus rhythm or atrial fibrillation.
- Overall 1-year survival rate with the device is 90%.

Transcatheter Ablation

This technique involves placing an electrode catheter in a heart chamber. It is placed adjacent to a critical portion of a reentrant circuit, which might include one of the pathways participating in AV nodal reentrant tachycardia or an accessory pathway in patients with Wolff-Parkinson-White syndrome, an automatic atrial focus, or a portion of the reentrant circuit adjacent to a scar in the ventricle in patients with ventricular tachycardia. Previously, direct current was passed through the catheter; the current exited the catheter tip and produced a 1-cm scar that was 2 to 3 mm in depth. Most ablations are now performed with radio-frequency energy, which passes through the catheter tip and heats the adjacent tissue; the result is a smaller scar with a lesion size that is easier to control.

- Catheter ablation: AV nodal reentrant tachycardia, accessory pathway in Wolff-Parkinson-White syndrome, automatic atrial focus, atrial flutter, and some cases of ventricular tachycardia.
- Catheter ablation is performed with radio-frequency energy passed through a catheter.

Radio-frequency energy used to treat an accessory pathway (Wolff-Parkinson-White syndrome) or reentrant tachycardia within the AV node is successful in 95% of cases. About 1% to 2% of patients have complications, including vascular injury where the catheters are placed, cardiac perforation, and infection. In addition, if the accessory pathway is close to the normal conduction system or if AV nodal reentrant tachycardia is ablated, there is a 5% risk of creating complete heart block that requires permanent pacing. Compared with previous surgical approaches for the treatment of similar tachycardias, the technique has reduced the hospital stay from 7 days to 1 to 2 days and the time to return to work or school from 6 to 8 weeks to 3 to 5 days. The cost is approximately 40% of the surgical cost.

- Catheter ablation is successful in 95% of cases of accessory pathway or reentrant tachycardia in the AV node.
- The complication rate is 1%-2%.
- Catheter ablation reduces hospital stay to 1-2 days.
- The cost is 40% of the surgical cost.

Catheter ablation is also used to achieve complete heart block in patients with supraventricular tachycardias (usually atrial fibrillation or atrial flutter) that are refractory to medications and associated with rapid ventricular rates. Either direct-current or radio-frequency ablation results in heart block in more than 95% of patients, and permanent pacing is then required. Such patients have significant symptomatic improvement because the heart rate is regular and they respond normally to exercise because of rate-responsive pacing. This technique trades tachycardia-associated problems for problems associated with permanent pacemaker implantation and follow-up.

- Catheter ablation achieves complete heart block in supraventricular tachycardias that are refractory to medication and associated with rapid ventricular rates.
- Catheter ablation results in heart block in >95% of patients; permanent pacing is then required.
- Symptoms improve significantly.

Antitachycardia Surgery

Endocardial resection is a standard technique for treating ventricular tachycardia associated with aneurysm. The border zone adjacent to a myocardial scar (including aneurysm) is generally the location for the reentrant circuit. This border zone is located with mapping systems at the time of operation and is then removed with a technique called subendocardial resection. The operative mortality rate is approximately 10%; arrhythmia is cured in 85% of survivors.

- Endocardial resection is an option for treating ventricular tachycardia associated with aneurysm.
- Operative mortality rate is 10%.
- Arrhythmia is cured in 85% of survivors.

Endocardial resection is also a standard technique for treating an accessory pathway or AV nodal reentrant tachycardia.

Either sharp dissection or cryoablation of the accessory pathway is used. Surgical success rates approach 95%. The surgical mortality rate is 1%, and the risk of heart block is 1% to 2%. For the most part, surgical techniques have been replaced by transcatheter radio-frequency ablation.

- Operation is standard for treating accessory pathway or AV nodal reentrant tachycardia.
- The success rate is 95%.
- The current therapeutic interventions in tachycardia are summarized in Table 3-12.

Table 3-12.—Summary of Tachyarrhythmia Therapy

Supraventricular tachycardia	Drug	Ablation	ICD	Surgery
AVNRT	+	++	-	-
AVRT	+	++	-	-*
EAT	+	+	-	-*
IAST	++	o	-	-
Typical A flutter	+	++	-	-*
AFib	++	o	o	+

Symbols: +, effective; ++, preferred; o, investigational; -, no indication; -*, few indications, can be effective.
A, atrial; AFib, atrial fibrillation; AVNRT, atrioventricular nodal reciprocating tachycardia; AVRT, atrioventricular reciprocating tachycardia; EAT, ectopic atrial tachycardia; IAST, inappropriate sinus tachycardia; ICD, implantable cardioverter defibrillator.

PART III
Paul A. Friedman, M.D.

SPECIFIC ARRHYTHMIA PROBLEMS

Sinus Node Dysfunction

Sinus node dysfunction, also called "sick sinus syndrome," includes sinus bradycardia, sinus pauses, tachycardia-bradycardia syndrome (Fig. 3-11), and sinus arrest. It usually is associated with conduction system disease and lack of an appropriate junctional escape focus during sinus pause or sinus bradycardia. The diagnosis is made from the medical history and results of ECG and Holter monitoring, which are the most useful diagnostic tests. Electrophysiologic testing is used to evaluate patients with a history consistent with sinus node disease in whom ECG or Holter monitoring has not shown the mechanism because of infrequent spells. Electrophysiologic testing has low sensitivity because patients may be in an increased adrenergic state in the laboratory and catecholamines prevent the sinus bradycardia or sinus pauses from being apparent. Prolonged monitoring with an event recorder is also useful for diagnosis.

- Sinus node dysfunction includes sinus bradycardia, sinus pauses, tachycardia-bradycardia syndrome, and sinus arrest.
- Sinus node dysfunction is associated with conduction system disease.
- The diagnosis is made from the history and the results of ECG and Holter monitoring.
- Electrophysiologic testing is used for patients in whom the mechanism of dysfunction is not shown by ECG or Holter monitoring.

Asymptomatic patients with sinus node dysfunction are followed without specific therapy. Symptomatic patients are usually treated with pacemakers. Often, patients with tachycardia-bradycardia have atrial fibrillation that at times presents with rapid ventricular rates and at other times with inappropriate, symptomatic bradycardia. Pacemakers are used to prevent the bradycardia, and drugs are used to slow conduction through the AV node and to prevent episodes of rapid ventricular rate.

- Asymptomatic patients with sinus node dysfunction: followed without specific therapy.
- Symptomatic patients with sinus node dysfunction: treated with pacemakers.

Conduction System Disorders

First-degree AV block results in a prolonged PR interval and is usually due to conduction delay within the AV node. In patients with associated bundle branch block, the conduction delay may be distal to the AV node in the His-Purkinje system. Patients with second-degree AV block of the Mobitz I (Wenckebach) variety have a gradual prolongation of the PR interval before the nonconducted P wave. The subsequent PR interval is shorter than the PR interval before the nonconducted P wave (Fig. 3-12 and 3-13). Also, the RR interval that encompasses the nonconducted P wave is shorter than two RR intervals between conducted beats. Wenckebach conduction often accompanies an inferior myocardial infarction, which results in ischemia of the AV node. This problem generally does not require pacing unless there are documented hemodynamic problems associated with the slow heart rate.

- First-degree AV block results in a prolonged PR interval.
- Second-degree AV block of Mobitz I type results in a gradual prolongation of the PR interval before the nonconducted P wave.
- Wenckebach conduction may accompany inferior myocardial infarction.
- Wenckebach conduction does not require pacing unless hemodynamic problems are associated with slow heart rate.

Second-degree AV block due to the Mobitz II mechanism

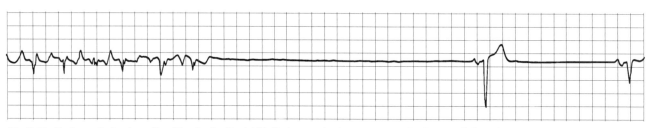

Fig. 3-11. Tachycardia-bradycardia with episode of atrial fibrillation terminating spontaneously; these are followed by a 4.5-second pause until sinus node recovers. (From MKSAP IX: Part C Book 1, 1992. American College of Physicians. By permission.)

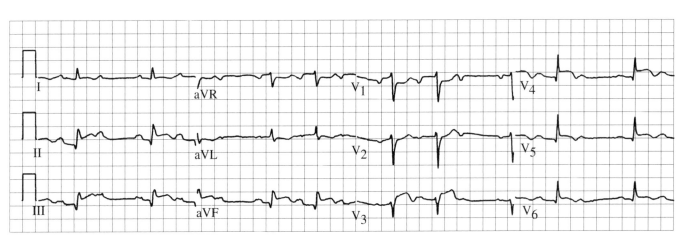

Fig. 3-12. 3:2 Mobitz I (or Wenckebach) second-degree atrioventricular block in a patient with acute inferior myocardial infarction.

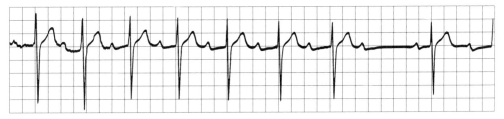

Fig. 3-13. Mobitz I second-degree atrioventricular block; note gradual PR prolongation. PR after nonconducted P wave is shorter than PR preceding nonconducted P wave.

is generally caused by conduction disease in the His-Purkinje system and is associated with bundle branch block (Fig. 3-14). This conduction abnormality is shown on the ECG as a sudden failure of a P wave to conduct to the ventricle, with no change in the PR interval either before or after the nonconducted P wave. This problem often heralds complete heart block, and strong consideration should be given to permanent pacing. *Complete heart block* is diagnosed when there is no relationship between the atrial rhythm and the ventricular rhythm and the *atrial rhythm is faster than the ventricular escape rhythm* (Fig. 3-15). The ventricular escape rhythm is either a junctional escape focus, with a conduction pattern similar to the conduction pattern seen during normal rhythm, or a ventricular escape focus, with a wide QRS conduction pattern. In most cases, complete heart block is treated with permanent pacing.

- Second-degree AV block of Mobitz II type is usually due to conduction disease in His-Purkinje system.
- It often heralds complete heart block; consider permanent pacing.
- Complete heart block: no relationship between atrial rhythm and ventricular rhythm, and atrial rhythm is faster than ventricular escape rhythm. Treatment: pacing.

Bifascicular block refers to left bundle branch block, right bundle branch block with left anterior fascicular block (marked left-axis deviation), or right bundle branch block with left posterior fascicular block (right-axis deviation). Bifascicular block is usually associated with underlying structural heart disease and has a 1% chance of progressing to complete heart block in asymptomatic persons. Patients presenting with syncope and bifascicular block may have intermittent complete heart block caused by their conduction system disease or ventricular tachycardia caused by the underlying myocardial disease. Permanent pacing can be used to treat syncope due to complete heart block, but syncope due to ventricular tachycardia is typically treated with an implantable defibrillator, although antiarrhythmic medications or surgery may be used, depending on the clinical situation. Patients with syncope and bifascicular block should undergo electrophysiologic testing (especially if the ejection fraction is decreased) to determine whether they have ventricular tachycardia, because this rhythm occurs in 40% of such patients. Although treatment with permanent pacing only does not decrease the risk of sudden death in these patients, it improves their syncope.

- Bifascicular block is usually associated with structural heart disease.

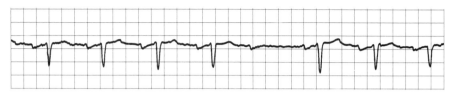

Fig. 3-14. Mobitz II second-degree atrioventricular block with no change in PR interval before or after nonconducted P wave.

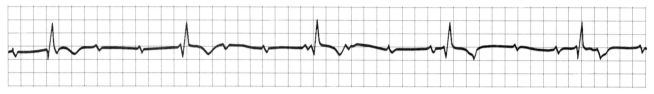

Fig. 3-15. Complete heart block with an atrial rate at 70 beats per minute and a ventricular escape rhythm at 30 beats/min.

- Bifascicular block progresses to complete heart block in 1% of asymptomatic persons.
- Permanent pacing is used to treat syncope in complete heart block.
- Syncope due to ventricular tachycardia is typically treated with an implantable defibrillator, although antiarrhythmic drugs or surgery may be used in some cases.
- Patients with syncope, bifascicular block, and ventricular tachycardia who receive only permanent pacing have improvement in syncope but no decrease in risk of sudden death.

High-degree AV block is diagnosed when there is a 2:1 or higher AV conduction block (Fig. 3-16). It might be caused by a Wenckebach or a Mobitz II mechanism. A Wenckebach mechanism is more likely if the QRS conduction is normal, and a Mobitz II-type mechanism is more likely if the QRS complex demonstrates additional conduction disease, such as bundle branch block.

Carotid Sinus Syndrome

Carotid sinus massage is performed to identify carotid sinus hypersensitivity (Fig. 3-17). Approximately 40% of patients older than 65 years have a hyperactive carotid sinus reflex (3-second pause or a decrease in blood pressure of 50 mm Hg), although most of these patients have no spontaneous syncope. Carotid sinus massage should be performed over the carotid bifurcation at the angle of the jaw in patients without evidence of carotid bruit on carotid auscultation or a history of cerebrovascular disease. Carotid sinus massage is performed with moderate pressure over the carotid bifurcation for 5 seconds while monitoring heart rate and blood pressure. Approximately 35% of patients with a hyperactive carotid sinus reflex have a pure cardioinhibitory component manifested only by a pause in ventricular activity exceeding 3 seconds. Fifteen percent

of patients have a pure vasodepressor component, with a normal heart rate maintained but a decrease in blood pressure greater than 50 mm Hg. Sixty percent of patients have a combined response, with both cardioinhibitory and vasodepressor components. In such patients, permanent pacing may prevent the cardioinhibitory response, but the vasodepressor response continues to produce symptoms.

- Carotid sinus massage is used to identify carotid sinus hypersensitivity.
- About 40% of patients >65 years have a hyperactive carotid sinus reflex (3-second pause or decrease in blood pressure of 50 mm Hg).

Occasionally, associated neck abnormalities, including lymph node enlargement, previous neck surgery, and regional tumor, result in carotid sinus syndrome. Surgical techniques to treat this condition are usually unsuccessful, and the primary form of therapy is AV sequential pacing for the cardioinhibitory component and elastic stockings for the vasodepressor component. On occasion, patients respond to anticholinergic medications.

Pacemaker Indication Summary

To summarize, pacemakers generally are indicated for symptomatic bradycardias. Commonly, these are AV block (second-degree Mobitz II, high-grade, or third-degree), sinus node dysfunction, and carotid sinus hypersensitivity. They usually are best documented by correlating the symptoms with ECG recording. In asymptomatic patients, pacing should be considered in complete heart block (particularly with escape <40 beats/min or pauses >3 seconds), Mobitz II block (especially associated with bi- or trifascicular block), and postoperative AV block.

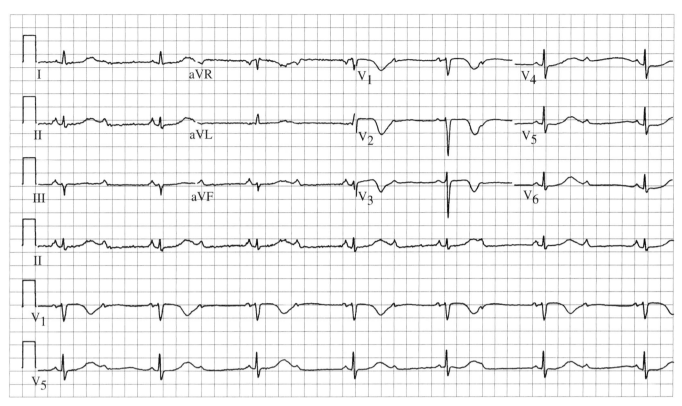

Fig. 3-16. High-grade 2:1 atrioventricular conduction block.

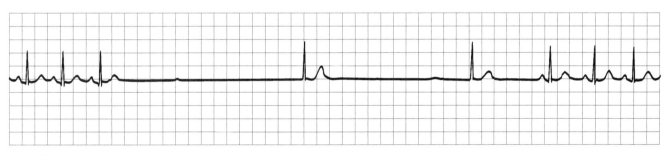

Fig. 3-17. Carotid sinus massage resulting in sinus pause with junctional escape beats before sinus rhythm returns.

- Pacing is indicated for symptomatic bradycardias due to second- or third-degree heart block, sinus node dysfunction, and carotid sinus hypersensitivity.
- Asymptomatic patients with complete heart block, Mobitz II AV block, or postoperative AV block should also be considered for pacing.

Atrial Flutter

Atrial flutter is identified by the characteristic sawtooth pattern of atrial activity at a rate of 240 to 320 beats/min. Patients with normal conduction systems maintain 2:1 AV conduction; thus, the ventricular rate is often close to 150 beats/min. Higher degrees of AV block (3:1 or higher) in the

absence of drugs to slow AV node conduction (digoxin, β-adrenergic blocker, calcium antagonist) imply AV conduction disease (Fig. 3-18). Patients with 2:1 AV conduction and a heart rate of 150 beats/min often have one of the flutter waves buried in the QRS complex. Carotid sinus massage results in increased AV block, revealing the flutter waves and establishing the diagnosis.

- Atrial flutter: atrial activity at 240-320 beats per minute.
- Ventricular rate is close to 150 beats/min.

Pharmacologic therapy for atrial flutter is used to slow AV nodal conduction and to control the ventricular rate or

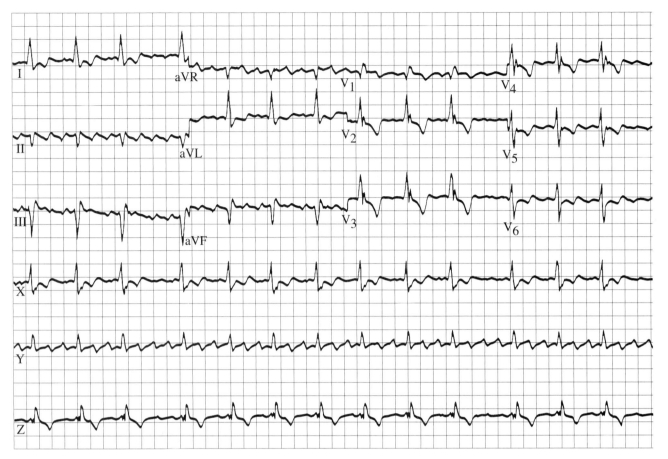

Fig. 3-18. Atrial flutter with 3:1 conduction in a patient with atrioventricular conduction disease.

to control the flutter itself. The same medications used to treat atrial fibrillation (discussed below) are used to treat atrial flutter. Success rates for the control of atrial flutter are 30% to 50%.

Nonpharmacologic therapy for typical atrial flutter has been well established. Unlike atrial fibrillation, which is composed of multiple reentrant wavelets that travel through the atria, typical atrial flutter consists of a single reentrant circuit that follows the tricuspid valve annulus (Fig. 3-19). This fixed reentrant pathway results in a surface ECG with very stable flutter waves (Fig. 3-18) and provides a target for ablation. Radio-frequency catheter ablation of this single circuit has a success rate greater than 90%. This procedure must not be confused with AV node ablation for atrial fibrillation. In atrial flutter ablation, a lesion is placed in the atrium to interrupt the flutter circuit; AV nodal conduction is not impaired and normal sinus rhythm (with no need for pacing) ensues. In AV node ablation for atrial fibrillation, the AV node (or His bundle) is ablated, preventing atrial impulses from reaching the ventricles, thus controlling ventricular rate; the atria,

however, continue to fibrillate, and because of the presence of AV block, a pacemaker is required.

- Typical atrial flutter ablation has a success rate greater than 90%.
- Atrial flutter can be associated with thromboembolism and probably should be treated similarly to atrial fibrillation with regard to anticoagulation.

Atrial Fibrillation

Atrial fibrillation is the most common arrhythmia encountered in clinical practice. Its frequency increases with age. Atrial fibrillation is characterized by continuous and irregular activity of the ECG baseline caused by swarming electrical currents in the atria. According to population-based studies, its prevalence is 5% among patients 65 years and older. Common causes and associated conditions include hypertension, cardiomyopathy, valvular heart disease (particularly mitral stenosis), sick sinus syndrome, Wolff-Parkinson-White syndrome (especially in young patients), alcohol use ("Holiday

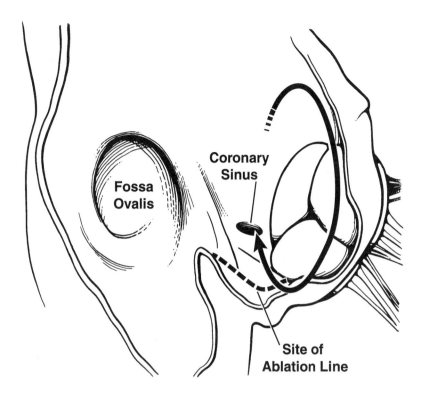

Fig. 3-19. View of the right atrium, with the tricuspid valve on the right. The atrial flutter circuit is confined to the path depicted by the circular arrow adjacent to the valve. An ablation lesion along the dashed line ("site of ablation line") interrupts the circuit, eliminating atrial flutter. In contrast to atrial flutter, atrial fibrillation has wandering wavefronts throughout the atria, which will not respond to the flutter ablation line.

heart"), and thyrotoxicosis. The presence of these conditions should be sought in the history and physical examination of patients with atrial fibrillation.

- Common causes of atrial fibrillation include hypertension, cardiomyopathy, valvular heart disease, sick sinus syndrome, Wolff-Parkinson-White syndrome, thyrotoxicosis, and alcohol use.
- Atrial fibrillation must be distinguished from atrial flutter (uniform flutter waves) and multifocal atrial tachycardia (isoelectric interval between PACs that have three or more different morphologies).

Therapy for Atrial Fibrillation

Therapy for atrial fibrillation can be divided into two broad categories: 1) ventricular rate control (by slow conduction through the AV node) with stroke prophylaxis (for ongoing atrial fibrillation) and 2) maintenance of sinus rhythm (rhythm control). The choice of the approach taken depends partly on the degree of the patient's symptoms, age and preference, and the coexisting conditions. Currently, it is not known whether one approach is superior; this issue is being evaluated by a multicenter trial.

- It is important to know which agents are useful for rate control and which for rhythm control (Table 3-13)

Rate Control and Anticoagulation

The three main categories of drugs used to blunt the AV nodal response in atrial fibrillation are digitalis glycosides, β-adrenergic blocking agents, and calcium channel blockers. These are summarized in Table 3-13. None of these agents has been shown to be effective in the prevention of recurrent atrial fibrillation. There is one exception: continuation of β-blockers after cardiac surgery may prevent recurrent atrial fibrillation.

Digoxin primarily has an indirect effect by increasing vagal tone and, thus, slowing AV nodal conduction. Because of its mechanism of action, digoxin is less effective than β-blockers or calcium channel blockers, particularly with exercise, when an increase in sympathetic tone results in more rapid AV nodal conduction. Thus, the optimal role for digoxin in atrial fibrillation is in patients with left ventricular dysfunction (because of the drug's positive inotropy) or as adjunctive therapy in patients receiving β-blockers or calcium channel blockers.

- Digoxin alone is no better than placebo for terminating atrial fibrillation.

Table 3-13.—Pharmacologic Therapy for Atrial Fibrillation

Agents	Comments
Control of ventricular rate	
β-Blockers (e.g., atenolol, metoprolol, propranolol, carvedilol)	Ideal postoperatively and in hyperthyroidism, acute MI, and chronic CHF (especially carvedilol)
Calcium channel blockers (verapamil, diltiazem)	Nifedipine, amlodipine, and felodipine are not useful for slowing AV conduction
Digoxin	Less effective than β-blockers and calcium channel blockers, especially with exercise
	Useful in heart failure
Maintenance of sinus rhythm	
Class IA: quinidine, diso-pyramide, procainamide	Enhance AV conduction—rate must be controlled before use
	Monitor QTc
Class IC: propafenone, flecainide	Slow AV conduction
	Often first choice for patients with normal heart
	Monitor QRS duration
Class III: sotalol, ami-odarone	Amiodarone is agent of choice for ventricular dysfunction and post-MI

AV, atrioventricular; CHF, congestive heart failure; MI, myocardial infarction.

- Digoxin is less effective than β-blockers or calcium channel blockers in controlling ventricular rate and is best used as an adjunctive agent or in the setting of impaired ventricular function.

β-Blockers such as propranolol, metoprolol, and atenolol are effective in slowing AV nodal conduction and may be particularly useful when atrial fibrillation complicates hyperthyroidism or myocardial infarction (in which case they reduce the risk of death from myocardial infarction). β-Blockers also have been shown to decrease the risk of postoperative myocardial infarction, making them well suited for postoperative atrial fibrillation. Carvedilol has been shown to decrease mortality in patients with chronic heart failure and may be a good choice in that setting. Esmolol, because of its intravenous formulation and short half-life, is particularly useful for acute management of atrial fibrillation.

- β-Blockers are effective in slowing ventricular rate in atrial fibrillation, but they do not terminate atrial fibrillation (though they may prevent it postoperatively).
- β-Blockers are particularly useful postoperatively and in hyperthyroidism, acute myocardial infarction, and chronic heart failure.

Calcium channel blockers are divided broadly into two groups: dihydropyridines (nifedipine, amlodipine, felodipine) and nondihydropyridines (diltiazem, verapamil). Dihydropyridine agents have little or no effect on AV nodal conduction and no role in the management of atrial fibrillation. Verapamil and diltiazem are both available as intravenous and oral preparations and are well suited for acute and chronic rate control. Also, both agents have negative inotropic effects and should be used cautiously in congestive heart failure.

- Diltiazem and verapamil are both effective for rate control in atrial fibrillation; nifedipine, amlodipine, and felodipine are not and have no role in the management of atrial fibrillation.

Adenosine is very effective at slowing AV nodal conduction; however, because of its short half-life, it has no role in the treatment of atrial fibrillation. It can be useful diagnostically by slowing ventricular rate transiently, permitting visualization of atrial activity if the diagnosis is in question.

Nonpharmacologic AV Nodal Rate Control

If the rate cannot be controlled pharmacologically or rhythm control medications (discussed below) are either ineffective or not well tolerated, catheter ablation of the AV junction is an alternative. For patients with chronic atrial fibrillation, a VVIR pacemaker is implanted, and for those with paroxysmal atrial fibrillation, dual-chamber pacemakers with mode switching functions are used. These permit the tracking of P waves during sinus rhythm and revert to VVIR (or DDIR) pacing when atrial fibrillation recurs. With this approach, the risk of thromboembolism is unchanged because the fibrillation itself persists in the atria; thus, appropriate stroke prophylaxis must be prescribed.

Rhythm Control

Rhythm control (maintenance of sinus rhythm) can control symptoms effectively. However, maintaining sinus rhythm has not been shown to decrease the likelihood of thromboembolism, nor has it been shown to prolong survival. In fact, some drugs used to prevent recurrences may cause new arrhythmias (proarrhythmias).

- Class IA agents (quinidine, procainamide, and disopyramide) can be associated with torsades de pointes, particularly at the time of reversion of atrial fibrillation to normal sinus rhythm, and should be initiated in a monitored setting.

- Class IA agents also enhance AV nodal conduction, so rate control agents should be given before their use to slow AV nodal conduction.
- Class IB agents (lidocaine, mexiletine, tocainide) have no significant effect in treating atrial fibrillation and should not be used for that purpose.
- For patients with a normal heart, class IC agents (propafenone, flecainide) are often a good first choice and often can be used safely in an outpatient setting (with ECG and treadmill testing at 3 days to exclude proarrhythmia).
- Amiodarone has been proven safe for post-myocardial infarction patients and those with systolic dysfunction and is preferable in these situations.

Stroke Prevention

Acute Cardioversion to Normal Sinus Rhythm

Electrical cardioversion from atrial fibrillation is commonly used to control atrial fibrillation. Current guidelines state that patients with atrial fibrillation lasting more than 2 days should receive anticoagulation before cardioversion. It has been demonstrated that several weeks of warfarin therapy before cardioversion can reduce the incidence of cardioversion-associated thromboembolism to 0% to 1.6% (compared with up to 7% in the absence of anticoagulation). Additionally, anticoagulation should be continued for 4 weeks after cardioversion because of the increased risk of thromboembolism in the weeks following cardioversion. Although few data are available about cardioversion in the absence of anticoagulation for atrial fibrillation of recent onset (less than 48 hours), current guidelines do not mandate anticoagulation in this setting. Although atrial flutter historically was thought to confer a very low risk, more recent data have contested this observation, suggesting that guidelines similar to those for atrial fibrillation should be followed.

- Patients with more than 2 days of atrial fibrillation must receive anticoagulation treatment for 3 weeks before and 4 weeks after cardioversion.
- An alternative approach for patients with more than 2 days of atrial fibrillation may be transesophageal echocardiography, with cardioversion (if no thrombus found) and 3-4 weeks of anticoagulation treatment subsequently, although this approach is less well validated.

Chronic Stroke Prevention

Patients with atrial fibrillation due to rheumatic valvular disease have a markedly increased risk of stroke and should receive warfarin therapy. Most patients encountered in clinical practice have nonrheumatic atrial fibrillation. A series of landmark studies has demonstrated that warfarin decreases the incidence of thromboembolism by 68% to 84% in this population. The risk of thromboembolism can be determined by clinical and echocardiographic risk factors, which should be used to guide treatment (Tables 3-14 and 3-15). The risk factors are advanced age, previous transient ischemic attack or stroke, history of hypertension, diabetes mellitus, and congestive heart failure. Echocardiographic risk factors included depressed left ventricular function and left atrial enlargement. Patients who are younger than 60 years and have no clinical heart disease or hypertension are at extremely low risk and require no treatment, although some physicians recommend aspirin. Thus, a strategy based on age and risk factors has emerged and is summarized in Table 3-15. Patients younger than 60 years (65 in some reports) with no risk factors can be given no therapy or aspirin. Patients older than 75 years or those with risk factors should receive warfarin. In patients treated with warfarin, the International Normalized Ratio (INR) should be maintained in the range of 2.0 to 3.0 (although 2.0 to 2.5 may be preferable in the older than 75 years group). INR values are preferable to prothrombin times for management because prothrombin time assays vary among laboratories.

- The clinical risk factors for stroke in nonrheumatic atrial fibrillation are age >75 years, previous transient ischemic attack or stroke, history of hypertension, diabetes mellitus, congestive heart failure—these should be known for board examination.
- Echocardiographic risk factors are depressed ventricular function and left atrial enlargement.
- Patients <60 years with structurally normal hearts and no hypertension are at low risk for thromboembolism and require no specific therapy.
- Warfarin should be used to maintain an INR of 2.0 to 3.0 (although 2.0-2.5 is preferable in the elderly).

Table 3-14.—Risk Factors for Thromboembolism in Nonrheumatic Atrial Fibrillation

Clinical risk factors	Echocardiographic risk factors
Advanced age (>65 yr)	Left ventricular dysfunction
Previous TIA or stroke	Left atrial enlargement
Hypertension	
Diabetes (in pooled analysis)	
Heart failure	
Other high-risk clinical settings	
Prosthetic heart valves	
Thyrotoxicosis	

TIA, transient ischemic attack.

Table 3-15.—Recommended Management of Patients With Nonrheumatic Atrial Fibrillation

Age, yr	Risk factors	Recommendations
<65	Present	Warfarin INR 2-3
	No risk factors	Aspirin or nothing
65-75	Present	Warfarin INR 2-3
	No risk factors	Warfarin or aspirin (based on discussion with patient of relatively low risk of stroke, decrease in risk with warfarin, monitoring needs, etc.)
>75		Warfarin INR 2-3 (but should be kept closer to 2.0-2.5 because of increased risk of hemorrhage in this age group)

INR, International Normalized Ratio.

- Studies have shown no difference between paroxysmal and chronic atrial fibrillation in stroke rate risk.

Supraventricular Tachycardia

Paroxysmal supraventricular tachycardia (PSVT) refers to cardiac arrhythmias of supraventricular origin using a reentrant mechanism with an abrupt onset and termination, a regular RR interval, and a narrow QRS complex, unless there is a rate-related or preexisting bundle branch block (Fig. 3-20). In patients with a normal QRS during sinus rhythm (lack of preexcitation), PSVT is due to reentry within the AV node in 60%, reentry using a concealed accessory pathway in 30%, and reentry in the sinus node or atrium in the remaining 10% (Fig. 3-21). Episodes usually respond to vagal maneuvers; if these fail, intravenously administered adenosine or verapamil terminates the arrhythmia in 90% of patients.

- PSVT is arrhythmia with an abrupt onset and termination.
- Acutely, PSVT usually responds to vagal maneuvers; if not, adenosine or verapamil terminates the arrhythmia in 90% of patients.

PSVT generally is not a life-threatening arrhythmia and only occasionally is associated with near-syncope or syncope. The rhythm is more serious when it is associated with significant heart disease, and cardiac decompensation results with the sudden increase in heart rate. This can occur in patients with congenital heart disease, cardiomyopathy, or ischemic heart disease. Patients with AV nodal reentrant tachycardia usually have simultaneous activation of the atrium and ventricle, in which case the atria contract against closed tricuspid and mitral valves (similar to pacemaker syndrome) and produce symptoms associated with atrial distention, including a fullness in the neck, hypotension, and polyuria. Hypotension and polyuria are due partly to the release of atrial natriuretic peptide.

- PSVT generally is not a life-threatening arrhythmia; it is often seen in an otherwise normal heart.
- PSVT is more serious when associated with heart disease.

Chronically, PSVT responds to most antiarrhythmic drugs, including drugs that suppress AV nodal conduction (digoxin, β-adrenergic blocker, and calcium antagonist), assuming that part of the reentrant circuit uses the AV node, and to drugs that slow conduction within the reentrant circuit, including class IA (quinidine, procainamide, disopyramide), IC (propafenone, flecainide), and III (amiodarone, sotalol) antiarrhythmic drugs.

Most forms of PSVT can be "cured" permanently with catheter ablation, with success rates greater than 90%. For young patients in whom β-blocker or calcium channel blocker therapy fails or who choose not to take them, catheter ablation is usually preferred over class I or class III antiarrhythmic drugs. For patients with PSVT and hypertension that require treatment, the best treatment is with β-blockers or calcium channel blockers, which might treat both conditions.

- PSVT responds to most antiarrhythmic drugs chronically.
- PSVT usually can be "cured" permanently with catheter ablation.

Multifocal atrial tachycardia is an automatic atrial rhythm diagnosed when three or more distinct atrial foci (P waves of different morphology) are present and the rate exceeds 100 beats/min (Fig. 3-22). The rhythm occurs primarily in patients with decompensated lung disease with associated hypoxia, increased catecholamines (exogenous and endogenous), atrial stretch, and local tissue acid-base and electrolyte disturbances. This rhythm is made worse by digoxin, which shortens atrial refractoriness, but does respond to improved oxygenation and slow channel blockade with verapamil or diltiazem.

- Digoxin worsens multifocal atrial tachycardia.
- Multifocal atrial tachycardia is best treated by correction of the underlying medical illnesses and calcium channel blockers.

Distinguishing Supraventricular Tachycardia With Aberrancy From Ventricular Tachycardia

A wide QRS tachycardia may be due to supraventricular tachycardia with aberrancy or to ventricular tachycardia. Useful findings to identify ventricular tachycardia are listed in Table 3-16.

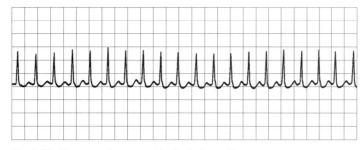

Fig. 3-20. Paroxysmal supraventricular tachycardia.

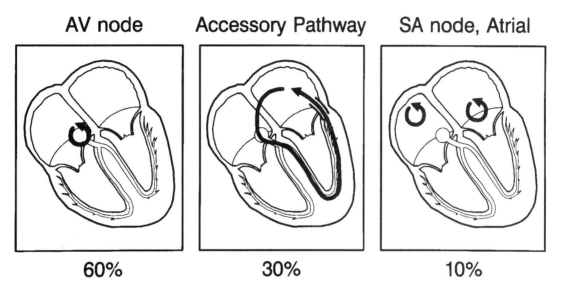

Fig. 3-21. Mechanisms of paroxysmal supraventricular tachycardia in patients with a normal ECG during sinus rhythm. AV, atrioventricular; SA, sinoatrial.

Approximately 85% of wide QRS tachycardias are ventricular in origin and are often well tolerated. The absence of hemodynamic compromise during tachycardia is not a clue that the tachycardia is supraventricular in origin. In patients with a wide QRS tachycardia and a history of ischemic heart disease (angina, myocardial infarction, Q wave on ECG), the tachycardia is ventricular in origin in 90% to 95%. Therefore, most wide QRS complex tachycardias are ventricular tachycardia (Fig. 3-23).

● About 85% of wide QRS tachycardias are ventricular in origin.
● In patients with wide QRS tachycardia and ischemic heart disease, tachycardia is ventricular in origin in 90%-95%.

Avoid intravenous administration of verapamil in patients with a wide QRS tachycardia unless the tachycardia is supraventricular in origin. Most patients with a wide QRS tachycardia have ventricular tachycardia, and verapamil causes hemodynamic deterioration that requires cardioversion in more than

half of the patients. The use of verapamil results in peripheral vasodilatation, further increase in catecholamines, and decreased cardiac contractility, all of which contribute to adverse hemodynamics.

● Avoid intravenously administered verapamil for wide QRS tachycardia.
● Verapamil causes hemodynamic deterioration requiring cardioversion in ventricular tachycardia.

Wolff-Parkinson-White Syndrome

This abnormality is defined as 1) symptomatic tachycardia, 2) a short PR interval (<0.12 second), 3) a delta wave, and 4) a prolonged QRS interval (>0.12 second).

In Wolff-Parkinson-White syndrome, normal activation of the ventricle is a fusion complex. Part of the activation is due to conduction over the accessory pathway, and the remaining activation is due to conduction through the normal His-Purkinje conduction system. Not all patients with preexcitation have a short PR interval. Normal PR conduction may occur if the

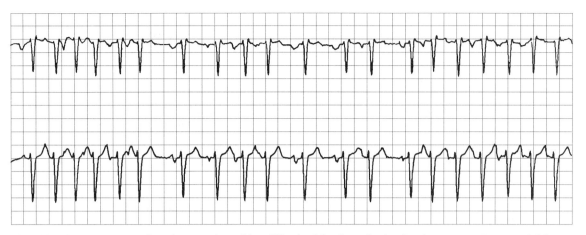

Fig. 3-22. Simultaneous recordings from a patient with multifocal atrial tachycardia showing three or more P waves of different morphology. (*Lower panel,* From MKSAP IX: Part C Book 1, 1992. American College of Physicians. By permission.)

accessory pathway is far removed from the AV node. In patients with a far left lateral accessory pathway, the heart is activated through the AV node before atrial activation reaches the accessory pathway. Thus, the PR interval may be normal before the onset of the delta wave.

Ventricular activation is abnormal in patients with Wolff-Parkinson-White syndrome. Infarction, ventricular hypertrophy, and ST-T wave changes should not be interpreted after the diagnosis is established, because these changes are usually due to the abnormal pattern of ventricular activation.

- In Wolff-Parkinson-White syndrome, the PR interval may be normal before the onset of the delta wave.
- Ventricular activation is abnormal in Wolff-Parkinson-White syndrome.

Preexcitation occurs in about 2 of 1,000 patients; tachycardia subsequently develops in 70%. Of patients with tachycardia, 70% have PSVT and 30% have atrial fibrillation. The atrial fibrillation often occurs after a short episode of PSVT.

Table 3-16.—Findings That Identify Ventricular Tachycardia

Evidence of AV dissociation with P waves "marching through" the QRS complexes
A QRS width >0.14 second if the tachycardia has a right bundle branch block pattern and >0.16 second if the tachycardia has a left bundle branch block pattern
Northwest axis (axis between -90° and -180°)
A different QRS morphology in patients with a preexisting bundle branch block
A history of structural heart disease

AV, atrioventricular.

Elimination of PSVT after surgery or catheter ablation generally eliminates problems with atrial fibrillation. The most serious rhythm disturbance is the onset of atrial fibrillation with rapid ventricular conduction over the accessory pathway resulting in ventricular fibrillation (Fig. 3-24). Most asymptomatic patients do not benefit from risk stratification with electrophysiologic testing, including induction of atrial fibrillation, unless they have a high-risk occupation. Patients who are asymptomatic have a negligible chance of sudden death, and in patients who are symptomatic, the incidence of sudden death is 0.0025 per patient-year.

- Preexcitation occurs in 2 of 1,000 patients; tachycardia develops in 70%.
- Of patients with tachycardia, 70% have PSVT and 30% have atrial fibrillation.
- Asymptomatic patients have a negligible chance of sudden death.
- In symptomatic patients, the incidence of sudden death is 0.0025 per patient-year.

Patients with Wolff-Parkinson-White syndrome may have either 1) a manifest accessory pathway resulting in preexcitation on the ECG (Fig. 3-25) due to antegrade conduction over the accessory pathway or 2) a concealed accessory pathway that is capable of conducting only in the retrograde direction, and, therefore, the surface ECG in sinus rhythm is normal. Both manifest and concealed accessory pathways have the same mechanism of reentrant tachycardia, in which antegrade conduction over the normal conduction system results in a normal QRS complex (unless there is rate-related bundle branch block) and conduction continues through the ventricle, returns retrogradely over the accessory pathway, and continues through the atrium to complete the reentrant circuit, termed "orthodromic

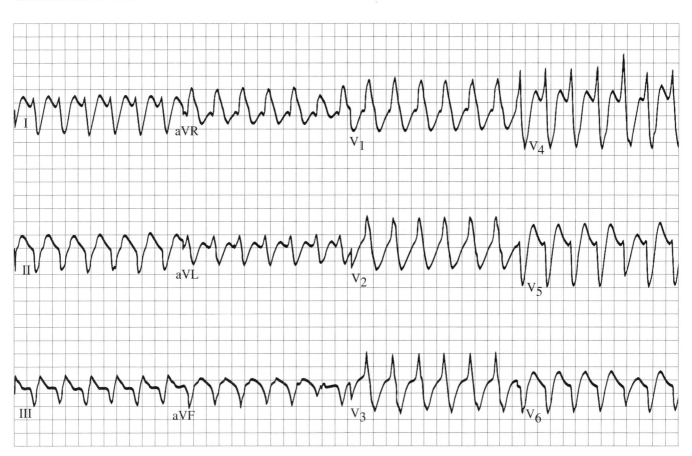

Fig. 3-23. Ventricular tachycardia with a wide QRS complex, northwest axis, and fusion complexes in a patient with normal blood pressure.

AV reentry" (Fig. 3-26). Five percent of patients may have reentrant tachycardia that goes in the reverse direction (antidromic AV reentry), in which ventricular activation over the accessory pathway activates the ventricle from an ectopic location; the result is a wide QRS complex tachycardia that is often confused with ventricular tachycardia (Fig. 3-27).

Electrophysiologic testing should be performed in patients with *symptomatic* Wolff-Parkinson-White syndrome. This testing identifies the pathway location, confirms that the pathway is an integral part of the reentrant circuit and not an innocent bystander (i.e., the arrhythmia is AV nodal reentry), and evaluates for a second accessory pathway that occurs in approximately 15% of patients.

Atrial Fibrillation in Wolff-Parkinson-White Syndrome

Atrial fibrillation in Wolff-Parkinson-White syndrome is of special interest because it can be life-threatening and requires therapy that is different from the usual treatment for atrial fibrillation. Patients with Wolff-Parkinson-White syndrome have an accessory pathway that can conduct electrical activity from the atrium to the ventricle, bypassing the AV node. Because the accessory pathway does not slow conduction in the same manner as the AV node, the ventricular response to atrial fib-

rillation can be extraordinarily and dangerously rapid. Also, wide, irregular, and rapid ventricular complexes are seen because activation down the accessory pathway does not use the normal His-Purkinje system (Fig. 3-24). The use of agents such as calcium channel blockers, β-blockers, or digoxin can result in an even more rapid ventricular response due to blocking of conduction down the AV node (which can limit concealed conduction into the pathway). Therefore, the agent of first choice is procainamide, which slows accessory pathway and intra-atrial conduction. Should a patient with Wolff-Parkinson-White syndrome and atrial fibrillation become hypotensive, cardioversion should be performed.

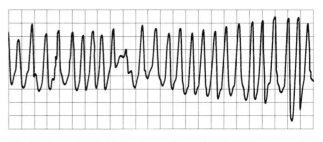

Fig. 3-24. Atrial fibrillation in a patient with Wolff-Parkinson-White syndrome shows wide QRS complex and irregular RR intervals.

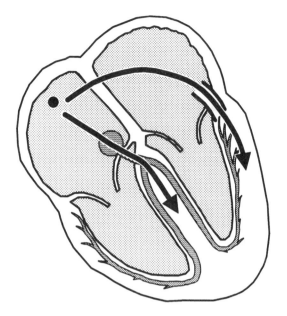

Fig. 3-25. Conduction of sinus impulse in Wolff-Parkinson-White syndrome. Ventricles are activated over the normal atrioventricular node–His-Purkinje system and accessory pathway; the result is a fusion complex (QRS and delta wave).

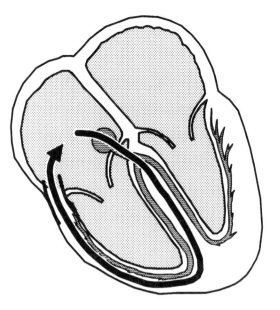

Fig. 3-26. Typical mechanism of supraventricular tachycardia in patients with Wolff-Parkinson-White syndrome; the result is a narrow QRS complex because ventricular activation is over the normal conduction system.

- Atrial fibrillation in Wolff-Parkinson-White syndrome should not be treated with digoxin, adenosine, β-blockers, or calcium channel blockers.
- In atrial fibrillation in Wolff-Parkinson-White syndrome, procainamide can be used to slow the ventricular rate (by slowing atrial and accessory pathway conduction) and to restore sinus rhythm.
- If the heart rate is rapid and there is hemodynamic compromise, perform cardioversion.

PSVT in patients with an accessory pathway often ends with vagal maneuvers or intravenously administered adenosine or verapamil. Additional episodes can be prevented with a β-adrenergic blocker, a calcium antagonist, and class IA (quinidine, procainamide, disopyramide), class IC (propafenone, flecainide), and class III (amiodarone, sotalol) antiarrhythmic drugs. Radio-frequency ablation is used to ablate the accessory pathway and to cure the tachycardia, thus eliminating the need for medical therapy.

- Additional PSVT is prevented with a β-adrenergic blocker, a calcium antagonist, and class IA, IC, and III antiarrhythmic drugs.
- Radio-frequency ablation is used to cure tachycardia and should be strongly considered for symptomatic patients.

Tachycardia-Mediated Cardiomyopathy

Supraventricular tachycardia, atrial fibrillation with a rapid ventricular rate, and ventricular tachycardia have been associated with cardiomyopathy. Treatment of the tachycardia has allowed cardiac performance to return to near normal. When patients present with heart failure and tachycardia is identified, determine whether the heart failure is causing the tachycardia or the tachycardia has caused the heart failure. Control of ventricular rate often improves ventricular function. In a patient with heart failure who has a rhythm with an abnormal P-wave axis, tachycardia-mediated cardiomyopathy should be suspected.

Ventricular Ectopy and Nonsustained Ventricular Tachycardia

Management of frequent ventricular ectopy and nonsustained ventricular tachycardia is predicated upon the underlying cardiac lesion. In patients with structurally normal hearts, the long-term prognosis is excellent and no specific therapy is warranted in the absence of symptoms. If symptoms are present, management includes reassurance, β-blockers or calcium channel blockers for disturbing symptoms, and, in rare cases of frequent monomorphic symptomatic ventricular ectopy, catheter ablation.

In patients with previous myocardial infarction, depressed ventricular function (ejection fraction ≤35%), and nonsustained ventricular tachycardia, electrophysiologic study can risk stratify, even in the absence of symptoms. In this population, if inducible tachycardia refractory to procainamide is present, mortality is decreased with the implantation of a defibrillator.

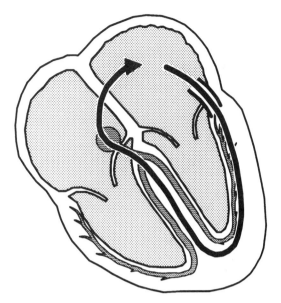

Fig. 3-27. Unusual mechanism of supraventricular tachycardia in patients with Wolff-Parkinson-White syndrome; the result is a wide QRS complex because ventricular activation is over an accessory pathway. This arrhythmia is difficult to distinguish from ventricular tachycardia.

The management of patients with dilated cardiomyopathy is not well defined, although amiodarone may be appropriate in some settings (it has been shown to decrease mortality in this population).

- Patients with a structurally normal heart and complex ectopy or nonsustained ventricular tachycardia have an excellent prognosis; management includes reassurance or, if bothersome symptoms persist, calcium channel bockers or β-blockers.
- Patients with depressed ventricular function and nonsustained ventricular tachycardia are at increased risk for sudden cardiac death; patients with previous myocardial infarction can be risk stratified with electrophysiologic study.

Ventricular Tachycardia and Fibrillation

Patients who present with ventricular tachycardia or fibrillation or who survive sudden cardiac death (out of hospital cardiac arrest who were successfully resuscitated) have lethal ventricular arrhythmias and a significant risk of recurrence. Survivors of sudden cardiac death have a risk of death approaching 30% in the first year after hospital dismissal. They should receive electrophysiologic-guided therapy, which improves outcome. For about 40% of patients, an antiarrhythmic drug is identified that prevents induction of ventricular tachycardia or fibrillation, and these patients have approximately a 5% chance of death at 1 year if dismissed with that medication. Patients in whom the baseline electrophysiologic study is negative or an

antiarrhythmic drug cannot be identified to prevent tachycardia continue to have an increased risk of sudden death and should be considered for antitachycardia surgery or an implantable cardioverter defibrillator. This device has reduced the recurrence rate of sudden death to 2% at 1 year and to 4% at 4 years; the overall mortality rate is 10% at 1 year and 20% at 4 years.

- Patients with ventricular tachycardia or fibrillation who survive sudden cardiac death have a significant risk of recurrence.
- Survivors of sudden cardiac death have a risk of death of 30% at 1 year after hospital dismissal.
- Electrophysiologic-guided therapy improves outcome.
- For 40% of patients, an effective antiarrhythmic drug can be identified.

Torsades de Pointes

This is a form of ventricular tachycardia with a characteristic polymorphic morphology described as a "twisting of the points" (torsades de pointes) (Fig. 3-10). The QT interval is prolonged, and the tachycardia is initiated by a late-coupled PVC. The arrhythmia is usually due to a medication (quinidine, procainamide, disopyramide, sotalol, tricyclic antidepressants), electrolyte disturbance (hypokalemia), or bradycardia (especially after myocardial infarction). After the tachycardia has been converted to sinus rhythm (electrically or spontaneously), treatment should be aimed at shortening the QT interval until the offending drug can be metabolized or the electrolyte disturbance or bradycardia corrected. Treatment options include temporary overdrive pacing, isoproterenol infusion, or magnesium. Patients with QT prolongation in the absence of medications, electrolytes, or bradycardia have a congenital form of this problem and are usually treated with a β-adrenergic blocker.

- Torsades de pointes is a form of ventricular tachycardia involving a prolonged QT interval.
- Torsades de pointes is usually due to a medication, an electrolyte disturbance, or bradycardia.
- Treatment includes temporary overdrive pacing, isoproterenol, or magnesium.

Ventricular Arrhythmias During Acute Myocardial Infarction

Prevention of myocardial ischemia and the use of β-adrenergic blockers are essential during and after acute myocardial infarction to decrease the frequency of life-threatening ventricular arrhythmias. Asymptomatic complex ventricular ectopy, including nonsustained ventricular tachycardia, should not be treated empirically in the acute phase of myocardial infarction because the risk of proarrhythmia outweighs the potential benefit of therapy for reducing the incidence of sudden cardiac death after hospital dismissal.

The results from amiodarone trials are mentioned above. The routine use of lidocaine or amiodarone in suppressing ventricular arrhythmias in the acute phase of myocardial infarction is not recommended.

Ventricular tachycardia and fibrillation occurring within 24 hours after myocardial infarction are independent risk factors for in-hospital mortality at the time of the acute myocardial infarction but are not risk factors for subsequent total mortality or mortality due to an arrhythmic event after hospital dismissal and do not require antiarrhythmic therapy.

Ventricular tachycardia and fibrillation occurring 24 hours or longer after an acute myocardial infarction in the absence of reinfarction are independent risk factors for increased total mortality and death due to an arrhythmic event after hospital dismissal. Patients should be assessed with electrophysiologic testing, and the treatment option is usually an implantable cardioverter defibrillator.

Episodes of refractory ventricular tachycardia and fibrillation during acute myocardial infarction should be treated with intravenously administered lidocaine, procainamide, bretylium, or amiodarone and patients should have adequate oxygenation and normal electrolyte values. Recent data suggest that amiodarone may be a reasonable choice if lidocaine fails to control arrhythmia. If these drugs are ineffective, alternative therapies to prevent recurrences of tachycardia include overdrive pacing if the tachycardia follows a bradycardia event, interaortic balloon pump, and coronary revascularization.

- Refractory ventricular tachycardia and fibrillation during acute myocardial infarction should be treated with intravenously administered lidocaine, procainamide, bretylium, or amiodarone.
- Alternative therapies are overdrive pacing and coronary revascularization.

Role of Pacing in Acute Myocardial Infarction

Among patients with an acute inferior myocardial infarction, 5% to 10% have Mobitz I second-degree or third-degree block in the absence of bundle branch block, and the site is usually in the AV node. This usually is transient, tends not to recur, and requires pacing only if there are symptoms as a result of bradycardia.

Bundle branch block occurs in 10% to 20% of patients with acute myocardial infarction; in half of these patients, it is present at the initial presentation, often representing preexisting conduction system disease. The appearance of a new bundle branch block is an indication for prophylactic temporary pacing.

Death in patients with myocardial infarction and bundle branch block is usually due to advanced heart failure and ventricular arrhythmias rather than to the development of complete heart block. Patients in whom transient complete heart block develops in association with a bundle branch block are at risk for recurrent complete heart block and should undergo permanent pacing. A new bundle branch block that never progresses to complete heart block is not an indication for permanent pacing.

- Death in patients with myocardial infarction and bundle branch block is due to advanced heart failure.
- New bundle branch block that never progresses to complete heart block is not an indication for permanent pacing.
- Second-degree (Mobitz II) with bilateral bundle branch block and third-degree AV block warrant pacing.

SYNCOPE

Syncope, defined as a transient loss of consciousness with spontaneous recovery, is a frequent clinical syndrome that requires medical evaluation. Its causes can be categorized as cardiovascular, noncardiovascular, and unexplained syncope, as summarized in Table 3-17. It is estimated that 30% of the cases of syncope have a cardiogenic cause (an arrhythmia),

Table 3-17.—Major Causes of Syncope

Cardiovascular	Noncardiovascular
Cardiogenic syncope	Neurologic
Structural heart disease	Metabolic
Coronary artery disease	Psychiatric
Rhythm disturbances	
Reflex syncope	
Vasovagal	
Carotid sinus hypersensitivity	
Situational	
Micturition	
Deglutition	
Defecation	
Glossopharyngeal neuralgia	
Postprandial	
Tussive	
Valsalva	
Oculovagal	
Sneeze	
Instrumentation	
Diving	
Post exercise	
Orthostatic hypotension	

From Shen W-K, Gersh BJ: Syncope: mechanisms, approach, and management. *In* Clinical Autonomic Disorders: Evaluation and Management. Edited by PA Low. Boston, Little, Brown and Company, 1993, pp 605-640. By permission of Mayo Foundation.

35% have a vasovagal cause, and 10% to 25% are related to a miscellaneous disorder such as orthostatic or situational syncope or seizures or are drug-related episodes. In 10% to 25% of cases, the cause is—and often remains—unknown.

The most important aspect of evaluation for syncope is the clinical history and physical examination. The initial history and physical examination provide the key information in 40% to 75% of the patients for whom a diagnosis is eventually established. The factors associated with increased cardiogenic causes for syncope are listed in Table 3-18. In patients with increased risk of cardiogenic syncope, electrophysiologic testing should be considered. If an arrhythmogenic cause (bradycardia or tachycardia) for syncope has been established by noninvasive tests such as ECG, Holter monitoring, or transtelephonic monitoring, electrophysiologic testing is not indicated unless other arrhythmias are suspected. In patients at low risk for cardiogenic syncope, a noninvasive approach should be considered.

Tilt table testing is effective in eliciting a vasovagal response. For diagnostic purposes, tilt table testing is indicated in patients with recurrent syncope without evidence of structural cardiac disease or in those with structural heart disease but after other causes of syncope have been excluded by appropriate testing. Tilt table testing generally is not indicated for patients with a single episode of syncope without injury or in a high-risk setting with clear-cut vasovagal clinical features.

After the diagnosis of syncope has been established, the treatment usually is straightforward. Pacemaker therapy is appropriate for sinus node dysfunction and AV conduction disease. Various treatment options for tachyarrhythmias are discussed above. Pharmacologic therapy can be effective in selected patients with significant symptomatic vasovagal syncope. These therapeutic options include β-blockers, anticholinergic drugs, vasoconstrictors, increased intravascular volume, and maneuvers to prevent venous pooling. Recent reports suggest that serotonin reuptake blockers may be effective in a subgroup of patients. Pacemaker therapy can be effective in preventing syncope in patients with a predominant cardioinhibitory subtype of vasovagal syncope and may be effective in patients with very frequent recurrent vasovagal syncope.

Table 3-18.—Risk Stratification in Patients With Unexplained Syncope

High-risk factors	Low-risk factors
Coronary artery disease, previous myocardial infarction	Isolated syncope without underlying cardiovascular disease
Structural heart disease	Younger age
Left ventricular dysfunction	Symptoms consistent with a vasovagal cause
Congestive heart failure	Normal ECG
Older age	
Abrupt onset	
Serious injuries	
Abnormal ECG (presence of Q wave, bundle branch block, or atrial fibrillation)	

ECG, electrocardiogram.
From Shen W-K, Gersh BJ: Syncope: mechanisms, approach, and management. *In* Clinical Autonomic Disorders: Evaluation and Management. Edited by PA Low. Boston, Little, Brown and Company, 1993, pp 605-640. By permission of Mayo Foundation.

PART IV
Rick A. Nishimura, M.D.

Coronary heart disease, principally myocardial infarction, accounts for approximately one of three deaths in the U.S., or nearly 600,000 deaths annually. The substantial reductions in the death rate from acute myocardial infarction that have occurred in the last 2 decades (Fig. 3-28) are attributed to efforts in primary prevention and new interventions in the treatment of myocardial infarction. The variable presentation of myocardial infarction includes asymptomatic patients; ones with angina, silent ischemia, unstable angina, or myocardial infarction; and sudden death.

- About 1/3 of the deaths annually in the U.S. are due to myocardial infarction.
- The substantial decrease in the last 2 decades in death from acute myocardial infarction is due to primary prevention and new treatments of myocardial infarction.

PREVENTION OF CORONARY HEART DISEASE

The known risk factors for coronary artery disease are tobacco abuse, serum cholesterol level, a lower serum high-density lipoprotein (HDL) cholesterol level, serum low-density lipoprotein (LDL) cholesterol level, hypertension, physical inactivity, obesity, diabetes mellitus, gender, and alcohol. Primary prevention includes modification of the following risk factors (N Engl J Med 326:1406-1416, 1992):

- Smoking more than doubles the incidence of coronary heart disease and increases mortality by 70%.
- The relative risk of smokers who have quit smoking decreases rapidly, approaching the levels of nonsmokers within 2-3 years.
- Plasma levels of total cholesterol and LDL cholesterol are important risk factors for coronary heart disease. This relationship is strongest at high levels of cholesterol.
- A 1% decrease in total serum cholesterol yields a 2%-3% decrease in the risk of coronary heart disease.
- Lowering increased plasma levels of LDL cholesterol slows progression and promotes regression of coronary atherosclerosis.
- Lowering increased plasma levels of LDL cholesterol prevents coronary events, presumably because of stabilization of lipid-laden plaques.
- The estimated decreased risk of myocardial infarction is 2%-3% for each 1-mm Hg decrease in diastolic blood pressure.
- The estimated decrease in the risk of myocardial infarction

with the maintenance of an active compared with sedentary lifestyle is 35%-55%.
- The adjusted mortality rates for coronary heart disease are two to three times higher in men with diabetes mellitus and three to seven times higher in women with diabetes mellitus.
- There are no definitive data to suggest that estrogen replacement in women prevents cardiovascular disease.
- Although heavy alcohol use increases the risk of cardiovascular disease, moderate consumption decreases the risk of heart disease.

Secondary prevention refers to efforts to prevent recurrent ischemic events in patients with known coronary artery disease. The role of antiplatelet agents, β-blockers, and angiotensin-converting enzyme (ACE) inhibitors is discussed below. Aggressive treatment of cholesterol levels is of value. The co-A reductase inhibitors reduce events after myocardial infarction to a greater degree than would be expected from their effect on atherosclerosis progression alone. This may be related to stabilization of lipid-rich plaques, which are prone to rupture.

In patients who have had a myocardial infarction and have increased levels of cholesterol (>220 mg/dL), treatment with a "statin" decreases overall mortality by 30% and disease mortality from coronary events by 42%.

In patients who have had a myocardial infarction and have "average" levels of cholesterol (cholesterol, <240; LDL, >125), treatment with a "statin" reduces the chance of fatal heart disease or recurrent myocardial infarction by 24%.

Current indications for instituting cholesterol-lowering therapy are as follows:

- Known coronary artery disease: LDL >100.
- Risk factors for coronary artery disease: LDL >130.
- Others: LDL >160.

MECHANISM OF ATHEROSCLEROSIS

The "response to injury" hypothesis is the most prevalent explanation of atherosclerosis (N Engl J Med 326:242-250, 1992). According to this hypothesis, chronic minimal injury to the arterial endothelium is caused mainly by a disturbance in the pattern of blood flow (type I injury), potentiated by high cholesterol levels, infections, and tobacco smoke. Type I injury leads to the accumulation of lipids and macrophages. The release of toxic products by macrophages produces type II injury, which is characterized by the adhesion of platelets. Macrophages and platelets with endothelial-release growth

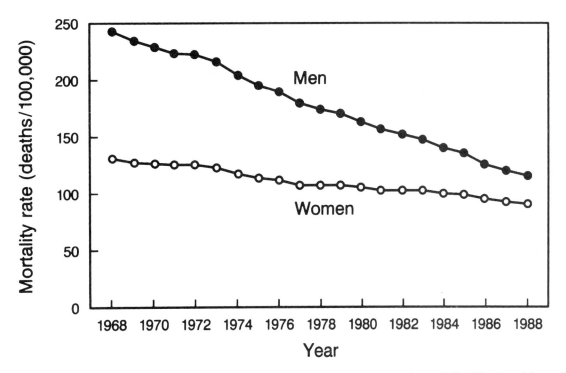

Fig. 3-28. Annual mortality rates from acute myocardial infarction among men and women in the United States, 1968-1988. (From Manson JE, Tosteson H, Ridker PM, Satterfield S, Hebert P, O'Connor GT, Buring JE, Hennekens CH: The primary prevention of myocardial infarction. N Engl J Med 326:1406-1416, 1992. By permission of the journal.)

factors cause migration and proliferation of smooth muscle cells, which form a fibrointimal lesion or lipid lesion. Disruption of a lipid lesion with a thin capsule causes type III damage, with thrombus formation. The thrombus may organize and contribute to the growth of the atherosclerotic lesion or become totally occluded, culminating in unstable angina or myocardial infarction (Fig. 3-29).

- The most prevalent explanation for atherosclerosis is the "response to injury" hypothesis.
- Type II injury is characterized by the adhesion of platelets.
- Type III damage is disruption of a lipid lesion leading to thrombus formation.
- Lipid-laden coronary artery lesions with less severe angiographic stenosis are more prone to rapid progression due to atherosclerotic plaque disruption.
- In up to two-thirds of cases of unstable angina or myocardial infarction, the lesion is a vessel with <50% stenosis.

CHRONIC STABLE ANGINA

Pathophysiology

In chronic stable angina, myocardial ischemia is caused chiefly by increased myocardial oxygen demand of the heart. Less important factors are perfusion pressure (aortic-to-right-atrial gradient), autoregulation (maintenance of coronary blood flow through a physiologic range of perfusion pressures), autonomic tone, and compressive effect (high left ventricular end-diastolic pressure decreases subendocardial flow). Normally, coronary blood flow can increase up to five times to meet myocardial oxygen demands of the heart. Ischemia occurs when flow reserve is inadequate, usually the result of fixed coronary artery disease. Resting blood flow does not cause ischemia unless vessel stenosis is greater than 95%. However, a decrease in flow reserve begins to occur with about 60% stenosis, which is the mechanism for ischemia with exercise. The four factors that determine myocardial oxygen consumption are heart rate, afterload, contractility, and wall tension [wall tension = (left ventricular radius) x (left ventricular pressure)]. With a dilated, poorly contractile left ventricle, the contribution of wall tension to myocardial oxygen consumption outweighs the other factors. The temporal sequence of events includes ischemia → diastolic dysfunction → regional wall motion abnormalities → electrocardiographic changes → pain.

- In chronic stable angina, myocardial ischemia is caused by increased myocardial oxygen demand.
- Normally, coronary blood flow can increase up to five times to meet myocardial oxygen demands.
- Resting blood flow does not cause ischemia unless stenosis is >95%.

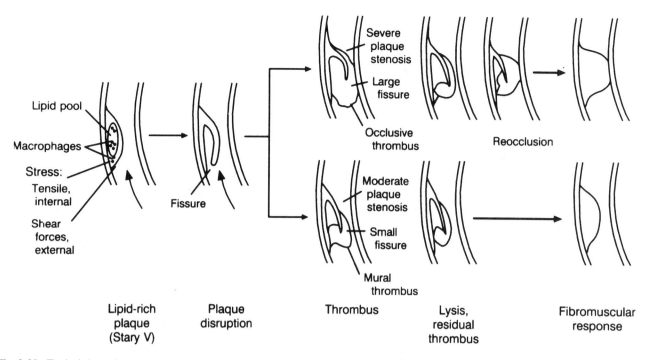

Fig. 3-29. Typical dynamic evolution of complicated disrupted plaque. Curved arrows indicate direction of blood flow. (From Fuster V, Badimon L, Badimon JJ, Chesebro JH: The pathogenesis of coronary artery disease and the acute coronary syndromes [First of two parts]. N Engl J Med 326:242-250, 1992. By permission of the journal.)

- Four factors of myocardial oxygen consumption: heart rate, afterload, contractility, and wall tension.
- The temporal sequence of events: ischemia → diastolic dysfunction → regional wall motion abnormalities → electrocardiographic changes → pain.

Symptomatic Chronic Coronary Artery Disease

Many patients have symptoms of angina pectoris during physical activity. The pain is described variously as "pressure," "burning," "stabbing," "ache," "hurt," or "shortness of breath." It can be substernal or epigastric and can radiate to the neck, jaw, shoulder, elbow, or wrist. In chronic stable angina, the pain lasts 2 to 30 minutes and is usually relieved by rest. It is generally precipitated by any activity that increases myocardial oxygen consumption. The physical signs occurring with the pain include onset of a fourth heart sound and mitral regurgitant murmur due to papillary muscle dysfunction. ST-segment depression may be found on the electrocardiogram (ECG), indicating subendocardial ischemia. The double product [(heart rate) x (systolic blood pressure)] is useful for defining myocardial oxygen demand. Nocturnal angina can be caused by unstable angina and also by increased wall tension with left ventricular dysfunction.

- The pain of angina pectoris during physical exercise is described in various ways.

- Physical signs occurring with the pain are a fourth heart sound and mitral regurgitant murmur due to papillary muscle dysfunction.
- The double product [(heart rate) x (systolic blood pressure)] is useful for defining myocardial oxygen demand.

Silent Ischemia

Silent ischemia is common in patients with symptomatic stable coronary artery disease, unstable angina, or after myocardial infarction. It is diagnosed by the presence of ST-segment depression in the absence of symptoms. Silent ischemia can occur either with an increase in myocardial oxygen consumption or at rest. The treatment is similar to that for chronic unstable angina; nitrates and β-blockers are effective agents. Whether percutaneous transluminal coronary angioplasty or coronary artery bypass grafting should be performed for silent ischemia alone is debated. The prognosis for this condition is the same as for symptomatic ischemia.

- Silent ischemia is common in patients with symptomatic stable coronary artery disease, unstable angina, or after myocardial infarction.
- Silent ischemia is diagnosed by the presence of ST-segment depression in the absence of symptoms.
- Treatment is similar to that for chronic unstable angina.

- Nitrates and β-blockers are effective therapeutic agents in silent ischemia.
- Whether coronary angioplasty or bypass grafting should be performed for silent ischemia is debated.
- The prognosis is the same for silent ischemia and symptomatic ischemia.

Ancillary Testing

Ancillary tests for coronary artery disease include measurement of left ventricular function, stress testing, and coronary angiography. Left ventricular function is the most important predictor of prognosis and should be measured in all patients by two-dimensional echocardiography, radionuclide angiography, or left ventricular angiography. Exercise testing is performed with the treadmill or bicycle exertion test in conjunction with ECG monitoring, thallium or technetium-sestamibi scanning (perfusion of myocardium), radionuclide angiography (left ventricular function), or echocardiography (left ventricular function) to check for ischemia. During a standard treadmill test (i.e., exercise with stepped increases in workload every 2-3 minutes), heart rate, blood pressure, and the onset of subjective symptoms are monitored. Continuous monitoring of cardiac rhythm and 12-lead ECG at 1-minute intervals are performed. The ECG is positive for ischemia if a flat ST-segment depression is 1 mm or greater. The ECG response is uninterpretable on the treadmill exertion test when there are resting T-wave abnormalities, left bundle branch block, left ventricular hypertrophy, paced rhythm, digoxin therapy, or mitral valve prolapse. For interpreting the results of this test, Bayes theorem is important. According to this theorem, the predictive value of a test depends on the prevalence of the disease in the population studied.

- The most important predictor of prognosis is left ventricular function.
- The ECG is positive for ischemia if there is a flat ST-segment depression ≥1 mm.
- T-wave abnormalities, left bundle branch block, left ventricular hypertrophy, paced rhythm, digoxin therapy, or mitral valve prolapse makes the ECG response to the treadmill exertion test uninterpretable.
- Bayes theorem—the predictive value of a test depends on the prevalence of the disease in the population studied.

The sensitivity and specificity of ECG treadmill exertion testing are about 70% and 75%, respectively. Thus, a young patient with atypical chest pain and no risk factors (A in Fig. 3-30) has a low pretest probability (5%) of coronary artery disease. If the test results are negative, the probability decreases to 3%. However, if the results are positive, the probability is less than 15%. In comparison, an older man (B in Fig. 3-30) with typical chest pain and multiple risk factors has a high pretest probability (90%) of coronary artery disease, and even with negative test results, the probability is higher than 70%. The treadmill exertion test should not be used to make the *diagnosis* of coronary artery disease.

Several different types of cardiac imaging modalities add to the sensitivity and specificity of ECG treadmill exertion testing. In thallium imaging, thallium-201 injected at peak exercise labels areas of perfusion; "cold spots" are nonperfused regions. Scanning is repeated 3 to 24 hours later. Persistent cold spots indicate previous infarction, and reperfused areas indicate ischemia. Single photon emission computed tomography (SPECT) thallium scanning (use of multiple tomographic planes) is more accurate than planar thallium scanning. In patients with left bundle branch block and severe left ventricular hypertrophy, thallium scanning gives false-positive results during exercise stress.

Sestamibi scanning uses an isotope with a half-life different from that of thallium. Also, because this isotope is more powerful than thallium, it is routinely used in women and obese patients to avoid artifact. However, the results are interpreted in the same way as those of thallium scanning, with "cold" spots indicating lack of perfusion.

In radionuclide angiography (multiple-gated acquisition scanning, MUGA), erythrocytes are labeled with technetium-99m and the left ventricular cavity is imaged during the cardiac cycle to measure, at rest and at peak exercise, left ventricular volume, ejection fraction, and regional wall motion

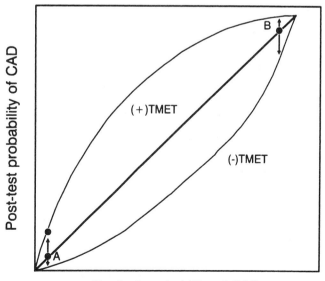

Fig. 3-30. The effect of Bayes theorem on the ability of treadmill exertion testing (TMET) to diagnose coronary artery disease (CAD). Representative patients A and B are described in the text.

abnormalities.   MUGA is positive if the ejection fraction decreases and/or new regional wall motion abnormalities appear. Because multiple cycles are gated, MUGA cannot be used with irregular rhythms. In exercise echocardiography, two-dimensional echocardiography is performed at rest and at peak exercise. Digital acquisition allows side-by-side comparisons of images from the same view. The test is positive for ischemia if global systolic function decreases and/or new regional wall motion abnormalities appear.

- The sensitivity and specificity of ECG treadmill exertion testing are about 70% and 75%, respectively.
- The treadmill exertion test should not be used to make the diagnosis of coronary artery disease.
- Thallium or sestamibi scanning gives false-positive results during exercise in patients with left bundle branch block and severe left ventricular hypertrophy.
- MUGA is positive if the ejection fraction decreases and/or new regional wall motion abnormalities appear.
- Two-dimensional echocardiography is positive for ischemia if global systolic function decreases and/or new regional wall motion abnormalities appear.

All these imaging modalities are more expensive than the ECG treadmill exertion test. Because Bayes theorem applies, imaging modalities should not be used for diagnosis of coronary artery disease over ECG treadmill testing except in cases of an uninterpretable ECG, or false-positive ECG results, or for localizing specific regions of ischemia (for future revascularization procedures).

Pharmacologic stress tests that provoke ischemia have been developed for patients who cannot exercise. These tests include the use of dipyridamole thallium, which redistributes flow away from ischemic myocardium. Adenosine thallium works in the same way as dipyridamole. In dobutamine echocardiography, the myocardial oxygen demand is increased. Pacing echocardiography increases heart rate.

Treadmill exertion testing identifies high-risk patients. High-risk patients are identified if the following are obtained on testing: less than stage I of the Bruce protocol, heart rate of less than 120 beats/min, ST-segment depression greater than 2 mm, ST-segment depression greater than 6 minutes' duration after stopping, decreased blood pressure, multiple perfusion defects, and a decrease in ejection fraction greater than 20%. In patients with poor prognostic factors, it is reasonable to proceed with coronary angiography to define the anatomy of the coronary arteries and the need for intervention. However, in patients who achieve a good work load without significant ST-segment depression and have appropriate blood pressure and heart rate responses, medical management may be indicated because of the excellent prognosis.

- The major usefulness of stress testing is to identify high-risk patients, not to diagnose coronary artery disease.
- The treadmill exertion test should not be performed on patients with either unstable angina or severe aortic stenosis.

Coronary Angiography

Although coronary angiography has many limitations, it is the standard method for defining the severity and extent of coronary artery disease. Subjective visual estimation of the percentage of stenosis may grossly underestimate the severity of the disease, especially if it is diffuse, because angiography outlines only the vessel lumen. The risk of serious complications of coronary angiography is less than 1%; they include vascular complications (1.0%), myocardial infarction (0.5%), stroke (0.5%), ventricular fibrillation (0.5%), and death (0.1%). Risk is greater in older patients or in those with severe left ventricular dysfunction, left main coronary artery disease, or other coexistent medical diseases.

- Coronary angiography is the standard method for defining the severity of coronary artery disease.
- Visual estimation of the percentage of stenosis may grossly underestimate disease severity.
- The risk of serious complications in coronary angiography is <1%.

Medical Therapy

The medical treatment for chronic stable angina should be given in a step-wise manner according to symptoms. Sublingual nitroglycerin should be given as needed. Long-acting nitrates should be added sequentially if symptoms continue. A first-line drug should be increased to the optimal dosage before a second or third drug is added. Nitrates relieve angina mainly by producing venodilatation, which decreases wall tension. β-Blockers are the most effective drugs for patients with coronary artery disease and should be the first-line drug of choice. β-Blockers relieve angina mainly by decreasing heart rate, reducing contractility, and decreasing (long-term) blood pressure (renin effect). β-Blockers are the most effective drugs for reducing the double product (heart rate x blood pressure) with exercise. β-Blockers may improve survival in some patients with known coronary artery disease, particularly those with depressed left ventricular systolic function.

Nitrate tolerance can occur with continuous exposure (use nitrate-free interval with dosing three times daily). Isosorbide dinitrate, at least 20 to 30 mg three times a day, needs to be used. β-Blockers should not be used if the patient has significant bronchospastic disease, congestive heart failure, or bradycardia. However β-blockers can and would be used in patients with left ventricular systolic dysfunction in the absence of overt heart failure. β-Blockers should be given at a dosage that keeps the resting heart rate less than 70 beats/min. Always look for treatable underlying factors contributing to ischemia (anemia, thyroid abnormalities, hypoxia). In patients with left ventricular dysfunction and nocturnal angina, diuretics and ACE inhibitors may be helpful in reducing wall tension.

Calcium channel blockers are effective in relieving angina by decreasing afterload, heart rate, and contractility; they may be used as a third-line drug (Table 3-19). However, short-acting calcium channel blockers, specifically the dihydropyridines, may increase mortality in patients with ischemic heart disease. This detrimental effect probably is not present with the longer acting calcium channel blockers in patients with normal systolic function, but the use of these agents should be avoided in patients with left ventricular systolic dysfunction. If a calcium channel blocker is required in patients with left ventricular systolic dysfunction, amlodipine should be used.

- The initial therapy for chronic stable angina is β-blockade with sublingual nitroglycerin as needed.
- Add long-acting nitrates sequentially if symptoms continue.
- Nitrates relieve angina by producing venodilatation, which decreases wall tension.
- β-Blockers relieve angina by decreasing heart rate, reducing contractility, and decreasing blood pressure.
- β-Blockers are the most effective drugs for reducing the double product.
- Nitrate tolerance can occur with continuous exposure.
- Do not use β-blockers if the patient has significant bronchospastic disease, congestive heart failure, or bradycardia.
- β-Blockers should be given at a dosage to keep the resting heart rate <70 beats/min.
- Look for treatable underlying factors contributing to ischemia.
- Diuretics and ACE inhibitors may be helpful in patients with left ventricular dysfunction and nocturnal angina.

- Short-acting calcium channel blockers should be avoided in patients with coronary artery disease.
- In patients with left ventricular dysfunction, all calcium channel blockers except amlodipine should be avoided.

Antiplatelet agents may be helpful in patients with chronic stable angina pectoris. A low dose of aspirin probably does not prevent progression of atherosclerosis, but it may prevent acute myocardial infarction in patients with known coronary artery disease. In two large primary prevention trials, aspirin produced a 33% decrease in the risk for first, nonfatal myocardial infarction in men (no convincing data exist about the use of aspirin in women). The role of aspirin in primary prevention of stroke or overall cardiovascular mortality is uncertain.

- A low dose of aspirin probably does not prevent progression of atherosclerosis but may prevent acute myocardial infarction in patients with known coronary artery disease.
- No convincing data exist about the use of aspirin in women.
- The role of aspirin in primary prevention of stroke or overall cardiovascular mortality is uncertain.

Catheter-Based Treatment

Percutaneous transluminal coronary angioplasty (PTCA) is the most common catheter-based intervention. PTCA is a combination of "splitting" the atheroma and stretching the noninvolved segment of artery. In experienced laboratories, the success rate is usually greater than 90%. However, there is a risk of emergency coronary artery bypass (1%-2%), myocardial infarction (2%-4%), and death (1%). These risks are increased in long, tubular, eccentric, and calcified lesions and also in older women. Restenosis is a major problem (30%-45% restenosis at 6 months). Antiplatelet agents given before PTCA may decrease the rate of acute closure but do not prevent restenosis. Class IIb-IIIa inhibitors may decrease acute events in high-risk patients. Other catheter-based therapies

Table 3-19.—Relative Effects of Calcium Channel Blockers

	Verapamil	Nifedipine	Diltiazem	Amlodipine
Decrease heart rate	+++	±	+	+
Decrease blood pressure	++	+++	++	++
Decrease contractility	+++	+	++	±
Side effects	Constipation	Edema	Least	Hypotension
	AV block	Hypotension		
Lowest effective dose	360 mg/day	90 mg/day	300 mg/day	10 mg/day

+, effective; ++, more effective; +++, most effective; ±, little effect.
AV, atrioventricular.

(atherectomy, Rotoblator, laser) have high restenosis rates similar to those of PTCA. These other catheter-based therapies are used in an attempt to prevent acute complications of balloon dilatation. Intracoronary stents are effective in treating acute dissections, a complication of PTCA. Stent placement will reduce the rate of restenosis compared with PTCA alone in selected patients with larger caliber vessels and good distal runoff. Thus far, no medical therapy has proved effective in preventing restenosis after PTCA or other catheter-based therapies.

- PTCA is a combination of splitting the atheroma and stretching the noninvolved segment of artery.
- The initial success rate is usually >90%.
- Restenosis is a major problem of PTCA (30%-45% restenosis at 6 months). Stents can reduce the rate of restenosis in selected patients.
- Antiplatelet agents reduce problems of acute events but do not prevent restenosis.
- No medical therapy is effective in preventing restenosis after PTCA.

Surgical Treatment

The surgical treatment for severely symptomatic patients with chronic stable angina is coronary artery bypass grafting (CABG) with either saphenous vein or internal mammary artery grafts. CABG provides excellent relief from symptoms (partial relief in >90% of patients and complete relief in >70%). In-hospital mortality after CABG varies widely from less than 1% to 30%. Mortality increases with age, poor ventricular function, female sex, left main coronary artery disease, unstable angina, and diabetes mellitus. Complications of CABG include sternal wound infection (especially in patients with diabetes mellitus), severe left ventricular dysfunction (from perioperative myocardial infarction or inadequate cardioprotection), and late constrictive pericarditis. The procedure is not without latent problems. Closure rates of saphenous vein grafts are 20% and 50% at 1 year and 5 years, respectively. The patency rate is higher for internal mammary arteries, possibly up to 90% patency at 5 years. A minithoracotomy with a left internal mammary artery-left anterior descending artery anastomosis may shorten hospitalization, but long-term follow-up is needed.

- CABG provides excellent relief from symptoms.
- CABG gives partial relief in >90% of patients and complete relief in >70%.
- In-hospital mortality after CABG varies widely from <1% to 30%.
- Mortality increases with age, poor ventricular function, female sex, left main coronary artery disease, unstable angina, and diabetes mellitus.

- Closure rates of saphenous vein grafts are 20% and 50% at 1 year and 5 years, respectively.

Several randomized trials have compared CABG with medical therapy, and the intermediate-term follow-up results are as follows:
- CABG does not prevent myocardial infarction.
- CABG does not uniformly improve left ventricular function.
- CABG does not decrease ventricular arrhythmias.
- CABG only improves survival in patients with 1) left main coronary artery disease, 2) three-vessel disease and moderately depressed left ventricular function, 3) three-vessel disease and severe symptoms of ischemia at a low workload, and 4) multivessel disease with involvement of the proximal left anterior descending artery. In all other subsets of patients, CABG should not be performed to improve survival.
- The indications for CABG versus medical therapy are 1) relief of symptoms in patients who have limiting symptoms unresponsive to medical management and 2) prolonging life in subsets of patients listed above.
- These recommendations were based on the randomized trials of CABG vs. medical therapy, which all had a small number of patients and limited use of internal mammary artery grafts. In larger meta-analyses, there was a survival benefit for CABG vs. medical therapy in all patients with three-vessel disease.

Medical Versus Catheter-Based Versus Surgical Therapy

The decision about which therapy to use for a patient with chronic, stable angina is an individual one and must be based on the patient's age, lifestyle, and personal preference. However, randomized trials have compared the medical, catheter-based, and surgical therapies, and their results help in guiding decisions on which therapy to use for a selected subset of patients. The following summarizes the results of these trials.

1. Medical therapy versus PTCA (one-vessel disease):
- PTCA has a similar or higher incidence of myocardial infarction and emergency CABG.
- PTCA does not decrease the future risk of myocardial infarction.
- PTCA does not improve resting left ventricular function.
- PTCA does not increase survival.

2. PTCA versus surgical therapy (multivessel disease—excluding left main coronary artery disease and totally occluded vessels):
- The rates of procedure-related mortality are similar (1%-2%).

- There are more procedure-related Q-wave infarctions with CABG than with PTCA (4.6% vs. 2.1%), but events are well tolerated.
- The duration of initial hospitalization is longer for CABG than for PTCA.
- The overall incidences of death or myocardial infarction are similar at 5-year follow-up (85%-90% free of death and 80% free of myocardial infarction).
- Patients undergoing CABG have less angina, require less antianginal medication, and are less likely to need a repeat revascularization procedure than those undergoing PTCA (8% vs. 54% at 5-year follow-up).
- In patients with diabetes mellitus, 5-year survival is higher with CABG than with PTCA (80% vs. 65%). Increased survival is associated with a patent left internal mammary artery-left anterior descending artery graft.

Postcardiotomy Syndrome

Postcardiotomy syndrome occurs 2 weeks to 2 years postoperatively and consists of fever, pericarditis, and increased sedimentation rate. Rarely, it can present as pericardial tamponade. It is probably an autoimmune process (associated with antimyocardial antibodies); treatment is with aspirin and nonsteroidal anti-inflammatory drugs. Postperfusion syndrome is also characterized by fever and pericarditis but is associated with increased values on liver function tests and atypical lymphocytes, presumably due to cytomegalovirus syndrome. In patients with fever and pleuritic chest pain postoperatively, measure the erythrocyte sedimentation rate and perform a special blood smear to check for postperfusion or postcardiotomy syndrome.

- Postcardiotomy syndrome occurs 2 weeks to 2 years postoperatively.
- It consists of fever, pericarditis, and increased sedimentation rate.
- It is probably an autoimmune process (associated with antimyocardial antibodies).
- Treatment—aspirin and nonsteroidal anti-inflammatory drugs.
- Postperfusion syndrome: fever, pericarditis, increased values on liver function tests, and atypical lymphocytes.
- Measure the erythrocyte sedimentation rate and perform a special blood smear in patients with fever and pleuritic chest pain postoperatively to check for postcardiotomy or postperfusion syndrome.

UNSTABLE ANGINA

The definition of unstable angina is 1) accelerating pattern of angina, 2) rest pain or prolonged episodes of pain, 3) new onset of rapidly progressive angina, or 4) nocturnal angina. The mechanism is probably plaque rupture, with platelet aggregation and subsequent thrombus formation. Coronary artery spasm may have a role. The vasomotor response of coronary arteries is regulated by endothelial-relaxing and endothelial-constricting factors, which are activated partly by platelets. The diagnosis of unstable angina is made on the basis of the medical history, ST-segment changes on ECG, and the absence of increased creatine kinase-MB fraction. It is important to diagnose unstable angina because it may be the prelude to acute myocardial infarction.

- Unstable angina is 1) accelerating pattern of angina, 2) rest pain or prolonged episodes of pain, 3) new onset of rapidly progressive angina, or 4) nocturnal angina.
- The mechanism is probably plaque rupture, with platelet aggregation and subsequent thrombus formation.
- Coronary artery vasomotor response is regulated by endothelial-relaxing and endothelial-constricting factors.
- The diagnosis is made on the basis of the medical history, ST-segment changes, and the absence of increased creatine kinase-MB fraction.

Treatment of unstable angina consists of immediate hospitalization with ECG monitoring. It is important to decrease the myocardial oxygen demand. First and foremost, unstable angina is treated with sedation (to decrease anxiety and catecholamine stimulation of the heart). β-Blockers, nitrates, and calcium channel blockers are effective in decreasing myocardial oxygen demand (see Chronic Stable Angina, page 89). Antiplatelet agents, such as aspirin, are effective in decreasing the incidence of progression to myocardial infarction and should be used in all patients. Heparin given intravenously also decreases the incidence of progression to myocardial infarction and should be used in all patients who are without any contraindication. The use of newer agents such as GP IIb/IIIa inhibitors, low molecular weight heparins, and antithrombins may help in improving outcome of patients with unstable angina.

- For unstable angina, immediate hospitalization with ECG monitoring.
- Decrease myocardial oxygen demand with β-blockers, nitrates, and calcium channel blockers.
- Antiplatelet agents are effective in decreasing the incidence of progression to myocardial infarction and should be used in all patients.
- Heparin given intravenously (or low-molecular-weight heparin given subcutaneously) should be used in all patients without any contraindication.

The work-up for unstable angina is controversial. Many cardiologists recommend coronary angiography to define coronary anatomy. Exercise testing is usually not performed.

However, this aggressive approach with angiography and PTCA or CABG has not been shown to prevent myocardial infarction or to prolong longevity in comparison with medical therapy. With medical therapy, there is a high crossover to revascularization therapy in the following 6 months.

- PTCA or CABG has not been shown to prevent myocardial infarction or to prolong longevity in patients with unstable angina but both are highly effective in relieving pain.

CORONARY ARTERY SPASM

The vasomotor tone of coronary arteries is important in the pathogenesis of coronary artery disease. Coronary artery vasoconstriction can be seen as a response to arterial injury. The endothelium affects vascular tone by releasing relaxing factors, for example, prostacyclin and endothelium-derived relaxing factor, that prevent vasoconstriction and platelet deposition. With dysfunctional endothelium, these factors are absent and the coronary arteries may be more prone to spasm. Most clinical episodes of coronary artery spasm occur superimposed on atherosclerotic plaques. However, patients may have primary coronary artery spasm and angiographically normal coronary arteries.

- Endothelium affects vascular tone by releasing relaxing factors, e.g., prostacyclin and endothelium-derived relaxing factor.
- With dysfunctional endothelium, coronary arteries may be more prone to spasm.
- Most episodes of spasm occur superimposed on atherosclerotic plaques.
- Patients may have primary coronary artery spasm and angiographically normal coronary arteries.

The typical presentation of coronary artery spasm consists of recurrent episodes of rest pain in association with ST-segment elevation, which reverses with administration of nitrates. Coronary angiography with ergonovine or methylergonovine challenge has been used to diagnose coronary artery spasm in these patients, but its sensitivity and specificity are unknown. The use of acetylcholine to provoke spasm may be useful because this directly examines the status of the endothelium. ST-segment elevation on the resting 12-lead ECG during an episode of rest pain is the standard criterion for diagnosing coronary artery spasm. Coronary artery spasm is treated with long-acting nitrates and/or calcium channel blockers.

- The typical presentation of coronary artery spasm is recurrent episodes of rest pain and ST-segment elevation that is reversed with nitrates.

- The standard criterion for diagnosis: spontaneous ST-segment elevation on resting 12-lead ECG during an episode of rest pain.

MYOCARDIAL INFARCTION

Background

Myocardial infarction accounts for a large percentage of morbidity and mortality in the U.S. in the 1990s. More than 500,000 people are admitted annually to a hospital because of myocardial infarction. However, more than 50% of people with myocardial infarction die before reaching the hospital. With the advent of coronary care units 3 decades ago, mortality from myocardial infarction was trimmed from 30% to 15% by treating ventricular arrhythmias. Beta-blockade has further decreased in-hospital and post-hospital mortality by 30% to 40%. In the late 1980s, reperfusion therapy was shown to further improve survival and has become standard care for selected patients with myocardial infarction. Currently, overall in-hospital mortality is 5% to 10%. After myocardial infarction, another 2% to 10% of patients die in the ensuing year.

- More than 50% of people with myocardial infarction die before reaching the hospital.
- By treating ventricular arrhythmias, mortality was trimmed from 30% to 15%.
- β-Blockade has reduced in-hospital and post-hospital mortality by 30%-40%.
- Thrombolytic therapy has reduced overall mortality to 5%-10%.

Pathogenesis

Acute transmural myocardial infarction is usually caused by sudden complete occlusion of a coronary artery. The mechanism of myocardial infarction is usually plaque rupture, leading to platelet aggregation and thrombus formation. Without collateral circulation, 90% of the myocardium supplied by an occluded artery is infarcted within 3 hours.

- The usual cause of acute transmural myocardial infarction is sudden complete occlusion of a coronary artery.
- The usual mechanism is plaque rupture, leading to platelet aggregation and thrombus formation.

Currently, two categories of myocardial infarction used clinically are based on the ECG. "ST-segment elevation (Q-wave) myocardial infarction" is diagnosed on the basis of chest pain with ST-segment elevation and subsequent development of Q waves. (This term replaces "transmural myocardial infarction," because not all myocardial layers are necessarily involved.) The likelihood of occlusive coronary artery thrombus at early coronary angiography is high (>85%). "Non-Q-wave myocardial infarction" is diagnosed on the basis of two of the following three criteria: 1) prolonged chest pain, 2) persistent ST-segment changes longer than 24 hours, and 3) increased creatine kinase-MB fraction. (This term replaces "subendocardial myocardial infarction.") The likelihood of an occlusive coronary artery thrombus is about 30% to 40%. In patients with non-Q-wave myocardial infarction, multivessel disease is likely because long-standing multivessel disease provides collaterals that prevent transmural injury.

- ST-segment elevation (Q-wave) myocardial infarction is diagnosed on the basis of chest pain with ST-segment elevation and subsequent Q waves.
- Q-wave myocardial infarctions are associated with larger infarctions and higher in-hospital mortality than non-Q-wave myocardial infarctions.
- Non-Q-wave myocardial infarctions have a higher risk for reinfarction, continued angina, and even post-hospital death.

Several new concepts have been developed in the past decade for examining patients with myocardial infarction. "Stunned myocardium" occurs when a coronary artery is completely occluded and then opened. If reperfusion occurs early enough, systolic contraction of the affected myocardium may remain decreased after the event, although the myocardium remains viable. Systolic contraction then returns hours to days later. Currently, no clinical test differentiates "stunned myocardium" from infarcted, dead myocardium. "Ischemia at a distance" occurs when infarction is in the distribution of one coronary vessel and ischemia with subsequent hypokinesis occurs in the distribution of a second vessel in which there is a high-grade stenosis. When this is seen on echocardiography, the prognosis is poor because of recurrent myocardial infarction and increased mortality. "Infarct remodeling" occurs mainly after large anteroapical myocardial infarctions. An area of infarction may undergo thinning, dilatation, and dyskinesis. This is associated with a higher incidence of congestive heart failure and post-hospital mortality. ACE inhibitors may help prevent infarct remodeling.

- Stunned myocardium—a coronary artery is completely occluded and then opened and transient akinesis of the myocardium occurs.
- Ischemia at a distance—infarction is in the distribution of one coronary artery, and ischemia and subsequent hypokinesis are in the distribution of a second vessel in which there is a high-grade stenosis.
- Infarct remodeling—occurs after large anteroapical myocardial infarctions.

- ACE inhibitors may help prevent infarct remodeling.

Presentation and Diagnosis

The typical presentation of myocardial infarction is anginal-sounding pain lasting longer than 30 to 45 minutes associated with ECG changes and elevated creatine kinase-MB fraction or troponin. However, more than 25% to 30% of myocardial infarctions are silent and present later as new ECG abnormalities or regional wall motion abnormalities. Silent myocardial infarctions occur especially in patients with diabetes mellitus and in the elderly. The increased incidence of myocardial infarction in the early morning is perhaps related to increased platelet aggregation. The pain of myocardial infarction mimics that of other diseases, for example, gastrointestinal or pericardial disease or musculoskeletal pain. Myocardial infarction may occur without ECG changes. Thus, all patients with ischemic-sounding pain should either be hospitalized or placed in a chest pain unit despite the lack of ECG changes.

- More than 25%-30% of myocardial infarctions are silent.
- Silent myocardial infarctions occur especially in patients with diabetes mellitus and in the elderly.
- Increased incidence of myocardial infarction in the early morning is perhaps related to increased platelet aggregation.
- The pain of myocardial infarction mimics that of other diseases.
- Myocardial infarction may occur without ECG changes.
- All patients with ischemic-sounding pain should be hospitalized or placed in a chest pain unit.

An increased creatine kinase-MB fraction, indicative of myocardial necrosis, confirms the clinical diagnosis of myocardial infarction. The peak values are at 12 to 20 hours. Thus, a negative creatine kinase-MB fraction at admission does not rule out myocardial infarction. Any creatine kinase-MB peak occurring earlier than 12 hours may indicate reperfusion. (SGOT and LDH levels, used in the past, have later peaks but currently are not used for the diagnosis of myocardial infarction.) Newer markers of myocardial infarction (myoglobin, troponin levels, creatine kinase isoforms) are available for the diagnosis of myocardial necrosis.

- An increased creatine kinase-MB fraction indicates myocardial necrosis.
- Negative creatine kinase-MB fraction at admission does not rule out myocardial infarction.
- Newer markers (myoglobin, troponin levels) may provide a more accurate diagnosis of myocardial infarction than creatine kinase.

Basic and Drug Treatments

Bed rest and sedation are essential and are beneficial in the acute stage of myocardial infarction for decreasing myocardial oxygen demand. Analgesics, particularly morphine, are beneficial for recurrent pain. Currently, prolonged bed rest is not recommended, and the effort to shorten hospitalization is increasing. Many physicians recommend a gradual increase in activity level over 3 to 6 days for an uncomplicated myocardial infarction. During the acute 3- to 4-day period, ECG monitoring is recommended for both tachyarrhythmias and bradyarrhythmias. Oxygen can be used at the initial presentation but has little benefit after 2 or 3 hours unless hypoxia is present. However, modest hypoxemia is not uncommon, even with uncomplicated myocardial infarction, and is due to ventilation/perfusion lung mismatch.

- Prolonged bed rest is not recommended.
- Oxygen should not be continued beyond 3 hours after the initial presentation unless hypoxia is present.

Heparin is important in treating acute myocardial infarction. It prevents 1) recurrent infarction, especially after thrombolytic therapy, 2) deep venous thrombosis, and 3) intracardiac thrombus formation. Intracardiac thrombus formation occurs in 40% of patients with anterior myocardial infarction, and almost 50% of these patients have a systemic embolic event. Thus, intravenous unfractionated heparin therapy is especially indicated in these higher risk patients. Low-molecular-weight heparin given subcutaneously may be more effective. Aspirin decreases recurrent infarction by 49% in patients not receiving thrombolytic therapy. It also reduces mortality when given in addition to thrombolytic therapy.

- Heparin is important in treating acute myocardial infarction.
- Heparin prevents recurrent infarction, deep venous thrombosis, and intracardiac thrombus formation.
- Intracardiac thrombus formation occurs in 40% of patients with anterior myocardial infarction.
- Aspirin decreases recurrent infarction by 49% in patients not receiving thrombolytic therapy.

Nitroglycerin is useful for a subset of patients with myocardial infarction—for those with heart failure (by decreasing wall tension) and for those with continued pain. In the early stages of myocardial infarction, nitroglycerin given intravenously should be used instead of long-acting nitrates given orally to prevent acute decreases in blood pressure. Intravenous nitroglycerin may reduce infarct size by decreasing wall tension and affecting "remodeling." Also, it may decrease susceptibility to ventricular fibrillation. If the mean blood pressure is greater than 80 mm Hg, intravenous nitroglycerin may

reduce mortality by 10% to 25%, specifically in patients with anterior myocardial infarction and poor left ventricular function. However, in patients with low blood pressure and those with inferior and right ventricular infarctions, nitroglycerin may decrease blood pressure too much and cause increased mortality. The dosage of intravenous nitroglycerin is a 15-μg bolus and an initial infusion of 10 μg/min. Intravenous infusion should be increased every 5 to 10 minutes until the blood pressure decreases 10% to 15%, up to a maximum of 150 to 200 μg/min. Mean blood pressure should be kept higher than 80 mm Hg. Nitrate intolerance occurs with infusions lasting longer than 24 hours. Do not use intravenous nitroglycerin in patients with low blood pressure or right ventricular infarction. Intravenous nitroglycerin may improve mortality in patients with large anterior myocardial infarctions and congestive heart failure.

- Nitroglycerin is useful for patients with heart failure and those with continued pain.
- Intravenous nitroglycerin may reduce infarct size by decreasing wall tension and affecting remodeling.
- Nitroglycerin may decrease susceptibility to ventricular fibrillation.
- Nitrate intolerance occurs with infusions longer than 24 hours.
- Do not use intravenous nitroglycerin in patients with low blood pressure or right ventricular infarction.
- Intravenous nitroglycerin may improve mortality in patients with large anterior myocardial infarctions and congestive heart failure.

β-Blockers are useful both in acute myocardial infarction and postmyocardial infarction setting. If given early, they decrease infarction size and in-hospital mortality. If given after myocardial infarction has been completed, β-blockers can reduce posthospital reinfarction and mortality. In an acute setting, the typical dosage of metoprolol is 5 mg given intravenously three times, 5 minutes apart, followed by 100 mg given orally twice daily. β-Blockers will also decrease pain and the incidence of ventricular fibrillation. The beneficial effects are probably multifactorial but include 1) decreased myocardial oxygen demand, 2) increased threshold for ventricular fibrillation, 3) decreased platelet aggregability, and 4) decreased sympathetic effects on the myocardium. β-Blockers are most beneficial in patients with large infarctions, that is, those at higher risk for complications. Acute intravenous β-blockers are also beneficial in patients undergoing thrombolytic therapy. β-Blockers are especially useful for patients with hyperdynamic circulation and continued postinfarction pain and should be given to patients presenting with less than 12 hours of pain who do not have contraindications, especially those with anterior myocardial infarction.

- Acute intravenous β-blockers decrease infarction size and in-hospital mortality.
- Acute intravenous β-blockers decrease the incidence of ventricular fibrillation.
- Contraindications to β-blockers are bradycardia, atrioventricular block, hypotension, severe heart failure, and inferior myocardial infarction with high vagal tone.

Calcium channel blockers have been used to treat myocardial infarction, but their routine use has *no* proven benefit. Routine use of verapamil and nifedipine has no benefit and may increase mortality. Diltiazem, 60 to 90 mg given every 6 hours within 72 hours after myocardial infarction, may prevent later reinfarction and recurrent angina in patients with non-Q-wave myocardial infarction; however, it probably increases mortality in patients with Q-wave myocardial infarction and depressed left ventricular function. Because most patients with non-Q-wave myocardial infarction at risk for later events will probably be identified and have a revascularization procedure performed, routine use of calcium channel blockers is not indicated. However, by producing coronary vasodilatation and decreasing myocardial oxygen demand, calcium channel blockers may be beneficial in treating postinfarction angina if beta-blockade is ineffective or cannot be used.

- Routine use of calcium channel blockers for myocardial infarction has no proven benefit.
- Routine use of verapamil and nifedipine may increase mortality.
- Calcium channel blockers may be beneficial for patients with postinfarction angina and those with non-Q-wave myocardial infarction.

In most patients, magnesium does not appear to have a role after myocardial infarction.

Treatment—Reperfusion Therapy

Early reperfusion therapy has had a tremendous impact on the treatment of acute myocardial infarction. Overall, mortality is decreased 27% ± 3% when reperfusion is given early. In more than 50,000 patients in ISIS-3 and GISSI-2 studies, the 35-day in-hospital mortality was only 10% with thrombolytic therapy. Time is of the essence when giving reperfusion therapy. The faster the reperfusion, the better the extent of myocardial salvage and the better the effect on mortality. Without collaterals, 90% of the myocardium at risk is infarcted within 3 hours after occlusion. Very early reperfusion has a major effect on direct myocardial salvage. In a study in which thrombolysis was given less than 90 minutes after the onset of pain, the mortality was 1%. In most U.S.

studies, the average time from pain onset to artery opening is 3.7 hours. The delay is in patient presentation (22%), transport (21%), in-hospital institution of the drug (35%), and reperfusion drug time (19%). Reperfusion at 2 to 6 hours salvages the peri-infarction zone, depending on the degree of collateral circulation. Thus, there is a lesser effect on myocardial salvage but an important effect on survival. The "open artery concept" describes a benefit in improvement in post-hospital mortality in the presence of an open artery after thrombolytic therapy, which is not reflected in improved ventricular function. The reason for this is unclear but may be related to improved electrical stability or prevention of ventricular remodeling.

- Overall, mortality is decreased 27% ± 3% when reperfusion is given early.
- In more than 50,000 patients, the 35-day in-hospital mortality was 10% with thrombolytic therapy.
- The faster the reperfusion, the better the extent of myocardial salvage.
- Without collaterals, 90% of the myocardium at risk is infarcted within 3 hours after occlusion.

Controversy exists about the effectiveness of intravenous thrombolytic therapy versus emergency PTCA in patients with acute myocardial infarction. After administration of thrombolytic therapy, emergency PTCA is not indicated in the absence of ongoing pain, because of a higher incidence of complications than in patients not undergoing emergency PTCA. The controversy is now about whether intravenous thrombolytic therapy should be given versus direct PTCA. Intravenous thrombolysis may not be as effective (65%-70%) in opening arteries as PTCA (90%) and there is a higher incidence of TIMI III flow after direct PTCA. However, this is counterbalanced by faster administration of intravenous thrombolysis and wider availability of the intravenous drug. Fewer than 10% of all hospitals have the capability for emergency PTCA. Late patency (>24 hours) is 70% to 80% for both methods. Thus, with the lack of available resources, intravenous thrombolytic therapy is the treatment of choice in most medical centers for patients with acute myocardial infarction. Emergency PTCA may be used in patients with 1) contraindication for intravenous thrombolysis, 2) cardiogenic shock, 3) continued ischemia after thrombolytic therapy, or 4) those with immediate access to a high volume catheterization laboratory.

- The effectiveness of intravenous thrombolytic therapy versus emergency primary PTCA in patients with acute myocardial infarction is controversial.
- After giving thrombolytic therapy, emergency PTCA is not indicated in the absence of ongoing pain.

- Intravenous thrombolysis may not be as effective (65%-70%) in opening arteries as PTCA (90%).
- Fewer than 10% of hospitals have the capability for emergency PTCA.
- Intravenous thrombolytic therapy is the treatment of choice in most medical centers for stable patients with acute myocardial infarction with no contraindications.

Thrombolytic therapy definitely is indicated for patients presenting within 6 hours after the onset of pain who have ST-segment elevation and no contraindication. It should be considered for patients up to 12 hours after the onset of symptoms with continued pain. Whether thrombolytic therapy should be given to patients later than 6 hours after pain onset who have no evidence of continued ischemia is unclear. It should also be given to patients presenting within 6 hours after pain onset and left bundle branch block. Thrombolytic therapy is not indicated for patients with pain and other ECG abnormalities (ST-segment depression) or patients after 12 hours without pain.

- Thrombolytic therapy definitely is indicated for patients presenting within 6 hours after the onset of pain who have ST-segment elevation and no contraindication.
- Thrombolytic therapy may be given to patients 6-12 hours after pain onset who have evidence of continued ischemia.
- Thrombolytic therapy is not indicated for patients with pain and other ECG abnormalities (ST-segment depression).
- Thrombolytic therapy is not indicated for patients after 12 hours without evidence of continued ischemia.

Contraindications to thrombolytic therapy include a history of bleeding, severe hypertension, recent stroke, diabetic hemorrhagic retinopathy, recent cardiopulmonary resuscitation, previous allergy to streptokinase, recent surgical procedure, suspected aortic dissection or pericarditis, and pregnancy. Major complications of intravenous thrombolysis include major bleeding (5%-6%), intracranial bleeding (0.5%), major allergic reaction (0.1%-1.7%), and hypotension (2%-10%). A higher incidence of myocardial rupture may occur in patients given thrombolytic therapy late (>12 hours after pain onset).

- Major complications of intravenous thrombolysis are major bleeding (5%-6%), intracranial bleeding (0.5%), major allergic reaction (0.1%-1.7%), and hypotension (2%-10%).
- A higher incidence of myocardial rupture may occur in patients given thrombolytic therapy late (>12 hours after pain onset).

Three agents are available for intravenous thrombolysis (Table 3-20). Streptokinase, a nonselective thrombolytic agent, combines with circulating plasminogen to split circulating and thrombus-bound plasminogen into plasmin, which splits fibrin. It lyses circulating fibrinogen and thus has systemic effects. The dosage is a 250,000-U bolus and 1.5×10^6 U in 1 hour. Tissue plasminogen activator (tPA) binds to preformed fibrin preferentially and lyses it without activating plasminogen in the general circulation. Thus, it has less effect on circulating fibrinogen and is "fibrin-specific." It has the fastest onset of action. The dosage is 100 mg over 90 minutes. Anistreplase (APSAC) is composed of anisoylated plasminogen and streptokinase bound together and inactivated by plasminogen. It requires spontaneous deacylation, which occurs in the plasma before the active streptokinase-plasminogen complex is generated, splitting plasminogen to plasmin. Thus, anistreplase is a more stable agent and may be given as a single intravenous bolus. The dosage is 30 U over 5 minutes. Newer plasminogen activators are being investigated.

In the large European trials, there was no proven benefit of one thrombolytic therapy over the others. In the GUSTO trial, there was a lower mortality rate when an accelerated dose of tPA was given with intravenous heparin than with streptokinase. Compared with streptokinase, tPA is more costly and has a slightly increased risk of cerebral hemorrhage, especially in the elderly. It is reasonable to give tPA preferentially to younger patients who present very early with a large myocardial infarction.

After intravenous thrombolysis, a high-grade residual lesion is usually present. Reocclusion or ischemia occurs in 15% to 20% of patients and reinfarction occurs in 2% to 3%. In the U.S., both heparin and aspirin are given after intravenous thrombolysis with the specific tissue plasminogen activators to prevent reinfarction. After tPA, heparin is given as a bolus injection, followed by a continuous infusion to keep the activated partial thromboplastin time at 50 to 70 seconds. The indication for coronary angiography or PTCA after intravenous thrombolysis is continued pain or ischemia documented on functional testing. There is no benefit from routine intervention in all patients.

- After intravenous thrombolysis, reocclusion or ischemia occurs in 15%-20% of patients and reinfarction occurs in 2%-3%.
- Both aspirin and heparin are given after intravenous thrombolysis to prevent reinfarction.
- The benefit is clear with aspirin but not with heparin.
- Streptokinase is the least expensive thrombolytic therapy.
- tPA is the most clot-specific thrombolytic therapy.
- The least amount of antigenicity is with tPA.

Acute Mechanical Complications of Myocardial Infarction

Cardiogenic shock after myocardial infarction has a high mortality, but with newer interventions, the mortality has decreased from 90% to 60%. However, it is important to determine the cause of cardiogenic shock. Although most cases are due to extensive left ventricular dysfunction, there are other causes, for example, right ventricular infarction and mechanical complications of myocardial infarction. Swan-Ganz catheterization and two-dimensional echocardiography may help in determining its cause (Table 3-21).

● Cardiogenic shock after myocardial infarction approaches 90% mortality.
● Most cases of cardiogenic shock are due to extensive left ventricular dysfunction.
● Swan-Ganz catheterization and two-dimensional echocardiography may help determine other causes of cardiogenic shock.

Right ventricular infarction occurs in up to 40% of patients with inferior myocardial infarction and is diagnosed by increased jugular venous pressure in the presence of clear lung fields. ST-segment elevation in a V_{4R} lead is diagnostic of a large right ventricular infarction and portends a high mortality rate. In extreme circumstances, right ventricular infarction can cause cardiogenic shock, because the right ventricle is not able to pump effectively enough blood to fill the left ventricle. Treatment includes large amounts of fluids given intravenously and infusion of dobutamine. If right ventricular infarction is recognized early, reperfusion therapy is indicated.

● Right ventricular infarction occurs in up to 40% of patients with inferior myocardial infarction.

Myocardial free wall rupture may occur and cause abrupt decompensation. Free wall rupture occurs in 85% of all ruptures. It occurs suddenly, usually 2 to 14 days after transmural myocardial infarction, most commonly in elderly hypertensive women. It usually presents as electromechanical dissociation or death. If rupture is contained in the pericardium, tamponade may occur. If the diagnosis can be made by emergency echocardiography, surgery should be performed. If the rupture is sealed off, pseudoaneurysm may occur; operation is required because of the high incidence of further rupture.

● Free wall rupture occurs in 85% of all ruptures.
● It occurs suddenly, usually 2-14 days after transmural myocardial infarction.

Table 3-20.—Thrombolytic Agents

Agent	Clot specific	Half-life	Allergic reaction	Dosage	Cost
Streptokinase	+	++	++	1.5×10^6 U/hr	+
tPA (tissue plasminogen activator)	+++	+	-	10-mg IV bolus, with 90 mg IV over 90 min	+++
APSAC (anisoylated plasminogen-streptokinase activator complex)	+	+++	+	30 U/5 min	++

-, none; +, some; ++, more; +++, most.

Table 3-21.—Diagnosis of Cause of Cardiogenic Shock

Cause	Swan-Ganz catheterization				2-Dimensional echocardiography
	RA	PAWP	CO		
Left ventricular dysfunction	↑	↑↑	↓↓		Poor left ventricle
Right ventricular infarction	↑↑	↓	↓↓		Dilated right ventricle
Tamponade	↑↑	↑↑	↓↓	End-equalization	Pericardial tamponade
PM rupture	↑	↑↑	↓↓	Large "V"	Severe mitral regurgitation
VSD	↑	↑↑	↑	Step-up	Defect seen
PE	↑↑	=	↓	PADP > PAWP	Dilated right ventricle

CO, cardiac output; PADP, pulmonary artery diastolic pressure; PAWP, pulmonary artery wedge pressure; PE, pulmonary emboli; PM, papillary muscle; RA, right atrial pressure; VSD, ventricular septal defect.

Papillary muscle rupture occurs in 5% of all ruptures and usually 2 to 10 days after myocardial infarction. It is associated with inferior myocardial infarction, because of the single blood supply to the posteromedial papillary muscle. Papillary muscle rupture is heralded by the sudden onset of dyspnea and hypotension. Although a murmur may be present, it may not be audible because of equalization of left atrial and left ventricular pressures. The diagnosis is made with echocardiography or Swan-Ganz catheterization, which demonstrates a large "V" wave on pulmonary artery wedge pressure. The treatment is intra-aortic balloon pumping and emergency operation.

- Papillary muscle rupture occurs in 5% of all ruptures.
- It usually occurs 2-10 days after myocardial infarction.
- It is associated with inferior myocardial infarction.
- It is heralded by sudden dyspnea and hypotension.
- It is diagnosed with echocardiography and Swan-Ganz catheterization.

Ventricular septal defects occur in 10% of all ruptures, usually 1 to 20 days after myocardial infarction. It is equally frequent in inferior and anterior myocardial infarctions. Ventricular septal defects associated with inferior myocardial infarctions have a poorer prognosis because of the serpiginous nature of the rupture and associated ventricular infarction. They are indicated by the sudden onset of dyspnea and hypotension. A loud murmur and systolic thrill are always present. The diagnosis is made with echocardiography or Swan-Ganz catheterization, which demonstrates a step-up in oxygen saturation from the right atrium to the pulmonary artery. Treatment is intra-aortic balloon pump and emergency operation.

- Ventricular septal defects occur in 10% of all ruptures.
- They are equally frequent in inferior and anterior myocardial infarctions.
- They are indicated by the sudden onset of dyspnea and hypotension.
- A ventricular septal defect almost always has a thrill and loud murmur.

Prehospital Dismissal Evaluation

To properly evaluate a patient with myocardial infarction before dismissal from the hospital, determine the predictors of mortality. These include status of the left ventricle, ventricular arrhythmias, and presence of continued myocardial ischemia.

Rehabilitation treadmill exertion testing should be performed in most patients after myocardial infarction to detect continued ischemia, particularly in those who did not have thrombolytic therapy. It is a low-risk test in properly selected patients and is performed 8 to 10 days after the infarction. It is usually a limited workload to 5 metabolic equivalents (METs)

or 70% of the maximum heart rate. High-risk patients identified by treadmill exertion testing have a greater than 1-mm ST-segment depression, a decrease in blood pressure, or an inability to achieve 4 METs on the exercise test. Imaging exercise tests may identify additional high-risk patients by demonstrating multiple areas of ischemia. Pharmacologic stress tests (dobutamine echocardiography, dipyridamole thallium scanning, or adenosine thallium scanning) may be useful in patients unable to exercise. The role of stress testing in patients after thrombolytic therapy is less clear because most of these patients do well without intervention.

- After myocardial infarction, most patients should undergo rehabilitation treadmill testing.
- It is a low-risk test in properly selected patients and is performed 8-10 days after the infarction.

ACE inhibitors should be given to all patients with large anterior myocardial infarctions to prevent infarct remodeling and expansion. In patients with an ejection fraction less than 40%, the administration of ACE inhibitors will prevent future congestive heart failure and improve mortality. The time to start ACE inhibitors is not settled. Acute, intravenous administration of ACE inhibitors within 24 hours after an infarction may be detrimental. However, oral ACE inhibitors given at least 2 or 3 days after the onset of myocardial infarction are beneficial.

Coronary angiography is indicated after myocardial infarction if the results of a rehabilitation treadmill exertion test are positive or postinfarction angina occurs.

- Coronary angiography is indicated if the results of a rehabilitation treadmill exertion test are positive or postinfarction angina occurs.

No randomized trials have examined the benefit of PTCA or bypass grafting after myocardial infarction. However, in high-risk patients (i.e., those with continued ischemia or positive results on the treadmill exertion test), it is reasonable to proceed with intervention. PTCA can be undertaken if there is a single-vessel high-grade lesion amenable to the procedure. CABG should be performed if there is left main or proximal three-vessel disease or two- or three-vessel disease that supplies a large portion of the myocardium, especially when associated with moderate depression in left ventricular function.

The following apply to patients who survive acute myocardial infarction:

- Aspirin decreases recurrent myocardial infarction by 31% and late mortality by 15%, more so in cases of non-Q-wave myocardial infarction.

- Warfarin may cause a similar decrease in mortality and reinfarction, but it is not used routinely in the U.S.
- "Statins" reduce recurrent events and mortality in patients with increased cholesterol levels (total cholesterol >200 mg/dL).
- "Statins" reduce recurrent events in patients with "average" cholesterol levels (LDL >125 mg/dL).
- β-Blockers improve survival after myocardial infarction.
- β-Blockers are most effective in high-risk patients (i.e., decreased left ventricular function and ventricular arrhythmias) and may not be required in low-risk patients.
- β-Blockers are also effective after thrombolytic therapy.
- Because antiarrhythmic agents are associated with increased mortality, they should not be used to suppress ventricular ectopy.
- ACE inhibitors decrease mortality after anterior myocardial infarction and depressed left ventricular function, presumably by inhibiting infarct remodeling.
- A rehabilitation program is essential for the patient's well-being and cardiovascular fitness.

PART V
Barry L. Karon, M.D.
Rick A. Nishimura, M.D.

DEFINITION

Heart failure is the clinical syndrome characterized by the inability of the heart to meet the metabolic demands of the body while maintaining normal ventricular filling pressures. Although the most common cause is left ventricular systolic dysfunction (as in dilated cardiomyopathy), other causes must be considered. To treat heart failure properly, the cause and precipitating factors must be identified. Backward heart failure is caused by increased filling pressure, which affects the pulmonary venous circulation and causes shortness of breath and paroxysmal nocturnal dyspnea. Increased filling pressure can also affect the systemic venous circulation and cause edema and ascites. Forward heart failure is caused by low cardiac output, which produces symptoms of fatigue and lethargy. Most patients will have a combination of the symptoms of backward and forward heart failure.

Myocardial dysfunction causing heart failure may manifest as impaired contractile function (systolic dysfunction) resulting in low stroke volume. Abnormal diastolic filling usually is present as well and is as important as systolic dysfunction in causing the signs and symptoms of heart failure. However, as many as one-third of patients who present with heart failure may have normal systolic function; diastolic dysfunction is predominantly the cause of their heart failure.

- Heart failure is the inability of the heart to meet the metabolic demands of the body while maintaining normal filling pressures.
- The most common cause of heart failure is left ventricular myocardial contractile dysfunction (systolic dysfunction).
- High ventricular filling pressures cause dyspnea and edema (backward heart failure).
- Reduced cardiac output (forward heart failure) causes fatigue and lethargy.
- Diastolic dysfunction is as important as systolic dysfunction in causing signs and symptoms of heart failure.
- Many patients with heart failure may have normal systolic function.

Ventricular diastolic function is a complex process. Three of its major components are relaxation, passive filling, and atrial contribution. Relaxation is an active energy-requiring process in which calcium is removed from the actin myosin filaments, causing contracted muscle to return to its original length. After relaxation, filling of the ventricle continues along the pressure gradient from the left atrium to the left ventricle (passive filling). The amount of filling during this phase is determined by left atrial pressure and left ventricular compliance; compliance is the increase in ventricular volume per unit of driving pressure. Thus, abnormally low compliance impairs filling and produces high end-diastolic pressure. The contribution from atrial contraction further increases ventricular volume by as much as 15% to 20% in normal subjects and 45% to 50% in those with abnormal ventricular relaxation and passive filling (Table 3-22).

- Three major components of ventricular diastolic function are relaxation, passive filling, and atrial contribution.
- Relaxation is impaired in ischemic or hypertrophied myocardium.
- Impaired ventricular compliance means higher pressures are needed to produce volume changes.

Table 3-22.—Abnormal Diastolic Function in Myocardial Disease

Phase	Influencing factors	Treatment
Relaxation	Ischemia, hypertrophy	Treat ischemia, hypertension
Passive filling	Myocardial compliance, heart rate	Slow heart rate
Atrial contraction	Atrial contraction, atrioventricular synchrony	Maintain sinus rhythm

- Atrial contraction takes on greater importance in patients with reduced ventricular relaxation or compliance.
- In most disease states, there is a combination of systolic and diastolic abnormalities.
- Treatment of diastolic dysfunction involves treating ischemia and hypertension, providing an adequate diastolic filling period, and maintaining atrioventricular synchrony.

ETIOLOGY

The mechanism and cause of heart failure must be defined to properly select therapy. A simple categorical framework is given in Table 3-23.

Clinically, the most common cause of heart failure is left ventricular myocardial contractile dysfunction. Because the treatment and prognosis are different for other causes of heart failure, accurate diagnosis is essential and is made on the basis of physical examination and noninvasive testing, such as echocardiography or radionuclide angiography.

PRECIPITATING FACTORS

The appearance or worsening of heart failure symptoms may merely represent natural disease progression. Often, however, one or more precipitating factors are responsible for symptomatic deterioration (Table 3-24). If these factors are not identified and corrected, symptoms of heart failure frequently return

Table 3-23.—Causes of Heart Failure and Treatment

Cause	Treatment
Myocardial	
Dilated cardiomyopathy (including ischemic)	Angiotensin-converting enzyme inhibitors, nitrates, digoxin, diuretics, nitrates and hydralazine in combination, transplantation, coronary revascularization, left ventricular aneurysmectomy, β-adrenergic blockers (carvedilol, metoprolol, bisoprolol), amlodipine
Hypertrophic cardiomyopathy	β-Adrenergic blockers, verapamil, disopyramide, surgical myectomy, dual-chamber pacing
Restrictive cardiomyopathy	Diuretics, heart transplant, treat underlying systemic disease
Pericardial	
Tamponade	Pericardiocentesis
Constrictive pericarditis	Pericardiectomy
Valvular	Valve repair or replacement
Hypertension	Antihypertensive treatment
Pulmonary hypertension	Heart-lung transplant, calcium channel blockers, prostacyclin infusion
High output	Correct underlying cause
Hyperthyroidism, Paget disease	
Arteriovenous fistula	

Table 3-24.—Precipitating Factors in Heart Failure

Diet (excessive sodium or fluid intake, alcohol)
Noncompliance with medication or inadequate dosing
Sodium-retaining medications (NSAIDs)
Infection (bacterial or viral)
Myocardial ischemia or infarction
Arrhythmia (atrial fibrillation, bradycardia)
Breathing disorders of sleep
Anemia
Metabolic (hyperthyroidism, hypothyroidism, chronic renal failure)
Pulmonary embolus

NSAIDs, nonsteroidal anti-inflammatory drugs.

after initial therapy. The most common precipitants are dietary indiscretion (sodium, fluid, alcohol) and medication noncompliance (cost, regimen complexity, patient understanding).

The evaluation of each patient with heart failure follows these steps: 1) a medical history (include sodium and fluid intake, medication use and compliance, and sleep history from bedroom partners), 2) chest radiography to look for pneumonitis, 3) electrocardiography and creatine kinase-MB or troponin blood tests to document the rhythm and seek ischemia or myocardial injury, and 4) culture specimens of blood, urine, and sputum as appropriate. Other tests should include determination of complete blood cell count and thyroid-stimulating hormone, creatinine, and arterial blood gas values (if pulmonary embolus is a clinical concern).

- For different causes of heart failure, treatment and prognosis are different.
- For every patient with heart failure, precipitating factors must be sought and treated.

ACUTE HEART FAILURE SYNDROMES

Acute heart failure syndromes usually present as pulmonary edema with or without shock. The most common cause is ischemic heart disease; less common causes include uncontrolled hypertension, progressive valvular disease, or infective endocarditis. Evaluation and treatment often proceed simultaneously. Testing includes hematologic studies; determination of electrolyte, cardiac enzyme, creatinine, and arterial blood gas values; chest radiography; electrocardiography; and echocardiography (if the mechanism of heart failure is clinically indeterminate). Initial treatment includes oxygen, intravenous loop diuretic, and morphine sulfate. Angiography should be considered for active ischemia or an evolving infarction.

DEFINITION OF CARDIOMYOPATHIES

The 1995 WHO Task Force on Cardiomyopathies defined them as disease of myocardium associated with cardiac dysfunction. Major categories are dilated, hypertrophic, restrictive, arrhythmogenic right ventricular, and unclassified cardiomyopathies. The task force also defined several specific cardiomyopathies, but pathophysiologically all of these behave as dilated, hypertrophic, or restrictive cardiomyopathies. The different anatomical and pathophysiologic processes for each cardiomyopathy are listed in Table 3-25.

DILATED CARDIOMYOPATHY

Etiology

The major abnormality in dilated cardiomyopathy is decreased systolic function (low ejection fraction) with enlargement of the left ventricular cavity and often increased left ventricular end-diastolic pressure due to coexistent diastolic dysfunction. The increased filling pressures and low cardiac output produce symptoms of shortness of breath and fatigue.

Table 3-25.—Anatomical and Pathophysiologic Processes for Each Cardiomyopathy

Type	Left ventricular cavity size	Left ventricular wall thickness	Systolic function	Diastolic function	Other
Dilated cardiomyopathy	↑	N/↑	↓	↓/N	
Hypertrophic cardiomyopathy	↓/N	↑	↑	↓	Left ventricular outflow obstruction
Restrictive cardiomyopathy	N/↑	N	N	↓	

↓, N, ↑, decreased, normal, increased, respectively.

A true dilated cardiomyopathy is indicated by left ventricular dysfunction without any known cause. Many of these are genetic; an affected family member can be identified in up to 30% of cases Other causes of severe left ventricular dysfunction include severe coronary artery disease ("hibernating myocardium"), multiple areas of previous infarction, uncontrolled hypertension, ethanol abuse, hyperthyroidism or hypothyroidism, postpartum cardiomyopathy, toxins and drugs, tachycardia-induced cardiomyopathy, infiltrative cardiomyopathy (i.e., hemochromatosis, sarcoidosis, or amyloidosis, but in amyloidosis, restrictive cardiomyopathy is more common), acquired immunodeficiency syndrome (AIDS), and pheochromocytoma.

- In dilated cardiomyopathy, the major abnormality is decreased systolic function (low ejection fraction).
- There is a genetic link in dilated cardiomyopathy (up to 30% of cases).
- Other causes of severe left ventricular dysfunction: severe coronary artery disease ("hibernating myocardium"), multiple areas of previous infarction, uncontrolled hypertension, ethanol abuse, hyperthyroidism or hypothyroidism, postpartum cardiomyopathy, toxins and drugs, tachycardia-induced cardiomyopathy, infiltrative cardiomyopathy (i.e., hemochromatosis, sarcoidosis, or amyloidosis), AIDS, and pheochromocytoma.

Clinical Presentation

The presentation of dilated cardiomyopathy is highly variable. The patient may be asymptomatic, in which case the diagnosis is made on basis of examination, chest radiography, ECG, or echocardiography. Patients may have symptoms of mild to severe heart failure (New York Heart Association functional class II-IV). Other patients may present with the sudden onset of a systemic embolus. Atrial and ventricular arrhythmias are common in dilated cardiomyopathy. If heart failure is present, the following may be found on physical examination: jugular venous pressure is increased (if there is right heart involvement), upstroke of the carotid artery is low volume, the left ventricular impulse is displaced and sustained with a rapid filling wave, third or fourth heart sounds are frequently audible, and apical systolic murmur of mitral regurgitation is present.

- Presentation of dilated cardiomyopathy is highly variable.
- Carotid volume is low, third heart sound is often present, and the apex is displaced and sustained.

ECG frequently shows left ventricular hypertrophy, intraventricular conduction delay, or left bundle branch block. Rhythm abnormalities may include premature atrial contractions, atrial fibrillation, premature ventricular contractions, or short bursts of ventricular tachycardia. The chest radiograph often shows left ventricular enlargement and pulmonary venous congestion. The diagnosis is made on the basis of reduced ejection fraction measured by echocardiography, radionuclide angiography, or left ventriculography.

- ECG shows left ventricular hypertrophy, intraventricular conduction delay, or left bundle branch block.
- Atrial and ventricular rhythm disturbances are common.
- Chest radiograph often shows left ventricular enlargement and pulmonary venous congestion.
- The diagnosis requires demonstration of reduced ejection fraction.

Evaluation

After the diagnosis of impaired left ventricular contractile function is made, treatable secondary causes of left ventricular dysfunction should be excluded. Sensitive thyroid-stimulating hormone level should be determined to exclude hyperthyroidism or hypothyroidism. Iron and iron-binding capacities (or ferritin level) should be measured to rule out hemochromatosis. The serum angiotensin-converting enzyme level should be measured. The metanephrine level should be measured if there is a history of severe labile hypertension or unusual spells. Ethanol or drug abuse must be documented.

In severe coronary artery disease, reversible left ventricular dysfunction can be caused by hibernating myocardium. In this situation, long-standing diffuse ischemia depletes adenosine triphosphate stores in myocardial cells, which are thus functionally inactive. However, with revascularization, left ventricular function may gradually improve. Identifying affected patients is difficult. Currently, the reference standard is positron emission tomography (PET), which can demonstrate metabolic activity. Stress echocardiography and radionuclide perfusion imaging are more widely available than PET and are also useful in identifying hibernating myocardium.

Tachycardia-induced cardiomyopathy can occur in patients with prolonged periods of tachycardia (usually atrial fibrillation, flutter, or incessant atrial tachycardia). The mechanism of this is unknown, but it is an important cause to establish because systolic dysfunction can be completely reversed after the tachycardia is treated.

- After depressed left ventricular function is diagnosed, seek treatable causes of reversible left ventricular dysfunction.
- Perform blood tests for thyroid dysfunction, sarcoid, and hemochromatosis—reversible causes of cardiomyopathy.
- Hibernating myocardium is a reversible cause of left ventricular dysfunction.
- Tachycardia-induced cardiomyopathy is reversible.

Some patients have left ventricular dysfunction caused by acute myocarditis. The natural history of these patients is unknown. Many patients develop permanent left ventricular dysfunction, whereas others experience improvement with time. Thus, it is necessary to measure left ventricular function 3 to 6 months after making the diagnosis. Although endomyocardial biopsy may help diagnose myocarditis, immunosuppressive therapy has not been demonstrated to improve outcome and should be reserved for patients with concomitant skeletal myositis or clinical deterioration despite standard pharmacologic therapy.

Pathophysiology

For understanding the treatment of heart failure associated with dilated cardiomyopathy, the hemodynamic, pathophysiologic, and biologic aspects of heart failure must be appreciated.

Preload can be thought of as the ventricular end-diastolic volume. The relationship of stroke volume to preload is shown on the Starling curve in Figure 3-31. *Afterload* is the tension, force, or stress acting on the fibers of the ventricular wall after the onset of shortening. Left ventricular afterload is increased by aortic stenosis and systemic hypertension but is decreased by mitral regurgitation. Importantly, afterload is increased by ventricular enlargement and therefore the compensatory preload adjustment to contractile dysfunction has a putative effect on stroke volume via its effects on afterload.

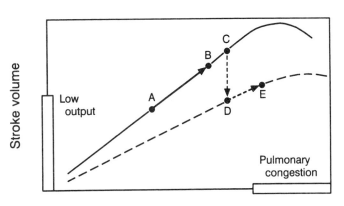

Fig. 3-31. Starling curve. Solid line is patient with normal contractility, and the dotted line is one with depressed systolic function. Normally, stroke volume depends on preload of the heart. Increasing preload increases stroke volume (A to B). Myocardial dysfunction causes a shift of the curve downward and to the right (C to D), causing a severe decrease in stroke volume, which leads to symptoms of fatigue and lethargy. The compensatory response to decrease in stroke volume is an increase in preload (D to E). Because the diastolic pressure-volume relationship is curvilinear, increased left ventricular volume produces increased left ventricular end-diastolic pressure, causing symptoms of pulmonary congestion. Note flat portion of the curve at its upper end; here, there is little increase in stroke volume for increase in preload.

Figure 3-32 illustrates the neurohumoral response to decreased myocardial contractility. Decreased cardiac output activates baroreceptors and the sympathetic nervous system. Sympathetic nervous system stimulation causes an increased heart rate and contractility. Alpha-stimulation of the arterioles causes an increase in afterload. The renin-angiotensin system is activated by sympathetic stimulation, decreased renal blood flow, and decreased renal sodium. This system in turn activates aldosterone, causing increased renal retention of sodium and, thus, more pulmonary congestion. A low rate of renal blood flow results in renal retention of sodium. An increased level of angiotensin II causes vasoconstriction and an increase in afterload. In congestive heart failure, the compensatory mechanisms that increase preload eventually cause a malcompensatory increase in afterload, in turn causing further decrease in stroke volume.

Finally, neurohormonal (adrenergic, angiotensin II) and other signaling pathways (endothelin, tissue necrosis factor-α, stretch, and wall stress) lead to altered myocyte gene expression (and thus impaired myocyte function) and progressive myocyte loss. These contribute to the progressive myocardial dysfunction and remodeling, which are the natural history of untreated myocardial dysfunction.

- Increase in preload causes increase in stroke volume.
- Increase in afterload causes decrease in stroke volume.
- Either increase in afterload or decrease in myocardial contractility can shift the Starling curve downward and to the right.
- Initial compensatory neurohormonal mechanisms lead to long-term increase in afterload with further decrease in stroke volume.
- The biologic aspects of myocyte dysfunction help explain the benefits of angiotensin-converting enzyme inhibitor and β-adrenergic blocker therapy.

Treatment

For treatment of dilated cardiomyopathy, it is important to diagnose and remove precipitating factors, as mentioned above. Treatment of congestive heart failure in patients with dilated cardiomyopathy should be based on the pathophysiologic mechanisms described above (Fig. 3-33).

Nonpharmacologic treatment is crucial to patient management. It includes sodium and fluid restriction, avoidance of alcohol, daily patient monitoring of weight, and regular aerobic exercise. Ongoing patient and family education and regular outpatient follow-up (often with nurse specialists) reduce heart failure exacerbations, emergency room visits, and hospitalizations.

The mainstays of therapy are angiotensin-converting enzyme (ACE) inhibitors. By blocking conversion of angiotensin I to

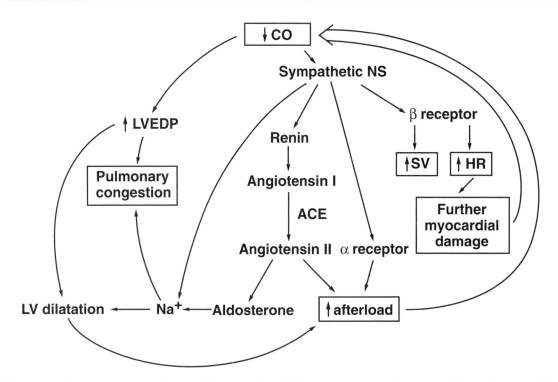

Fig. 3-32. Neurohumoral response to decreased myocardial contractility. ACE, angiotensin-converting enzyme; CO, cardiac output; HR, heart rate; LV, left ventricle; LVEDP, left ventricular end-diastolic pressure; NS, nervous system; SV, stroke volume.

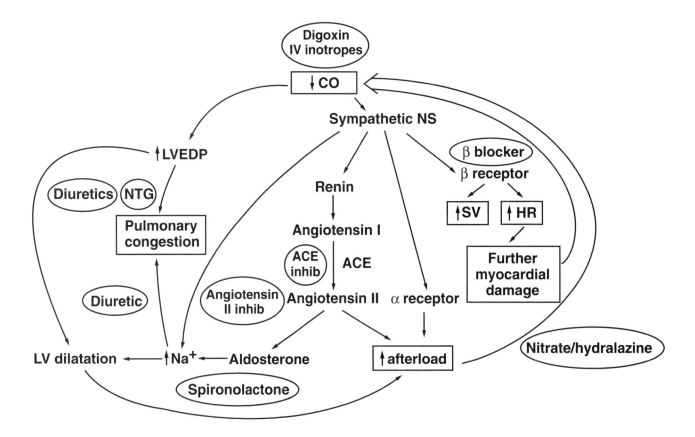

Fig. 3-33. The effect of various drugs used to treat heart failure in patients with dilated cardiomyopathy. IV, intravenous; NTG, nitroglycerin. Other abbreviations as in Figure 3-32.

angiotensin II, ACE inhibitors decrease afterload by inhibition of angiotensin II and decrease sodium retention by inhibition of aldosterone. ACE inhibitors also directly affect myocyte gene expression, growth, and remodeling. Overall, ACE inhibitors provide symptomatic improvement in patients with New York Heart Association (NYHA) functional class II-IV failure and improve mortality in patients with moderate and severe heart failure. In asymptomatic patients, ACE inhibitors prevent onset of heart failure and reduce the need for hospitalization.

- ACE inhibitors decrease afterload, decrease sodium retention, and directly reduce adverse biologic effects on myocytes.
- ACE inhibitor use decreases mortality in patients with moderate and severe heart failure.
- ACE inhibitors symptomatically improve patients with NYHA class II-IV heart failure symptoms.
- In asymptomatic patients, ACE inhibitors reduce the incidence of heart failure and reduce the need for hospitalization.

ACE inhibitors are given initially in small doses because of possible hypotensive effects. Dosage should be titrated up as tolerated on the basis of symptoms, blood pressure, and potassium and creatinine measurements. Even if a patient is clinically compensated on a low or intermediate ACE inhibitor dose, upward dose adjustment as tolerated is beneficial. For optimal ACE inhibitor doses to be achieved, the diuretic dose may need downward adjustment. Common side effects of ACE inhibitors include hypotension, hyperkalemia, azotemia, cough, angioedema (mild or severe), and dysgeusia.

- ACE inhibitor doses are initially low but should be titrated upward; concomitant diuretic dose may need reduction.
- ACE inhibitor side effects: hypotension, hyperkalemia, azotemia, cough, angioedema, and dysgeusia.

Although less well studied than ACE inhibitors, direct angiotensin II receptor blockers provide similar hemodynamic benefits to patients with dilated cardiomyopathy. They cause less cough and angioedema than ACE inhibitors and should be tried in patients who cannot tolerate ACE inhibitors because of these bradykinin-mediated side effects

Drugs that directly affect contractility include digoxin and phosphodiesterase inhibitors (milrinone and amrinone). Digoxin provides symptomatic relief when the ejection fraction is <40%, but it does not improve survival. Because digoxin is excreted by the kidneys, its dosage needs to be decreased with increased levels of creatinine and in older patients. The typical dosage is 0.25 mg/day but should be decreased to 0.125

mg/day if creatinine clearance is less than 70 mL/min-m^2 body surface area. In patients with chronic renal failure, digoxin dose is adjusted on the basis of trough digoxin levels. Because of drug-to-drug interaction, digoxin dosage should be decreased with concomitant administration of quinidine, verapamil, and amiodarone. Although short-term parenteral inotropic agents (milrinone and amrinone) may improve symptoms, long-term use increases mortality and therefore should be used transiently and only in severe cases of congestive heart failure.

- Digoxin and phosphodiesterase inhibitors (milrinone and amrinone) directly affect contractility.
- Digoxin dosage needs to be decreased in azotemic and older patients.
- Digoxin dosage should be decreased with concomitant administration of quinidine, verapamil, and amiodarone.

Diuretics should be used only in patients with symptoms of pulmonary congestion or physical evidence of fluid overload. Regular diuretic use causes neurohumoral activation and electrolyte imbalances. Mild fluid overload is initially treated with thiazide diuretics if renal function is normal. Loop diuretics are needed if there is significant fluid overload, renal dysfunction, or fluid overload resistant to thiazides. Occasionally, a combination of thiazides and loop diuretics is needed for severe fluid retention. The addition of spironolactone can help in patients with hypokalemia and may provide additional benefit by blocking aldosterone-mediated sodium retention.

Nitrates reduce preload and afterload through venodilatation. They also are anti-ischemic agents, may improve endothelial function, and combat ventricular remodeling. They should be given with a nitrate-free interval to prevent nitrate tolerance. Hydralazine may potentiate nitrate therapy by reducing nitrate tolerance when they are used in combination.

- Diuretics and nitrates reduce pulmonary congestion.
- Nitrates reduce preload and afterload.
- Nitrate tolerance is best avoided by providing a nitrate-free interval.

With reduced afterload, stroke volume improves, as do symptoms. The combination of high-dose nitrates and hydralazine provides symptomatic improvement and improved mortality in patients with heart failure. However, the rate of intolerance to the necessary doses of medications is high, and their demonstrated mortality benefit is less than that achieved with ACE inhibitors.

- Stroke volume improves with reduced afterload.
- Combination of nitrates and hydralazine improves symptoms and mortality.

β-Adrenergic blockers have now been shown to be beneficial (symptoms, ejection fraction, mortality) as an adjunct to standard therapy with ACE inhibitors, digoxin, and diuretics in the treatment of patients with dilated cardiomyopathy. Although they may acutely have unwanted hemodynamic effects (negative inotropes, attenuation of heart rate response that may be maintaining cardiac output in the setting of reduced stroke volume), they provide long-term (may take up to 6 months) benefit by modifying the unfavorable biologic effects of enhanced adrenergic tone. These drugs should not be given to patients with decompensated heart failure and are most useful for patients with NYHA class II or III symptoms. Their role in asymptomatic left ventricular dysfunction is uncertain. Initial dosing should be low, clinical follow-up should be close, and upward titration of the β-blocker dose should be slow and cautious. Well-studied β-blockers in patients with heart failure include metoprolol, carvedilol, and bisoprolol (although only carvedilol currently has the approval of the Food and Drug Administration for the treatment of heart failure).

- β-Blockers have been studied as adjunctive therapy to ACE inhibitors, digoxin, and diuretics.
- β-Blockers provide long-term ventricular function benefit and slow or reverse pathologic remodeling in dilated cardiomyopathy.
- β-Blockers need to be given carefully to avoid left ventricular decompensation.

A 48-hour infusion of dobutamine may give symptomatic relief, but the effect is often temporary and mortality may be increased. The infusion should be given with continuous ECG monitoring to look for arrhythmia. The usual dosage is 10 to 25 µg/kg per minute to get the resting heart rate 15 to 20 beats per minute above baseline. Dobutamine may replenish low catecholamine stores. This therapy is reserved for severely symptomatic patients who are unresponsive to other therapies; they may receive continuous outpatient infusions.

- 48-Hour infusion of dobutamine may give temporary symptomatic relief.
- Dobutamine may cause increased mortality.

Amlodipine is safe in patients with dilated cardiomyopathy and may provide a survival benefit in patients with idiopathic dilated cardiomyopathy. First-generation calcium channel blockers (verapamil, diltiazem, nifedipine), however, are relatively contraindicated because of their negative inotropic effects.

Anticoagulation with warfarin is recommended for patients in atrial fibrillation and those with intracardiac thrombus or a history of systemic or pulmonary thromboembolism.

- Anticoagulation with warfarin is recommended in patients with atrial fibrillation, intracardiac thrombus, or a history of thromboembolism.

The prognosis for patients with dilated cardiomyopathy varies with functional class. Even with standard therapy, patients who have mild to moderate heart failure have a 40% mortality at 4 years, whereas patients with severe heart failure have a 1-year mortality of up to 35%. Patients with asymptomatic left ventricular systolic dysfunction do well initially but have a 40% mortality at 7 years, a finding emphasizing the need to treat these patients aggressively with ACE inhibitors. Heart transplantation is the procedure of choice for patients with severe dilated cardiomyopathy and severe symptoms. With successful transplantation, the 1-year survival is 90%. The major contraindication for transplantation in an otherwise healthy patient is a high pulmonary arteriolar resistance. In the United States, donor availability is the major limiting factor. Long-term complications after heart transplantation include rejection, infection, hypertension, hyperlipidemia, malignancy, and accelerated coronary vasculopathy.

- After symptoms are severe, 1-year mortality is 35% for patients with dilated cardiomyopathy, even with optimal medical therapy.
- Patients with asymptomatic dilated cardiomyopathy have increased mortality.
- The procedure of choice for some of these patients is heart transplantation. With successful transplantation, 1-year survival is 90%.

Recapitulation of Drug Therapy of Heart Failure
- ACE inhibitors improve symptom status and mortality in patients with symptomatic dilated cardiomyopathy.
- ACE inhibitors prevent deterioration and subsequent hospitalizations in patients with asymptomatic dilated cardiomyopathy.
- The combination of high-dose nitrates and hydralazine improves symptoms and survival (though survival benefit is less than with ACE inhibitors), but intolerance to the high doses limits their usefulness.
- Nitrates should be used with a nitrate-free interval to prevent nitrate tolerance.
- Digoxin is useful for symptomatic treatment of patients with dilated cardiomyopathy but provides no survival benefit.
- Phosphodiesterase inhibitors and prolonged infusion of dobutamine directly increase contractility and may improve symptoms transiently, but they probably increase mortality.
- β-Blockers are beneficial when given (in addition to ACE inhibitors, digoxin, and diuretics) to patients with NYHA class II-III heart failure.

HYPERTROPHIC CARDIOMYOPATHY

Etiology

Hypertrophic cardiomyopathy is a genetically and phenotypically heterogeneous family of disorders characterized by defects involving myocyte proteins with hypertrophy as a compensatory response. There is usually dynamic left ventricular outflow tract obstruction, but 20% to 40% of patients have no obstruction. The diagnosis is currently based on the echocardiographic finding of severe hypertrophy of the myocardium in the absence of a secondary cause, such as hypertension, aortic stenosis, chronic renal failure, or infiltrative disease (although in the future it will increasingly become a diagnosis made with genetic testing). Because hypertrophic cardiomyopathy is a hereditary disease, all patients should have their first-degree relatives screened, and genetic counseling is advised for potential parents.

- Hypertrophic cardiomyopathy is a heterogeneous family of disorders of myocyte proteins with compensatory myocardial hypertrophy.
- Dynamic left ventricular outflow tract obstruction occurs in 60%-80% of patients.
- Diagnosis is based on the echocardiographic finding of severe myocardial hypertrophy in the absence of a secondary cause.
- Family screening and genetic counseling are advised.

Symptoms

Hypertrophic cardiomyopathy has several different manifestations. There appears to be a bimodal age distribution of presentation. Young males (usually in the teens or early 20s) have a high propensity for syncope and sudden death. Older patients (in the 50s and 60s) present with symptoms of shortness of breath and angina and may have a better prognosis than young patients. The classic presentation of the younger group is a young athlete undergoing a physical examination to participate in sports who is found to have a heart murmur or left ventricular hypertrophy on ECG. The classic presentation of the older group is an elderly woman in whom pulmonary edema develops after noncardiac surgery and whose condition worsens with diuresis, afterload reduction, and inotropic support (all of which worsen dynamic left ventricular outflow tract obstruction). The classic symptom triad is syncope, angina, and dyspnea (symptoms similar to those of valvular aortic stenosis). Some hypertensive patients have a small hyperdynamic left ventricle with hypertrophy and dynamic left ventricular outflow tract obstruction—"hypertensive-hypertrophic cardiomyopathy." Although the pathophysiology is the same as in hypertrophic cardiomyopathy, these patients are not at increased risk for sudden death and ventricular fibrillation.

There is a 1.5% per year incidence of evolution from hypertrophic to dilated cardiomyopathy. This may reflect either the natural history or a superimposed secondary process such as ischemia. The treatment of a "burnt-out hypertroph" is then the same as that for other dilated cardiomyopathies.

- The classic presentation of hypertrophic cardiomyopathy is the triad of angina, syncope, and dyspnea.
- Bimodal distribution of presentation: young males with high incidence of sudden death and older patients with dyspnea and angina.
- Prognosis for older patients may be better than for younger patients.
- Patients with hypertension may have hypertrophy and dynamic left ventricular outflow tract obstruction similar to those of patients with hypertrophic cardiomyopathy.

Pathophysiology

Signs and symptoms of hypertrophic cardiomyopathy are caused by four major abnormalities: diastolic dysfunction, left ventricular outflow tract obstruction, mitral regurgitation, and ventricular arrhythmias.

Diastolic dysfunction is caused by many mechanisms. Severe hypertrophy and increased muscle mass produce decreased compliance so that there is increased pressure per unit volume entering the left ventricle during diastole. Marked abnormality in calcium metabolism causes abnormal ventricular relaxation. High afterload due to left ventricular tract obstruction also delays ventricular relaxation. All these events cause increased left ventricular diastolic pressure, which leads to angina and dyspnea.

In many patients, dynamic left ventricular tract obstruction is caused by the hypertrophied septum encroaching into the left ventricular outflow tract. This subsequently "sucks in" the anterior leaflet of the mitral valve (systolic anterior motion), creating left ventricular outflow tract obstruction. Because of this pathophysiologic process, dynamic outflow tract obstruction increases dramatically with decreased preload, decreased afterload, or increased contractility.

Systolic anterior motion of the mitral valve distorts the mitral valve apparatus during systole and may cause significant mitral regurgitation. The degree of mitral regurgitation is also dynamically influenced by the degree of left ventricular outflow tract obstruction. Patients with severe mitral regurgitation usually have severe symptoms of dyspnea.

Because of cellular disarray in patients with hypertrophic cardiomyopathy, the electrical conduction system is dispersed, leading to a high propensity for ventricular arrhythmias. The frequent occurrence of ventricular arrhythmias may cause sudden death or syncope.

- A major pathophysiologic abnormality in patients with hypertrophic cardiomyopathy is diastolic dysfunction.
- Left ventricular outflow tract obstruction and mitral regurgitation are caused by distortion of the mitral valve apparatus (systolic anterior motion), and they are dynamically influenced by preload, afterload, and contractility.
- The propensity for ventricular arrhythmias causing syncope and sudden death is high.

Examination

Hypertrophic cardiomyopathy is suspected on the basis of abnormal carotid artery upstroke and left ventricular impulse. The carotid artery upstroke is very rapid compared with that of patients with aortic stenosis. If left ventricular outflow tract obstruction is significant, carotid artery upstroke has a bifid quality. The left ventricular impulse is always very sustained, indicating significant left ventricular hypertrophy. It frequently has a palpable "a" wave. Patients with significant left ventricular outflow tract obstruction may have a triple apical impulse. The first heart sound is normal, and the second heart sound is paradoxically split. A loud systolic ejection murmur indicates left ventricular outflow tract obstruction. The murmur changes in intensity with changes in loading conditions (Table 3-26). A holosystolic murmur of mitral regurgitation may be present; it increases in intensity with increases in the dynamic left ventricular outflow tract obstruction. Maneuvers affect the mitral regurgitant murmur of hypertrophic obstructive cardiomyopathy differently than other mitral regurgitant murmurs. When mitral regurgitation is not due to hypertrophic obstructive cardiomyopathy, it increases with increasing afterload and varies little with changes in contractility and preload. When mitral regurgitation is due to hypertrophic cardiomyopathy, however, increased afterload decreases the dynamic left ventricular outflow obstruction and thus the amount of secondary mitral regurgitation.

In patients with hypertrophic obstructive cardiomyopathy, the ejection murmur increases in intensity, whereas the arterial pulse volume decreases on the beat following a premature ventricular contraction. This is called the Brockenbrough sign, and it is due to increased contractility and decreased afterload. In contradistinction, in patients with fixed left ventricular outflow obstruction (e.g., aortic stenosis), both the murmur intensity and the pulse volume increase with the beat following a premature contraction.

- Diagnosis of hypertrophic cardiomyopathy is suspected by palpating a sustained left ventricular impulse and rapid upstroke of the carotid artery.
- The outflow murmur intensity and carotid upstroke change with changes in loading conditions of the heart.
- In hypertrophic obstructive cardiomyopathy, the secondary

Table 3-26.—Dynamic Left Ventricular Outflow Tract Obstruction

Increased obstruction
Decreased afterload
Amyl nitrite
Vasodilators
Increased contractility
Postpremature ventricular contraction beat
Digoxin
Dopamine
Decreased preload
Squat-to-stand
Nitrates
Diuretics
Valsalva maneuver (strain phase)
Decreased obstruction
Increased afterload
Handgrip
Stand-to-squat
Decreased contractility
β-Blockers
Verapamil
Disopyramide
Increased preload
Fluids

mitral regurgitation murmur changes in the same direction as that of the left ventricular outflow obstruction murmur under different loading conditions. This differs from the auscultatory findings when mitral regurgitation is due to other conditions.

Diagnostic Testing

Patients with hypertrophic cardiomyopathy almost always have an abnormal ECG, which shows significant left ventricular hypertrophy (Fig. 3-34). Because ECG abnormalities may precede echocardiographically detected phenotypic expression, surveillance echocardiography is appropriate in patients with suspicious results of electrocardiography. Apical hypertrophic cardiomyopathy is a variant of hypertrophic cardiomyopathy in which the hypertrophy is localized at the apex of the left ventricle. Although patients with apical hypertrophic cardiomyopathy do not have outflow tract obstruction (no murmur or secondary mitral regurgitation), they do have diastolic dysfunction and a predisposition to ventricular arrhythmias. The ECG in these patients typically has large, diffuse, symmetrical T-wave inversions across the precordium (Fig. 3-35).

Hypertrophic cardiomyopathy is diagnosed with echocardiography, which shows severe hypertrophy of the myocardium

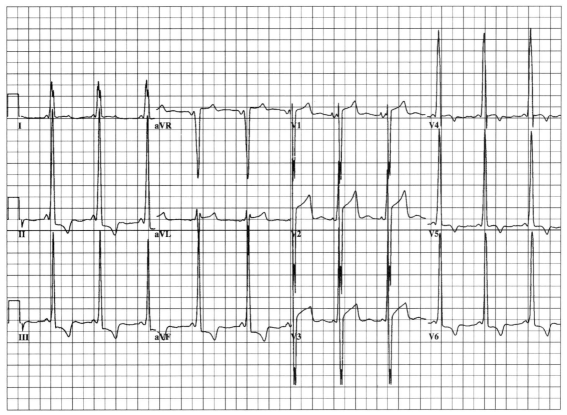

Fig. 3-34. Electrocardiogram in hypertrophic cardiomyopathy showing marked left ventricular hypertrophy.

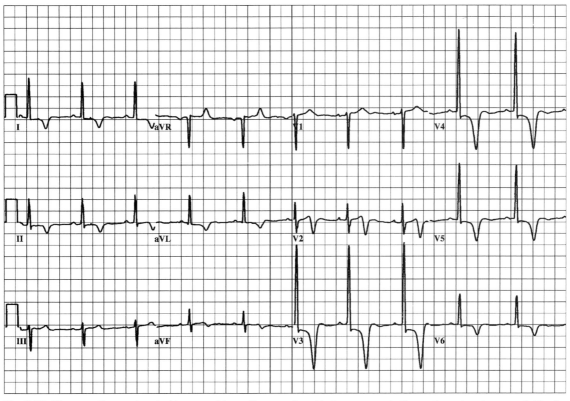

Fig. 3-35. Electrocardiogram in apical hypertrophic cardiomyopathy with deep symmetric T-wave inversions in precordial leads.

(left ventricular wall thickness >16 mm in diastole) without any known cause. Formerly, asymmetric septal hypertrophy was required for the diagnosis, but it is now recognized that hypertrophy can be in any part of the myocardium. Doppler echocardiography can be used to diagnose left ventricular outflow tract obstruction, measure its severity, and detect mitral regurgitation. Cardiac catheterization is no longer necessary for diagnosing dynamic left ventricular outflow tract obstruction because all diagnostic data can be obtained by two-dimensional and Doppler echocardiography.

Sudden death is a problem in patients with hypertrophic cardiomyopathy. Because of a strong assocation between ventricular arrhythmias and sudden death, 48- to 72-hour Holter monitoring is recommended for all patients with hypertrophic cardiomyopathy. Predictors of sudden death include a personal or family history of sudden death, left ventricular hypertrophy, ventricular tachycardia at electrophysiologic study, young male, history of syncope, and nonsustained ventricular tachycardia. Genetic markers may identify patients with a strong propensity for sudden death. In most patients, carefully supervised stress testing also is indicated to search for ventricular tachycardia, to objectify symptom threshold, and to evaluate the variables contributing to symptoms.

- ECG usually shows evidence of left ventricular hypertrophy in cases of hypertrophic cardiomyopathy.
- Apical hypertrophy is suspected by the presence of large symmetric inverted T-waves in precordial leads on ECG.
- Diagnosis of hypertrophic cardiomyopathy is made with echocardiography, which shows hypertrophy in absence of any known cause.
- Predictors of sudden death: personal or family history of sudden death, young male, history of syncope, nonsustained ventricular tachycardia, massive left ventricular hypertrophy, and sustained ventricular tachycardia at electrophysiologic study.
- 48- to 72-Hour Holter monitoring recommended for all patients with hypertrophic cardiomyopathy.

Treatment

Treatment of Symptomatic Patients

For symptomatic patients with hypertrophic cardiomyopathy, initial treatment is with drugs that decrease contractility in an attempt to decrease left ventricular outflow tract obstruction (Fig. 3-36). The most effective medication is a high dose of β-adrenergic blockers (>240 mg equivalent of propranolol/day). Although verapamil may be used if β-adrenergic blockade fails, it may cause sudden hemodynamic deterioration in patients with high resting left ventricular outflow tract gradients because of its vasodilating properties.

Disopyramide may improve symptoms by decreasing left ventricular outflow tract obstruction, but anticholinergic side effects limit its use. All drugs that reduce afterload or preload and those that increase contractility must be avoided in patients with hypertrophic cardiomyopathy. Cautious diuretic use for volume overloaded states is permitted.

Surgical myectomy is reserved for patients who are severely symptomatic despite optimal medical therapy and produces dramatic symptomatic relief. Mortality associated with this procedure is less than 5% overall in experienced centers and less than 1% in patients younger than 40 years. Its complications are rare but include complete heart block, aortic regurgitation, and ventricular septal defect. Myectomy is a highly operator-dependent procedure and should be performed only at medical centers that specialize in this procedure. Catheter ablation of the septum by alcohol infusion is an as yet experimental surrogate for the operative procedure.

Dual-chamber pacing is an accepted alternative to myectomy for patients with hypertrophic cardiomyopathy and severe left ventricular outflow tract obstruction. Dual-chamber pacing can produce a reduction in gradient and symptomatic improvement in some patients. More studies need to be completed before recommending dual-chamber pacing for *all* patients with symptomatic hypertrophic obstructive cardiomyopathy.

Whether to treat asymptomatic patients with nonsustained ventricular tachycardia is a controversial subject (Fig. 3-37). No antiarrhythmic agent is uniformly effective, and any may make the arrhythmia worse. In selected patients with multiple risk factors for sudden death, empiric amiodarone or an automatic implantable cardiac defibrillator might be chosen. In patients who have already had an out-of-hospital arrest, the treatment of choice is an automatic implantable cardiac defibrillator.

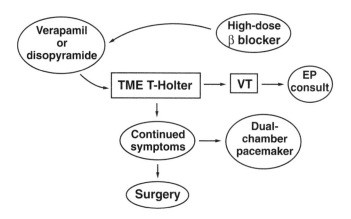

Fig. 3-36. Treatment of symptomatic patients. EP, electrophysiologic; TMET, treadmill exertion test; VT, ventricular tachycardia.

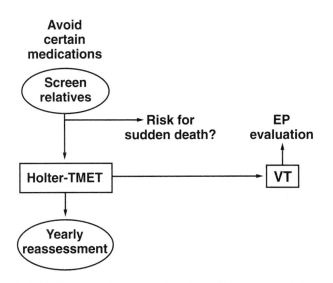

Fig. 3-37. Treatment of asymptomatic patients. Abbreviations as in Figure 3-36.

- β-Adrenergic blockade is treatment of choice for patients with symptomatic hypertrophic cardiomyopathy.
- Verapamil may cause sudden hemodynamic deterioration in patients with high resting left ventricular outflow tract obstruction.
- Surgical myectomy is reserved for severely symptomatic patients unresponsive to medical therapy.
- Dual-chamber pacing is an accepted treatment strategy, but its role relative to medical management or surgical myectomy is not known.
- No antiarrhythmic agent is uniformly effective, and any may worsen the arrhythmia.
- Automatic implantable cardiac defibrillator is treatment of choice for patients with out-of-hospital arrest.

RESTRICTIVE CARDIOMYOPATHY

Definition

The primary abnormality in restrictive cardiomyopathy is diastolic dysfunction. Diastolic dysfunction causes abnormal left ventricular filling such that a greater than usual increase in filling pressure is required to fill the ventricle. This is reflected back to the pulmonary and systemic circulations, causing symptoms of shortness of breath and edema. In addition, the ventricle cannot fill adequately to meet its preload requirements, thus resulting in low cardiac output (Starling mechanism), fatigue, and lethargy. Normal myocardial contractile function is maintained in most patients with restrictive cardiomyopathy. However, at the end stage of the disease, there can be loss of contractile function as well.

- In restrictive cardiomyopathy, primary abnormality is diastolic dysfunction.
- Diastolic dysfunction means a greater pressure per unit volume is required to fill the ventricle, causing dyspnea and edema.
- Left ventricle cannot fill to meet its preload requirements, causing low output, fatigue, and lethargy.

The cause of primary restrictive cardiomyopathy is unknown. There are two major categories: idiopathic restrictive cardiomyopathy and endomyocardial fibrosis. In idiopathic restrictive cardiomyopathy, there is progressive fibrosis of the myocardium. Familial cases, often with peripheral myopathy as well, have been reported. Endomyocardial fibrosis is probably an end stage of eosinophilic syndromes in which there is intracavitary thrombus filling of the left ventricle. This restricts filling and causes increased diastolic pressures. This fibrosis also may involve the mitral valve, causing severe mitral regurgitation. There may be two different forms of endomyocardial fibrosis: active inflammatory eosinophilic myocarditis in temperate zones and chronic endomyocardial fibrosis in tropic zones.

Diseases that cause infiltration of the myocardium (such as amyloid) have a presentation and pathophysiology similar to those of primary restrictive cardiomyopathy. Signs and symptoms similar to those of restrictive cardiomyopathy also may develop after radiation therapy, anthracycline chemotherapy, and heart transplantation. Although other infiltrative diseases (sarcoid, hemochromatosis) initially may mimic restrictive cardiomyopathy, they usually have progressed to a dilated cardiomyopathy by the time they cause cardiac symptoms.

- Restrictive cardiomyopathy may be idiopathic or due to infiltrative diseases (amyloid).
- Endomyocardial fibrosis is probably an end stage of eosinophilic syndromes.
- Secondary fibrosis may involve mitral valve, causing severe mitral regurgitation.

Signs and Symptoms

Patients with restrictive cardiomyopathy usually present with edema, dyspnea, ascites, and low output symptoms. Atrial arrhythmias due to passive atrial enlargment are frequently present, and the patient may present with atrial fibrillation. Jugular venous pressure is almost always increased, with rapid X and Y descents. The precordium is quiet, and heart sounds are soft. There may be an apical systolic murmur of mitral regurgitation and a left sternal border murmur of tricuspid regurgitation. A third heart sound may be present. Dullness at the bases of the lungs is consistent with bilateral pleural effusions. ECG is usually low or normal voltage with atrial arrhythmias. Chest radiography shows pleural effusions with normal cardiac silhouette or atrial enlargement.

- Restrictive cardiomyopathy: biventricular failure, dyspnea, edema, and low output symptoms.
- Atrial arrhythmias are frequently present.
- Jugular venous pressure is increased, with rapid X and Y descents.

Diagnosis

Restrictive cardiomyopathy is diagnosed with echocardiography. Typical findings are normal left ventricular cavity size and function and marked enlargement of both atria. If there is right heart failure, the inferior vena cava is enlarged. Echocardiography is usually nonspecific about the cause except in two instances. First, in amyloid heart disease, echocardiography demonstrates thickened myocardium with a scintillating appearance as well as pericardial effusion and thickened regurgitant valves. Second, in endomyocardial fibrosis, there is an apical thrombus (without underlying apical akinesis) or thickening of the endocardium under the mitral valve, which often tethers the valve, causing mitral regurgitation. Cardiac catheterization shows elevation and end-equalization of all end-diastolic pressures. A typical "square-root sign" or "dip and plateau" pattern consistent with early rapid filling is present. Endomyocardial biopsy usually is not helpful unless there is a systemic disease that has caused infiltration of the myocardium (i.e., amyloid).

- Restrictive cardiomyopathy is diagnosed with echocardiography.
- Typical findings: normal left ventricular cavity size and function and marked enlargement of both atria.
- Amyloid heart disease: thickened myocardium with scintillating appearance, pericardial effusion, valvular regurgitation.
- Endomyocardial fibrosis: thrombus in left ventricular apex (without apical akinesis) or posterior mitral leaflet tethering causing mitral regurgitation.

Treatment

There is no medical treatment for idiopathic restrictive cardiomyopathy. Diuretics decrease filling pressures and give symptomatic relief, but this may be at the expense of further decreasing cardiac output. Digoxin usually is not helpful, because systolic contractility is maintained. Heart transplantation is the only proven therapy for patients with severe restrictive cardiomyopathy. Corticosteroids and cytotoxic drugs are appropriate during the early stages of eosinophilic endocarditis. Endomyocardial fibrosis can be surgically resected and the mitral valve can be replaced, although mortality is significant.

- There is no medical treatment for idiopathic restrictive cardiomyopathy.
- Diuretics decrease filling pressures.
- Digoxin usually is not helpful.
- Heart transplantation is only proven therapy.
- Medical therapy is used for early stages of eosinophilic endocarditis, and operation is used for endomyocardial fibrosis in selected cases.

It is important to differentiate restrictive cardiomyopathy from constrictive pericarditis. Both have similar presentations and findings on clinical examination and diagnostic studies. However, in constrictive pericarditis, pericardiectomy produces symptomatic improvement and, frequently, survival. Therefore, exploratory thoracotomy may be indicated in patients with normal left ventricular systolic function, large atria, and severe elevation of diastolic filling pressures if doubt remains after anatomic (fast computed tomography) and other tests (fast computed tomography, echocardiography, cardiac catheterization).

- It is important to differentiate restrictive cardiomyopathy from constrictive pericarditis.
- In constrictive pericarditis, pericardiectomy produces symptomatic improvement and may prolong survival.

QUESTIONS

Multiple Choice (choose the one best answer)

1. A 58-year-old woman with known rheumatic valve disease has been followed by you for the last 3 years. During her most recent visit she does not describe any change in symptoms, but on physical examination you notice the absence of the previously noted opening snap. Which of the following physical signs would *not* be expected to accompany such a finding?
   a. Increased jugular venous pulse compared with that in previous examination
   b. Accentuated right ventricular lift
   c. Accentuated carotid upstroke
   d. Accentuated "a" wave in the jugular venous pulse
   e. Diastolic rumble

2. A 40-year-old previously healthy man presents to the emergency room with an episode of right-sided numbness. He has not seen a physician for the past 10 years and denies any previous medical history. Physical examination reveals a 3/6 systolic and 2/6 diastolic murmur suggestive of mild combined aortic valve disease. Which of the following examinations may yield the underlying pathophysiologic mechanism most expeditiously?
   a. An eye examination
   b. Echocardiography
   c. Head computed tomography
   d. Electrocardiography
   e. Examination of peripheral pulses

3. A patient is referred to you because of the possibility of significant aortic stenosis. Which of the following physical findings would make you question this diagnosis?
   a. Carotid upstroke significantly parvus and tardus
   b. The arterial or central pulse is bisferiens
   c. Displaced and forceful apical impulse
   d. Presence of the A_2 component of the second heart sound
   e. A late peaking systolic murmur, followed by a 3/6 diastolic murmur

4. Which of the following statements is true?
   a. A loud first heart sound is often noted in severe calcific mitral stenosis
   b. A third heart sound in a young patient suggests aortic valve disease due to a bicuspid aortic valve
   c. A fourth heart sound indicates systolic dysfunction
   d. The loss of an opening snap in a patient with known mitral valve disease is suggestive of a reduction in the mitral valve gradient
   e. The preservation of the A component of the second heart sound suggests mild rather than severe aortic stenosis

5. A 28-year-old woman complains of atypical chest pain. On auscultation of the heart, you notice a brief 2/6 systolic murmur at the apex. Which of the following maneuvers or phenomena points to organic mitral regurgitation rather than mitral valve prolapse?
   a. Carotid sinus massage
   b. Handgrip with an increase in murmur loudness
   c. Valsalva maneuver with an increase in the murmur loudness
   d. Squatting leads to a decrease in the murmur intensity
   e. A decrease in the murmur after an extrasystole

6. A 36-year-old patient with Hodgkin disease treated 10 years ago develops shortness of breath. Which of the following signs would *not* be expected?
   a. Angina
   b. Peripheral edema
   c. Loud systolic murmur
   d. Three-component murmur
   e. Fatigue

7. Which of the following patients with amyloidosis is most likely *not* to have cardiac involvement?
   a. A 74-year-old man with insidious onset of dyspnea
   b. A 40-year-old woman with a family history of early death from congestive heart failure
   c. A 50-year-old patient having chronic dialysis as a result of chronic renal failure
   d. A 37-year-old patient with amyloidosis of the tongue, kidney, and liver
   e. A 52-year-old man with increased pre-albumin

8. Which of the following statements is correct regarding prosthetic valves?
   a. The older the patient, the faster calcification occurs in bioprosthetic valves
   b. Tissue valves last longer in the mitral than aortic position
   c. Tissue valves are resistant to systemic carcinoid disease due to special coating
   d. Mechanical valves have a longer durability
   e. Hemolysis most often occurs because of malfunction of mechanical valve prosthesis

9. Determination of the left ventricular ejection fraction is the most commonly used test to characterize left ventricular function. Which of the following statements is true?
   a. Contrast ventriculography is the most accurate method to determine the left ventricular ejection fraction

b. First-pass radionuclide angiography relies on certain assumptions about the shape of the left ventricle and the contraction pattern

c. Magnetic resonance imaging (MRI) is faster than electron beam computed tomography (EBCT) for acquiring the images

d. All of the above answers are correct

e. None of the above answers are correct

10. You are asked to see a 64-year-old patient for preoperative evaluation. He is scheduled to undergo laparoscopic cholecystectomy. Four years ago, he had an inferior myocardial infarction, followed by triple-bypass surgery. He has remained symptom-free since the surgery and exercises 30 minutes on a stationary bicycle 5 times a week, but he still has several cardiac risk factors, including a low high-density lipoprotein cholesterol value of 34 mg/dL, an increased low-density lipoprotein cholesterol value of 156 mg/dL, and a strong family history of coronary artery disease. What would you recommend as further workup?

a. No further workup, patient cleared for surgery

b. A blood pool radionuclide angiogram to determine the left ventricular function (ejection fraction)

c. An echocardiogram to assess left ventricular function and regional wall motion abnormalities

d. Stress thallium test to assess the degree of ischemia

e. Coronary angiography with left ventriculography

11. Which of the following physical findings is not usually associated with secundum atrial septal defect in young patients?

a. Systolic ejection murmur

b. Diastolic rumble that increases with inspiration

c. Fixed split of second heart sound

d. Third heart sound

e. Right ventricular lift or heave

12. Which of the following statements is true?

a. Secundum atrial septal defect (ASD) is usually associated with anomalous pulmonary venous return

b. Sinus venosus ASD is usually associated with a cleft mitral valve

c. Secundum ASD does not require antibiotic prophylaxis

d. In most patients with ASD, atrial fibrillation will not develop until the 8th decade

13. What is the most common adult congenital heart disease?

a. Secundum atrial septal defect

b. Patent ductus arteriosus

c. Bicuspid aortic valve

d. Ventricular septal defect

14. A 15-year-old patient with Down syndrome presents with increasing dyspnea on exertion and fatigue. Physical examination shows a slight sternal lift, a widely split S_2 (no appreciable movement of split with respiration), a grade 3/6 holosystolic murmur (radiates across the axilla), and a soft, long apical diastolic rumble. Electrocardiography shows sinus rhythm, a PR interval of 240 ms, left-axis deviation, and a right bundle branch block. Chest radiography suggests left atrial and right ventricular enlargement. What is the most likely diagnosis?

a. Restrictive (small) ventricular septal defect

b. Secundum atrial septal defect

c. Primum atrial septal defect

d. Primum atrioventricular septal defect with a cleft mitral valve

15. A 35-year-old man is referred for evaluation of long-standing hypertension. Examination shows grade 3/6 systolic ejection murmur. Electrocardiography shows left ventricular hypertrophy with strain. Echocardiography suggests bicuspid aortic valve and confirms ventricular hypertrophy (without significant stenosis or regurgitation). What is the next most appropriate step?

a. Refer the patient for magnetic resonance imaging of thoracic aorta

b. Treatment with β-adrenergic blocker

c. Reassurance and follow-up in 5 years

d. Genetic counseling

16. Which of the following requires antibiotic prophylaxis?

a. A patient with secundum atrial septal defect having a dental extraction

b. A patient with ligated patent ductus arteriosus having dental extraction

c. A patient with click and murmur consistent with mitral valve prolapse having a dental extraction

d. A patient with bicuspid aortic valve having transesophageal echocardiography

17. A 45-year-old woman has a large ventricular septal defect and Eisenmenger syndrome. All of the findings would be expected *except*:

a. Loud P_2

b. Loud systolic murmur

c. Cyanosis

d. Decrescendo diastolic murmur

e. Hemoglobin value of 19 mg/dL

18. All of the following associations are correct *except*:

a. Noonan syndrome and pulmonary stenosis

b. Down syndrome and primum atrioventricular septal defect

   c. Coarctation and Turner syndrome

   d. Down syndrome and mitral valve prolapse

19. A 44-year-old father of two young children presents with a 6-month history of dyspnea, leg edema, orthopnea, paroxysmal and nocturnal dyspnea, and carpal tunnel syndrome. An echocardiogram obtained elsewhere shows a massive increase in left ventricular wall thickness (especially in the septum), thickening of all four cardiac valves, a small pericardial effusion, restrictive physiology in the diastolic filling pattern, and an inducible gradient in the outflow tract of 40 mm Hg. On the basis of this echocardiogram, his physician started therapy with atenolol, 100 mg orally twice a day. However, his symptoms progressed over the ensuing weeks and he presents now for a second opinion. The electrocardiogram is shown. The most likely diagnosis is:

   a. Hypertrophic cardiomyopathy

   b. Amyloidosis/restrictive cardiomyopathy

   c. Neither

   d. Both

20. A 40-year-old woman presents with a history of carcinoid heart disease. All of the following features might be found on physical examination *except*:

   a. Prominent "v" wave in jugular venous wave profile

   b. Holosystolic murmur that increases with inspiration

   c. Diminished carotid upstrokes

   d. Pulsatile liver

21. What is the most common mechanism for cardiac arrhythmias?

   a. Abnormal automaticity

   b. Triggered activity

   c. Atrial fibrillation

   d. Reentry

   e. Parasystole

22. Which of the following conditions or drugs does not enhance automaticity?

   a. Increased sympathetic tone

   b. Increased parasympathetic tone

   c. Ischemia

   d. Isoproterenol

23. A 45-year-old woman has occasional (4 episodes in 6 months) palpitations lasting up to 10 minutes. During each episode, she experiences heart pounding, diaphoresis, and chest tightness. She is otherwise very active and does not have any history of cardiac disease. Which of the following tests may provide the best diagnostic approach?

   a. Holter monitoring

   b. Treadmill exercise test

   c. Transtelephonic event recorder

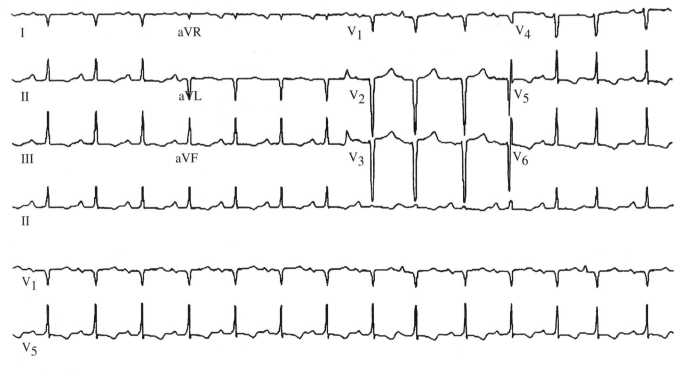

Question 19

d. Electrophysiologic testing
e. Coronary angiography

24. Which of the following variables is not associated with increased risk of ventricular arrhythmia?
    a. Increased heart rate variability
    b. Presence of nonsustained ventricular tachycardia or Holter monitoring
    c. Presence of late potentials on signal-averaged ECG
    d. Inducible ventricular tachycardia during electrophysiologic testing

25. A 65-year-old man has experienced two syncopal episodes in the last week. Both episodes occurred without warning and lasted 2 to 3 minutes, with immediate recovery. His medical history is significant for coronary artery disease and myocardial infarction, with an ejection fraction of 30%. What is the most appropriate diagnostic evaluation?
    a. Computed tomography of head
    b. Carotid ultrasonography
    c. Holter monitoring
    d. Electrophysiologic testing
    e. Transtelephonic event recording

26. Permanent pacemaker therapy is clearly indicated in which one of the following conditions?
    a. A 3-second pause recorded on cardiac monitoring while the patient was starting amiodarone therapy for paroxysmal atrial fibrillation
    b. Resting heart rate of 40 beats/min in an asymptomatic 70-year-old man with known coronary disease
    c. Presyncope and syncope in a 75-year-old woman with Parkinson disease and orthostatic hypotension
    d. Intermittent 3° atrioventricular block in a 50-year-old woman with near syncope

27. In the setting of renal insufficiency, dosing should be adjusted in which of the following drugs?
    a. Amiodarone
    b. Sotalol
    c. Propafenone
    d. Lidocaine

28. Which of the following drugs is least effective in maintaining sinus rhythm in patients with paroxysmal atrial fibrillation?
    a. Quinidine
    b. Lidocaine
    c. Sotalol
    d. Amiodarone
    e. Propafenone

29. Which of the following statements is correct?
    a. Suppression of premature ventricular complexes (PVCs) results in improved survival
    b. Suppression of PVCs decreases the risk of sudden cardiac death
    c. Class IC antiarrhythmic agents are effective in suppressing PVCs and nonsustained ventricular tachycardia but increase mortality in patients with coronary artery disease and previous myocardial infarction
    d. Amiodarone should routinely be given to patients with frequent PVCs and nonsustained ventricular tachycardia

30. A 25-year-old man has recurrent palpitations correlated with a regular narrow complex tachycardia at a rate of 200 beats/min. He has been intolerant of β-blockers and calcium channel blockers in the past. What is the most appropriate therapeutic approach at this time?
    a. Continue observation
    b. Antitachycardia pacemaker
    c. Electrophysiologic evaluation and ablation
    d. Defibrillator implantation
    e. Amiodarone

31. A 78-year-old man describes having had several dizzy spells over the past few weeks. He also passed out once suddenly without warning. He has no previous history of cardiac disease, takes no medications, and has been active walking several miles a day with no symptoms of breathlessness or chest pain. Holter monitoring was performed and a rhythm strip during an episode of dizziness is shown in the figure. The appropriate next step is:
    a. Arrange for permanent pacemaker implantation
    b. Perform an electrophysiologic study
    c. Perform coronary angiography
    d. Perform a treadmill exercise test
    e. None of the above

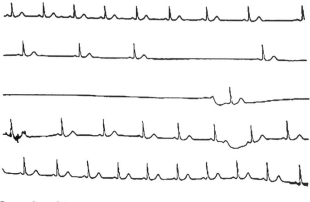

Question 31

32. A 24-year-old pregnant woman is admitted to the hospital for dehydration after protracted morning sickness. While the patient is being monitored, the rhythm shown in the figure is noted. You are consulted. The next appropriate step would be:
    a. Observation
    b. Immediate placement of a temporary pacemaker
    c. Implantation of a permanent pacemaker
    d. Infusion of aminophylline
    e. Emergency echocardiography

33. All the following suggest the diagnosis of ventricular tachycardia *except* for:
    a. P waves that "march through" the QRS complexes
    b. Right bundle branch block pattern with R' taller than R (i.e., rsR' pattern)
    c. Northwest axis (axis between -90° and -180°)
    d. A different QRS morphology in patients with preexisting bundle branch block
    e. A history of structural heart disease

34. A 56-year-old man complained of palpitations. The electrocardiographic results are shown in the figure. Which of the following statements is true?
    a. Adenosine terminates this rhythm
    b. For successful cardioversion, 200 J or more are required
    c. Radio-frequency ablation is more than 90% effective
    d. Propafenone has no effect on this rhythm
    e. β-Blockers are not effective for the control of the ventricular heart rate

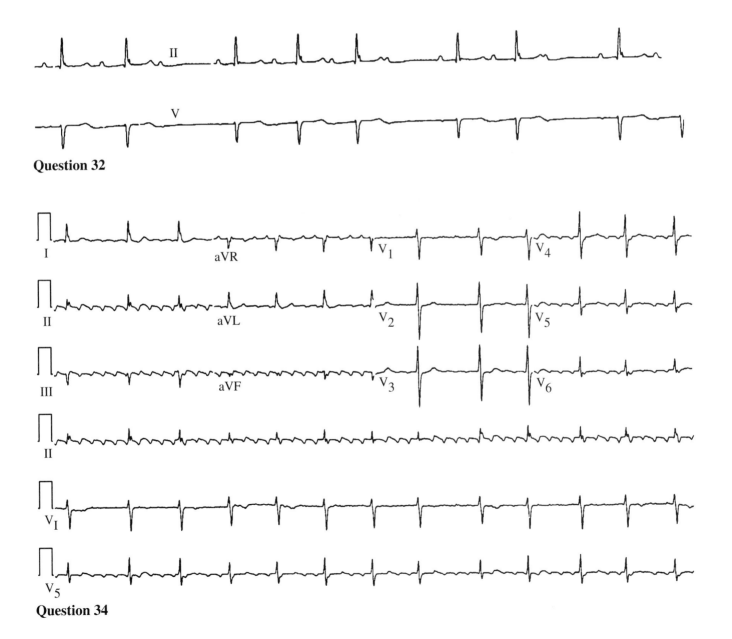

Question 32

Question 34

35. A patient has had palpitations for 8 days. The electrocardiographic results are shown. Which of the following is *not* a risk factor in this patient for stroke?
    a. Hypertension
    b. Previous cerebrovascular accident
    c. An ejection fraction of 30%
    d. Female gender, age older than 75 years
    e. All are risk factors

36. For the patient in question 35, which of the following is *not* an appropriate course of action?
    a. Check electrolytes and thyroid function
    b. Begin warfarin treatment, and plan on cardioversion in 1 month
    c. Begin β-blocker therapy
    d. Begin heparin infusion, and immediately perform cardioversion
    e. All of above

37. A 64-year-old man who had a myocardial infarction 4 years ago generally has been well. At 10:00 a.m. this morning, he developed palpitations while hunting. He walked 1 mile to his car and drove himself to the emergency room, where electrocardiography was performed (see figure). He has had no chest pain or shortness of breath and feels mildly dizzy. His blood pressure is 95/70 mm Hg and the pulse is rapid and regular. Which of the following is true?
    a. Cannon A waves are *not* present on examination
    b. Adenosine is the treatment of choice
    c. Immediate cardioversion is required
    d. Lidocaine infusion is appropriate therapy
    e. Ventricular tachycardia is not present because a pulse is palpable

38. A 28-year-old woman with no history of cardiac disease was sitting in class when she felt the sudden onset of palpitations and marked dizziness. The episode lasted for 1 hour. The symptoms subsided spontaneously. The next day, electrocardiography was performed (see figure). The appropriate next step is:
    a. Reassure the patient
    b. Perform an exercise treadmill test
    c. Perform a tilt table test
    d. Perform an electrophysiologic study
    e. Perform coronary angiography

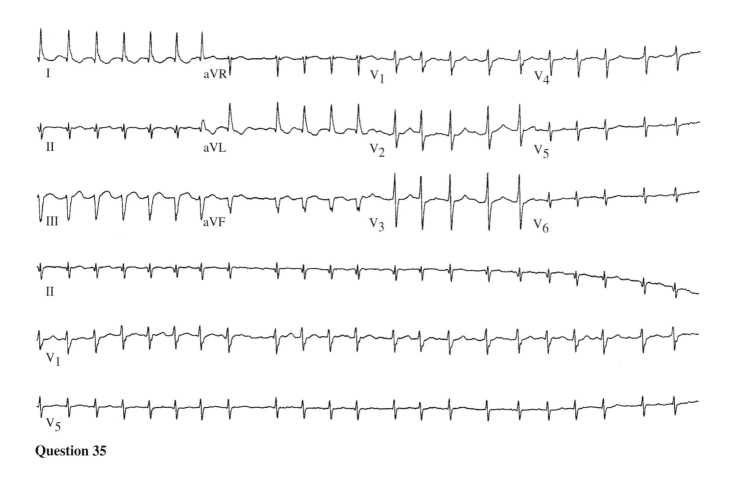

Question 35

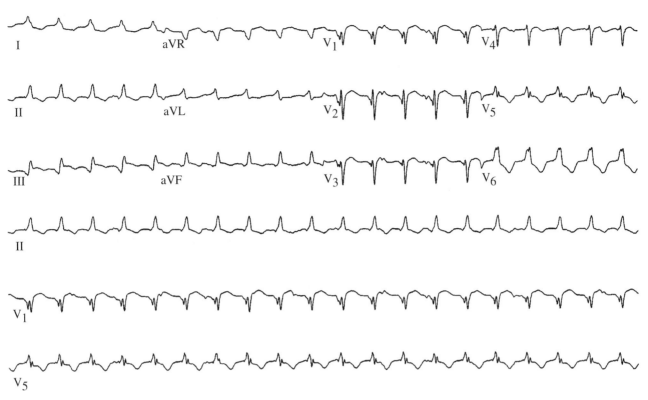

Question 37

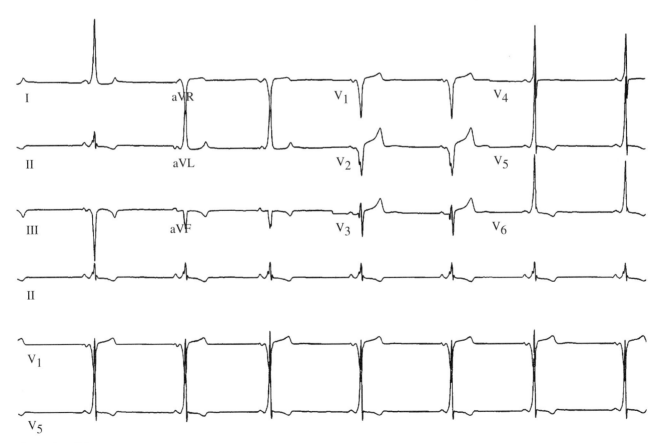

Question 38

39. A 26-year-old medical student was observing a cesarean section when he began to feel warm, clammy, and nauseated, and then he lost consciousness. He came to promptly and felt embarrassed, weak, and "washed out" for the next several hours. There are no focal neurologic deficits. The results of physical examination and electrocardiography are normal. The appropriate next step is:
   a. Reassure the patient
   b. Perform a tilt table test
   c. Perform an electrophysiologic study
   d. Perform computed tomography of head and electroencephalography
   e. Perform a treadmill exercise test

40. A 45-year-old man suddenly developed palpitations, chest heaviness, and difficulty breathing. He came to the emergency department and electrocardiography was performed (see figure). All of the following are true *except:*
   a. Carotid sinus massage or Valsalva maneuvers frequently terminate the arrhythmia
   b. Adenosine terminates the arrhythmia
   c. Lidocaine terminates the arrhythmia
   d. β-Blocker therapy is effective for the long-term management of this arrhythmia
   e. Radio-frequency ablation is effective for the long term

41. A 65-year-old man presents with 4 hours of severe chest pain. Electrocardiography shows ST-segment elevations in V_1-V_4. What is the most likely cause of his problem?
   a. Coronary spasm
   b. Coronary embolism
   c. Increased MVo_2 demand
   d. Coronary dissection
   e. Plaque rupture

42. A 65-year-old man who had a myocardial infarction 2 years earlier presents with depression. He has no symptoms of angina. His blood pressure is 120/70 mm Hg and his pulse is 60. His total cholesterol is 220 and LDL is 130. He exercises daily, is at his ideal weight, and follows a low-fat diet. The only medication he takes is aspirin. What should be done?
   a. Continued observation
   b. Start treatment with a "statin"
   c. Start treatment with a "resin"
   d. Start treatment with a β-blocker
   e. Echocardiography

43. A 50-year-old man presents with 2 hours of typical angina pectoris at rest. He has had a myocardial infarction. Examination findings include pulse, 90; blood pressure, 105/70 mm Hg; jugular venous pressure, 12 cm H_2O; and a soft S_3. Electrocardiography shows ST-segment depression in V_3-V_6. Which of the following is the best therapy at this time?
   a. Metoprolol 5 mg IV x 3
   b. Streptokinase 1 million U over 1 hour
   c. Diltiazem CD 180 mg orally
   d. Enalapril 5 mg IV over 10 minutes
   e. IV NTG to decrease blood pressure to less than 100 mm Hg

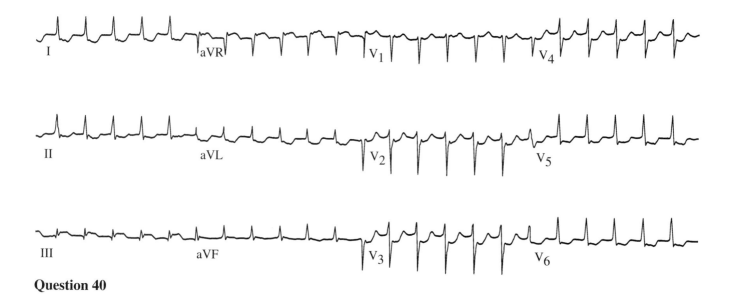

Question 40

44. A 28-year-old internal medicine resident presents with sharp stabbing chest pain at rest before taking a board examination. He has no risk factors for coronary artery disease, and the physical examination and electrocardiographic findings are normal. On a treadmill exercise test, he goes 10 minutes but has a 1-mm flat ST-segment depression in lead V_5. Which of the following is the next best thing to do?
    a. Dobutamine echocardiography
    b. Coronary angiography
    c. Adenosine thallium scan
    d. Reassurance only
    e. Exercise multiple-gated acquisition scanning (MUGA)

45. In which of the following patients would coronary artery bypass grafting prolong life?
    a. A 74-year-old man with stable angina and an ejection fraction of 30%, 80% stenosis of mid-left anterior descending artery, 70% stenosis of right coronary artery, and 70% stenosis of circumflex coronary artery
    b. A 62-year-old woman with stable angina and an ejection fraction of 60%, 90% stenosis of mid-left anterior descending artery, 30% stenosis of right coronary artery, and 40% stenosis of circumflex coronary artery
    c. A 55-year-old man with a recent anterior MI, ejection fraction of 40%, 95% stenosis of mid-left anterior descending artery, and minimal right coronary artery and circumflex coronary artery disease
    d. A 46-year-old man with unstable angina and ejection fraction of 50%, 99% stenosis of mid-left anterior descending artery, and 99% stenosis of right coronary artery
    e. None of the above

46. For a patient with a high-grade lesion of the mid-left anterior descending artery and stable class II angina, which of the following is true?
    a. Percutaneous transluminal coronary angioplasty (PTCA) should be done to prevent myocardial infarction
    b. PTCA should be done to prolong life
    c. Coronary artery bypass grafting should be done to prevent myocardial infarction
    d. Restenosis with PTCA can be reduced with aspirin
    e. PTCA and medical therapy are comparable for the hard end points of death and myocardial infarction

47. Which of the following interventions has not been found to reduce mortality and/or prevent myocardial infarction in a 60-year-old man with a previous myocardial infarction, stable exertional angina, a low-density lipoprotein level of 160 mg/dL, an ejection fraction of 40% and a 90% stenosis of the right coronary artery with an occluded circumflex artery.
    a. Percutaneous transluminal coronary angioplasty and stent
    b. A "statin"
    c. Aspirin
    d. Angiotensin-converting enzyme inhibitor
    e. None of the above

48. Which is the earliest manifestation of myocardial ischemia?
    a. Contraction abnormalities
    b. Angina pectoris
    c. Relaxation abnormalities
    d. ST-segment depression
    e. Elevated left ventricular end-diastolic pressure

49. A 65-year-old man presents with 4 hours of chest pain and a 3-mm ST-segment elevation in the inferior leads. Heart rate is 80 beats/min and blood pressure is 140/90 mm Hg. Which of the following should not be given?
    a. Aspirin, 325 mg
    b. Lopressor, 5 mg IV x 3
    c. Diltiazem, 60 mg orally
    d. Streptokinase, 1 million U over 90 minutes
    e. Heparin, 5,000-U bolus and a drip

50. A 44-year-old man presents with an inferior myocardial infarction that occurred 2 days earlier. He now has progressive hypotension, tachycardia, and oliguria. On physical examination, jugular venous pressure is 18 cm H_2O and the lung fields are clear. Which of the following should *not* be done?
    a. Furosemide given IV
    b. 2D-echocardiography
    c. V_{4R} electrocardiography
    d. Fluids given IV
    e. Low dose of dopamine

51. A 63-year-old man is seen in the office because of subacutely worsening dyspnea on exertion. He has idiopathic dilated cardiomyopathy with an ejection fraction of 35%. He had stable New York Heart Association (NYHA) class II symptoms until approximately 1 month previously; he now has a productive cough as well as dyspnea at 1 block or 1 flight of stairs. He denies chest pain, use of over-the-counter medications, or change in sodium, fluid, or alcohol intake. He has been compliant with his chronic regimen of enalapril and furosemide. Examination reveals a pulse of 92 beats per minute with frequent premature beats, blood pressure 126/80 mm Hg, and a normal jugular venous

pressure. There is a sustained, enlarged apical impulse, paradoxical splitting of the second heart sound, and a third heart sound. The lungs are clear to auscultation. There is no hepatomegaly or peripheral edema. Which of the following is the most appropriate next step?

a. Treadmill exercise test with tomographic thallium scintigraphy
b. Electrocardiography and chest radiography
c. Refer for coronary angiography
d. Begin therapy with carvedilol and slowly titrate the dose upward every 2 weeks as tolerated
e. Substitute lisinopril for enalapril

52. A previously healthy 68-year-old woman presents to the office with recent onset of dyspnea on exertion but no other symptoms. Examination reveals a heart rate of 150 beats per minute and blood pressure of 110/70 mm Hg. The jugular venous pressure is normal; the carotid arteries are low volume. The apex is displaced and enlarged. There is a gallop but no murmur. Chest radiography shows cardiomegaly with clear lung fields. Electrocardiography shows atrial flutter with 2:1 block and a normal QRS morphology. Echocardiography shows left ventricular enlargement and an ejection fraction of 25%. All of the following are appropriate except:

a. Schedule dipyridamole-technetium tomographic perfusion scanning
b. Begin digoxin therapy, 0.25 mg/day
c. Begin captopril therapy, 6.25 mg three times a day
d. Begin warfarin therapy
e. Electrical cardioversion on an outpatient basis the next day

53. A 58-year-old man presents in the office with light-headedness. He has known ischemic left ventricular dysfunction and an ejection fraction of 27%. A month previously he had his regular checkup and was doing well with digoxin (0.25 mg/day), furosemide (40 mg/day), and lisinopril (10 mg/day). Two weeks previously he was seen in the emergency room because of peripheral edema and a 5-pound weight gain. At that time, his furosemide dosage was increased to 40 mg twice a day. Three days ago he was seen in the outpatient clinic because of fatigue. His lisinopril dose was increased to 20 mg/day. Now he has light-headedness intermittently during the day but he denies chest pain, dyspnea on exertion, or edema. Supine blood pressure is 100/70 mm Hg and pulse is 64 beats per minute. Upright he becomes dizzy and the blood pressure is 70/40 mm Hg while the pulse increases to 80 beats per minute. The jugular veins are not visualized, the lungs are clear, and there is no edema. There is a third heart sound but no

murmurs. The most appropriate next step would be:
a. Decrease the lisinopril dose to 10 mg/day and follow up in 3 days
b. Order echocardiography
c. Discontinue the use of furosemide and follow up in 2 weeks
d. Decrease the furosemide dose to 40 mg/day and follow up in 3 days
e. Refer the patient to an otorhinolaryngologist for electronystagmography and consideration of canalith repositioning

54. The digoxin dosage should empirically be halved with the initiation of which one of the following drugs?
a. Disopyramide
b. Amiodarone
c. Flecainide
d. Sotalol
e. Propafenone

55. A 60-year-old man is referred because of newly diagnosed nonobstructive hypertrophic cardiomyopathy. He has no symptoms, but a murmur was heard on a work physical examination and echocardiography showed concentric severe left ventricular hypertrophy, an ejection fraction of 65%, and mild mitral regurgitation. He has no personal or family history of cardiac disease and he is not receiving any medications. His examination reveals a blood pressure of 150/85 mm Hg and a pulse of 80 beats per minute. There is no jugular venous distention, the carotid upstroke is normal, the apical impulse is normal, and there are no gallops. There is a II/VI apical holosystolic murmur in addition to a short III/VI systolic ejection murmur along the left sternal border. After a premature beat, the intensity of the ejection murmur increases. Chest radiography is normal. The electrocardiogram is shown. You would next recommend which of the following?
a. Blood and urine immunoelectrophoresis
b. Genetic counseling
c. β-Adrenergic blocker therapy
d. 24-Hour Holter monitoring
e. 48-Hour Holter monitoring

56. A 42-year-old woman with hypertrophic obstructive cardiomyopathy is hospitalized because of increasing dyspnea and orthopnea. She had been stable for years while receiving metoprolol, 100 mg twice a day. Recently your partner increased her metoprolol dosage to 150 mg twice a day because of dyspnea. She felt worse and now is admitted from the emergency room. Examination reveals mild dyspnea at rest, blood pressure of 130/85 mm Hg,

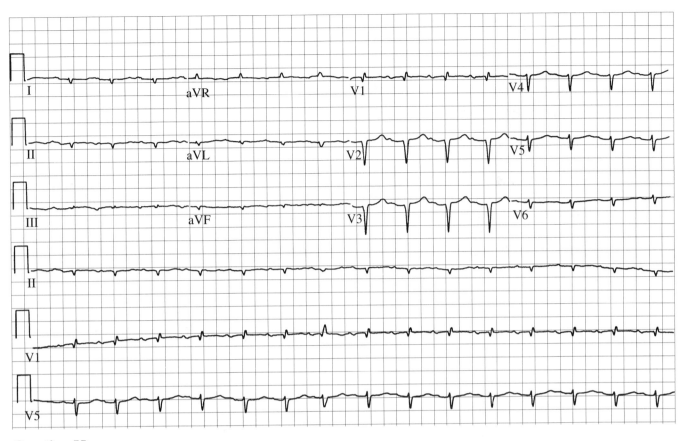

Question 55

pulse 60 beats per minute, mild expiratory wheezing, and bibasilar crackles. The carotid upstrokes are hyperdynamic and bifid. The apex is sustained. There is a harsh III/VI systolic ejection murmur at the base and a III/VI holosystolic murmur at the apex. A soft third heart sound is present. The electrocardiogram shows atrial fibrillation with a ventricular rate of 59 beats per minute. Chest radiography shown pulmonary venous hypertension with a small right pleural effusion. Which of the following is *not* an appropriate next step.

a. Reduce the metoprolol dosage to 100 mg twice a day, begin oral theophylline and inhaled steroid therapy, and dismiss with outpatient follow-up in 3 days

b. Order echocardiography to assess the left ventricle and mitral valve

c. Begin intravenous heparin therapy

d. Order a single dose of furosemide, 20 mg intravenously

e. Reduce the metoprolol dosage to 100 mg twice a day

57. A 48-year- old woman has chronic mild dyspnea on exertion and was hospitalized elsewhere 3 months earlier because of severe dyspnea and peripheral edema. She was treated in the intensive care unit for 24 hours for heart failure and responded well to intravenous diuretics. Data from a pulmonary artery catheter at that time revealed the following data at initial placement:

Cardiac index 2.8 L/min per m^2
Right ventricle 43/17 mm Hg
Pulmonary capillary wedge pressure 18 mm Hg
Right atrium 18 mm Hg
Pulmonary artery 41/22 mm Hg

Her ejection fraction by radionuclide angiography was 63%, and the electrocardiogram and myocardial enzyme values were normal. Currently, she has dyspnea at 1 flight of stairs, sleeps with two pillows because of reflux symptoms, and has moderate ankle edema. Her past medical history is notable for Hodgkin disease treated with mantle radiation when she was 19 years old, a breast biopsy negative for malignancy at age 41, and hypertriglyceridemia. Her current medications are furosemide, 40 mg/day; potassium chloride, 20 mEq/day; gemfibrozil, 600 mg twice a day; and an estrogen/progesterone combination. She smokes one pack of cigarettes per day but wishes to stop. Examination reveals a blood pressure of 115/80 mm Hg, pulse 84 beats per minute, and jugular venous distention with prominent descents. Examination of the heart, lungs, and abdomen is normal. There is moderate bilateral pitting edema. Chest radiography shows upper normal heart size, small bilateral pleural effusion, and prominent pulmonary venous vascularity. The electrocardiogram is normal. The creatinine is 0.8 mg/dL, and the potassium level is 4.1 mg/dL. All of the following are appropriate *except:*

a. Echocardiography
b. Cine computed tomography of the chest
c. Refer for coronary angiography and right ventricular biopsy
d. Increase the furosemide dosage to 40 mg twice a day and double the potassium chloride dose
e. Arrange an appointment for the patient with the local nicotine dependence multidisciplinary clinic

58. Which of the following *decreases* outflow tract obstruction in patients with hypertrophic obstructive cardiomyopathy?

a. Change from a squat to stand position
b. Disopyramide
c. Digoxin
d. Amyl nitrite inhalation
e. Isosorbide dinitrate

59. Which of the following statements about digoxin use is *true*?

a. It is a better inotrope in nonischemic than in ischemic cardiomyopathy
b. It provides no benefit to patients with left ventricular dysfunction who are in sinus rhythm
c. The most common manifestation of digitalis toxicity is visual blurring
d. The DIG trial demonstrated a survival benefit in patients

with left ventricular dysfunction who received digoxin instead of placebo
e. Digoxin decreases the likelihood that patients with left ventricular dysfunction will be admitted to the hospital because of congestive heart failure

60. An 82-year-old woman is referred for evaluation and management of congestive heart failure. She has chronically reduced mobility due to her age and diffuse degenerative joint disease. She has a 1-month history of bilateral lower extremity edema that improved only minimally with an outpatient trial of hydrochlorothiazide and triameterene. She was hospitalized briefly and her edema resolved with bed rest and furosemide. After dismissal, however, the edema has returned despite furosemide use (40 mg twice a day). She denies dyspnea (in the setting of minimal activity), orthopnea, or paroxysmal nocturnal dyspnea. Examination reveals an elderly woman in no distress. Her heart rate is 72 beats per minute and regular, blood pressure is 140/75 mm Hg, and the jugular venous pressure is low. The precordium is quiet, heart sounds are distant, and there are neither murmurs nor gallops. There is moderate bilateral, symmetric pitting edema of the feet, ankles, and calves. The electrocardiogram is normal. Chest radiography shows normal heart size and pulmonary vascularity. Which of the following is the most appropriate next step?

a. Ultrasound evaluation of the leg veins
b. Double the furosemide dose
c. Radionuclide angiography (MUGA scan) to measure ejection fraction
d. Ventilation-perfusion scan
e. Begin angiotensin-converting enzyme inhibitor therapy

ANSWERS

1. Answer c.

The "new" absence of the opening snap indicates progressive calcification of the mitral valve and thus progression of the mitral stenosis. This would lead to increased pulmonary pressure; that is, answers a, b, and d correspond with an increase in pulmonary pressure, which is common in worsening mitral stenosis. The diastolic rumble, a murmur that increases in loudness with an increase in the gradient between the left atrium and ventricle, would intensify. Because the mitral stenosis impedes left ventricular filling, the output will likely diminish, leading to a "parvus" carotid pulse, not an accentuation.

2. Answer e.

This case should evoke a stepwise logical approach. This young patient has experienced a temporary central sensory deficit and has combined aortic valve disease (stenosis and regurgitation). In the absence of any previous medical history (specifically rheumatic fever), the aortic stenosis/regurgitation is likely due to a deformed valve. The most common cause in this patient's age group is a bicuspid aortic valve. This, in turn, is associated in about 10% with coarctation of the aorta, which can result in significant upper extremity hypertension. Confirmation of a significant radial-femoral delay (checking both pulses simultaneously) or upper and lower extremity blood pressure measurements to confirm a significant (>25-30 mm Hg) difference would strongly suggest the presence of aortic coarctation.

3. Answer c.

Answers a, b, c, and e are classic findings in advanced aortic stenosis; however, the A_2 component of the second heart sound diminishes and is ultimately absent with progression of the aortic stenosis.

4. Answer e.

The first heart sound constitutes mitral valve closure followed by tricuspid valve closure. To be audible, the valve leaflets have to retain pliability. Once the valve becomes "frozen," as in the case of severe calcific mitral stenosis, the initially loud sound diminishes in intensity. The third heart sound is normal in patients younger than 30 years because of the dynamic relaxation with fast tensing of the chordae tendineae. A fourth heart sound results from a stiff, not failing, ventricle and thus represents diastolic rather than systolic dysfunction. The loss of the opening snap is a corollary to diminution of the first heart sound with progressive mitral leaflet calcification. Conversely, preservation of the A component of the second heart sound suggests pliable rather than completely immobile aortic cusps.

5. Answer b.

The carotid sinus massage would lead to only a temporary small decrease in the heart rate in healthy people. It is not a maneuver used in the differential diagnosis of mitral regurgitation vs. mitral valve prolapse. The handgrip leads to increased peripheral resistance and subsequently more mitral regurgitation. Squatting and Valsalva are maneuvers with opposite consequences. Squatting increases peripheral resistance and thus would lead to an increase in the mitral regurgitant murmur. The converse is true for the Valsalva maneuver.

6. Answer c.

Answers b, d, and e are all part of the symptom complex of constrictive pericarditis. Although less common with mediastinal mantle radiation than with radiation therapy after breast cancer, x-ray induced coronary artery disease may still occur. Radiation does not induce valvular destruction.

7. Answer c.

All forms of amyloidosis can involve the heart, leading ultimately to irreversible heart failure. The senile form of systemic amyloidosis (answer a) is most commonly associated with cardiac involvement. In early systemic amyloidosis (answer d), cardiac involvement is also common. In familial amyloidosis (answers b and e), infiltrative cardiomyopathy is present in approximately 50% of cases. In secondary amyloidosis due to renal failure, tuberculosis, rheumatoid arthritis, or chronic infection, amyloid deposit in the heart is not common.

8. Answer d.

Tissue valves calcify as easily, if not more rapidly, than native valves, especially in young patients. They are not immune to destruction by carcinoid disease and last longer in the aortic position, probably due to the extensive motion of the mitral valve annulus during the cardiac cycle. Mechanical valves are more durable; long-term results are currently best with Starr-Edwards prostheses despite the "simple" design. However, hemolysis is worse with large perivalvular leaks.

9. Answer e.

Contrast ventriculography (conventional and echocardiography) relies on assumptions of left ventricular shape and contraction to extrapolate end-diastolic and end-systolic volumes. In contrast, first-pass and blood pool radionuclide angiography count the concentration of isotopes in the left ventricular cavity, independent of shape and contraction pattern. Image acquisition is much slower with MRI than EBCT; however, precision is excellent in both techniques.

10. Answer a.

The patient is scheduled for minor surgery. Despite the

presence of cardiovascular risk factors and a history of coronary artery disease, myocardial infarction, and bypass surgery, he is asymptomatic without evidence of congestive heart failure and angina in the presence of a regular exercise program. He is at a very low risk of a perioperative event and does not require any workup at this time.

11. Answer d.

The classic finding of atrial septal defect on physical examination is a "fixed-split" second heart sound. However, systolic flow murmurs are common because of the increased flow through the pulmonary artery (never more than grade 3/6). Less commonly, a tricuspid diastolic flow rumble can be heard. This indicates a large shunt. Right ventricular lifts also are associated with volume overload of the right side. Early diastolic filling sounds are rare and late findings associated with right ventricular failure. All of the findings on physical examination are right-sided because the defect causes volume overload of the right side of the heart.

12. Answer c.

Patients with secundum ASD do not require antibiotic prophylaxis for subacute bacterial endocarditis; sinus venosus and ostium primum do require prophylaxis. It is the most common ASD (70% of all ASDs). Sinus venosus ASD is associated with anomalous pulmonary venous return because it is high in the atrial septum. Ostium primum ASD is low and usually associated with a cleft in the mitral valve and mitral (sometimes tricuspid) regurgitation. If the defect is uncorrected, patients often develop symptoms of dyspnea, right heart failure, and atrial fibrillation by the fifth decade.

13. Answer c.

Bicuspid aortic valve occurs in 1% to 2% of the adult population. The second-most common is secundum ASD. Ventricular septal defect is the most common congenital defect of childhood. Occasionally, mitral valve prolapse is cited as a "congenital defect" and is far more common than the others.

14. Answer d.

Primum atrioventricular septal defect is the most common congenital defect associated with Down syndrome. It classically is present with a cleft mitral valve. This explains the physical examination findings of a fixed-split S_2, volume overload of the right ventricle (sternal lift), and severe mitral regurgitation (holosystolic murmur with diastolic rumble indicating increased flow across the mitral valve). The electrocardiogram is very characteristic of primum defect, first-degree atrioventricular block, left-axis deviation, and right bundle branch block. A primum atrial septal defect or restrictive ventricular septal defect would not produce the murmurs heard on this examination.

Ventricular septal defect also would not cause the fixed split S_2 or electrocardiographic findings. Patients with Eisenmenger syndrome should have cyanosis and signs of pulmonary hypertension. Secundum atrial septal defect typically does not have the mitral regurgitation or electrocardiographic findings of this patient.

15. Answer a.

The patient has hypertension at a young age and now a bicuspid valve. An exhaustive search to rule out coarctation must be done. Seventy percent of patients with coarctation have a bicuspid aortic valve. Although standard echocardiography may help diagnose the coarctation, it is not always well seen on this examination. Further testing with transesophageal echocardiogram, digital subtraction angiography, magnetic resonance imaging, or computed tomography is necessary.

16. Answer c.

According to current guidelines, patients with murmurs should have prophylaxis for dental procedures. Patients with secundum atrial septal defects have not been shown to be at increased risk of endocarditis. Diagnostic procedures, including transesophageal echocardiography and gastroscopy, do not require prophylaxis.

17. Answer b.

Eisenmenger syndrome produces irreversible pulmonary hypertension due to long-standing left-to-right shunt. This eventually results in shunt reversal and loss of classic systolic murmur. Pulmonary hypertension produces a loud P_2 and pulmonary incompetence, causing the descrescendo diastolic murmur. Cyanosis produces significant erythrocytosis and increased hemoglobin levels, often in the high teens or 20s.

18. Answer d.

Down syndrome is associated with partial atrioventricular canal or primum defect, which is commonly associated with cleft mitral valve, not mitral valve prolapse.

19. Answer b.

The patient presents with both right- and left-sided symptoms. His echocardiogram has some features of hypertrophic cardiomyopathy, including a dynamic left ventricular outflow tract obstruction; however, his clinical history and electrocardiogram give the diagnosis away. With his very thickened walls and normal voltage on his electrocardiogram, he cannot have hypertrophic cardiomyopathy, because the voltage should be increased. In addition, it is unusual, although not impossible, for patients with hypertrophic cardiomyopathy to present with such severe symptoms of right-sided heart failure, which are common for patients with restrictive cardiomyopathies. On echocardiography, the predominant pathophysiology is restrictive hemodynamics. In hypertrophic cardiomyopathy, most patients have a marked diastolic relaxation abnormality. This case also points out that patients without hypertrophic cardiomyopathy may present with dynamic left ventricular outflow tract obstruction. This is further evidenced by the patient's marked deterioration after the administration of atenolol for a presumed diagnosis of hypertrophic cardiomyopathy. This is another clue that the diagnosis was wrong.

20. Answer c.

The dominant lesion in this patient with carcinoid tumors is tricuspid regurgitation. This will be associated with a large "v" wave on jugular venous profile—pulsatility of the liver when severe. Right-sided valvular involvement is predominant because the serotonin-like substance that causes the valve disease is metabolized in the lungs. However, if there is a shunt (intracardiac patent foramen ovale or intrapulmonary) or lung metastasis, then left-sided valves may be involved.

21. Answer d.

It has been estimated that 80% to 90% of clinical arrhythmias are mediated by a reentry mechanism.

22. Answer b.

Increased parasympathetic tone inhibits automaticity. Increased sympathetic tone, ischemia, and isoproterenol enhance automaticity.

23. Answer c.

Because of the infrequent and rather benign nature of her symptoms, a transtelephonic event recorder is the best diagnostic approach to document the presumed rhythm disturbance correlated with her symptoms.

24. Answer a.

Decreased heart rate variability is associated with increased risk of ventricular arrhythmias. Nonsustained ventricular tachyarrhythmias, late potentials, and inducible ventricular tachycardia are predictors of clinical ventricular arrhythmias.

25. Answer d.

The patient's presentation suggests cardiogenic syncope in the setting of coronary disease and compromised ejection fraction. Electrophysiologic testing is the diagnostic approach of choice. Syndrome of a neurologic cause would be extremely uncommon without any neurologic sequelae. Because of the higher likelihood for cardiogenic syncope, noninvasive monitoring would be less desirable.

26. Answer d.

High-degree atrioventricular (AV) block (Mobitz II 2° AV block and 3° AV block) correlated with symptoms belongs to the class I indication for permanent pacing. In the absence of any symptoms, permanent pacing is not usually indicated. A permanent pacemaker is not indicated for orthostatic hypotension.

27. Answer b.

Sotalol is excreted exclusively by the renal route. Other drugs, such as amiodarone, propafenone, and lidocaine, are metabolized predominantly by the liver.

28. Answer b.

Lidocaine is not effective in treating supraventricular arrhythmias, including atrial fibrillation.

29. Answer c.

Cardiac Arrhythmia Suppression Trial (CAST) showed that class IC agents (flecainide, encainide, and moricizine) are effective in suppressing premature ventricular complexes and nonsustained ventricular tachycardia in patients with coronary artery disease, myocardial infarction, and compromised ejection fraction (EF <40%). However, increased mortality was noted in the treatment groups when compared with the placebo.

30. Answer c.

The patient has recurrent symptomatic supraventricular tachycardia. He has been intolerant of pharmacologic therapy. The best therapeutic approach at this time would be an electrophysiologic evaluation and radio-frequency ablation. The procedure will likely provide 95% probability in successfully ablating the arrhythmogenic source. The procedure is associated with 1% to 2% complications.

31. Answer a.

The patient has sinus node dysfunction. This syndrome can include sinus bradycardia, sinus pauses, episodes of tachycardia (often atrial fibrillation), and sinus arrest. It often is associated with conduction system disease and failure of an adequate junctional escape. Although asymptomatic patients with sinus node dysfunction can be followed without specific therapy, in this patient, symptomatic pauses are clearly documented. These are effectively treated by permanent pacing. Although an electrophysiologic study is highly specific for sinus node dysfunction, it is not very sensitive, likely because of differences in the autonomic state at the time of the study compared with at the patient's normal activities. There is no role for coronary angiography, nor is a treadmill exercise test needed. The diagnosis of sinus node dysfunction is made best with a history and the results of electrocardiography and Holter monitoring.

32. Answer a.

This 24-year-old woman demonstrates second-degree atrioventricular block, type I (Wenckebach). Wenckebach block typically occurs in the atrioventricular node, especially when it is associated with a narrow QRS complex, as in this tracing. It is characterized by a gradual prolongation of the PR interval before the nonconducted P wave and a subsequent PR interval that is shorter than the PR interval before the nonconducted P wave. This pattern of gradual prolongation results in telltale group beating of the QRS complexes. Atrioventricular node Wenckebach is a benign condition that can be associated with hypervagotonic states such as nausea, pain, and vomiting. It is also seen in inferior myocardial infarction, in which case it results from ischemia of the atrioventricular node. In this setting, it does not require pacing unless there is documented hemodynamic compromise associated with the bradycardia, and it often resolves.

33. Answer b.

P waves "march through" the QRS complexes indicating atrioventricular dissociation. In the setting of a wide complex tachycardia, it is very specific for ventricular tachycardia. A right bundle branch block pattern with R' taller than R (rsR') is not very specific for ventricular tachycardia. It can also be seen with functional bundle branch block due to a rapid heart rate or premature atrial contractions. The presence of a northwest axis and a different QRS morphology in patients with preexisting bundle branch block are both suggestive of ventricular tachycardia. A history of structural heart disease, and in particular previous myocardial infarction or surgery involving ventricular incisions, significantly increases the likelihood that a wide complex tachycardia is ventricular in origin.

34. Answer c.

The rhythm shown is atrial flutter. This rhythm involves intra-atrial reentry in a circuit that is parallel to the tricuspid valve annulus. The administration of adenosine will result in transient atrioventricular node block and clear demonstration of the persistent atrial flutter waves in most cases, but it will not terminate the intra-atrial reentry itself. Adenosine may in some cases cause atrial flutter to degenerate into atrial fibrillation because of its shortening of the atrial effective refractory period. Atrial flutter is a very organized rhythm and can frequently be cardioverted with less than 50 J. Atrial flutter ablation is successful in more than 90% of cases. A linear radio-frequency lesion is placed between the tricuspid valve annulus and the inferior vena cava, interrupting the reentrant circuit. Propafenone, a class IC agent, is effective in atrial flutter, although the recurrence rate at 1 year may exceed 50% Although β-blockers do not control the atrial flutter itself, by increasing the degree of atrioventricular block, they slow the ventricular rate.

35. Answer e.

The electrocardiogram shows atrial fibrillation, which is characterized by an irregular baseline without clear-cut P waves and an irregularly irregular ventricular response. Several studies have demonstrated that the risk of cerebrovascular accident in patients with nonrheumatic atrial fibrillation is increased with hypertension, previous cerebrovascular accident, and a decreased ejection fraction. It is also increased in women older than 75. Men with structurally normal hearts under the age of 60 are considered to have "lone atrial fibrillation," which carries a very low risk of thromboembolism and requires no specific antithrombotic therapy.

36. Answer d.

This patient has atrial fibrillation, which according to the history has persisted for 4 days. Patients with more than 24 to 48 hours of atrial fibrillation should be anticoagulated for 3 or 4 weeks before elective cardioversion to diminish the risk of stroke. Emerging evidence suggests that intravenous heparin followed by transesophageal echocardiography, and cardioversion if no atrial thrombus is present, is an acceptable alternative approach. In this setting, however, continuous anticoagulation for at least 4 weeks after cardioversion is required to prevent post-cardioversion thromboembolism. Beginning a heparin infusion followed by immediate cardioversion is not an appropriate action. Checking electrolytes and thyroid function tests to screen for predisposing factors for atrial fibrillation is appropriate. β-Blockers are effective in controlling the ventricular rate by limiting the number of atrial signals that can successfully penetrate the atrioventricular node and activate the ventricles. β-Blockers or calcium channel blockers in general are more effective than digoxin in controlling the ventricular response in atrial fibrillation. β-Blockers, calcium channel blockers, and digoxin have not been shown to terminate atrial fibrillation.

37. Answer d.

The electrocardiogram shows ventricular tachycardia with a wide complex tachycardia in a patient with structural heart disease and atrioventricular dissociation as seen by the P waves that march through the QRS complexes. Many patients with a remote myocardial infarction who develop ventricular tachycardia do so because of a reentrant rhythm around a fixed scar in the absence of recurrent infarction. Cannon A waves are caused by atrial contraction against closed atrioventricular valves due to atrioventricular dissociation and are frequently present in the presence of ventricular tachycardia. Adenosine is not effective in treating this arrhythmia. The patient is hemodynamically stable and immediate cardioversion is not required. A trial of medical therapy with lidocaine infusion under close monitoring is appropriate. The presence of a palpable pulse does *not* exclude ventricular tachycardia—this is a dangerous misconception.

38. Answer d.

The electrocardiogram shows a Wolff-Parkinson-White pattern with a short PR interval and a delta wave due to ventricular preexcitation from an accessory pathway with antegrade conduction. Patients with symptomatic Wolff-Parkinson-White syndrome should undergo electrophysiologic testing to identify the pathway location, confirm that the pathway is an integral part of the reentrant circuit, and determine the risk of rapid atrial fibrillation. Also, catheter ablation can provide a permanent cure more than 95% of the time. There is no need for a tilt table test, coronary angiography, or treadmill testing in this patient.

39. Answer a.

This patient has classic vasodepressor syncope associated with a typical prodrome of warmth, diaphoresis, nausea, and the subsequent sensation of fatigue and malaise lasting for several hours or even a day. There are no findings to suggest significant cardiovascular or neurologic illness warranting further evaluation.

40. Answer c.

This tracing shows a supraventricular narrow complex tachycardia. The small deflections in the tail end of the QRS complex in lead V_1 likely reflect retrograde atrial activity. When retrograde atrial activity is seen within 90 ms of the QRS onset, then the mechanism is almost always atrioventricular node reentrant tachycardia. This rhythm frequently responds to carotid sinus massage or Valsalva maneuvers, and these should be attempted. If they fail, intravenous adenosine or verapamil terminates the arrhythmia in 90% of patients. Lidocaine has no role in the treatment of supraventricular arrhythmias. β-Blocker therapy is effective for long-term management of this arrhythmia. Radio-frequency ablation is successful in more than 95% of cases in permanently curing this arrhythmia and is frequently the treatment of choice in symptomatic younger patients to avoid the need for lifelong medical therapy.

41. Answer e.

The most common cause of an acute ischemic coronary syndrome is rupture of an unstable plaque. Coronary spasm can also cause rest angina but is relatively uncommon in the U.S. Coronary embolism and coronary dissection are seen very infrequently. Increased myocardial oxygen demand will produce a non-Q-wave myocardial infarction in the presence of significant fixed coronary disease, but this will not produce ST-segment elevation.

42. Answer b.

In a patient with known coronary artery disease, low-density lipoprotein cholesterol should be lowered to <100 mg/dL. There is no need to start treatment with a β-blocker if the blood pressure is controlled and the patient is asymptomatic.

43. Answer e.

In a patient presenting with prolonged chest pain and ST-segment depression, an evolving non-Q-wave myocardial infarction must be ruled out. Because there is no ST-segment elevation, thrombolytic therapy has not been shown to be effective. The primary cause of increased myocardial oxygen demand must be determined. In a patient with a third heart sound and increased jugular venous pressure, the increase in wall tension is the major component of increased myocardial oxygen demand. Metoprolol, which is a selective β-blocker, may make the patient worse because of its negative inotropic properties. Diltiazem should never be given to a patient with coronary artery disease and left ventricular dysfunction. Although an angiotensin-converting enzyme inhibitor would be beneficial in the long term, intravenous enalapril can cause too rapid a decrease in blood pressure. Intravenous nitroglycerin is the optimal treatment to lower myocardial oxygen demand.

44. Answer d.

In this patient, there is an extremely low pretest probability of coronary artery disease. Therefore, even a "positive" treadmill exertion test will result in a low post-test probability. No further tests are required for this patient with atypical chest pain and no risk factors. Reassurance only is the proper treatment.

45. Answer a.

Coronary artery bypass grafting will prolong life in only a subset of patients. This includes patients with left main coronary artery disease or those with three-vessel disease and depressed left ventricular systolic function.

46. Answer e.

This patient has single-vessel disease and class II angina pectoris. Catheter-based therapy, consisting of percutaneous transluminal coronary angioplasty (PTCA), has not been shown to prevent myocardial infarction or to prolong life. Similarly, in patients with one-vessel disease, coronary artery bypass grafting does not prevent myocardial infarction or prolong life. No medical therapy has been shown to reduce restenosis following

PTCA. Randomized trials have shown that PTCA and medical therapy are comparable for the hard end points of death and myocardial infarction.

47. Answer a.

In patients with stable exertional angina, the only interventions that reduce mortality and/or prevent myocardial infarction are the institution of a "statin" agent in patients with hyperlipidemia or the institution of aspirin. In patients with an ejection fraction less than or equal to 40%, an angiotensin-converting enzyme inhibitor has been shown to reduce mortality. Percutaneous transluminal coronary angioplasty and stent do not reduce mortality and/or prevent myocardial infarction in this subgroup of patients.

48. Answer c.

The earliest manifestation of myocardial ischemia is relaxation abnormality. In the "ischemic cascade," the steps are relaxation abnormality, contraction abnormality, electrocardiographic abnormality, and angina pectoris.

49. Answer c.

This patient presents with an inferior myocardial infarction and 4 hours of chest pain. Proper treatment includes the initiation of treatment with salicylates, intravenous β-blocker, heparin, and a thrombolytic agent. Calcium channel blockers have not been shown to be effective in patients with ST-segment elevation myocardial infarction.

50. Answer a.

This patient with a recent inferior myocardial infarction has evidence of right ventricular infarction. Two-dimensional echocardiography should be performed to document the cause of his hypotension. A V_{4R} lead in the electrocardiogram will also be useful in documenting the presence of a right ventricular infarction. The treatment for this patient is fluids to increase left ventricular filling pressures and intravenous dopamine to increase right ventricular contractility.

51. Answer b.

When a patient has new or worsening congestive heart failure, precipitating causes should be sought. If compliance historically is not an issue, the most common precipitants include ischemia, infection, or dysrhythmia. Noninvasive tests to evaluate the rhythm (e.g., new atrial fibrillation) and to confirm heart failure changes (as opposed to pulmonary infection masquerading as heart failure) are appropriate. Exercise stress testing or angiography should not be done until patients are better compensated. β-Adrenergic blockers should not be used for patients with acutely decompensated heart failure. Substitution of one angiotensin-converting enzyme inhibitor

for another is usually done to combat side effects, improve compliance, or decrease cost but does not change treatment efficacy.

52. Answer e.

It would be appropriate to treat newly recognized left ventricular dysfunction with digoxin and angiotensin-converting enzyme inhibitor therapy. Despite the absence of angina, coronary artery disease is a frequent cause of left ventricular dysfunction in a 68-year-old, and a screening test for ischemia, such as perfusion imaging, is appropriate. The risk of atrial thrombus in this situation is not negligible; atrial flutter, especially with concomitant left ventricular dysfunction of indeterminate duration, justifies therapeutic anticoagulation. If there were severe hemodynamic compromise, emergency electrical cardioversion could be justified. Alternatively, transesophageal echocardiography-guided elective cardioversion is an option. However, in a compensated situation, elective cardioversion should be done under the protective cover of adequate systemic anticoagulation.

53. Answer d.

The findings fit best with symptomatic orthostatic hypotension, likely as a result of the increase of diuretic dose in addition to the increase in angiotensin-converting enzyme inhibitor dose. Given the absence of findings of fluid overload (by examination and chest radiography), it is preferable to decrease the diuretic dose while maintaining aggressive angiotensin-converting enzyme inhibitor therapy. Timely follow-up is necessary, however, to confirm that the desired effect has been obtained.

54. Answer b.

The digoxin dosage should be decreased when the drug is given concurrently with amiodarone, quinidine, or verapamil. Although other drugs may have minimal pharmacokinetic interactions with digoxin, only these three predictably increase the digoxin blood level significantly. The combination of digoxin with other antiarrhythmic drugs may cause additive chronotropic or conduction abnormalities, but this is judged during the course of treatment and does not routinely result in an empiric downward adjustment of the dose.

55. Answer a.

The examination and electrocardiogram do not fit with a diagnosis of hypertrophic cardiomyopathy. The finding of thick ventricular walls on echocardiography in combination with low voltage on the electrocardiogram suggests amyloid cardiomyopathy, hence the immunoelectrophoreses. It is normal for systolic ejection murmurs to become louder after pauses, and this finding is not diagnostic for obstructive cardiomyopathy. In hypertrophic obstructive cardiomyopathy, not only does the murmur get louder but also simultaneously the carotid upstroke is diminished.

56. Answer a.

This patient has new signs and symptoms of congestive heart failure in addition to wheezing in the setting of a recent increase in β-adrenergic blocker dose, hypertrophic obstructive cardiomyopathy, atrial fibrillation, and a mitral regurgitant murmur. Because she felt worse after the metoprolol dose was increased, its dose should be lowered. Either new left ventricular dysfunction or a new or increased degree of mitral regurgitation might cause the change in her symptoms; because these are treated differently, echocardiography is justified. New atrial fibrillation can cause heart failure in obstructive cardiomyopathy because of the loss of atrial contractility and needs to be addressed; heparin therapy is begun while the strategy to manage the atrial fibrillation is formulated. Although diuretics are relatively contraindicated in hypertrophic obstructive cardiomyopathy, a small dose can be carefully given to patients presenting with congestive heart failure (if there is hemodynamic embarrassment, replacement fluid can be given). Because of the multiple issues of congestive heart failure and the wheezing (bronchospasm versus heart failure) and atrial fibrillation, dismissal of this patient would be inappropriate. In addition, theophylline treatment is contraindicated because its positive inotropic action may aggravate the outflow tract obstruction.

57. Answer c.

The symptoms and physical findings are those of biventricular heart failure. The outside pulmonary artery catheter data and radionuclide angiogram suggest a primary diastolic dysfunction. Historically, this might be pericardial or myocardial disease due to previous radiation. An echocardiogram could confirm normal ventricular function and assessing the pericardium and myocardium. Ultrafast computed tomography is excellent to assess pericardial thickening. Given the persistent fluid overload, an increase in diuretic dose is appropriate. In the absence of either angina or evidence of ischemia, coronary angiography is not indicated. Right ventricular endomyocardial biopsy is usually not helpful for distinguishing restrictive cardiomyopathy from pericardial disease. Although an infiltrative cardiomyopathy is possible, other noninvasive screening tests should precede the ultimate decision regarding right ventricular biopsy.

58. Answer b.

Measures that decrease preload or afterload and measures that increase contractility will all *increase* the degree of outflow tract obstruction. Changing from a squat to standing position decreases preload, as does isosorbide dinitrate and amyl nitrite inhalation. The digoxin is a positive inotrope. Therefore, all of these measures cause increases in outflow tract obstruction. Disopyramide, however, is a negative inotrope and therefore decreases the degree of outflow tract obstruction.

59. Answer e.

Digoxin is an equally potent inotrope in ischemic and nonischemic ventricular dysfunction. Benefit has been established in patients who remain in sinus rhythm. Common side effects include fatigue and dysrhythmia. Visual changes can occur and most commonly are an alteration of color as opposed to blurring. The DIG trial demonstrated a decrease in hospitalization in patients with heart failure. Fewer patients died of heart failure, but this was offset by an increase in the number of patients receiving digoxin who died an arrhythmic death. Therefore, the net effect on survival was neutral.

60. Answer a.

The patient's sole symptom is edema, without symptoms to suggest left-sided heart failure. The examination shows edema despite normal jugular venous pressure, suggesting that the problem may not be due to increased right-sided filling pressures. Electrocardiography does not suggest left ventricular dysfunction, and chest radiography does not suggest left-sided heart failure. In this setting and given the failure to respond to empiric treatment, further evaluation of the return of fluid from the legs to the right heart is appropriate and can noninvasively be done by ultrasound evaluation of veins for clot and for venous competence. Increasing the furosemide dose may be effective but has failed already in this patient's management and would not help explain what is happening physiologically. Radionuclide angiography measures left ventricular ejection fraction, which is not likely to be useful in a patient without abnormalities of the left heart on standard clinical grounds and without symptoms of left heart failure. Venous disease including deep venous thrombosis is very possible without pulmonary embolization, and a ventilation-perfusion scan would not help in this regard. There are no cardiac physical findings of pulmonary hypertension to suggest the possible presence of pulmonary emboli, nor has the patient had suggestive symptoms. Without evidence of ventricular dysfunction or hypertension, angiotensin-converting enzyme inhibitor therapy is not indicated.

NOTES

CHAPTER 4

CLINICAL PHARMACOLOGY AND TOXICOLOGY

Thomas F. Bugliosi, M.D.

EPIDEMIOLOGY

Most exposures to poison (67%) reported to the American Association of Poison Control Centers in 1997 occurred in persons younger than 19 years. Overall, accidental poisoning outnumbers intentional poisoning in all age groups. However, if only fatal cases are considered (786 in 1997), most occurred in adults, and suicide was the cause in 53%. It is important to remember that the vast majority of all poisonings are not deadly, and most patients do well with good supportive care (Am J Emerg Med 16:443-497, 1998)

- Most exposures to poison are in persons <19 years.
- Accidental poisoning outnumbers intentional poisoning.
- Vast majority of poisonings are not deadly.
- Fatal poisonings are more common in adults, and suicide is the single most common cause.

DIAGNOSIS

Clinical

Any patient who presents with an altered mental status should be considered to have taken an overdose. The history provided by the patient is often unreliable, and every effort should be made to interrogate family, friends, paramedics, and law enforcement officers present at the scene. Ask them to bring in pill remnants and containers.

- Patient with altered mental status should be considered to have taken overdose.
- History given by patient is often unreliable.

The next step is a thorough general examination. Many of the most frequent poisonings produce classic physical signs and symptoms, and you should be familiar with these. The findings associated with various agents are listed below.

- Many poisonings produce classic physical signs and symptoms.

Anticholinergic syndrome (atropine, belladonna alkaloid, tricyclic antidepressants, antipsychotics, medications for Parkinson disease, and antihistamines):

Dry skin and mucous membranes
Hyperthermia
Flushing
Tachycardia
Hypertension
Mydriasis
↓ Salivation
↓ Sweating
Ileus
Urinary retention
Anxiety/confusion
Seizures
Mnemonic: "Red as a beet, hot as a hare, dry as a bone, blind as a bat, and mad as a hatter."

Cholinergic syndrome (organophosphate poisoning):

Sweating
Salivation
Lacrimation
Miosis
Bradycardia
Vomiting
Diarrhea
Wheezing
Muscle cramps/fasciculations
Altered mental status
Acronym is "SLUDGE": *S*alivation, *L*acrimation, *U*rination, *D*efecation, *G*astrointestinal upset, *E*mesis

Opiates (for example, morphine, codeine, heroin, methadone):

Miosis
Respiratory depression

Drowsiness
Nausea/vomiting
Pulmonary edema
Seizures
Classic triad is depressed mental status, depressed
    respiration, miosis.
Barbiturates (for example, pentobarbital, phenobarbital):
    Central nervous system depression
    Respiratory depression
    Bradycardia
    Hypotension
    Hypothermia
    Areflexia
    Pulmonary edema
    Blisters
    Pupils variable
Stimulants (amphetamines, cocaine, aminophylline):
    Central nervous system excitation/agitation
    Seizures
    Hypertension
    Tachycardia
    Hallucinations
    Arrhythmias/cardiovascular collapse
    Mydriasis
Substance withdrawal:
    Agitation
    Confusion
    Mydriasis
    Tachycardia
    Hypertension
    Nausea
    Vomiting
    Abdominal pain
    Seizures

Laboratory Evaluation

Toxicologic Screening

Many misconceptions exist regarding the utility of
the standard drug screen. Many commonly encountered
drugs cannot be easily detected. The predictive value of
a negative toxicologic test is only 40%. Of the drugs
that can be detected, quantitative results can be obtained
in only 5%-10% of cases. When quantitative results
can be measured, they often correlate poorly with clinical signs and symptoms. Most qualitative tests require
urine samples, and most quantitative tests require serum
samples.

- Predictive value of negative toxicologic test is only 40%.
- Quantitative results useful in only 5%-10% of cases.

- Most qualitative tests require urine samples; most quantitative tests require serum samples.
- Treat the patient on the basis of symptoms and signs, not
  results of toxicologic screening.

Quantitative drug levels have important therapeutic implications in only a handful of cases:
    Acetaminophen
    Salicylates
    Theophylline
    Methanol
    Ethylene glycol
    Iron
    Lithium
    Seizure medications (for seizure prophylaxis)
    Carbon monoxide
    Methemoglobin

Arterial Blood Gases

Perhaps the most useful ancillary blood test that can be
performed is the arterial blood gas analysis. This not only
will give critical acid-base information but also can diagnose
specific poisonings such as carbon monoxide and methemoglobin.

- Arterial blood gas analysis is very useful test.

Osmolar Gap

This is calculated as the difference between the osmolarity
as measured by freezing point depression and the calculated
osmolarity.

- Calculated osmolarity $= 2\,[Na^+] + \dfrac{BUN}{2.8} + \dfrac{Glucose}{18}$
  (BUN, blood urea nitrogen).
- Osmolar gap $=$ measured osmolarity - calculated osmolarity.
- If osmolar gap >10, consider acetone, ethanol, methanol,
  ethylene glycol, isopropanol, and diuretics (mannitol,
  glycerol, or sorbitol).

Anion Gap

The anion gap can be extremely useful in patients with
suspected overdose.

Anion gap $= Na^+ - (Cl^- + HCO_3^-)$; normal gap is 8-12 mEq.

A decreased anion gap can occur in patients with hyper-
magnesemia, bromide or lithium ingestion, or hypoalbuminemia. An increased anion gap can occur in patients who
have ingested methanol, ethylene glycol, propylene glycol,
salicylates, strychnine, isoniazid, paraldehyde, phenformin,
carbon monoxide, cyanide, or iron. Nontoxicologic causes

of an increased anion gap include uremia, diabetic ketoacidosis, and lactic acidosis.

- Iron ingestion is a cause of increased anion gap that is often forgotten.
- Acetaminophen, narcotics, hallucinogens, and stimulants generally do not cause an increased anion gap.

ESSENTIALS OF CARE

Care of the poisoned patient can be divided into 1) supportive care, 2) prevention of further absorption, 3) enhancement of excretion, and 4) administration of a specific antidote.

Supportive Care

Any patient who presents with an altered mental status or confusing symptom complex should be evaluated for drug overdose. Secure airway, breathing, and circulation (ABCs). If a cervical spine injury is a possibility, maintain cervical spine precautions. Most patients will do well with careful attention to the ABCs, including endotracheal intubation if necessary. Intravenous access and cardiac monitoring should be initiated. Confused, agitated, or violent patients require close observation and possibly physical restraints.

- Any patient with altered mental status should be evaluated for drug overdose.
- Secure airway, breathing, circulation (ABCs).
- Establish intravenous access and cardiac monitoring.

Dextrose (D_{50}) was once considered "standard" care of patients with altered mental status. A growing body of evidence, however, suggests that increased glucose concentrations may worsen the functional recovery of patients with brain injury not related to hypoglycemia. Therefore, every patient with altered mental status should have a quick fingerstick blood glucose determination. Dextrose should be administered to patients with documented hypoglycemia. In addition, administer 100 mg thiamine intramuscularly to alcoholic patients.

- Increased glucose concentrations may worsen functional recovery in patients with brain injury not related to hypoglycemia.
- Every patient with altered mental status should have quick fingerstick blood glucose determination.
- Alcoholic patients should be treated with 100 mg thiamine intramuscularly.

Naloxone was also considered standard care of patients with altered mental status. Naloxone has been reported to cause pulmonary edema in a few anecdotal case reports. Patients with hypoventilation, miosis, or other signs of narcotic abuse who present with altered mental status should be given 2 mg naloxone by intravenous push. Naloxone can also be given subcutaneously or intramuscularly or by endotracheal tube. Remember that many narcotics have longer half-lives than naloxone, so all patients require prolonged monitoring for resedation. The dose of naloxone may need to be repeated.

- Naloxone has been reported to rarely cause pulmonary edema.
- Naloxone 2 mg intravenously should be given in patients with hypoventilation, miosis, or signs of narcotic abuse.
- All patients require prolonged monitoring for resedation.

Prevention of Further Absorption

Many toxins can be absorbed through the skin, and decontamination of the skin is mandatory in such cases. Gastric emptying can be accomplished with induced emesis or gastric lavage utilizing a large-bore (36- to 40-French) tube. In general, there has been a significant trend away from these treatments for several reasons:

- No studies prove that these efforts positively influence outcome.
- Recent studies have shown that activated charcoal alone may be superior to either induced emesis or gastric lavage, and it seems to cause fewer complications.
- Gastric emptying is time-consuming in a busy emergency department.
- Either method of gastric emptying removes only about 30% of ingested material.

Induced Emesis

Syrup of ipecac is the only acceptable emetic. It acts centrally (medulla) and peripherally. Vomiting usually occurs within 20 minutes. The usual adult dose is 30 mL, which may be given again in 30 minutes if vomiting has not occurred.

An indication for ipecac is ingestion of a potentially toxic substance in the home setting in persons older than 6 months. Contraindications are nontoxic ingestions, caustic ingestions, hydrocarbon ingestions, age younger than 6 months, altered mental status, poor gag reflex, seizures, and substance likely to alter mental status rapidly (for example, tricyclics). Complications are prolonged vomiting, Mallory-Weiss tear, aspiration pneumonia, intracranial hemorrhage, and delayed charcoal administration.

- Ipecac is the only acceptable emetic.
- Usual adult dose is 30 mL; may be repeated in 30 minutes.
- Aspiration is major concern with ipecac.
- Patient must be alert and likely to stay that way.

Gastric Lavage

This is accomplished with the patient in the left lateral decubitus position; a large-bore orogastric tube is used. A cuffed endotracheal tube should be placed before procedure if patient has altered mental status, depressed gag reflex, or seizures. Indications are recent (<1 hour) ingestion of a potentially toxic substance, substances not well bound by charcoal, or toxic substances that delay gastric emptying. Contraindications are nontoxic ingestions, caustic ingestions, and patients who present more than 1 hour after ingestion (except in cases of potentially delayed gastric emptying). Complications are aspiration pneumonia, perforation of esophagus or stomach, and inadvertent tracheal intubation.

• Before gastric lavage, cuffed endotracheal tube should be placed if patient has altered mental status, depressed gag reflex, or seizures.

Activated Charcoal

Activated charcoal is emerging as the treatment of choice for most poisonings. It is an inert compound that binds to most substances. The dose is generally 1 g/kg body weight. This may be given as a slurry down an orogastric tube or nasogastric tube, or the patient can drink it. Charcoal is generally ineffective for absorbing small ionic compounds such as lithium, magnesium, arsenic, and alcohols. In addition, charcoal should not be given in cases of caustic ingestions because the caustic substances are poorly bound by activated charcoal, and the subsequent endoscopic view will be obscured. Pulse charcoal in which 50 g of charcoal is given every 2 to 4 hours has theoretical value in overdoses involving drugs that undergo enterohepatic circulation (for example, barbiturates, meprobamate, carbamazepine, theophylline, phenytoin, tricyclics). Data are not conclusive, however, and the complication rate is increased. Administration of cathartics after charcoal administration has not been proved to be effective.

• Activated charcoal emerging as treatment of choice for most poisonings.
• Dose is 1 g/kg body weight.
• Charcoal generally ineffective for absorbing small ionic compounds such as lithium, magnesium, arsenic, alcohols.
• Charcoal should not be given for caustic ingestion.

Enhancement of Excretion

Several methods may enhance excretion: forced diuresis, alkaline or acid diuresis, hemodialysis, and hemoperfusion. A brief review of volume of distribution is necessary to understand the limited role enhancement of excretion plays in most overdoses.

The volume of distribution (V_d) is defined as that volume of fluid into which a drug seems to distribute with the concentration equal to that in plasma. It is a hypothetical volume only. It does not refer to any physiologic space. When V_d is large (>1 liter/kg), the tissue concentration is large (and vice versa).

$$V_d = \frac{A \text{ (amount ingested)}}{C \text{ (plasma concentration)}}$$

The V_d can be used to predict the serum level of a drug if the amount ingested is known. For example, if a 70-kg patient ingested 50 100-mg tablets of phenytoin ($V_d = 0.75$ liter/kg), the plasma level can be predicted:

$$V_d = \frac{A}{C} \qquad V_d = 0.75 \text{ liter/kg x } 70 \text{ kg} = 52.5 \text{ liters}$$

$$52.5 \text{ liters} = \frac{5,000 \text{ mg}}{C} = 95 \text{ mg/liter}$$

Drugs are eliminated by first order, zero order, or combination kinetics. First-order elimination is how the kidney handles toxins. A constant fraction of the drug is eliminated per unit time. The higher the plasma concentration, the greater the amount of drug excreted per unit time. Zero-order elimination is how the liver handles toxins. This type of elimination involves saturable enzymes that, when saturated, allow only for a constant amount of drug to be eliminated. Once enzymes are saturated, serum levels can increase dramatically. Examples include phenytoin, salicylates, and ethanol. Combination elimination occurs with salicylates, phenytoin, and ethanol. These drugs switch their elimination from first-order to zero-order elimination.

• First-order elimination is how kidney handles toxins.
• Zero-order elimination is how liver handles toxins.
• Combination elimination occurs with salicylates, phenytoin, ethanol in the therapeutic range.

Forced Diuresis

Most attempts at increasing drug elimination by forced diuresis (thereby increasing urine flow) are not successful. In general, for many drugs, elimination by renal excretion is not dependent on urine flow rates. In addition, drugs that are highly protein-bound or have a large volume of distribution (V_d) are not affected by forced diuresis.

• Most attempts at forced diuresis are not successful.
• Drugs that are highly protein-bound are not affected by forced diuresis.

Urine Alkalinization

Weak acids such as salicylates, phenobarbital, and isoniazid are ionized in a more alkaline medium. Promoting an alkaline urine by alkalinizing a patient slows reabsorption of weakly acidic compounds because they will exist as anions that do not readily cross lipid membranes. As a result, urinary clearance is increased. An alkaline diuresis is accomplished by adding 1 ampule of $NaHCO_3$ to 1 liter of 0.45 normal saline and monitoring urine pH.

Urine Acidification

Although several drugs (for example, amphetamines and phencyclidine) may have their elimination enhanced by acidifying the urine, this is not recommended because of the possibility of acute renal tubular necrosis caused by rhabdomyolysis.

- Urine acidification not recommended because of possibility of acute renal tubular necrosis.

Hemodialysis

Hemodialysis has very limited application in drug overdoses. Suitable substances should be of small molecular weight and soluble, have limited protein and lipid binding, and have a small volume of distribution (V_d). The driving force is the concentration gradient of unbound, ultrafiltrable solute.

Hemodialysis is indicated in some cases of the following overdoses (depending on patient's condition): ethylene glycol, methanol, lithium, salicylates, bromide. Hemodialysis is not indicated for overdoses of tricyclic antidepressants, antihistamines, benzodiazepines, digitalis, phenothiazines, opiates, or ethchlorvynol.

Hemoperfusion

Hemoperfusion is accomplished by pumping a patient's blood through an extracorporeal cartridge containing adsorbent particles (activated charcoal, carbon, or polystyrene resin). The factors that limit toxin removal in hemodialysis are not as important in hemoperfusion.

Hemoperfusion is indicated in some cases of ingestions of phenobarbital, other barbiturates, diphenylhydantoin, and theophylline. The major rate-limiting factors are the affinity of the adsorbent for the toxin and the rate of blood flow through the circuit. Complications include thrombocytopenia, leukopenia, hypoglycemia, and hypocalcemia. Most overdoses can be managed without hemodialysis or hemoperfusion. Applications must be considered on an individual basis.

- In hemoperfusion, major rate-limiting factors are affinity of adsorbent for toxin and rate of blood flow through circuit.
- Complications include thrombocytopenia, leukopenia, hypoglycemia, hypocalcemia.
- Most overdoses can be managed without hemodialysis or hemoperfusion.

Administration of an Antidote

There are specific antidotes for only a few agents involved in overdoses. Even when a specific antidote is available, it is often not needed, and supportive care is all that is necessary. A partial list of antidotes is included in Table 4-1.

CYCLIC ANTIDEPRESSANTS

Overdose with cyclic antidepressants (for example, imipramine, amitriptyline, desipramine, doxepin) is one of the most serious types of overdose; it causes approximately 25% of all deaths due to poisoning. They are rapidly absorbed and readily distributed to body tissues and fat. In fact, tissue levels may be much higher than plasma levels. Cyclic antidepressants have a high degree of protein binding (85% to 99%) and a huge volume of distribution (V_d) (that is, not removed by hemodialysis or hemoperfusion). Increasing pH increases protein binding; thus, less free drug is available to exert its effect.

- Overdose with cyclic antidepressants one of most serious types of overdose.
- Causes about 25% of all deaths due to poisoning.
- Cyclic antidepressants are rapidly absorbed and readily distribute to body tissues and fat.
- They have high degree of protein binding.

Table 4-1.--Antidotes for Agents Associated With Overdose

Drug/toxin	Antidote
Acetaminophen	N-Acetylcysteine
Anticholinergics	Physostigmine
Benzodiazepines	Flumazenil
Carbon monoxide	Oxygen
Cyanide	Amyl nitrite, sodium nitrite, sodium thiosulfate
Ethylene glycol	Ethanol, fomepizole
Iron	Deferoxamine
Isoniazid	Pyridoxine
Methanol	Ethanol
Narcotics	Naloxone
Nitrites	Methylene blue
Organophosphates	Atropine Pralidoxime
Tricyclics	Sodium bicarbonate

From Bryson PD: Comprehensive Review in Toxicology. Second edition. New York, Raven Press, 1989, p 11. By permission of Taylor & Francis.

Table 4-2.--Effects of Tricyclic Antidepressants

Action	Clinical findings
1. Quinidine-like effect	↓ Myocardial contractility
	↑ Myocardial conduction
	Increased P-R and Q-T intervals
	Widened QRS
	Ventricular arrhythmia
	Hypotension
2. Anticholinergic	Supraventricular tachycardia, hyperthermia, mydriasis, anxiety, hallucinations, seizures, coma, death
3. Block reuptake of norepinephrine	↓ Myocardial contractility
	Hypotension
	Bradycardia
4. Antihistamine	

Tricyclics (most cyclic antidepressants have three rings) have four main actions (Table 4-2):
1. Class IA antiarrhythmic effects (quinidine-like)
2. Anticholinergic activity
3. Block reuptake of norepinephrine in central nervous system
4. Antihistamine (H_1 and H_2 antagonist)

Toxic effects vary, but rapid deterioration is common. Ventricular arrhythmias, seizures, hypotension, and respiratory depression are some of the more dangerous side effects to anticipate. Maprotiline (Ludiomil) is a tetracyclic antidepressant that causes more seizures but fewer cardiovascular side effects. Remember, cardiotoxicity is the main cause of death associated with cyclic antidepressants.

- Toxic effects vary, but rapid deterioration is common with overdose of cyclic antidepressants.

Treatment of patients who have overdosed on cyclic antidepressants first includes securing the ABCs. Because seizures or rapid deterioration is common, many patients require endotracheal intubation. Do not induce vomiting. After ABCs are secured, gastric lavage is indicated even if several hours have elapsed since ingestion because the anticholinergic effects cause delayed gastric emptying. Activated charcoal is recommended and, because of enterohepatic circulation, pulse charcoal may be of benefit. Cardiac monitoring is needed for all patients for a minimum of 24 hours.

- Seizures or rapid deterioration is common with overdose of cyclic antidepressants.
- Do not induce vomiting.
- Activated charcoal is recommended.

Treatment of specific complications is outlined below:
1. Cardiotoxicity: Alkalinization causes more cyclic antidepressant to be protein-bound, leaving less free drug to exert its effect. It may be the best treatment of most forms of cardiovascular toxicity and can narrow widened QRS complexes, abolish arrhythmias, and improve perfusion. The goal is a serum pH of about 7.5. Dysrhythmias should be treated with alkalinization. Lidocaine and phenytoin are both reasonable choices for ventricular arrhythmias. Bretylium has an effect similar to that of the tricyclics and should be avoided. Class IA agents (quinidine, procainamide, and disopyramide) should be avoided.
2. Seizures: After alkalinization, diazepam and phenytoin are used, as for other patients with seizures. Refractory seizures should be treated with phenobarbital or general anesthesia.
3. Hypotension: After crystalloid fluid challenge and alkalinization, you may need catecholamine pressors such as epinephrine, norepinephrine, or phenylephrine. Isoproterenol, dobutamine, and low-dose dopamine should be avoided because they may worsen hypotension through unopposed β-adrenergic effect. (Cyclic antidepressants produce strong α-adrenergic blockade.)
4. Anticholinergic toxicity: Physostigmine can reverse the anticholinergic effects of cyclic antidepressants, but its use is controversial. It has a low therapeutic:toxic ratio and can produce cholinergic crises. Its use should be limited to patients with severe hypertension, seizures, or dysrhythmias not responsive to other forms of therapy.

- Lidocaine and phenytoin are reasonable choices for ventricular arrhythmias.

- Refractory seizures should be treated with phenobarbital or general anesthesia.
- For hypotension, avoid isoproterenol, dobutamine, and low-dose dopamine.
- Physostigmine can reverse anticholinergic effects of cyclic antidepressants; it has low therapeutic:toxic ratio and can produce cholinergic crises.

ACETAMINOPHEN

Acetaminophen is the active metabolite of phenacetin and is a common over-the-counter antipyretic analgesic available in many forms. It is rapidly absorbed. Toxicity is from a minor metabolite formed via the cytochrome P450 system. Actually, most of an acetaminophen dose is conjugated with glucuronic acid and sulfate and then excreted by the kidneys. Only a very small amount is metabolized by the cytochrome P450 system. In cases of overdose, however, the sulfate and glucuronide conjugating systems are saturated, so more metabolism occurs through the cytochrome P450 system. Under normal circumstances, the metabolite of this system is conjugated with hepatic glutathione and excreted. In the case of overdose, however, hepatic glutathione is rapidly depleted and the metabolite binds to hepatocytes, producing cell death.

- Acetaminophen is active metabolite of phenacetin.
- It is rapidly absorbed.
- In acetaminophen overdose, sulfate and glucuronide conjugating systems are saturated, so more metabolism occurs through cytochrome P450 system.
- In overdose, metabolite binds to hepatocytes, producing cell death.

Hepatotoxicity, the main complication of acetaminophen overdose, can be predicted accurately with a nomogram (Fig. 4-1). This is based on the estimate that 15 g of acetaminophen in a single ingestion causes hepatotoxicity in an adult. For safety, and because patients with chronic liver disease have less glutathione stores, 7.5 g is used for the nomogram. Remember that patients taking phenobarbital and alcohol have stimulated cytochrome P450 systems and are more likely to experience toxicity at any given dose.

- Hepatotoxicity is main complication of acetaminophen overdose.

Treatment of acetaminophen overdose requires precise determination of the time of ingestion and quantified serum levels of acetaminophen. For patients who are in the "toxic" range on the nomogram, treatment with N-acetylcysteine is indicated. N-Acetylcysteine provides a -SH group for the toxic intermediary to bind to, thus sparing the hepatocytes. N-Acetylcysteine is given orally in the United States, but it has been used intravenously in other countries for years, and it should be given within 24 hours of ingestion. The loading dose of 140 mg/kg is followed by 70 mg/kg every 4 hours for 17 doses. The odor is offensive, and it may be best to give it through a nasogastric tube.

- For patients in toxic range of acetaminophen overdose, treatment with N-acetylcysteine is indicated.
- Treatment should be given within 24 hours of ingestion.

There is some debate regarding the initial treatment of acetaminophen overdose. There is theoretical concern that if activated charcoal is given initially, it may also bind the antidote (N-acetylcysteine). In practice, however, this is not a major concern, and because activated charcoal binds acetaminophen well, most investigators recommend it. Induced emesis should be avoided because prolonged vomiting may delay giving N-acetylcysteine if it is found to be indicated.

SALICYLATES

Salicylates are weak acids that are rapidly absorbed and have a small volume of distribution (V_d, 0.2 liter/kg). Although the half-life is short (15 minutes) under normal conditions, in case of overdose the half-life may be prolonged to 20 hours. Overall, the number of accidental ingestions has decreased, and most toxicity is now related to chronic salicylate use. A 50% increase in the daily dose of aspirin can result in a 300% increase in plasma level. As salicylate levels increase, a typical pattern of acid-base disturbances occurs:

$$\text{Respiratory} \rightarrow \text{Respiratory} \rightarrow \text{Metabolic acidosis}$$

Respiratory → Respiratory → Metabolic acidosis
alkalosis   alkalosis   (anion gap)
                 +
          Metabolic acidosis
            (anion gap)

This pattern may be accelerated in children. About the only abnormality that does not occur is metabolic alkalosis.

- In salicylate overdose, half-life may be prolonged to 20 hours.
- Most toxicity is now related to chronic salicylate use.
- 50% increase in daily dose of aspirin can result in 300% increase in plasma level.

Other symptoms and signs of salicylate overdose are listed in Table 4-3.

An elderly patient who is confused and has a high anion gap

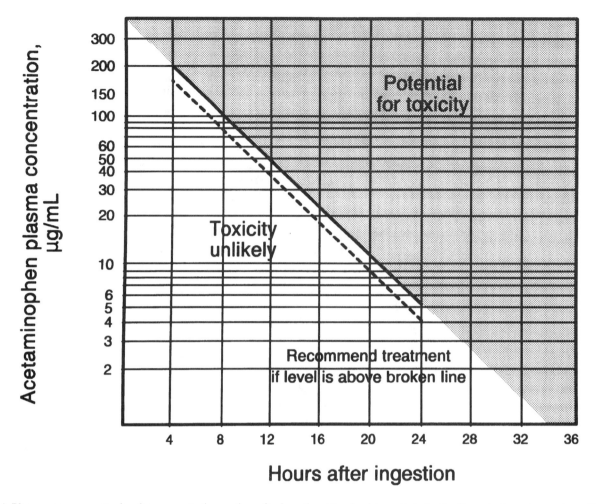

Fig. 4-1. Plasma or serum acetaminophen concentration vs. time after ingestion. Graph relates only to levels after a single acute overdose. Broken line represents 25% allowance below solid line; it is included to allow for possible errors in acetaminophen assays and estimated time from ingestion of overdose. (From Chiang WK, Wang RY: Evaluation and management of acute acetaminophen toxicity. Emerg Med Reports 14:83-90, 1993 and from McNeil Consumer Products Co., as adapted from Rumack BH, Matthews H: Acetaminophen poisoning and toxicity. Pediatrics 55:871-876, 1975. By permission of American Health Consultants, McNeil Consumer Products Co., and Pediatrics.)

metabolic acidosis or unexplained respiratory alkalosis may have salicylate toxicity. This is a common presentation. Salicylate intoxication can cause noncardiogenic pulmonary edema.

Treatment includes usual supportive care and activated charcoal. Consider gastric lavage if the duration since ingestion is less than 1 hour. Fluids should be given to correct losses and to promote diuresis. Potassium levels need to be monitored carefully. Alkalinization increases urinary excretion of salicylates dramatically and may prevent salicylates from crossing the blood-brain barrier (ion trapping). Hemodialysis is used in certain cases, such as renal failure, noncardiogenic pulmonary edema, persistent or progressive central nervous system manifestations, and deterioration despite adequate supportive care and alkaline diuresis.

- Treatment of salicylate overdose: activated charcoal, fluids

to correct losses and promote diuresis, monitoring of potassium levels, alkalinization to increase urinary excretion, hemodialysis in some cases.

THEOPHYLLINE

Theophylline is approximately 50% protein-bound, and about 90% of excretion occurs through liver metabolism. Metabolism is increased with cigarette smoking and use of phenobarbital or phenytoin. Metabolism is decreased with erythromycin, cimetidine, propranolol, ciprofloxacin, and heart failure or liver disease. The clinical presentation of theophylline toxicity depends not only on the amount of drug ingested but also on whether the patient is chronically maintained on theophylline. Patients who chronically take theophylline have more toxicity, in general, than their counterparts at the same serum level.

Table 4-3.--Clinical and Laboratory Abnormalities in Salicylate Overdose

Central nervous system	Gastrointestinal	Pulmonary	Renal	Miscellaneous
Tinnitus	Nausea	Tachypnea	Tubular	Hyperpyrexia
Delirium	Vomiting	Noncardiogenic	necrosis	Hypokalemia
Stupor	Gastritis	pulmonary edema		Hypoglycemia
Coma				Platelet dysfunction
Seizures				Acid-base
				disturbances

- Theophylline is 50% protein-bound; 90% of excretion is through liver metabolism.
- Patients who chronically take theophylline have more toxicity than their counterparts at same serum level.

Symptoms of theophylline toxicity are nausea and vomiting, agitation, tachypnea, cardiac arrhythmia (atrial fibrillation, multifocal atrial tachycardia, ventricular tachycardia, ventricular fibrillation), and seizures. Seizures increase mortality and may be first manifestation. Hypokalemia, hypophosphatemia, and hyperglycemia also occur.

Treatment includes routine supportive decontamination procedures. Pulse charcoal is strongly suggested. Hemoperfusion is indicated for patients with increasing serum levels or seizures from sustained-release products and for patients whose condition is deteriorating despite appropriate initial management. Although levels do not correlate well with toxicity, if the plasma level is more than 40 μg/mL in chronic overdose or more than 80 μg/mL in acute overdose, consider hemoperfusion. Levels should be checked frequently during treatment.

IRON

Iron poisoning is a common cause of pediatric ingestion emergencies. It is much less common in adults. Toxicity may occur at doses of 20 to 60 mg/kg. Lethal dose is 60 to 80 mg/kg of elemental iron.

Clinically, several phases are encountered in overdose:
Phase I (gastrointestinal symptoms 1/2 to 6 hours): nausea, vomiting, hematemesis, abdominal pain, diarrhea
Phase II (6 to 24 hours): latent period, patient seems to improve. Anion gap metabolic acidosis
Phase III (systemic toxicity): altered mental status, seizures, hepatic/renal failure, coagulopathy, death
Phase IV (late complications): gastrointestinal obstruction
Initial treatment includes standard supportive care and gastric emptying. Some authors recommend gastric lavage be performed with $NaHCO_3$, which converts iron to a less

absorbable salt. This practice is controversial and not thoroughly investigated. Activated charcoal may be given but is of questionable value. Overall, iron is fairly resistant to various stomach decontamination regimes.

Patients suffering from significant iron overdose should have adequate crystalloid fluid resuscitation. Deferoxamine is a chelating agent that enhances iron elimination by producing a water-soluble substance (ferrioxamine) that can be excreted by the kidneys. It is administered intravenously at a rate of 15 mg/kg per hour. Deferoxamine should be given in any moderately or severely symptomatic patient regardless of iron levels, if serum iron level is more than 350 μg/dL, or in any patient whose serum iron level is greater than total iron-binding capacity.

A word of caution is in order in regard to treating patients for iron overdose. First, although iron tablets often are seen on abdominal radiograph, their absence is not a guarantee that a significant iron overdose has not occurred. Second, a patient who presents to the emergency department in phase II (latent period) may appear well despite having taken a serious overdose. Finally, do not withhold chelation therapy in moderately or severely symptomatic patients while waiting for determination of serum iron levels.

- Deferoxamine is a specific chelating agent for iron.
- Serum iron levels should not be solely relied on in determining need for deferoxamine therapy.
- A normal abdominal radiograph does not exclude severe iron overdose.

LITHIUM

In general, lithium has a low therapeutic index. In acute intoxication, serum levels may not accurately reflect the severity of overdose. Early signs of toxicity are nausea and vomiting, dysarthria, and hand tremor. Later signs are ataxia, fasciculations, hyperreflexia, confusion, seizures, coma, and cardiotoxicity (rare).

Charcoal is not used for treatment because it does not absorb lithium. Rehydration with normal saline is helpful (lithium can cause nephrogenic diabetes insipidus). Alkalinization of the urine can increase renal excretion of lithium. Hemodialysis should be considered for patients with renal failure, for patients with deterioration after appropriate treatment, or if serum lithium levels exceed 4 mEq/L.

β-ADRENERGIC BLOCKERS

Extremely small doses of β-adrenergic blockers can produce life-threatening reactions. Blood levels are not helpful. Clinical findings include bradycardia (many rhythm types), hypotension, peripheral cyanosis, pulmonary edema, altered mental status, and many electrocardiographic abnormalities.

The treatment of β-adrenergic blocker overdose includes gastric lavage rather than emesis induction because β-adrenergic blockers taken in large quantity exert their effects quickly. Activated charcoal should also be administered. The hypotension and bradycardia are often refractory to usual therapies, including dopamine, epinephrine, and atropine. Intravenous glucagon seems to be the most consistent agent for reversing the toxic effects of β-adrenergic blocker overdose. Glucagon is given as an intravenous bolus (0.05-0.15 mg/kg) followed by a continuous infusion at 2-5 mg/hour.

- Glucagon is most consistent agent for reversing β-adrenergic blocker toxicity.

DIGITALIS

Clinical manifestations of digitalis toxicity include both cardiac and noncardiac symptoms. Toxic effects of digitalis in patients receiving chronic therapy can occur at any serum level. Acute overdoses of digitalis are rare but usually severe.

Noncardiac signs and symptoms are nausea, vomiting, abdominal pain, confusion, hallucinations, occasionally seizures, visual disturbances (many), and hyperkalemia. Cardiac symptoms are junctional tachycardia, ventricular premature contractions, ventricular tachycardia, ventricular fibrillation, atrial flutter, atrial fibrillation, and all types of atrioventricular block. Although hypokalemia increases the risk of toxicity in patients chronically taking digitalis, hyperkalemia is a complication of acute digitalis overdose.

Treatment includes supportive care with cardiac monitoring, and gastric emptying if ingestion was recent. Treat dangerous hyperkalemia with intravenous glucose, insulin, and bicarbonate. *Avoid* calcium in cases of digitalis toxicity. Atropine may be effective for bradycardias, as may external

pacemakers. Treat stable ventricular arrhythmias with lidocaine or phenytoin. Magnesium sulfate may be beneficial. Digoxin immune Fab (ovine) (Digibind) is digoxin-specific antibody fragments that have been induced in sheep. It acts by binding digoxin molecules, making them incapable of binding at their receptor, the Na^+K^+-ATPase. Its use should be reserved for severe intoxication. It is given intravenously, and its dose is titrated to clinical effect. Many vials are often required. Because serum digoxin levels reflect both bound and unbound drug, they may actually increase over several hours.

- Avoid calcium in digitalis toxicity.
- Atropine may be effective for bradycardias.
- Lidocaine or phenytoin is preferred agent for ventricular irritability.
- Digoxin-specific Fab fragments reserved for severe intoxication.

CYANIDE

Cyanide binds to iron in cytochrome oxidase, and the result is cellular hypoxia. It does not combine with the iron in hemoglobin. Cyanide is used in many industries, and the natural environment contains various cyanogenic glycosides that, when broken down and ingested, can release cyanide.

- Cyanide binds to iron in cytochrome oxidase.
- It does not combine with the iron in hemoglobin.

Clinical symptoms with inhalation (symptoms within seconds) are dry, burning throat, air hunger, hyperpnea, apnea, seizures, and death. Symptoms with ingestion (symptoms delayed) are nausea, vomiting, confusion, vertigo, giddiness, seizures, and cardiac dysrhythmias.

The diagnosis of cyanide overdose must initially be made clinically because rapid deterioration leading to death can occur well before any laboratory confirmation can be obtained. The history may provide clues to occupational cyanide exposure (electroplating, metallurgy, etc.), intentional cyanide exposure (suicide attempt), or accidental ingestion (apricot, plum, or peach pits). The odor of bitter almonds or peach pits is diagnostic of cyanide poisoning. Finally, altered mental status and tachypnea but no cyanosis suggest cyanide overdose.

Treatment includes supplemental high-flow 100% oxygen. If cyanide is ingested, consider gastric lavage and charcoal. Nitrite-thiosulfate is the therapy of choice in cyanide overdose. The nitrite causes creation of methemoglobin, which allows cyanide to bind to this rather than the cytochromic system. Thiosulfate then converts this to thiocyanate, which can be excreted by the kidney.

OPIOIDS

Opioids include many drugs that often are abused in society (for example, morphine, heroin, methadone, codeine, propoxyphene, opium, fentanyl, meperidine). Morphine, opium, and codeine are the only natural (opium-derived) opioids. All other opioids require minor or major chemical alterations to produce.

Clinical features of opioid overdose are drowsiness, lethargy, respiratory depression, coma, nausea, vomiting, miosis, ileus, urinary retention, and pulmonary edema.

- Morphine, opium, and codeine are natural opioids.
- Heroin and methadone cause pulmonary edema.
- Classic opioid triad: respiratory depression, pinpoint pupils, coma.

Opioid ingestions are associated with other drugs in 90% of cases, and 95% of all emergency room visits by opioid abusers are for infections or trauma (not overdose). Thiamine, 100 mg intramuscularly, is given. If the blood glucose level is less than 80 mg/dL, 50 mL of dextrose (D_{50}, push) is given. Naloxone (Narcan), 2 mg by intravenous bolus, is given and repeated as necessary. A continuous infusion is occasionally required. Naloxone can be given intravenously, intramuscularly, or subcutaneously or by endotracheal tube. Many opioids have a longer half-life than naloxone, so prolonged monitoring for resedation is necessary.

- 90% of opioid ingestions are associated with other drugs.
- Patients successfully treated with naloxone require prolonged monitoring.

COCAINE

Although legally classified as a narcotic, cocaine is the only naturally occurring local anesthetic. When abused, it may be injected intravenously or subcutaneously, swallowed, smoked, or applied to oral or genital mucous membranes. Cocaine is cut with many substances, some of which have toxicity of their own.

Clinical features of cocaine use are excitement, euphoria, restlessness, nausea, vomiting, headache, seizures, tachycardia or hypertension, hypoventilation, psychosis, and mydriasis. Serious effects are malignant hyperthermia, seizures, and ventricular tachycardia.

The treatment of cocaine overdose is generally supportive. Seizures may be treated with diazepam and phenytoin. Propranolol can be used for severe hypertension or tachycardia, although some authors prefer labetalol (an α- and β-adrenergic blocker), which would not cause unopposed α-stimulation. Haloperidol can be used for hallucinations, although some authors prefer benzodiazepines.

In an attempt to smuggle cocaine, some patients have swallowed balloons or condoms filled with it ("body packers"). If an abdominal radiograph demonstrates this, consideration should be given to endoscopic or surgical removal.

AMPHETAMINES

Amphetamines are noncatechol sympathomimetic adrenergic agents that have more central nervous system stimulant activity than catecholamines. Symptoms of intoxication include tachycardia, headache, hypertension, euphoria, mydriasis, anxiety, hypothermia, seizures, diaphoresis, hallucinations, and arrhythmias. The hypertension and cardiac arrhythmias may be severe.

In general, emesis or lavage is not helpful for treatment. Phentolamine (α-adrenergic blocker) or labetalol (α- and β-blocker) should be used to treat hypertensive crisis. Haloperidol is used for psychosis and agitation.

BENZODIAZEPINES

Benzodiazepines are a frequent cause of overdose (accidental, intentional, and iatrogenic) in adults. The associated morbidity and mortality are directly related to respiratory and central nervous system depression. In the past several years, an antagonist (flumazenil, Romazicon) has become available in the United States.

Flumazenil is a relatively pure antagonist with limited agonist or inverse agonist properties. It effectively antagonizes the neurologic, behavioral, and respiratory depressant effects of benzodiazepines. The initial dosage is 0.2 mg intravenously over 30 seconds. Subsequent dosages of 0.3 to 0.5 mg intravenously over 30 seconds can be given until desired effects are achieved or cumulative dose of 3 mg is given. Adverse reactions, including nausea, vomiting, dizziness, and, rarely, seizures, can occur, especially if cyclic antidepressants were also ingested. Two other problems can occur: 1) the precipitation of a withdrawal-type syndrome if the patient chronically uses benzodiazepines, and 2) resedation is very common, so prolonged monitoring is required.

Endotracheal intubation and ventilation is the treatment of choice for hypoventilatory patients. The exact role of flumazenil in benzodiazepine overdose has yet to be determined.

- For benzodiazepine overdose, endotracheal intubation and ventilation is used in hypoventilatory patients.
- Flumazenil can effectively reverse benzodiazepine-induced central nervous system and respiratory depression, but its role in overdose situations is unclear.

ALCOHOLS AND GLYCOLS

Ethanol, isopropyl alcohol (rubbing alcohol), methanol (wood alcohol), and ethylene glycol all produce an osmolar gap (see page 138). Methanol and ethylene glycol produce a large anion gap metabolic acidosis (serum bicarbonate level usually <10 mEq/L). Ethylene glycol produces calcium oxalate crystalluria. Isopropyl alcohol produces ketones but no acidosis.

Ethanol

Ethanol is the most abused drug. It is metabolized by liver alcohol dehydrogenase through zero-order kinetics (that is, enzymes that are saturable). Blood alcohol levels are a poor predictor of level of impairment and anticipated morbidity. Clinical findings are slurred speech, ataxia, nystagmus, dulled sensory perception, tachycardia, hypoventilation, hypothermia, and coma.

Because alcoholics also experience trauma, hypoglycemia, and life-threatening infections, part of treatment is to be vigilant. Observation until the patient is sober is a good general rule. Thiamine, 100 mg intramuscularly, can be given. If the blood glucose value is less than 80 mg/dL, 50 mL of dextrose is given. Naloxone, 2 mg intravenously, should be given if any signs of narcotic overdose are present. Severe intoxication occasionally requires endotracheal intubation and gastric lavage (especially if multiple drugs are ingested).

- Alcoholics also experience trauma, hypoglycemia, life-threatening infection.
- General rule, observe patient until he or she is sober.
- If blood glucose value <80 mg/dL, give 50 mL dextrose.

Isopropyl Alcohol

Isopropyl alcohol is rubbing alcohol. It can cause toxicity by ingestion or inhalation, but it is not absorbed through the skin. On an equal-dose basis, it is more toxic than ethyl alcohol, causing more central nervous system depression. It is also metabolized by alcohol dehydrogenase, the end products being acetone, CO_2, and H_2O. Thus, it produces an osmolar gap and ketosis without significant metabolic acidosis.

- Isopropyl alcohol is rubbing alcohol.
- More toxic than ethyl alcohol.
- Produces osmolar gap and ketosis without significant metabolic acidosis.

Clinical effects are the same as those of ethanol; other effects are hemorrhagic gastritis, hypotension, rhabdomyolysis, hepatocellular toxicity, and breath with a sweet odor.

Treatment is generally supportive, as for ethanol. Only in extremely rare cases is hemodialysis considered (for example, severe coma or isopropyl alcohol level >400 mg/dL).

Methanol

Methanol (wood alcohol) is metabolized by liver alcohol dehydrogenase to formaldehyde and formic acid (toxicity). Thus, it produces an osmolar gap and an impressively elevated anion gap metabolic acidosis. In fact, serum bicarbonate levels may reach 3 mEq/L. There is a latent period of 8 to 72 hours, and then visual symptoms (blurred vision, photophobia, papilledema), central nervous system effects (confusion, lethargy, coma), abdominal pain, nausea, and vomiting develop.

- Methanol produces osmolar gap and elevated anion gap metabolic acidosis.

Gastric lavage and activated charcoal are used for treatment. Ethanol has a greater affinity for alcohol dehydrogenase and, thus, helps prevent the formation of toxic metabolites. The goal is to achieve an ethanol level of 100 mg/dL. There are many dosing regimens. Hemodialysis works well and should be considered if methanol level is more than 50 mg/dL or if patient has deteriorated on ethanol therapy. Thiamine, other vitamins, magnesium, and glucose are given as needed. Bicarbonate therapy is controversial and should be guided by blood gas values.

- For methanol intoxication, gastric lavage and activated charcoal are used for treatment.
- Hemodialysis works well.
- Bicarbonate therapy is controversial.

Ethylene Glycol

Ethylene glycol is commonly found in antifreeze and many other products. It is also metabolized by liver alcohol dehydrogenase to its toxic metabolites. Clinically, ethylene glycol overdose affects the central nervous system (ataxia, nystagmus, seizures, coma, papilledema), kidney (calcium oxalate crystals, acute tubular necrosis), and gastrointestinal tract (abdominal pain, nausea, vomiting). Late effects are pulmonary edema and cardiac failure. Similar to methanol, ethylene glycol produces an osmolar gap and an impressive anion gap metabolic acidosis.

- Ethylene glycol found in antifreeze.
- Produces an osmolar gap and impressive anion gap metabolic acidosis.
- Produces calcium oxalate crystalluria.

Treatment is similar to that for methanol toxicity, that is, ethanol and hemodialysis if the ethylene glycol level is more than 50 mg/dL or there is clinical deterioration on ethanol therapy. Recently, a competitive inhibitor of the enzyme alcohol dehydrogenase was approved for use in cases of ethylene glycol ingestion (fomepizole). Theoretically, this antidote accomplishes the same thing as ethanol but with fewer undesirable side effects.

ORGANOPHOSPHATES

The inhibition of acetylcholinesterase by organophosphates results in increased cholinergic activity. Carbamates are also inhibitors of acetylcholinesterase, but they cause less toxicity because their binding is reversible. Clinical findings of pesticide overdose are bradycardia, lacrimation, salivation, sweating, urinary incontinence, wheezing, fecal incontinence, and miosis. Delayed effects are fasciculations, tachycardia, mydriasis, and hypertension.

Evaluation of patients includes determination of both serum (easier) and red blood cell (more accurate) cholinesterase levels.

- Organophosphates inhibit acetylcholinesterase.

Treatment includes establishment of an airway. Atropine, 2 to 4 mg, is given as needed. The stabilized patient is fully decontaminated by removing clothing and irrigating. Charcoal is used depending on route of contamination. Pralidoxime (Protopam, 2-PAM) reactivates cholinesterase and reverses cholinergic and nicotine effects. Dosage in adults is 1 g over 15 minutes.

- Treatment of pesticide toxicity includes atropine, 2-4 mg as needed.
- Pralidoxime also used.

CARBON MONOXIDE POISONING

Carbon monoxide is the leading cause of toxin-related death. It is a colorless, odorless, nonirritating gas that reversibly displaces oxygen in hemoglobin to produce carboxyhemoglobin (COHb). Symptoms are often vague and misdiagnosed.

Although at time of exposure COHb level can correlate with symptoms, the COHb level after initiation of treatment with 100% oxygen can be deceptively low (Table 4-4). Diagnosis is established from the history (especially if 100% oxygen administered) and from COHb levels.

- In carbon monoxide poisoning, carboxyhemoglobin level at exposure can correlate with symptoms, but after treatment with 100% oxygen, level can be deceptively low.

Treatment is administration of 100% oxygen (decreases half-life of COHb by 400%). The use of hyperbaric oxygen is somewhat controversial. It may prevent delayed neurologic sequelae, but controlled studies are lacking. Consider it for patients in coma, those with neurologic deficits, chest pain, or acidosis, or in pregnant patients. COHb value more than 30% may also be an indication, but the decision should be based on the clinical picture.

METHEMOGLOBINEMIA

Methemoglobinemia is an abnormal, nonfunctioning ferric hemoglobin ($HbFe^{3}+$) that cannot bind oxygen. It is caused by hereditary diseases (rare) but also by drugs of abuse such as amyl nitrite and isobutyl nitrite. These are used for short-term "rush" effect and as orgasm enhancers.

Diagnosis is based on the finding of chocolate-brown cyanosis unrelieved by oxygenation and arterial blood gases with low saturation but normal arterial oxygen partial pressure.

Treatment includes supplemental oxygen. Methylene blue acts as a cofactor in methemoglobinemia reductase system. Its use is reserved for patients with hypoxic symptoms or methemoglobin levels more than 30%. It may cause hemolysis in high doses.

Table 4-4.--Relationship of Carboxyhemoglobin Levels to Clinical Presentation

COHb, %	Signs and symptoms
0	None
10	Headache
20	Headache, dyspnea
30	Nausea, dizziness, impaired judgment
40	Confusion, syncope
50	Coma, seizures
60	Hypotension, respiratory failure
70	Death

QUESTIONS

Multiple Choice (choose the one best answer)

1. An 18-year-old woman is brought to the emergency department approximately 30 minutes after taking an unknown quantity of imipramine tablets. Emergency medical services personnel report a 2-minute seizure en route. On arrival, the patient is postictal with a Glasgow Coma score of 7. Her blood pressure is 90/60 mm Hg, and pulse is 130 beats/min. Her respirations are 12/min. She has an intravenous line of .9 normal saline in place. Your initial management sequence should be:
   a. Immediately place patient in the left lateral decubitus position and begin gastric lavage with a large-bore orogastric tube while initiating alkalinization of the patient's blood.
   b. Place an 18-F nasogastric tube and give activated charcoal (1 g/kg) immediately. Initiate alkalinization of the patient's blood.
   c. Perform endotracheal intubation with an appropriately sized cuffed endotracheal tube. After verifying tube position, perform gastric lavage with a large-bore orogastric tube. Follow up with activated charcoal (1 g/kg). Initiate alkalinization of the patient's blood.
   d. Give 30 mL of syrup of ipecac and begin alkalinization of patient's blood.
   e. Begin alkalinization of patient's blood and arrange for emergency hemodialysis.

2. An inmate from a local prison is brought to the emergency department after ingesting a large amount of "homemade" liquor. He is unconscious and responds only minimally to painful stimuli. His blood pressure is 110/90 mm Hg and pulse is 110 beats/min. His respirations are 12/min.

   Laboratory evaluation shows:

Sodium	135 mEq/L
Potassium	4.5 mEq/L
Chloride	95 mEq/L
HCO_2	10 mEq/L
Blood urea nitrogen	15 mg/dL
Glucose	100 mg/dL
Serum osmolality	300 mosm/kg

   Calcium oxalate crystals are seen in the urine. This patient has most likely taken an overdose of:
   a. Ethanol
   b. Methanol
   c. Isopropyl alcohol
   d. Ethylene glycol
   e. Aspirin

3. Hemodialysis may be useful in each of the following overdose situations *except*:
   a. Cyclic antidepressants
   b. Methanol
   c. Ethylene glycol
   d. Aspirin
   e. Lithium

4. A 50-year-old man has ingested 100 tablets of diphenhydramine in a suicide attempt. You would expect all of the following signs *except*:
   a. Mydriasis
   b. Tachycardia
   c. Dry, flushed, warm skin
   d. Hypertension
   e. Excessive salivation

5. A 19-year-old man is brought in by emergency medical services personnel after taking an overdose of an unknown substance. His past medical history includes only seizures. He is comatose with no response to painful stimuli. His blood pressure is 100/80 mm Hg, and pulse is 50 beats/min. Respiratory rate is 8/min, temperature is 34.8°C. He is areflexic, and you note bilateral rales on lung auscultation. You suspect:
   a. Barbiturate overdose
   b. Opiate overdose
   c. Amphetamine overdose
   d. Cyclic antidepressant overdose
   e. Antihistamine overdose

6. In which of the following overdose situations is a quantitative drug level most important?
   a. Aspirin
   b. Acetominophen
   c. Methanol
   d. Ethylene glycol
   e. Theophylline

7. Which of the following statements regarding gastric lavage is true?
   a. Gastric lavage should be performed on any patient who has taken a potentially dangerous overdose within the past 6 to 8 hours.
   b. Gastric lavage is quick, is without complications, and greatly speeds up the administration of activated charcoal.
   c. Gastric lavage can remove up to 75% of an ingested substance if accomplished in a timely manner.
   d. Gastric lavage should be reserved for patients who have taken a potentially dangerous overdose within

the past 1 or 2 hours. It should be accomplished *after* the airway has been assessed and secured, if necessary, with a cuffed endotracheal tube.

e. Gastric lavage should be accomplished using an 18-F nasogastric tube.

8. Which of the following statements concerning the cause of overdose is true?
   a. Most overdoses are not fatal and occur in children.
   b. Most overdoses are fatal and occur in adults.
   c. Most overdoses occur at the workplace.
   d. Most fatal overdoses occur in the very young (younger than 2 years).
   e. Most fatal overdoses are the result of accidental ingestion.

9. Which of the following statements regarding activated charcoal administration in overdose situations is *not* true?

a. Activated charcoal is emerging as the treatment of choice for most overdoses.
b. Activated charcoal is given in a dose of 1 g/kg body weight.
c. Single-dose activated charcoal is generally regarded as causing fewer complications than pulse charcoal therapy.
d. Activated charcoal binds small ionic compounds such as lithium and iron well.
e. Charcoal can be given as a slurry down an orogastric or nasogastric tube, or the patient can drink it.

10. Hemoperfusion should be considered in overdoses of:
    a. Aspirin
    b. Theophylline
    c. Acetaminophen
    d. Lithium
    e. Ethylene glycol

ANSWERS

1. Answer c.

Cyclic antidepressants can cause a rapid decrease in a patient's level of consciousness. Before gastric lavage, patients with altered mental status, a depressed gag reflex, or seizures should be intubated with an appropriately sized cuffed endotracheal tube. Syrup of ipecac should be avoided because of a high likelihood of aspiration. Hemodialysis is ineffective for removing cyclic antidepressants because of the large volumes of distribution and high protein binding.

2. Answer d.

The patient has both an osmolar gap (19) and an increased anion gap (20) metabolic acidosis. You would suspect either ethylene glycol or methanol as the cause of his unconsciousness. Further evidence in favor of ethylene glycol ingestion is provided by the calcium oxalate crystals present in the urine.

3. Answer a.

To be a suitable candidate for hemodialysis, a patient must have overdosed on a substance of small molecular weight and a small volume of distribution. The substance also must have limited protein and lipid binding. Tricyclic antidepressants have large volumes of distribution and high degrees of protein binding; thus, hemodialysis is impractical.

4. Answer e.

Antihistamines are one of the compounds known to produce the anticholinergic syndrome. All of the choices listed are signs of the anticholinergic syndrome *except* excessive salivation. This actually occurs in the cholinergic syndrome.

5. Answer a.

The areflexic coma, hypothermia, and pulmonary edema are clues that this patient has taken a barbiturate overdose. His past history of seizure also points to this possibility because he may have access to barbiturates. Opiate overdose would not be expected to produce the areflexia or this marked degree of hypothermia unless other factors were present. Amphetamines, cyclic antidepressants, and antihistamines would produce tachycardia, hypertension, and, often, hyperthermia.

6. Answer b.

Quantitative drug levels have important therapeutic implications in only a few situations. Frequently, therapy must begin before the drug level is complete (for example, methanol and ethylene glycol), or the quantitative drug level may not correlate well with toxicity (for example, aspirin and theophylline). In acetaminophen overdose, quantitative drug levels are extremely important and can correlate well with subsequent liver damage. There is the added benefit of a therapeutic "window," allowing for administration of the antidote *N*-acetylcysteine to be guided by drug levels most of the time.

7. Answer d.

Gastric lavage is a time-consuming procedure that, under ideal conditions, removes less than 40% of an ingested material. It should be done only when a patient arrives in the emergency department 1 or 2 hours after ingesting a potentially toxic substance. Many complications are associated with gastric lavage.

8. Answer a.

Most overdoses are not fatal and occur in children. Fatal overdoses are a very small fraction of total overdoses (<1%), and these are usually in adults who intentionally took a drug either to commit suicide or in a "recreational" fashion.

9. Answer d.

Activated charcoal is emerging as the treatment of choice in most cases of overdose. It can be given with a nasogastric or orogastric tube, or the patient can drink the dose (1 g/dL). Single-dose activated charcoal is less likely to cause aspiration or ileus. Unfortunately, some compounds such as alcohols or small ionic compounds are not well bound.

10. Answer b.

Hemoperfusion is indicated in some overdoses of barbiturate, diphenylhydantoin, and theophylline preparations. Hemodialysis is indicated in some overdoses of aspirin, ethylene glycol, methanol, lithium, and bromide. Neither method is indicated in acetaminophen overdose.

CHAPTER 5

CRITICAL CARE MEDICINE

Steve G. Peters, M.D.
William F. Dunn, M.D.

Critical Care Medicine encompasses multidisciplinary aspects of the management of severely ill patients. All areas of medicine may have relevance for critically ill patients, but this review focuses on aspects of cardiopulmonary monitoring and life support, technological interventions, and disease states typically managed in the intensive care unit (ICU).

A few general tips for preparing for the board examination: 1) Stress the acute care of common life-threatening conditions. Review a general manual or textbook of medical therapeutics. 2) Try to identify important areas with which you are less familiar or experienced. Also, review situations encountered in major hospitals of large U.S. cities, for example, complications of alcohol, drug overdose, and trauma. 3) Common things are commonly tested, but be aware of unusual causes or features of common conditions, for example, adult respiratory distress syndrome (ARDS) as a result of thrombotic thrombocytopenic purpura. 4) In reviewing drugs, stress common agents that have serious toxic effects, for example, antihypertensive agents, theophylline, antibiotics, immunosuppressive agents, and antidepressants. 5) Know the indications for (and complications of) common invasive procedures, for example, pulmonary angiography, cardiac catheterization, and hemodialysis. 6) Know the current advanced cardiac life support guidelines.

- Stress acute care of common life-threatening conditions.
- Identify important areas with which you are less familiar or experienced.
- Be aware of unusual causes or features of common conditions.
- Know the indications for (and complications of) invasive procedures.
- Know the advanced cardiac life support guidelines.

RESPIRATORY FAILURE

Effective functioning of the respiratory system requires normal central nervous system control, neuromuscular transmission and bellows function, and gas exchange at the alveolar-capillary level. Respiratory failure may result from disease at any of these levels.

Physiologic Definitions and Relationships

Lung Volumes

TLC = total lung capacity—the total volume of gas in the chest at the end of a maximal inspiration. VC = vital capacity—the volume of a maximal breath (expired or inspired). V_T = tidal volume—the volume of a normal breath. FRC = functional residual capacity—lung volume at the end of a normal expiration. It reflects the relaxation point of the respiratory system or the point at which outward recoil of the chest wall is balanced by inward recoil of the lungs. Compliance (C) of the lungs or respiratory system is defined by the change in volume (ΔV) for a given change in pressure (ΔP).

$$C_{STATIC} = \frac{\Delta V}{\Delta P}$$

where ΔV is measured in liters (L) and ΔP in cm H_2O. Emphysema causes the loss of recoil and, thus, increased compliance. Most other disease states, particularly interstitial diseases, fibrosis, pulmonary edema, and ARDS, cause decreased compliance (i.e., "stiff" lungs, or increased transpulmonary pressure for a given volume change).

- Normal compliance = 0.2 L/cm H_2O.
- Emphysema causes the loss of recoil and increased compliance.
- Interstitial diseases, fibrosis, pulmonary edema, and ARDS cause decreased compliance.

Resistance (R) to air flow is defined by the change in pressure (ΔP) for a given change in flow ($\Delta \dot{V}$)

$$R = \frac{\Delta P}{\Delta \dot{V}}$$

where ΔP is measured in cm H_2O and $\Delta \dot{V}$ in L/s. Common causes of increased airway resistance include bronchospasm and airway secretions.

- Common causes of increased airway resistance: bronchospasm and airway secretions.

The total pressure required to inflate the respiratory system (spontaneously or with a mechanical ventilator) is the pressure required to overcome elastic recoil (primarily due to lungs and chest wall) plus the pressure to overcome flow resistance (primarily due to airways/endotracheal tube):

$$P_{inflation} = \frac{\Delta V}{C_{ST}} + R \times \Delta \dot{V}$$

(Elastic Load)   (Resistive Load)

Gas exchange requires alveolar ventilation for the elimination of carbon dioxide, oxygen uptake across the alveolar-capillary membrane, and the delivery of oxygen to tissues. Hypoxemia may result from a decrease in the inspired partial pressure of oxygen (e.g., high altitude, including air travel), hypoventilation, ventilation-perfusion ($\dot{V}/Q$) mismatch, shunting, or diffusion barrier. Estimation of the alveolar-arterial gradient (A-a) for oxygen is essential in analyzing the cause of hypoxemia. Important relationships include the following:

The partial pressure of carbon dioxide ($Paco_2$) in the blood is directly proportional to the amount of carbon dioxide produced ($\dot{V}co_2$), and inversely proportional to alveolar ventilation ($\dot{V}A$):

$$Paco_2 = k \frac{\dot{V}co_2}{\dot{V}A}$$

Alveolar ventilation is equal to total ventilation ($\dot{V}E$) minus dead space ventilation ($\dot{V}D$). Thus, physiologic dead space is defined by the portion of a breath that does not participate in gas exchange. Dead space volume (V_D) may be anatomical (conducting airways) or alveolar (areas of ventilation that receive no perfusion):

$$\dot{V}A = \dot{V}E - (V_D \times f)$$

where f = breaths/min.

$$\frac{V_D}{V_T} \text{ normally is } <0.25 - 0.30$$

$$\frac{V_D}{V_T} = \frac{Paco_2 - P_Eco_2}{Paco_2}$$

(Bohr Equation)

where P_Eco_2 is the partial pressure of expired carbon dioxide. The dead space-to-tidal volume ratio is calculated by measuring the partial pressure of carbon dioxide in an arterial blood ($Paco_2$) gas sample and an expired gas sample (P_Eco_2). The greater the dead space, the greater the difference between $Paco_2$ and P_Eco_2.

- Physiologic dead space is defined by the portion of breath not participating in gas exchange.
- Increased dead space leads to decreased CO_2 elimination (or increased respiratory drive to eliminate the increase in CO_2 burden).

Alveolar gas consists of inspired gases saturated with water vapor. The alveolus also contains carbon dioxide delivered from the blood. The sum of the partial pressures of all gases present equals the ambient barometric pressure. The alveolar air equation defines this relationship:

$$PAO_2 = FIO_2 (P_B - P_{H_2O}) - \frac{Paco_2}{R}$$

where PA is alveolar partial pressure, PB is barometric pressure (about 760 mm Hg at sea level), P_{H_2O} is water vapor pressure (47 mm Hg), and R is the respiratory quotient ($\dot{V}co_2/\dot{V}o_2$, normally about 0.8). The simplified equation is

$$PAO_2 = FIO_2 (P_B - 47) - \frac{Paco_2}{0.8}$$

Breathing room air ($FIO_2 = 0.21$) at sea level:

$$PAO_2 = 150 - \frac{40}{0.8}$$

or normal PAO_2 is approximately equal to 100 mm Hg.

The A-a oxygen difference is defined by PAO_2 minus Pao_2, which is normally less than 10 to 20 mm Hg when breathing room air. The A-a gradient normally increases to approximately 50 to 100 mm Hg as the FIO_2 increases from 0.21 to 1.0. Hypoxemia due to hypoventilation is characterized by increased $Paco_2$ and decreased Pao_2 but by a relatively normal A-a gradient. Hypoxemia due to ventilation-perfusion mismatch shows an increased A-a gradient. A shunt is defined by perfusion in the absence of ventilation (i.e., $\dot{V}/Q = 0$). With a pure shunt, Pao_2 does not increase even though FIO_2 is increased to 100%. Normal shunt fraction is less than 3% to 5% of total cardiac output. The shunt fraction is measured on

100% oxygen and is expressed as:

$$\frac{Q_s}{Q_t} = \frac{Cc'o_2 - Cao_2}{Cc'o_2 - C\overline{v}o_2} = \frac{P(A-a)o_2 \times 0.003}{P(A-a)o_2 \times 0.003 + (Ca-C\overline{v})o_2}$$

The content of oxygen in the blood is the total amount of oxygen bound to hemoglobin (Hgb) plus the amount dissolved.

$$O_2 \text{ content: } C_xO_2 = \underset{\text{(Bound)}}{1.34 \times Hgb \times S_xO_2} + \underset{\text{(Dissolved)}}{0.003 \times P_xO_2}$$

where x may equal arterial, venous, capillary, etc.

Under steady state conditions, the amount of oxygen used by the tissues equals the amount taken up by the lungs. The oxygen uptake, $\dot{V}o_2$, can be defined by amount of oxygen leaving the lungs in pulmonary venous blood minus the amount of oxygen coming into the lungs in the pulmonary arteries. This should be familiar as the Fick equation:

$$\dot{V}o_2 = CO\,(Cao_2 - C\overline{v}o_2)$$

where CO is cardiac output.

- Hypoxemia due to hypoventilation: increased $Paco_2$, decreased Pao_2, normal A-a gradient.
- Shunt is defined by perfusion in absence of ventilation, i.e., $\dfrac{\text{Ventilation}}{\text{Perfusion}} = 0$.
- The normal shunt fraction is <3%-5% of total cardiac output.
- A shunt leads to hypoxemia that shows little improvement after supplemental oxygen.

Many applications of the Fick equation are important in managing critically ill patients. One application involves continuous monitoring of mixed venous oxygen saturation by a specialized type of pulmonary artery catheter. Expressing oxygen content in terms of saturation and rearranging the Fick equation to solve the $S\overline{v}o_2$ yields the following:

$$S\overline{v}o_2 = Sao_2 - \frac{\dot{V}o_2}{CO \times Hgb \times 1.34}$$

Note that decreased mixed venous oxygen saturation may be due to decreased arterial saturation, increased oxygen consumption, decreased cardiac output, or decreased hemoglobin. Certain disease states, particularly early sepsis, may be characterized by normal or increased mixed venous oxygen saturation, because cardiac output initially increases, along with impaired oxygen uptake by the tissues. Later in sepsis, mixed venous $S\overline{v}o_2$ typically decreases because of decreased oxygen delivery.

- Decreased mixed venous oxygen may be due to: decreased arterial saturation, increased oxygen consumption, decreased cardiac output, or decreased hemoglobin.
- Early sepsis: normal or increased mixed venous oxygen saturation.

Under normal circumstances, oxygen demand by the tissues is met by the supply. Oxygen delivery is defined by cardiac output times arterial oxygen content, i.e.,

$$O_2 \text{ delivery} = CO \times Cao_2$$

Although cardiac output may decrease, $\dot{V}o_2$ of the tissues may be maintained by increased oxygen extraction.

- Oxygen delivery = cardiac output x arterial oxygen content.

ACID-BASE BALANCE AND ARTERIAL BLOOD GASES

The production of acid byproducts is the normal result of cellular metabolism. An acid is defined as a hydrogen ion, $[H^+]$, or proton donor. A base accepts protons. The dissociation constant (K) for an acid (HA) may be defined as

$$K = \frac{[H^+][A^-]}{[HA]}$$

Buffer systems minimize the changes in pH associated with the addition of acid or base. For carbonic acid:

$$H_2O + CO_2 \overset{}{\longleftrightarrow} H_2CO_3 \overset{K}{\longleftrightarrow} H^+ + HCO_3^-$$

$$\text{and } K = \frac{[H^+][HCO_3^-]}{[H_2CO_3]}$$

The Henderson-Hasselbalch equation:

$$pH = pK + \log \frac{[HCO_3^-]}{[H_2CO_3]}$$

where $pH = -\log[H^+]$ and $pK = -\log K$. The pK for carbonic acid is 6.1. $[H_2CO_3]$ is often measured by taking $0.03 \times Paco_2$ (i.e., dissolved carbon dioxide). So the Henderson-Hasselbalch equation can be rewritten as

$$pH = 6.1 + \log \frac{[HCO_3^-]}{0.03 \times Paco_2}$$

Hydrogen ions are buffered by several mechanisms in different body fluid compartments. In plasma and interstitial fluid, bicarbonate is the major buffer, with proteins and phosphate compounds contributing to a lesser extent. In erythrocytes, hemoglobin is the major buffer, but bicarbonate contributes approximately 30% and phosphate 10% of the buffering capacity. The kidney eliminates organic acid and also contributes by 1) reabsorption of bicarbonate from tubular fluids, 2) formation of titratable acid, and 3) elimination of [H$^+$] as ammonium ions.

- Bicarbonate is the major buffer in plasma and interstitial fluid.
- In erythrocytes, hemoglobin is the major buffer.
- The kidney eliminates organic acid and reabsorbs bicarbonate from tubular fluids.

Given the importance of the carbonic acid-bicarbonate system, many acid-base problems involve some method for solving variables of the Henderson-Hasselbalch equation. Because pK is constant, given two of the three values for pH, P_{CO_2}, and HCO_3^-, the missing variable can be calculated. Graphic displays are commonly used; two of the variables are plotted at constant values (isopleths) for the third variable (the Davenport diagram is an example).

Patterns of Acid-Base Disorder

Respiratory Acidosis

Acute respiratory acidosis is defined by rapid development of carbon dioxide retention (Pa_{CO_2} >45 mm Hg) with a concomitant decrease in pH (<7.35). Common causes include respiratory depression by drugs such as narcotics, central nervous system injury, acute diaphragm or neuromuscular weakness, severe parenchymal respiratory failure, and cardiac failure. Because carbon dioxide diffuses quickly into cells and the cerebrospinal fluid, the physiologic effects of the acidosis may occur rapidly. Confusion, obtundation, and signs of cerebral edema are commonly observed. Chronic respiratory acidosis is typically seen in patients with severe chronic obstructive lung disease (particularly chronic bronchitis or bronchiectasis) and in other states associated with chronic alveolar hypoventilation. Chronic respiratory acidosis may be compensated partly by renal mechanisms, that is, increased reabsorption of bicarbonate and excretion of acid in the urine.

- Acute respiratory acidosis: rapid onset of carbon dioxide retention with concomitant decrease in pH.
- Chronic respiratory acidosis is typically seen in patients with severe chronic obstructive lung disease or other states associated with chronic alveolar hypoventilation.

Respiratory Alkalosis

Acute respiratory alkalosis is the result of a rapid decrease in Pa_{CO_2} due to hyperventilation. Hyperventilation is usually associated with anxiety or pain. Other important causes are early shock states, pulmonary embolism, other causes of hypoxemia, hyperthermia, salicylate intoxication, liver failure, and disorders of the central nervous system. Patients with unexplained hypocapnia should be evaluated for these disorders. In mechanically ventilated patients, respiratory alkalosis may result from inadvertent over-ventilation, that is, excessive tidal volume and/or respiratory rate, especially in a volume preset assist-control ventilator mode.

- Respiratory alkalosis is the result of alveolar hyperventilation.
- Common causes include anxiety, pain, shock, pulmonary embolism, hypoxemia, fever, salicylate overdose, liver failure, and mechanical over-ventilation.

Metabolic Acidosis

Metabolic acidosis results from the accumulation of organic acids such as lactate, pyruvate, or keto acids. Acidosis may develop by increased acid production or decreased renal excretion of acid. Conditions causing metabolic acidosis are further characterized by the anion gap, that is,

$$[Na^+] - ([Cl^-] + [HCO_3^-])$$

with a normal value of 8 to 14 mEq/L.

A normal anion gap or non-anion gap acidosis is characterized by an increase in chloride balancing the loss of bicarbonate. Causes include gastrointestinal losses of bicarbonate, that is, diarrhea, urinary diversion procedures, or intestinal fistulas. Renal losses of bicarbonate (renal tubular acidosis) are also associated with a normal anion gap. Causes of acidosis associated with other anions—increased anion gap disorders—are diabetic ketoacidosis, lactic acidosis, uremia, and toxins (ethylene glycol, methanol, paraldehyde, and salicylate).

- Metabolic acidosis: result of accumulation of organic acids, e.g., lactate, pyruvate, keto acids.
- Normal anion gap or non-anion gap acidosis is characterized by increase in chloride balancing loss of bicarbonate.
- Increased anion gap disorders: diabetic ketoacidosis, lactic acidosis, uremia, toxins (ethylene glycol, methanol, paraldehyde, salicylate, isoniazid, cyanide, toluene).

Metabolic Alkalosis

Primary metabolic alkalosis is characterized by increased bicarbonate and pH. Hypokalemia and hypochloremia are commonly associated and further perpetuate the alkalosis. Common causes are volume contraction states, particularly those associated with the loss of chloride and hydrogen ion (vomiting and nasogastric suctioning). Diuretic therapy and mineralocorticoids are also common contributing factors. Although respiratory compensation (hypoventilation) for metabolic alkalosis might seem counterproductive, it can occur and may contribute to hypoxemia. As with other acid-base disorders, therapy is directed at the underlying cause, but support with volume and potassium and chloride replacement are important.

- Primary metabolic alkalosis is characterized by increased bicarbonate and pH.
- Hypokalemia and hypochloremia are commonly associated and further perpetuate alkalosis.
- Common causes are volume contraction states, particularly those associated with further loss of chloride and hydrogen ion (vomiting, nasogastric suctioning).

Mixed Acid-Base Disorders

Mixed disorders are characterized by a combination of the primary abnormalities described above or by a primary disorder and compensatory changes in $PaCO_2$ or bicarbonate. For example, combined respiratory and metabolic acidosis may occur in patients with depressed respiration and tissue hypoperfusion, as would occur with severe shock, after cardiorespiratory arrest, or with status epilepticus. In these situations, pH is severely depressed and immediate therapy is necessary. Treatment includes assisted ventilation plus measures to improve cardiac output and organ perfusion. Sodium bicarbonate might be given for severe acidemia (pH <7.0-7.1), but treatment must be directed at the underlying cause of the primary disorder.

- Combined respiratory and metabolic acidosis leads to severe acidemia.
- Treatment should be directed at the underlying disorder.

Respiratory acidosis and metabolic alkalosis typically occur in patients with chronic obstructive pulmonary disease (COPD) or chronic alveolar hypoventilation. Secondary bicarbonate retention may be augmented by concomitant corticosteroid therapy or diuretics. Because a given blood gas measurement showing increased $PaCO_2$ and increased bicarbonate (with pH near 7.4) could occur by many mechanisms, the clinical history is essential for determining the most likely pathophysiology. If patients with chronic hypercarbia are mechanically ventilated, there is a risk of severe alkalemia if the ventilator settings are adjusted to "normalize" the $PaCO_2$ at approximately 40 mm Hg without recognizing the chronic compensatory nature of the increase in bicarbonate.

- Respiratory acidosis plus metabolic alkalosis is seen most commonly in patients with chronic respiratory insufficiency plus bicarbonate retention.

Metabolic acidosis and respiratory alkalosis may occur in patients with tissue hypoperfusion and respiratory stimulation, as is commonly seen with early shock states, sepsis, and liver or renal failure. This pattern is also typical of salicylate intoxication.

- Metabolic acidosis and respiratory alkalosis are commonly seen with shock states, sepsis, or salicylate overdose.

Metabolic and respiratory alkalosis rarely occurs in spontaneously breathing patients but can develop quickly with mechanical ventilation. This usually is the result of a disorder causing respiratory alkalosis, as described above, combined with a metabolic alkalosis induced by volume contraction, gastric suctioning, hypokalemia, diuretics, or corticosteroids. Seizures and/or cardiac arrhythmias may result from severe alkalemia. Treatment usually requires replacement of volume, potassium, and chloride.

CLINICAL APPROACH TO ARTERIAL BLOOD GASES

There are many ways to assess problems of acid-base balance and gas exchange. When interpreting arterial blood gases, the following approach is useful:

1. Consider the pH. Are conditions normal (pH 7.35-7.45), acidemic (<7.35), or alkalemic (>7.45)?
2. Assess $PaCO_2$. Does the $PaCO_2$ change (from 40 mm Hg) account for the pH change (from 7.40)? Evaluation of this relationship requires calculation, graphic display, or a rule of thumb, such as: an acute change in $PaCO_2$ of 10 mm Hg should be associated with a pH change in the opposite direction of approximately 0.08 unit. If an abnormal pH can thus be accounted for by the change in $PaCO_2$, a simple acute respiratory disturbance is present. If not, a mixed acid-base disorder is defined.
3. The change in bicarbonate, that is, base deficit or excess, should confirm the conditions already defined by pH and $PaCO_2$.
4. Consider PaO_2. If hypoxemia is present, estimate the A-a gradient. If this is normal and $PaCO_2$ is increased, hypoventilation alone should account for the hypoxemia. There should be no significant associated pulmonary parenchymal radiographic infiltrate. The A-a gradient should be increased in conditions of ventilation-perfusion mismatching, shunting, or diffusion barrier.
5. Compare the PaO_2 and the arterial saturation, SaO_2. The SaO_2 should correspond to the expected values for a normal oxygen-hemoglobin dissociation curve. If saturation is lower than expected, consider the presence of other hemoglobin forms, for example, carboxyhemoglobin or methemoglobin.

As examples, use the algorithm above to match the following arterial blood gases with the clinical scenarios listed below.

	pH	$Paco_2$	HCO_3^-	Pao_2 (room air)	Sao_2
A.	7.35	60	32	50	85%
B.	7.50	46	34	85	94%
C.	7.18	70	26	55	89%
D.	7.28	31	15	110	99%
E.	7.38	30	18	105	75%

1. 20-year-old woman with diabetic ketoacidosis
2. 20-year-old man with acute narcotic overdose
3. 60-year-old man 1 week after an abdominal operation, with continuous nasogastric suction and diuretic therapy
4. 60-year-old woman with severe emphysema
5. 60-year-old man with carbon monoxide intoxication
(Answers: 1. D, 2. C, 3. B, 4. A, 5. E)

- Consider the pH.
- Assess $Paco_2$.
- Change in bicarbonate should confirm the conditions already defined by pH and $Paco_2$.
- Consider Pao_2 and A-a gradient.

Airway Management

Endotracheal intubation allows control of the airway, ability to deliver specific inspired oxygen and positive pressure ventilation, and protection from aspiration. Indications for intubation include airway protection in cases of obstruction or loss of normal gag and cough reflexes, central nervous system injury or sedation with loss of normal controls of ventilation, and any cause of respiratory failure requiring positive pressure-assisted ventilation. Oral-tracheal intubation is usually achieved through direct visualization with a laryngoscope. In experienced hands, this procedure should be relatively quick and safe. Complications may include vomiting and aspiration, hypoxemia during the procedure, and inadvertent intubation of the esophagus. The major contraindication for laryngoscopic intubation is an unstable cervical spine (due to trauma or degenerative conditions such as rheumatoid arthritis). In such cases, fiberoptic intubation (passing a tube over a bronchoscope) or tracheostomy may be necessary. In semiconscious and spontaneously breathing patients, nasotracheal intubation may be accomplished "blindly" and may be more comfortable for patients. Complications include bleeding, obstruction of sinus drainage with sinusitis, and damage to nasal structures.

- Endotracheal intubation allows control of the airway.
- Contraindication: unstable cervical spine (trauma or rheumatoid arthritis).

- In semiconscious, spontaneously breathing patients, nasotracheal intubation may be an alternative.

In emergency situations in which airway control is required, cricothyrotomy may be lifesaving. This procedure involves identification and puncture of the cricothyroid membrane. In patients requiring prolonged mechanical ventilation or airway support, the timing of tracheostomy is controversial. The use of high-volume low-pressure endotracheal tube cuffs has decreased the frequency of tracheal injury and stenosis caused by prolonged intubation. Tracheostomy has the advantages of decreased laryngeal injury, increased patient comfort, ease of suctioning, and, in certain patients, allowance for oral ingestion and speech. Complications may include tracheal injury and stenosis, bleeding, tracheoesophageal fistula, and possibly increased bronchial or pulmonary infections. Tracheostomy is commonly considered in patients who have needed or are expected to need intubation and mechanical ventilation for longer than 2 to 4 weeks.

- In emergency situations, cricothyrotomy may be lifesaving.
- High-volume low-pressure endotracheal tube cuffs have decreased frequency of tracheal injury and stenosis.
- Tracheostomy is for patients who have needed or are expected to need intubation and mechanical ventilation for >2-4 weeks.

Mechanical Ventilation

Mechanical ventilation may be valuable in various conditions of respiratory failure, including loss of respiratory control, neuromuscular or respiratory pump failure, and disorders of gas exchange. Many specific variables have been suggested (although they may not be absolute) as criteria for ventilator support and are listed in Table 5-1.

Complications of Mechanical Ventilation

Complications of mechanical ventilation may relate to airway access, physiologic responses to positive pressure, and

Table 5-1.—Criteria for Ventilator Support

Respiratory rate >30/min
Minute ventilation >10 L/min
Maximal inspiratory pressure < -20 cm H_2O
Vital capacity <10 mL/kg
Pao_2 <60 mm Hg with Fio_2 >0.60
Pao_2/Fio_2 <100-150
$P(A-a)O_2$ >300 mm Hg on Fio_2 1.0
Vd/Vt >0.60
$Paco_2$ >50 mm Hg

complications related to other organ systems. Examples are given in Table 5-2.

Other complications, such as pulmonary embolism or malnutrition, may also reflect the underlying disease state. Management of these complications requires ongoing surveillance and recognition. Diagnosis of pneumonia may be difficult in patients receiving mechanical ventilation because pulmonary infiltrates are frequently present, tracheal secretions may be colonized by bacteria, and signs such as fever and leukocytosis are frequently blunted. Prophylaxis is commonly given to reduce stress-related gastritis and ulceration. H_2-Blockers may increase colonization of the respiratory tract by gram-negative bacteria. Sucralfate or frequent use of antacids is an alternative. The hemodynamic complications of increased intrathoracic pressure may be overcome by fluid administration; however, there is often a coexisting condition of capillary leak and pulmonary edema that may worsen.

- Diagnosis of pneumonia may be difficult in patients receiving mechanical ventilation.
- Prophylaxis is commonly given to reduce stress-related gastritis and ulceration.
- H_2-Blockers may increase colonization of respiratory tract by gram-negative bacteria; sucralfate or frequent use of antacids is an alternative.

An important and occasionally subtle complication of positive pressure ventilation is called "intrinsic positive end-expiratory pressure" (PEEP), "auto-PEEP," "breath stacking," or "dynamic hyperinflation." This refers to a phenomenon of inadequate time during the expiratory phase of the respiratory cycle, so that a mechanically assisted breath is delivered before passive expiration of the lungs is complete. Thus, a new machine breath is delivered before the previous breath is completely exhaled. This may worsen hyperinflation, increase intrathoracic pressure, reduce venous return and worsen the

Table 5-2.— Complications of Mechanical Ventilation

Airway injury, bleeding, infection
Ventilator malfunction—leaks, power loss, incorrect settings, or alarm failures
Barotrauma; pneumothorax; interstitial, subcutaneous, or mediastinal air
Decreased right ventricular filling, increased right ventricular afterload, decreased cardiac output, hypotension
Gastrointestinal tract bleeding, stress gastritis, ulceration
Decreased urine output
Alteration in intracranial pressure

---

associated complications (e.g., barotrauma), especially in patients with airway obstruction. Intrinsic PEEP may exist in spontaneously breathing patients with obstructive airway disease, but the effect is most significant in mechanically ventilated patients. Treatment typically involves optimizing bronchodilator therapy and altering the ventilator cycle to allow maximal expiratory time.

"Modes of mechanical ventilation" refers to the pattern of cycling of the machine breath and its relation to the spontaneous breaths of the patient. Volume preset assist-control mode is defined by a machine-assisted breath for every inspiratory effort by the patient. If no spontaneous breaths occur during a preset time interval, a controlled breath of predetermined tidal volume will be delivered by the ventilator. The backup rate should determine the minimal minute ventilation the patient will receive. The advantage of the assist-control mode is that it should allow maximal rest for the patient and maximal control of ventilation. The disadvantage is that hyperventilation and/or air trapping can occur in patients making rapid inspiratory efforts.

Volume preset intermittent mandatory ventilation (IMV) allows a preset number of machine-assisted breaths of a given tidal volume. Between machine breaths, patients may breathe spontaneously. The IMV mode was developed as a mode of weaning patients, such that the number of mechanical breaths delivered could be gradually decreased, thus allowing for increasing spontaneous ventilation. However, recent trials have shown that this mode of weaning is inferior to weaning via T-piece trials or pressure support ventilation.

- Assist-control mode: machine-assisted breath for every inspiratory effort by the patient (amandated minimal frequency is set by the physician).
- Assist-control mode advantage: allows maximal rest for patient and maximal control of ventilation.
- Assist-control mode disadvantage: hyperventilation and/or air trapping in patients making rapid inspiratory efforts.
- IMV: allows preset number of machine-assisted breaths of a given tidal volume.
- Between machine breaths, patients may breathe spontaneously.
- IMV appears to be inferior to other weaning techniques (T-piece trials or pressure support).

Pressure support may be used to assist spontaneously breathing patients, with or without IMV breaths. In this technique, for each inspiratory effort by the patient, the ventilator delivers a high rate of flow of inspired gas, up to a preset pressure limit. This pressure support occurs only during the spontaneous inspiratory effort, so that the rate and pattern of respiration are determined by the patient.

- With pressure support ventilation, for each inspiratory effort of the patient, the ventilator delivers a high flow of inspired gas, up to preset pressure limit.

PEEP is intended to increase functional residual capacity, recruit partially collapsed alveoli, improve lung compliance, and improve ventilation-perfusion matching. An adverse effect of PEEP is an excessive increase in intrathoracic pressure with decreased cardiac output. Overdistention of lung units may also worsen gas exchange because of ventilator-induced lung injury. At levels of PEEP greater than 10 to 15 cm H_2O, barotrauma is of particular concern. The optimal, or best, PEEP may be defined as the lowest level of PEEP needed to achieve satisfactory oxygen delivery at a nontoxic FIO_2.

- PEEP: to increase functional residual capacity, recruit partially collapsed alveoli, improve lung compliance, improve ventilation-perfusion matching.
- Adverse effect of PEEP: excessive increase in intrathoracic pressure with decreased cardiac output.
- Overdistention of lung units may also worsen ventilation-perfusion matching and gas exchange.
- Optimal, or best, PEEP: lowest level of PEEP needed to achieve satisfactory oxygenation at a nontoxic FIO_2.

Pulmonary oxygen toxicity appears to be the result of direct exposure to high tensions of inspired oxygen or alveolar oxygen. For adults, oxygen toxicity is not believed to be a major clinical concern below an FIO_2 of 0.40 to 0.50. Higher levels of inspired oxygen may be associated with acute tracheobronchitis (most likely an irritant effect). After several days of exposure, a syndrome of diffuse alveolar damage and lung injury may develop. The pathologic picture may resemble that of ARDS.

- Pulmonary oxygen toxicity: result of direct exposure to high tensions of inspired oxygen or alveolar oxygen.
- Syndrome of diffuse alveolar damage and lung injury may develop.

ADULT RESPIRATORY DISTRESS SYNDROME

Diffuse lung injury with acute hypoxic respiratory failure may result from various injuries. Acute lung injury is a frequent primary cause of critical illness and may occur as a complication or a coexisting feature of multisystem disease. Mortality from all causes averages about 50%. Existing therapies do not significantly alter overall mortality in established ARDS. Recent emphasis is on identification of patients at high risk for acute lung injury and on possible early interventions. ARDS is commonly defined as diffuse acute lung injury that has the following major features: diffuse pulmonary infiltrates,

severe hypoxemia due to shunting and ventilation-perfusion mismatch, and normal or low pulmonary capillary wedge pressure (i.e., noncardiogenic pulmonary edema). Criteria for the diagnosis of ARDS are listed in Table 5-3.

- Diffuse lung injury with hypoxic respiratory failure may result from various injuries.
- Mortality from all causes averages about 50%.
- Existing therapies do not significantly alter overall mortality in established ARDS.

ARDS was initially described as a post-traumatic or shock-induced injury, but it occurs with various states, as outlined in Table 5-4.

Relative risks of developing ARDS have been estimated from studies of predisposed groups. The greatest frequency is among patients with sepsis (approximately 40%), gastric aspiration (30%), multiple transfusions (25%), pulmonary contusion (20%), disseminated intravascular coagulation (20%), pneumonia requiring ICU management (12%), and trauma with long-bone or pelvic fractures (5%).

The pathophysiology of ARDS depends on damage to the alveolar-capillary unit. The earliest histologic changes are endothelial swelling, followed by edema and inflammation. Mononuclear inflammation, loss of alveolar type I cells, and protein deposition in the form of hyaline membranes may occur within 2 or 3 days. Fibrosis may develop after days or weeks of the process. Damage to type II alveolar epithelial cells leads to loss of surfactant. The surfactant that is produced may also be inactivated by proteins present in the airways. Alveolar filling and collapse cause intrapulmonary shunting and ventilation-perfusion mismatch with hypoxemia.

Table 5-3.— Criteria for Diagnosis of Adult Respiratory Distress Syndrome

Appropriate setting
Pulmonary injury, shock, trauma
Acute event
Clinical respiratory distress, tachypnea
Diffuse pulmonary infiltrates on chest radiography
Interstitial and/or alveolar pattern
Hypoxemia
PaO_2/FIO_2 ratio <150
Decreased compliance of respiratory system
<50 mL/cm H_2O
Exclude
Chronic pulmonary disease accounting for clinical picture
Left ventricular failure (most series require pulmonary artery wedge measurement <18 mm Hg)

Table 5-4.—Disorders Associated With Adult Respiratory Distress Syndrome

Shock	Any cause
Sepsis	Lung infections, other bacteremic or endotoxic states
Trauma	Head injury, lung contusion, fat embolism
Aspiration	Gastric, near-drowning, tube feedings
Hematologic	Transfusions, leukoagglutinin, intravascular coagulation, thrombotic thrombocytopenic purpura
Metabolic	Pancreatitis, uremia
Drugs	Narcotics, barbiturates, aspirin
Toxic	Inhaled—O_2, smoke Irritant gases—NO_2, Cl_2, SO_2, NH_3 Chemicals—paraquat
Miscellaneous	Radiation, air embolism, altitude

Death from ARDS usually is not due to isolated hypoxemic respiratory failure. The most frequent causes of mortality are complications of infection, sepsis syndrome, and failure of other organ systems. In addition to clinical risk factors listed above, specific variables associated with mortality include fewer than 10% band forms on peripheral blood smear, persistent acidemia, bicarbonate less than 20 mEq/L, and blood urea nitrogen greater than 65 mg/dL. Therefore, the systemic effects associated with ARDS may be important to outcome.

- Death from ARDS usually is not due to isolated hypoxemic respiratory failure.
- Infection, sepsis syndrome, and failure of other organ systems are the usual causes of mortality.
- Variables associated with mortality: <10% band forms on peripheral blood smear, persistent acidemia, bicarbonate <20 mEq/L, blood urea nitrogen >65 mg/dL.

The traditional therapy of ARDS involves optimization of physiologic variables and supportive management of associated complications. Measures include optimization of gas exchange and hemodynamics, nutrition, ambulation, and control of infections. Hypoxemia is typically corrected with positive pressure ventilation with supplemental oxygen and PEEP. PEEP provides potential benefits of increased lung volume and lung compliance and improvement in ventilation-perfusion relationships. Maintaining PEEP at a level adequate to prevent repetitive opening and closing of gravitationally dependent lung units (i.e., above "closing volume") may be helpful

in limiting tissue sheer forces that can potentiate capillary injury and, thus, worsen the degree of diffuse alveolar damage. Beyond an optimal level of PEEP, an increase in intrathoracic pressure may be associated with decreased venous return, increased pulmonary vascular resistance, decreased left ventricular filling, and a corresponding decrease in cardiac output.

Limiting the degree of alveolar distention during peak inflation may limit the potential for alveolar disruption, with the subsequent development of barotrauma complications (i.e., microscopic "volutrauma"). This is commonly done by providing tidal volumes of limited size, either via a volume preset or a pressure-targeted mode of ventilation. The use of PEEP levels chosen so that the lung volume is maintained above closing volume and tidal volumes chosen to prevent alveolar disruption is termed the "protective ventilatory strategy" of ventilatory management in ARDS. Supportive management of associated complications includes screening for underlying infections and early antibiotic therapy. Selective bowel decontamination by oral or nasogastric administration of a combination of nonabsorbable antibiotics may decrease the colonization of the airway by gram-negative organisms (reported to decrease the incidence of pneumonia in patients receiving mechanical ventilation).

- Hypoxemia is typically corrected with positive pressure ventilation with supplemental oxygen and PEEP.
- A "protective ventilatory strategy" in ARDS is designed to limit tissue sheer forces at low lung volumes and alveolar disruption at high lung volumes.
- Screen for underlying infections and early antibiotic therapy.
- Selective bowel decontamination may decrease the colonization of airway by gram-negative organisms.

Because increased capillary permeability allows greater intravascular fluid leak at any given hydrostatic pressure, attempt to limit intravascular volume to that necessary for systemic perfusion. However, associated shock states may demand volume expansion or increased inotropic support. Crystalloids can provide adequate filling pressures in patients with shock states, but large volumes may be required. Specific applications for colloids in ARDS include blood products (e.g., for coagulopathies or anemia). Supplemental nutrition is typically provided throughout the course of critical illness. Many patients with ARDS have associated multiorgan injury and may have ileus and/or gastrointestinal dysfunction precluding enteral feedings. Such feedings are recommended if tolerated. The consequences of malnutrition may include impairment of respiratory muscle function, depressed ventilatory drive, and limitation of host defenses. Mobilization, ambulation, and ventilator weaning are carried out as early as practical.

- Crystalloids can provide adequate filling pressures in patients with shock states.
- Many patients with ARDS have associated multiorgan injury.

Pharmacologic therapies have been directed against proposed biochemical and cellular mechanisms of ARDS. The presumed pathogenesis of acute lung injury is centered on the role of polymorphonuclear leukocytes. Activation of complement by many stimuli associated with lung injury may lead to recruitment and activation of neutrophils, which may injure endothelium by releasing proteolytic enzymes and liberating toxic oxygen species (e.g., hydrogen peroxide, hydroxyl radical, singlet oxygen, superoxide). Bronchoalveolar lavage fluid from patients with established ARDS and from high-risk patients may show increased numbers of cells, predominantly neutrophils. (Normal lavage fluid contains about 93% alveolar macrophages, with 5% to 7% lymphocytes and few neutrophils.) The percentage of neutrophils is correlated with the abnormalities of gas exchange and alveolar protein content. However, experimental lung injury may occur in the absence of neutrophils, and typical ARDS is seen in severely neutropenic patients. Thus, other mechanisms presumably have a role. Arachidonic acid metabolites are implicated in many biochemical events associated with acute lung injury. Arachidonic acid is released from cell membranes by phospholipases. Arachidonate may then be metabolized via the lipoxygenase pathway to leukotriene compounds or via the cyclooxygenase pathway to prostaglandins or thromboxane. These compounds are potentially crucial in the pathogenesis of acute lung injury. Thromboxane A_2, a potent vasoconstrictor, induces platelet aggregation. Prostacyclin, or PGI_2, has the opposite effects on smooth muscle and platelet aggregation and is a potential therapeutic agent for ARDS. PGE_1, a prostaglandin, relaxes vascular and bronchial smooth muscle and inhibits neutrophil chemotaxis.

- Acute lung injury: presumed pathogenesis centers on polymorphonuclear leukocytes.
- Neutrophils may injure endothelium by releasing proteolytic enzymes and liberating toxic oxygen species.
- Experimental lung injury may still occur in the absence of neutrophils.
- Arachidonic acid metabolites are implicated in many biochemical events associated with acute lung injury.
- Thromboxane A_2: potent vasoconstrictor, induces platelet aggregation.
- PGE_1: relaxes vascular and bronchial smooth muscle and inhibits neutrophil chemotaxis.

Potential therapeutic and prophylactic agents have been directed against steps in arachidonate pathways. Corticosteroids

decrease cell membrane disruption and have other anti-inflammatory properties. Specifically, no differences in mortality have been observed in prospective, randomized studies of ARDS patients receiving methylprednisolone or placebo. However, limited trials have suggested that there may be benefit in using corticosteroid therapy in the fibroproliferative phase of ARDS. Trials of corticosteroids in sepsis have also shown no difference in overall mortality. Corticosteroids may delay the resolution of secondary infections; a greater number of deaths related to secondary infection after corticosteroids has been observed.

- Corticosteroids decrease cell membrane disruption and have other anti-inflammatory properties.
- However, in early-phase ARDS, corticosteroids are potentially harmful and have no proven benefit.
- Corticosteroids may reduce the time to resolution of fibroproliferative (late-phase) ARDS.
- In sepsis, no difference has been shown in overall mortality with corticosteroids.

Nonsteroidal anti-inflammatory drugs (NSAIDs), for example, ibuprofen and indomethacin, block cyclooxygenase and thromboxane formation. In animal models of acute lung injury and septic shock, NSAIDs have beneficial effects if used prophylactically. However, no benefit is known for established ARDS. Other mediators, particularly those associated with sepsis, may be important factors in the pathogenesis of acute lung injury. Endotoxin, a complex lipopolysaccharide, may activate complement; it has been associated with neutrophilic alveolitis. Monoclonal antiendotoxin antibodies are reported to have beneficial effects in some patients with sepsis, but controlled trials have failed to show improved overall survival.

The prognosis for recovery of lung function in patients who survive ARDS is good. Studies of survivors have shown nearly normal lung volumes and airflow 6 to 12 months after the illness, with mild impairment in gas exchange—decreased diffusing capacity, desaturation with exercise, or widened A-a gradient. Therefore, the incentive is strong to continue aggressive measures in the patients with otherwise reversible organ dysfunction.

- Prognosis for the recovery of lung function in patients surviving ARDS is good.
- Mild decreases in oxygenation and diffusing capacity are typically observed after 6-12 months.

CARDIOPULMONARY RESUSCITATION

General clinical algorithms for standardized responses to cardiac dysrhythmias or arrest should be reviewed. Ideally, in ICUs, cardiorespiratory problems should be prevented or anticipated and recognized quickly.

Basic Life Support

Airway Control

Relieve obstruction. Remove any foreign bodies. If not dislodged or obstructing, dentures may improve the seal of a face mask. However, dentures are usually removed before endotracheal intubation.

Suction (saliva, emesis, blood). A rigid suction catheter is most useful. Use head-tilt, chin-lift, or forward thrust of the jaw to open the posterior pharynx. The oropharyngeal or nasopharyngeal airway may help maintain patency and facilitate suctioning and mask ventilation.

Supply a high rate of flow of supplemental oxygen. Ventilation is usually begun with a bag-valve-mask technique. Because a combined respiratory and metabolic acidosis is common, hyperventilation should be carried out to the extent possible.

Endotracheal intubation provides better control of the airway for ventilation, oxygenation, and suctioning and should be performed as soon as practical during the resuscitation effort. However, the best possible ventilation and oxygenation should be provided before any attempt at intubation, and efforts should be limited to 15 to 30 seconds before resuming mask ventilation.

For chest compressions, a 5:1 compression-to-ventilation ratio is recommended for two-person resuscitation. Check the femoral pulse for effectiveness of compressions. Monitoring of expired carbon dioxide (capnometry) by various devices is used to assess the adequacy of ventilation and to confirm endotracheal (versus esophageal) intubation. Under conditions of controlled ventilation and cardiac resuscitation, expired carbon dioxide may be an indicator of effective chest compressions (i.e., by Fick equation for CO_2—$\dot{V}CO_2 = CO \times (C\bar{v}\text{-}Ca)\, CO_2$. CO_2 delivery to the lungs depends on adequate cardiac output.

- Relieve obstruction.
- Oropharyngeal or nasopharyngeal airway may help maintain patency.
- Supply a high rate of flow of supplemental oxygen.
- Endotracheal intubation: better control of the airway for ventilation.

Electrical Therapy

Ventricular fibrillation is the most common rhythm in sudden cardiac arrest. The time to defibrillation is the most important factor determining successful resuscitation. In monitored patients in ICUs, defibrillation typically should be the first treatment, with other life support efforts initiated only after immediate attempts at electrical conversion. Electrical pacing may be useful in some cases of bradycardia and heart block.

- Ventricular fibrillation is the common rhythm in sudden cardiac arrest.
- Time to defibrillation is the most important factor determining successful resuscitation.
- In monitored patients in ICUs, defibrillation should typically be the first treatment.

Drug Therapy

Several recent trends and changes in recommendations about drug use are noteworthy. Electrical defibrillation is the treatment of choice for ventricular fibrillation. As additional therapy, lidocaine and bretylium have similar results in clinical outcome. Because bretylium may have adverse hemodynamic effects (hypotension), lidocaine is the recommended first-line therapy.

Sodium bicarbonate is still often used despite potential adverse effects and the lack of documented efficacy. A rapid bolus of sodium bicarbonate may induce osmotic and ionic shifts and, by generating carbon dioxide, may transiently worsen intracellular acidosis. Currently, bicarbonate is recommended only after another initial treatment has been established and if persistent metabolic acidosis and/or hyperkalemia is documented.

- Bicarbonate is recommended only after another initial treatment has been established.

Calcium may provide positive inotropic effects and vasoconstriction, but benefits in cardiac arrest have not been confirmed. Current indications for calcium include calcium channel blocker toxicity, acute hyperkalemia, or hypocalcemia.

- Indications for calcium: calcium channel blocker toxicity, acute hyperkalemia, hypocalcemia.

Epinephrine is administered during resuscitation from cardiac arrest for documented effects of peripheral vasoconstriction and improved coronary artery and cerebral blood flow during cardiopulmonary resuscitation. Epinephrine should also increase contractility in the beating heart. However, myocardial oxygen consumption may also increase, and automaticity and arrhythmias may be promoted. The optimal dose of epinephrine is debated. Blood flow may increase to a greater extent at doses higher than the standard 1 mg recommended for adult humans. A high dose of epinephrine (about 0.2 mg/kg) increases coronary artery perfusion in humans. Outcome and complications between standard and high doses of epinephrine:

no additional toxicity but no improvement in survival. Standard doses and interval should remain the routine.

- High dose of epinephrine (about 0.2 mg/kg) increases coronary artery perfusion in humans, but controlled trials have not shown increased long-term survival.

VASCULAR ACCESS AND HEMODYNAMIC MONITORING

Central Venous Catheterization

The first choice for access in stable patients requiring intravenous therapy is the peripheral veins. However, in ICUs, central venous catheterization is often necessary for the following indications: lack of adequate peripheral veins, need for hypertonic or phlebitic medications or solutions, need for long-term access, measurement of central pressures, and access for procedures (hemodialysis, cardiac pacing). Relative contraindications include inexperience of the practitioner, coagulopathy, inability to identify landmarks, infection or burn at the entry site, and thrombosis of the proposed central venous site. Central venous catheters are usually placed over a guidewire (modified Seldinger technique). Complications of central venous catheterization include infections, cardiac arrhythmias, pneumothorax, air embolism, catheter or guidewire embolism, catheter knotting, bleeding, and other potential complications of needle or catheter misplacement.

- Central venous catheterization is often necessary.
- Contraindications: inexperienced practitioner, coagulopathy, inability to identify landmarks, infection or burn at the entry site, thrombosis of proposed central venous site.

- Complications: infections, cardiac arrhythmias, pneumothorax, air embolism, catheter or guidewire embolism, catheter knotting, bleeding.

Catheter-related infections are usually attributed to the migration of bacteria from the skin along the catheter tract. Catheter-related infection is usually defined by more than 15 colonies (CFU/mL) on semiquantitative culture of the catheter tip. Catheter-related bacteremia is defined by similar growth and blood cultures positive for the same organism. Risk factors include infected catheter site or cutaneous breakdown, multiple manipulations, the number of catheter lumens, and the duration of use of the same site (particularly after 3-4 days). Treatment should include catheter removal and replacement at another site if necessary.

- Catheter-related infections usually are attributed to migration of bacteria from the skin along the catheter tract.
- Risk factors: infected catheter site or cutaneous breakdown, multiple manipulations, number of catheter lumens, duration of use of same site.

Pulmonary Artery Catheterization

Although common use (or overuse) of pulmonary artery catheterization is criticized, data from pulmonary artery catheterization may aid diagnosis and therapy in many disorders encountered in ICUs. Physiologic data that may be obtained are listed in Table 5-5.

Clinical conditions for which hemodynamic data may be useful include shock states, pulmonary edema, oliguric renal failure, indeterminate pulmonary hypertension, and myocardial and valvular disorders. Intravascular volume may be assessed more accurately, and effects of therapeutic interventions

Table 5-5.—Hemodynamic Data Obtained With Pulmonary Artery Catheterization

Variable	Normal value
Right atrial pressure (RAP)	2-8 mm Hg
Pulmonary arterial pressure (PAP)	16-24/5-12 mm Hg
Pulmonary capillary wedge pressure (PCWP)	5-12 mm Hg
Cardiac output (CO)	4-6 L/min
Cardiac index (CI = CO/body surface area)	2.5-3 L/min per m^2
Stroke volume (SV = CO/heart rate)	50-100 mL/beat
Stroke volume index (SVI = SV/body surface area)	35-50 mL/m^2
Systemic vascular resistance [SVR = (blood pressure - RAP)/CO]	10-15 mm Hg/L per min (x80 to convert to 800-1,200 dyne • s/cm^5)
Pulmonary vascular resistance [PVR = (PAP - PCWP)/CO]	1.5-2.5 mm Hg/L per min (100-200 dyne • s/cm^5)

(volume, vasodilator therapy, or inotropes) may be evaluated. Mixed venous oxygen saturation may also be measured, as indicated above. This may be particularly useful in assessing the effects of PEEP on oxygen delivery (i.e., improving arterial saturation but potentially decreasing cardiac output).

Complications of pulmonary artery catheterization include arrhythmias, right bundle branch block, complete heart block in patients with preexisting left bundle branch block, vascular or right ventricular perforation, thrombosis and embolism, catheter knotting, infection, and pulmonary infarction or rupture due to persistent wedging or overdistention of the balloon.

A recent retrospective case-control study found that the use of a pulmonary artery catheter was associated with higher mortality than no catheter in patients with similar severity of illness. However, the causes of this observation remain uncertain, and catheter use is still a common clinical practice.

- Complications of pulmonary artery catheterization: arrhythmias, right bundle branch block, complete heart block in patients with preexisting left bundle branch block, vascular or right ventricular perforation, thrombosis and embolism, catheter knotting, infection, pulmonary infarction or rupture due to persistent wedging or overdistention of the balloon.

The use of pulmonary capillary wedge pressure (PCWP) as an indicator of left ventricular end-diastolic pressure assumes a continuous hydrostatic column from pulmonary capillary to the left atrium. Although digital displays of PCWP are usually available, the pressure wave should be examined for potential artifacts and for the degree of respiratory variation. Because varying intrathoracic pressure may be sensed by the pulmonary artery catheter, recorded PCWP should be obtained at end-expiration. Even with these measures, PCWP may be influenced by airway pressure—thus, not accurately reflecting ventricular filling pressure—especially with high levels of PEEP.

- PCWP is an indicator of left ventricular end-diastolic pressure.
- PCWP may be influenced by airway pressure, especially with high levels of PEEP.

SHOCK STATES

Shock is defined by evidence of end-organ hypoperfusion, usually (but not necessarily) associated with hypotension. A common classification is cardiogenic (decreased cardiac output), hypovolemic (decreased blood volume), and septic (variable cardiac output, decreased systemic vascular resistance). All forms of shock may be characterized by hypotension, tachycardia, tachypnea, altered mental status, decreased urine output, and lactic acidosis. The clinical history often helps determine the diagnosis, for example, blood loss, trauma, myocardial infarction, systemic infection. Compared with other causes, septic shock is often characterized by relatively warm extremities and normal or increased cardiac output.

- Shock is defined by evidence of end-organ hypoperfusion, usually associated with hypotension.
- Common classification: cardiogenic, hypovolemic, and septic.
- Shock is characterized by hypotension, tachycardia, tachypnea, altered mental status, decreased urine output, and lactic acidosis.
- Septic shock is often characterized by relatively warm extremities and normal or increased cardiac output.

Sepsis syndrome is typically defined by a known or presumed source of infection associated with fever (or hypothermia) and leukocytosis (or leukopenia) *and* evidence of systemic effects, including hypotension, decreased urine output, or metabolic acidosis. After a rapid initial assessment, treatment is directed at the presumed source, for example, volume (blood loss, hypovolemia), vasodilator, or inotropic therapy (cardiogenic) or fluids, antibiotics, and drainage of any infected space (sepsis). If the response to the initial therapy is inadequate, and especially if intravascular volume status is uncertain clinically, pulmonary artery catheterization may be useful. For example, if the wedge pressure remains less than 12 to 15 mm Hg, further volume support and/or erythrocytes should be administered. If the wedge pressure is greater than 18 to 20 mm Hg and there is evidence of cardiac dysfunction, a vasodilator (nitroprusside) and diuretic therapy might be considered. If "hyperdynamic" indices are observed, that is, increased cardiac output and low peripheral resistance, fluids should first be given to achieve a high-normal wedge pressure. Low doses of dopamine, 2 to 5 μg/kg per minute, may improve renal perfusion. *After* volume support has been given and tissue perfusion is still inadequate, careful administration of vasoconstrictors (norepinephrine) may improve organ perfusion. Septic shock is commonly associated with multiorgan injury.

Multisystem organ failure typically is defined as acute dysfunction of two or more organ systems lasting longer than 2 days. Sepsis is the most common cause. The pathogenesis is attributed to the hemodynamic and immunologic effects of endotoxin, cytokines (tumor necrosis factor [TNF-α]), interleukins (IL-1, IL-2, IL-6, IL-8), platelet activating factor, arachidonic acid metabolites, polymorphonuclear leukocyte-derived toxic products, and myocardial depressant factors. Corticosteroids have no known benefit and potential adverse effects in patients with sepsis syndrome, with or without ARDS.

- Sepsis syndrome typically is defined by known or presumed source of infection associated with fever (or hypothermia) and leukocytosis (or leukopenia) and evidence of systemic effects (hypotension, decreased urine output, metabolic acidosis).
- Treatment is directed at the presumed source.
- Septic shock is commonly associated with multiorgan injury.
- Multisystem organ failure: acute dysfunction of two or more organ systems lasting >2 days.
- Pathogenesis is attributed to hemodynamic and immunologic effects of endotoxin, cytokines (TNF-α), IL-1, IL-2, IL-6, IL-8, platelet activating factor, arachidonic acid metabolites, polymorphonuclear leukocyte-derived toxic products, and myocardial depressant factors.
- Corticosteroids have no known benefit.

Mortality in patients with sepsis and multiorgan failure may be greater than 70% to 90%. Adverse risk factors include age older than 65 years, continued systemic signs of sepsis, persistent deficit in oxygen delivery, and preexisting renal or liver failure. Physiologic scoring systems (e.g., APACHE) may predict outcome more accurately for patient subgroups.

- Mortality in patients with sepsis and multiorgan failure may be >70%-90%.

DISEASE SEVERITY SCORING SYSTEMS

The use of a severity-of-illness scoring system is increasingly prevalent in ICUs. These systems may define quantitative overall risks for *populations* of patients. An accurate quantifiable description of the pretreatment status of critically ill patients can allow improved precision in the evaluation and implementation of new therapies (i.e., clinical research). Furthermore, these systems can be of great use in quality assurance measures. In the most systems, however, the most appropriate roles in individual case management remain unclear. The types of clinical scoring systems have ranged from simple counts of failing organs to highly sophisticated methods incorporating (acute and chronic) clinical and physiologic measures into proprietary logistic regression prediction equations derived from multi-institutional patient databases.

The Glasgow Coma Scale (GCS) was initially developed in the early 1970s as a triage tool for patients with head injury. This scoring system assigns a weighted point score for three behavioral responses: eye opening (1 to 4 points), best verbal response (1 to 5 points), and best motor response (1 to 6 points). Thus, the range of GCS scores is 3 to 15 points: severe dysfunction = 3 to 8 points, moderate dysfunction = 9 to 12 points,

and mild dysfunction = 12 to 14 points. The GCS system has been shown to correlate with mortality and the level of ultimate brain function in patients with traumatic brain injury. Because of its efficacy and simplicity, GCS has been used within other scoring systems.

Several multisystem scoring systems have been developed for use in critically ill patients. Although a detailed review of these systems is beyond the scope of this text, these systems include, among others, the Acute Physiology and Chronic Healthy Evaluation (APACHE) system, Simplified Acute Physiology Score (SAPS), the Mortality Probability Model (MPM) and the Therapeutic Intervention Scoring System (TISS).

- Severity scoring systems attempt to quantify overall risk for *populations* of patients.
- Severity scoring systems can be of great use in a clinical research and quality assurance functions.
- The best role for most scoring systems in the care of *individual* patients remains undefined.

ETHICS IN THE ICU

The principles listed in Table 5-6 provide a framework for assessing ethical issues in the ICU. However, the potential for conflict frequently arises because patients often are unable to participate in their own care, many family members may be involved, and the medical staff may disagree about the prognosis and proposed interventions.

Recent legal opinions have supported the concept that a competent person may refuse life-sustaining therapy. Decision making for incompetent patients is more controversial, and living-will legislation has been designed partly to address such conflicts.

- A competent person may refuse life-sustaining therapy.
- Decision making for incompetent patients is more controversial; living-will legislation has been designed partly to address such conflicts.

"Do Not Resuscitate" orders have become increasingly common and important in recent years. Guidelines of the American Medical Association include

1. Consent to cardiopulmonary resuscitation is presumed unless the patient (or patient's surrogate) has expressed in advance the wish not to be resuscitated or if, in the judgment of the treating physician, an attempt to resuscitate the patient would be futile. Resuscitation efforts should be considered futile if they cannot be expected either to restore cardiac or respiratory function or to achieve the expressed goals of the patient.

Table 5-6. --Principles for Assessing Ethical Issues in Intensive Care Units

Beneficence—acting in the patient's benefit by sustaining life, treating illness, and relieving pain

Nonmaleficence—do no harm

Autonomy—fundamental right to self-determination

Informed consent—providing factual and adequate information for competent patients to make decisions about their care

Substituted judgment—ability of a family member, guardian, or other surrogate to make decisions on behalf of the patient on the basis of what he or she believes the patient would have chosen if competent

Social justice—allocation of medical resources according to need (note that this concept implies overt health care rationing and may conflict with perceived individual rights)

Advance directives—living will: designed for persons to express their wishes regarding life-sustaining treatment at such time when they are deemed terminally ill and no longer able to participate in such decisions; typically there is provision or request for denial of specific life-support measures and designation of a surrogate decision maker.

2. The appropriateness of cardiopulmonary resuscitation should be discussed with patients at risk for cardiopulmonary arrest, preferably in the outpatient setting or early during hospitalization, and the resuscitation status should be reassessed periodically.
3. The physician is ethically obligated to honor the resuscitation preferences of the patient or surrogate except when this would mandate use of futile therapeutic efforts (potential conflicts may arise in the application of this principle).
4. "Do Not Resuscitate" orders should be entered in the medical record.
5. "Do Not Resuscitate" orders affect the administration of cardiopulmonary resuscitation only; other therapeutic interventions should not be influenced by the order.

Withholding Life Support Versus Withdrawal of Existing Support

Recent deliberations and court rulings have supported the concept that withholding and withdrawing of life support are essentially equivalent. In general, an irreversible or terminal illness is considered a prerequisite for withdrawal of support, but the interpretation may vary widely.

QUESTIONS

Multiple Choice (choose the one best answer)

1. A 37-year-old man with a history of rheumatoid arthritis receiving long-term salicylate therapy comes to the emergency department with a 3-day history of intermittent melena followed by syncope. On examination, he is pale and tachycardic (pulse, 120), blood pressure is 85/40 mm Hg, hemoglobin is 5.6 g/dL; mean corpuscular volume is 73.5 fL (normal, 81-95). Emergent endoscopy reveals a duodenal ulcer with a visible vessel, without active bleeding. Six units of erythrocytes and 4 L of 0.9% saline are transfused during the first 6 hours of hospitalization. Another 4 units of erythrocytes and 2 L of saline are required 2 days later for recurrent hemorrhage despite aggressive acid inhibition therapy. One day after his second hemorrhage, the following laboratory values were obtained: aspartate aminotransferase (AST), 67 U/L

(normal, 12-31); hemoglobin, 10.5 g/dL; prothrombin time, 18 s (INR = 1.8); partial thromboplastin time, 47 seconds (normal, 21-33); fibrinogen, 130 mg/dL (normal, 175-350); and platelet count, 73,000/µL. D-dimer and factor VIII levels were normal. The most likely cause of the observed coagulation abnormality is:
   a. Disseminated intravascular coagulation
   b. Superimposed liver failure due to "shock liver"
   c. Dilutional coagulopathy
   d. Salicylate toxicity
   e. Vitamin K deficiency

2. A chronically malnourished 58-year-old alcoholic is admitted to the intensive care unit with a severe right lower lobe pneumonia following a generalized seizure. While receiving O_2 by 15 L/min non-breather mask, arterial blood gas values were $PaCO_2$, 95 mm Hg; $PaCO_2$, 55; and pH, 7.28. Possible factors that could potentiate respiratory muscle

weakness in this patient include all the following *except*:
a. Hyperkalemia
b. Hypokalemia
c. Hypocalcemia
d. Hypophosphatemia
e. Increased ventilatory load prompting respiratory muscle fatigue

3. A 17-year-old woman was admitted via the emergency department 4 hours after ingesting 75 100-mg amitriptyline tablets. On examination, she was somnolent, blood pressure was 70/40 mm Hg, and the pulse was 120/min. The QRS duration was 170 ms. Urine output was minimal during the first hour of management. All the following are appropriate in her management *except*:
a. Inotropic support with dopamine
b. Sodium bicarbonate administration
c. Nasogastric lavage, followed by activated charcoal administration
d. Intravenous hydration with 0.9% saline
e. Immediate intubation

4. A 19-year-old man with a history of depression and previous drug overdose was admitted to the intensive care unit after being brought to the emergency department by friends 6 hours after he had ingested 50 of his mother's 0.25-mg digoxin (Lanoxin) tablets and complained of abnormal vision, following which he had a generalized seizure. The patient was confused and complained of nausea. He was diaphoretic and tachycardic at 120 beats/min, with ectopy. Blood pressure was 90/55 mm Hg. Electrocardiography showed junctional tachycardia with ventricular premature contractions. The serum level of potassium was 6.7 mEq/L. Which one of the following is true?
a. The presence of hyperkalemia is reassuring regarding the risk of digitalis toxicity
b. Calcium gluconate, 1 ampule (90 mg) is indicated immediately
c. The patient should receive digoxin immune Fab (Digibind) intravenously
d. Hyperkalemia of digitalis intoxication is not affected by glucose and insulin infusion
e. Digitalis intoxication is treated primarily with hemodialysis

5. Proinflammatory cytokines in sepsis include all the following *except*:
a. Interleukin-1
b. Interleukin-6
c. Interleukin-8

d. Interleukin-10
e. Tumor necrosis factor-α

6. Causes of distributive shock include all the following *except*:
a. Sepsis
b. Pericardial tamponade
c. Bilateral adrenal hemorrhage
d. Anaphylaxis
e. Liver failure

7. Which of the following statements is true concerning adult respiratory distress syndrome (ARDS)?
a. Overall mortality approximates 80%
b. It is characterized by increased lung compliance
c. It is associated with a decrease in the ratio of dead space to tidal volume (Vd/Vt)
d. It may be caused by pancreatitis
e. The most frequent cause of mortality is ventilatory insufficiency

8. While ice fishing, a 16-year-old Minnesota boy was submerged in a recently frozen lake for approximately 40 minutes. On rescue by emergency personnel, he was asystolic and remained so during the 30-minute transport to the emergency department, during which continuous resuscitative efforts were made. On arrival, the core temperature was 28°C (82.4°F). Which of the following is the best initial management plan?
a. Cease resuscitative efforts
b. Intubation, warmed humidified oxygen, and cardiopulmonary bypass
c. Place the patient in a 40°C room, and apply hot blankets, continuing resuscitation
d. Continue resuscitation for another 30 minutes; if unsuccessful, discontinue
e. Apply blankets and warm bladder irrigation during resuscitation

9. Which of the following is correct regarding pressure support ventilation?
a. Respiratory rate is set by the physician
b. Increases in respiratory system resistance tend to produce increases in alveolar ventilation
c. Mean inspiratory flow is set by the physician
d. Tidal volume is set by the physician
e. Reductions in respiratory system compliance tend to produce reductions in alveolar ventilation

10. Assist control (AC) volume preset ventilation is characterized by which one of the following?

a. A minimum minute ventilation level defined by the set frequency and tidal volume
b. A variable tidal volume defined by the patients' respiratory efforts
c. Presence of intrinsic PEEP in all patients
d. Reductions in minute ventilation are induced by respiratory secretions/atelectasis
e. Requirement for sedation and paralysis in most patients

11. A 65-year-old 70-kg man with chronic obstructive pulmonary disease (COPD) (FEV_1, 1.0 L) is admitted with acute dyspnea associated with a COPD exacerbation following a viral illness. He is intubated for respiratory distress with acute and chronic respiratory acidosis and placed on an assist control (AC) mode of ventilation with 0.85 L tidal volume, FIO_2 = 0.60, rate = 12. You are called 2 hours later by the nurse because of hypotension. The plateau airway pressure is 40 cm H_2O. The patient's respiratory rate is 16. Oximetric saturation is 92%. The trachea is midline. Neck veins are distended. Breath sounds are distant but equal bilaterally. Which one of the following is the probable cause for this patient's acute deterioration?
   a. Acute pulmonary embolism
   b. Myocardial infarction
   c. Dynamic hyperinflation with auto-PEEP
   d. Mucus plugging of the right mainstem bronchus
   e. Pericardial tamponade

12. Concerning weaning of patients from mechanical ventilation, which one of the following is true?
   a. Intermittent mandatory ventilation (IMV) mode is inferior to other modes of weaning such as pressure support or T-piece trials
   b. Measurement of $P_{0.1}$ is at least as predictive as f/v_T ratio in predicting weanability from mechanical ventilation
   c. Doxapram is frequently useful as an adjunctive agent in weaning from mechanical ventilation
   d. Endotracheal tube size has little potential effect on work of breathing
   e. Intrinsic PEEP refers to an increase in end-expiratory pressure imposed by active expiration by the patient

13. Concerning the diagnosis of pulmonary embolism in patients in an intensive care unit, all of the following are true *except*:
   a. Ventilation-perfusion lung scanning is of limited use in establishing a diagnosis
   b. In patients with acute pulmonary embolism, noninvasive leg studies may be expected to be normal in at least 30% of patients
   c. Contrast computed tomography (electron beam or spiral computed tomography) is equally useful in the diagnosis of central or peripheral pulmonary emboli
   d. The presence of intracerebral metastases is a contraindication to thrombolytic therapy
   e. The incidence of intracranial hemorrhage in patients with pulmonary embolism treated with thrombolysis is approximately 2%

14. The following laboratory and hemodynamic values were obtained for a patient admitted to the intensive care unit:
    Hemoglobin, 10.0 g/dL
    pH, 7.39
    Blood pressure (systolic/diastolic/mean), 160/70/100 mm Hg
    Central venous pressure, 10 mm Hg
    Right ventricular pressure (systolic/diastolic/mean), 30/4/13 mm Hg
    Pulmonary artery pressure, 30/18/22 mm Hg
    Pulmonary capillary wedge pressure, 18 mm Hg
    Cardiac output, 5.4 L/min
    PaO_2, 60 mm Hg
    SaO_2, 90%
    The patient's body surface area is 1.8 m^2. The patient's systemic vascular resistance index is?
    a. 30 dynes • s • cm^{-5}
    b. 1,303 dynes • s • cm^{-5}
    c. 1,870 dynes • s • cm^{-5}
    d. 2,400 dynes • s • cm^{-5}
    e. 2,640 dynes • s • cm^{-5}

15. In the preceding question, the patient's oxygen delivery ($\dot{D}O_2$) would be approximately:
    a. Not calculable with the data provided
    b. 550 mL/min
    c. 650 mL/min
    d. 750 mL/min
    e. 800 mL/min

16. PaO_2, 87 mm Hg   Sodium, 145 mEq/L
    $PaCO_2$, 22 mm Hg   Chloride, 108 mEq/L
    pH, 7.47   Calcium, 9.8 mEq/L
    HCO_3^-, 14 mEq/L
    The above data are most consistent with which of the following diagnoses?
    a. Acute salicylate intoxication
    b. Acute meperidine overdose

c. Postlaparotomy nasogastric suction for 3 days

d. Acute hyperventilation syndrome

e. Acute liver necrosis

17. An 18-year-old woman comes to the emergency department complaining of abdominal pain. She is 35 weeks pregnant. Examination reveals an anxious-appearing gravid woman. Blood pressure is 145/82 mm Hg; pulse is 110/min; and the respiratory rate is 26/min, with shallow respirations. An arterial blood gas reveals:

Pao_2, 88 mm Hg   pH, 7.44

$Paco_2$, 28 mm Hg HCO_3^-, 18 mEq/L

The above data are most consistent with:

a. Acute pulmonary embolism

b. Diabetic ketoacidosis

c. Pyelonephritis

d. Acute salicylate intoxication

e. Physiologic effects of pregnancy

18. A 24-year-old man is brought to the emergency department obtunded after an acute overdose of heroin. He is receiving supplemental oxygen. Arterial blood gas values are as follows: Pao_2, 60 mm Hg; $Paco_2$, 80 mm Hg; pH, 7.07. Assuming a baseline bicarbonate concentration of 24 mEq/L, the expected bicarbonate level would now be:

a. 20 mEq/L

b. 24 mEq/L

c. 28 mEq/L

d. 32 mEq/L

e. 36 mEq/L

19. Pao_2, 85 mm Hg   Sodium, 140 mEq/L

$Paco_2$, 40 mm Hg   Potassium, 4.8 mEq/L

pH, 7.40   Calcium, 9.8 mEq/L

HCO_3^-, 24 mEq/L   Phosphorus, 5 mEq/L

BUN, 59 mg/dL   Chloride, 96 mEq/L

                                          Glucose, 180 mg/dL

What acid-based disturbance is depicted by the above values?

a. None

b. Respiratory acidosis and metabolic alkalosis

c. Respiratory acidosis and metabolic acidosis

d. Respiratory alkalosis and metabolic acidosis

e. Metabolic acidosis and metabolic alkalosis

20. All the following are of use in treating severe hyperkalemia *except*:

a. Glucose/insulin infusion

b. Intravenous magnesium

c. Intravenous sodium bicarbonate

d. Albuterol via nebulizer

e. Intravenous calcium

ANSWERS

1. Answer c.

Massive transfusion is usually defined as the replacement of at least a single blood volume within a 12-hour period and frequently leads to a clinically significant dilutional coagulopathy unless appropriate coagulation factors, calcium, and platelets are monitored and replaced as indicated. This patient did not experience hypotension to the degree usually associated with "shock liver" physiology. Patients with massive transfusion in the absence of disseminated intravascular coagulation are, like patients with liver failure, unlikely to have increased levels of D-dimers or decreased levels of factor VIII.

2. Answer c.

Although hypocalcemia is a common finding in such a scenario, it is not associated with respiratory muscle weakness. Hypocalcemia is usually asymptomatic, although when severe (or occurring rapidly) it may cause muscular spasms, laryngeal stridor, QT prolongation, and neurologic sequelae, including seizures. All the other choices are known potentiators of respiratory muscle weakness.

3. Answer a.

Because the mechanism of action of tricyclic antidepressants is by blockade of catecholamine reuptake in presynaptic nerve terminals, direct-acting pressor agonists rather than indirect agents (such as dopamine) in addition to intravenous hydration are more appropriate for initial pressor support. The prolonged QRS is diagnostic in this scenario for amitriptyline-induced cardiac conduction abnormality, with associated increased mortality; sodium bicarbonate decreases drug bioavailability and reduces cardiac mortality. Nasogastric lavage and activated charcoal administration are used to decrease absorption. Intubation of this patient is appropriate for airway control in the face of altered mental status.

4. Answer c.

The patient has a life-threatening ingestion of digoxin. Digoxin immune Fab (Digibind) is indicated for life-threatening digoxin intoxication. Hyperkalemia is a marker of toxicity due to digoxin-induced Na-K ATP-ase inhibition. Dangerous hyperkalemia is treated with glucose, insulin, and sodium bicarbonate. However, calcium administration should be avoided, because it may potentiate digoxin toxicity. Hemodialysis is not of benefit in digitalis intoxication because of the high volume of distribution of digoxin.

5. Answer d.

Interleukins-1, -6, and -8 and tumor necrosis factor-α are proinflammatory cytokines; interleukin-10 is an anti-inflammatory cytokine that modulates the inflammatory response.

6. Answer b.

Distributive shock is characterized by a high cardiac output, normal left ventricular filling, and decreased systemic vascular resistance. All the responses are causes of distributive shock physiology except cardiac tamponade, which is a cause of obstructive shock.

7. Answer d.

Adult respiratory distress syndrome (ARDS) is characterized by reduced lung compliance and increased V_D/V_T. Overall mortality is approximately 40% to 50%; the most frequent cause of death is complicating sepsis. Pancreatitis is one of the many known causes of ARDS.

8. Answer b.

This patient has a severe hypothermic injury. Active rewarming is indicated in patients with a core temperature <28°C or cardiac arrest. Techniques for active core rewarming include heated humidified oxygen, heated intravenous fluids, pleural lavage, peritoneal lavage, gastric/rectal lavage, arteriovenous or venovenous rewarming, and cardiopulmonary bypass.

9. Answer e.

Pressure support ventilation is a ventilatory mode in which the physician sets the pressure target, PEEP, and F_{IO_2}. The patient's respiratory drive and respiratory system mechanics determine inspiratory and expiratory time, respiratory frequency, and flow rates. An increase in respiratory system compliance (as would occur after clearing of lobar atelectasis) would tend to produce increased alveolar ventilation, whereas reductions in lung compliance (e.g., atelectasis), tend to produce a decrease in alveolar ventilation. An increase in resistive load would tend to produce a decrease in alveolar ventilation.

10. Answer a.

Assist control volume preset ventilation is characterized by the tidal volume and (minimal) respiratory rate set by the physician; the ventilation is augmented by the patient triggering additional breaths/min, given at the preset tidal volume. In the absence of airway obstruction, the presence of intrinsic PEEP is very uncommon at standard settings. Because tidal volume and (minimal) respiratory frequency are physician-defined, reductions in lung compliance do not decrease minute ventilation.

11. Answer c.

This patient was given a large tidal volume (12 mL/kg) in an assist control mode of volume pre-set ventilation. This choice of ventilator strategy may not allow for adequate expiratory time, thereby increasing end-expiratory lung volume (dynamic hyperinflation) and end-expiratory pressure ("intrinsic PEEP" or "auto-PEEP"). The associated decrease in effective venous return due to the increased intrathoracic pressure will predispose to hypotension.

12. Answer a.

Two prospective randomized trials have shown that IMV weaning is inferior to other methods. The f/v_T ratio has been found to be the best bedside discriminator between patients who are successfully weaned and those who are not. Small endotracheal tube diameters may have a dramatic effect in increasing work of breathing. Doxapram is rarely useful in weaning patients from mechanical ventilation.

13. Answer c.

Because of the underlying cardiopulmonary disease or the presence of mechanical ventilation, ventilation-perfusion lung scanning is frequently of little or no use in patients in the intensive care unit. Leg studies (invasive or noninvasive) are negative in at least 30% of patients with pulmonary embolism and should never be relied upon alone in ruling out pulmonary embolism. Thrombolytic therapy for pulmonary embolism has a mean reported incidence of 2% and is contraindicated in patients with known intracerebral metastases. Electron beam or spiral computed tomographic scans (with contrast) are less sensitive for peripheral, as compared with central, pulmonary emboli.

14. Answer d.

Systemic vascular index (SVRI) is defined as:

$$SVRI = \frac{MAP - CVP}{CI} \times 80$$

Cardiac index is defined as:

$$\frac{CO}{BSA}$$

15. Answer c.

Oxygen delivery ($\dot{D}O_2$) in mL/min is defined as $\dot{D}O_2 = CaO_2$.

16. Answer a.

The acid-based disorder depicted is that of concomitant metabolic acidosis and respiratory alkalosis, which is the typical finding of salicylate intoxication. Meperidine overdose would be expected to cause an acute respiratory acidosis; nasogastric suction would cause a primary metabolic alkalosis; acute hyperventilation would cause an acute respiratory alkylosis; and acute liver insufficiency can cause an acute or chronic respiratory alkalosis.

17. Answer e.

The arterial blood gas results shown indicate a chronic (compensated) respiratory alkalosis with a mildly widened alveolar-arterial gradient. This is expected with late-stage pregnancy.

18. Answer c.

The patient is experiencing an acute respiratory acidosis. For every $Paco_2$ increase of 10 mm Hg, there is an acute increase in bicarbonate concentration of 1 mEq/L. This is *not* due to renal compensation but to the mass action effect on serum bicarbonate induced by the increase in carbon dioxide concentration as shown by the formula:

$$CO_2 + H_2O \longleftrightarrow H_2CO_3 \longleftrightarrow H^+ + HCO_3^-$$

19. Answer e.

The presence of metabolic acidosis in this data set is only evident by the presence of an increased anion gap:

$$[Na^+] - ([Cl^-] + [HCO_3^-]) = 20 \text{ mEq/L}$$

However, the anticipated decrease in the serum level of bicarbonate is offset by a concomitant metabolic alkalosis, thereby normalizing the serum bicarbonate concentration and pH.

20. Answer b.

Glucose/insulin infusion, inhaled albuterol, and sodium bicarbonate act in reducing hyperkalemia through potassium redistribution. Intravenous calcium acts through a membrane antagonism effect. Intravenous magnesium has no role in the therapy of hyperkalemia.

CHAPTER 6
DERMATOLOGY

Marian T. McEvoy, M.D.

GENERAL DERMATOLOGY

Skin Cancer

Nonmelanoma skin cancers (basal cell, squamous cell) are the most common malignancy in the United States population; more than 600,000 cases occur each year. Basal cell carcinomas outnumber squamous cell carcinomas by a ratio of 4:1. The incidence of non-melanoma skin cancer is increasing rapidly, and an additional 12 million new cases of non-melanoma skin cancer are expected during the next 50 years. The increasing incidence of nonmelanoma skin cancer has been attributed to a combination of increased exposure to ultraviolet light, changes in clothing style, increased longevity, and ozone depletion.

Both basal cell and squamous cell carcinomas tend to occur on sun-exposed areas. Basal cell carcinomas are commonly slow growing and locally invasive. They often invade vital structures and can cause significant disfigurement. Basal cell carcinomas tend not to metastasize to regional lymph nodes. Squamous cell carcinomas, alternatively, can metastasize to regional lymph nodes, and approximately 2% of all squamous cell carcinomas lead to death. Fortunately, nonmelanoma skin cancers are highly curable; the cure rate is 90% if they are detected and treated early.

- Basal cell carcinoma and squamous cell carcinoma occur on sun-exposed skin.
- Cure rate is 90% with early detection and treatment.

Malignant Melanoma

An estimated 32,000 new cases of malignant melanoma and 8,000 new cases of melanoma in situ were diagnosed in the United States in 1994. The incidence of malignant melanoma is increasing rapidly in the United States. At the current rate, malignant melanomas will develop during the lifetime of 1 of every 105 Americans born in 1993 (approximately 1%). In contrast, the risk in 1980 was 1 in 250, and the risk in 1936 was only 1 in 1,500. If the incidence of malignant melanoma continues to increase at the current rate, by the year 2000 the lifetime risk for development of melanoma will increase to 1 in 75.

Risk factors for the development of malignant melanoma include fair skin, blond hair, freckling, intermittent sunlight exposure with blistering sunburns during childhood or adolescence, and genetic predisposition. The "familial atypical mole-melanoma syndrome" is transmitted by an autosomal dominant gene. This is characterized by a predisposition to dysplastic nevi and cutaneous melanomas. Patients with non-familial dysplastic nevi also have an increased risk for development of malignant melanoma. Other risk factors that have been identified include a personal or family history of melanoma, a personal or family history of nonmelanoma skin cancer, a large number of benign pigmented nevi, giant pigmented congenital nevus, immunosuppression, human immunodeficiency virus (HIV) positivity, and the use of tanning beds. Many primary melanomas occur on non-sun-exposed sites such as the back, scalp, and nails.

The key to improved survival with malignant melanoma has been early diagnosis. The most important prognostic feature of malignant melanoma is tumor thickness; this is defined as the measurement from the stratum granulosum to the deepest tumor cell in the histologic section and is referred to as the Breslow thickness. The 5-year survival rate approaches 100% in patients with lesions less than 0.75 mm thick, approximately 94% for lesions 0.76 to 1.50 mm, 84% for lesions 1.5 to 2.25 mm, 77% for lesions 2.26 to 3.00 mm, and 46% for lesions more than 3 mm. The 5-year survival rate is approximately 36% in patients with lymph node metastasis and 5% in patients with extranodal metastasis. Clark's levels of invasion (level 1, intraepidermal tumor only; level 2, tumor extending into papillary dermis; level 3, tumor pushing on papillary dermal-reticular dermal junction; level 4, lesion has invaded reticular dermis; level 5, invasion into subcutaneous fat) are not used for prognostic classification. Other factors such as sex and anatomic site have sometimes been cited as criteria of independent prognostic significance.

- The key to improved survival rate with malignant melanoma is early diagnosis.
- Most important prognostic feature is tumor thickness (Breslow thickness).

Stage I malignant melanoma consists of the cutaneous lesion without lymph node involvement, stage II consists of the primary skin lesion plus lymph node involvement, and stage III represents distant metastasis. The recommended management of stage I malignant melanoma is surgical. The previous recommendation of a 5-cm margin of excision for all types of malignant melanoma has been revised. Although "wide" excision of malignant melanoma is still the standard of treatment, excision margins more than 3 cm are no longer advocated. For excision of a thin melanoma (<1 mm thick), a 1-cm margin is generally recommended, and a 2- to 3-cm margin is advised for thicker lesions. Elective lymph node dissection does not improve outcome in patients with stage I disease. For stage II disease, excision of the primary skin lesion and regional lymph node dissection are usually recommended. Again, early diagnosis is the key to management, as no form of adjuvant therapy has been shown to improve survival in patients with advanced disease.

- Surgical management of stage I malignant melanoma consists of excision with tumor-free margins of 1-3 cm.

Sentinel node biopsy, whereby the draining lymph node is identified (by dye injection) and sampled, improves the prognosis for intermediate and thick melanomas on the limbs. With melanomas on the head and neck and trunk, sampling of the sentinel node is more complex and the decision to perform this procedure needs to be individualized on the basis of melanoma thickness and other prognostic factors.

Prevention of Melanoma and Nonmelanoma Skin Cancer

Dermatologists encourage regular use of sunscreens with a sun protection factor (SPF) of at least 15. Sunlight exposure during the first 18 years of life accounts for up to 80% of cumulative lifetime sun exposure. Therefore, sunscreen use is particularly important in children and adolescents. Persons with light skin types and outdoor workers need to be particularly vigilant with sun protection. Because the prognosis with melanoma and nonmelanoma skin cancer improves with early diagnosis, these lesions need to be recognized by health care workers and the general public alike.

Cutaneous T-Cell Lymphoma

Forms of cutaneous T-cell lymphoma are mycosis fungoides and Sézary syndrome. Mycosis fungoides generally manifests as discrete or coalescing patches, plaques, or nodules on the skin. Mycosis fungoides may progress to involve lymph nodes and viscera. From the time of extracutaneous involvement, the median duration of survival has been estimated at 2.5 years. The course of patients with patch- or plaque-stage cutaneous lesions, without extracutaneous disease, is less predictable, but the median duration of survival is approximately 12 years. Sézary syndrome is characterized by generalized erythroderma, keratoderma of the palms and soles, and a Sézary cell count of more than $1,000/mm^3$ in the peripheral blood. Most patients have severe pruritus.

- Mycosis fungoides and Sézary syndrome are forms of cutaneous T-cell lymphoma.
- Mycosis fungoides may progress to involve lymph nodes and viscera.
- Median survival for patients with mycosis fungoides is 12 years; from time of extracutaneous involvement, it is 2.5 years.

Both mycosis fungoides and Sézary syndrome are characterized by the presence of Sézary cells (lymphocytes with hyperchromatic and convoluted nuclei) involving the epidermis (epidermotrophism) and dermis. Immunohistochemical stains of cutaneous lesions demonstrate that these neoplastic T cells usually express CD3 and CD4 antigens, and molecular genetic studies reveal clonal rearrangement of the T-cell receptor gene in lymphocyte populations from skin biopsy, lymph node, and peripheral blood specimens of patients with cutaneous T-cell lymphoma.

- Mycosis fungoides and Sézary syndrome are T-cell lymphomas characterized by presence of Sézary cells in skin and peripheral blood.

Treatment of cutaneous T-cell lymphoma includes topical nitrogen mustard, psoralen with ultraviolet-A light (PUVA), radiotherapy (electron beam, orthovoltage), and systemic chemotherapy. Interferon, retinoids, and other agents have also been used. Most recently, extracorporeal photopheresis has become popular in the treatment of cutaneous T-cell lymphoma. After ingestion of 8-methoxypsoralen, the patient's leukocytes are exposed to ultraviolet light A and then reinfused.

Psoriasis

Psoriasis occurs in approximately 1% to 2% of the population of the United States. Onset of lesions is most common in the third decade of life, and about a third of patients have a family history of psoriasis. The cutaneous disease is usually chronic, and the most common presentation is with papules and plaques covered with a silvery scale. Patterns of psoriasis include psoriasis vulgaris with large plaque-like lesions on the trunk and limbs and classic involvement of the elbows and knees. Guttate psoriasis is an acute form of psoriasis which often follows streptococcal throat infection and presents with small lesions (5-10 mm in diameter) of psoriasis on the trunk and limbs. Other, less common forms of psoriasis include pustular psoriasis, which may be localized to the hands and feet or may be generalized. Approximately 50% of patients have nail abnormalities, most commonly onycholysis, pitting, and oil spots. Lesions of psoriasis are characterized by koebnerization, which is a term used to describe the induction of lesions at sites of trauma.

- Onset of psoriasis lesions is in the third decade of life.
- One-third of patients have family history.
- 50% of patients have nail abnormalities.

The treatment of psoriasis includes topical steroids, topical tar preparations, and phototherapy. Newer forms of treatment of localized psoriasis include a topical synthetic vitamin D analogue, calcipotriene, and a topical retinoid, tazarotene.

Systemic agents used in the treatment of psoriasis include methotrexate, acitretin, and cyclosporine.

Ultraviolet Light

Natural sunlight may be divided into ultraviolet-B (UVB, 280-320 nm), ultraviolet-A (320-400 nm), and visible light. UVB radiation is responsible for the sunburn reaction. In treating inflammatory dermatoses, UVB has been used most commonly in combination with tar, as in the Goeckerman therapy of psoriasis. The therapeutic wavelength for the treatment of psoriasis has been identified, and narrow-band UVB units (311 nm) have been recently introduced in the United States. UVB may also benefit atopic dermatitis, lichen planus, and certain other inflammatory dermatoses.

PUVA

PUVA consists of ingestion of psoralen followed by exposure of the skin to ultraviolet-A light. PUVA has most commonly been used for therapy of generalized psoriasis, but it is also effective in the treatment of various dermatoses, including lichen planus, mycosis fungoides, urticaria pigmentosa, and vitiligo. PUVA therapy is associated with minimal or no systemic side effects. The main side effect of PUVA therapy is an increased risk (>12 times) of cutaneous squamous cell carcinoma in patients who have received long-term therapy.

- PUVA is commonly used for therapy of generalized psoriasis.
- PUVA is associated with minimal or no systemic side effects.
- Main side effect with PUVA is increased risk of cutaneous squamous cell carcinoma.

Atopic Dermatitis

The atopic diathesis is manifested by one or more of the following: atopic dermatitis, asthma, and allergic rhinitis or conjunctivitis. Atopic dermatitis often presents in the neonatal period with scaling and erythema of the scalp and face, later spreading to the trunk. The distribution is often extensor in the older infant, and by the age of approximately 3 years the more classic flexural distribution is observed. In adolescence, facial involvement (perioral, eyelid, and forehead) is common. Generalized flares of eczema can occur at any age.

Disturbances in cell-mediated immunity lead to an increased incidence of bacterial and viral infections. Secondary infection with *Staphylococcus aureus* presents as a weeping, crusting dermatitis (impetiginization). Eczema herpeticum is the term used to describe a secondary infection with the herpes simplex virus, which may be generalized. Infections with the human papilloma virus and molluscum contagiosum are also more common and the lesions are more numerous in patients with atopic dermatitis.

- Eczema herpeticum, a generalized herpes simplex virus infection, may occur in patients with atopic dermatitis.

Allergic Contact Dermatitis

Allergic contact dermatitis is a form of localized or generalized dermatitis that results from exposure to an antigen. This is a type 4 hypersensitivity reaction (delayed, cell-mediated). Recognition of antigens by T-lymphocytes requires participation of Langerhans cells, which are the "antigen-presenting" cells of the epidermis. During investigation of the cause of allergic contact dermatitis, one must consider the anatomical location of the cutaneous lesions and environmental exposure to allergens, including occupational, household, and recreational contactants.

- Allergic contact dermatitis is type 4 hypersensitivity reaction (delayed, cell-mediated).
- Langerhans cells are "antigen-presenting" cells of epidermis.

Patch testing is performed by applying various substances to the patient's back; each substance is under a small aluminum disk covered with adhesive tape. These are left on the patient's back for 48 hours, and the results are interpreted at 48 and 96 hours. Positive reactions occur most often to the following antigens: nickel sulfate, potassium dichromate, thimerosal, paraphenylenediamine, ethylenediamine, neomycin sulfate, benzocaine, thiuram, and formalin.

Nickel sulfate allergies are mainly associated with jewelry. Paraphenylenediamine is present in hair dyes and other cosmetics; *para*-aminobenzoic acid (PABA) in sunscreens is immunologically related to paraphenylenediamine. Potassium dichromate sensitivity is one of the most common types of occupational allergic contact dermatitis and occurs in construction workers exposed to cement, leathers, and certain paints. Formaldehyde is a common preservative in cosmetics and shampoos. Neomycin sulfate and benzocaine are components of many topical antimicrobial and analgesic preparations. Thimerosal is a commonly used preservative in contact lens solutions and in some intramuscular injections. Thiuram is a rubber accelerator and fungicide and therefore may correlate with occupational dermatitis or dermatitis related to wearing shoes containing rubber.

- Nickel sulfate allergies are associated with jewelry.
- Potassium dichromate sensitivity occurs in construction workers exposed to cement, leathers, certain paints.
- Formaldehyde is a common preservative in cosmetics and shampoos.

Acne Vulgaris

Acne vulgaris is one of the most common problems seen in clinical dermatology. Acne occurs physiologically at puberty with varying degrees of severity. In some persons, acne persists into the second and third decades of life. The pathogenesis of acne is multifactorial; inheritance, increase in sebaceous gland activity, hormonal influences, disturbances of keratinization, and bacterial infection have all been implicated. The primary lesions of acne are noninflammatory and include microcomedones, closed comedones (whiteheads), and open comedones (blackheads). The secondary or inflammatory lesions include papules and pustules, nodules, and cysts. Acne may be divided into grades 1, 2, and 3 based on the clinical findings. Comedonal acne (grade 1) is treated with agents that cause dryness and peeling and help to eliminate comedones. Such agents include topical tretinoin (Retin A) and benzoyl peroxide. Treatment of papular or pustular acne (grade 2) is the same with the addition of topical or systemic antibiotics. Cystic acne (grade 3) is treated with systemic antibiotics; when it is severe and extensive or unresponsive to conventional therapy, isotretinoin (Accutane) is the treatment of choice.

Systemic Retinoids

Isotretinoin (13-*cis*-retinoic acid) is a synthetic vitamin A derivative used primarily for the treatment of severe nodulocystic acne vulgaris. The mechanism of action of 13-*cis*-retinoic acid in acne is probably multifactorial, including improvement in keratinization, decrease in sebum production, and decrease in inflammation. A 20-week course at a dosage of approximately 1 mg/kg per day is the standard regimen.

- Isotretinoin is used for treatment of severe acne vulgaris.

The greatest risk associated with use of systemic retinoids is teratogenicity. Before isotretinoin is prescribed, female patients must be counseled on this side effect and use reliable contraception during therapy and for at least 1 month after use of the drug is discontinued.

- Greatest risk with use of systemic retinoids is teratogenicity.

The systemic retinoids are associated with various side effects, including xerosis, dermatitis, cheilitis, sticky skin, peeling skin, epistaxis, conjunctivitis, hair loss, and nail dystrophy. Symptoms of arthralgias and myalgias may also occur. Most patients develop some degree of hyperlipidemia, including hypertriglyceridemia and hypercholesterolemia. Other laboratory abnormalities include elevation of liver enzyme values and leukopenia. Skeletal hyperostosis may occur, particularly in association with long-term use.

- Side effects of systemic retinoids include xerosis, dermatitis, cheilitis, sticky skin, peeling skin, epistaxis, conjunctivitis, hair loss, nail dystrophy.

Acitretin is effective for treatment of pustular psoriasis, erythrodermic psoriasis, and generalized chronic plaque-type psoriasis. It has been used successfully as a single agent and in combination with PUVA therapy. Because of the risk of teratogenicity, conception is not recommended for at least 3 years after acitretin therapy.

Autoimmune Bullous Diseases

Bullous pemphigoid is the most common autoimmune bullous disease. The disease predominantly occurs in elderly patients and usually presents with large, tense bullae on erythematous bases with a predilection for flexural areas (plate 6-1). Lesions are often generalized but may be localized. The most common histologic pattern is a subepidermal bulla with eosinophils, although there is a subset of patients with neutrophil-rich lesions, noninflammatory lesions, or eosinophilic spongiosis without evidence of blisters histologically.

- Bullous pemphigoid is the most common autoimmune bullous disease.
- Occurs predominantly in elderly patients.
- Presents as large, tense bullae with predilection for flexural areas.

Immunofluorescence testing is important for diagnosis of bullous pemphigoid. Direct immunofluorescence testing of perilesional skin shows deposition of C3 in a linear pattern at the basement membrane zone in almost all cases and of IgG in more than 90%. Indirect immunofluorescence testing of serum demonstrates IgG anti-basement-membrane zone antibodies in approximately 70% of cases. Routine indirect immunofluorescence testing of serum in patients suspected to have autoimmune bullous diseases is usually performed with monkey esophagus as substrate. The sensitivity of detection of anti-basement-membrane zone antibodies is increased by use of sodium chloride (NaCl)-split human skin as substrate. In addition, use of NaCl-split skin as substrate for indirect immunofluorescence testing is useful in distinguishing between bullous pemphigoid and epidermolysis bullosa acquisita, a rare blistering disease with a similar clinical presentation. On NaCl-split skin substrate, basement membrane zone antibodies from patients with bullous pemphigoid localize to the epidermal side (roof) of the substrate, or occasionally to both the roof and the floor of the substrate, whereas basement membrane zone antibodies from patients with epidermolysis bullosa acquisita localize to the dermal side (floor) of the substrate. This procedure often obviates immunoelectron microscopy to distinguish between bullous pemphigoid and epidermolysis bullosa acquisita.

- Immunofluorescence testing important for diagnosis of bullous pemphigoid.
- Almost all cases have deposition of C3 and IgG in linear pattern at basement membrane zone.

Immunoelectron microscopy of bullous pemphigoid lesions demonstrates deposition of IgG at the lamina lucida and hemidesmosomes.

Treatment of bullous pemphigoid includes systemic corticosteroids, dapsone, azathioprine, and cyclophosphamide. In general, bullous pemphigoid requires less immunosuppressive therapy than does pemphigus. Also in contrast to pemphigus, the titer of circulating antibodies does not correlate with disease activity.

Epidermolysis bullosa acquisita is another subepidermal bullous disease. It is characterized clinically by blisters or erosions induced by trauma, which predominantly occur on acral locations. A small subset of patients have generalized lesions, which clinically may be difficult to distinguish from bullous pemphigoid. The histologic pattern is a subepidermal bulla, with or without eosinophils or neutrophils.

- Epidermolysis bullosa acquisita characterized by blisters or erosions induced by trauma.
- Occurs predominantly on acral sites.

Direct immunofluorescence testing reveals a pattern similar to that in bullous pemphigoid, namely, deposition of IgG and C3 in a linear pattern at the basement membrane zone. In contrast to bullous pemphigoid, C3 may be absent or IgG may be the dominant immunoreactant. Indirect immunofluorescence testing of serum on monkey esophagus substrate demonstrates IgG anti-basement-membrane zone antibodies in 25% to 50% of patients; these antibodies localize to the dermal side (floor) of NaCl-separated human skin substrate. In patients who lack circulating antibodies, the NaCl-split skin technique may be applied to skin biopsy tissue from the patient. Epidermolysis bullosa acquisita tends to be resistant to immunosuppressive therapy.

- On direct immunofluorescence, epidermolysis bullosa acquisita shows deposition of IgG and C3 in a linear pattern at the basement membrane zone.
- Epidermolysis bullosa acquisita tends to be resistant to immunosuppressive therapy.

Cicatricial pemphigoid is characterized by mucosal lesions, with limited or no cutaneous lesions. The disease predominantly affects oral and ocular mucous membranes, and less frequently the genital, pharyngeal, or upper respiratory mucosa. This disease is also known as benign mucous membrane pemphigoid, which is often a misnomer because untreated ocular involvement may lead to blindness. Patients may present with oral erosions or diffuse gingivitis.

- Cicatricial pemphigoid affects oral and ocular mucous membranes, and less frequently genital, pharyngeal, or upper respiratory mucosa.

Direct immunofluorescence testing of mucosal tissue shows deposition of C3 and IgG in a linear pattern at the basement membrane zone, as in bullous pemphigoid. There may be IgA deposition, in addition to IgG and C3, in approximately 20% of patients. The diagnostic yield of oral mucosal tissue is better than that of conjunctiva. Serum rarely contains IgG anti-basement-membrane zone antibodies demonstrable on monkey esophagus substrate. Use of NaCl-split human skin or oral mucosa as substrate increases the sensitivity of detection of circulating anti-basement-membrane zone antibodies.

- In cicatricial pemphigoid, direct immunofluorescence shows deposition of C3 and IgG in linear pattern at basement membrane zone.

Treatment of cicatricial pemphigoid is similar to that of bullous pemphigoid, with systemic corticosteroids, dapsone, azathioprine, or cyclophosphamide. Cyclophosphamide has been used particularly in patients with ocular involvement.

Herpes gestationis, also referred to as pemphigoid gestationis, consists of intensely pruritic urticarial papules, plaques, or blisters usually occurring in the latter half of pregnancy. The lesions are histologically characterized by a subepidermal bulla with eosinophils.

- Herpes gestationis consists of intensely pruritic urticarial papules, plaques, or blisters.

Direct immunofluorescence testing of perilesional skin demonstrates deposition of C3 in a linear pattern at the basement membrane zone. In contrast to bullous pemphigoid, IgG is deposited at the basement membrane zone in only 30% to 40% of cases. Direct immunofluorescence testing is particularly useful because the other dermatoses of pregnancy (such as pruritic urticarial papules and plaques of pregnancy, PUPP) are negative by immunofluorescence testing. The serum from approximately half of patients with herpes gestationis contains the "HG factor," which is a complement-fixing IgG anti-basement-membrane zone antibody. IgG1 is the major subclass in serum and tissue from patients with herpes gestationis, whereas it is IgG4 in patients with bullous pemphigoid. The circulating antibody crosses the placenta, and the baby born to a mother with herpes gestationis may develop a transient blistering eruption during the neonatal period.

- In herpes gestationis, direct immunofluorescence shows deposition of C3 in a linear pattern at the basement membrane zone.

Linear IgA bullous dermatosis is characterized by vesicles or blisters on erythematous bases in a generalized distribution with a high rate of mucosal involvement. There is no association with gluten-sensitive enteropathy. *Chronic bullous disease of childhood* is immunologically identical to linear IgA bullous dermatosis of adults. Both diseases have clinical and histologic features in common with dermatitis herpetiformis and bullous pemphigoid. The histologic pattern is a subepidermal bulla with features of dermatitis herpetiformis or pemphigoid.

The diseases are characterized by the direct immunofluorescence finding of IgA deposition in a linear pattern at the basement membrane zone, with or without C3 or IgG deposition. Circulating IgA anti-basement-membrane zone antibodies, usually in low titer, are better demonstrated with use of NaCl-split skin as substrate than with monkey esophagus as substrate. Treatment of linear IgA bullous dermatosis and chronic bullous disease of childhood includes systemic corticosteroids, dapsone, and sulfapyridine.

- In linear IgA bullous dermatosis and chronic bullous disease

of childhood, direct immunofluorescence shows IgA deposition in a linear pattern at the basement membrane zone.

Dermatitis herpetiformis (plate 6-2) is characterized by extremely pruritic, grouped vesicles occurring predominantly over the elbows, knees, buttocks, back of the neck and scalp, and low back, usually beginning in the third or fourth decade of life. The characteristic histologic pattern in skin biopsy tissue consists of papillary stuffing with neutrophils underlying a microvesicle. Virtually all patients have some degree of gluten-sensitive enteropathy, although it is usually low-grade and subclinical. This association is important in terms of management of dermatitis herpetiformis. Dermatitis herpetiformis is also associated with thyroid disease.

- In dermatitis herpetiformis, virtually all patients have some degree of gluten-sensitive enteropathy.

The hallmark of the diagnosis of dermatitis herpetiformis is the direct immunofluorescence finding of IgA deposits in a stippled, granular, or clumped pattern, concentrated in papillary bodies and along the basement membrane zone. It is recommended that skin biopsy specimens be obtained from an area 0.5 to 1 cm away from an active lesion. IgA deposits tend to persist in the skin over time. A small percentage of patients who strictly adhere to a gluten-free diet may show diminution in IgA deposits after many years, but IgA deposits in the skin are unaffected by pharmacologic therapy. The serum of patients with dermatitis herpetiformis may contain IgA anti-reticulin and IgA anti-endomysial antibodies. IgA anti-endomysial antibodies and IgA anti-reticulin antibodies are found in approximately 70% of patients with dermatitis herpetiformis or celiac disease and in close to 100% of such patients who have grade III or IV gluten-sensitive enteropathy. Testing for IgA anti-endomysial antibodies is useful for both diagnosis and management of dermatitis herpetiformis, although these antibodies correlate with the degree of gluten-sensitive enteropathy rather than the skin lesion per se.

- In dermatitis herpetiformis, direct immunofluorescence shows IgA deposits in stippled, granular, or clumped pattern.
- Testing for IgA anti-endomysial antibodies is useful for diagnosis and management.

The mainstay of treatment of dermatitis herpetiformis consists of dapsone and a gluten-free diet. Patients who strictly adhere to a gluten-free diet may have a decreased need for dapsone. Patients must adhere to the diet for at least 8 months before its effect is seen. The titer of IgA anti-endomysial antibodies decreases during strict adherence to a gluten-free diet.

Systemic corticosteroids are not helpful in the treatment of dermatitis herpetiformis.

● Treatment of dermatitis herpetiformis: dapsone and gluten-free diet.

Bullous eruption of systemic lupus erythematosus shares clinical and histologic features with dermatitis herpetiformis. The blisters were therefore originally thought to represent the coexistence of dermatitis herpetiformis and lupus erythematosus, but they are now established as a distinct subset of lupus.

Direct immunofluorescence testing demonstrates deposition of IgG, IgM, IgA, or C3 in a linear or granular pattern at the basement membrane zone, similar to the classic "lupus band." Indirect immunofluorescence testing of serum may show IgG anti-basement-membrane zone antibodies; testing on NaCl-split skin substrate reveals a pattern identical to that of serum from patients with epidermolysis bullosa acquisita—staining of the floor (dermal side) of separated skin.

● In bullous eruption of systemic lupus erythematosus, direct immunofluorescence shows deposition of IgG, IgM, IgA, or C3 in a linear or granular pattern at basement membrane zone.

The clinical variants of *pemphigus* include pemphigus vulgaris and pemphigus foliaceus (with subsets pemphigus erythematosus and fogo selvagem, the latter being an endemic form of pemphigus that occurs in South America). There is also a drug-induced variant of pemphigus, particularly associated with D-penicillamine, captopril, or other thiol-containing medications.

● A drug-induced variant of pemphigus is associated with D-penicillamine.

More than 50% of patients with pemphigus vulgaris present with oral lesions, and more than 90% have oral mucosal involvement at some point in the course of the disease. Pemphigus vulgaris is characterized by coalescing blisters and erosions, often with generalized involvement. In contrast, pemphigus foliaceus, considered to represent the "superficial" variant of pemphigus, may present with superficial scaling-crusting lesions of the head and neck area (in a seborrheic dermatitis-like pattern) or generalized distribution (plate 6-3). The histologic hallmark of pemphigus is the presence of acantholysis (detachment of intercellular adhesion resulting in rounded keratinocytes). Pemphigus vulgaris is characterized by an intraepidermal bulla in a suprabasilar location. Pemphigus foliaceus involves acantholysis at the granular layer.

● The histologic hallmark of pemphigus is the presence of acantholysis.

All types of pemphigus are characterized by the deposition of IgG and C3 at the intercellular space (epidermal cell surface) on direct immunofluorescence testing (intercellular substance antibody, ICS). Indirect immunofluorescence testing demonstrates IgG anti-ICS antibodies in approximately 90% of cases. The titer of IgG anti-ICS antibodies is useful in both diagnosis and management of pemphigus. IgG in pemphigus is predominantly IgG4.

● All types of pemphigus are characterized by direct immunofluorescence finding of IgG and C3 deposition at the epidermal cell surface.
● Titer of IgG anti-ICS antibodies is useful in diagnosis and management.

Pemphigus antibodies are pathogenic in that they have been demonstrated to induce acantholysis in vitro and in animal models.

● Pemphigus antibodies induce acantholysis.

High-dose corticosteroids are generally required to control pemphigus. Various "steroid-sparing" immunosuppressive agents have been used, including azathioprine, cyclophosphamide, gold, and dapsone.

● High-dose corticosteroids generally are required to control pemphigus.

Erythema Multiforme

This is an acute, usually self-limited eruption of maculopapular, urticarial, occasionally bullous lesions characterized by "iris" or "target" morphology (plate 6-4). A subset of patients with erythema multiforme may have recurrent lesions. When erythema multiforme presents with extensive cutaneous and mucosal lesions, it is referred to as Stevens-Johnson syndrome. Various etiologic factors have been implicated in erythema multiforme. The most commonly cited precipitating factor is viral infection, particularly herpes simplex virus. This is responsible for a significant percentage of recurrent erythema multiforme. Other infectious agents that have been noted to cause erythema multiforme include *Mycoplasma pneumoniae* and *Yersinia enterocolitica*. Drugs have been reported to induce erythema multiforme, particularly sulfonamides, barbiturates, and anticonvulsants. Erythema multiforme may be associated with underlying connective tissue disease or malignancy. A small subset of patients with erythema multiforme have disease limited to the oral mucosa. Erythema multiforme tends to involve the lips, buccal mucosa, and tongue, in contrast to pemphigus vulgaris, which typically involves the pharynx, buccal mucosa, and tongue, and pemphigoid, which most often involves gingivae. Neither pemphigus nor pemphigoid tends to involve the lips.

- Most commonly cited precipitating factor is viral infection, particularly herpes simplex.
- Other agents: *Mycoplasma pneumoniae* and *Yersinia enterocolitica*.
- Drugs also induce erythema multiforme: sulfonamides, barbiturates, anticonvulsants.

Erythema Nodosum

Erythema nodosum typically presents as tender, erythematous, subcutaneous nodules localized to the pretibial areas. The lesions may be acute and self-limited or chronic, lasting for months up to years. The most common cause is streptococcal pharyngitis. Other infectious agents that have been implicated in the development of erythema multiforme include *Yersinia enterocolitica*, *Coccidioides*, and *Histoplasmosis*. Drug-induced erythema nodosum is most often associated with oral contraceptives and sulfonamides. Other associations with erythema nodosum include sarcoidosis, inflammatory bowel disease, and Behçet syndrome.

- The most common cause of erythema nodosum is streptococcal pharyngitis.
- Drug-induced erythema nodosum is most often associated with oral contraceptives and sulfonamides.
- Other associations: sarcoidosis, inflammatory bowel disease, Behçet syndrome.

Drug Reactions

The morphologic spectrum of reactions that may be induced by medications is broad, and hundreds of drugs may produce a given cutaneous reaction. Types of cutaneous lesions induced by drugs include morbilliform maculopapular eruptions, acnefolliculitis, necrotizing vasculitis, vesiculobullous lesions, erythema multiforme, erythema nodosum, fixed drug eruptions, lichenoid reactions, photosensitivity reactions, pigmentary changes, and hair loss.

Approximately 2% of hospitalized patients have cutaneous drug reactions, and penicillin, sulfonamides, and blood products are responsible for approximately two-thirds of such reactions. The most common types of clinical presentations (in descending order of frequency) are exanthematous or morbilliform eruptions, urticaria or angioedema, fixed drug eruption, and erythema multiforme. Stevens-Johnson syndrome, exfoliative erythroderma, and photosensitive eruptions are less common. Urticarial drug reactions are most often

related to aspirin, penicillin, or blood products. Photoallergic reactions are most often associated with sulfonamides, thiazides, griseofulvin, or phenothiazines. Phototoxic (sunburn-like, nonimmunologic) reactions may be induced by tetracyclines. Chronic use of chlorpromazine may be associated with slate-gray discoloration of sun-exposed skin, and amiodarone has been associated with slate-blue discoloration of sun-exposed areas, particularly the face. Antimalarial drugs induce yellow pigmentation or blue-gray pigmentation, depending on the compound used.

- 2% of hospitalized patients have cutaneous drug reactions.
- Penicillin, sulfonamides, and blood products are responsible for about two-thirds of drug reactions.
- Urticarial drug reactions are most often related to aspirin, penicillin, and blood products.
- Photoallergic reactions are most often associated with sulfonamides, thiazides, or phenothiazines.
- Phototoxic reactions may be induced by tetracyclines.

Exanthematous or morbilliform eruptions are the most common type of cutaneous drug reaction. This type of eruption usually begins within a week of onset of therapy, but it may occur more than 2 weeks after initiation of the drug or up to 2 weeks after use of the drug has been discontinued. Ampicillin, penicillin, and cephalosporins are commonly associated with morbilliform eruptions. A fixed drug eruption is one or several lesions that recur at the same anatomic location on rechallenge with the medication. The genital and facial areas are common sites of involvement. Phenolphthalein, barbiturates, salicylates, and oral contraceptives have been implicated in the cause of fixed drug eruptions.

- Exanthematous or morbilliform eruptions are the most common cutaneous drug reaction.
- A fixed drug eruption is one or several lesions that recur at the same location on rechallenge.
- Phenolphthalein, barbiturates, salicylates, and oral contraceptives are implicated in fixed drug eruptions.

Lichenoid drug eruptions are morphologically similar to lichen planus (with violaceous papules of the skin) and have most often been associated with gold and antimalarial drugs, although various medications may induce this type of reaction.

CUTANEOUS SIGNS OF UNDERLYING MALIGNANCY

Cutaneous metastasis occurs in 1% to 5% of patients with metastatic neoplasms. The types of malignancy metastatic to the skin reflect the most common types of visceral carcinoma, in particular, lung, breast, kidney, gastrointestinal, melanoma, and ovary. Lesions usually present on the scalp, face, or trunk.

- Cutaneous metastasis occurs in 1%-5% of patients with metastatic neoplasms.
- Lesions usually present on scalp, face, trunk.

Paget disease of the nipple is an erythematous, scaly, or weeping eczematous eruption of the areola. Virtually all patients with Paget disease have an underlying ductal carcinoma of the breast. In contrast, *extramammary Paget disease*, a morphologically similar eruption that usually occurs in the anogenital region, is associated with underlying carcinoma in only about 50% of cases. Extramammary Paget disease may be associated with underlying cutaneous adnexal carcinoma or with underlying visceral carcinoma (particularly of the genitourinary or distal gastrointestinal tracts).

- Patients with Paget disease have underlying ductal carcinoma of breast.
- Extramammary Paget disease is associated with underlying carcinoma in only 50% of cases.

Acanthosis nigricans (plate 6-5) consists of velvety hyperpigmentation of the intertriginous regions, particularly the axillae and groin. It has been associated with adenocarcinoma of the gastrointestinal tract, particularly the stomach, and insulin-resistant diabetes. Acanthosis nigricans may also be associated with obesity or certain medications (such as prednisone and nicotinic acid) or have an autosomal-dominant variant.

- Acanthosis nigricans is associated with adenocarcinoma of the gastrointestinal tract, particularly the stomach.
- May also be associated with obesity, certain medications, and insulin-resistant diabetes.

Pyoderma gangrenosum (plate 6-6) consists of ulcers with irregular, undermined, inflammatory, violaceous borders that heal with cribriform scarring. The lesions are most commonly associated with inflammatory bowel disease or rheumatoid arthritis. The bullous form of pyoderma gangrenosum is associated with malignancy of the hematopoietic system, particularly leukemia.

- Pyoderma gangrenosum is most commonly associated with inflammatory bowel disease or rheumatoid arthritis.
- The bullous form is associated with leukemia.

The skin lesions of *glucagonoma syndrome (necrolytic migratory erythema)* (plate 6-7) consist of erosions, crusting, and peeling involving the perineum and perioral areas, but may be generalized. The syndrome also includes stomatitis, glossitis (beefy tongue), anemia, diarrhea, and weight loss. It is associated with an islet cell (α) tumor of the pancreas.

- Glucagonoma syndrome consists of erosions, crusting, and peeling involving the perineum and perioral areas.
- It is associated with islet cell tumor of the pancreas.

Leser-Trélat syndrome consists of sudden onset of numerous seborrheic keratoses, and it may be associated with underlying malignancy.

Torre (Muir-Torre) syndrome consists of multiple sebaceous tumors of the skin associated with visceral carcinomas. These tumors are sebaceous adenomas, sebaceous epitheliomas, or sebaceous carcinomas. Patients may have one or numerous lesions. In addition, keratoacanthomas of the skin are also part of this syndrome. Of the underlying malignancies, carcinoma of the colon is the most common, although breast, hematologic, and other malignancies have been observed. The inheritance pattern is autosomal dominant.

- Torre syndrome consists of multiple sebaceous tumors of the skin associated with visceral carcinomas.
- Carcinoma of the colon is the most common underlying malignancy.

Cowden syndrome has autosomal dominant inheritance. Cutaneous abnormalities include trichilemmomas, verrucous papules, and oral fibromas. The syndrome is associated with thyroid and breast carcinoma. There is an increased incidence of fibrocystic disease of breast and thyroid adenoma.

- Cowden syndrome has autosomal dominant inheritance.
- Cutaneous abnormalities: trichilemmomas, verrucous papules, oral fibromas.

Gardner syndrome is a hereditary (autosomal dominant) form of colonic polyposis. Clinical features include adenomatous polyps of the colon, osteomas of the skull and face, scoliosis, soft tissue tumors (including dermoids, lipomas, and fibromas), and sebaceous (epidermal inclusion) cysts of the face and scalp. There is a high incidence of colonic carcinoma. In approximately 60% of patients, adenocarcinoma of the colon develops by age 40 years, and malignancies of other sites have been associated with this syndrome, including adrenal, ovarian, and thyroid.

- Gardner syndrome is a hereditary (autosomal dominant) form of colonic polyposis.
- Clinical features: soft tissue tumors, sebaceous cysts of face.

- There is a high incidence of colonic carcinoma.

Acquired ichthyosis has most often been associated with Hodgkin disease, but it has been reported with other types of lymphoma, multiple myeloma, and various carcinomas.

- Acquired ichthyosis is associated with Hodgkin disease.

Paraneoplastic acrokeratosis of Bazex consists of psoriasiform lesions of the hands, feet, ears, and nose, onychodystrophy, and carcinoma of the upper respiratory system, pharynx, or esophagus.

- Paraneoplastic acrokeratosis of Bazex consists of psoriasiform lesions and carcinoma of the upper respiratory system.

Hirsutism may reflect androgen excess due to an adrenal or ovarian tumor.

Hypertrichosis represents increase in hair unrelated to androgen excess, such as hypertrichosis lanuginosa acquisita (growth of soft downy hairs). It has been associated with carcinoid tumor, adenocarcinoma of the breast, lymphoma, gastrointestinal malignancy, and other types of neoplasms.

Erythema gyratum repens presents with a striking pattern of concentric erythematous bands in a "wood grain" pattern almost universally associated with underlying malignancy. The classic association is with breast carcinoma, but other types of malignancy have been reported.

- Erythema gyratum repens classically is associated with breast carcinoma.

Sweet syndrome (acute febrile neutrophilic dermatosis) has skin lesions that consist of erythematous plaques and nodules, most commonly located on the extremities and face. The association is with leukemia, particularly acute myelocytic or acute myelomonocytic leukemia.

- Sweet syndrome is associated with leukemia.

Generalized pruritus is the presentation for many cutaneous and systemic disorders. Pruritus may be the presenting symptom in lymphoma.

- Pruritus may be the presenting symptom in lymphoma.

In *dermatomyositis*, the pathognomonic skin lesions are Gottron papules (plate 6-8) involving the skin over the joints of the fingers, elbows, and knees. Poikilodermatous lesions or erythematous macular-papular eruptions may diffusely involve the face, particularly the periorbital area ("heliotrope rash" [plate 6-9]), and the trunk and extremities. The cutaneous lesions are photosensitive. The disease is characterized by proximal myositis. Although creatine phosphokinase and aldolase levels are usually increased in patients with myositis, it is important to verify the diagnosis by obtaining an electromyogram and a muscle biopsy specimen. Dermatomyositis is associated with an increased incidence of underlying malignancy.

- Dermatomyositis may involve the periorbital area ("heliotrope rash") or the dorsal aspect of the hands (Gottron papules).
- Lesions are photosensitive.
- Characterized by proximal myositis.

Multiple mucosal neuromas syndrome is associated with autosomal dominant inheritance. The main features include neuromas of the skin or mucosa (anterior tongue, lips, eyelids, conjunctiva), medullary carcinoma of the thyroid, pheochromocytoma, and parathyroid adenoma.

- Multiple mucosal neuromas syndrome: medullary carcinoma of thyroid, pheochromocytoma, parathyroid adenoma.

Cutaneous *amyloidosis* may present clinically as macroglossia (plate 6-10), waxy papules on the eyelids or nasolabial folds, pinch-purpura, and postproctoscopic purpura (plate 6-11). Multiple myeloma may be associated with amyloid.

- Amyloidosis may be associated with multiple myeloma.

Tylosis is a rare disorder characterized by palmar-plantar keratoderma associated with esophageal carcinoma. It has autosomal dominant inheritance.

- Tylosis is associated with esophageal carcinoma.

The *autoimmune bullous diseases* are a heterogeneous group of disorders characterized by antibody deposition at the basement membrane zone or epidermis. An association with malignancy has been demonstrated in several of these disorders.

- Pemphigus is associated with thymoma with or without myasthenia gravis.
- Paraneoplastic pemphigus presents with clinical and histologic features of pemphigus and erythema multiforme and is associated with lymphomas and leukemia.
- Patients with dermatitis herpetiformis rarely develop intestinal lymphoma.

- Epidermolysis bullosa acquisita is associated with amyloidosis and multiple myeloma.
- Bullous pemphigoid has not been associated with an increased risk of underlying malignancy.

DERMATOLOGY: AN INTERNIST'S PERSPECTIVE

Respiratory

The skin is involved in 15% to 35% of patients with *sarcoidosis*. Lesions may present as 1) lupus pernio (erythematous swelling of the nose), 2) translucent papules around the eyes and nasolabial folds, 3) annular lesions with central atrophy, 4) nodules on the trunk and extremities, and 5) scar sarcoid. Acute sarcoidosis may present with a combination of erythema nodosum, bilateral hilar lymphadenopathy, fever, and arthralgias (Löfgren syndrome).

- Skin is involved in 15%-35% of patients with sarcoidosis.
- Lesions may present as lupus pernio (erythematous swelling of nose).

Erythema nodosum (plate 6-12) is a reactive condition that may be associated with acute sarcoidosis. Erythema nodosum typically presents as tender, erythematous, subcutaneous nodules localized to pretibial areas. The lesions may be acute and self-limited or chronic, lasting for months up to years.

- Erythema nodosum may be associated with acute sarcoidosis.

In *Wegener granulomatosis*, cutaneous involvement occurs in more than 50% of patients and is manifested by cutaneous infarction, ulceration, hemorrhagic bullae, purpuric papules, or urticaria. A skin biopsy may show hypersensitivity vasculitis or granulomatous vasculitis.

- In Wegener granulomatosis, cutaneous involvement occurs in >50% of patients.
- Manifestations: ulceration, hemorrhagic bullae, purpuric papules, urticaria.

Churg-Strauss granulomatosis/allergic granulomatosis syndrome is characterized by combination of adult-onset asthma, peripheral eosinophilia, and pulmonary involvement with recurrent pneumonia or transient infiltrates. Skin lesions have been reported in up to 60% of patients and consist of palpable purpura, cutaneous infarcts, and subcutaneous nodules.

- Skin lesions of Churg-Strauss granulomatosis occur in up

to 60% of patients.
- Skin lesions include palpable purpura, cutaneous infarct, and subcutaneous nodules.

In *relapsing polychondritis*, there is episodic destructive inflammation of cartilage of the ears, nose, and upper airways. There may be associated arthritis and ocular involvement. In the acute stage, the ears may be red, swollen, and tender. Later, they become soft and flabby. Nasal chondritis may lead to saddle-nose deformities. Relapsing polychondritis is mediated by antibodies to type II collagen.

- Relapsing polychondritis: episodic destructive inflammation of cartilage of ears, nose, upper airways.
- Nasal chondritis may lead to saddle-nose deformities.

Cardiovascular

In several syndromes, lentigines have been associated with cardiac abnormalities. These include the *LEOPARD*, *NAME*, and *LAMB* syndromes.

- LEOPARD syndrome (Moynahan syndrome): *l*entigines, *e*lectrocardiographic changes, *o*cular hypertelorism, *p*ulmonary stenosis, *a*bnormal genitalia, *r*etardation of growth, *d*eafness.
- NAME syndrome: *n*evi, *a*trial myxoma, *m*yxoid neurofibromas, *e*philides.
- LAMB syndrome: *l*entigines, *a*trial myxoma, *m*ucocutaneous myxomas, *b*lue nevi.

Pseudoxanthoma elasticum may be transmitted by autosomal dominant or autosomal recessive inheritance. Yellow xanthoma-like papules are seen on the neck (plucked-chicken skin), axillae, groin, and abdomen. Angioid streaks may be seen in the fundus. Skin biopsy shows degeneration of elastic fibers. Systemic associations include stroke, myocardial infarction, peripheral vascular disease, and gastrointestinal hemorrhage.

- Pseudoxanthoma elasticum is associated with stroke, myocardial infarction, peripheral vascular disease, and gastrointestinal hemorrhage.

Ehlers-Danlos syndrome includes 10 subgroups that vary in severity and systemic associations. Cutaneous findings are skin hyperextensibility with hypermobile joints and fish-mouth scars. Angina, peripheral vascular disease, and gastrointestinal bleeding may be associated.

- Ehlers-Danlos syndrome is associated with angina, peripheral vascular disease, and gastrointestinal bleeding.

Erythema marginatum is one of the diagnostic criteria for acute rheumatic fever. This uncommon eruption occurs on the trunk and is characterized by erythematous plaques with rapidly mobile serpiginous borders.

- Erythema marginatum is one of the diagnostic criteria for acute rheumatic fever.

Gastrointestinal

Osler-Weber-Rendu syndrome (hereditary hemorrhagic telangiectasia), with autosomal dominant inheritance, is manifested by cutaneous and mucosal telangiectasias. Frequent nosebleeds and gastrointestinal bleeds may be a presenting feature. Pulmonary arteriovenous malformations and central nervous system angiomas are also features of this syndrome.

- Osler-Weber-Rendu syndrome has autosomal dominant inheritance.
- Features: nosebleeds, gastrointestinal bleeds, pulmonary arteriovenous malformations, central nervous system angiomas.

Acrodermatitis enteropathica is an inherited (autosomal recessive) or acquired disease characterized by zinc deficiency (failure of absorption or failure to supplement). The clinical features include angular cheilitis, a seborrheic dermatitis-like eruption, erosions, blisters, and pustules, with skin lesions particularly involving the face, hands, feet, and perineum. Alopecia and diarrhea are other features of this syndrome.

- Acrodermatitis enteropathica: inherited (autosomal recessive) or acquired disease.
- Characterized by zinc deficiency (failure of absorption or failure to supplement).

Peutz-Jeghers syndrome is an inherited (autosomal dominant) syndrome of intestinal polyposis. Patients have hamartomas, mostly involving the small bowel, with slightly increased risk of developing carcinoma. Cutaneous lesions include macular pigmentation (freckles) of the lips, periungual skin, fingers, and toes and pigmentation of the oral mucosa.

- Peutz-Jeghers syndrome is inherited (autosomal dominant) syndrome of intestinal polyposis.
- An increased risk of developing carcinoma was recently recognized.

Dermatitis herpetiformis (plate 6-2) is an immune-mediated bullous disease that presents with intensely itchy vesicles on extensor surfaces (elbows, knees, buttocks, scapula). Gluten-sensitive enteropathy occurs in up to 70% of patients.

- Dermatitis herpetiformis is an immune-mediated bullous disease.
- Gluten-sensitive enteropathy occurs in up to 70% of patients.

Extensive *aphthous ulceration* may be associated with Crohn disease or gluten-sensitive enteropathy.

- Aphthous ulceration may be associated with Crohn disease or gluten-sensitive enteropathy.

Pyoderma gangrenosum (plate 6-6) presents with ulceration, predominantly on the lower extremities, with inflammatory undermined borders. The lesions heal with cribriform scarring. The phenomenon whereby lesions occur at sites of trauma is known as pathergy—the occurrence of the disease at sites of trauma is classic. Systemic disease associations include inflammatory bowel disease (ulcerative colitis more commonly than Crohn disease), rheumatoid arthritis, and paraproteinemia.

- Pyoderma gangrenosum occurs at sites of trauma.
- Associated diseases are inflammatory bowel disease (ulcerative colitis more than Crohn disease), rheumatoid arthritis, paraproteinemia.

Cutaneous Crohn disease may present as skin nodules with granulomatous histology. Other manifestations include pyostomatitis vegetans (granulomatous inflammation of the gingivae), granulomatous cheilitis, oral aphthous ulceration, perianal skin tags, and perianal fistulae.

- Manifestation of Crohn disease: pyostomatitis vegetans (granulomatous inflammation of gingivae).

Bowel bypass syndrome presents with a flu-like illness with fever, malaise, arthralgias, myalgias, and inflammatory papules and pustules on the extremities and upper trunk. The disease is recurrent and episodic and occurs in up to 20% of patients after jejunoileal bypass. The condition responds to antibiotics or to reversal of the bypass procedure.

- Bowel bypass syndrome: flu-like illness, inflammatory papules and pustules.
- Occurs in up to 20% of patients after jejunoileal bypass.

Gardner syndrome and *glucagonoma syndrome* are described on page 181.

Nephrology

Partial lipodystrophy is associated with C3 deficiency and the nephrotic syndrome.

Uremic pruritus is associated with end-stage renal disease and responds to ultraviolet B therapy.

Neurocutaneous

Fabry disease is an X-linked recessive disorder due to deficiency of the enzyme α-galactosidase A. The skin changes consist of numerous vascular tumors (angiokeratomas) that develop during childhood and adolescence. Corneal opacities are present in 90% of patients. Systemic manifestations include paresthesias and pain due to involved peripheral nerves, renal insufficiency, and vascular insufficiency of the coronary and central nervous system.

- Fabry disease is a recessive disorder due to deficiency of α-galactosidase A.
- Systemic manifestations: paresthesias, renal insufficiency, vascular insufficiency.

The clinical features of *ataxia-telangiectasia* include cutaneous and ocular telangiectasia, cerebellar ataxia, choreoathetosis, IgA deficiency, and recurrent pulmonary infections.

Tuberous sclerosis may be inherited in an autosomal dominant pattern (25%) or may occur sporadically (new mutation). Predominant cutaneous lesions include hypopigmented macules, adenoma sebaceum, subungual or periungual fibromas, and shagreen patch (connective tissue nevus) (plate 6-13). This syndrome is associated with epilepsy (80%) and mental retardation (60%). Rhabdomyomas may occur in the heart in childhood. Angiomyolipomas occur in the kidneys in up to 80% of adults with this syndrome.

- Tuberous sclerosis may be inherited in an autosomal dominant pattern or be sporadic.
- It is associated with epilepsy (80%) and mental retardation (60%).
- Angiomyolipomas occur in kidneys in up to 80% of affected adults.

Neurofibromatosis (von Recklinghausen disease) (plate 6-14) occurs in 1 in 3,000 births. Inheritance is autosomal dominant, and approximately 50% of cases are new mutations. The major signs of the disease are café-au-lait spots, axillary freckling (Crowe sign), neurofibromas, and Lisch nodules of the iris.

- Neurofibromatosis is autosomal dominant.
- Major signs: café-au-lait spots, axillary freckling, neurofibromas.

Neurofibromatosis has various clinical manifestations, as reflected in the Ricardi classification:

1. Classic: Neurofibromas, café-au-lait spots, Lisch nodules of iris, chromosome 17, positive family history.
2. Central: Bilateral acoustic neuromas, few neurofibromas, few café-au-lait spots, *no Lisch nodules*, chromosome 22, positive family history.
3. Mixed: Features of no. 1 and no. 2, central nervous system tumors, positive family history.
4. Variant: Variable family history, diffuse café-au-lait spots, neurofibromas, with or without central nervous system tumors.
5. Segmental or dermatomal: Neurofibromas or café-au-lait spots, skin involvement only, negative family history.
6. Multiple café-au-lait spots: Skin involvement only, negative family history, no neurofibromas.
7. Late onset: Cutaneous disease for more than 30 years.
8. Other: Clinical syndromes not fitting the above classifications.

The associated central nervous system tumors include acoustic neuromas, optic gliomas, and meningiomas. Other associated tumors include pheochromocytoma, neuroblastoma, and Wilms tumor. Café-au-lait spots and neurofibromas frequently occur in the absence of neurofibromatosis. The diagnostic criteria for neurofibromatosis include two or more of the following:

1. Six or more café-au-lait macules more than 0.5 cm in greatest diameter in prepubertal patients, or more than 1.5 cm in diameter in adults.
2. Two or more neurofibromas of any type, or one plexiform neurofibroma.
3. Freckling of skin in axillary or inguinal regions.
4. Optic gliomas.
5. Lisch nodules.
6. An osseous lesion such as sphenoid dysplasia or thinning of long bone cortex with or without pseudarthrosis.
7. A first-degree relative with neurofibromatosis that meets the above diagnostic criteria.

Sturge-Weber-Dimitri syndrome is characterized by capillary angioma (port-wine stain) in the distribution of the upper or middle branch of the trigeminal nerve. There may be associated meningeal angioma in the same distribution. Intracranial tramline calcification, mental retardation, epilepsy, contralateral hemiparesis, and visual impairment may be associated.

- Sturge-Weber-Dimitri syndrome characterized by capillary angioma in distribution of upper or middle branch of trigeminal nerve.
- Associated features: intracranial calcification, mental retardation, epilepsy, contralateral hemiparesis, visual impairment.

Klippel-Trenaunay-Weber syndrome is the constellation of hemangiomas in a dermatomal distribution with associated arteriovenous malformation.

Cobb syndrome is a noninherited disorder in which port-wine stain or angiokeratoma occurs in a dermatomal distribution associated with spinal cord angioma within one or two segments of the cutaneous lesions.

Sneddon syndrome involves extensive livedo reticularis and cerebrovascular accidents, possibly as manifestation of the antiphospholipid syndrome.

Cerebral granulomatous angiitis is a sequela of ophthalmic herpes zoster and is responsible for the combination of ophthalmic zoster followed by a delayed contralateral hemiplegia (weeks to months; average, 8 weeks).

Rheumatology: Cutaneous Associations of Arthritis

Psoriatic arthritis occurs in 4% to 5% of patients with psoriasis. Several different patterns of arthritis are seen and are well summarized in the Moll and Wright classification. An asymmetric oligoarthritis occurs in 70% of patients. This group includes patients with "sausage digits" and monoarthritis. The second most common presentation is a symmetric arthritis clinically similar to rheumatoid arthritis, which occurs in 15% of patients with psoriatic arthritis. Distal interphalangeal involvement, arthritis mutilans, and a spinal form of arthritis similar to ankylosing spondylitis each occur in 5% of patients with psoriatic arthritis.

- Psoriatic arthritis occurs in 4%-5% of patients with psoriasis.
- Asymmetric oligoarthritis is most common.
- 5% of patients have ankylosing spondylitis.

Reiter syndrome consists of the triad of urethritis, conjunctivitis, and arthritis. The disease usually affects young men. Two-thirds of patients have skin lesions, namely, circinate balinitis, consisting of erythematous plaques of the penis, and keratoderma blennorrhagicum, a pustular psoriasiform eruption of the palms and soles. Most patients are HLA-B27 positive.

- Reiter syndrome triad: urethritis, conjunctivitis, arthritis.
- Most patients are HLA-B27 positive.

Multicentric reticulohistiocytosis may affect the skin, mucosa, joints, bones, and viscera. Most patients have skin lesions and arthritis. Skin lesions consist of red-brown papules and nodules, most commonly located on the dorsal aspects of hands and face. Approximately half of all patients have mucosal lesions, particularly of the lips, buccal mucosa, tongue, gingiva, or nose. The arthritis consists of severely destructive and mutilating involvement, particularly of the interphalangeal joints of the hands ("opera glass hand" or "telescope fingers"), knees, wrists, hips, ankles, feet, elbows, and spine. Multicentric reticulohistiocytosis has also been associated with underlying malignancy.

- Multicentric reticulohistiocytosis involves skin lesions and arthritis.
- May be associated with underlying malignancy.

Erythema chronicum migrans is an annular, sometimes urticarial, erythematous lesion presenting as a manifestation of Lyme disease. The lesion develops subsequent to, and surrounding the site of, a tick bite. Lesions are single in 75% of patients and multiple in 25%. Other acute features of Lyme disease include fever, headaches, myalgias, arthralgias, and lymphadenopathy. The tick, *Ixodes dammini*, contains a spirochete, *Borrelia burgdorferi*, that is responsible for the syndrome. Arthritis is a late complication of Lyme disease. Weeks or months after the initial illness, patients may develop meningoencephalitis, peripheral neuropathy, myocarditis, atrioventricular node block, or destructive erosive arthritis.

- Erythema chronicum migrans presents as a manifestation of Lyme disease.
- Lesion develops subsequent to and surrounding the site of tick bite.
- Lesions are single in 75% and multiple in 25%.

In *rheumatoid arthritis,* nodules occur over the extensor surfaces of joints, most commonly on the dorsal hands and elbows. Rheumatoid vasculitis with ulceration may occur in the setting of rheumatoid arthritis with a high circulating rheumatoid factor.

During the late stages of *gout,* tophi (urate deposits with surrounding inflammation) occur in the subcutaneous tissues. Improved methods of treatment account for the decrease in the incidence of tophaceous gout in recent years.

- Gouty tophi occur in subcutaneous tissues.

In *lupus erythematosus* (LE), cutaneous abnormalities occur in approximately 80% of patients. LE can be classified into acute cutaneous LE (malar rash, generalized maculopapular eruption, or bullous LE), subacute cutaneous LE, and chronic cutaneous LE (localized discoid LE, generalized discoid LE, and lupus panniculitis).

- In LE, cutaneous abnormalities occur in 80% of patients.

Skin lesions are present in up to 85% of patients with acute systemic LE. A butterfly rash with erythema involving the nose and cheeks is characteristic. Erythematous papules and plaques also may occur on the dorsal aspect of the hands, and the skin overlying the interphalangeal and metacarpal phalangeal joints is spared. Maculopapular erythema also may occur on sun-exposed areas.

Subacute cutaneous LE (plate 6-15) usually presents with generalized annular or polycyclic plaques. The lesions may appear papulosquamous or vesiculobullous. Subacute cutaneous LE is characterized by the presence of anti-Ro (anti-SSA) antibodies in serum and photosensitivity. These antibodies cross the placenta, and children born to mothers with subacute cutaneous LE may develop congenital heart block or a transient photodistributed skin eruption during the neonatal period.

- Subacute cutaneous LE presents with annular or polycyclic plaques.
- Subacute cutaneous LE is characterized by the presence of anti-Ro (anti-SSA) antibodies and photosensitivity.

Discoid LE (plate 6-16) is characterized by erythematous papules and plaques with follicular hyperkeratosis and scaling. Localized discoid LE is usually not associated with systemic LE. Generalized discoid LE or disseminated discoid LE refers to lesions involving the head and neck area or the trunk and extremities. Discoid LE most commonly affects the face, scalp, and ears. Although most patients with discoid LE lack manifestations of systemic LE, approximately 25% of patients with systemic LE have had cutaneous lesions of discoid LE at some point during the course of their illness.

- Discoid LE is characterized by erythematous papules and plaques with follicular hyperkeratosis and scaling.
- Discoid LE most commonly affects the face, scalp, ears.
- 25% of patients with systemic LE have had cutaneous manifestations of discoid LE.

The "lupus band test" refers to the finding of immunoglobulin and complement at the basement membrane zone of skin biopsy tissue as determined by direct immunofluorescence testing. In biopsy of lesional tissue from discoid LE or systemic LE, immunoglobulin and complement are demonstrable at the basement membrane zone in more than 90% of patients. Only 50% to 60% of patients with subacute cutaneous LE have a positive lupus band test of lesional skin. The lupus band test is positive in nonlesional skin (normal-appearing, non-sun-exposed skin, typically buttock) from 50% of patients with systemic LE and is associated with an increased incidence of renal disease.

Circulating antinuclear antibodies are demonstrable in most patients with systemic LE and subacute cutaneous erythematosus, but they are present in only a small percentage of patients with discoid LE. A homogeneous antinuclear antibody pattern tends to correlate with the diagnosis of systemic LE, peripheral (rim) pattern correlates with lupus nephritis, speckled anticentromere pattern is associated with the CREST variant of scleroderma (CREST: *c*alcinosis cutis, *R*aynaud phenomenon, *e*sophageal dysmotility, *s*clerodactyly, and *t*elangiectasia), nucleolar pattern usually correlates with the diagnosis of scleroderma and uncommonly with lupus, and the particulate pattern is associated with various connective tissue diseases, including LE. In addition to association with subacute cutaneous LE, anti-Ro (anti-SSA) antibodies are associated with Sjögren syndrome, LE with C2 deficiency, and neonatal LE.

The term "scleroderma" encompasses a spectrum of disease ranging from generalized multisystem disease to localized cutaneous disease. The systemic end of the spectrum is represented by progressive systemic sclerosis and the CREST syndrome. The middle area of the spectrum is represented by eosinophilic fasciitis and linear scleroderma, which may have systemic involvement. Localized scleroderma (also known as morphea) may be a single plaque or may be multiple plaques in a generalized distribution.

Systemic scleroderma consists of diffuse sclerosis associated with smoothness and hardening of the skin, with masklike face and microstomia. Sclerodactyly, periungual telangiectasia, hyperpigmentation, and cutaneous calcification may be observed. Esophageal, pulmonary, renal, and cardiac involvement may be associated with systemic scleroderma. The CREST syndrome (plate 6-17) is associated with circulating anticentromere antibodies.

- Systemic scleroderma may include sclerodactyly, periungual telangiectasia, hyperpigmentation, and cutaneous calcification.

Eosinophilic fasciitis manifests as tightly bound thickening of the skin and underlying soft tissue of the extremities. Other features include arthralgias, hypergammaglobulinemia, and peripheral blood eosinophilia.

- Eosinophilic fasciitis manifests as tightly bound thickening of skin and underlying soft tissue of extremities.

Morphea manifests as discrete sclerotic plaques with white shiny center and erythematous or violaceous periphery. Localized or linear scleroderma may have various presentations depending on extent, location, and depth of sclerosis. Most lesions are characterized by sclerosis and atrophy associated with depression or "delling" of the soft tissue; underlying bone may be affected in linear scleroderma.

- Morphea manifests as discrete sclerotic plaques with white shiny center.
- Underlying bone may be affected in linear scleroderma.

Hematologic

Graft-versus-host disease (GVHD) most commonly occurs after bone marrow transplantation and represents the constellation of skin lesions, diarrhea, and liver function abnormalities. GVHD occurs in 60% to 80% of patients who undergo allogeneic bone marrow transplantation.

- GVHD commonly occurs after bone marrow transplantation.
- Includes skin lesions, diarrhea, liver function abnormalities.

GVHD generally occurs in two phases. Acute GVHD begins 7 to 21 days after transplantation, and chronic GVHD begins within months to 1 year after transplantation. One or both phases may occur in the same patient. Acute GVHD results from attack of donor immunocompetent T lymphocytes and null lymphocytes against host histocompatibility antigens. Chronic GVHD results from immunocompetent lymphocytes that develop in the recipient.

The cutaneous abnormalities of acute GVHD include pruritus, numbness or pain of the palms and soles, an erythematous macular-papular eruption of the trunk, palms, and soles, and blisters that, when extensive, resemble toxic epidermal necrolysis. Acute GVHD also includes intestinal abnormalities resulting in diarrhea and liver function changes.

- Cutaneous abnormalities of GVHD: pruritus, numbness or pain of palms and soles, erythematous macular-papular eruption of trunk, palms, and soles.

Chronic GVHD mainly affects skin and liver. Early chronic GVHD is characterized by a lichenoid reaction consisting of cutaneous and oral lesions that resemble lichen planus, with coalescing violaceous papules on the skin and white reticulated patches on the buccal mucosa. Late chronic GVHD is characterized by cutaneous sclerosis, poikilodermatous-reticulated lesions, and scarring alopecia. The histologic pattern of GVHD includes lymphocytes in proximity to dyskeratotic keratinocytes, so-called satellite cell necrosis. The cutaneous infiltrate is composed predominantly of suppressor/cytotoxic T cells.

- Chronic GVHD: lichenoid reaction consisting of cutaneous and oral lesions.

Mastocytosis (mast cell disease) can be divided into four groups, depending on the age at onset and the presence or absence of systemic involvement: 1) urticaria pigmentosa arising in infancy or adolescence without significant systemic involvement, 2) urticaria pigmentosa in adults without significant systemic involvement, 3) systemic mast cell disease, and 4) mast cell leukemia.

The cutaneous lesions may be brown to red macules, papules, nodules, or plaques that urticate on stroking. Less commonly, the lesions may be bullous, erythrodermic, or telangiectatic. The systemic manifestations are due to histamine release and consist of flushing, tachycardia, and diarrhea.

- Cutaneous lesions of mastocytosis: brown to red macules, papules, nodules, or plaques that urticate on stroking.
- Systemic manifestations—flushing, tachycardia, diarrhea—due to histamine release.

Necrobiotic xanthogranuloma—indurated plaques with associated atrophy and telangiectasia with or without ulceration—may occur on the trunk or periorbital areas. Serum electrophoresis shows an IgGκ paraproteinemia or multiple myeloma.

Endocrine

Diabetes Mellitus

Several dermatologic disorders have been described in diabetes.

Necrobiosis lipoidica diabeticorum (plate 6-18) classically occurs on the shins and presents as yellow-brown atrophic telangiectatic plaques that occasionally ulcerate. Two-thirds of patients have diabetes.

- Necrobiosis lipoidica diabeticorum occurs on the shins.
- Two-thirds of patients have diabetes.

Granuloma annulare is an asymptomatic eruption consisting of small, firm, flesh-colored or red papules in an annular configuration (plate 6-19) (less commonly nodular or generalized). The association with diabetes is disputed.

- Granuloma annulare consists of small, firm, flesh-colored or red papules in an annular configuration.

Rarely, patients with poorly controlled diabetes present with spontaneously occurring *subepidermal blisters* (bullosa diabeticorum) on the dorsal aspects of the hands and feet.

The *stiff hand syndrome* has been reported in juvenile-onset insulin-dependent diabetes. Patients have limited joint mobility and tight waxy skin on the hands. There is an increased risk of subsequent renal and retinal microvascular disease.

- Stiff hand syndrome: increased risk of subsequent renal and retinal microvascular disease.

In *scleredema,* there is an insidious onset of thickening and stiffness of the skin on the upper back and posterior neck. The condition is more common in middle-aged men with diabetes. The diabetes is often long-standing and poorly controlled.

- Scleredema is more common in middle-aged men with diabetes.
- Diabetes is often long-standing and poorly controlled.

Thyroid
Pretibial myxedema and thyroid acropachy are cutaneous associations of Graves disease.

Metabolic

The *porphyrias* are a group of inherited or acquired abnormalities of heme synthesis. Each type is associated with deficient activity of a particular enzyme. The porphyrias are usually divided into three types: erythropoietic, hepatic, and mixed.

Erythropoietic porphyria (Günther disease) is a hereditary form (autosomal recessive) characterized by marked photosensitivity, blisters, scarring alopecia, hirsutism, red-stained teeth, hemolytic anemia, and splenomegaly. The skin lesions are severely mutilating. Onset is in infancy or early childhood.

- Erythropoietic porphyria is autosomal recessive.
- Skin lesions are severely mutilating.

Erythropoietic protoporphyria is an autosomal dominant syndrome that usually begins during childhood. It is characterized by variable degrees of photosensitivity and a marked itching, burning, or stinging sensation that occurs within minutes after sun exposure. It is associated with deficiency of ferrochelatase.

- Erythropoietic protoporphyria is autosomal dominant.
- It is associated with deficiency of ferrochelatase.

Porphyria cutanea tarda, one of the hepatic porphyrias, is an acquired or hereditary (autosomal dominant) disease associated with a defect in uroporphyrinogen decarboxylase. The disease may be precipitated by exposure to toxins (such as chlorinated phenols or hexachlorobenzene), alcohol, estrogens, iron overload, and infection with hepatitis C. Porphyria cutanea tarda usually presents in the third or fourth decade of life. Clinical manifestations include photosensitivity, skin fragility, erosions and blisters (particularly on dorsal surfaces of the hands) (plate 6-20), hyperpigmentation, milia, hypertrichosis, and facial suffusion. Some patients develop sclerodermoid skin changes. The diagnosis is confirmed by the finding of elevated porphyrin levels in the urine. Treatment includes phlebotomy and low-dose chloroquine.

- Porphyria cutanea tarda is acquired or inherited (autosomal dominant).
- It is associated with a defect in uroporphyrinogen decarboxylase.
- It may be precipitated by exposure to toxins or infection with hepatitis C.

Pseudoporphyria is a porphyria cutanea tarda-like clinical syndrome induced by drugs, including tetracycline, furosemide, and nalidixic acid, or by hemodialysis. The clinical features resemble those of porphyria cutanea tarda, but there is usually no demonstrable biochemical abnormality of porphyrin metabolism.

- Pseudoporphyria is induced by drugs (tetracycline, furosemide, nalidixic acid) or by hemodialysis.

Acute intermittent porphyria ("Swedish porphyria") lacks skin lesions and is characterized by acute attacks of abdominal pain or neurologic symptoms.

- Acute intermittent porphyria lacks skin lesions.
- It involves acute attacks of abdominal pain or neurologic symptoms.

Variegate porphyria (mixed porphyria) also follows autosomal dominant inheritance. Variegate porphyria is characterized by cutaneous abnormalities that are similar to those of porphyria cutanea tarda and by acute abdominal episodes, as in acute intermittent porphyria. Variegate porphyria tends to be precipitated by drugs, such as barbiturates and sulfonamides.

- Variegate porphyria is autosomal dominant.
- It tends to be precipitated by drugs, such as barbiturates and sulfonamides.

NAIL CLUES TO SYSTEMIC DISEASE

Onycholysis consists of distal and lateral separation of the nail plate from the nail bed. Onycholysis may be due to psoriasis, infection (such as *Candida* or *Pseudomonas*), a reaction to nail cosmetics, or a drug reaction. Drugs that have been noted to induce onycholysis include tetracycline and chlorpromazine. Association with thyroid disease (hyperthyroidism more than hypothyroidism) has also been observed.

- Onycholysis may be due to psoriasis, infection (*Candida* or *Pseudomonas*), nail cosmetics, or drug reaction.

Pitting is a common feature of psoriatic nails. Pits have also been associated with alopecia areata.

Twenty-nail dystrophy is most often associated with lichen planus or alopecia areata.

Terry nails consist of whitening of the proximal or entire nail as a result of changes in the nail bed. This abnormality is associated with cirrhosis.

- Terry nail is associated with cirrhosis.

Muehrcke lines consist of white parallel bands associated with hypoalbuminemia.

- Muehrcke lines are associated with hypoalbuminemia.

"Half-and-half" nails (Lindsay nails) are nails in which the proximal half is white and the distal half is red. This abnormality may be associated with renal failure.

- "Half-and-half" nails may be associated with renal failure.

Yellow nails are associated with chronic edema, pulmonary disease, pleural effusion, chronic bronchitis, bronchiectasis, and lung carcinoma.

Beau lines are transverse grooves in the nail associated with high fever, systemic disease, and drugs.

Koilonychia (spoon nails) is associated with iron deficiency anemia, but it may also be idiopathic, familial, or related to trauma.

- Koilonychia is associated with iron deficiency anemia.

Blue-colored lunula is associated with hepatolenticular degeneration (Wilson disease) and argyria.

Mees lines are white bands associated with arsenic.

- Mees lines are associated with arsenic.

CUTANEOUS MANIFESTATIONS OF HIV INFECTION

Primary infection with human immunodeficiency virus (HIV) results in a flu-like illness and an exanthem in 30% to 60% of patients. The exanthem may be morbilliform or pityriasis rosea-like. Oral ulceration and erosions and erosive esophagitis also may occur at this stage. The acute exanthem and enanthem are self-limited and often go undiagnosed.

In the early stage of the disease, cutaneous manifestations include genital warts, genital herpes, psoriasis, and mild seborrheic dermatitis. With symptomatic HIV infection (CD4 count of 200-400), both infections and inflammatory dermatoses occur more frequently. These include psoriasis, oral hairy leukoplakia, candidiasis, herpes zoster, herpes simplex, tinea pedis, and onychomycosis. In patients with a family history of atopy, atopic dermatitis may be a manifestation at this stage.

As the CD4 count decreases to less than 200, patients present with a disseminated fungal infection, herpes zoster, persistent herpes simplex, bacilliary angiomatosis, and molluscum contagiosum. *Bacillary angiomatosis* consists of one or more vascular papules or nodules caused by a *Rickettsia*-like organism related to *Rochalimaea quintana*. Eosinophilic folliculitis, a pruritic eruption primarily involving the head, neck, trunk, and proximal extremities, is characteristic of symptomatic HIV infection.

With advanced HIV infection (CD4 counts of <50), overwhelming infection is characteristic. Infectious agents include cytomegalovirus, *Cryptococcus*, *Acanthamoeba*, and extensive molluscum contagiosum.

Oral hairy leukoplakia is caused by Epstein-Barr virus infection of the oral mucosa and usually occurs in patients with advanced HIV infection.

Molluscum contagiosum, a common viral infection of otherwise healthy children, has been observed in 10% to 20% of patients with HIV infection.

- Molluscum contagiosum is observed in 10%-20% of patients with HIV infection.

Epidemic Kaposi sarcoma usually presents as oval papules or plaques oriented along skin lines of the trunk, extremities, face, and mucosa. This presentation is in contrast to that of classic Kaposi sarcoma in elderly patients, which occurs predominantly on the distal lower extremities. Kaposi sarcoma-herpes simplex virus (human herpes virus 9) has been identified in tissue from patients with both epidemic and classic Kaposi sarcoma.

- Epidemic Kaposi sarcoma: oval papules or plaques along skin lines of trunk, extremities, face, mucosa.
- It is most commonly associated with HIV infection.

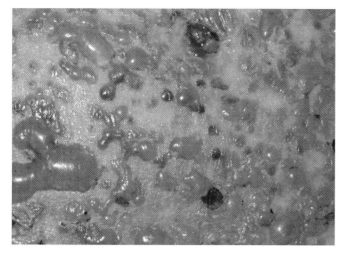

Plate 6-1. Bullous pemphigoid.

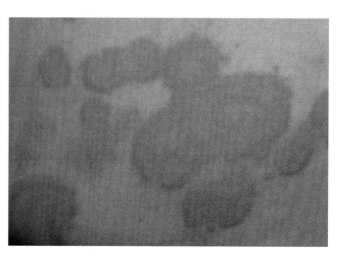

Plate 6-2. Dermatitis herpetiformis.

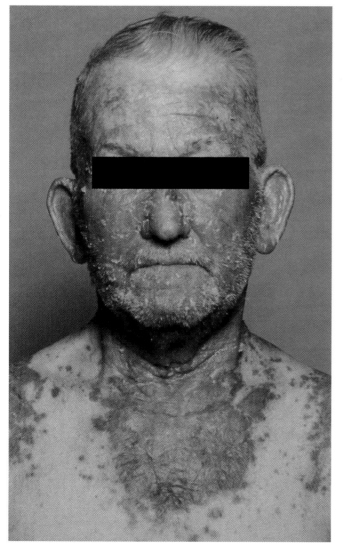

Plate 6-3. Pemphigus foliaceus.

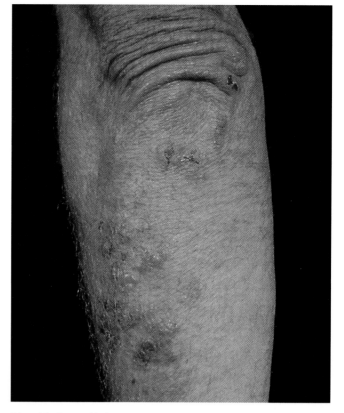

Plate 6-4. Erythema multiforme.

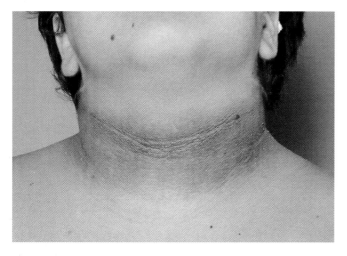

Plate 6-5. Acanthosis nigricans.

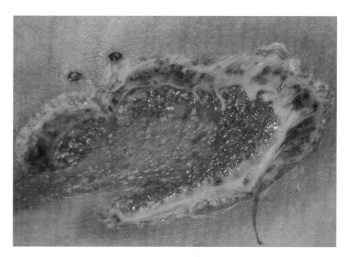

Plate 6-6. Pyoderma gangrenosum.

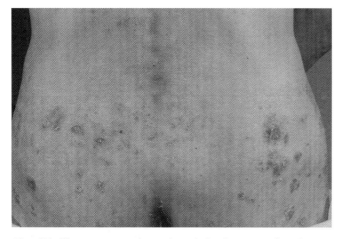

Plate 6-7. Glucagonoma syndrome (necrolytic migratory erythema).

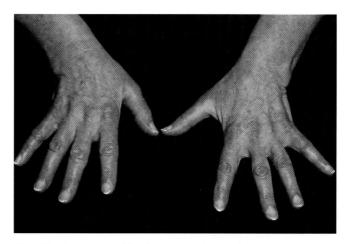

Plate 6-8. Dermatomyositis: Gottron papules.

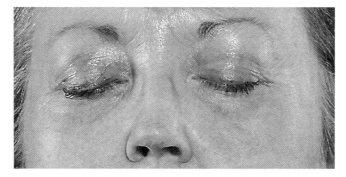

Plate 6-9. Dermatomyositis: heliotrope discoloration.

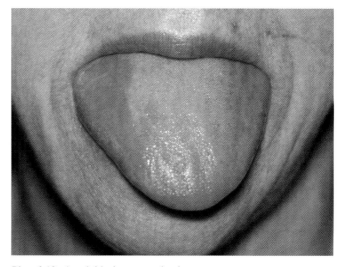

Plate 6-10. Amyloidosis: macroglossia.

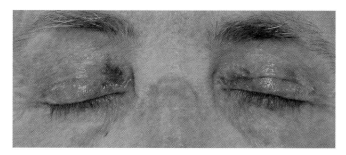

Plate 6-11. Amyloidosis: postproctoscopic purpura.

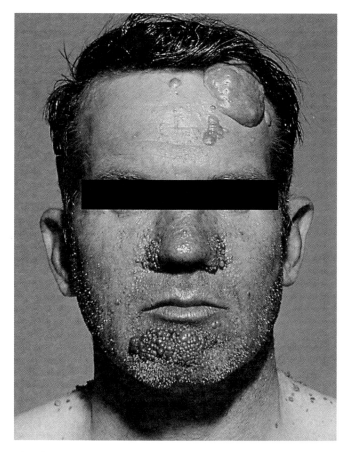

Plate 6-13. Tuberous sclerosis: adenoma sebaceum and forehead plaque.

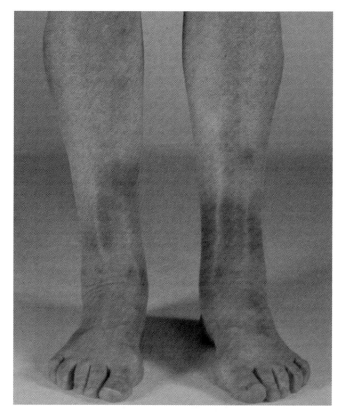

Plate 6-12. Erythema nodosum.

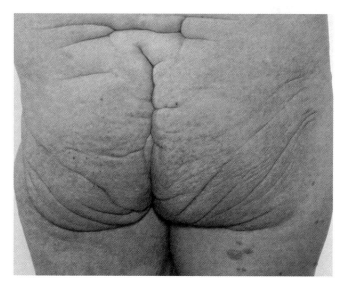

Plate 6-14. Neurofibromatosis: plexiform neurofibroma.

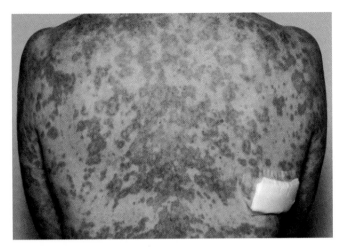

Plate 6-15. Subacute cutaneous lupus erythematosus.

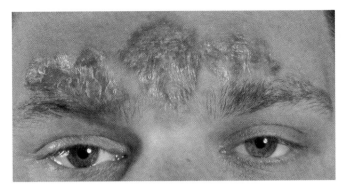

Plate 6-16. Discoid lupus erythematosus.

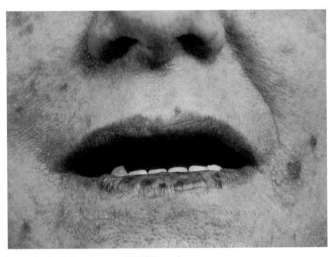

Plate 6-17. Scleroderma: CREST syndrome.

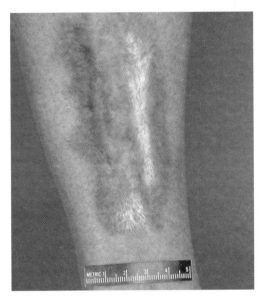

Plate 6-18. Necrobiosis lipoidica diabeticorum.

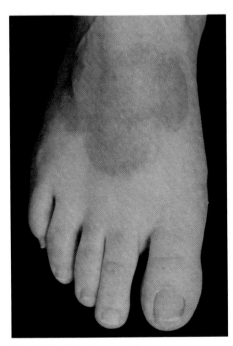

Plate 6-19. Granuloma annulare.

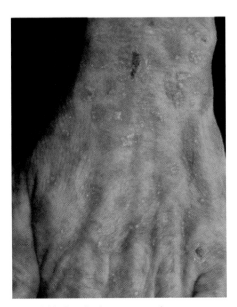

Plate 6-20. Porphyria cutanea tarda.

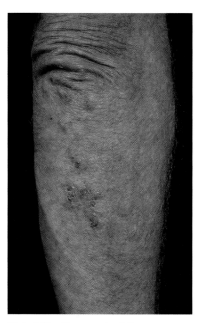

Plate 6-21. (See question 1.)

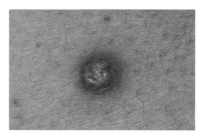

Plate 6-22. (See question 3.)

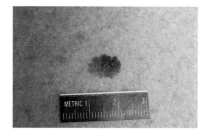

Plate 6-23. (See question 4.)

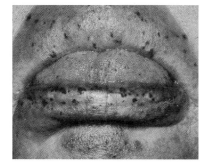

Plate 6-24. (See question 6.)

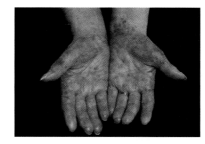

Plate 6-25. (See question 7.)

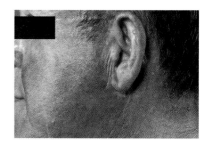

Plate 6-26. (See question 8.)

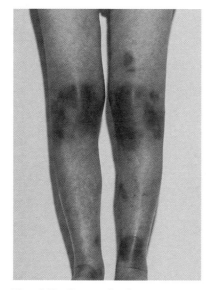

Plate 6-27. (See question 9.)

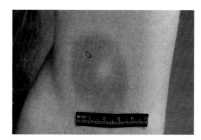

Plate 6-28. (See question 10.)

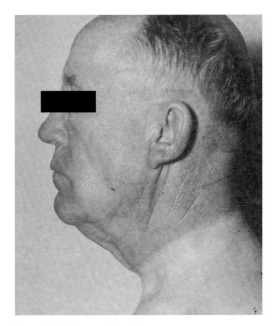

Plate 6-29. (See question 11.)

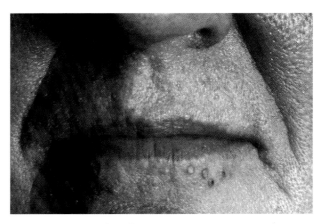

Plate 6-30. (See question 12.)

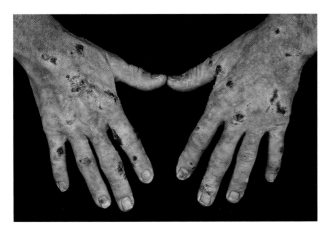

Plate 6-31. (See questions 13 and 14.)

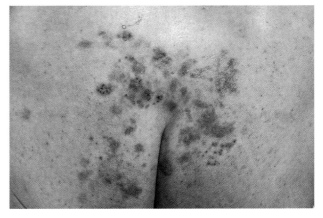

Plate 6-32. (See question 15.)

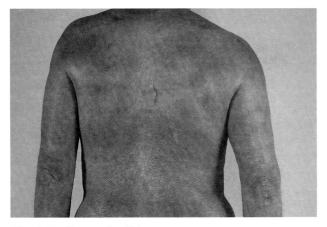

Plate 6-33. (See question 17.)

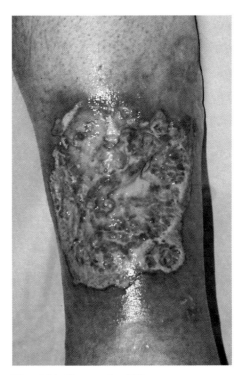

Plate 6-34. (See question 18.)

QUESTIONS

Multiple Choice (choose the one best answer)
1. A 25-year-old white man presents with itching on the elbows (plate 21) and buttocks. Examination reveals excoriations and vesicles. The most likely diagnosis is:
   a. Herpes simplex
   b. Pinworms
   c. Dermatitis herpetiformis
   d. Bullous pemphigoid
   e. Pemphigus

2. The patient described in question 1 should be screened for:
   a. Thymoma
   b. Acquired immunodeficiency syndrome (AIDS)
   c. Gluten-sensitive enteropathy
   d. Hypogammaglobulinemia
   e. Lyme disease

3. A 12-year-old boy is referred by his wrestling coach with raised papules on the inner thighs and buttocks (plate 22). What is the diagnosis?
   a. Impetigo
   b. Molluscum contagiosum
   c. Herpes gladiatorum
   d. Chickenpox
   e. Folliculitis

4. A 20-year-old man is seen for pre-employment screening. The pigmented lesion shown on plate 23 is noted on physical examination. What would you advise?
   a. Observation
   b. Shave biopsy
   c. Excisional biopsy
   d. Curettage
   e. Liquid nitrogen therapy

5. The most likely diagnosis in the patient described in question 4 is:
   a. Benign nevus
   b. Spitz nevus
   c. Pigmented actinic keratosis
   d. Seborrheic keratosis
   e. Melanoma

6. A 45-year-old woman (see plate 24) presents to the emergency department for the third time this month with severe epistaxis. On the basis of your examination, you diagnose:
   a. Physical abuse
   b. CREST syndrome
   c. Alcoholism
   d. Osler-Weber-Rendu syndrome
   e. Disseminated vascular coagulopathy

7. through 11. Match the clinical photographs shown in plates 25 through 29 (questions 7 through 11, respectively) with the causative drug.
   a. Amiodarone
   b. Hydrochlorothiazide
   c. Phenytoin
   d. Oral contraceptives
   e. Phenolphthalein-containing laxative

12. A 35-year-old woman presents for breast screening. She has a strong family history of breast carcinoma. On facial examination, you note papules (plate 30). What is the diagnosis?
    a. Dermal nevi
    b. Muir-Torre syndrome
    c. Cowden syndrome
    d. Gardner syndrome
    e. Adenoma sebaceum

13. A 60-year-old construction worker complains of fragile skin with slow-healing ulcers. Examination of his hands shows the changes shown on plate 31. What is the diagnosis?
    a. Cement dermatitis
    b. Impetigo
    c. Psoriasis
    d. Porphyria cutanea tarda
    e. Discoid lupus erythematosus

14. Which of the following is a precipitating factor for the condition shown in plate 31?
    a. Hepatitis C
    b. Streptococcal infection
    c. Lithium
    d. Potassium dichromate
    e. Gold therapy

15. A male who is positive for human immunodeficiency virus (HIV) complains of having diarrhea for the past 4 days. Plate 32 shows the findings on perianal examination. What is the diagnosis?
    a. Herpes simplex virus
    b. Human papillomavirus
    c. Irritant dermatitis
    d. Extramammary Paget disease
    e. Pemphigus

16. Kaposi sarcoma has been linked to infections with:
   a. Herpes simplex virus (HSV)1
   b. HSV2
   c. Human herpes virus 8
   d. Epstein-Barr virus
   e. Cytomegalovirus

17. A 70-year-old man presents with itching and chills. Physical examination shows generalized erythroderma (plate 33). The differential diagnosis includes each of the following *except*:
   a. Sézary syndrome
   b. Cutaneous T-cell lymphoma
   c. Psoriasis
   d. Dermatomyositis
   e. Dermatitis

18. A 36-year-old schoolteacher presents with a leg ulcer of recent onset (plate 34). On the basis of your examination, which of the following is the most likely diagnosis?
   a. Cryoglobulinemia
   b. Calciphylaxis
   c. Venous stasis
   d. Atherosclerosis obliterans
   e. Pyoderma gangrenosum

19. Which of the following diseases is associated with hepatitis C?
   a. Pyoderma gangrenosum
   b. Porphyria cutanea tarda
   c. Erythema nodosum
   d. Erythema multiforme
   e. Psoriasis

ANSWERS

1. Answer c.

Dermatitis herpetiformis presents with intensely pruritic vesicles on the elbows, buttocks, and knees. In patients with pinworms, small excoriations may be seen in the perianal region but not on the buttocks. Patients with bullous pemphigoid tend to have large, tense bullae with a predilection for flexural regions. Pemphigus presents with erosions and crusting and does not have any predilection for the buttock or elbow areas. Herpes simplex tends to be localized to one body area rather than multiple sites, as in this patient.

2. Answer c.

Gluten-sensitive enteropathy is associated with dermatitis herpetiformis. Thymoma may be seen in patients with pemphigus.

3. Answer b.

Molluscum contagiosum is characterized by umbilicated papules. The papules contain the causative pox virus and spread rapidly to contiguous surfaces. Bullous impetigo presents with blisters that are rapidly eroded, leaving crusts and erosions. Herpes gladiatorum is a herpes simplex infection and presents with grouped vesicles on the involved area. In chickenpox, there are usually widespread lesions with vesicles and crusts in various stages of evolution. Folliculitis presents with yellow pustules.

4. Answer c.

Because the lesion in plate 23 is suspicious for malignant melanoma, an excisional biopsy is recommended. This will give ample tissue, which can be step-sectioned to give a reliable depth should the lesion prove to be melanoma. The pitfall with the shave biopsy technique is that the lesion may not be completely removed, and it is then impossible to assess the depth of the lesion and recommend appropriate excision margins.

5. Answer e.

This lesion shows characteristics of malignant melanoma with variegation in pigment and irregular outline in addition to large size. A benign nevus, in contrast, would be evenly pigmented and symmetrical with smooth borders. The Spitz nevus is a red to pink papule. Pigmented actinic keratosis would be unusual on this body site and clinically presents with a scaly, pigmented lesion. Seborrheic keratosis would have a verrucous quality.

6. Answer d.

Osler-Weber-Rendu syndrome often presents with epistaxis or gastrointestinal bleeding, and the clinical clue is extensive telangiectasias on the face and mucosal surface.

7. Answer c.

Phenytoin may cause erythema multiforme, Stevens-Johnson syndrome, or toxic epidermal necrolysis. The photograph shows erythema multiforme with palmar involvement.

8. Answer a.

Amiodarone causes a distinctive slate-gray discoloration on sun-distributed areas.

9. Answer d.

Oral contraceptives are one of the recognized drugs in precipitating erythema nodosum.

10. Answer e.

Phenolphthalein-containing laxatives are the most common cause of a fixed drug eruption.

11. Answer b.

Hydrochlorothiazide causes photosensitivity, which presents as a sunburn-type reaction.

12. Answer c.

Cowden syndrome is characterized by cutaneous tumors that are derived from the hair follicles. Benign and malignant diseases of the breast and thyroid are associated with this syndrome.

13. Answer d.

Porphyria cutanea tarda presents with blistering on sun-exposed areas, skin fragility, and slow healing. In female patients, hirsutism also may be an early manifestation. Cement dermatitis may also be found in builders. This presents as a generalized, erythematous, weeping, itchy eruption often involving the hands and other exposed areas. Impetigo presents with localized yellow, crusted lesions. Psoriasis and discoid lupus erythematosus manifest as papulosquamous lesions on the dorsum of the hands.

14. Answer a.

Hepatitis C, alcohol, iron overload, and estrogen therapy are recognized precipitants of porphyria cutanea tarda. Lithium may precipitate or flare psoriasis. Potassium dichromate is the allergen in cement dermatitis.

15. Answer a.

Herpes simplex infection may present with widespread vesicles and erosions, particularly in the setting of HIV infection. Warts caused by the human papillomavirus are also common. In this setting, a wart presents with warty papules and fungating growths. Irritant dermatitis, extramammary Paget disease, and pemphigus all present with erythema, erosion, and weeping.

16. Answer c.

Human herpes virus 8 has been identified in specimens with Kaposi sarcoma from patients with or without HIV infection.

17. Answer d.

Generalized erythroderma is often associated with itching and chills. There is a wide differential diagnosis for this, including Sézary syndrome, cutaneous T-cell carcinoma, psoriasis, and atopic and contact dermatitis. Dermatomyositis presents with an erythema usually confined to sun-exposed areas. Skin biopsy and peripheral blood studies will be helpful in determining the diagnosis in this patient.

18. Answer e.

This ulcer shows a purulent base with undermined borders and is characteristic of pyoderma gangrenosum. Cryoglobulinemia presents with vasculitis with palpable purpura and areas of ulceration on the extremities. Calciphylaxis occurs in patients with renal failure and is manifested by tissue infarction, often involving the thighs or buttocks. Venous stasis may be associated with ulceration on the medial aspect of the ankles bilaterally with surrounding stasis dermatitis. Atherosclerosis obliterans presents with infarctive lesions on the limbs with a background of pallor due to decreased arterial profusion.

19. Answer b.

Porphyria cutanea tarda may be precipitated by hepatitis C infection. Erythema nodosum and erythema multiforme are both reactive phenomena but neither has been specifically associated with hepatitis C. Psoriasis flares are associated with streptococcal infection.

NOTES

CHAPTER 7

ENDOCRINOLOGY

Charles F. Abboud, M.D.

HYPOTHALAMIC-PITUITARY DISORDERS

The anterior pituitary cells and their hormones, the hypothalamic regulators of these hormones, and the major clinical hypothalamic-pituitary syndromes are outlined in Table 7-1.

Hypopituitarism

Etiology

Hypopituitarism usually results from deficiency of anterior pituitary hormones or, rarely, from tissue resistance to the actions of these hormones. The deficiency of anterior pituitary hormones may be a consequence of primary pituitary disease, hypothalamic or pituitary stalk disease, or an extrasellar disorder.

Primary pituitary disease is associated with loss of anterior pituitary cells. The common causes of primary pituitary hypopituitarism are pituitary tumors and surgical or radiotherapeutic ablation of the pituitary. Infrequent causes include pituitary infarction, as in postpartum pituitary necrosis (Sheehan syndrome) or after pituitary apoplexy, and lymphocytic hypophysitis.

Hypothalamic-hypopituitarism can result from hypothalamic or pituitary stalk disease associated with loss of hypophysiotropic regulatory hormones of anterior pituitary cells. Primary hypothalamic diseases are relatively rare and include genetic (Kallmann syndrome), traumatic (accidental, surgical, or radiotherapeutic), inflammatory/infiltrative (tuberculosis, sarcoidosis, histiocytosis X), vascular (bleeding disorders, coagulopathy, vasculitis), and neoplastic disorders, whether primary (glioma, ependymoma, hamartoma, gangliocytoma) or metastatic (neoplasms such as breast or lung).

Functional hypothalamic disorders are common and include 1) functional GnRH suppression related to disorders of weight, exercise, psychiatric disorder, systemic disease or endocrinopathy such as hyperprolactinemia and thyroid, or adrenal disorder, and uncompensated diabetes mellitus; 2) functional GH lack seen in emotional deprivation syndrome; 3) functional ACTH lack seen after withdrawal of prolonged

supraphysiologic glucocorticoid therapy; and 4) functional TSH lack seen for a few weeks after correction of a hyperthyroid state. A structural hypothalamic disorder is not evident in a functional hypothalamic disorder, and normal endocrine function is ultimately restored after the management/removal of the cause.

Extrasellar disorders impinge on and impair the function of the hypothalamic-pituitary unit. These include craniopharyngioma and other developmental cysts, optic glioma, meningioma, nasopharyngeal carcinoma or sphenoid sinus mucocele, and carotid artery aneurysms.

- Hypopituitarism can result from primary pituitary disorders, hypothalamic/pituitary stalk disorders, or extrasellar disorders.
- Most common causes of primary hypopituitarism: pituitary tumors and surgical or radiotherapeutic ablation.
- Postpartum pituitary necrosis is common when obstetrical care is suboptimal.
- Most common causes of hypothalamic hypopituitarism: reversible functional disorders, accidental or surgical or radiotherapeutic trauma, and infiltrative disorders.
- Most common cause of hypopituitarism due to extrasellar disorder: craniopharyngioma.

Clinical Features

Hypopituitarism can present with features of deficiency of one or more anterior pituitary hormones. The clinical picture depends on the age at onset, hormone(s) affected, extent and duration of deficiency, and acuteness of the process (Table 7-1). The most common presentation is that of a chronic process of insidious onset.

Hypopituitarism in Adults

Gonadotropin deficiency—The features are those of loss of the steroidogenic and gametogenic functions of the gonads. In women, these features include infertility, oligo/amenorrhea,

Table 7-1.—The Hypothalamic-Pituitary Hormones: Functions and Clinical Syndromes

Hormone	GH	PRL	LH/FSH	ACTH/LPH/END	TSH	ADH or AVP
Anterior-pituitary cell	Somatotroph	Lactotroph	Gonadotroph	Corticotroph	Thyrotroph	Supraoptic and para-ventricular nuclei
Regulation (the dominant regulators are italicized)	*GHRH (+)* GHRIH (-)	*DA (-)* TRH, VIP (+)	*GnRH (+)* DA, opioids (-)	*CRH (+)* AVP (+)	*TRH (+)* GHRIH, DA (-)	Plasma osmolality (osmo-receptors) and blood volume (volume- and baro-receptors)
Secretion	Episodic Sleep-related surge	Episodic Sleep-related surge	Phasic in life Episodic Cyclic in women in reproductive age	Episodic Diurnal Stress-responsive	Episodic Minimal diurnal change	Exquisitely sensitive to changes in plasma osmolality
Physiologic functions	IGF-I mediated growth Intermediary metabolism	Lactogenesis Others (?)	Initiation and maintenance of sexual/ reproductive functions	ACTH: Initiation and maintenance of cortisol production by adrenal cortex Pigmentary effects LPH/END: (?)	Initiation and main-tenance of T_4/T_3 secretion by the thyroid gland	Maintenance of plasma osmolality Maintenance of blood volume and pressure
Deficiency in adult	Syndrome of GH deficiency?	Loss of postpartum lactation	Hypogonad-otropism	Secondary cortisol deficiency	Secondary hypo-thyroidism	Central diabetes insipidus
Deficiency in child	Shortness of stature Hypoglycemia	Not recognized	Hypogonad-otropism in the adolescent	Secondary cortisol deficiency	Secondary hypo-thyroidism	Central diabetes insipidus
Hypersecretion in adult	Acromegaly	Hyperpro-lactinemic syndrome	No distinct syndrome	Cushing disease	TSH-induced hyper-thyroidism	SIADH
Hypersecretion in child	Gigantism	Hyperpro-lactinemic syndrome in the adolescent	Precocious puberty	Cushing disease	TSH-induced hyper-thyroidism	SIADH

ACTH, corticotropin; AVP, arginine vasopressin or antidiuretic hormone; CRH, corticotropin-releasing hormone; DA, dopamine; END, β-endorphin; FSH, follicle-stimulating hormone; GH, growth hormone; GHRH, GH-releasing hormone; GHRIH, GH-releasing inhibiting hormone or somatostatin; GnRH, gonadotropin-releasing hormone; LH, luteinizing hormone; LPH, β-lipotropin; PRL, prolactin; SIADH, syndrome of inappropriate ADH (AVP); TRH, thyrotropin-releasing hormone; TSH, thyrotropin; VIP, vasoactive intestinal peptide.

loss of libido, vaginal dryness and dyspareunia, involution of the uterus and genitalia, and atrophy/loss of secondary sex characteristics. In men, these features include loss of libido, potency impairment, infertility, atrophy/loss of secondary sex characteristics, atrophy of the testes and prostate, and, occasionally, gynecomastia. In both sexes, fine wrinkling of the skin may be seen radially around the mouth or eyes and osteoporosis may occur.

ACTH deficiency—The features of ACTH deficiency result primarily from cortisol lack and loss of the pigmentary functions of ACTH and related peptides. Such features may include ill health, anorexia, weight loss, gastrointestinal disturbances, rheumatologic aches and pains, hypoglycemia, hyponatremia, propensity to adrenocortical crises, pallor, and inability to tan or maintain a tan. Characteristically, the features of mineralocorticoid deficiency are absent because aldosterone secretion depends on the renin-angiotensin system, not ACTH. Therefore, hyperkalemia and hypovolemia with orthostatism are typically absent.

TSH deficiency—TSH deficiency results in lack of thyroid hormone and the characteristic features of slowing of emotional, mental, and physical functions. The thyroid gland is atrophic.

Prolactin deficiency—The inability to lactate because of prolactin deficiency is seen only in women in the postpartum state.

Growth hormone deficiency—The features of GH deficiency in adults include ill health and asthenia, fatigue, muscle weakness, osteopenias, obesity, psychosocial difficulties, and increased cardiovascular risk.

- Gonadotropin deficiency: failure of production of sex steroids and gametes; main features are hypogonadism and infertility.
- ACTH deficiency: cortisol deficiency and loss of pigmentary effects of ACTH and related peptides. Cortisol lack: chronic ill health, hypoglycemia, hyponatremia, and propensity to adrenocortical crises. Aldosterone secretion is basically normal; hyperkalemia and hypovolemia are characteristically absent.
- TSH deficiency: hypothyroidism and absence of goiter.
- Prolactin deficiency: failure of lactation in postpartum women.
- GH deficiency: ill-defined syndrome of asthenia, weakness, and ill health.

The Acute Presentations of Hypopituitarism

Adrenocortical crisis may be precipitated by 1) withdrawal of prolonged suppressive glucocorticoid therapy without proper glucocorticoid coverage in the period needed for recovery of the hypothalasmic-pituitary-adrenal axis, 2) pituitary surgery without optimal glucocorticoid stress coverage, 3) acute medical/surgical illness in a patient with unrecognized or poorly managed cortisol lack, 4) pituitary apoplexy, and 5) thyroid hormone replacement in a patient with associated unrecognized ACTH deficiency.

Other acute presentations are fasting hypoglycemia syndrome (decreased hepatic neoglucogenesis because of lack of cortisol and GH), hyponatremic syndrome (renal water conservation because of decreased GFR and unchecked ADH secretion and action), and increased sensitivity to central nervous system (CNS) depressants (decreased metabolism and clearance because of lack of ACTH and TSH).

- Acute presentations of hypopituitarism: adrenocortical crisis, fasting hypoglycemia syndrome, hyponatremic syndrome, and increased sensitivity to CNS depressants.

Diagnosis

The diagnosis of hypopituitarism requires documenting the presence of hypopituitarism and delineating its cause. For nontrophic hormones, the use of provocative tests is essential for the diagnosis of hormone deficiency in the appropriate clinical setting (e.g., suspected GH deficiency in a child). For trophic hormones, the diagnosis of hormone deficiency rests on evaluating target gland function. If target gland failure is present, trophic hormone levels are required to distinguish between primary failure of the target gland and failure due to hypothalamic-pituitary disease.

- In diagnosing hypopituitarism: hypopituitarism must be documented and its cause delineated.
- For GH, use a provocative test in the appropriate clinical setting.
- For the trophic hormones: evaluate target gland function if target gland failure is present, additional studies are needed to distinguish between primary failure of the target gland and failure due to hypothalamic-pituitary disease.

Endocrine Evaluation

1. Gonadotropin-axis. *Males:* low sperm count, low serum testosterone level, and inappropriately low serum LH and FSH levels. *Females:* low serum estradiol level and inappropriately low serum LH and FSH levels. Provocative tests for LH and FSH using GnRH or clomiphene are rarely needed in clinical practice.

- Males: low sperm count, low serum testosterone, and inappropriately low serum LH and FSH levels.
- Females: low serum estradiol and inappropriately low serum LH and FSH levels.

2. ACTH-adrenocortical axis. In chronic ACTH lack, the adrenal cortices are atrophic and typically do not show

a cortisol secretory response to the short-acting exogenous ACTH test (cosyntropin test). If a hypocortisol state is present, the diagnosis of primary adrenocortical failure is supported by presence of hyperpigmentation and mineralocorticoid deficiency and is documented by increased serum level of ACTH or lack of adrenocortical responsiveness to prolonged exogenous ACTH stimulation. In adrenocortical failure due to hypothalamic-pituitary disease, there is pallor, loss of tanning ability, absence of mineralocorticoid deficiency, inappropriately low serum level of ACTH, and adrenal responsiveness to prolonged exogenous ACTH stimulation (a stepwise cortisol secretory response). Other provocative tests, including insulin-hypoglycemia and metyrapone tests, document pituitary ACTH-adrenal unresponsiveness.

- Cosyntropin test, the short ACTH test, usually shows absence of cortisol secretory response.
- Adrenocortical failure due to hypothalamic-pituitary disease: pallor, loss of tanning ability, absence of mineralocorticoid deficiency, inappropriately low serum level of ACTH, and adrenal responsiveness (stepwise response) to prolonged exogenous ACTH stimulation.
- Insulin-hypoglycemia or metyrapone tests show adrenal unresponsiveness.

3. TSH-thyroid axis. Low serum level of free thyroxine (FT_4) (or free thyroxine index [FTI]) and an inappropriately "normal" or low serum level of TSH. In hypothyroid patients, a high serum level of TSH or the presence of goiter points to primary hypothyroidism, and an inappropriately low serum level of TSH confirms the diagnosis of TSH deficiency.

- TSH deficiency: low serum level of FT_4 or FTI and an inappropriately "normal" or low serum TSH.

4. Growth hormone. a) *Provocative tests:* low serum level of GH unresponsive to challenge by provocative tests. *Screening tests:* sleep or exercise. *Definitive tests:* insulin-hypoglycemia, L-dopa, arginine, or clonidine. Insulin hypoglycemia is the standard test; other tests are used if insulin hypoglycemia is not safe (e.g., in the elderly or in those with CNS or ischemic myocardial disorder). b) *Serum insulin growth factor (IGF)-I:* low IGF-I levels can be seen in GH deficiency or nutritional disorders.

- Low serum levels of GH are unresponsive to stimulation; low serum levels of IGF-I.

5. Prolactin. Provocative tests for PRL are not needed in clinical practice.

- Low serum level of PRL.

"Anatomical" Evaluation

This includes imaging of the hypothalamic-pituitary region (computed tomography [CT] or magnetic resonance imaging [MRI]) and neuro-ophthalmologic evaluation to assess visual fields, visual acuity, and optic disks.

- Anatomical evaluation: imaging with CT or MRI and neuro-ophthalmologic evaluation.

Etiologic Diagnosis

In determining the cause of hypopituitarism, suspected functional causes must be removed or corrected. Normalization of pituitary function after correction of a functional cause lends support to "functional" hypopituitarism. If the functional causes are excluded, or if hypopituitarism persists despite removal or correction of a functional cause, evaluation for organic hypothalamic-pituitary disease is mandatory. This evaluation is based on the clinical setting and appropriate endocrine and anatomical studies.

- In determining the cause of hypopituitarism: suspected functional causes must be removed or corrected.
- Next, evaluate for organic hypothalamic-pituitary disease based on the clinical setting and appropriate laboratory and radiologic studies.

Therapy in Adults

Therapy includes correction, if possible, of the cause and, when applicable, administration of the hormone(s) of the target gland(s) or, in selected cases, pituitary hormones.

- Therapy: treat cause and, if needed, administer pituitary hormones or target gland hormones.

1. ACTH deficiency. Glucocorticoid replacement is critical. Dosage: hydrocortisone, 10-20 mg in early a.m. and 5-10 mg in early p.m. for adults (or equivalent dosage of glucocorticoid analogs such as prednisone). Instruct patients about need for dose modification during acute illness. In patients with combined ACTH-TSH lack, initiate glucocorticoid therapy before thyroid hormone therapy to avoid thyroid hormone-induced increased need for cortisol and precipitation of acute adrenocortical crisis.

- Instruct patients about dose modification during acute illness.

- In patients with combined ACTH-TSH lack, initiate glucocorticoid therapy before thyroid hormone therapy.

  2. TSH deficiency. The drug of choice is T_4 (page 221). Initiate therapy with a low dose and gradually increase it over a period of weeks (unless the TSH deficiency is of recent onset, when one can start with an average replacement dose). Assess the adequacy of therapy by the feeling of well-being and serum level of free T_4. Do not use serum TSH levels to monitor the adequacy of T_4 dosage, because they are characteristically low in untreated persons.

- T_4 is the drug of choice.
- Initiate therapy with a low dose and gradually increase it over a period of weeks.
- Do not use sTSH levels to monitor the adequacy of therapy. Use the patient's clinical state and a measurement of free thyroxine or FTI.

  3. Gonadotropin deficiency. a) Sex steroid therapy—*In females*, conjugated estrogens, 0.6-1.25 mg (or equivalent) daily. Use progestational agents for a woman with intact uterus: medroxyprogesterone acetate, 10 mg daily for days 1-12 of each month (see page 253). *In males*, long-acting testosterone parenteral preparation (testosterone enanthate or cypionate), 100-200 mg every 2-3 weeks or, alternatively, testosterone transdermal patches (page 247). The goal is to restore full androgenicity. In both sexes, delay therapy in puberty to avoid premature closure of epiphyses and to allow maximal linear growth. Evaluate psychosexual needs and patient's lifestyle to assess the impact of therapy. Assess status of the prostate in middle-aged and elderly men before therapy and follow annually. b) For restoration of fertility, FSH/LH (or GnRH therapy in patients with hypothalamic disorders) may be indicated.

- In hypogonadal females, use estrogen therapy, e.g., conjugated estrogens; use supplemental progestational agents for women who have their uteri.
- In hypogonadal males, use long-acting parenteral testosterone esters or transdermal testosterone patches.
- In adolescents, delay sex hormone therapy as long as possible to avoid premature closure of the epiphyses.
- For restoration of fertility, consider the use of exogenous gonadotropins or, if feasible, GnRH therapy in patients with hypothalamic disease.

  4. GH deficiency. In GH-deficient adults, GH therapy in the short term enhances the sense of well-being,

normalizes body composition, increases muscle strength and exercise capacity, increases bone mineral density, and improves cardiac function. GH therapy may be considered for those with hypothalamic-pituitary disease and a poor GH response to a standard stimulus. Several recombinant human GH preparations are available. The usual dose is 5 to 10 µg/kg body weight subcutaneously. The goal of therapy is to restore serum IGF-I to normal levels and to avoid side effects. The long-term effects of such therapy are unknown, and thus a benefit-risk profile cannot be determined.

Pituitary Tumors

Pituitary tumors can be "microadenomas" (≤10 mm) or "macroadenomas" (>10 mm) in size, "sellar" or "sellar/extrasellar" in extent, and "functioning" or "nonfunctioning" in type. *Functioning pituitary tumors* include prolactinomas (40%-50%), GH tumors (10%-15%), ACTH tumors (10%-15%), and TSH tumors (<5%). *Nonfunctioning tumors* (30%-40%) include the gonadotropinomas and null cell adenomas. Pituitary tumors can be sporadic or part of multiple endocrine neoplasia type I (MEN I).

- Tumor size: microadenoma (≤10 mm) or macroadenoma (>10 mm).
- Tumor extent: sellar or sellar/extrasellar.
- Tumor may be functioning or nonfunctioning.
- Tumor may be isolated or part of MEN I.

Clinical Features

The usual presentation is that of a chronic slowly evolving disorder. Mass effects include headaches and evidence of tumor extension beyond the confines of the sella. *Superior extension* of the tumor may cause 1) chiasmal syndrome, with impaired visual acuity and visual field defects; 2) hypothalamic syndrome, with vegetative disturbance in thirst, appetite, satiety, sleep, and temperature regulation and with the endocrine disorder of diabetes insipidus or syndrome of inappropriate ADH; 3) obstructive hydrocephalus; and 4) frontal lobe dysfunction. *Lateral extension* of the tumor may cause impairment of cranial nerves III, IV, V, and VI, with diplopia, facial pain, and temporal lobe dysfunction. *Inferior extension* of the tumor may lead to a nasopharyngeal mass or cerebrospinal fluid (CSF) rhinorrhea.

Endocrine effects include the following. 1) *Hypersecretory states*: hyperpituitarism can lead to gigantism/acromegaly (GH excess), hyperprolactinemic syndrome (PRL excess), Cushing disease and Nelson-Salassa syndrome (ACTH excess), and thyrotoxicosis (TSH excess). Generally, LH/FSH and α subunit excess are clinically silent. 2) *Hypopituitarism* caused by destruction of the pituitary gland by tumor growth.

3) *Endocrine associations* of pituitary tumors include MEN I, that is, parathyroid tumor or hyperplasia (primary hyperparathyroidism), endocrine pancreas tumor or hyperplasia (various endocrine pancreatic syndromes), other endocrine gland tumors (thyroid, adrenal), and lipomas.

Rarely, pituitary tumors can present acutely with pituitary apoplexy, which may be the first clinical expression of the underlying tumor.

- Mass effects: headaches and extrasellar effects due to tumor extension beyond the sella.
- Endocrine effects: due to hypersecretory states or to hypopituitarism.
- Endocrine associations of pituitary tumors: MEN I.
- Pituitary apoplexy may complicate the course or may be the initial presentation of the tumor.

Diagnosis

The presence of a pituitary tumor is suggested by the clinical features and by the findings of CT or MRI of the pituitary region. Neuro-ophthalmologic evaluation, including assessment of visual acuity, visual fields, and optic disks, is important, particularly if a suprasellar extension is present. Endocrine evaluation includes evaluation for hormonal excess (see below under the specific functioning pituitary tumor syndromes) or hormonal lack and for the presence of any associated MEN I. A diagnosis of a pituitary tumor is made if the sellar mass is associated with anterior pituitary hormone excess (except for mild hyperprolactinemia, which can occur with other masses in the area and "stalk effect"). Otherwise, the diagnosis is confirmed at surgical exploration.

- Pituitary tumor: presence is suggested by clinical assessment and CT and MRI findings.
- Neuro-ophthalmologic evaluation is important, particularly with suprasellar extension.
- Endocrine evaluation should assess for hormonal excess or lack and the presence of any associated MEN I.
- Diagnosis: the presence of a hyperfunctioning state (except modest hyperprolactinemia, which can occur with any pituitary mass associated with suprasellar extension and the "stalk effect") and tissue diagnosis at surgery.

Treatment

Therapy Directed at the Tumor

Pituitary tumors generally are treated with surgical excision or irradiation. Drug therapy is available for PRL-, GH-, or TSH-producing tumors. Medical therapy is used most commonly as primary therapy for prolactinomas; also, it can be a useful adjunct to ablative therapy. Conservative noninterventional therapy can be an option if the tumor is small and has no effect on quality/quantity of life.

- Treatment: surgical excision, irradiation, or drug therapy.
- Drug therapy: option of primary therapy for prolactinomas; drug therapy can also be a useful adjunctive therapy in the treatment of GH or TSH tumors.
- Noninterventional therapy: an option when the tumor is small and nonfunctioning or for a microprolactinoma not associated with clinical features that impinge on the quality of life.

Surgery

Transsphenoidal surgery is the operation of choice for most tumors. The transcranial operation is reserved for tumors with a large suprasellar extension. Surgical morbidity and mortality and the available neurosurgical expertise should be considered. In good hands, morbidity is less than 1% for microadenomas and less than 4% for macroadenomas (bleeding, infection, transient diabetes insipidus, CSF rhinorrhea), and mortality is less than 1%. Persistence/recurrence of the tumor is less than 20% to 30% for microadenomas and 50% to 70% for macroadenomas.

Radiotherapy

Radiotherapy can be delivered by conventional means, heavy particles, or stereotactic means such as a gamma knife. Issues to be considered are long latent period (few months to years), postradiation hypopituitarism (30%-40% of patients, but less so with the highly focused gamma-knife modality), and potential for CNS damage (rare) or development of CNS tumors (very rare).

Drug Therapy

Dopamine agonists (bromocriptine or cabergoline in the U.S.) are used for the management of prolactinomas or GH-producing tumors. Somatostatin analog (octreotide) is used mainly for the management of GH- or TSH-producing tumors. Consider the efficacy, long-term safety, and cost.

Follow-Up

Follow-up is essential for all therapeutic options to monitor persistence or recurrence of the tumor, the development of hypopituitarism in patients treated surgically or radiotherapeutically, and the possible occurrence of other aspects of MEN I in familial cases.

Prolactinoma and the Hyperprolactinemic Syndrome

Pituitary tumors associated with hyperprolactinemia may be prolactinomas, "mixed" tumors (e.g., GH- and PRL-producing tumors), or nonfunctioning tumors with a suprasellar extension and "stalk effect." In stalk-effect hyperprolactinemia, impingement of the mass on the pituitary stalk interferes with the access of hypothalamic dopamine to the anterior pituitary and allows for disinhibition of prolactin secretion by normal lactotrophs.

- Pituitary tumors associated with hyperprolactinemia: prolactinomas, mixed tumors, or any tumor/mass lesion with a suprasellar extension and stalk effect.

Clinical Features

Prolactinomas usually present with manifestations of hyperprolactinemia and, occasionally, pituitary mass effects.

Endocrine effects include effects of hyperprolactinemia—*in women*, galactorrhea, ovulatory and menstrual dysfunction (short luteal phase or anovulation leading to infertility), oligo/amenorrhea and hypogonadism, hyperandrogenic manifestations (hirsutism or acne), and decreased libido; *in men*, libido and potency impairment, oligospermia (infertility), and, rarely, galactorrhea or gynecomastia; and *in adolescents*, delayed puberty.

In men, the recognition of hyperprolactinemia frequently is delayed because decreased libido and impaired potency may be dismissed by the patient and physician and attributed to psychiatric factors. In those harboring a pituitary tumor, marked hyperprolactinemia and a macroprolactinoma are usual at the time of presentation.

Neurologic effects are caused by the mass effect of the pituitary tumor.

- Endocrine effects: the effects of hyperprolactinemia, associated pituitary dysfunction, and associated MEN I.
- Hyperprolactinemia exerts its clinical effects on GnRH secretion, the breasts, and adrenal cortices.
- *In women*, ovulatory/menstrual dysfunction, galactorrhea, hirsutism; *in men*, decreased libido and impotence; *in adolescents*, delayed sexual maturation.
- In males, recognition of hyperprolactinemia is frequently delayed; macroprolactinoma usually is present at diagnosis.

Diagnosis

Differential Diagnosis

It is important to differentiate prolactinoma from other causes of hyperprolactinemia and from other pituitary area masses. Hyperprolactinemia can be physiologic or pathologic in origin. *Physiologic hyperprolactinemia* is seen in pregnancy and the postpartum state and conditions of stress such as surgery or acute illness. *Pathologic hyperprolactinemia* can be eutopic or ectopic in production. Eutopic hyperprolactinemia occurs in the context of primary pituitary disease

or may be due to hypothalamic/stalk disease, resulting in loss of dopaminergic influence and disinhibition of prolactin secretion by normal lactotrophs (organic and functional hypothalamic/stalk disease). Ectopic hyperprolactinemia (very rare) has been reported with hypernephroma, gonadoblastoma, and ovarian teratomas.

Primary pituitary causes of hyperprolactinemia include prolactinoma, "mixed tumors," nonfunctioning pituitary tumors with suprasellar extension and stalk effect, hypophysitis, and primary empty sella. *Hypothalamic/stalk disorders* can be functional or organic in nature. *Functional hypothalamic disorders* lead to hyperprolactinemia because of interference with the synthesis, secretion, or action of dopamine or other hypothalamic regulators of prolactin secretion. These disorders include 1) drugs such as neuroleptics, antidepressants, some antihypertensives, narcotics, H_2-receptor blockers, verapamil, and estrogens; 2) primary hypothyroidism (15%-30%); 3) chest wall irritative lesions such as herpes zoster, other types of dermatitis, and thoracotomy; 4) renal failure; and 5) cirrhosis or hepatic encephalopathy. *Organic hypothalamic disorders* include traumatic disorders such as surgery or irradiation, inflammatory disorders such as sarcoidosis or histiocytosis X, or neoplastic disorders such as craniopharyngioma, optic glioma, meningioma, or metastases such as those from the breast or lungs.

- Hyperprolactinemia may be physiologic or pathologic.
- Physiologic hyperprolactinemia is seen in pregnancy, postpartum state, and under stress.
- Pathologic hyperprolactinemia may be eutopic (pituitary) or ectopic (extrapituitary) in origin.
- Pituitary causes: most common is prolactinoma.
- Hypothalamic causes: functional or organic. Functional disorders include use of drugs, primary hypothyroidism, chest wall lesions, and chronic renal or hepatic failure. Organic causes include hypothalamic disorders of various etiologies.

Diagnostic Approach

1. Rule out pregnancy. A pregnancy test is an essential part of the work-up of any female of reproductive age.
2. Check serum level of PRL. a) Serum levels of prolactin greater than ten times normal (>200 ng/mL) establish the diagnosis of prolactinoma. However, prolactinomas, particularly microprolactinomas, may be associated with lower prolactin levels. b) If serum level of prolactin is less than ten times normal (<200 ng/mL), rule out functional causes, that is, exclude drugs, irritative lesion of the chest wall, primary hypothyroidism, and chronic renal failure. If a functional cause is present, remove it or treat if possible. If hyperprolactinemia does not resolve in

about 3 months, evaluate for hypothalamic-pituitary disease. c) If a functional cause is not present, rule out organic hypothalamic-pituitary disease by CT or MRI and by evaluating other pituitary functions and the visual fields if necessary. Diagnostic possibilities include pituitary tumor, other organic hypothalamic-pituitary disease, and "idiopathic" hyperprolactinemia.

The major differential diagnosis is between a macroprolactinoma and a nonprolactinoma mass associated with stalk-effect hyperprolactinemia. The differentiation has therapeutic implications because prolactinoma is usually treated with dopamine agonists and a nonprolactinoma with suprasellar extension is treated surgically. A serum prolactin level greater than 200 ng/mL points to a prolactinoma, and a level less than 75 ng/mL points to a nonprolactinoma mass. A value between 75 and 200 ng/mL requires, if feasible, a trial of dopamine agonist therapy. Tumor mass regression with this therapy points to a prolactinoma, and the absence of tumor regression indicates need for surgical therapy.

If a discernible cause is not found after a thorough evaluation, the hyperprolactinemia is considered to be of indeterminate origin. Follow-up evaluation is critical in these patients because some of them may harbor microadenomas or other hypothalamic-pituitary space-occupying lesions that are below the limit of radiologic detection, and follow-up examinations may show evidence of a mass. The serum level of PRL should be checked every 6 to 12 months and CT or MRI should be repeated in 1 or 2 years or earlier if deemed necessary by the development of new symptoms.

Therapy

Treatment of Microprolactinoma or Idiopathic Hyperprolactinemia

Treatment is indicated for management of infertility, hypogonadism, significant galactorrhea, and hirsutism or to meet the patient's desire. Treatment options include dopamine-agonist therapy with bromocriptine or cabergoline, and transsphenoidal surgery for microprolactinoma (surgery can be used as primary therapy or for those intolerant or resistant to dopamine-agonist therapy). Otherwise, observe and check the serum level of PRL annually and perform CT or MRI every 2 or 3 years.

Treatment of Macroprolactinoma

Therapy is indicated for all patients because of the threat of the mass lesion and the effects of hyperprolactinemia. Drug therapy with a dopamine-agonist is the preferred treatment. Surgical excision or radiotherapy is reserved for the drug-intolerant or drug-resistant cases (10%-20% for bromocriptine; 3%-7% for cabergoline).

Dopamine Agonists

Bromocriptine is a dopamine agonist that suppresses hyperprolactinemia and restores gonadal function (70%-80%); it may decrease tumor size (<50%). Its effect can be dramatic. It is not antimitotic. It is costly and can have side effects, which usually are minimal and include nausea, fatigue, nasal stuffiness, and postural hypotension. Its long-term safety is unknown. The usual dose for prolactinoma is 5.0 to 7.5 mg/day. To prevent or to minimize the side effects, bromocriptine treatment is started with a small dose (1.25-2.5 mg) taken with food and at bedtime; the dose is increased in steps every 3 to 5 days. Bromocriptine is a temporizing therapy, and discontinuation of its use usually leads to resumption of tumor growth and endocrine dysfunction.

Cabergoline has been introduced recently into the U.S. market. It is a potent dopamine agonist, is convenient to use (0.25-0.5 mg orally once or twice weekly), and has better efficacy and tolerability than bromocriptine.

- Bromocriptine: dopamine agonist that suppresses hyperprolactinemia and restores gonadal function (70%-80%). It may decrease tumor size (<50%).
- Cabergoline: an alternative dopamine-agonist.
- Discontinuation of the use of the dopamine-agonist usually leads to resumption of tumor growth and endocrine dysfunction.

Dopamine agonist therapy and pregnancy—Restoration of gonadal function and fertility is a major goal of drug therapy. The use of the drug should be stopped at the earliest sign of pregnancy. In pregnancy, the risk of tumor growth for microprolactinoma is less than 5% and for macroprolactinoma, 20%-40%. Observe patients closely, especially if they have macroprolactinomas, and periodically perform clinical and visual field evaluations. If tumor growth is suspected, confirm with MRI of the head. If significant tumor growth complicates pregnancy, consider surgical excision or reinstituting bromocriptine therapy.

- Use of bromocriptine should be stopped at earliest sign of pregnancy.
- During pregnancy, the risk of tumor growth for microprolactinoma is <5% and for macroprolactinoma, 20%-40%.
- If significant tumor growth complicates pregnancy, consider surgical excision or reinstituting bromocriptine therapy.

Surgical Treatment for Prolactinomas

The surgical cure rates for microadenomas and macroadenomas are 60% to 80% and 0% to 30%, respectively.

GH Tumors: Acromegaly/Gigantism

Etiology

The cause usually is a pituitary disorder, GH-producing pituitary tumors (>99%). Rarely, acromegaly may be caused by ectopic GH-producing tumors or hypothalamic or extrahypothalamic GHRH-producing tumors.

Clinical Features

The clinical presentations are related to GH/IGF-I excess, the pituitary tumor, and the associations of acromegaly. *Excess GH/IGF-I* leads to gigantism in a child and to characteristic acromegalic features in an adult, hyperhidrosis, heat intolerance, increased skin porosity and oiliness, carbohydrate intolerance (20%), and, rarely, frank diabetes mellitus, hypercalciuria, hyperphosphatemia, acroparesthesias, nerve entrapment syndromes, myopathy, hypertension or cardiomyopathy, Raynaud phenomenon, fibromas or acanthosis nigricans, and sleep apnea.

Mass-related manifestations include hypopituitarism, hyperprolactinemia (which may be caused by a stem cell tumor, mixed tumor, or stalk effect of the extrasellar extension of a large GH-producing macroadenoma), and anatomical effects related to extrasellar extension.

The associations of acromegaly include diffuse or nodular goiter, thyrotoxicosis (which may be related to mixed GH/TSH tumor, associated Graves disease, or multinodular toxic goiter), and MEN I. In patients with acromegaly, there appears to be a two- to threefold increase in the development of malignant tumors, and a three- to eightfold excess risk of colon cancer and premalignant colon polyps. Currently, it seems prudent to use colonoscopy to evaluate all patients with acromegaly at diagnosis and then at 2- or 3-year intervals.

- Clinical presentation of GH-producing tumors: related to GH/IGF-I excess, the pituitary tumor, and to associations of acromegaly.
- Acromegaly is associated with increased risk of premalignant colon polyps, colon cancer, and other malignancies: screen with colonoscopy at diagnosis and every 2 or 3 years.

Endocrine Diagnosis

A random serum level of GH may be helpful. Values <1 ng/mL exclude acromegaly, and those >50 ng/mL confirm acromegaly. Values in the range of 2 to 50 ng/mL are nondiagnostic. *Test of GH suppressibility*—Perform an oral glucose tolerance test with GH responses; nonsuppressible GH during an oral glucose tolerance test is the reference standard test. GH levels will not suppress to <1 ng/mL in active acromegaly. *Serum IGF-I (somatomedin C)*—Increased levels confirm the diagnosis of acromegaly (if one excludes physiologic elevations of pregnancy and adolescence).

Radiologic Diagnosis

When the diagnosis is documented biochemically, proceed with imaging of the sella (CT or MRI). If a pituitary tumor is not delineated (a rare event), measure serum GHRH levels to exclude a GHRH-producing tumor and search for evidence of an ectopic GH-producing tumor.

- Random serum level of GH may be helpful: a value <1 ng/mL excludes the diagnosis, and a value >50 ng/mL confirms the diagnosis.
- Glucose tolerance test-GH suppressibility test: failure of GH to suppress to <1 ng/mL is diagnostic of acromegaly.
- Serum IGF-I (somatomedin C): IGF-I is increased in all patients with active acromegaly.
- When acromegaly is documented biochemically, proceed with imaging the sella. If no tumor is visible, measure serum level of GHRH and look for evidence of an ectopic GH-producing tumor.

Therapy

Pituitary Tumor

Surgical adenomectomy is the treatment of choice (page 206) and the cure rate is 40% to 80% depending on the size of the tumor. For postoperatively persistent disease, consider radiotherapy plus interim pharmacologic therapy (either bromocriptine or octreotide or both). Radiotherapy has been used as primary ablative therapy; drug therapy can be given in the interval while awaiting the full effects of radiotherapy.

Radiation therapy has a cure rate of 70% after 10 years; hypopituitarism can occur in up to 50% of patients in 10 years; other morbidity is rare. The major disadvantage of radiotherapy is its long latent period (months to years) before it controls disease activity.

The usual dose of bromocriptine is 5 to 20 mg/day or higher; it can normalize GH/IGF-I in less than 10% and lead to tumor shrinkage in less than 10%. This is a temporizing therapy. The experience with cabergoline is limited. Octreotide is an effective therapeutic option; the average dose is 100-200 µg/8 hr given subcutaneously; it can normalize GH/IGF-I in 80% of patients and lead to tumor shrinkage in 30% to 50%. The side effects of octreotide include nausea, flatulence, mild malabsorption, cholelithiasis (10% of patients), and impairment of glucose tolerance. This, too, is a temporizing therapy. Gallbladder ultrasonography is performed initially and repeated at 1- or 2-year intervals.

- Therapy of choice: surgical excision. For persistent disease: radiotherapy plus interim pharmacologic therapy.
- Radiation therapy may be used as alternative ablative therapy.

- Drug therapy: octreotide, bromocriptine, or both; temporizing; mainly used while awaiting the full effects of primary or adjunctive radiotherapy.

Ectopic GH or GHRH Tumor

Surgical resection is the therapy of choice. For persistent disease, consider octreotide.

ACTH-Producing Tumors

These are discussed below in the section on Cushing syndrome (page 238).

Gonadotropin-Producing Tumors

These tumors constitute the largest fraction of nonfunctioning pituitary tumors. Although more than 80% are able to synthesize the gonadotropins and/or their subunits, increased serum levels of FSH, LH, or their subunits are found in less than 35% of patients. Clinically, the tumors are macroadenomas at presentation; they may present at any age but usually in middle-aged or elderly persons, predominantly in males. Extrasellar effects dominate the clinical picture, and some degree of hypopituitarism is usually present. The tumor mass may be associated with stalk-effect hyperprolactinemia. CT or MRI reveals the sellar mass with extrasellar extension. Currently, no effective medical therapy is available. Treatment is usually surgical, with or without postoperative irradiation. Endocrine replacement therapy is given for management of hypopituitarism.

Thyrotropin-Producing Tumors

The characteristic clinical presentations of primary TSH tumors are diffuse goiter and hyperthyroidism. Other presentations include extrasellar mass effects and hypopituitarism. Laboratory evaluation reveals that, in a thyrotoxic patient, the sTSH value is normal or high, α-glycoprotein subunit levels are high, and TSH responsiveness to TRH is absent. CT or MRI shows a sellar mass with or without extrasellar extension. *The major differential diagnosis is Graves disease*. In TSH-producing tumors, and in contrast to Graves disease, one finds equal sex incidence, absence of ophthalmopathy/dermopathy, and normal or high sTSH values in the presence of hyperthyroidism. Treatment options include ablation (surgically or with irradiation), pharmacologic therapy with octreotide, and ancillary measures for the management of thyrotoxicosis.

Pituitary Incidentaloma

This is a relatively common entity. Autopsy studies suggest that 10% to 20% of persons harbor small pituitary tumors. CT or MRI of the head performed for nonendocrine reasons shows mass lesions in the sella larger than 3 mm in 4% to 20% of cases. Potential threats to health include functioning pituitary tumors and those incidentalomas with actual or potential mass effects. The diagnostic approach includes screening for functioning pituitary tumors and the delineation of mass effects (extrasellar effects and hypopituitarism). Screening for functioning pituitary tumors includes prolactin, IGF-I, 1 mg-overnight dexamethasone suppression test or 24-hour urinary free cortisol, free T_4 and TSH, and measurement of FSH, LH, and their subunits. Finding a functioning pituitary tumor that can cause morbidity or mortality (all such tumors except the small microprolactinoma in a postmenopausal female or microgonadotropinoma) or the presence of an incidentaloma larger than 1 cm in diameter dictates active intervention. Otherwise, observe and repeat the imaging study in 6 to 12 months and, later, at less frequent intervals. An increase in the size of the incidentaloma requires surgical intervention.

Miscellaneous Pituitary Disorders

Craniopharyngioma

Craniopharyngioma is a slow-growing encapsulated squamous cell tumor originating from remnants of Rathke pouch. It is the most common tumor in the pituitary region in childhood but can occur at any age. Two-thirds of the tumors are suprasellar, and one-third originate in or extend into the sella. Most are cystic, and some are solid or mixed. These tumors have a propensity to calcification. The clinical presentation includes obstructive hydrocephalus, hypothalamic syndrome (diabetes insipidus/hyperprolactinemia), chiasmal defects, hypopituitarism, or calcification in or around the sella, as seen incidentally on radiography. Radiography shows calcification in intrasellar or suprasellar regions (75% of children; 25% of adults). CT or MRI reveals a solid or cystic mass, calcification (CT), and low attenuation values (cholesterol content).

Therapy—Surgical excision is possible for only small craniopharyngiomas. Larger craniopharyngiomas are decompressed. A ventriculoperitoneal shunt is used for obstructive hydrocephalus. Other treatments include postoperative radiotherapy and management of endocrine dysfunction.

Pituitary Apoplexy

This refers to hemorrhagic infarction of the pituitary gland, with or without underlying disease. The usual clinical setting is that of a pituitary tumor, irradiated pituitary tumor, pregnancy, anticoagulation therapy, increased intracranial pressure, vascular disease (e.g., diabetes mellitus), or vasculitis (e.g., temporal arteritis). Clinical features: 1) Asymptomatic if small or gradual bleeding. 2) Acute if sudden or large hemorrhage—severe headache, ophthalmoplegia, visual defects, meningismus, depressed sensorium, and acute adrenocortical crisis. Death may occur. Diagnosis is made on the basis of the characteristic clinical, radiologic, and surgical findings. Therapy includes neurosurgical decompression and hormonal support.

Late sequelae may include hypopituitarism, secondary empty sella syndrome, or regression of hypersecretory syndrome in infarcted functioning pituitary tumor.

Lymphocytic Hypophysitis

This is presumed to be of autoimmune origin. It usually occurs in association with other autoimmune endocrinopathies and affects adults, predominantly women, especially during pregnancy and the postpartum period. The clinical presentation may include hypopituitarism or the presence of a sellar mass associated with hyperprolactinemia. The major differential diagnoses are prolactinoma and Sheehan syndrome. The diagnosis depends on the associations and the results of surgical exploration. No specific therapy is available. Hormonal replacement is given as needed.

Vasopressin Deficiency: Diabetes Insipidus

Etiology

Renal water output is dependent on the presence of AVP and a responsive distal nephron. Therefore, diabetes insipidus (DI) may result from one of two pathophysiologic defects: 1) decreased production of AVP in response to normal osmotic stimulation and 2) decreased responsiveness of the renal distal nephron to AVP (nephrogenic, or vasopressin-resistant, DI). Decreased production of AVP in response to normal osmotic stimulation results most commonly from organic disorders of the anterior hypothalamus, median eminence, or upper stalk (hypothalamic, neurogenic, central, or vasopressin-sensitive DI). Infrequently, it results from functional suppression of AVP production by the ingestion of excessive volumes of fluid (primary polydipsia or dipsogenic DI) and, rarely, from enhanced deactivation of the hormone by circulating degrading enzymes (vasopressinases) or AVP antibodies.

Hypothalamic DI may result from genetic or acquired disorders of the anterior hypothalamus, median eminence, or upper pituitary stalk. Genetic disorders are rare. Acquired disorders include traumatic (closed head trauma or neurosurgery), inflammatory/granulomatous (sarcoidosis, tuberculosis, or histiocytosis X), primary neoplasms such as craniopharyngioma, germinoma, and optic glioma, or metastatic neoplasms primarily from the breast or lung. Idiopathic hypothalamic DI is probably the most common cause of the syndrome and may be an autoimmune disorder.

Nephrogenic DI also may be caused by genetic or acquired disorders, the most common being chronic renal disease, electrolyte abnormalities (hypercalcemia or hypokalemia), and AVP-antagonist drugs such as lithium and demeclocycline.

Dipsogenic DI may be idiopathic or associated with psychosis or, rarely, organic disorders of the anterior hypothalamus such as sarcoidosis or neoplasms.

- DI may result from decreased production of or renal unresponsiveness to AVP.
- Hypothalamic DI: genetic or acquired loss of AVP-secreting neurons. Commonest cause is idiopathic DI. Other causes include traumatic, idiopathic, and neoplastic primary or metastatic neoplasms.
- Nephrogenic DI: genetic or acquired renal unresponsiveness to AVP. Common causes: chronic renal disease, hypercalcemia, hypokalemia, and use of AVP-antagonists.
- Dipsogenic DI: inappropriate excessive fluid intake and functional suppression of AVP secretion. May be idiopathic, psychogenic, or organic in cause.

Clinical Features

The clinical manifestations include those of DI and the etiologic disorder. 1) Polyuria and polydipsia, often with preference for ice-cold water, are characteristic. Nocturia is usually present, and enuresis may be the presenting complaint in children. 2) An abrupt onset of symptoms usually points to central DI. 3) Absence of nocturia, variable intensity or intermittency of symptoms, and a 24-hour urine output greater than 18 L suggest primary polydipsia. It is important to remember that because patients with hypothalamic or nephrogenic DI rely on their thirst mechanism to regulate water balance, no other ill effects may be seen unless the patient becomes unconscious for any reason, is unable to obtain fluids, or develops an impaired thirst mechanism. In such circumstances, extreme hyperosmolar dehydration and a hypertonic encephalopathy may develop. Cortisol and, to a lesser extent, thyroid hormones are necessary for the renal excretion of a water load by dampening AVP secretion and action. In patients with hypothalamic DI, the development of hypopituitarism may mask hypothalamic DI, which becomes apparent only after adequate cortisol replacement.

- DI is characterized by polyuria (2.5-20 L/day) and polydipsia, often with preference for ice-cold water.
- Abrupt onset of symptoms usually suggests central DI, and absence of nocturia suggests primary polydipsia.
- When thirst sensation is impaired or access to water is restricted, hyperosmolar state may ensue and may be complicated by hypertonic encephalopathy and circulatory collapse.
- Cortisol is necessary for the kidney's ability to excrete a water load. Cortisol deficiency may mask DI, and DI may become apparent after cortisol replacement.

Endocrine Diagnosis

The diagnosis depends on a careful and complete clinical evaluation, the use of random plasma and urine osmolality levels, and the use of provocative tests. The induction of plasma hyperosmolality (either by water deprivation or administration of hypertonic saline) is used to assess the patient's ability to produce AVP and to respond to it. The patient's response can be assessed indirectly by measurements of urine volume and osmolality before and after the administration of exogenous AVP or directly by measurements of plasma levels of AVP in addition to plasma and urine osmolalities.

Although the diagnosis of severe DI of any cause can be straightforward, the diagnostic process often is made difficult because the disorder may be only partial in extent and prolonged periods of polyuria, regardless of the primary cause, may decrease the maximal urine-concentrating ability "renal medullary washout," adding in effect a nephrogenic DI component to the basic disease process.

1) Check *random plasma osmolality* (or *serum level of Na*) and *urine osmolality* values under conditions of ad lib fluid intake. In a patient with polyuria and dilute urine, a random plasma osmolality greater than 295 mOsm/kg points to either neurogenic or nephrogenic DI, whereas a plasma osmolality less than 280 mOsm/kg points to primary polydipsia. 2) If plasma osmolality is between 280-295 mOsm/kg, a water dehydration test is indicated. A plasma osmolality greater than 295 mOsm/kg in the water ad lib state or at the end of a water dehydration test (or a serum sodium value >143 mEq/L) and urine osmolality less than 150 mOsm/kg exclude primary polydipsia and point to central or nephrogenic DI. Administer 5 units of aqueous AVP or 1 μg desmopressin (DDAVP) subcutaneously and collect urine for osmolality 30, 60, and 120 minutes later. A post-AVP or desmopressin urine osmolality greater than 150% of the preinjection osmolality points to central DI; if less than 150% of preinjection osmolality, it points to nephrogenic DI. 3) A partial response to water deprivation, with a urine osmolality greater than 300 mOsm/kg, can occur in partial neurogenic or nephrogenic DI as well as in primary polydipsia. In this circumstance, it is necessary to collect plasma for AVP assay at the end of the dehydration test in addition to determining plasma and urine osmolalities. The results are plotted on nomograms.

- Obtain random plasma and urine osmolality values: a random plasma osmolality >295 mOsm/kg points to neurogenic or nephrogenic DI. These can be differentiated by the response to exogenous AVP. A random plasma osmolality <280 mOsm/kg, in an untreated patient, points to primary polydipsia.
- Otherwise, a provocative osmolar test is needed: water deprivation test or administration of hypertonic saline.
- Absence of response to water deprivation (urine osmolality <300 mOsm/kg) points to either complete neurogenic or nephrogenic DI. The diagnosis is determined by assessing the response to exogenous AVP.
- A partial response to water deprivation (urine osmolality >300 mOsm/kg) may occur in any type of DI. Measure

plasma AVP and plot plasma AVP against plasma osmolality or urine osmolality and use standard nomograms.

Etiologic Diagnosis

Look for clinical evidence of hypothalamic-pituitary or systemic disorders, perform MRI, examine the visual fields, and assess anterior pituitary functions. The most common causes of central DI are idiopathic DI, trauma (accidental or neurosurgical), metastases from breast or lung tumors, and hypothalamic area tumors. Systemic diseases with hypothalamic or stalk involvement must be considered.

Therapy

Always treat the underlying cause. However, in central DI, this seldom restores AVP secretion; therefore, DI is usually irreversible. There is no need for drug therapy in patients with mild DI (urine output, 2-5 L/day) who have free access to water. For more significant degrees of central DI, which interferes with the patient's life pursuits or sleep, desmopressin is the drug of choice. In contrast to AVP, desmopressin has a much longer duration of action and is devoid of pressor or uterine effects. It is administered by nasal insufflation or spray in a dose of 5 to 10 μg once or twice daily or orally (0.1-0.8 mg/day in divided doses). For patients who are unconscious or allergic to nasal desmopressin, the drug can be given parenterally (1-2 μg subcutaneously or intravenously 1 or 2 times daily). For patients with partial central DI, AVP agonists such as chlorpropamide (100-500 mg/day) and carbamazepine (400-600 mg/day) may be used. Thiazides are the only treatment available for nephrogenic DI. Psychiatric assessment and therapy are needed for patients with psychogenic primary polydipsia. *Follow-up:* In some cases of "idiopathic DI," a discernible cause may become evident in up to 4 years of follow-up.

- Therapy, whenever possible, is directed at the cause.
- Mild central DI: free access to water.
- Moderate to severe central DI: desmopressin.
- For partial central DI, use AVP agonists such as chlorpropamide, 250-500 mg/day.
- For nephrogenic DI: thiazides are only treatment available.

AVP (ADH) Excess

Etiology

AVP excess, in the absence of a hyperosmolar stimulus, may be appropriate when it occurs in response to hypovolemia or hypotension and inappropriate when it occurs in the absence of a hypovolemic/hypotensive stimulus. The syndrome of inappropriate ADH (SIADH) can result from exogenous or endogenous disorders.

Exogenous AVP excess may result from the inappropriate administration of AVP, its analogs such as desmopressin, or oxytocin. *Endogenous AVP excess* may originate from a eutopic hypothalamic or an ectopic extrahypothalamic source. *Eutopic AVP excess* may be a consequence of 1) CNS/hypothalamic disorders of various causes (such as traumatic, inflammatory, degenerative, vascular, or neoplastic disorders), 2) the use of agonist drugs that enhance AVP secretion or action (chlorpropamide, carbamazepine, vincristine, vinblastine, cyclophosphamide, phenothiazines, monoamine oxidase inhibitors, tricyclic antidepressants, and clofibrate), and 3) neurogenic influences such as pain or nausea. *Ectopic extrahypothalamic AVP excess* may result from 1) malignancies (cancer of the bronchus, pancreas, ureter, prostate or bladder, lymphoma, leukemia, thymoma, or mesothelioma) or 2) benign pulmonary disorders (pneumonia, lung abscess, empyema or pneumothorax, tuberculosis, cystic fibrosis, and the use of positive-pressure ventilation).

Pathophysiology

Continued water intake and AVP hypersecretion in the absence of a hyperosmolar stimulus leads to 1) increased renal water retention, hyponatremia, and hypo-osmolality of body fluids in the face of an inappropriately concentrated urine; 2) expansion of body fluid compartments, including extracellular fluid volume; 3) homeostatic adjustments that promote "renal escape" and natriuresis, including increased GFR, increased atrial natriuretic hormones, and suppression of the renin-angiotensin-aldosterone axis. Natriuresis exacerbates plasma hypo-osmolality, thus explaining the absence of edema despite an expanded extracellular fluid volume.

- Physiologic or appropriate AVP hypersecretion occurs in response to plasma hyperosmolality or hypovolemia/hypotension.
- Pathophysiologic or inappropriate AVP excess occurs in the absence of physiologic stimuli and can have either an exogenous or endogenous cause. Endogenous AVP excess can be of a eutopic-hypothalamic or ectopic-extrahypothalamic source.
- SIADH is characterized by hypervolemia, hyponatremia, and hypo-osmolality of body fluids, inappropriately concentrated urine, natriuresis, absence of edema, and low serum creatinine and uric acid levels (a result of increased GFR).

Clinical Features

The clinical features are a composite of the effects of the underlying disorder and those of the hyponatremic syndrome that depend on the degree and the rapidity of its development. Patients with SIADH may be asymptomatic if the hyponatremia is mild or has developed gradually over weeks and months. When patients are symptomatic, the most frequent symptoms are lethargy, fatigue, ill health, anorexia, nausea and vomiting, and irritability or confusion. Severe or rapidly developing hyponatremia can lead to a behavioral change, a change in the level of consciousness, or seizures.

- Clinical features depend on the degree and rapidity of the development of hyponatremia and range from the asymptomatic to a neurologically impaired state.

Diagnosis

1) Confirm true hyponatremia. Exclude pseudohyponatremia associated with hyperlipidemia or hyperlipoproteinemia (clinical and biochemical features and normal plasma osmolality indicate pseudohyponatremia). 2) Exclude hyperosmolar states and loss of intracellular water to the hyperosmolar extracellular fluid, as in hyperglycemia and the use of mannitol (plasma glucose, history of mannitol use, and increased plasma osmolality). 3) In the absence of advanced renal failure, the differential diagnosis is between SIADH and appropriate AVP excess associated with decreased cardiac output (volume and pressure stimuli). 4) Establish the appropriateness or inappropriateness of AVP hypersecretion. Exclude appropriate AVP excess (fluid sequestration and edema in congestive heart failure or nephrosis or in cirrhosis and ascites [clinical picture], renal and extrarenal fluid losses [findings of hypovolemia], and hypothyroidism and hypocortisol states [appropriate endocrine tests]). 5) If the findings point to SIADH, identify the cause. Consider an exogenous source. If not, search for a eutopic or ectopic source of AVP hypersecretion.

The major diagnostic challenge is to differentiate SIADH from subclinical hypovolemia. Consider urine sodium concentration, serum creatinine or uric acid levels, and plasma renin activity and aldosterone level. In contrast to findings in SIADH, subclinical hypovolemia is associated with a urine sodium less than 20 mEq/L, increased serum creatinine and uric acid levels, and an increased plasma renin activity and plasma aldosterone level.

- Confirm true hyponatremia and exclude hyperosmolar states, advanced renal failure, and states of appropriate AVP excess.
- Major diagnostic challenge is to differentiate SIADH from subclinical hypovolemia: consider urinary sodium, serum creatinine and uric acid, and plasma renin activity and aldosterone.

Therapy

Therapy for SIADH includes identifying and managing the underlying disorder, restricting water intake to 800 to 1,000 mL daily and monitoring the patient's weight and serum sodium level, and if necessary, giving an AVP antagonist (demeclocycline, 900-1,200 mg/day). Lithium is not recommended because of its potential serious side effects. If acute neurologic sequelae are present, give hypertonic saline intravenously, 200 to 300 mL of 5% NaCl over 3 to 4 hours. Achieve a gradual increase in serum Na (do not exceed 0.5 mEq/hr or 12 mEq/24 hr). Continue giving hypertonic saline until the neurologic symptoms cease and a "safe" serum Na level of 120 mEq/L is reached. Rapid correction of hyponatremia can lead to central pontine myelinolysis, which often is fatal.

- Therapy: identify and treat the underlying disorder and manage the hyponatremia.
- Therapy for hyponatremia: water restriction and, if needed, an AVP antagonist (demeclocycline).
- Acute neurologic sequelae: hypertonic saline to increase serum Na by 0.5 mEq/ hr to control symptoms and achieve a "safe" serum Na of 120 mEq/L.
- Rapid correction of hyponatremia can lead to potentially fatal central pontine myelinolysis.

DISORDERS OF THE THYROID GLAND

Laboratory Assessment of the Thyroid Axis

Several thyroid tests are available to define abnormalities in thyroid function, size, or structure and to aid in delineating an etiologic diagnosis. Clinicians should be aware that abnormal findings on these tests can also be seen in euthyroid patients with nonthyroidal illness or with altered thyroid hormone transport and metabolism.

- Interpretation of thyroid function tests: consider thyroid function, altered thyroid hormone transport and metabolism, and effects of nonthyroidal illness.

1. Serum T_4. Serum T_4 concentrations (normal value, 5-11 μg/dL) are determined by three factors: thyroid function, concentration and binding affinity of thyroid hormone-binding proteins, and the rate of T_4 clearance. *Decreased serum T_4* occurs in hypothyroidism; euthyroid patients with low serum concentration of binding proteins (androgen and anabolic steroid therapy, glucocorticoid excess, chronic liver disease, acromegaly, use of niacin or asparaginase, genetic TBG [thyroxine-binding globulin] deficiency); and conditions associated with the presence of binding inhibitors (as in nonthyroidal illness and the use of drugs such as salicylates, other nonsteroidal anti-inflammatory drugs [NSAIDs], and furosemide). *Increased serum T_4* occurs in thyrotoxicosis; euthyroid patients with

increased TBG (estrogen use, pregnancy, acute hepatitis, acute intermittent porphyria, perphenazine use, and familial TBG excess); patients with familial genetic excess in albumin or prealbumin-binding protein; peripheral resistance to thyroid hormones; conditions associated with decreased T_4 clearance (euthyroid sick syndrome and use of drugs such as amiodarone, oral cholecystographic agents, or propranolol); and presence of anti-T_4 antibodies, as in some patients with Hashimoto thyroiditis.

2. Serum T_3. The determinants of serum T_3 concentrations are thyroid function, extrathyroidal deiodination of T_4 to T_3 in peripheral tissues, and concentrations and binding affinities of thyroid hormone-binding proteins. *Decreased serum T_3* occurs in hypothyroidism; euthyroid state in neonates and the elderly; nonthyroidal illness; patients with caloric deprivation; use of drugs (such as propranolol, glucocorticoids, certain iodinated contrast agents, and amiodarone) that block the T_4 to T_3 conversion; and states with decreased TBG levels (see above). *Increased serum T_3* occurs in thyrotoxicosis, euthyroid patients with TBG excess (see above), and peripheral hormone resistance. The only clinical indication for measuring serum T_3 concentration is the diagnosis of T_3 toxicosis in a patient with clinical manifestations of hyperthyroidism who has a normal serum T_4 concentration.

3. Free T_4. The principal determinant of the free T_4 serum concentrations is thyroid function. *Decreased free T_4* occurs in hypothyroidism and nonthyroidal illness. *Increased free T_4* occurs in hyperthyroidism, nonthyroidal illness, and peripheral hormone resistance.

4. Assessment of thyroid hormone-binding proteins. This can be done directly with radioimmunoassays or, more commonly, indirectly with the T_3 resin-uptake test (RT_3U). The RT_3U test is an indirect measurement of the unoccupied T_4-binding sites on the binding proteins. The normal range is 30% to 40%. A decrease in T_4 binding sites and, therefore, an increase in RT_3U is seen in hyperthyroidism, low TBG states, and in the presence of binding inhibitors as in nonthyroidal illness or with the use of certain drugs (see above). An increase in T_4 binding sites and, thus, a decrease in RT_3U is seen in hypothyroidism and high TBG states. It is clear that serum T_4 must be evaluated in conjunction with the RT_3U test. Concordant results of serum T_4 and RT_3U point to abnormalities in thyroid function, whereas discordant results point to binding-protein abnormalities. A high serum T_4 level and RT_3U point to hyperthyroidism, and a low serum T_4 level and RT_3U point to hypothyroidism. A high serum T_4 level and a low RT_3U point to high TBG states, whereas low serum T_4 level and high RT_3U point to low TBG states.

5. Free thyroxine index. FTI represents the product of serum T_4 and RT_3U. It is an indirect measurement of free T_4 and correlates well with the clinical state and with free T_4 concentrations. *Decreased FTI* occurs in hypothyroidism and nonthyroidal illness. *Increased FTI* occurs in hyperthyroidism, nonthyroidal illness, peripheral hormone resistance, genetic albumin and prealbumin-binding protein excess, and anti-T_4 antibodies.

6. Serum TSH (normal value, 0.5 to 4.0 mU/L). The sensitivity of currently available TSH assays is 0.05 to 0.1 mU/L, and this sensitivity clearly delineates low-normal from suppressed or low values. *Increased TSH* occurs in primary hypothyroidism (low serum T_4 and T_3 levels), in which TSH values are usually greater than 20 mU/L; subclinical hypothyroidism (normal serum T_4 and T_3 levels), in which TSH values are between 4 and 20 mU/L; during recovery from nonthyroidal illness (serum T_4 and T_3 levels are low or low normal); and in TSH-producing tumor or peripheral resistance to thyroid hormones (serum T_4 and T_3 levels are high). *Decreased TSH* occurs in hyperthyroidism of any cause (high serum T_4 and T_3 levels) except that due to TSH-producing tumors, subclinical hyperthyroidism (normal serum T_4 and T_3 levels), central hypothyroidism (low serum T_4 and T_3 levels), nonthyroidal illness (low T_3 and normal or low T_4 levels), and use of certain drugs (somatostatin, dopamine, glucocorticoids).

Serum sTSH is the single best test of thyroid function and can be used as a thyroid function screening test in outpatients. Normal sTSH values imply, in most instances, absence of thyroid dysfunction (the only exceptions are hyperthyroidism due to TSH-tumor and central hypothyroidism when the TSH levels may be "inappropriately" normal relative to the prevailing serum concentrations of T_4 and T_3). An abnormal TSH should prompt measurement of free T_4 or FTI. In patients with an increased TSH, a low free T_4 or FTI points to primary hypothyroidism and a high free T_4 or FTI points to a TSH-producing tumor or to peripheral resistance to thyroid hormone. In patients with a low or undetectable TSH, an increased free T_4 or FTI points to hyperthyroidism of any cause (except that due to TSH tumors), and a low free T_4 or FTI points to central hypothyroidism or a nonthyroidal illness.

7. Thyroid scanning. Thyroid scanning may be performed with pertechnetate or isotopes of radioiodine. The main indications for thyroid scanning are evaluation of nodular goiter, an adjunct to fine needle aspiration in the evaluation of the "suspicious" nodule (when cytopathologic differentiation between follicular adenoma or carcinoma is difficult), evaluation of a retrosternal mass to document its thyroidal origin, delineation of thyroid agenesis or dysgenesis or ectopic thyroid in struma ovarii, and detection of metastatic disease in the postoperative evaluation and follow-up of patients with differentiated thyroid cancer.

8. Radioactive iodine (^{131}I) uptake. In the U.S., the normal 24-hour uptake is 10% to 25%. A 24-hour ^{131}I uptake study is indicated for etiologic diagnosis of hyperthyroidism to distinguish those hyperthyroid states associated with a low radioiodine uptake (silent or subacute thyroiditis, exogenous hyperthyroidism, or ectopic hyperthyroidism [struma ovarii]); pre-^{131}I treatment of thyrotoxicosis to aid in dose calculations; and management and follow-up of differentiated thyroid malignancy.

9. Serum thyroglobulin. Thyroglobulin levels (normal value, 2-25 µg/L) may be increased in many benign or malignant thyroid disorders. Indications for measurement of serum thyroglobulin are 1) as a tumor marker in the follow-up of patients with differentiated thyroid carcinoma and 2) the differentiation between silent thyroiditis and exogenous hyperthyroidism. In both these conditions, radioiodine uptake is low, but the serum thyroglobulin levels are high in silent thyroiditis and low in exogenous hyperthyroidism.

10. TSH receptor-stimulating immunoglobulins (TSI). These are immune markers of Graves disease and are helpful in differentiating euthyroid ophthalmopathy from other causes of proptosis, in predicting remission/relapse in thiourea-treated patients with Graves disease, and in predicting possible occurrence of neonatal thyrotoxicosis in an infant to be born to a pregnant woman with past or present Graves disease.

11. Antithyroglobulin and antimicrosomal (antiperoxidase) antibodies. These are used as indicators of autoimmune thyroid disease. The antimicrosomal antibodies are more specific but less sensitive than the antithyroglobulin antibodies. High titers occur in more than 90% of patients with Hashimoto thyroiditis and modestly increased titers are found in primary atrophic hypothyroidism and in Graves disease. Low titers can also be seen in patients with other autoimmune disorders, such as systemic lupus erythematosus and rheumatoid arthritis. The absence of these antibodies does not exclude the presence of autoimmune thyroid disease.

12. Thyroid ultrasonography. Potential indications for this test include assessment of thyroid size and configuration when thyroid palpation is difficult, assessment of the size and consistency of nodule(s) in patients with a nodular goiter, and follow-up of patients with thyroid cancer to assess local recurrence or cervical lymph node metastases.

Hyperthyroidism

Etiology

Excess thyroid hormone(s) may be derived from an endogenous or exogenous source. Endogenous hyperthyroidism is caused by either a thyroidal (eutopic) or extrathyroidal (ectopic) disorder. Eutopic hyperthyroidism can result from a primary thyroid disorder or from abnormal regulation of the thyroid gland. Primary thyroid disorders that cause hyperthyroidism include autonomous nodular goiter (single or multiple nodules); follicular disruptive inflammatory process, as in subacute or painless silent thyroiditis; and metastatic follicular thyroid cancer. Abnormal regulation of the thyroid gland that leads to hyperthyroidism occurs in thyroid-stimulating immunoglobulins (TSI)-dependent hyperthyroidism seen in Graves disease, TSH-dependent hyperthyroidism occurring in association with TSH tumors or selective pituitary resistance to thyroid hormones, and human chorionic gonadotropin (hCG)-dependent hyperthyroidism seen in association with trophoblastic disease. Ectopic hyperthyroidism occurs in struma ovarii. Exogenous hyperthyroidism is common and results from the administration (pharmacologic or surreptitious) of supraphysiologic doses of T_4 and/or T_3.

The commonest cause of hyperthyroidism in the U.S. is Graves disease (60%-80%). Other frequent causes include toxic nodular goiter, silent and subacute thyroiditis, and exogenous hyperthyroidism. Other causes are rarely seen in practice.

- Hyperthyroidism may be exogenous or endogenous in origin.
- Endogenous hyperthyroidism may be eutopic (thyroidal) or ectopic (extrathyroidal) in origin.
- Eutopic hyperthyroidism may result from a primary thyroid disorder or from abnormal regulation of the thyroid.
- The commonest cause of hyperthyroidism in the U.S. is Graves disease.

Clinical Features

The common features of hyperthyroidism include 1) nervousness, irritability, and emotional lability; 2) hypermetabolism, heat intolerance, and warm moist skin; 3) palpitations, tachycardia, arrhythmias (particularly atrial fibrillation in the elderly), and dyspnea on exertion; 4) fatigue and muscle weakness, especially of proximal muscles; 5) weight loss despite increased appetite and caloric intake; 6) hyperdefecation; 7) hair loss or change in texture, pruritus, and onycholysis; and 8) menstrual irregularities and infertility. Grittiness in the eyes, excessive lacrimation, photophobia, diplopia, eye protrusion, and, rarely, decrease in visual acuity are symptoms of Graves ophthalmopathy.

Goiter is present in most patients, but it may not be seen in the elderly, in exogenous hyperthyroidism, or in struma ovarii. The characteristics of the goiter depend on the underlying thyroid disorder (see below). Examination of the eyes may show the noninfiltrative findings that may be seen in hyperthyroidism of any cause (retraction of the upper lid, stare, and lid lag) or the infiltrative findings of Graves disease (puffiness of the lids, conjunctival injection and chemosis, proptosis, extraocular muscle weakness, decreased visual acuity).

Uncommon manifestations include 1) apathetic hyperthyroidism of the elderly, in whom the dominant expressions are cardiac manifestations (tachyarrhythmias and congestive heart failure), profound weakness, loss of appetite and weight, apathy, and listlessness; 2) organ dominance such as proximal myopathy, chronic diarrhea, or osteoporosis; 3) gynecomastia in young adult males; 4) disorders associated with Graves disease (myasthenia gravis, hypokalemic periodic paralysis, or other autoimmune disorders such as Addison disease or pernicious anemia).

- The usual clinical features of hyperthyroidism reflect increased metabolism, a hyperdynamic cardiovascular system, and the catabolic effects of excess thyroid hormones.
- The presence of goiter and its characteristics vary according to the cause.
- Eye findings may be noninfiltrative (in hyperthyroidism of any cause) or infiltrative (specific for Graves disease).
- Uncommon manifestations include apathetic hyperthyroidism in the elderly, organ dominance, gynecomastia, and disorders associated with Graves disease.

Diagnosis of Hyperthyroidism

The diagnosis of hyperthyroidism depends on assessment of the clinical features and the findings of increased serum levels of thyroid hormone(s) and evidence of thyroid dysregulation. The most common expression of thyroid dysregulation is the finding of suppressed TSH. The two critical tests are the measurement of the serum concentration of free T_4 and TSH.

An increased serum free T_4 level is diagnostic of hyperthyroidism if a nonthyroidal illness can be excluded. Normal free T_4 values do not exclude hyperthyroidism and should prompt the determination of serum T_3 levels to establish the diagnosis of T_3 toxicosis. Suppressed TSH level is seen in all types of hyperthyroidism except the types caused by rarely occurring TSH tumors and selective pituitary resistance to thyroid hormones. A low serum TSH level by itself is not diagnostic of hyperthyroidism and can be seen in a few normal elderly patients, the first trimester of pregnancy, the use of certain drugs (glucocorticoids, dopamine, or somatostatin), and in euthyroid patients with a nonthyroidal illness. The finding of a low serum TSH level in the presence of normal levels of thyroid hormones points to subclinical hyperthyroidism.

- The two critical tests: serum free T_4 and TSH.
- Increased free T_4: hyperthyroidism, acute nonthyroidal illness, and tissue resistance to thyroid hormones.
- Normal free T_4: consider T_3 toxicosis and check serum T_3 level.
- Suppressed TSH: all cases of hyperthyroidism except those due to rare TSH tumor or selective pituitary resistance to thyroid hormones.
- Suppressed TSH may be seen in euthyroid states: the elderly, the first trimester of pregnancy, the use of certain drugs, and nonthyroidal illness.
- Subclinical hyperthyroidism: suppressed TSH and normal serum levels of free T_4 and T_3.

Etiologic Diagnosis

Graves Disease

Graves disease is an autoimmune, multisystem disease characterized by the triad of hyperthyroidism, diffuse goiter, and mesenchymal extrathyroidal manifestations of ophthalmopathy, dermopathy, and thyroid acropachy. These manifestations can occur singly or in combination. Although it is seen most often in young females, it can occur at any age and in either sex. There is a strong familial predisposition. The immediate cause of the hyperthyroid state is the production of thyroid-stimulating autoantibodies that bind to the TSH receptor. The disease is characterized by remissions and relapses. The goiter is usually two to three times normal size, diffuse, smooth, and somewhat firm. Of the patients, 20% (especially the elderly) may not have a goiter. (For the eye findings, see page 216.) Localized pretibial myxedema (raised thickened peau d'orange changes usually affecting the dorsum of the feet and legs) occurs in patients who either have or have had Graves eye disease. Thyroid acropachy may accompany the dermal changes.

- Graves disease: autoimmune multisystem disease with a strong familial predisposition.
- Characteristic triad: hyperthyroidism, diffuse goiter, mesenchymal extrathyroidal effects (ophthalmopathy, dermopathy, acropachy).
- Immediate cause of hyperthyroidism: production of thyroid-stimulating antibodies.
- 20% of patients, especially elderly, may not have goiter.

Toxic Multinodular Goiter

Toxic multinodular goiter, a disease of the elderly, occurs in patients who have had a long-standing simple nodular goiter with autonomy in one or more nodules. The hyperthyroidism usually is less severe than that of Graves disease and may be characterized by the dominance of organ-specific manifestations. The goiter usually is large, nodular, and asymmetrical; it may be difficult to palpate in some patients because of either a short neck or a substernal extension.

- Toxic multinodular goiter: disease of the elderly, usually occurs in patients with long-standing simple nodular goiter with autonomy in one or more nodules.
- Hyperthyroidism may be characterized by dominance of organ-specific manifestations, particularly cardiovascular and muscular.
- Goiter may be difficult to palpate because of short neck or substernal extension.

Toxic Adenoma

Toxic adenoma is caused by a hyperfunctioning autonomous follicular adenoma and is seen most often in middle-aged women. The solitary nodule is >3 cm in diameter, easily palpable, and firm. Radioisotope scan shows intense uptake in the nodule, with no uptake in the rest of the gland.

- Solitary nodule: >3-cm diameter, easily palpable, firm.
- Radioisotopic scan: intense uptake in nodule and suppressed uptake in the rest of the gland.

Thyroiditis

Thyrotoxicosis can occur in thyroiditis because of unregulated release of colloid, and its stored thyroid hormones from the inflamed, disrupted thyroid follicles. It is transient and lasts a few weeks, until the hormone stores are depleted. A short period of hypothyroidism may ensue until the thyroid gland recovers. Thyroiditis-induced thyrotoxicosis can be caused by subacute thyroiditis and painless lymphocytic thyroiditis.

- Transient hyperthyroidism of a few weeks' duration can occur in thyroiditis through the release of stored hormone from disrupted thyroid follicles.
- Transient hypothyroidism may occur during the recovery period.
- It can be seen in subacute thyroiditis and in painless lymphocytic thyroiditis.

Exogenous Hyperthyroidism

Exogenous hyperthyroidism can result from prescribed or factitial ingestion of supraphysiologic doses of T_4 and/or T_3, ingestion of iodides in susceptible persons, or ingestion of ground meat contaminated with thyroid tissue. Factitial thyrotoxicosis should be suspected in thyrotoxic patients without a palpable goiter and who have suppressed ^{131}I uptake. Low serum levels of thyroglobulin differentiate this disorder from the hyperthyroidism of silent painless thyroiditis.

- Causes: prescribed or factitiously ingested thyroid hormone(s), ingestion of iodides in susceptible persons, ingestion of ground meat contaminated with thyroid tissue.
- Absence of goiter and suppressed radioiodine uptake in a thyrotoxic patient should prompt consideration of factitial thyrotoxicosis.
- Serum thyroglobulin may be used to differentiate exogenous hyperthyroidism from silent thyroiditis.

Summary of Diagnostic Approach

1) Clinical evaluation: look for goiter and its characteristics; look for Graves ophthalmopathy. An infiltrative ophthalmopathy points to Graves disease. 2) Hyperthyroidism and diffuse goiter: Graves disease, painless thyroiditis, and TSH-induced hyperthyroidism. The suppressed TSH excludes TSH-induced hyperthyroidism. Radioiodine uptake results are critical in the differential diagnosis, that is, high uptake in Graves disease and low uptake in silent thyroiditis. 3) Hyperthyroidism with nodular goiter: multinodular (toxic multinodular goiter), single nodule larger than 3 cm (toxic nodule), confirm "hot" nodule with thyroid scanning. 4) Painful tender goiter: subacute thyroiditis, confirm by high erythrocyte sedimentation rate and low radioiodine uptake. 5) Hyperthyroidism in a patient who does not have a palpable thyroid: think of exogenous (low radioiodine uptake, low serum thyroglobulin) and ectopic hyperthyroidism (struma ovarii, uptake in the pelvic mass).

Therapy

Therapy depends on the cause of the thyrotoxic state, the state of the patient and severity of illness, and the preference of the physician. Available options include the following.

Thionamides

Methimazole and propylthiouracil (and carbimazole, which is used outside the U.S.) block thyroid hormone formation and may decrease the production of thyroid-stimulating immunoglobulins. In addition, propylthiouracil decreases peripheral T_4 to T_3 conversion. They do not cause irreversible changes in the thyroid gland and their effect is temporary and lasts only while the drugs are being given. Indications: *Thionamides are given to control the thyrotoxic state (of any cause except that of thyroiditis and exogenous hyperthyroidism) and, in Graves disease, with the hope that the disease will enter a spontaneous remission during drug therapy.* Administration: Therapy is initiated with either methimazole, 20 to 30 mg daily as a single dose, or with propylthiouracil, 100 to 150 mg/8 hr.

Improvement is evident in 1 or 2 weeks, and euthyroidism is usually achieved in 6 to 8 weeks. The dose is adjusted to achieve a euthyroid state. Maintenance doses are then given to maintain euthyroidism. In Graves disease, therapy is continued for 6 to 12 months, and then the use of the drug is discontinued. More than 50% of patients have recurrence of the hyperthyroidism, usually within the first 3 to 6 months. *Side effects* are uncommon (<5%). Remember the serious side effects of agranulocytosis, vasculitis, hepatitis, and aplastic anemia (<0.2%-0.5%). Agranulocytosis can develop abruptly within a few hours. Both drugs can cross the placenta and, if given in high doses, can block the fetal thyroid.

- Methimazole and propylthiouracil: block thyroid hormone formation and may decrease production of thyroid-stimulating immunoglobulins.
- Propylthiouracil: decreases T_4 to T_3 conversion.
- The antithyroid drug is given to control hyperthyroidism. In Graves disease, treat for 6-12 months; discontinue therapy and assess patient periodically for recurrence.
- Serious side effects: agranulocytosis, vasculitis, hepatitis, and aplastic anemia (<0.2%-0.5%).
- Agranulocytosis can develop abruptly within a few hours.
- Thionamides can cross the placenta and, in high doses, can block the fetal thyroid.

Radioiodine

Indications—Radioiodine therapy is an effective ablative therapy. It does not carry the risk of thyroid carcinogenesis or leukemogenic potential and does not lead to malformations in subsequent pregnancies. [131]I can be given to the young and old, with the only absolute contraindication being pregnancy. However, in practice, most physicians avoid its use in very young patients. *Administration*—The usual dose is 100 to 200 μCi/g (estimated weight). Lower doses are less likely to relieve hyperthyroidism and do not obviate eventual hypothyroidism. *Efficacy*—Improvement occurs in 4 or 5 weeks, and the maximal effect from a given dose of ^{131}I is obtained in 2 or 3 months. Of the patients treated with such a dose, 80% to 90% are rendered euthyroid or hypothyroid. The dose can be repeated in patients with persistent disease. In those rendered euthyroid, follow-up every 6 to 12 months is indicated; 2% to 5% of patients per year develop hypothyroidism. *Side effects*—Its major drawback is the almost certain eventual development of ^{131}I-induced hypothyroidism. Radiation painful thyroiditis may appear in 7 to 10 days; it may worsen the thyrotoxic state and may lead to enlargement of the gland and potential obstructive/compressive symptoms, particularly in those with a substernal goiter. Because of the risk of aggravating thyrocardiac disease in elderly patients or in patients with impaired cardiac reserve, it is best to render these patients euthyroid with antithyroid drug therapy before administering [131]I. Some authorities believe that radioiodine therapy may worsen Graves ophthalmopathy.

- [131]I: a safe and effective ablative therapy. It is the preferred treatment for adults in the U.S.
- Only absolute contraindication: pregnancy.
- Maximal effect is obtained in 2-3 months; 80%-90% of patients are rendered euthyroid or hypothyroid. Major drawback is the eventual development of ^{131}I-induced hypothyroidism.
- Radiation painful thyroiditis may appear in 7-10 days. It may cause transient worsening of the hyperthyroid state; the enlargement of the gland may worsen obstructive/compressive symptoms, particularly in patients with substernal goiter.
- Elderly thyrotoxic patients or those with impaired cardiac reserve: use antithyroid drugs to render patient euthyroid and then give radioiodine therapy.

Surgery

As a therapeutic option, subtotal thyroidectomy is considered for 1) patients with large compressive/obstructive glands, 2) thyrotoxic patients with thyroid nodules that are suspicious on fine needle aspiration, 3) patients with Graves disease who are young or pregnant, and 4) patients in whom antithyroid therapy fails and who refuse radioiodine. To prevent thyrotoxic crisis and excessive bleeding from the overactive friable gland, it is customary to render the patient euthyroid with antithyroid drug therapy and then to give iodides for 7 to 10 days preoperatively. Damage to the recurrent laryngeal nerves or parathyroid glands should be a rare occurrence in experienced hands (<1%-2%).

- Subtotal thyroidectomy: considered for thyrotoxic patients with large goiters, suspicious nodules; patients with Graves disease who are young or pregnant; and patients in whom antithyroid therapy fails and who refuse radioiodine.
- Preoperative preparation: it is customary to use antithyroid drugs to render the patient euthyroid and then to give iodides for 7-10 days.

Supportive Therapy

Iodides, usually as potassium iodide (SSKI) or iodine (Lugol solution), are given as 5 to 10 drops/day. Iodides block hormone secretion and, in some patients, synthesis. Organic iodides also block peripheral T_4 to T_3 conversion. Potential indications include preoperative preparation of thyrotoxic patients for subtotal thyroidectomy, patients with actual or impending thyrotoxic crisis, and a temporary expedient while awaiting full effect of radioiodine therapy.

β-Blockers should be used only as adjunctive therapy. Propranolol is used most commonly in a dose of 40 to 120 mg/day in divided dosage. Such therapy only controls the adrenergic manifestations of hyperthyroidism and may also decrease the conversion of T_4 to T_3. The major uses of these drugs are in severe hyperthyroidism and while awaiting the effects of more definitive therapy. These drugs should not be used alone in the preoperative preparation of thyrotoxic patients, because they do not prevent thyrotoxic crisis. They are contraindicated in patients with asthma or congestive heart failure.

Summary of Management

1. Graves disease—Options are antithyroid drugs or radioiodine. Radioiodine therapy often is preferred (unless the patient is pregnant or very young, in which case surgical excision or antithyroid drugs may be used).
2. Severe hyperthyroidism—Antithyroid drugs until euthyroid, then ^{131}I or surgical excision.
3. Toxic single nodule—Surgical excision or radioiodine.
4. Toxic multinodular goiter—Surgical excision or radioiodine plus temporizing antithyroid drug therapy.
5. Silent thyroiditis—Symptomatic supportive therapy with β-blockers.
6. Subacute thyroiditis—Symptomatic supportive therapy with β-blockers, steroids can be used in severe cases.
7. Tumor-induced (struma, hydatidiform, or TSH tumor)—Surgical excision.

Thyrotoxic Crisis

This state of severe hyperthyroidism is seen in untreated or inadequately treated hyperthyroid patients undergoing surgical treatment or who have acute intercurrent illness. It is characterized by extreme irritability, delirium, hyperpyrexia, tachycardia, hypotension, vomiting, diarrhea, prostration, and coma. Untreated, it is fatal. Start treatment promptly without waiting for confirmation of diagnosis: 1) propylthiouracil to block thyroid hormone synthesis, 2) sodium iodide to inhibit release of thyroid hormones, 3) propranolol to decrease conversion of T_4 to T_3, and 4) supportive therapy, including glucocorticoid support. After recovery, plan for definitive therapy of the thyrotoxic state.

Thyrotoxicosis in Pregnancy

In normal pregnancy, T_4 and T_3 levels increase, RT_3U is decreased, FTI is normal, and sTSH may be decreased modestly. An increase in FTI and sTSH less than 0.1 mU/mL indicates thyrotoxicosis. [131]I uptake test is absolutely contraindicated. For Graves thyrotoxicosis in pregnancy, most physicians rely on antithyroid drug therapy. Surgical excision may be an option after the first trimester. Radioiodine therapy is absolutely contraindicated. Antithyroid drugs cross the placenta, but maternal T_4 and T_3 do not cross the placenta. Give antithyroid drugs in the smallest dose necessary to control the disease. β-Blockers should not be given. Inorganic iodides cross the placenta and may block the fetal thyroid.

Hypothyroidism

Etiology

Hypothyroidism can be a consequence of either decreased hormone production or peripheral tissue resistance to the actions of thyroid hormones. Decreased hormone production, which accounts for almost all cases, can result from either thyroid gland disease (thyroprivic or primary hypothyroidism) or loss of trophic stimulation by TSH, resulting from hypothalamic-pituitary disease (trophoprivic or central hypothyroidism). Primary hypothyroidism accounts for more than 90% of all causes.

Primary hypothyroidism can be organic or functional and either permanent or reversible. The commonest causes of organic permanent hypothyroidism in iodine-replete areas of the world are Hashimoto thyroiditis, spontaneous atrophic hypothyroidism (a variant of autoimmune thyroiditis), and hypothyroidism that follows radioiodine treatment of hyperthyroidism, surgical thyroidectomy, or radiation therapy for neck malignancies. Reversible primary hypothyroidism may be seen transiently during the course of subacute or silent thyroiditis. Functional reversible primary hypothyroidism is seen with the use of goitrogens such as iodides, lithium, and thioureas. Primary hypothyroidism may be clinical (low serum T_4 and T_3 levels and increased serum TSH) or subclinical (normal T_4 and T_3 levels and increased TSH levels). Subclinical hypothyroidism may or may not progress to florid hypothyroidism.

Central hypothyroidism may occur in the context of hypopituitarism resulting from organic hypothalamic-pituitary disease or it may occur as an isolated TSH deficiency of indeterminate cause. Functional reversible TSH suppression occurs after the withdrawal of exogenous thyroid hormone(s) therapy or after the correction of the hyperthyroid state; it lasts for a few weeks and resolves spontaneously.

- Hypothyroidism usually results from decreased hormone production and rarely from tissue resistance to thyroid hormones.
- Decreased production of thyroid hormones may be due to primary thyroid disorder or to central hypothalamic-pituitary disease. Hypothyroidism is usually permanent but may be reversible.
- The common causes of primary hypothyroidism are Hashimoto thyroiditis, atrophic thyroiditis, radioiodine therapy, thyroidectomy, neck irradiation.
- Reversible hypothyroidism may be seen with the use of goitrogens or transiently in subacute or silent thyroiditis.

- TSH deficiency may be isolated or part of a more generalized hypopituitarism.
- Transient TSH deficiency may occur during recovery from endogenous or exogenous hyperthyroidism.

Clinical Features

The clinical features include those of thyroid hormone deficiency and the etiologic disorder.

Features related to thyroid hormone deficiency vary and depend on the severity and duration of the deficiency. These include 1) mental, emotional, and physical slowing; 2) hypometabolism, bradycardia, cold intolerance, and weight gain; 3) dryness of the skin and hair and brittleness of the nails; 4) aches and pains, fatigue, muscle weakness, and muscle cramps; 5) tendency to constipation; 6) daytime somnolence; 7) facial puffiness and pallor; 8) carpal tunnel syndrome; and 9) normocytic anemia.

Uncommon manifestations are 1) neuropsychiatric (dementia, dysarthria, deafness, cerebellar ataxia, peripheral neuropathy, or psychoneurosis/psychoses); 2) cardiopulmonary (hypertension, cardiomegaly/failure, pericardial/pleural effusions, or respiratory depression); 3) gastrointestinal (ileus or ascites); 4) genitourinary (potency impairment in males and menorrhagia, dysmenorrhea, or amenorrhea/galactorrhea in females); 5) musculoskeletal (arthritis or cramps/stiffness); 6) hematologic (macrocytic anemia, pernicious anemia [associated autoimmune disease] or microcytic anemia [iron deficiency]); 7) endocrine (growth retardation, abnormalities of sexual maturation, galactorrhea, associated autoimmune endocrinopathies, or SIADH); and 8) metabolic/laboratory findings (hyperlipidemia, hypercalcemia, hyperuricemia, or increased aspartate aminotransferase, lactate dehydrogenase, or creatine phosphokinase).

Associations of autoimmune thyroiditis include other autoimmune endocrinopathies such as Addison disease, type 1 diabetes mellitus, hypoparathyroidism, pernicious anemia, and a positive family history.

Examination of the thyroid reveals, depending on the underlying cause, a diffuse goiter or an atrophic thyroid. In severe and prolonged hypothyroidism, electrocardiography reveals sinus bradycardia, low-voltage complexes, and ST-T-wave abnormalities.

- Clinical features: those of hypothyroidism itself and of the etiologic disorder.
- The presentations of hypothyroidism are protean: it affects every body system and organ.

Diagnosis

Documentation of Hypothyroidism

Low blood levels of thyroid hormone are key to the diagnosis. Reliance is placed on measurements of free T_4 or

FTI. A low free T_4 or FTI is diagnostic of hypothyroidism, if a nonthyroidal illness is excluded. A high free T_4 or FTI is seen in hypothyroid patients with peripheral tissue resistance to thyroid hormones. Serum measurements of T_3 are not helpful in the diagnosis of hypothyroidism: T_3 production by extrathyroidal tissues depends on many nonthyroidal influences, a low T_3 level can be seen in many euthyroid patients with nonthyroidal illness, and serum T_3 levels may be normal in hypothyroid patients.

Delineation of Cause of Hypothyroid State

It is critical to delineate whether the hypothyroidism is primary or central, because 1) central hypothyroidism may be caused by a serious disorder such as a hypothalamic or pituitary mass lesion that can be associated with increased morbidity and mortality and 2) TSH deficiency may be associated with other hormone deficiencies of hypopituitarism. Should the hypothyroidism be of central origin, cortisol deficiency should be looked for and, if found, treated with cortisol replacement *before* the institution of thyroid hormone therapy, otherwise thyroid hormone therapy may trigger an acute adrenocortical crisis. *Serum TSH measurement is critical for this delineation.* A high TSH level in a hypothyroid patient points to primary hypothyroidism, but a "normal" or low TSH points to central hypothyroidism. The presence of a goiter in a hypothyroid patient is indicative of primary hypothyroidism. A small or atrophic gland, however, may be seen in primary or central hypothyroidism.

Hashimoto thyroiditis is usually associated with a diffuse bosselated firm goiter and a high titer of antimicrosomal (antiperoxidase) antibodies. Hypothyroidism occurring after radioiodine therapy, thyroid surgery, or radiation therapy to the neck or hypothyroidism occurring transiently during the course of subacute or silent thyroiditis is usually obvious from a careful clinical evaluation. A careful drug inquiry is required to exclude goitrogen-induced hypothyroidism. The finding of central hypothyroidism usually prompts MRI of the head and assessment of the other pituitary functions.

- Obtain free T_4 or FTI and TSH measurements.
- Normal free T_4 or FTI and TSH levels exclude hypothyroidism.
- Low free T_4 or FTI and increased TSH levels are diagnostic of primary hypothyroidism if the recovery phase from a nonthyroidal illness is excluded.
- Normal free T_4 or FTI and increased TSH levels indicate subclinical primary hypothyroidism.
- Low free T_4 or FTI and "normal" or low TSH levels in a hypothyroid patient indicate central hypothyroidism. MRI of the head and pituitary function tests should be performed.
- High free T_4 or FTI and TSH levels in a clinically hypothyroid patient point to peripheral tissue resistance to thyroid hormone.
- Clinical evaluation and judicious use of laboratory tests are key to determining the cause.
- Remember the causes of reversible hypothyroidism; inquire about exposure to goitrogens.

Therapy

Synthetic T_4 is the drug of choice. T_4 is well absorbed from the gastrointestinal tract (>90%). It has a half-life of 7 days, which allows single daily dosing, stable serum T_4 levels, and stable physiologic serum T_3 levels from the conversion of T_4 to T_3 by the peripheral tissues. Dosage and administration—the usual daily replacement dose is 1.6 μg T_4/kg; the average dose is 0.1 mg/day. Start with a low dose (except in young patients or if hypothyroidism is of recent onset, when one can start with the average replacement dose) such as 0.025 mg/day and increase slowly every few weeks by 0.025 mg/day. The goals of therapy are to normalize TSH in primary hypothyroidism and to normalize free T_4 or FTI in central hypothyroidism.

In patients with primary hypothyroidism receiving previously documented adequate therapy, an increase in sTSH may indicate substandard medication, poor compliance, malabsorption (e.g., concomitant use of bile acid sequestrant therapy, ferrous sulphate or sucralfate), ongoing progressive thyroid disease, pregnancy, or increased hormone clearance (phenytoin, rifampin). A decrease in sTSH in a patient with primary hypothyroidism previously treated adequately may indicate reduced requirements of aging, patient's self-induced overmedication, regeneration of autonomous thyroid remnant, or decreased clearance. Therefore, it is important to assess sTSH annually or as indicated by patient's symptoms, not only to ensure compliance but to determine whether an adjustment in the dose is indicated. T_4 replacement therapy usually is lifelong, unless the hypothyroidism is transient or reversible.

- Synthetic T_4 is the drug of choice. Start low and increase slowly (except in young patients or if hypothyroidism is of recent onset).
- Monitor TSH and clinical response in primary hypothyroidism.
- Monitor clinical response and serum level of T_4 in central hypothyroidism.
- In primary hypothyroidism, check TSH annually or whenever clinical state warrants to assess adequacy of therapy.
- Give T_4 either 1 hour before or 4 hours after a concomitantly used medication that may interfere with T_4 absorption in the intestine (bile acid sequestrants).

Miscellaneous Circumstances

Thyroxine Replacement in Pregnancy

In primary hypothyroid patients who had been receiving adequate T_4 therapy before conception, 75% have increased sTSH during pregnancy and need an increase in the T_4 dosage (probably related to increased clearance of T_4 and increase in serum concentration of TBG). Assess TSH levels periodically during pregnancy, and adjust T_4 dosage as necessary to maintain a normal sTSH. The T_4 dose is reduced to the prepregnancy level in the postpartum period.

Thyroxine Replacement Therapy in Hypothyroid Patients With Angina

Start low, 12.5 or 25 µg/day, and increase slowly every 6 to 8 weeks to full replacement, if tolerated. If angina worsens, reduce or discontinue drug treatment. About 40% of treated patients cannot tolerate the full T_4 replacement dosage. Treat symptomatic coronary artery disease as appropriate. The hypothyroid state does not contraindicate urgent anesthesia or surgery. Start replacement therapy as soon as cardiac status has been stabilized.

Surgery in Hypothyroid Patients

Generally, surgery is well tolerated by these patients. Because drug degradative and excretory functions may be slowed, there is need for a decrease in the dosing of anesthetics, sedatives, or narcotics. Be vigilant about the serum concentration of sodium, because hypothyroid patients cannot excrete a water load efficiently because of inappropriate ADH excess state and reduced GFR. Also, keep in mind that hypothyroid patients mount a lesser febrile response to postoperative infection.

Subclinical Hypothyroidism

This is a condition in which the sTSH is minimally elevated, between 5 and 10 mIU/L (normal, 0.4-5.0 mIU/L), in a patient who is clinically euthyroid and has a normal free T_4 level or FTI. It is a relatively common disorder and affects 5% to 15% of elderly persons, particularly women. It also can be seen in inadequately treated patients with primary hypothyroidism and in patients who have been treated with radioiodine or have had subtotal thyroidectomy for Graves disease. These patients usually are asymptomatic or have minimal nonspecific symptoms. Replacement therapy generally is recommended for symptomatic patients and those at risk for progressive disease. Progression to overt hypothyroidism is likely if the patient has Hashimoto thyroiditis or has been treated with radioiodine or surgery for Graves disease.

Myxedema Crisis

This occurs in patients with severe hypothyroidism and is either spontaneous or precipitated by an acute illness, exposure to cold, or use of sedatives or opiates. It carries a high mortality (20%-50%). The onset is gradual, with progressive stupor culminating in coma. Seizures may occur, and hypothermia, hypotension, hypoventilation, hyponatremia, and hypoglycemia may be present. Most often, the patients are elderly and have overt hypothyroidism.

Perform confirmatory blood tests and start treatment promptly. Do not wait for the laboratory results. Institute supportive therapy and give aggressive thyroid hormone therapy. Conserve body heat; do not warm externally. Conserve vital functions; consider tracheal intubation and ventilatory support if respiratory depression occurs. Cautiously maintain hydration and hemodynamic functions and watch for hyponatremia (SIADH). Give T_4, 2 µg/kg intravenously over 5 to 10 minutes and 100 µg/24 hr intravenously thereafter. Support the patient with glucocorticoids in high doses (hypothyroidism may have slowed down adrenal responsiveness, and there may be associated Addison disease).

Thyroiditis

Hashimoto Thyroiditis

Hashimoto thyroiditis, an autoimmune disorder with a familial predisposition, is a common disease, particularly in middle-aged and elderly patients and predominantly in women. It is the most common cause of primary hypothyroidism. *Goiter*—Variable size, rubbery to firm, and usually diffuse (may be nodular). *Thyroid function*—Euthyroidism or hypothyroidism (frank or subclinical) and, rarely, hyperthyroidism indistinguishable from Graves disease. May present with postpartum painless thyroiditis. *Thyroid antibodies* are positive and in high titers: antimicrosomal (antiperoxidase) antibodies (95%); antithyroglobulin antibodies (50%-60%). *Management*—T_4 therapy (replacement therapy for subclinical or overt hypothyroidism and suppressive therapy to decrease the size of a large diffuse goiter) and surgery (for large obstructive goiters).

Painless Lymphocytic Thyroiditis (Silent Postpartum Thyroiditis)

This probably is a variant of Hashimoto thyroiditis. It occurs most commonly in females, especially in the postpartum period. Typical scenario—Hyperthyroid phase, followed by hypothyroid phase and eventual restoration of euthyroidism. Either dysfunction may occur independently of the other. In the hyperthyroid phase, FTI is increased, sTSH is suppressed, ^{131}I uptake is low, and antithyroid antibody levels are normal or modestly increased. There is absence of ophthalmopathy or dermopathy. The disease is self-limiting but has a tendency to recur in subsequent pregnancies. No treatment is required in most patients. However, β-blockers may be used in the hyperthyroid phase and temporary T_4 therapy may be used in the hypothyroid phase. Chronic autoimmune thyroiditis with goiter or hypothyroidism, or both, develops in 40% to 50% of patients in 5 to 10 years

Subacute Painful Thyroiditis (de Quervain Thyroiditis)

De Quervain thyroiditis probably is a viral thyroiditis. Its onset is gradual or abrupt. It is characterized by a painful tender goiter that usually is diffuse but may be unilateral. It usually is associated with fever, malaise, myalgia, and a history of an upper respiratory tract infection. Hyperthyroidism of a few weeks' duration may be present in 50% of patients. De Quervain thyroiditis may be followed by transient hypothyroidism, but ultimate restoration of function is the rule. A marked increase in the erythrocyte sedimentation rate is a characteristic feature; FTI is increased and sTSH is suppressed in the hyperthyroid phase and ^{131}I uptake is suppressed. The illness is self-limited but may be characterized by remissions and relapses. Treat moderate disease with NSAIDs, and treat severe disease with short-term glucocorticoid therapy. *The major differential diagnosis is with hemorrhage into a thyroid nodule*: abrupt onset of pain, tender nodule, absence of systemic features, normal erythrocyte sedimentation rate, normal thyroid function, normal ^{131}I uptake and cold nodule on scan, and resolution after a few days.

Goiter

Multinodular Euthyroid Goiter

Etiology—Benign (sporadic multinodular goiter or Hashimoto thyroiditis) or malignant (primary carcinoma, metastatic carcinoma, or lymphoma).

Diagnostic approach—If any nodule is dominant, manage as a single nodule (see below). If any feature suggests malignancy, tissue diagnosis (fine needle aspiration) and surgical therapy are needed. If onset is gradual and progression is slow, the differential diagnosis is benign multinodular goiter vs. Hashimoto thyroiditis. Check for antimicrosomal antibodies.

Single or Dominant Thyroid Nodule

Etiology—Benign nodules include adenoma, cyst, focal thyroiditis, benign multinodular goiter with dominant nodule, and remnant hyperplasia (postsurgical ablation). Malignant nodules are classified as primary (thyroid follicle, either differentiated [papillary or follicular] or undifferentiated [anaplastic], parafollicular C cell [medullary carcinoma]) and secondary (metastatic or lymphoma).

Diagnostic approach—Identify any factors that increase suspicion of malignancy: young age, male, rapid growth, invasive characteristics, history of irradiation, family history of thyroid cancer, or appearance while patient is receiving suppressive doses of thyroid hormone. Determine serum sTSH: suppressed sTSH suggests a hyperfunctioning nodule that is likely benign, and an increased sTSH should prompt consideration of focal autoimmune thyroiditis as the cause of the nodule.

Fine needle aspiration is the most important diagnostic step. It is a safe and effective outpatient procedure (sensitivity for detection of thyroid malignancy is 95%-98%). Interpretation of the aspirated tissue by an experienced cytopathologist is critical for the usefulness of the procedure. 1) *Benign aspirate*: observe and recheck in 4 to 6 months and then periodically. 2) *Suspicious aspirate*: request a thyroid isotope scan. If there is a "hot nodule," observe or ablate; if a "cold nodule," surgical excision. 3) *Malignant aspirate*: surgical excision. 4) *Nondiagnostic aspirate* (10%): repeat fine needle aspiration or make a decision based on the clinical assessment.

Thyroid Cancer

Differentiated Thyroid Cancer

Papillary cancer is the commonest type of thyroid cancer (50%-60% of cases). Its incidence peaks in early adulthood and again in late adulthood. Dissemination is typically to lymph nodes; other sites of metastases include the lungs and bone. The usual presentation is with a thyroid mass or cervical lymphadenopathy or the cancer can be found incidentally in surgically excised thyroid glands.

Follicular carcinoma (20% of cases) spreads preferentially by a hematogenous route. The neoplastic follicles can trap iodine and synthesize thyroid hormones. The usual presentation is with a thyroid mass or metastatic deposits in the lungs, bones, or brain. Rarely, if the tumor burden is large, follicular carcinoma can lead to thyrotoxicosis.

Undifferentiated *anaplastic carcinoma* usually presents in the elderly with a rapidly progressive thyroid mass. It has a poor prognosis, and longevity is <6 to 9 months.

Prognosis—In patients with differentiated cancer, the 20-year cause-specific mortality rate varies between less than 5% and 15%, with papillary cancer having the best prognosis. Factors associated with a poorer prognosis include old age, male sex, large size of primary tumor, invasiveness and extracapsular spread of the tumor, higher histologic grade, and the presence of distant metastases (metastases to the cervical lymph nodes do not affect prognosis).

Therapy—Surgical excision is the definitive therapy. Several factors are important. 1) Multicentricity occurs in 25% to 50% of all differentiated cancers, 2) recurrence rates tend to be lower in patients who have more extensive surgery, and 3) total thyroidectomy is to be avoided, if possible, to minimize the risks of postoperative hypoparathyroidism or damage to the recurrent laryngeal nerve. Surgical excision is usually in the form of either lobectomy with or without subtotal contralateral lobectomy or near total thyroidectomy. The affected lymph nodes are selectively excised.

Postoperative management—Patients in the low risk groups are treated with suppressive doses of T_4. Those at a higher risk undergo radioiodine imaging at 4 to 6 weeks postoperatively, with 30 to 70 mCi of ^{131}I given to ablate the thyroid remnant (or a larger dose if metastases are found) and then suppressive T_4 therapy is initiated. T_4 suppressive therapy is given to reduce the incidence of tumor recurrence. For the low risk group, the goal is a TSH value between 0.1 and 0.4 mIU/L and for the high risk group, less than 0.1 mIU/L.

Follow-up—Patients are evaluated in 3 to 6 months and then at yearly intervals. Chest radiography, serum TSH and thyroglobulin, and neck ultrasonography are performed at each visit. Most differentiated thyroid cancers, regardless of whether they trap iodine, synthesize and secrete thyroglobulin. Serum thyroglobulin can be used as a marker of recurrent/persistent disease. In a patient who has little or no thyroid tissue and is receiving suppressive T_4 therapy, the serum thyroglobulin level should be from less than 5 to 10 ng/mL; a higher level nearly always indicates persistent/recurrent disease. [131]I imaging is indicated in patients with evidence of recurrent or metastatic disease. Otherwise, it is repeated every 3 to 5 years in high-risk patients. Late recurrences are treated, depending on location, with either surgery or [131]I. Radiotherapy is given for local bony painful metastasis. The treatment of anaplastic carcinoma is palliative.

- Papillary cancer: the most common (50%-60%). It spreads to lymph nodes and has the best prognosis. Presentation: thyroid mass, cervical lymphadenopathy, found incidentally in excised thyroid glands.
- Follicular carcinoma (20%): spreads preferentially by hematogenous route. Presentation: thyroid mass, metastatic deposits. It can lead to thyrotoxicosis (rare).
- Anaplastic carcinoma: usually presents in the elderly with rapidly progressive thyroid mass. Prognosis is very poor.
- Surgical excision is the definitive therapy. Suppressive doses of T_4 are used (monitored by sTSH).
- Follow-up: serum TSH, thyroglobulin, neck ultrasonography, and chest radiography. [131]I imaging is done if there is evidence of recurrent/persistent disease or every 3-5 years in the high risk group.
- Recurrences are treated, depending on location, with surgery or [131]I.

Miscellaneous Thyroid Disorders

Nonthyroidal Illness Syndrome

Definition—Patients who are hospitalized for systemic illness, psychiatric disorders, or trauma frequently have abnormalities in thyroid hormone(s) levels in the absence of identifiable intrinsic thyroid disease. These abnormalities do not appear to have a functional impact and revert to normal with recovery from the associated illness. They do not require therapy. 1) *The low T_3-normal T_4 variant* is the most common variant and is due to decreased 5'-deiodinase activity; this results in decreased extrathyroidal conversion of T_4 to T_3 and increased reverse T_3. The levels of T_4 and TSH are normal. 2) *The low T_3-low T_4 variant* occurs in patients who have more severe illness; in addition to low T_3 levels, these patients have a low T_4 level, which results from decreased T_4 binding or displacement. The TSH level may be normal or low because of the central effects of the illness and may be mildly increased, less than 20 µU/mL, during recovery. 3) *The high T_4 variant* is probably due to decreased T_4 clearance and is seen in patients with liver disease, particularly acute hepatitis, or psychiatric illness, particularly manic-depressive disorders. The T_3 levels are low or normal and TSH is variable.

Diagnosis—The major challenge in sick hospitalized patients is to distinguish the effects of nonthyroidal illness from those of intrinsic thyroid disease. The laboratory features associated with nonthyroidal illness may suggest central hypothyroidism (low T_4 and normal or low TSH levels), primary hypothyroidism (low T_4 and modestly increased TSH levels seen during recovery), or hyperthyroidism (high T_4 and low TSH levels). Helpful features in the differential diagnosis include clinical evaluation (goiter, extrathyroidal manifestations of Graves disease, hypothalamic-pituitary mass effects, or hypopituitarism), consideration of the serum level of T_3 and TSH, and observation of the course of the illness: 1) a high serum T_3 level points to hyperthyroidism and excludes nonthyroidal illness, 2) TSH greater than 20 µU/mL points to primary hypothyroidism, 3) TSH less than 0.03 µU/mL points to hyperthyroidism, and 4) the features of nonthyroidal illness resolve with recovery from the acute illness, whereas those of intrinsic thyroid disease persist beyond such recovery.

Excess Iodides and the Thyroid

Normal persons can adapt to excess iodides and maintain a euthyroid state because, initially, of Wolff-Chaikoff effect and, later, decreased trapping of iodine. In persons with impaired thyroid autoregulation, iodide excess can lead to either hyperthyroidism or hypothyroidism. It is important to consider iodide effects in the appropriate setting and to monitor thyroid function, particularly in the elderly (high prevalence of Hashimoto thyroiditis and nodular goiters and difficulty detecting thyroid dysfunction in this age group).

Amiodarone—It is stored in fat and may provide excess iodides for months after the discontinuation of therapy. It may lead to hyperthyroidism in two ways: by iodide excess in patients with autonomous thyroids and by drug-induced thyroiditis.

Lithium and the Thyroid

Lithium and the Thyroid

Lithium has antithyroid actions: it decreases the secretion and the synthesis of thyroid hormones. The use of lithium can be associated with the development of goiter and hypothyroidism, particularly in patients with underlying autoimmune thyroid disease. Rarely, the use of lithium has been associated with the development of *hyperthyroidism*, probably because of the coincidental activation of autoimmune thyroid disease.

- Lithium: can be associated with development of goiter and hypothyroidism.

DISORDERS OF THE PARATHYROID AND ENDOCRINE BONE

Primary Hyperparathyroidism

Etiology

Primary hyperparathyroidism is the most common parathyroid disorder, with a prevalence of 0.1% to 0.5%. The disease mostly affects persons older than 50 years and is two or three times more common in females. It is caused by a single adenoma in 80% of patients, multiple adenomas in 5%, hyperplasia of all four glands in 15%, and, very rarely, by a parathyroid carcinoma in fewer than 1%. The adenoma may be ectopic in location in 6% to 10% of patients and may be found in the thyroid, thymus, or mediastinum. The disease may be sporadic or familial; the familial form may be a part of MEN I (in association with tumors of the anterior pituitary and endocrine pancreas) or MEN IIA (in association with medullary carcinoma of the thyroid and pheochromocytoma). The usual parathyroid lesion in familial hyperparathyroidism is hyperplasia.

- Primary hyperparathyroidism is a common disorder that may be sporadic or familial.
- Parathyroid adenoma is the usual cause.
- Hyperplasia is uncommon except in the familial form.
- Familial primary hyperparathyroidism may occur alone or be associated with MEN I or MEN IIA.

Clinical Features

More than 50% of patients with primary hyperparathyroidism are asymptomatic and identified by multichannel chemical testing. When present, symptoms result from the effects of hypercalcemia on cellular functions and the deposition of calcium salts in tissues. Symptoms may include the following. 1) Renal: polyuria, polydipsia due to hypercalcemia-induced nephrogenic diabetes insipidus, renal colic, nephrolithiasis, and chronic renal failure. Primary hyperparathyroidism is found in 5% of patients with a first renal stone and in 15% with recurrent stones. 2) Neuromuscular: fatigue, weakness, myopathy, impairment of consciousness, confusion, depression, and hyporeflexia. 3) Gastrointestinal: anorexia, nausea, vomiting, and constipation; hypercalcemia may be associated with peptic ulcer and pancreatitis. 4) Cardiovascular: hypertension and arrhythmias; hypercalcemia potentiates the cardiac effects of digitalis. Electrocardiography (ECG) may show shortened QT intervals. 5) Skeletal: osteopenia, osteitis fibrosa cystica with bone pain, deformities, and pathologic fractures. 6) Metastatic calcification: band keratopathy or nephrocalcinosis. Also, primary hyperparathyroidism has known associations with chondrocalcinosis and pseudogout. Hypercalcemic crisis is infrequent and may be the presenting feature in the elderly and in those with parathyroid carcinoma. The dominant manifestations are those of dehydration and hypotension, abdominal pain, nausea and vomiting, pyrexia, and altered level of consciousness.

- Primary hyperparathyroidism is commonly asymptomatic and detected serendipitously in multichannel blood screening.
- When the disease is symptomatic, the symptoms may involve several organ systems.
- Clinical features may include renal, neuromuscular, gastrointestinal, cardiovascular, and skeletal components.
- Hypercalcemic crisis is rare.
- Known associations include peptic ulcer, pancreatitis, and pseudogout.

Laboratory Features

Hypercalcemia is the cardinal laboratory feature; it may be mild and intermittent. *Hypophosphatemia*—the serum level of phosphate is usually low but may be normal. (Note that the serum phosphate level may be low in any hypercalcemic state and that a high serum phosphate level in a hypercalcemic patient points to renal insufficiency or to non-PTH-dependent hypercalcemia.) *Urine calcium* is usually normal or modestly increased; in a hypercalcemic patient, a low urinary level of calcium is seen in familial hypocalciuric hypercalcemia and with the use of thiazides, whereas significant hypercalciuria (>400 mg/24 hr) usually points to a nonparathyroid cause. Serum PTH is usually increased (90% of patients); it may be "normal" in 10% of patients, but it is always inappropriately increased for the degree of hypercalcemia. Immunoradiometric assay of PTH is the most reliable assay. The ECG may show a short QT interval or arrhythmia.

Radiologic Features

Primary hyperparathyroidism is associated with osteopenia and characteristic skeletal changes, which include 1) subperiosteal bone resorption that is noted especially on the radial borders of the phalanges in radiographs of the hands, 2) "salt and pepper" findings in lateral radiographs of the skull, and 3) osteitis fibrosis cystica (fibrous replacement of the resorbed bone, which may present with bone pain, tenderness, deformity, or fracture). Renal findings include stones and their effects and nephrocalcinosis.

- The cardinal laboratory findings are hypercalcemia and an increased or "inappropriately normal" serum PTH level.
- Hypercalcemia may be mild and intermittent; a low serum phosphate level is nonspecific.
- Serum PTH: increased in 90% of patients; normal in 10%, but inappropriate for the prevailing level of serum calcium.
- Urine calcium is usually normal or minimally increased.
- Radiology: Skeletal—osteopenia and characteristic skeletal findings of subperiosteal bone resorption, "salt and pepper" skull, and osteitis fibrosa cystica. Renal—calcium-containing stones or nephrocalcinosis.

Diagnosis

Diagnosis rests on the documentation of hypercalcemia and the demonstration that primary hyperparathyroidism is its cause. It is important to remember that primary hyperparathyroidism is a common disorder and may coexist with other causes of hypercalcemic syndrome.

When interpreting a total serum calcium value, consider the factors that determine the distribution of calcium between the bound and ionized fractions (plasma protein concentration and acid-base balance among others). Pay particular attention to the concentration of albumin, the major calcium-binding protein in the blood. If the albumin level is abnormal, a correction factor is applied: for each 1 g/dL change in albumin concentration from normal, the total calcium changes by 0.8 mg/dL in the same direction. If hypercalcemia is mild, confirm it with blood collected in the fasting state and without prolonged venous stasis.

- Serum total calcium should be considered in relation to the serum albumin levels.
- An abnormal value for serum calcium requires confirmation.

Differential Diagnosis

Primary hyperparathyroidism is the most common cause of hypercalcemia in ambulatory patients. The major diagnostic challenge is to distinguish it from other hypercalcemic states. Fundamentally, hypercalcemia can result from increased bone resorption, increased intestinal absorption, or decreased urinary excretion of calcium. More than one mechanism may be involved in a disorder. From a clinical standpoint, the causes can be categorized as either PTH-dependent or PTH-independent.

Other Causes of Parathyroid-Dependent Hypercalcemia

Familial Hypocalciuric Hypercalcemia

This is an autosomal dominant disorder; the gene mutation has been mapped to the long arm of chromosome 3. The distinctive features are uncomplicated asymptomatic mild hypercalcemia in a relatively young patient, with normal or slightly elevated PTH, a low urinary calcium, and a positive family history. The diagnosis is strongly supported by a calcium-to-creatinine clearance ratio less than 0.01. Parathyroid surgery is unjustified because the disease is benign and uncomplicated and it usually is not curative unless a complete parathyroidectomy is done and hypoparathyroidism ensues. Family screening is important. Hypercalcemia may be detected in affected family members before age 10 years.

Thiazides

Mild hypercalcemia may be seen in some patients receiving thiazide therapy and may be multifactorial (dehydration, decreased renal calcium clearance, and, possibly, increase in PTH secretion). The mild hypercalcemia usually resolves within a few weeks after the discontinuation of drug therapy. Thiazide hypercalcemia is more likely to occur in patients with underlying mild primary hyperparathyroidism and in those with increased bone turnover and hypercalciuria (e.g., Paget disease and thyrotoxicosis).

Lithium

Hypercalcemia occurs in 10% of patients who take lithium. Lithium increases the set-point of calcium inhibition of parathyroid secretion. The hypercalcemia is reversible if the treatment with lithium is discontinued.

Parathyroid-Independent Hypercalcemia

Hypercalcemia of Malignancy

Hypercalcemia of malignancy is common, often develops acutely, and may be severe. It is the commonest cause of hypercalcemia in hospitalized patients and is caused by either local destructive skeletal neoplastic effects or humoral factors from a remote neoplasm. Increased levels of PTH-rP are seen in most patients with humoral hypercalcemia of malignancy. Serum PTH is characteristically suppressed.

Vitamin D Intoxication

Hypercalcemia, hypercalciuria, renal insufficiency, and soft tissue calcification follow prolonged ingestion of vitamin D or its metabolites in high dosages. This occurs most commonly during therapy with vitamin D, but it also may occur as part of a fad food regimen or from surruptitious use by patients with psychiatric disease. The condition may persist for months after treatment with vitamin D_2 has been discontinued because the vitamin is stored in fat. Levels of $1,25(OH)_2D$ are increased. Response to glucocorticoids is prompt. Hypercalcemia is also seen in hypervitaminosis A.

Sarcoidosis, Other Granulomatous Disorders, and Some Lymphomas

The hypercalcemia in these disorders is vitamin D-dependent and may occur in up to 15% of patients; hypercalciuria is even more common. Granulomas and lymphomas have 1-hydroxylase and can autonomously generate calcitriol, $1,25(OH)_2D$, from circulating $25(OH)D$. The serum levels of $25(OH)D$ are normal, and those of $1,25(OH)_2D$ are increased. The hypercalcemia is responsive to glucocorticoid therapy.

Other Endocrinopathies

In hyperthyroidism, bone turnover is enhanced, with bone resorption exceeding bone formation and resulting in hypercalcemia (25% of patients) and hypercalciuria (50%). The hypercalcemia is reversible and resolves with the treatment of thyrotoxicosis. In Addison disease, hypercalcemia is frequent and related to dehydration and an increase in the protein-bound fraction; it is reversible with glucocorticoid therapy.

Immobilization

Immobilization may result in hypercalcemia in patients with rapid bone turnover, such as adolescents and patients with Paget disease.

Milk-Alkali Syndrome

This results from a combination of high calcium intake and absorbable alkali. It is characterized by hypercalcemia, alkalosis, renal failure, hypocalciuria, and soft tissue calcification. It is preventable.

- Rule out laboratory error and factitial causes. Correct for serum albumin or determine the ionized calcium value.
- The most critical laboratory test is assay of serum PTH, optimally by a two-site immunometric method.
- Suppressed PTH: parathyroid-independent hypercalcemia. Increased PTH-related protein: humoral hypercalcemia of malignancy. Increased $1,25(OH)_2D$: granulomatous disorder or some type of lymphoma.
- High serum PTH level: primary hyperparathyroidism.
- "Normal" or "minimally elevated" serum level of PTH: primary hyperparathyroidism, thiazides, lithium, familial hypocalciuric hypercalcemia; family history, benign clinical course, and low urinary concentration of calcium point to familial hypocalciuric hypercalcemia.

Therapy

Surgical therapy by an experienced endocrine surgeon is the treatment of choice. This may consist of adenomectomy in patients with a parathyroid adenoma or a subtotal parathyroidectomy, leaving about 50 mg of parathyroid tissue, in patients with parathyroid hyperplasia. Alternatively, total parathyroidectomy can be performed, transplantation of some of the excised tissue to either the sternocleidomastoid muscle or forearm, from where it can be removed at a later date should hypercalcemia persist or recur. Problems may arise because of variation in site and the number of glands. Some parathyroid glands may lie within the thyroid gland or in the superior mediastinum. Reversible mild asymptomatic hypocalcemia may occur in the early postoperative period. Significant and prolonged hypocalcemia may occur in the "bone-hunger" syndrome.

Conservative therapy may be indicated in cases of mild uncomplicated disease, especially in the elderly. Medical therapy for chronic hypercalcemia usually is not effective. Options include oral phosphate and, in postmenopausal women, estrogen therapy.

- Surgery is the therapy of choice unless the disease occurs in the elderly and is mild and uncomplicated. Medical therapy is ineffective.
- Surgery: excision of the adenoma or excision and autotransplantation of the hyperplastic glands.
- Localization studies usually are reserved for patients with persistent or recurrent hyperparathyroidism.

Management of Hypercalcemic Crisis

Treatment of the Primary Cause

When feasible, treatment of the primary cause, such as parathyroid adenomectomy for primary hyperparathyroidism or medical management of thyrotoxicosis, is the most important therapeutic option. Glucocorticoids are the drugs of choice for the hypercalcemia of Addison disease and in vitamin D excess, either of exogenous or endogenous origin (sarcoidosis and other granulomatous disorders). These drugs also are effective in some malignancies, such as multiple myeloma, certain lymphomas, and breast cancer with metastasis. Indomethacin or aspirin as anti-prostaglandins are usually ineffective.

Nonspecific Therapy

Nonspecific therapy is designed to decrease bone resorption and enhance renal excretion of calcium. Currently, optimal management consists of volume expansion and calciuresis, which provide an early but transient hypocalcemic effect, and use of bisphosphonates, which provide a more substantial and prolonged effect.

- Nonspecific therapy: to decrease bone resorption and increase renal excretion.
- Volume expansion, calciuresis, and use of bisphosphonates: the preferred methods of treatment.

Volume expansion and calciuresis—Volume expansion and the promotion of urinary calcium excretion by the administration of saline solution and loop diuretics form the cornerstone of the emergency management of hypercalcemia and can reduce serum calcium levels by 1 to 3 mg/dL. This therapy is temporizing and may not be useful in patients with significant renal failure. It is important not to initiate diuresis until volume repletion and electrolyte balance are achieved. Careful monitoring is vital, particularly of the level of hydration and electrolyte balance and of cardiac and renal functions.

- Volume expansion and calciuresis form the cornerstone of therapy.
- Consider the severity of the hypercalcemia, the age of the patient, and the state of cardiac and renal functions.
- Do not initiate forced saline diuresis until volume repletion is achieved. Watch for volume or electrolyte abnormalities.

Drug therapy—*Bisphosphonates* are "first-line therapy" in the management of severe hypercalcemia. *Pamidronate* is the bisphosphonate used most widely in the U.S. for the management of hypercalcemia. It is an extremely potent antiresorptive agent that is given as a single intravenous dose of 30 to 90 mg. Pamidronate is effective in 24 to 48 hours (in 70% to >90% of patients) and normalizes the serum calcium level in most patients and for weeks or months. Side effects include low-grade fever (20% of patients), hypocalcemia (10%), and, uncommonly, hypophosphatemia, hypomagnesemia, and reversible hepatic injury.

Calcitonin, an alternative choice, has a direct antiresorptive effect on osteoclasts and promotes calciuresis. It has a rapid onset of action (few hours) and is safe. It is administered in a dose of 2 to 8 IU/kg intravenously, intramuscularly, or subcutaneously every 6 hours. However, its effect is modest and variable, and tachyphylaxis often develops within a few days. Side effects include nausea, flushing, and skin rash.

Plicamycin (mithramycin), another alternative, inhibits osteoclastic resorption. A dose of 15 to 25 mg/kg is given over a period of 4 to 24 hours. The effect is rapid (24-48 hours) and may last for 5 to 7 days; it normalizes calcium in 40% to 60% of patients. Side effects include thrombocytopenia and qualitative platelet defects, renal insufficiency, and liver abnormalities.

Gallium nitrate (Ganite), an inhibitor of osteoclastic bone resorption, may be administered in a dose of 200 mg/m^2 of body surface area in 1 L of fluid daily for 5 consecutive days. Therapy achieves eucalcemia in 75% of patients, and the effect may last 7 to 10 days. Side effects include nausea, hypotension, and renal insufficiency.

- Bisphosphonates are potent antiresorptive agents and are the drugs of choice in the management of severe hypercalcemia.
- Pamidronate is the bisphosphonate most frequently used in the U.S. When given as a single intravenous dose of 30-90 mg, it is rapidly effective and can normalize serum calcium in most patients. Its effect is prolonged for days to weeks. Common side effects include low-grade fever and low serum levels of calcium, phosphate, and magnesium.
- Calcitonin: safe but has a modest and transient effect.
- Plicamycin is effective (40%-60%) and has a rapid effect that may last for 5-7 days. Gallium nitrate is effective (75%); its effect may last 7-10 days.
- Dialysis is reserved for patients with renal failure.

Hypoparathyroidism

Etiology

Parathyroid deficiency may result from 1) hypoparathyroidism, in which PTH production by the parathyroid glands is decreased because of an organic or functional disorder, and 2) pseudohypoparathyroidism, in which the parathyroid glands and PTH production are normal but there is target-tissue (renal and skeletal) resistance to PTH action.

Hypoparathyroidism may result from inadvertent surgical damage to the parathyroid glands during thyroidectomy, radical neck dissection, or surgical management of primary hyperparathyroidism. This is the most common cause of organic hypoparathyroidism; it may be transient or permanent, and it may appear shortly or in a few months or years after the surgical insult. Occasionally, hypoparathyroidism may result from other organic disorders: autoimmune, infiltrative (hemochromatosis or Wilson disease), or congenital (DiGeorge syndrome). Idiopathic hypoparathyroidism often appears as a familial disorder and may have an autoimmune basis. It occasionally accompanies other endocrine deficiency states. Hypomagnesemia is a cause of functional and reversible hypoparathyroidism; it decreases the secretion and action of PTH.

- Surgical hypoparathyroidism: may result from inadvertent damage to parathyroid glands and may be transient or permanent.
- Hypoparathyroidism may occasionally result from other organic parathyroid disorders: autoimmune, infiltrative, congenital.

- Idiopathic hypoparathyroidism: often appears as a familial disorder; may have an autoimmune basis.
- Hypomagnesemia: decreases secretion and action of PTH; an important cause of functional and reversible hypoparathyroidism.

Pseudohypoparathyroidism is an inherited disorder characterized by end-organ resistance to PTH action due to a receptor or postreceptor mechanism. Type IA: defect in Gs subunit of the receptor; characteristic features are short stature, round face, obesity, short neck, short metacarpals and metatarsals, subcutaneous calcification, mild mental retardation. *Pseudopseudohypoparathyroidism* is a variant disorder with the same characteristic physical features but without the biochemical abnormalities.

Clinical Features

PTH deficiency leads to decreased mobilization of calcium from bone, decreased renal distal tubular calcium reabsorption, decreased proximal renal tubular phosphate excretion, and decreased renal generation of $1,25(OH)_2D$ because of decreased activity of 1-hydroxylase. The composite effect is one of hypocalcemia and hyperphosphatemia.

Hypocalcemia may be asymptomatic and detected only by biochemical screening. When present, the symptoms of hypocalcemia reflect not only its degree but also the rate of its development. 1) Neuromuscular: paresthesias and muscle spasms, such as carpopedal spasms, laryngeal stridor, and convulsions. Apathy, lethargy, and depression may occur. Specific neurologic sequelae include basal ganglia calcification, extrapyramidal manifestations, and benign intracranial hypertension. 2) Gastrointestinal: abdominal pain, nausea, vomiting, and malabsorption. 3) Cardiovascular: prolonged QT interval and congestive heart failure resistant to standard therapy but responsive to normalization of serum level of calcium. 4) Other effects: premature cataracts, alopecia, and mucocutaneous candidiasis. Children may have enamel hypoplasia and failure of secondary dentition. The signs of Chvostek and Trousseau are characteristic of hypocalcemia, although they rarely can be elicited in normal persons.

Laboratory Features

The biochemical characteristics of parathyroid deficiency are hypocalcemia and hyperphosphatemia in the presence of normal renal function. In hypoparathyroidism, serum PTH, in the face of hypocalcemia, is low or undetectable, whereas in pseudohypoparathyroidism the PTH levels are characteristically high. In a hypocalcemic patient, low serum phosphate favors vitamin D deficiency, and high phosphate levels, in the presence of normal renal function, point to hypoparathyroidism.

Radiologic Features

These include basal ganglia calcification and the skeletal features characteristic of pseudohypoparathyroidism, that is, short metacarpals or metatarsals, subcutaneous calcifications, and exostoses.

- Symptoms of hypocalcemia reflect not only its degree but also the rate of its development.
- Neuromuscular: tetany, carpopedal spasms, laryngeal stridor, and convulsions.
- CNS: basal ganglia calcification, extrapyramidal manifestations, benign intracranial hypertension.
- Cardiovascular: prolonged QT; congestive heart failure resistant to standard therapy but responsive to restoration of eucalcemia.
- Signs: Chvostek and Trousseau.
- Laboratory features: hypocalcemia and hyperphosphatemia in the presence of normal renal function. In hypocalcemic patients, PTH is low in hypoparathyroidism and increased in pseudohypoparathyroidism.
- Radiologic features: basal ganglia calcification; radiologic features characteristic of pseudohypoparathyroidism.

Diagnosis

Differential Diagnosis

The hallmark of PTH deficiency is hypocalcemia, and the main differential diagnoses are those of other conditions associated with hypocalcemia. Basically, hypocalcemia may result from decreased secretion of PTH or from PTH resistance, from decreased production of vitamin D or from vitamin D resistance, and from other miscellaneous disorders associated with a decrease in mobilization of calcium from bone or an increase in calcium deposition in tissues.

Vitamin D deficiency may be caused by nutritional, malabsorptive, liver, or renal disorders that lead to decreased production of $1,25(OH)_2D$ or by vitamin D resistance, a rare disorder. In vitamin D deficiency, hypocalcemia triggers secondary hyperparathyroidism; the serum PTH levels are high and excess PTH leads to phosphaturia and hypophosphatemia (except when GFR is decreased, as in vitamin D deficiency associated with renal failure).

In acute or chronic renal failure, hypocalcemia is multifactorial, resulting from hyperphosphatemia and decreased $1,25(OH)_2D$.

Increased deposition of calcium and phosphate into bone overwhelms the ability of the parathyroids to maintain calcium homeostasis. This may occur in osteoblastic metastases seen most commonly with prostatic cancer and in "hungry bone" syndrome seen in patients who recently have had parathyroidectomy for the treatment of hyperparathyroidism associated with extensive osteitis fibrosa cystica.

Increased deposition of calcium salts in soft tissues occurs with inappropriate intravenous phosphate therapy or in acute pancreatitis.

- The differential diagnosis is that of other causes of hypocalcemic syndrome.
- Vitamin D deficiency: decreased production or tissue resistance.
- Acute or chronic renal failure.
- Increased skeletal or extraskeletal deposition of calcium and phosphate.

Diagnostic Approach

Exclude laboratory error and pseudohypocalcemia (correct the total calcium for the prevailing albumin levels or determine ionized calcium level). Confirm hypocalcemia by repeated measurements.

The clinical evaluation and determination of serum creatinine and magnesium levels will identify renal failure and magnesium deficiency states.

Assay of serum PTH is the next critical diagnostic step. In a hypocalcemic patient, a low serum PTH titer is diagnostic of hypoparathyroidism. A high serum level of PTH points to vitamin D deficiency or pseudohypoparathyroidism. The clinical findings, the characteristic phenotype and family history, and the unresponsiveness to exogenous PTH identify patients with pseudohypoparathyroidism.

The next step involves assays for serum 25(OH)D and 1,25(OH)$_2$D. Low plasma levels of 25(OH)D are seen in nutritional, malabsorptive, or hepatic causes of vitamin D deficiency; a low or normal plasma 1,25(OH)$_2$D is seen in renal failure, and a high plasma 1,25(OH)$_2$D is seen in vitamin D tissue-resistance.

Therapy

If hypocalcemia is severe or acute in development, urgent treatment is indicated to prevent tetany, laryngeal stridor, or convulsions, and provision of calcium intravenously is essential. If the disease is chronic and less urgent, oral calcium and vitamin D therapy are the cornerstones of treatment.

Urgent therapy—Intravenous calcium is essential for therapy. Calcium gluconate, 10 to 20 mL of 10% solution (90 mg elemental calcium per 10 mL) is infused over 5 to 10 minutes. The serum calcium level is maintained between 7.0 and 8.5 mg/dL by a subsequent calcium infusion (10-15 mg/kg infused every 4-6 hours). It is critical to monitor the patient's clinical status and to measure serum calcium every 2 to 6 hours. Intravenous calcium may be hazardous in patients receiving digitalis.

Chronic therapy—Treatment is directed at the underlying cause. Oral calcium is given in the dose of 2.0 to 3.0 g elemental calcium per day (calcium carbonate is 40%, calcium citrate is

21%, and calcium gluconate is 9% elemental calcium). Ergocalciferol, or vitamin D$_2$, is given in the dose of 50,000 to 100,000 U/day. It has a slow on-effect (4-8 weeks) and a slow off-effect (6-18 weeks). Alternatively, one can prescribe dihydrotachysterol (0.125 mg/day) or, particularly in vitamin D deficiency of renal failure, calcitriol, or 1,25(OH)$_2$D (0.25-2.0 µg/day), which has a rapid on-effect (1-2 days) and a rapid off-effect (1-2 days). Useful adjuncts include a thiazide diuretic to reduce the risk of significant hypercalciuria and oral phosphate binders.

It is critical to monitor therapy closely. Overtreatment results in hypercalciuria, hypercalcemia, renal stones, and nephrocalcinosis. Therapeutic doses are adjusted to keep the serum calcium level just below the lower limits of normal, around 8.5 mg/dL, and urine calcium less than 300 mg/24 hr. Vitamin D toxicity is treated with discontinuation of the vitamin, adequate hydration, and, if needed, glucocorticoid therapy.

- Urgent therapy: for severe or acutely developing hypocalcemia. Relies on intravenous calcium.
- Chronic therapy: relies on oral calcium and vitamin D or its analogs.
- Monitoring of therapy: essential to ensure adequacy and to avoid overtreatment.

Osteoporosis

Osteoporosis refers to a metabolic bone disorder that is characterized by decreased bone mass per unit volume of bone and defective skeletal architecture that leads to increased bone fragility and propensity to fractures with minimal trauma. A classification by the World Health Organization has been introduced recently. Osteopenia is defined as a bone mass value 1 to 2.5 SD below the young adult mean. Osteoporosis is defined as a bone mass value more than 2.5 SD below the young adult mean, whether a fracture is present or not.

Etiology

Osteoporosis results from a long-term imbalance between resorption and formation that favors resorption. It is a generalized disorder but is most prominent in skeletal areas of high bone turnover, such as trabecular and endosteal surfaces. Osteoporosis may be an idiopathic skeletal disorder or caused by recognized disease entities.

Idiopathic osteoporosis is divided into *postmenopausal, or type I, osteoporosis*, which is characterized by high bone turnover and affects dominantly the trabecular bone (leading to vertebral and distal forearm fractures) and *senile, or type II, osteoporosis*, which occurs in women and men after age 70 and affects both trabecular and cortical bone. Type II osteoporosis is associated with fractures of the femoral neck, proximal humerus, tibia, and pelvis.

Secondary osteoporosis is seen in endocrinopathies (hypogonadism, hyperparathyroidism, endogenous or exogenous hyperthyroidism, and hypercortisolinism); nutritional disorders (calcium deficiency, protein malnutrition, vitamin C deficiency, and alcoholism); gastrointestinal disorders (cirrhosis, malabsorption, and postgastrectomy state); neoplastic disorders (multiple myeloma, leukemia, lymphoma, and systemic mastocytosis); and genetic abnormalities of bone collagen (homocystinuria, Ehlers-Danlos syndrome, and osteogenesis imperfecta). It also is associated with certain drugs (corticosteroids, heparin, methotrexate, GnRH analogs, lithium, and cyclosporine), and with immobilization (generalized or localized).

- Osteoporosis may be primary or secondary.
- Primary osteoporosis: postmenopausal (type I) and senile (type II).
- Postmenopausal osteoporosis: high bone turnover rate; primarily trabecular bone in the axial skeleton; vertebral and distal forearm fractures are characteristic.
- Senile osteoporosis: in the elderly; low bone turnover; appendicular and axial skeletons; hip fracture is characteristic.
- Secondary osteoporosis: endocrine, nutritional, gastroenterologic, neoplastic, genetic, drug-induced, or immobilization.

Clinical Features

Fracture

The dominant feature is the occurrence of fracture with minor trauma. The fracture can be axial (vertebral) or appendicular. Osteoporotic fractures heal normally. After several vertebral fractures, shortening of stature and spinal deformity may occur (kyphoscoliosis, loss of lumbar lordosis, and dowager's hump). Mechanical, chronic, low back pain results from muscle/tendon/ligament sprains and from degenerative joint disease.

Laboratory Features

The serum levels of calcium, phosphate, and alkaline phosphatase are normal in osteoporosis. Any abnormality of these levels is related to the etiologic disorder or associated disorder, such as osteomalacia. The serum level of alkaline phosphatase may be increased slightly during healing of an osteoporotic fracture.

Radiologic Features

The characteristic features are a decrease in bone density and the occurrence of fracture with minimal trauma. Lateral spine radiographs show loss of horizontal trabeculae and apparent prominence of the vertical trabeculae, Schmorl nodes,

biconcavity of the vertebrae, and reduction in vertebral height because of wedge or crush fractures. Bone mineral density can be assessed by single photon absorptiometry of the distal forearm or calcaneous, dual energy X-ray absorptiometry of the lumbar vertebrae or the hips, and quantitative CT of trabecular bone in the lumbar vertebrae. (Ultrasound pulse velocity-attenuation through accessible bone may become a useful technique in the future.) The results can be expressed in two ways: a T score, which relates bone mineral density to that of the young adult normal range, and a Z score, which relates bone mineral density to that of a similar age group. The T score is more useful in evaluating the risk of fractures. A decreased bone mineral density generally parallels the risk of fractures. Every 1 SD decrease in bone mineral density below the mean for young adults doubles the fracture risk.

- Occurrence of fracture with minimal trauma.
- Normal serum levels of calcium, phosphate, and alkaline phosphatase.
- Alkaline phosphatase may be increased minimally in the presence of a healing fracture.
- Bone mineral density: essential for the diagnosis of osteopenia and osteoporosis; a decrease in its value parallels the risk of fractures.

Diagnosis

The diagnosis of osteoporosis is based on the finding of low bone mass with or without fractures and the exclusion of other causes of osteopenia, principally osteomalacia, multiple myeloma, and metastatic disease.

Diagnosis Before a Fracture Occurs

Diagnosis before the occurrence of a fracture rests on the finding of low bone mass by bone mineral density. Currently, bone mineral density measurements are indicated only when knowledge of the results will make a difference in therapeutic approach: in menopausal women who are reluctant to use estrogen replacement; in patients with primary hyperparathyroidism and mild uncomplicated hypercalcemia to assess need for surgical therapy; to make a decision and conduct follow-up for patients in whom long-term glucocorticoid therapy is contemplated; and in patients who have radiologic evidence of previous vertebral fracture to assess whether osteoporosis is present.

Diagnosis in a Patient Who Has Sustained a Fracture With Minimal Trauma

Consider the clinical setting, and use laboratory and radiologic tools judiciously. 1) *Exclude osteomalacia*—In osteomalacia, in contrast to osteoporosis, there are bone pain, proximal muscle weakness, biochemical abnormalities (serum levels of calcium, phosphate, or alkaline phosphatase), and pseudofractures. It is important to remember that both metabolic bone disorders may coexist. 2) *Exclude malignancy*, particularly multiple myeloma or metastatic disease. 3) *Exclude other bone disorders* such as Paget disease and vertebral osteomyelitis. In osteoporosis, bone scans identify recent fractures but are otherwise negative; localized increased uptake in the absence of fractures may indicate Paget disease or neoplasm. Bone biopsy (after a double tetracycline label) is indicated in osteopenia in all men, black women, and premenopausal white women when the cause is undetermined to confirm the diagnosis of osteoporosis and to rule out osteomalacia and other bone diseases. 4) *Rule out secondary causes of osteoporosis* by history, physical examination, and appropriate laboratory and radiologic investigations. The endocrine tests that are required include serum calcium (and, if necessary, PTH), sTSH, screen for Cushing syndrome with 1-mg overnight dexamethasone suppression test or 24-hour urinary free cortisol, and serum estradiol or testosterone and serum LH and FSH to rule out hypogonadism. Tests to rule out myeloma and malabsorption are important.

.

- Diagnosis in a patient without a fracture: bone mineral density.
- Diagnosis in a patient who has sustained a fracture with minimal trauma: the diagnosis is one of exclusion. Exclude osteomalacia, malignancy, and other bone disorders such as Paget disease.
- Differential diagnosis of osteomalacia is important: in osteoporosis, there is no pain in the absence of fracture, no proximal weakness, no biochemical abnormalities, and no pseudofractures.
- Osteoporosis is confirmed: exclude secondary causes.

Therapy

Prevention

Prevention includes estrogen replacement in women at and beyond menopause and provision of adequate calcium and vitamin D supplementation, particularly in the elderly. In women, at least 1,000 mg/day of calcium in the estrogen-replete woman and 1,500 mg/day in the estrogen-deficient woman. In men, 1,000 mg/day in men ages 24 to 65 and 1,500 mg/day thereafter. Other measures include regular exercise with good mechanical loading of the spine, avoidance of alcohol and tobacco abuse, and rapid correction of bone-depleting states such as hypogonadism and thyrotoxicosis. When estrogen therapy is contraindicated or refused, alendronate (a bisphosphonate), 5 mg/day, may be used.

- Prevention: estrogen replacement in menopausal and postmenopausal women; adequate calcium and vitamin D intake;

regular weight-bearing exercise, avoidance of life habits that are known bone depleters, and rapid correction of bone-depleting states.

Management of Established Disease

The goals of therapy are to decrease bone resorption and/or to enhance bone formation. Estrogen, calcium, calcitonin, and the bisphosphonate alendronate are the only drugs approved for reduction of bone resorption.

Estrogen replacement is the therapy of choice for prevention and treatment of established osteoporosis in women who do not have contraindications to its use. It decreases bone resorption and decreases the incidence of osteoporotic fractures by 50%. Estrogen is started as early as possible after the onset of the estrogen-deficient state and is continued for at least 10 to 15 years and, preferably, for life. It can be given orally, transdermally, topically, or by injection. Progestin is added if the patient has an intact uterus to reduce the risk of endometrial hyperplasia/endometrial carcinoma. Progestin can be added sequentially or continuously. Endometrial biopsy is indicated for women who have pretreatment irregular bleeding or who have unscheduled or severe bleeding develop during therapy. Yearly breast examination and mammography are indicated because of the possibility of a small increase in the risk of breast cancer and because of the trophic effect that estrogen may have on the tumor.

- Estrogen replacement: therapy of choice for prevention and treatment of established osteoporosis in women who do not have a contraindication to its use.
- Start early and give for at least 10-15 years, if not for a lifetime.
- Add progestin for women who still have their uterus.
- Consider endometrial sampling: women with pretreatment irregular bleeding or with unscheduled bleeding during therapy.
- Yearly breast examination and mammography.

Calcitonin is an approved antiresorptive agent (this effect is greatest in patients with high bone turnover). In the past, it was given parenterally, but nasal calcitonin was approved recently in the U.S. to treat osteoporosis. The recommended dose is 200 IU, a nasal puff in one nostril per day. It is effective in increasing bone mass in the axial, but not in the appendicular, skeleton. Nausea and flushing, the side effects of parenteral calcitonin, are not seen with the intranasal form, and tachyphylaxis does not occur. Its long-term efficacy is not known. In addition to its antiresorptive effect, calcitonin has a potent analgesic effect.

- Nasal calcitonin: effective in increasing axial but not appendicular skeleton; tachyphylaxis does not occur; long-term efficacy is not known; has an analgesic effect.

Alendronate is an oral bisphosphonate that was approved recently for use in the U.S. to treat osteoporosis. It has a potent antiresorptive effect when given in a dose of 10 mg/day. It is effective on the axial and appendicular skeleton, increases bone mass by 5% to 8%, and reduces the risk of vertebral (and probably also of appendicular) fractures. Its long-term skeletal effects and safety are unknown. The most significant and, fortunately, rare side effects are esophagitis, ulceration, and necrosis. It should be given in the morning with a glassful of water and on an empty stomach (any food or other drink may interfere with intestinal absorption), and the patient should not lie down for 30 to 60 minutes after the dose.

- Alendronate: potent effective bisphosphonate; antiresorptive; reduces incidence of fractures by 50%; long-term efficacy and safety are undocumented.
- Infrequent but potentially serious pill-induced esophagitis.

Currently, no therapy is available to stimulate bone formation effectively and safely. Fluoride can increase bone formation, but it is associated with inadequate mineralization and increased incidence of appendicular fractures and cannot be recommended. In females, androgens may have unacceptable androgenic side effects; these agents are indicated only in the treatment of hypogonadal males with osteoporosis.

Osteomalacia

Osteomalacia is a metabolic bone disorder in adults characterized by defective mineralization of newly formed bone matrix and accumulation of unmineralized osteoid. The equivalent disorder in children, in which bone matrix and cartilage are affected by defective mineralization, is rickets.

Etiology

The prerequisites for normal mineralization of bone include 1) normal calcium/phosphate product in the extracellular fluid; 2) normal osteoblast (and, in children, chondrocyte) function to synthesize normal matrix, to regulate concentrations of calcium/phosphate at the mineralization sites, and to optimize pH for deposition of calcium and phosphate on the mature osteoid; and 3) absence of mineralization inhibitors. Osteomalacia results when any or a combination of these prerequisites are not met.

Osteomalacia may be a consequence of vitamin D deficiency, phosphate deficiency, defects in bone mineralization, or defects in the bone matrix. *Vitamin D deficiency* results from decreased availability through 1) low intake (in the U.S., this occurs mainly in alcoholics and in institutionalized elderly patients); 2) malabsorption, which may be related to intestinal bypass, adult celiac disease, postgastrectomy state, or cholestasis; and 3) decreased exposure to the sun. Other causes include

decreased liver production of 25(OH)D because of decreased synthesis (liver disease, or with the use of drugs such as isoniazid) or increased metabolism to inactive compounds (as with the use of phenytoin, phenobarbital, or rifampin). Still other causes of vitamin D deficiency are decreased renal production of $1,25(OH)_2D$ (renal failure, renal tubular disorders, use of drugs such as ketoconazole or isoniazid, aging, and congenital deficiency of 1-hydroxylase enzyme [vitamin D-dependent rickets, type I]) and end-organ resistance to vitamin D (vitamin D-dependent rickets, type II). In the U.S., the most common causes of vitamin D deficiency are malabsorption, liver disease, end-stage renal disease, and aging.

Phosphate deficiency may result from decreased availability (nutritional or from the use of phosphate binders) or increased renal loss due to renal tubular phosphate leak. The latter is seen in hereditary X-linked hypophosphatemia, acquired tubular phosphate leak (tumor-induced osteomalacia), and a more generalized tubular defect (Fanconi syndrome) that may be hereditary or acquired. Tumor-induced osteomalacia is seen with tumors of mesenchymal origin and in prostate and breast cancer. It is mediated by a hormonal factor, phosphatonin, elaborated by the tumor.

Defects in bone mineralization may occur in hypophosphatasia, with the use of bisphosphonates or fluoride, or in aluminum, strontium, or cadmium toxicity.

Defects in bone matrix occur in fibrogenesis imperfecta ossium.

- Osteomalacia: defective mineralization and accumulation of unmineralized osteoid.
- Etiology: vitamin D deficiency, phosphate deficiency, and rare disorders of bone mineralization and the bone matrix.
- In the U.S., the most common causes of vitamin D deficiency are malabsorption, liver disease, end-stage renal disease, and aging.

Clinical Features

The clinical features are a composite of the features related to osteomalacia and those related to the etiologic disorder. Typical features related to osteomalacia include diffuse bone pain and tenderness, generalized but mostly proximal muscle weakness and a waddling gait, and occurrence of fractures. Associated features may include hypocalcemic features in vitamin D deficiency and rhabdomyolysis seen with severe hypophosphatemia.

- Diffuse bone pain and tenderness; muscle weakness (particularly proximal); waddling gait; propensity to fracture.

Biochemical Features

These features depend on the cause. Serum alkaline phosphatase level is usually increased in all types except hypophosphatasia. The findings of *osteomalacia related to vitamin D deficiency* include low serum calcium level and compensatory secondary hyperparathyroidism: serum calcium level is low or low-normal, PTH is increased, serum phosphate level is low, urine calcium is low, and plasma vitamin D levels are abnormal [low plasma 25(OH)D in nutritional, malabsorptive, or hepatic causes; low or low-normal plasma $1,25(OH)_2D$ in renal failure; and high plasma $1,25(OH)_2D$ in vitamin D-tissue resistance]. *Osteomalacia related to phosphate lack* typically includes hypophosphatemia, normal serum calcium level, normal PTH, and normal 25(OH)D. Plasma $1,25(OH)_2D$ may be low. In *osteomalacia related to defective mineralization or abnormal osteoid*, the serum calcium and phosphate levels are normal.

- Serum alkaline phosphatase: increased in all types of osteomalacia except hypophosphatasia.
- Vitamin D deficiency: low or normal serum calcium level; secondary hyperparathyroidism; low serum phosphate and urinary calcium. Assays of vitamin D: low 25(OH)D in malabsorption or nutritional or hepatic cause; low or low-normal $1,25(OH)_2D$ in renal failure; high $1,25(OH)_2D$ in vitamin D resistance.
- Phosphate lack: hypophosphatemia; normal serum calcium, PTH, and 25(OH)D levels.
- Osteomalacia due to disorders of bone mineralization or bone matrix: normal serum calcium and phosphate levels.

Radiologic Features

Standard radiologic investigations usually show a mild decrease in bone density associated with coarsening of the trabeculae. Radiologic features of secondary hyperparathyroidism also may be seen. In later stages, bone deformity or vertebral collapse may occur. In some patients with long-standing osteomalacia, increased bone density may be seen because of the abundance of unmineralized osteoid. There is radiologic evidence of pseudofractures (Looser zones or milkman fractures). These distinctive skeletal features of osteomalacia refer to ribbon-like zones of rarefaction that usually are symmetrical and oriented perpendicularly to the bone surface and may range in length from a few millimeters to several centimeters. They are found most commonly in pubic rami, the medial aspect of the femur near the femoral head, scapulae, and metatarsals.

- Pseudofractures: distinctive radiologic feature.

Diagnosis

Osteomalacia is suspected in the presence of suggestive symptoms and biochemical or radiologic abnormalities that occur in the context of a clinical setting associated with osteomalacia.

The differential diagnosis includes osteoporosis (see above) and Paget disease (bone pain is not generalized but localized to the affected bone, normal serum calcium and phosphate and increased alkaline phosphatase, and distinctive radiologic features).

The definitive diagnosis is made on the basis of bone biopsy findings following double tetracycline labeling. Increased unmineralized osteoid is pathognomonic of osteomalacia.

The etiologic diagnosis is based on consideration of the clinical setting, the appropriate use of laboratory and radiologic studies as dictated by a presumptive diagnosis, and the features characteristic of osteomalacia.

- Suspect osteomalacia: bone pain in the absence of fracture; elevated alkaline phosphatase; low or low-normal serum calcium or low phosphate; clinical setting. Pseudofractures are characteristic.
- Definitive diagnosis: characteristic bone biopsy findings.
- Define the cause.

Therapy

Effective therapy is based on the identification of the etiologic disorder and, when feasible, its proper management, and the provision of adequate extracellular calcium and phosphate levels at the mineralization front. This usually is achieved by calcium and vitamin D supplementation in states of calcium lack and by phosphate supplementation and administration of $1,25(OH)_2D$ in phosphopenic states [hypophosphatemic states are associated with decreased renal 1-hydroxylase activity and decreased production of $1,25(OH)_2D$]. *Calcium supplementation*—An oral calcium preparation providing 1,000 to 2,000 mg of elemental calcium daily. *Vitamin D supplementation*—Nutritional deficiency: vitamin D_2 2,000 to 4,000 IU/day until healing of the osteomalacia, and then 400 IU/day; malabsorption and liver disorders: vitamin D_2 25,000 to 50,000 IU/day; anticonvulsant-induced vitamin D lack: vitamin D_2 4,000 IU/day; and renal insufficiency: $1,25(OH)_2D$ 0.5 to 3.0 µg/day. *Phosphate supplementation*—Oral neutral phosphate, 1 to 2 g/day.

The goals of therapy are healing of bone, resolution of symptoms, and normalization of serum calcium, phosphate, and alkaline phosphatase levels and urine calcium. Monitor for complications of therapy, including hypercalciuria, hypercalcemia, and renal impairment. Hypercalciuria is the first sign of overdosage.

- Treat the cause; provide adequate mineral supplementation and vitamin D.
- Monitor therapy for complications: hypercalciuria, hypercalcemia, and renal impairment.

Paget Disease

Paget disease affects 3% of the population older than 45 years. It is a focal monostotic or polyostotic bone disorder characterized by disorganized bone remodeling, structurally weakened bone, and skeletal pain and deformities. The sites of predilection are the sacrum, spine, femur, tibia, skull, and pelvis. Pagetoid bone is enlarged and evolves through three phases: the lytic phase, the mosaic pattern, and the sclerotic phase. Genetic factors and a slow-virus infection may have a role in pathogenesis.

Clinical Features

Most patients are asymptomatic and present incidentally with the finding of increased alkaline phosphatase or of a radiologic abnormality. The two main symptoms are pain and deformity. The pain may be related to pagetoid involvement, degenerative changes in adjoining joints, or the development of osteosarcoma. The deformity may affect the long bones, skull, or spine. Alkaline phosphatase level is the most useful marker for disease activity, its extent, and response to therapy.

Complications—The most common complications of pagetic lesions are traumatic and pathologic fractures. The fractures may be complete or incomplete (fissure fractures). There is increased incidence of bone tumors. These occur in less than 1% of cases manifested by increased pain, with or without an enlarging mass at pagetic sites. Sarcomas are the most common tumors and are most frequent in the pelvis, femur, humerus, skull, and facial bones. These tumors have a poor prognosis. Neurologic complications are caused by impingement of nerves by the enlarging bone or by interference with the blood supply, e.g., cranial nerve II, V, VII, and VIII dysfunction due to involvement of the skull, invagination of the base of the skull by the cervical vertebrae (platybasia), and possibly hydrocephalus. Nerve impingement or ischemia occurs with involvement of the spine. High-output congestive heart failure is rare but can occur when more than 20% of the skeleton is affected. Hypercalciuria and hypercalcemia can occur with immobilization or fracture because of unopposed increase in bone resorption. Hypercalcemia in an ambulatory patient should suggest the presence of another disorder, such as primary hyperparathyroidism.

- Common complications: traumatic and pathologic fractures.

Diagnosis

Paget disease should be strongly suspected when a markedly increased alkaline phosphatase level is seen in healthy older patients with normal plasma calcium levels. Bone scan is the most sensitive test in identifying pagetic bone lesions; these appear as focal areas of markedly increased uptake or "hot" spots. Suspected pagetic areas should be evaluated further with plain radiographs to provide evidence of lytic areas, fissure fractures, extent of deformity, and information about adjacent joints.

Therapy

The objectives of therapy are to relieve symptoms and to treat or prevent complications. Medical therapy consists of the use of antiresorptive drugs. *Intravenous pamidronate* is first-line therapy because of its superior efficacy and minimal side-effect profile. It is given in a single dose of 60 to 90 mg in an infusion over 4 hours and has a sustained effect for 12 to 18 months. Reduction or normalization of alkaline phosphatase occurs in 50% to 75% of patients. The dose can be repeated if necessary with equal efficacy. Side effects include flu-like symptoms, hypocalcemia (prevented by giving 1,000 mg/day of oral calcium for 1 or 2 weeks after treatment). *Alternative treatments*: oral alendronate, salmon calcitonin, and etidronate. *Monitoring therapy*: serum alkaline phosphatase. Elective orthopedic surgery may be needed; if so, pretreat with antiresorptives to reduce bleeding and postoperative hypercalcemia. Urgent neurosurgery for CNS compressive disease; antiresorptives are given concomitantly.

DISORDERS OF THE ADRENAL GLANDS

Adrenocortical Failure

Etiology

Adrenocortical failure results most commonly from a decrease in production of adrenal hormone(s). It is caused very rarely by target tissue-resistance to adrenal hormone(s). It may involve the zona fasciculata/reticularis (cortisol and sex-steroid deficiency) or the zona glomerulosa (aldosterone deficiency), singly or in combination. Decreased production of adrenocortical hormone(s) may be a consequence of adrenocortical disease (primary failure) or trophic hormone loss (secondary failure).

Primary Adrenocortical Failure, Addison Disease

This is associated usually with deficiency of all three hormones. It may result from 1) organ-specific autoimmune adrenalitis; 2) granulomatous adrenalitis such as tuberculosis or histoplasmosis; 3) bilateral adrenal hemorrhage in the setting of anticoagulant use, trauma, or sepsis (particularly meningococcemia); 4) acquired immunodeficiency syndrome (cytomegalovirus or mycobacterial infection); 5) metastatic malignancies; 6) congenital adrenal enzyme deficiency; or 7) use of steroidogenesis-blocking drugs such as aminoglutethimide or o,p′-DDD. In the U.S., the most common causes are autoimmune adrenalitis and bilateral adrenal hemorrhage. In adrenal failure associated with infections, the failure may be due to the combined effects of adrenalitis and the use of drugs that inhibit steroidogenesis, such as ketoconazole, or those that accelerate cortisol clearance, such as rifampin and phenytoin.

Secondary Adrenocortical Failure

Secondary failure is conventionally defined as adrenocortical failure due to lack of ACTH; therefore, it affects cortisol and sex-steroid production but leaves aldosterone secretion basically intact. Lack of ACTH may occur as an isolated deficiency or, more commonly, in association with other features of hypopituitarism. It may be seen in association with pituitary tumors, hypothalamic or extrasellar disease, surgery or irradiation to the hypothalamic-pituitary region, or head injury. Functional central ACTH deficiency, the most common cause of ACTH lack, is a consequence of suppression of the axis by the prolonged use of glucocorticoids in pharmacologic doses for nonendocrine purposes. The deficiency becomes clinically manifest after withdrawal of the glucocorticoid therapy.

Hypoaldosteronism can occur independently of cortisol deficiency. It may result from a primary disorder of the zona glomerulosa or it may be secondary to angiotensin II deficiency. The latter may be a consequence of renin deficiency, or angiotensin converting enzyme deficiency.

- Adrenocortical failure: most commonly results from decreased production of its hormones.
- Primary adrenocortical failure: deficiency involves cortisol, sex steroids, and aldosterone. It has many organic and functional causes; in the U.S., it most commonly is due to autoimmune adrenalitis and bilateral adrenal hemorrhage; worldwide, tuberculosis adrenalitis is common.
- Secondary adrenal failure: due to ACTH lack; affects production of cortisol and sex steroids; aldosterone secretion is basically intact; most commonly due to functional suppression of the axis by prolonged glucocorticoid therapy. ACTH lack also may be a consequence of hypopituitary syndrome.
- Hypoaldosteronism: may occur independently; may result from primary adrenocortical disorder or impairment of the renin-angiotensin II axis.

Clinical Features

The clinical features depend on 1) the extent of hormone deficiency, whether partial or complete; 2) whether one or all hormones are involved; 3) the rapidity of development of the deficiency; and 4) when present, the changes in the levels of circulating ACTH.

The usual presentation is that of a chronic slowly evolving disorder. 1) *Cortisol deficiency*: decreased vitality, energy,

and stamina; muscle weakness; anorexia, weight loss, nausea, vomiting, or diarrhea (may mimic abdominal malignancy); mood changes; hyponatremia, fasting hypoglycemia, transient hypercalcemia, anemia, lymphocytosis, and eosinophilia. 2) *Aldosterone deficiency*: hypovolemia, hypotension, and orthostatism; and hyperkalemia, hyperchloremic acidosis, and azotemia. 3) *Androgen deficiency*: not significant in males; associated with decreased libido and thinning of sexual hair in females. 4) *ACTH-related symptoms*: ACTH excess in Addison disease is associated with hyperpigmentation. Pallor and the inability to tan result from ACTH deficiency in hypothalamic-pituitary disease.

In Addison disease, the adrenocortical hormone deficiency is global, and serum ACTH levels are high. In ACTH lack, serum ACTH levels are low, cortisol and sex steroids are deficient, aldosterone secretion is intact (except in long-standing severe cases when the response to salt depletion may be slightly impaired), and hyperkalemia and azotemia are absent; however, hyponatremia may occur because of the loss of the restraining influence of cortisol on ADH secretion and action. In renin-angiotensin axis impairment, only aldosterone secretion is lacking.

Acute Adrenocortical Failure or Adrenal Crisis

Adrenal crisis is suggested in the presence of dehydration, hypotension, or shock out of proportion to severity of the current illness, nausea, vomiting with a history of anorexia and weight loss, abdominal pain (may mimic acute abdomen), unexplained fever, hyponatremia, hyperkalemia, azotemia, hypercalcemia, eosinophilia, and hypoglycemia. It often is precipitated by the occurrence of an intercurrent illness in a patient with unrecognized adrenocortical failure or who recently had glucocorticoid therapy withdrawn or in a patient who has sustained bilateral hemorrhage of the adrenals.

- Addison disease: usually presents as a chronic slowly evolving syndrome; manifestations are a composite of the effects of cortisol, sex steroids, aldosterone lack, and ACTH excess.
- Adrenocortical crisis: 1) intercurrent illness in a patient with unrecognized adrenocortical failure or with known disease who did not increase cortisol replacement appropriately or 2) adrenal hemorrhage bilaterally.

Diagnosis

Endocrine Diagnosis

The diagnosis is confirmed most reliably and effectively by the cosyntropin (Cortrosyn) test, which assesses the cortisol response to a synthetic, rapidly acting ACTH (250 μg). The normal response to cosyntropin is an increase in plasma cortisol greater than 7 μg/dL from baseline value or to an absolute value greater than 18 μg/dL.

An impaired response to cosyntropin establishes adrenocortical failure but does not delineate its type. Definition of whether the failure is primary or secondary in type rests on the measurement of serum ACTH: a high ACTH level points to Addison disease and a low or "inappropriately normal" level indicates secondary failure. If ACTH assays are not available, the differentiation rests on the long ACTH stimulation test: continued unresponsiveness indicates Addison disease and a stepwise response points to secondary failure.

A normal response to cosyntropin rules out Addison disease but does not exclude ACTH lack, which is either partial or of recent onset. If the diagnosis is still suspected, a metyrapone or insulin-hypoglycemia test is performed: a normal response excludes adrenocortical failure; an impaired response in a patient who has a normal response to cosyntropin points to secondary failure. A low-dose cosyntropin test (1 μg) has recently been advocated as a reliable alternative for the diagnosis of recent or partial ACTH lack.

- Perform the cosyntropin test.
- Subnormal cortisol response: establishes the diagnosis of adrenocortical failure. Cannot differentiate Addison disease from failure due to hypothalamic-pituitary disease. This differentiation is based on serum ACTH measurements or, if not available, on the long ACTH stimulation test.
- Normal cortisol response: excludes Addison disease. Does not rule out secondary adrenocortical failure that is partial or of recent onset. A metyrapone test or an insulin-hypoglycemia test is important for such diagnosis.

Etiologic Diagnosis

In Addison disease, an etiologic diagnosis depends on clinical assessment and a search for other autoimmune disorders, infections, and neoplasms. In secondary failure, assessment of other pituitary functions and MRI or CT of the head are performed.

- After the diagnosis is established, search for the cause.

Therapy

Primary adrenocortical failure requires glucocorticoid and mineralocorticoid replacement therapy, whereas secondary failure requires only glucocorticoid replacement. Patient education is a critical component of therapy: the need for disciplined daily life-long therapy, the manner of dosage adjustments during acute illness, the use of injectable glucocorticoids in circumstances when oral replacement therapy is not possible, and the use of an identification bracelet or necklace.

Primary Adrenocortical Failure

Glucocorticoid therapy: hydrocortisone (10-20 mg in a.m. and 5-10 mg in early p.m.) or prednisone (5 mg in a.m. and 0-2.5 mg in early p.m.). The adequacy of therapy is assessed by the patient's sense of well-being, the decrease in pigmentation, and the absence of manifestations of excessive glucocorticoid replacement; ACTH levels are not always reliable for monitoring the adequacy of therapy. *Mineralocorticoid therapy*: fludrocortisone, 0.05 to 0.2 mg orally and liberal salt intake. The adequacy of replacement is monitored by measurement of the supine and standing blood pressure, presence of edema, serum potassium level, and, if needed, plasma renin activity.

- Primary adrenocortical failure requires glucocorticoid and usually mineralocorticoid therapy.
- Secondary failure requires only glucocorticoid therapy.
- Patient education is a critical component of effective management.
- Therapy for primary adrenocortical failure: hydrocortisone, 20 mg in a.m. and 10 mg in early p.m., or equivalent; fludrocortisone, 0.05-0.2 mg orally; liberal salt intake.

Acute Illness Coverage

In mild-to-moderate acute illness, the glucocorticoid dosage is doubled or tripled and given at such dosage for the duration of the illness. In the presence of severe illness or vomiting, the patient needs to use parenteral dexamethasone (4 mg intramuscularly) and seek prompt medical help. For minor procedures performed under local anesthesia and for most radiologic procedures, no special preparation is required. For moderately stressful procedures such as endoscopy, hydrocortisone (100 mg intravenously) or another glucocorticoid in equivalent dosage should be given 1 hour before the procedure. For major surgery, 100 mg hydrocortisone is given intravenously before the induction of anesthesia and repeated every 6 to 8 hours for the first 24 hours; the dose then is tapered at a rate that depends on the patient's recovery (usually a decrease of dosage by 50%/day to maintenance levels). Hydrocortisone, in the stress-dosage mentioned, has an adequate mineralocorticoid effect.

- Glucocorticoid replacement needs to be modified in acute medical or surgical illness and when oral therapy is not possible.

Management of Adrenal Crisis

Prompt management is critical. 1) Establish intravenous access: draw blood for measuring electrolytes, glucose, plasma cortisol level, and serum ACTH level. 2) Do not wait for the results but institute management as soon as the diagnosis is suspected. Promptly infuse saline/dextrose to restore blood and extracellular fluid volume; give hydrocortisone, 100 mg every 6 hours; specific mineralocorticoid therapy usually is not necessary because hydrocortisone in these large doses will have a mineralocorticoid effect. 3) Use other supportive measures as needed. 4) After the patient's condition is stabilized, continue infusions, but at a lower rate. 5) Search for and treat possible infections and precipitating causes. 6) After the patient's condition has stabilized, switch the glucocorticoid therapy to dexamethasone (it will not interfere with plasma cortisol measurements) and perform the cosyntropin stimulation test to initiate the adrenocortical diagnostic process. Taper glucocorticoids to a maintenance level and begin mineralocorticoid replacement, if needed, after saline infusion is stopped.

- Prompt management is critical. Draw blood for measurement of electrolytes, glucose, plasma cortisol, and serum ACTH.
- Do not wait for results. Institute management as soon as the diagnosis is suspected.
- Parenteral glucocorticoids are critical. Ensure adequate fluid, electrolytes, and volume replacement. Search for and treat any underlying precipitating disorder such as infection.
- After stabilization, continue infusions at a lower rate. Perform the cosyntropin test.
- With recovery, taper glucocorticoid therapy to maintenance dosage and, in patients with primary failure, add mineralocorticoid replacement.

Cushing Syndrome

Etiology

Cushing syndrome may be of exogenous or endogenous origin. *Exogenous Cushing syndrome* is the most common cause of the syndrome. It may be the consequence of the therapeutic chronic use of supraphysiologic doses of cortisol or, more commonly, of its analogs such as prednisone, in the management of inflammatory, allergic, or neoplastic disorders. It rarely is caused by the surreptitious use of these agents.

Endogenous Cushing syndrome is caused by cortisol overproduction by the adrenal cortex. It may result from a primary adrenal, autonomous, and non-ACTH-dependent disorder. Such disorders include 1) an adrenal adenoma (a small <3 cm diameter differentiated tumor) that produces a "pure glucocorticoid excess" syndrome, 2) an undifferentiated adrenal carcinoma (usually >6 cm in diameter) that is inefficient in steroidogenesis and produces (in addition to cortisol) large quantities of adrenal androgens, or 3) the rare macronodular or micronodular adrenal hyperplasia.

- Endogenous Cushing syndrome: may result from a primary adrenal, autonomous, and non-ACTH-dependent disorder.

Another cause of endogenous Cushing syndrome is a secondary adrenal disorder due to excessive secretion of ACTH, the *ACTH-dependent Cushing syndrome*. This, in turn, may be caused by 1) a pituitary corticotroph-cell adenoma or, rarely, hyperplasia, so-called *Cushing disease*. The adenoma usually is small; more than 50% of these tumors are not detected on MRI. 2) *Ectopic ACTH-producing tumors*: these usually are rapidly growing malignant tumors of the lung, thymus, pancreas, or pheochromocytoma or medullary carcinoma of the thyroid. Alternatively, they may be indolent and be caused by bronchial carcinoids. 3) Very rarely, by *CRH-producing tumors* such as bronchial carcinoids, medullary cancer of the thyroid, and metastatic prostate carcinoma.

The most common causes of endogenous Cushing syndrome are Cushing disease (60%), adrenal tumors (25%), and ectopic-ACTH tumors (15%).

- Exogenous glucocorticoid therapy is the most common cause of Cushing syndrome.
- Endogenous Cushing syndrome is best classified into ACTH-independent and ACTH-dependent disorders.
- ACTH-independent disorders: adrenal tumors (25%) and, rarely, nodular hyperplasias.
- ACTH-dependent disorders: Cushing disease (60%), ectopic-ACTH disorders (15%), and, rarely, ectopic-CRH tumors.

Clinical Features

The clinical features of Cushing syndrome include the following:

1. Features of cortisol excess. These are the dominant features of the syndrome and may present in two ways. a) The usual features are those of chronic indolent cortisol excess (weight gain and central obesity; thin skin, easy bruisability, wide violaceous striae; plethora; muscle weakness; osteoporosis; and, in growing children or adolescents, cessation of linear growth; lanugo hair; hypertension; insulin resistance and secondary diabetes; hypercalciuria and renal stones; and propensity to fungal infections). b) Other features are those of severe and rapidly evolving cortisol excess as seen in the usual ectopic-ACTH malignant tumor, in which the manifestations may be dominated by weight loss, weakness, secondary diabetes, and the mineralocorticoid effects of hypertension, edema, and hypokalemia. The disorder may be too short in duration to allow the development of the more classic features of chronic cortisol excess.

2. Features of adrenal-androgen excess. These may be modest and lead to acne, hirsutism, and menstrual irregularities as in the usual cases of Cushing disease and ACTH-producing bronchial carcinoids or they may

be more severe and lead to virilization as in adrenal carcinoma. These features may be absent in patients with glucocorticoid-producing adrenal adenoma.

3. Features of ACTH excess. When produced in significant quantities, as in the usual malignant causes of ectopic-ACTH tumors, the excess may lead to hyperpigmentation.

4. Anatomical effects of the underlying tumor. These include extrasellar effects with pituitary macroadenomas, bronchopulmonary effects of lung cancer, and abdominal pain caused by adrenocortical carcinoma or metastatic effects of malignant causal tumors.

5. Infrequently, the clinical manifestations of cortisol excess are subtle, and the causal tumor presents initially as an incidental radiologic abnormality such as a pituitary or an adrenal incidentaloma.

- Features of cortisol excess dominate the picture; variably one may see the features of adrenal-androgen excess, ACTH excess, and the mass effects of the underlying tumor. Occasionally, attention may be drawn to the syndrome by the finding of a pituitary or an adrenal incidentaloma.
- Features of cortisol excess are usually chronic and slowly evolving, giving rise to the typical cushingoid features; with malignant ectopic-ACTH tumors, the clinical features may be dominated by weight loss, weakness, edema, hyperkalemia, hypertension, and secondary diabetes.

Diagnosis

Identification of Cushing Syndrome

The best screening tests for Cushing syndrome are the 1-mg overnight dexamethasone suppression test and urinary free cortisol. The reference-standard confirmatory test is the 2-day 2-mg/day low-dose dexamethasone suppression test. The demonstration of abnormal dexamethasone suppressibility or a significantly increased urinary free cortisol point to a diagnosis of Cushing syndrome, but only after alcoholism, depression, and acute illness have been excluded.

The 1-mg dexamethasone suppression test is a reliable screening test. The normal response is a plasma cortisol value less than 5 mg/dL. Patients with Cushing syndrome usually have values greater than 10 mg/dL. False-positive test results occur in 13% of patients with simple obesity and in 25% of chronically ill patients. Other causes of false-positive responses include acute illness, depression, estrogen use, pregnancy, and the use of drugs that can accelerate dexamethasone metabolism (phenytoin and barbiturates).

Urinary free cortisol is increased in more than 97% of patients with Cushing syndrome. However, it can also be increased in acute illness, trauma, surgery, alcoholism, and depression. Importantly, it can be modestly increased in simple obesity, but a value greater than 300 µg/24 hr usually points to Cushing syndrome.

The 2-mg low-dose dexamethasone suppression test is the standard test for the diagnosis of Cushing syndrome. False-positive results can be seen in patients with acute illness, severe stress, alcoholism, or depression and with the use of drugs known to accelerate dexamethasone metabolism.

- Screening tests: 1-mg dexamethasone test or urinary free cortisol (most reliable).
- Definitive test: urinary free cortisol >300 µg/24 hr or failure of normal suppression in the 2-mg 2-day low-dose dexamethasone suppression test.
- Exclude acute illness, alcoholism, and depression.

Etiologic Diagnosis

The critical tests include the serum ACTH level to differentiate between ACTH-dependent and ACTH-independent causes. Plasma ACTH levels are suppressed (<20 pg/mL) in patients with adrenal tumors, "normal" (20-80 pg/mL) or modestly increased (<200 pg/mL) in those with Cushing disease or ectopic-ACTH caused by bronchial carcinoids; and very high (>200 pg/mL) in most patients with the usual ectopic-ACTH tumor.

Another test is the 8-mg (2 mg qid for 2 days or 8 mg overnight) high-dose dexamethasone suppression test to distinguish between causes resistant to feedback inhibition (adrenal tumors and most ectopic ACTH tumors) from those that are partially autonomous and suppressible (Cushing disease and some patients with bronchial carcinoids).

Also important is radiologic assessment for tumor localization: pituitary, adrenal, or ectopic.

Patients with bronchial carcinoids may be indistinguishable clinically and biochemically from patients with Cushing disease. If CT or MRI of the sella and CT of the chest do not show any abnormality, resort to petrosal sinus selective venous sampling with CRH provocative testing. A central-to-peripheral ACTH gradient greater than 3:1 points to Cushing disease. Petrosal sinus sampling is very helpful in localizing the side that harbors the pituitary tumor, but only in a person who has not had surgery.

- The most important tests to delineate the cause: serum ACTH, the 8-mg high-dose dexamethasone suppression test, and radiologic evaluation.
- Cushing syndrome caused by adrenal tumor: low/undetectable ACTH level, nonsuppressible hypercortisol state, and an adrenal mass found on abdominal CT.
- Cushing syndrome caused by ectopic ACTH tumor: evident ectopic tumor, rapid clinical course, very high ACTH levels (>200 pg/mL), and nonsuppressibility.
- Cushing disease: ACTH values are normal/moderately increased (<200 pg/mL), hypercortisol state is dexametha-

sone-suppressible in >66% of patients, and CT/MRI of the sella may show a pituitary tumor. About 50% of patients have normal sellar radiographic features and about 33% have dexamethasone-nonsuppressibility.

- Patients with bronchial carcinoids: may be indistinguishable clinically and biochemically from patients with Cushing disease.
- If CT/MRI of the sella and CT of the chest show no abnormality, resort to petrosal sinus selective venous sampling with CRH provocative testing.

Therapy

1. Cushing disease: the treatment of choice is transsphenoidal surgical adenomectomy or subtotal hypophysectomy. For postoperative persistent disease, the therapeutic options include a) pituitary radiation therapy and the interim use of steroidogenesis-blockers such as ketoconazole or b) bilateral adrenalectomy and postoperative pituitary irradiation to reduce the risk of development of Nelson-Salassa syndrome (a usually progressive ACTH-pituitary tumor featuring hyperpigmentation and tumor-extrasellar effects).
2. Adrenal adenoma: unilateral adrenalectomy.
3. Adrenal carcinoma: unilateral adrenalectomy; o,p'-DDD, and steroidogenesis blockers are indicated for persistent or recurrent disease.
4. Ectopic-ACTH tumor: tumor excision; if incurable, steroidogenesis blockers are used for the short term. Bilateral adrenalectomy is recommended for tumors with a more indolent course.

   In all cases of Cushing syndrome, surgical excision of the causative tumor is followed by a period of cortisol lack caused by the suppressed hypothalamic-pituitary adrenal axis. It may take up to 1 or 2 years for the axis to recover; during this period, the patient needs glucocorticoid replacement therapy. If bilateral adrenalectomy is performed, the patient will need life-long glucocorticoid and mineralocorticoid replacement.

- A period of suppression of the normal axis follows the removal of the causative tumor and may last up to 1-2 years. During this period, treat with glucocorticoids, as in adrenocortical failure.
- Bilateral adrenalectomy: life-long glucocorticoid and mineralocorticoid replacement.

Primary Aldosteronism

Etiology

Primary aldosteronism results from the autonomous renin-angiotensin-independent disorder of the zona glomerulosa. It may be caused by aldosterone-producing adenoma (65%), idiopathic bilateral hyperplasia (30%), unilateral adrenal hyperplasia (<5%), adrenocortical carcinoma (<3%), and, very rarely, the familial disorder glucocorticoid-remediable aldosteronism.

Clinical Features

Most patients present with hypertension and hypokalemia. The hypertension can be mild to severe (malignant hypertension is extremely rare). Hypokalemia is typically unprovoked, but it may be provoked significantly and rapidly by the use of diuretic therapy. Most patients are asymptomatic, but a few may complain of the effects of hypokalemic alkalosis (fatigue and muscle weakness, paresthesias, orthostatic hypotension, nephrogenic diabetes insipidus, and glucose intolerance). Edema typically is absent. A subset of patients with primary aldosteronism have normokalemia (see below).

- Presentation: usually asymptomatic hypertension and unprovoked or easily provoked hypokalemia.
- Absence of edema because of "escape" from the salt-retaining effects; no escape occurs from the potassium and hydrogen ion-losing state.

Diagnosis

The diagnosis of primary aldosteronism rests on documenting autonomous aldosterone hypersecretion and on defining the underlying cause. Classically, primary aldosteronism results in hypertension, hypokalemia from inappropriate renal potassium loss, and suppressed plasma renin activity. Aldosterone secretion is excessive and autonomous of regulation by the renin-angiotensin system.

Endocrine Diagnosis

1. *Hypokalemia* is a classic finding in primary aldosteronism; however, it may be absent, and it is nonspecific. Patients with primary aldosteronism who typically have unprovoked hypokalemia may be normokalemic under the following circumstances: salt restriction and unavailability of sodium at the distal tubule for exchange with potassium or use of aldosterone receptor blockers and potassium-sparing diuretics such as spironolactone. Also, there is a subset of patients with normokalemic primary aldosteronism. Hypokalemia may be induced in any hypertensive patient by potassium loss from a gastrointestinal disorder (vomiting, diarrhea, or laxative abuse) or renal disorder (diuretics, other types of mineralocorticoid excess, or intrinsic renal disease). *Inappropriate kaliuresis*: check urinary potassium. In a patient with hypokalemia, a urinary potassium greater than 30 mEq/24 hr points to renal potassium wasting and increases the suspicion of aldosteronism.

2. Delineation of aldosterone excess and its nature. The best screening procedure is to obtain plasma aldosterone (PA) and renin activity (PRA) measurements and to calculate the *PA/PRA ratio* (PA in ng/dL and PRA in ng/mL per hr). *It is important to correct hypokalemia before measurements of aldosterone levels, because hypokalemia may reduce the aldosterone production in primary aldosteronism.* An increased PA and a suppressed PRA with a PA/PRA ratio greater than 20 points to the likelihood of primary aldosteronism. The diagnosis is confirmed by the demonstration of nonsuppressibility of aldosterone production (saline loading test or captopril test). An increased PA and an increased PRA with a PA/PRA ratio of less than 10 point to secondary aldosteronism. A low PA and a low PRA point to another mineralocorticoid as the cause of hypertension and hypokalemia.

- Unprovoked or easily provoked hypokalemia is characteristic.
- Exclude extrarenal potassium loss: check urinary potassium, a value >30 mEq/L in a patient with hypokalemia points to renal potassium-losing state, which includes mineralocorticoid excess.
- Patients with primary aldosteronism may have normokalemia: salt restriction (provoke by salt-loading), use of potassium-sparing diuretic (discontinue medication and recheck in 8 weeks).
- Best screening test: plasma aldosterone and plasma renin activity and calculating the PA/PRA ratio.
- PA/PRA ratio: >20 in primary aldosteronism; <10 in secondary aldosteronism.
- Confirm diagnosis: demonstrate autonomy of aldosterone production (saline loading fails to suppress aldosterone production).

Etiologic Diagnosis

The major challenge is differentiating between an aldosterone-producing adenoma and bilateral adrenal hyperplasia. This differentiation has important therapeutic implications. An aldosterone-secreting adenoma is treated surgically by unilateral adrenalectomy. However, bilateral hyperplasia is treated medically by the use of an aldosterone antagonist (see below). Modalities used to make this differentiation include CT of the adrenals, iodocholesterol scan, and selective venous sampling. CT of the adrenals is the most frequently used modality. An adrenal mass usually points to an aldosterone-producing adenoma. However, CT may be misleading because adenomas are small tumors and many may be missed, an adrenal mass seen on CT may not be an aldosteronoma but an adrenal incidentaloma, and the mass may be a hyperplastic nodule in macronodular bilateral adrenal hyperplasia. Selective venous sampling is the most accurate localizing procedure. A unilateral gradient points to an aldosteronoma, and the absence of a gradient points to bilateral hyperplasia. However, this procedure is difficult and requires radiologic expertise.

- The major differential diagnosis in primary aldosteronism: is the cause an adenoma or bilateral hyperplasia?
- The most reliable localizing test is selective venous sampling; a unilateral gradient points to an adenoma. The test is difficult and requires expertise.
- CT may demonstrate an adrenal mass, but there are several pitfalls.
- Iodocholesterol scanning may also be helpful.

Glucocorticoid-remediable hyperaldosteronism is a very rare familial autosomal dominant disorder in which the defect is chimeric gene duplication whereby the enzyme 11-hydroxylase in the zona fasciculata is fused with aldosterone synthetase. This allows the expression of the aldosterone synthetase effect in the zona fasciculata and the production of aldosterone under the regulation of ACTH and not angiotensin II. It becomes manifest in childhood or adolescence with the typical picture of primary aldosteronism. The diagnosis is based on the young age of the patient, a positive family history, an elevated 24-hour-urinary 18-hydroxycortisol and 18-oxotetrahydrocortisol (18-hydroxylated metabolites of hydrocortisone), and the dexamethasone-suppressibility of the clinical and biochemical features.

Differential Diagnosis

The major differential diagnoses are to distinguish these patients from those with the hypertensive variants of secondary aldosteronism and those with other causes of mineralocorticoid hypertension.

Secondary aldosteronism associated with hypertension results from increased renin production as a consequence of renal artery stenosis, malignant hypertension, or a renin-producing tumor. Plasma renin activity, angiotensin II, and aldosterone production are increased, and patients present with renin-dependent hyperaldosteronism with hypertension and hypokalemia.

Mineralocorticoid-induced hypertension, caused by excess mineralocorticoid other than aldosterone, is seen in deoxycorticosterone-producing tumor, an 11- or 17-hydroxylase congenital adrenal hyperplasia, Cushing syndrome, and genetic or acquired (use of licorice or chewing tobacco) deficiency of the enzyme 11-hydroxysteroid-dehydrogenase. This enzyme is present in the distal renal tubule and catalyzes the local biologic inactivation of hydrocortisone to cortisone. Such inactivation prevents hydrocortisone from binding to the mineralocorticoid receptor and functioning as a mineralocorticoid at the renal tubule. Deficiency of this enzyme, relative or absolute, leads to increased hydrocortisone levels at the distal tubule and to hydrocortisone-induced mineralocorticoid effect. In all these disorders, hypertension and hypokalemia occur, with suppressed plasma renin activity and suppressed production of aldosterone.

- Secondary aldosteronism: hypertension, hypokalemia, increased aldosterone, increased plasma renin activity.
- Other types of mineralocorticoid-induced hypertension: hypertension, hypokalemia, low aldosterone, suppressed plasma renin activity.

Therapy

Surgical unilateral adrenalectomy is the treatment of choice for aldosteronoma or unilateral hyperplasia unless the patient is a poor surgical risk. Surgery corrects the hypokalemia (100%) and normalizes or significantly improves the hypertension in about 70% of patients. Patients with persistent postoperative hypertension should be treated with standard antihypertensive drug therapy.

Medical treatment is indicated for the management of bilateral adrenal hyperplasia and for patients with aldosteronoma who are poor surgical risks. (Surgical treatment in hyperplasia requires bilateral adrenalectomy to normalize the serum potassium level but it rarely restores blood pressure to normal levels.) This consists of dietary salt restriction and the use of potassium-sparing diuretics. Spironolactone, an aldosterone antagonist, is given in a dose of 25 to 100 mg/8 to 12 hours. It restores normokalemia and normalizes blood pressure in most patients. Adverse effects include gastrointestinal upset, menstrual irregularity, and, in men, gynecomastia and impaired libido and potency. Women of childbearing age who take spironolactone should use oral contraceptives, because the drug may cause feminization of the male fetus through its androgen-blocking effects. Men may be treated more conveniently with amiloride (10-20 mg/day) or triamterene (50-150 mg/day). In glucocorticoid-remediable hyperaldosteronism, dexamethasone may be given in the dose of 1 mg/day.

- Surgery: unilateral adrenalectomy for patients with aldosteronoma unless the patient refuses surgery or is a poor surgical risk.
- Medical therapy: for patients with hyperplasia and for those with aldosteronoma who are poor surgical risks or who refuse surgery.
- Medical treatment: dietary salt restriction and potassium-sparing diuretics. Spironolactone, an aldosterone antagonist, is most commonly used.

- In glucocorticoid-remediable hyperaldosteronism: dexamethasone, 1 mg/day.

Pheochromocytoma

Etiology

Pheochromocytomas are chromaffin tumors that usually arise in the adrenal medulla, infrequently along the sympathetic chain in the abdomen, thorax, or neck and rarely in sympathetic tissue in the walls of the urinary bladder. They are important because 1) although rare and occurring in less than 1% of all hypertensive disorders, they usually present with a distinctive recognizable clinical syndrome, are curable, and, if untreated, can be lethal; 2) 10% of the tumors are malignant; and 3) 10% of the tumors are familial. More than 90% of the tumors are sporadic, adrenal in location, unilateral, and benign. Familial pheochromocytomas are more likely to be intra-adrenal, bilateral, and malignant. Extra-adrenal tumors are usually located in the abdomen. Less than 1% of pheochromocytomas are located in the chest or neck. Pheochromocytomas generally secrete both epinephrine and norepinephrine. Epinephrine-secreting tumors are located in either the adrenal medulla or in the organs of Zuckerkandl. Pheochromocytomas can secrete catecholamines persistently or episodically. Dopamine secretion occurs mostly with undifferentiated malignant tumors.

Clinical Features

Pheochromocytomas can be asymptomatic and discovered incidentally on abdominal imaging. More commonly, they are suspected because of the presence of 1) hypertension, particularly if it is labile, paroxysmal, or refractory to treatment; 2) paroxysmal symptoms of headaches, palpitations, sweating, anxiety with a feeling of impending doom, and pallor; 3) heat intolerance, sweating, and weight loss; 4) unexplained abdominal or chest pain; 5) orthostatic hypotension or unexplained shock after trauma, surgery, or parturition; 6) paradoxical response to some antihypertensive therapy (e.g., hydralazine, reserpine, guanethidine, or β-blockers); and 7) family history of pheochromocytoma, MEN IIA (Sipple syndrome: pheochromocytoma, medullary cancer of the thyroid, and primary hyperparathyroidism) or MEN IIB (mucosal neuroma syndrome: medullary cancer of the thyroid, pheochromocytoma, mucosal neuromas, alimentary ganglioneuromatosis, and marfanoid habitus), or von Hippel-Lindau disease, or neurofibromatosis. In most patients, the paroxysmal symptoms are stereotyped and vary only in severity or frequency. The common symptoms are headache, palpitations, and sweating; absence of all three in a hypertensive patient strongly points away from pheochromocytoma. Laboratory features include hemoconcentration, hyperglycemia, and, occasionally, hypercalcemia.

- Pheochromocytomas can be asymptomatic; discovered incidentally on abdominal imaging. More commonly, they are suspected because of hypertension or paroxysmal symptoms.
- Common symptoms: headache, palpitations, and sweating. Absence of all three symptoms in a hypertensive patient strongly points away from pheochromocytoma.
- Symptoms may be paroxysmal. In most patients, the paroxysmal symptoms are stereotyped and vary only in severity or frequency.
- Other presentations: heat intolerance, sweating, weight loss, unexplained abdominal or chest pain, paradoxical response to some antihypertensive agents, orthostatic hypotension, unexplained shock.
- Family history of pheochromocytoma, MEN IIA or MEN IIB, or other neuroectodermal syndromes.

Diagnosis

The diagnosis of pheochromocytoma proceeds in three steps: 1) to document catecholamine hypersecretion, 2) to exclude other disorders associated with hypertension and catecholamine excess, and 3) to localize the pheochromocytoma.

Endocrine Diagnosis

Endocrine diagnosis is based principally on urinary measurements of free catecholamines and their urinary metabolites, metanephrines, and vanillylmandelic acid. No one measurement is clearly superior to the others, and, in practice, the three measurements are made on the same 24-hour urine collection. (In all urine collections, creatinine is measured to ensure the adequacy of the collection. Among the drugs that can interfere with the usefulness of the assays are catecholamine-containing drugs, α-methyldopa, labetalol, monoamine oxidase inhibitors, and adrenergic blockers.) Normal values in a hypertensive, or otherwise symptomatic, patient are sufficient to exclude the diagnosis. Increased values are compatible with pheochromocytoma (see below). In borderline cases, the urinary studies can be repeated. In patients who have paroxysmal symptoms, the diagnostic yield can be significantly increased by initiating collection during or shortly after a paroxysm.

Plasma catecholamines generally are used as adjuncts to urinary studies. They must be obtained under strict conditions: basal state, supine position, and special collection tools. They represent secretion over a short period of time and are most useful if obtained during a paroxysm or in conjunction with provocative or suppression tests. A value greater than 2,000 ng/L is obtained in most patients with pheochromocytoma. A value less than 500 ng/L excludes the diagnosis. A value between 500 and 2,000 ng/L dictates the use of a provocative test (see below).

Demonstration of increased values of urinary catecholamines and their metabolites in a hypertensive patient establishes the diagnosis of pheochromocytoma only if confounding drugs are excluded and medical conditions associated with hypertension and hypersecretion of catecholamines are excluded (severe stress, intercurrent illness, acute myocardial ischemia, abrupt withdrawal of clonidine, drug and food interaction with monoamine oxidase inhibitors, excessive use of sympathomimetic amines).

The *glucagon provocative test* is potentially hazardous and has no place in routine evaluation. Occasionally, it may be useful for normotensive patients with a history of paroxysmal symptoms suggestive of pheochromocytoma. In these patients, the provocative test needs to be done under strictly monitored circumstances and only after α-blockade has been instituted to prevent adverse cardiovascular effects. Plasma catecholamine levels greater than 2,000 pg/mL within 3 to 5 min after the intravenous administration of 1 mg of glucagon point to the presence of pheochromocytoma. The *clonidine suppression test* has limited usefulness. A 50% decrease in plasma catecholamines within 3 hours after the administration of 0.3 mg of clonidine points away from pheochromocytoma.

- Document catecholamine hypersecretion. Check urinary catecholamines or metabolites. Normal values in a hypertensive patient exclude the diagnosis. In patients with paroxysmal symptoms, the diagnostic yield is increased significantly by initiating collection during or shortly after a paroxysm.
- Increased values in hypertensive patients establish the diagnosis only if other disorders associated with hypertension and catecholamine excess are excluded (severe stress, intercurrent illness, acute myocardial ischemia, or abrupt withdrawal of clonidine).
- Plasma catecholamines: adjuncts to urinary studies; most useful if obtained during a paroxysm or in conjunction with provocative or suppression tests.
- The glucagon provocative test is potentially hazardous and has no place in routine evaluation. Clonidine suppression test has limited usefulness.

Radiologic Localization

CT and MRI of the abdomen (and, if findings are negative, the pelvis, thorax, and neck) are the mainstay of radiologic localization. They have a sensitivity and specificity greater than 90%. CT has better spatial resolution. MRI is better at characterizing the mass, with pheochromocytomas showing high-signal intensity on T_2-weighted images. MRI is considered the radiologic procedure of choice. *Labelled ^{123}I-metaiodobenzylguanidine (^{123}I-MiBG)* is taken up by the neoplastic chromaffin tissue (adrenal or extra-adrenal) and can be used as an adjunct to CT or MRI. Its advantages are that it can be used for whole-body scanning and is better at delineating extra-adrenal tumors and metastases. It may be helpful even in delineating preclinical adrenal medullary hyperplasia. The disadvantages include a higher false-negative rate and the requirement of several days for completion.

- Radiologic localization of the pheochromocytoma is attempted only after biochemical confirmation.
- CT or MRI of the abdomen (if negative findings, image the pelvis and thorax): the mainstays of radiologic localization.
- MRI is the radiologic procedure of choice. Pheochromocytomas appear as high-intensity signal masses on T_2-weighted images.
- Labelled ^{123}I-MiBG is taken up by neoplastic chromaffin tissue; used as adjunct to CT or MRI.

Therapy

Surgical excision of the tumor is curative. Medical treatment is used in preoperative preparation to diminish perioperative morbidity and mortality and on a chronic basis in surgical failures. α-Adrenergic blockade is the cornerstone of medical therapy and should be instituted as soon as the diagnosis is made. Phenoxybenzamine is the drug of choice to control the hypertension and to restore plasma volume. Start with a dose of 10 mg twice daily and increase every few days until the desired effect is obtained. Its major side effect is postural hypotension. Alternate drugs include prazosin, terazosin, labetalol, nifedipine, and angiotensin-converting enzyme (ACE) inhibitors. β-Adrenergic blockers may be necessary to control tachyarrhythmias; these drugs should be used only after adequate α-blockade to prevent exacerbation of the hypertension. Propranolol, 10 mg 3 to 4 times daily, is usually adequate. *For hypertensive emergencies*, phentolamine, an α-blocker, is the drug of choice and can be given in 5- to 10-mg doses every 5 to 15 minutes as needed. Alternatively, nitroprusside or labetalol can be used. For an inoperable pheochromocytoma, add metyrosine, a competitive inhibitor of tyrosine hydroxylase, to the treatment.

Postoperatively, in the surgically cured patient, the urinary catecholamines and metabolites normalize in 2 weeks. Long-term follow-up is important to assess for persistence, recurrence, or development of other manifestations of MEN IIA or IIB.

- Surgical excision of the tumor is curative.
- Medical treatment: 1) preoperative preparation to diminish perioperative morbidity and mortality and 2) on a chronic basis in surgical failures.
- α-Adrenergic blockade: the cornerstone of medical therapy. It should be instituted as soon as the diagnosis is made.
- β-Blockade: may be necessary to control tachyarrhyth-

mias; use only after adequate α-blockade.
- For hypertensive emergencies: use phentolamine (an α-blocker).
- Long-term follow-up: important to assess for persistence, recurrence, and development of other manifestations of MEN IIA or IIB.

An Incidentally Discovered Adrenal Mass (Incidentaloma)

Etiology

Small (1-6 cm) adrenal masses are found in up to 9% of unselected autopsies and in fewer than 2% of all abdominal CT studies. Most of these are nonfunctioning adenomas; a few are functioning adenomas or carcinomas of the adrenal cortex or medulla. Metastatic disease to the adrenal glands is common. Identification of the nature of the mass is important: nonfunctioning adenomas are harmless, a functioning adenoma or a carcinoma requires surgery, and a metastasis requires oncologic care.

Diagnosis

The diagnosis of a functioning adrenal tumor rests on clinical evaluation, the use of screening tests, and, when appropriate, confirmatory tests. Hormonal evaluation should screen all patients for pheochromocytoma (24-hour urinary metanephrines, fractionated catecholamines, and vanillylmandelic acid) and Cushing syndrome (urinary free cortisol or an overnight dexamethasone suppression test). Screening for aldosteronoma is appropriate only in the setting of hypertension with or without hypokalemia (PA/PRA ratio). An androgen-producing, or a feminizing, adrenal tumor needs to be considered only in the setting of clinical findings suggestive of sex-steroid overproduction.

With the exception of an adrenal myelolipoma, which is benign and has characteristic fat-density images, CT does not differentiate between benign and malignant neoplasms. The best CT discriminating factor between a nonfunctioning benign and malignant tumor is the size of the mass. Most adrenocortical adenomas are less than 4 cm in diameter and the incidence of carcinoma in masses larger than 6 cm is more than 35%. Needle aspiration of a solid or mixed solid cystic mass cannot distinguish between a benign or a malignant adrenal neoplasm. Needle aspiration of a pheochromocytoma is potentially hazardous. The only place for needle aspiration in the diagnosis of an adrenal mass is in the clinical setting suggestive of adrenal metastases. Pheochromocytoma has to be excluded before the aspiration diagnosis.

Therapy

It is important to identify a pheochromocytoma or a cortisol-producing adenoma before any proposed surgical management of the adrenal mass. Unsuspected pheochromocytoma carries the risk of anesthetic/surgical acute catecholamine release. Few patients with a cortisol-producing adrenal tumor are asymptomatic and do not have the physical stigmata of Cushing syndrome and removal of the unsuspected cortisol-producing tumor may be followed by an adrenal crisis. (With cortisol excess, even if subclinical, ACTH is suppressed and the contralateral adrenal cortex is atrophic. Such patients need perioperative and postoperative cortisol replacement until recovery of the ACTH-adrenal axis, which may require 1-3 years.)

Surgery is indicated for a functioning adrenal tumor, an adrenal mass larger than 6 cm in diameter, and when needle aspiration (performed in the appropriate clinical setting) shows a bloody return.

Observation and follow-up: every patient with an adrenal mass that is not resected should have a repeat CT scan within 3 to 6 months to assess for growth of the mass. If the mass size is stable after 3 to 6 months, additional scans are performed in 12 and 24 months after the diagnosis. Every mass lesion that increases in size during the observation period must be surgically excised after appropriate biochemical studies are performed.

- Exclude pheochromocytoma and a subclinical cortisol-producing tumor before any proposed surgery for an adrenal mass.
- Surgical excision is indicated for functioning adrenal mass, large solid or solid-cystic mass (>6 cm), and cystic masses with blood contents on CT-guided needle aspiration.
- Otherwise, observation is indicated with repeat scans done in 3-6, 12, and 24 months. Increase in size of the mass at any time dictates surgical removal after appropriate screening endocrine tests.

THE TESTIS

Male Hypogonadism

Male hypogonadism refers to the clinical presentations resulting from testosterone deficiency. Such deficiency usually is associated with defects in spermatogenesis and infertility. However, spermatogenic failure may exist independently of any testosterone deficiency.

Etiology

Testosterone deficiency may result from decreased testosterone production by the testes or target tissue resistance to testosterone action. Decreased testosterone production may be the consequence of primary testicular failure (hypergonadotropic hypogonadism) or LH deficiency resulting from a central hypothalamic-pituitary disorder (hypogonadotropic hypogonadism).

Among the causes of primary hypergonadotropic testicular failure are genetic disorders such as Klinefelter syndrome; traumatic disorders such as those resulting from physical, radiotherapeutic, or chemotherapeutic agents; inflammatory disorders such as those due to mumps or autoimmune endocrinopathy; and degenerative disorders such as myotonia dystrophica.

Central hypogonadotropism may be a consequence of functional hypothalamic hypogonadotropism, as in constitutional delay in puberty, or the use of neuroleptic or antidepressant drugs, nutritional disorders, systemic illness, stress, or other endocrinopathies such as hyperprolactinemia, hyperestrogenic states, thyroid, or adrenal disorders. It also may result from organic disorders of the hypothalamic-pituitary unit. In organic disorders of the hypothalamic-pituitary unit, hypogonadotropism may occur alone, as in Kallmann syndrome, or as a part of a multitropic or pantropic hypopituitarism.

Androgen resistance may be genetic or acquired. Genetic androgen resistance may be complete resistance, as in testicular feminization, or partial resistance, as in 5 α-reductase deficiency or Reifenstein syndrome. Acquired androgen resistance may occur with the use of the androgen receptor blockers such as spironolactone or flutamide.

- Testosterone deficiency may result from decreased testosterone production or target tissue resistance.
- Decreased testosterone production may result from primary testicular failure (hypergonadotropic failure) or central hypothalamic pituitary disorder (hypogonadotropic failure).
- Primary testicular failure is a consequence of organic diseases of the testes.
- Central hypogonadotropism may result from functional or organic hypothalamic disorders or from organic diseases of the anterior pituitary gland.
- Target tissue resistance to testosterone action may be genetic or acquired.

Clinical Features

Men

The clinical presentations of hypogonadism in men include decreased libido and potency, decreased ejaculate volume, infertility, decreased energy and stamina, decreased sexual hair growth, and gynecomastia. Hot flushes may occur if the testosterone deficiency has a rapid onset. In men with chronic or severe testosterone deficiency, physical findings may include the classic hypogonadal facies (with pallor and fine wrinkling around the mouth and eyes), altered feminine-like fat distribution, testicular atrophy, decrease in prostate size, osteoporosis, and gynecomastia.

- Characteristic presentations include: decreased libido, potency impairment, decrease in ejaculate volume, gynecomastia, and secondary osteoporosis.
- In severe cases: characteristic facies, loss of secondary sex characteristics, and testicular and prostate atrophy.

Adolescents

Hypogonadism in adolescents presents as failure of sexual and physical maturation. Sexual infantilism is associated with absence of the pubertal growth spurt, eunuchoid habitus (ratio of upper [crown to pubis]-to-lower [pubis to floor] segment is <1 and the ratio of span to height is >1), high-pitched voice, poor muscle development, and female pattern of fat distribution. The testes are small and soft, less than 2 cm long, and less than 2 mL in volume; gynecomastia may be present. Note that small firm testes in a hypogonadal male should suggest the presence of Klinefelter syndrome and the association of anosmia/hyposmia with sexual infantilism should point to Kallmann syndrome. It is important to remember that eunuchoidism occurs only in the presence of normal growth hormone secretion; therefore, it is not seen in pubertal hypogonadism that occurs in the context of hypopituitarism.

- Pubertal hypogonadism: failure of sexual and physical maturation, eunuchoidism, and small testes.

Diagnosis

The diagnosis is suspected on the basis of the clinical picture and is confirmed by the finding of low serum levels of testosterone. Low serum levels of testosterone may reflect hypogonadism or sex hormone-binding globulin abnormalities. Low serum levels of free testosterone define hypogonadism. When convenient and possible, a semen analysis is performed. In almost all cases, a normal semen analysis indicates a normal hypothalamic-pituitary-gonadal axis.

The etiologic diagnosis is suspected on the basis of the clinical picture and is confirmed by measurements of the serum levels of LH and FSH. In primary testicular failure, the serum levels of FSH and LH are increased (hypergonadotropic hypogonadism). Additional tests are not indicated except for karyotype (to confirm Klinefelter syndrome or its variants or mosaics) or evaluation for other endocrinopathies (in patients with autoimmune testicular failure). In central hypothalamic-pituitary hypogonadism, serum levels of LH and FSH are low or "inappropriately normal" relative to the low level of serum testosterone (hypogonadotropic hypogonadism). The presence of pubertal hypogonadotropism, hyposmia or anosmia, and a positive family history point to Kallmann syndrome. Otherwise, hypogonadotropism dictates a complete clinical evaluation, determination of serum prolactin level and other pituitary function tests, and an MRI of the head to exclude mass lesions or other organic forms of hypothalamic-pituitary disease. It is important to consider functional hypogonadotropism in patients with isolated hypogonadotropism and negative MRI findings.

- Suspicion depends on clinical evaluation and the characteristic finding of low serum levels of testosterone. When feasible, a semen analysis is helpful; a normal analysis excludes hypogonadism.
- Low serum levels of testosterone may reflect hypogonadism or sex hormone-binding globulin abnormalities. Check free testosterone. Low free testosterone defines hypogonadism.
- Serum levels of LH and FSH: determine whether the hypogonadism is primary testicular (hypergonadotropic) or secondary to hypothalamic-pituitary (hypogonadotropic) disease.
- The cause of hypergonadotropism is usually obvious from the clinical setting.
- Hypogonadotropic hypogonadism should prompt assessment of the other pituitary functions, MRI of the head, and consideration of functional hypogonadotropism.

In the evaluation of delayed puberty, the challenge is to distinguish constitutional delay of puberty from disorders of the gonadal axis. The clinical setting and assessment of testicular volume are critical for such an evaluation. If the testicular volume is greater than 4 mL, it is safe to suspect that puberty probably has begun; observation and reassurance are indicated. If the volume is less than 4 mL, serum levels of testosterone, LH, and FSH are indicated to document the gonadal axis failure and to determine the level of impairment. In hypergonadotropic hypogonadism, the diagnosis depends on the clinical setting and karyotype. In the evaluation of hypogonadotropism, the presence of anosmia/hyposmia, other midline congenital defects, and a positive family history point to Kallmann syndrome. If smell sensation is normal, assessment of the other pituitary functions and CT or MRI of the head are indicated. Factors pointing to constitutional delay of puberty include the absence of other pituitary function abnormalities, negative findings on imaging studies, and a positive family history of delayed but eventually normal puberty; full pubertal development appears on follow-up examination. The presence of other pituitary function abnormalities and abnormal CT or MRI findings point to organic hypothalamic-pituitary disorder.

- Clinical setting and assessment of testicular volume are critical for evaluation of delayed puberty.
- If testicular volume is >4 mL, puberty has begun and observation is advised.
- If the volume is <4 mL, check serum levels of testosterone, LH, and FSH.

- In hypergonadotropism, diagnosis depends on the clinical setting and karyotype.
- In hypogonadotropism, evaluate the sense of smell; anosmia or hyposmia point to Kallmann syndrome.
- If smell sensation is normal, check other pituitary functions and image (CT/MRI) the pituitary area to exclude mass lesions or other organic hypothalamic-pituitary disorder.

Therapy

Androgen Therapy

In adults, androgen therapy is aimed at restoring and maintaining androgenic functions. In hypogonadal pubertal males, it is designed to initiate and induce full pubertal development. It is important to remember that systemic testosterone cannot produce the high intratesticular levels of testosterone required to stimulate spermatogenesis. In patients with hypogonadotropism, gonadotropin- or GnRH-therapy may be used to induce spermatogenesis and to restore fertility. Therapy is expensive and requires multiple injections for gonadotropin therapy and pump administration for GnRH.

Androgen replacement may be given in the form of parenteral long-acting 17-hydroxyl esters of testosterone (enanthate or cypionate esters). They are effective and safe. The usual dose for an adult male is 200 mg intramuscularly every 10 to 30 days. Aggressive testosterone therapy in pubertal patients may lead to premature closure of the epiphyses and compromise adult height. The dose is 50 to 100 mg/2 weeks given intramuscularly and is generally increased to full replacement over a number of months.

Transdermal testosterone, as a scrotal or nonscrotal patch, is applied on a daily basis (3 to 6 mg/day). This therapy is associated with stable physiologic serum testosterone concentrations.

Oral preparations available in the U.S. are all 17α-alkylated derivatives of testosterone. They are less effective, more costly, and can be associated with the potentially serious side effects of hepatotoxicity, induction of peliosis hepatis, and hepatic tumors. Methyltestosterone is given in a dose of 25 to 50 mg daily by mouth or 10 to 25 mg daily buccally. Fluoxymesterone is given orally in a dose of 5 to 10 mg daily.

Absolute contraindications to androgen therapy include androgen-dependent tumors of the prostate and male breast. Relative contraindications include mental retardation, psychopathy, and obstructive prostatism. Side effects include acne, mild weight gain, edema, increased erythropoiesis, and induction or worsening of obstructive sleep apnea. Androgens may worsen obstructive uropathy due to benign prostatic hypertrophy. Because prostate cancer is an androgen-dependent tumor, an annual prostate examination and serum prostate-specific antigen (PSA) level is recommended for all patients receiving androgen therapy.

- In adults, the aims of androgen therapy are to restore and maintain androgenic function. In hypogonadal pubertal males, the objectives are to initiate and induce full pubertal development.
- Androgen replacement: intramuscular testosterone enanthate or cypionate or transdermal testosterone.
- Aggressive testosterone therapy in pubertal patients may lead to premature closure of the epiphyses and compromise adult height.
- Oral preparations: all 17α-alkylated derivatives of testosterone. They can have potentially serious side effects.
- Absolute contraindications for testosterone therapy are androgen-dependent tumors of the prostate and male breast.
- Testosterone therapy may induce erythropoiesis and aggravate sleep apnea and obstructive prostatism. An annual prostate examination and serum PSA level are recommended.

Selected Disorders of Male Hypogonadism

Klinefelter Syndrome

The basic defect in this common sex chromosome anomaly (1:400-500) is the presence of one or more extra X chromosomes. The classic karyotype is 47,XXY. Variants include XXYY, poly X plus Y, and mosaicism. It is characterized by the development at puberty of seminiferous tubule hyalinization and clumping and varying levels of dysfunction of the Leydig cells. The syndrome is characterized by small firm testes, gynecomastia, varying degrees of testosterone deficiency and eunuchoidism, azoospermia, increased gonadotropin levels, and a positive buccal smear. (The clinical picture may differ in variants and mosaics. If more than one X chromosome is present, the incidence of mental retardation and somatic abnormalities is increased. In mosaics, the clinical manifestations are less severe; if an XY line is present, fertility may be possible.) Patients with Klinefelter syndrome have a slightly increased incidence of diabetes mellitus, chronic obstructive pulmonary disease, autoimmune disorders, varicose veins, malignancy of the breast, lymphoma, and germ cell neoplasm. Diagnosis is established by karyotyping of blood lymphocytes or testicular tissue. Infertility in classic Klinefelter syndrome is irreversible. Testosterone therapy is given for androgen deficiency, and reduction mammoplasty is performed if the gynecomastia is a source of emotional distress. Because of increased risk of breast cancer, an annual breast examination is recommended.

- Klinefelter syndrome: the basic defect is one or more extra X chromosomes.
- The classic karyotype is 47,XXY.
- Klinefelter syndrome is characterized pathologically by seminiferous tubule hyalinization and clumping and varying levels of Leydig cell dysfunction.
- Clinical findings: small firm testes, gynecomastia, varying degrees of testosterone deficiency and eunuchoidism, azoospermia, increased gonadotropin levels, and positive buccal smear. The clinical picture may differ in variants and mosaics.
- Confirmation: karyotyping of blood lymphocytes or testicular tissue.
- Therapy: in classic Klinefelter syndrome, infertility is irreversible. Testosterone therapy is given for androgen deficiency.

Kallmann Syndrome

This syndrome is characterized by isolated hypogonadotropism and associated anosmia/hyposmia. It is a congenital disorder, often familial, that is related to maldevelopment of the olfactory lobes and the GnRH-producing cells. (GnRH neurons, as well as the olfactory bulbs, develop originally in the epithelium of the olfactory placode and then migrate to their ultimate location in the hypothalamus and anterior cranial fossa, respectively. This neural migration is subserved by migration-facilitating proteins. Genetic defects in these proteins lead to anosmia and hypogonadotropic hypogonadism characteristic of the syndrome.) Patients present with delayed puberty. Sexual infantilism, eunuchoidism, and, occasionally, a micropenis are present. Anosmia or hyposmia is present in 80% of patients. Other midline defects such as cleft lip or palate, color blindness, cryptorchidism, and skeletal abnormalities may also be present. Laboratory evaluation reveals hypogonadotropic hypogonadism; other pituitary functions are normal. MRI of the head is negative. Therapy includes 1) androgen replacement for sexual development and maintenance of sexual functions and secondary sex characteristics and 2) GnRH or gonadotropin therapy for restoration of fertility potential.

- Kallmann syndrome: a syndrome of isolated hypogonadotropism and associated anosmia/hyposmia. It is a congenital disorder, often familial, and related to maldevelopment of the olfactory lobes and GnRH-producing cells.
- The clinical presentation is that of sexual infantilism. Anosmia or hyposmia is present in 80% of patients.
- Laboratory evaluation: hypogonadotropic hypogonadism; other pituitary functions are normal. MRI of the head is negative.
- Therapy: androgen replacement. GnRH or gonadotropin therapy are required for restoration of fertility.

Impotence

Etiology

Impotence is defined as the persistent inability to attain or to maintain an erection adequate for the successful conclusion of vaginal penetration. It may or may not be associated with impairment of libido or ejaculation. Testosterone is essential for the initiation and maintenance of libido and for facilitation of the psychic-neurogenic-vascular erectile responses. Derangements of any of these factors, singly or in combination, can result in potency impairment.

The etiology includes 1) penile disorders such as trauma or Peyronie disease; 2) vascular disorders, the most common cause of impotence in men older than 50 years, such as penile vascular insufficiency, corporeal venous leaks, and Leriche syndrome; 3) neurogenic disorders such as stroke, anterior lobe syndromes, spinal cord injury, multiple sclerosis, peripheral neuropathy related to diabetes mellitus or alcoholism, and damage to the penile nerve supply during radical prostatectomy; 4) endocrine disorders such as diabetes mellitus (multifactorial), hypogonadism, hyperprolactinemic states, thyroid or adrenal disorders; 5) systemic disorders; 6) psychogenic disorders, the most common cause of impotence in young men, which may be due to performance anxiety, marital conflict, fear of pregnancy or sexually transmitted diseases, and the various causes of major psychiatric illness; 7) various drugs such as antiandrogens, antihypertensives, antidepressants, and antipsychotics; and 8) substance or alcohol abuse.

- Potency is dependent on psychic, neurologic, vascular, and hormonal factors acting in concert on a normal genital apparatus.
- Potency impairment results from disorders of these interrelationships, singly or in combination.

Diagnosis

A complete medical history and clinical evaluation and appropriate tests are usually adequate to exclude alcohol or drug use; urogenital, neurologic, or vascular disorders; diabetes mellitus and autonomic neuropathy; and a psychiatric disorder. Potency impairment of abrupt onset, that is transient, intermittent, or selective, favors a psychogenic cause.

The next step is to evaluate the endocrine state by measuring the serum levels of testosterone, estradiol, LH and FSH, prolactin, and FTI.

If the endocrine studies are negative, further evaluations are performed as indicated by the clinical setting: 1) nocturnal penile tumescence and resistance to buckling, 2) noninvasive penile blood pressure and flow measurement with duplex ultrasonography (the penile/brachial index), 3) pharmaco-cavernosometry and cavernosography, 4) neurologic evaluation (bulbocavernous reflex latency and somatosensory evoked response of the dorsal nerve), and 5) psychiatric assessment.

- A complete clinical evaluation and few laboratory tests can exclude alcohol, drugs, urologic, neurologic, and vascular disorders, diabetes mellitus, and autonomic neuropathy.
- Endocrine evaluation includes the measurement of serum levels of testosterone, prolactin, and free thyroxine. Abnormal results dictate further evaluation to delineate the cause of the endocrinopathy.
- Objective indices of physiologic, vascular, or neurologic factors and a psychiatric consultation may be indicated.

Therapy

Treatment is directed, when appropriate, at the underlying cause(s) such as testosterone therapy for hypogonadism, dopamine-agonist therapy for hyperprolactinemia, avoidance of drugs and substance abuse, and psychosexual counselling. Other options of therapy include self-administration of vasodilator therapy (intracavernous vasodilator therapy with prostaglandin E_1, papaverine, phentolamine [or a combination— avoid in patients with significant venous leaks, unstable cardiac state, or a history of transient ischemic attacks]) or intraurethral administration of alprostadil. Sildenafil (Viagra) has recently been approved for the treatment of potency impairment. It blocks the enzyme cyclic GMP phosphodiesterase (type 5); the resultant increase in cyclic GMP intensifies and prolongs the nitric oxide-induced vasodilatation underlying penile tumescence. It can be given in a dose of 25 to 100 mg 1 hour before sexual activity. Side effects are related to the vasodilatory properties and are similar to those associated with the use of nitrates. Myocardial infarction and death have rarely been associated with the use of the drug. It is best avoided in patients with a history of coronary artery disease, especially those taking nitrates. The use of vacuum devices should not be used in patients who are prone to priapism or in those taking anticoagulants or those with bleeding tendency. Surgical therapy includes the use of a rigid, malleable, or inflatable penile prosthesis (risk of prosthesis infection particularly in diabetics and patients with spinal cord injury or urinary tract infection) and vascular reconstructive procedures for arterial occlusive disease or for venous leaks.

- Treatment is directed at the identified underlying cause(s).
- Nonspecific options include pharmacologic, mechanical, and surgical treatment.

Gynecomastia

Etiology

Gynecomastia refers to a benign enlargement of the male breast caused by an increase in glandular and stromal tissues. It is the most common disorder of the male breast, accounting for more than 85% of male breast masses. The basic mechanism of gynecomastia is relative estradiol excess, which can result from the following: 1) decreased androgen effect caused by a decrease in androgen production (aging, primary or central testicular failure, or use of inhibitors of testosterone biosynthesis such as ketoconazole), an increase in androgen-binding (hyperthyroidism or liver failure) or androgen-receptor blocker (use of spironolactone, cimetidine, or flutamide); 2) absolute increase in E_2 production (Klinefelter syndrome, adrenal cancer, Leydig cell tumor, or hCG-producing tumor); 3) increased estrogen precursor availability (androgen-secreting tumors, exogenous androgen use, or hyperthyroidism); 4) exogenous estrogen effect (digitalis or synthetic estrogens); and 5) displacement of estrogen from sex hormone-binding globulin and increased free estradiol (ketoconazole and spironolactone). Gynecomastia may result from a trivial cause or may be an early sign of serious illness. In all cases, the physician has to attempt to identify a specific cause. In healthy young pubertal males, the most likely cause is transient physiologic gynecomastia. Anabolic steroid use and Klinefelter syndrome may account for a small number of cases. All other causes are rare in this age group. In adults, the two most common causes are drugs and alcohol-related liver disease. Less common causes include recovery from malnutrition or other serious chronic illness. Rarely encountered are ectopic hCG-producing tumors, feminizing adrenal and testicular tumors, and pituitary tumors. In about 10% of cases, the cause of gynecomastia is indeterminate.

- The basic pathophysiologic mechanism is an increase in the estrogen/androgen ratio.
- Increased estrogen/androgen ratio may result from androgen deficiency, exposure to exogenous estrogen, or an endogenous increase in estrogen production.
- Gynecomastia may result from a benign or sinister cause. It is always important to attempt to identify a specific cause.
- In young pubertal males, the most likely cause is physiologic gynecomastia.
- In adults, the most common causes are drugs and alcohol-related liver disease.
- In about 10% of cases, the cause of gynecomastia is indeterminate or idiopathic.

Clinical Features

The clinical presentations are those of the gynecomastia itself and its etiologic disorder. Patients usually present with breast enlargement that may be unilateral or bilateral. Tenderness may be noted in about one-third of patients. Actual pain is rare. Rarely, a patient may complain of associated galactorrhea. Gynecomastia is identified by its firmness, fine nodularity, central location posterior to the areola from which it spreads radially, and well-defined outer border. The size can vary from a small subareolar button to that of the normal female breast. It usually is bilateral and symmetrical, but there may be pronounced asymmetry.

- The clinical features are those of gynecomastia itself and the etiologic disorder.
- Breast enlargement is the usual symptom; a painful tender gynecomastia of recent onset deserves evaluation.
- Gynecomastia: firm, centrally located mass with well-defined borders situated behind the areola, from which it spreads radially.

Diagnosis

If gynecomastia is bilateral, exclude pseudogynecomastia (fatty enlargement). If unilateral, it is important to exclude cancer of the breast. Signs that should arouse suspicion of malignancy include eccentric location relative to the areola, unusual firmness, fixation, ulceration, bloody discharge from the nipple, and the presence of axillary lymphadenopathy. Mammography and excisional biopsy may be necessary for definitive diagnosis.

A complete medical history, physical examination, and appropriate laboratory studies should rule out physiologic, pharmacologic, alcohol-related, and refeeding types of gynecomastia. Endocrine tests should include measurement of the serum levels of testosterone, E_2, LH and FSH, β-hCG, sTSH, dehydroepiandrosterone sulfate, and PRL. If needed, karyotyping should be performed.

- If gynecomastia is bilateral, rule out pseudogynecomastia. If unilateral, rule out tumors.
- Signs that arouse suspicion of malignancy: eccentric location relative to the areola, unusual firmness, fixation, ulceration, bloody discharge from the nipple, and axillary lymphadenopathy.
- Complete medical history, physical examination, appropriate laboratory studies to rule out physiologic, pharmacologic, alcohol-related, and refeeding types of gynecomastia.
- Endocrine tests: testosterone, E_2, LH and FSH, β-hCG, sTSH, dehydroepiandrosterone sulfate, and PRL (karyotype is added when appropriate).

Endocrine Diagnostic Approach

Determine β-hCG and LH and FSH levels. 1) An increased β-hCG points to an hCG-secreting tumor. 2) High serum LH and FSH levels point to primary testicular failure. Confirm by low serum level of testosterone. 3) Low levels of LH and FSH should prompt consideration of androgen- or estrogen-producing tumor, exogenous sex steroid use, and hypogonadotropism, including that associated with hyperprolactinemia. Inquire about the use of sex steroids. If negative, check serum testosterone and E_2 levels. A low level of free testosterone implies hypogonadotropism and should prompt a complete hypothalamic-pituitary evaluation. A high level of E_2 should prompt evaluation for feminizing adrenal or testicular tumors. 4) If the serum levels of LH, FSH, and sex steroids are normal, an underlying endocrinopathy is unlikely. These patients can be observed and reevaluated periodically.

- A useful endocrine diagnostic approach is to start with measuring the serum levels of β-hCG, LH, and FSH. Normal values exclude a serious underlying disorder.
- A high level of β-hCG points to a β-hCG-producing tumor.
- High LH and FSH levels: primary testicular failure.
- Low LH and FSH levels: exclude use of sex steroids; measure serum levels of testosterone and estradiol.
- Low testosterone level: hypogonadotropic hypogonadism; evaluate as for hypopituitarism.
- High E_2 level: look for estrogen-producing tumor.
- Normal LH and FSH levels: an endocrinopathy is unlikely.

Therapy

Therapy may include reassurance, correction of underlying disorders, tamoxifen (usually not helpful), and cosmetic surgery.

THE OVARY

Amenorrhea

Primary amenorrhea is present when menarche has not occurred by age 16 in a young female with normal secondary sex characteristics or by age 14 in the absence of secondary sex characteristics. Secondary amenorrhea is present when a woman with previously established menstrual function experiences the absence of menstruation for a period greater than three of her previous cycle intervals or for 6 months.

Etiology

The requirements for normal regular menstrual function are normal cyclic secretion of hypothalamic GnRH, normal cyclic secretion of the pituitary gonadotropins LH and FSH, normal ovarian follicular apparatus that responds to cyclic gonadotropin stimulation by ovulation and production of estrogen and progesterone in a cyclic fashion, and normal endometrium capable of responding to E_2 (follicular proliferative endometrium) and progesterone (luteal secretory endometrium) and then to their declining concentrations by the initiation of menstrual shedding.

Amenorrhea can be physiologic or pathologic. The commonest causes of amenorrhea are *physiologic* (pregnancy, lactation, and prepubertal and perimenopausal states). *Pathologic amenorrhea* may result from 1) a functional or organic hypothalamic disorder leading to loss of cyclic GnRH production; 2) organic pituitary disorder resulting in loss of the gonadotrope population; 3) organic ovarian disorder resulting in loss of the follicular apparatus, or in anovulation, and loss of the normal sequential E_2 and progesterone secretion; and 4) organic uterine disorders and loss of the endometrium or genital tract disorders preventing egress of the shed endometrium. The common causes of primary amenorrhea are gonadal dysgenesis (45% of cases), constitutional delay of puberty (20%), and müllerian agenesis (15%). The commonest causes of secondary amenorrhea are polycystic ovarian syndrome (30%), ovarian failure (10%), hypothalamic dysfunction (40%), and pituitary disease (20%).

- Amenorrhea can result from impaired function of any component of the hypothalamic-pituitary-gonadal axis or from an anatomical abnormality of the genital tract.
- The commonest causes of amenorrhea are physiologic: pregnancy, postpartum lactation, and prepubertal and perimenopausal states.
- The common causes of primary amenorrhea: gonadal dysgenesis, constitutional delay in puberty, and müllerian agenesis.
- The commonest causes of secondary amenorrhea: ovarian disorders, hypothalamic dysfunction, and pituitary disease.

Primary Amenorrhea

Outflow tract abnormalities are uncommon causes of primary amenorrhea. Developmental anomalies include imperforate hymen, isolated absence of the uterus, and vaginal aplasia or atresia. Ovarian disorders, including developmental and acquired disorders, account for most of the causes of primary amenorrhea. Hypothalamic-pituitary disease can cause gonadotropin deficiency and amenorrhea by 1) destruction of pituitary gonadotrophs or the hypothalamic GnRH cell population by organic diseases of various origins or 2) functional suppression of these cells, commonly by a nutritional or a psychiatric disorder, prolonged heavy exercise, systemic illness, and other endocrinopathies such as uncontrolled diabetes mellitus, hyperprolactinemic states, and thyroid and adrenal disorders. Organic hypothalamic-pituitary disease due to various causes is an uncommon cause of primary amenorrhea. In young adults, craniopharyngioma is the most common space-occupying lesion; prolactinomas occur in this age group but are rare.

- Outflow tract disorders are rare causes and include developmental abnormalities.
- Ovarian disorders are the most common cause of primary amenorrhea; they may be genetic or acquired.
- Hypothalamic-pituitary disease: it may be organic and caused by destructive processes affecting the endocrine hypothalamus or the anterior pituitary or it may be functional and caused by functional suppression of GnRH secretion by nutritional or psychiatric disorders, systemic disease, and other endocrinopathies.

Secondary Amenorrhea

Acquired *outflow tract abnormalities* are rare causes of secondary amenorrhea. Such disorders include 1) postabortive or postpartum endometritis; 2) overzealous dilatation and curettage, with destruction of the endometrial basal layer, formation of adhesions and obliteration of the endometrial cavity (Asherman syndrome); and 3) endometrial atrophy related to prolonged use of progestational agents or resulting from treatment of endometriosis.

Ovarian disorders are common causes of secondary amenorrhea. The most common disorder is polycystic ovary syndrome (see Hirsutism). Ovarian destructive processes are an uncommon cause of secondary amenorrhea and premature menopause. These processes include autoimmune oophoritis as part of polyendocrine autoimmune disease, various forms of mosaic gonadal dysgenesis that lead to premature exhaustion of the complement of ovarian follicles, abdominal irradiation, chemotherapy with such agents as cyclophosphamide and vincristine, and ovarian tumors that cause secondary amenorrhea by hormonal abnormalities (hypersecretion of estrogen, androgen, or hCG) or, if bilateral, by destruction of the ovarian tissue.

Hypothalamic-pituitary disorders are the most common pathologic causes of secondary amenorrhea and may be either functional or organic. *Functional hypogonadotropism* results from hypothalamic dysfunction caused by a defect in the cyclic center, inhibition of the mid-cycle surge of GnRH and LH, and the failure of ovulation. Mild disorders of GnRH release may be triggered by situational stresses or mild weight loss: FSH secretion is low-normal, E_2 production continues, the endometrium is proliferative, and exogenous progesterone leads to withdrawal bleeding. Moderate or severe disorders of GnRH release may occur with severe weight loss, severe emotional stresses, competitive athletics, systemic disease, thyroid disorders, uncontrolled diabetes mellitus, or a hyperandrogenic state caused by an adrenal or ovarian disorder. Under these circumstances, estrogen levels are low, the endometrium is atrophic, and exogenous progesterone does not lead to withdrawal bleeding. In *organic hypothalamic-pituitary disorder*, hypogonadotropism can be the only manifestation or it can occur in association with other pituitary function abnormalities. Hypogonadotropism can occur as a result of pituitary disorders, hypothalamic disorders, or disorders of extrasellar structures impinging on the hypothalamic-pituitary unit. Hyperprolactinemia is a common cause of secondary amenorrhea, accounting for 25% to 40% of all cases. Postpartum pituitary necrosis (Sheehan syndrome), previously a common cause, has declined in incidence with improvement in obstetric care.

- Acquired outflow tract abnormalities are uncommon causes of secondary amenorrhea.
- Ovarian disorders: common causes of secondary amenorrhea. The most common disorder is polycystic ovary syndrome. Ovarian destructive processes are an uncommon cause of secondary amenorrhea and premature menopause.
- Hypothalamic-pituitary disorder: the most common pathologic cause of secondary amenorrhea. It may be functional or organic.

Clinical Features

In addition to amenorrhea, findings of a hypoestrogenic state may be present: decreased vaginal secretions and dyspareunia, hot flushes, osteopenia, and lack of development or loss of the secondary sex characteristics. Other findings are those related to the etiologic disorder, such as hyperandrogenic features, expressible or spontaneous galactorrhea, shortness of stature or Turner stigmata, thyroid dysfunction and goiter, or other manifestations of hypopituitarism.

Diagnosis

Diagnostic Approach to Secondary Amenorrhea

1. Rule out physiologic amenorrhea: pregnancy test (β-hCG).
2. Rule out genital tract outflow disorders: evaluate clinical setting, particularly a history of overzealous dilatation and curettage preceding the amenorrhea. In outflow disorders, the progesterone test and estrogen/progesterone test do not result in withdrawal bleeding. Confirmation requires hysteroscopy or hysterosalpingogram.
3. Rule out a hyperandrogenic state: suspicion of a hyperandrogenic state is based on clinical finding and is confirmed by increased serum levels of testosterone or dehydroepiandrosterone sulfate.
4. Rule out disorders of the hypothalamic-pituitary gonadal axis. Measure the serum levels of E_2, LH, and particularly FSH to distinguish ovarian from hypothalamic-pituitary disorders. a) Low serum E_2 and increased FSH and LH levels point to primary ovarian failure. A karyotype is necessary in patients younger than 30 years. In the

absence of any readily apparent cause for ovarian failure such as trauma, chemotherapy, or radiotherapy, an autoimmune disorder should be considered. Appropriate tests for other evidence of autoimmune endocrinopathy such as sTSH, antimicrosomal antithyroid antibodies, and cosyntropin stimulation tests are indicated. b) Low serum levels of E_2 and inappropriately low levels of LH and FSH point to a hypothalamic-pituitary disorder. Rule out a functional disorder; if present, correct it; if periods resume, the diagnosis is functional disorder. If functional disorder is not present, or if its correction does not lead to the resumption of menstrual function, proceed with further tests. Rule out organic hypothalamic-pituitary disease. These include measurements of serum PRL and other pituitary hormones and imaging (CT or MRI) of the sella.

If an identifiable organic disease is found, treat it appropriately, but if no such organic disease is found, consider the amenorrhea to be of indeterminate cause and pursue long-term follow-up; an identifiable cause may become apparent in months or years.

- Rule out: physiologic amenorrhea (pregnancy test), genital tract outflow disorders (clinical evaluation, hysteroscopy), and hyperandrogenic state (clinical, serum levels of testosterone and dehydroepiandrosterone sulfate).
- Measure serum levels of E_2, LH, and FSH to distinguish ovarian from hypothalamic-pituitary disease.
- Low serum levels of E_2 and increased levels of FSH and LH: primary ovarian failure. Obtain a karyotype if the patient is <30 years old.
- Low serum levels of E_2 and inappropriately low levels of FSH and LH: hypothalamic-pituitary disorder. Rule out a functional disorder; rule out organic hypothalamic-pituitary disease.
- If no organic disease, consider amenorrhea to be of indeterminate cause and pursue long-term follow-up.

Diagnostic Approach to Primary Amenorrhea

The diagnostic approach starts with careful assessment of pubertal development and the secondary sex characteristics.

1. If the sex characteristics are those of an adult female and pregnancy test results are negative, consider outflow obstruction (imperforate hymen or vaginal atresia), genital tract anomalies (such as müllerian agenesis), or androgen insensitivity (e.g., testicular feminization). A pelvic examination is a critical clinical evaluation. Normal pelvic findings should prompt an evaluation similar to that for secondary amenorrhea. Absence of the uterus should prompt determining the serum level of testosterone: normal female testosterone level points to müllerian agenesis and a high

male serum testosterone level points to androgen insensitivity. An intact hymen or transverse vaginal septum points to outflow tract congenital disorder.

2. If hyperandrogenic manifestations are present, proceed with the same work-up as for hyperandrogenic syndrome.

3. If sexual infantilism is present, check serum FSH concentrations: a high FSH level points to primary gonadal failure and dictates a karyotype assessment; a normal or low FSH level points to hypogonadotropic hypogonadism and a hypothalamic-pituitary disorder: the differential diagnosis is between delayed puberty, Kallmann syndrome, functional hypothalamic disease, and organic hypothalamic or pituitary disorder. Evaluation of the sense of smell, a careful clinical evaluation, a family history, MRI of the head, and assessment of serum prolactin and other pituitary functions are the basis for the diagnostic differentiation.

- Evaluate secondary sex characteristics.
- Adult female sex characteristics and negative pregnancy test: consider outflow obstruction, genital tract anomalies, and androgen insensitivity.
- Presence of sexual infantilism indicates a disorder of the hypothalamic-pituitary gonadal axis. The most important test is measuring the serum level of FSH.
- Sexual infantilism with a high serum FSH level points to primary ovarian failure: the most likely diagnosis is gonadal dysgenesis. A karyotype is indicated.
- Sexual infantilism with a normal or low serum FSH level points to a hypothalamic-pituitary disorder: consider delayed puberty, functional hypothalamic disease, Kallmann syndrome, and other organic hypothalamic or pituitary disease.

Therapy

Management is directed at the underlying disorder and restoration of a eugonadal state. It is important to identify and to treat the cause, such as reversing the cause of functional hypogonadotropism, surgical treatment of pituitary tumors, and bromocriptine therapy for hyperprolactinemic disorders. If successful treatment of the cause is not possible, estrogen replacement and, when required and feasible, restoration of ovulation and fertility potential are indicated.

- It is important to identify and to treat the cause.
- If successful treatment of the cause is not possible: estrogen replacement therapy and, when needed and feasible, restoration of ovulation and reproductive potential.

Estrogen Replacement

The goals of estrogen therapy include control of vasomotor instability, prevention of genitourinary atrophy, preservation of secondary sex characteristics, prevention of osteoporosis, reduction of the risk of coronary artery disease (probable), and restoration of a sense of well-being. *Absolute contraindications* to estrogen therapy include known or suspected estrogen-dependent neoplasm (breast or uterus), cholestatic hepatic dysfunction, active thromboembolic disorder, history of thromboembolic disorder associated with previous estrogen use, neuro-ophthalmologic vascular disease, and undiagnosed vaginal bleeding.

Estrogen replacement therapy must be individualized and administered only after a thorough discussion with the patient about the pros and cons of the therapy. Therapy is initiated as soon as possible after the diagnosis of estrogen deficiency and is continued indefinitely or until the cause has been reversed. No estrogen preparation is superior to the other, and the cardioprotective effect of transdermal E_2 is unproved. Supplemental progestin is indicated only for women who have a uterus; medroxyprogesterone acetate is preferred rather than 19-nortestosterone derivatives, because it is less likely to lower HDL-C levels. Before estrogen therapy is initiated, it is advisable to give medroxyprogesterone acetate, 10 mg daily for 10 to 14 days. If no withdrawal bleeding occurs, an atrophic endometrium is present (after ruling out pregnancy in appropriate setting) and estrogen therapy can be initiated. However, if withdrawal bleeding occurs, the endometrium is estrogen-primed and consideration should be given to performing endometrial biopsy to rule out endometrial hyperplasia before initiating estrogen replacement therapy.

- The goal of estrogen therapy is to restore the euestrogenic state.
- Exclude the absolute contraindications.
- Individualize the therapy. Give it only after thoroughly discussing the pros and cons. The patient should be helped in making an informed decision.
- Initiate therapy as soon as the diagnosis of hypoestrogenism is made.
- Continue therapy indefinitely unless the cause is reversed or a significant side effect or contraindication develops.
- Use progestin supplementation in women who have a uterus.

Estrogen therapy can be administered orally, parenterally, topically, or transdermally. In the U.S., oral and transdermal modes of therapy are used most commonly. In women with a uterus and who need supplemental progestin, the therapy can be given sequentially or in combination. In sequential therapy, estrogen may be given as conjugated equine estrogen (or equivalent) in a dose of 0.625 mg daily in patients older than 45 years (or 0.9-1.25 mg in those younger than 45 years) on days 1 to 25 of each month and supplemented with a progestin, such as medroxyprogesterone acetate in a dose of 10 mg/day, days 14 to 25 of each month. Such sequential therapy results in predictable cyclic withdrawal bleeding in 50% to 60% of patients. For unpredictable bleeding, endometrial biopsy is indicated. The goal of combination therapy is to induce endometrial atrophy and amenorrhea and is preferred by patients who find cyclic withdrawal bleeding inconvenient or unacceptable. Conjugated equine estrogen is given in the same doses daily (or another estrogen formulation in equivalent dosage) and medroxyprogesterone acetate in a dose of 2.5 mg daily. Most patients can expect irregular spotting in the early months but become amenorrheic in 4 to 6 months. Any vaginal bleeding after 6 months should be evaluated promptly.

- There are many forms of estrogen administration. In the U.S., oral and transdermal therapy are the most commonly used.
- Sequential therapy results in predictable cyclic withdrawal bleeding in 50%-60% of patients. For unpredictable bleeding: endometrial biopsy.
- Combination therapy: induce endometrial atrophy and amenorrhea in those who find cyclic withdrawal bleeding inconvenient or unacceptable.

Complications of estrogen replacement include increased risk of endometrial cancer, which is dose- and duration-dependent (4x-8x); such cancer is usually stage I, with no excess mortality. This risk is prevented by progestin supplementation. Another possible complication is a slightly increased risk of breast cancer; the weight of present evidence indicates no such increased risk. Pretreatment breast examination and mammography (and annually thereafter) are essential. Another complication is increased risk of surgical gallbladder disease.

- Complications of estrogen replacement therapy: increased risk of endometrial cancer, possibly slightly increased risk of breast cancer, and increased risk of surgical gallbladder disease.

Ovulation Induction

Hypogonadal women who desire fertility can be given clomiphene citrate, exogenous gonadotropin, or GnRH therapy. The drug of choice for hyperprolactinemic infertility is the dopamine-agonist bromocriptine.

Selected Disorders Associated With Amenorrhea

Turner 45/XO Gonadal Dysgenesis

This is the most common cause of primary amenorrhea. It is estimated to affect 1 in 3,000 newborn females and is characterized by fibrous gonadal streaks, female phenotype, short

stature, skeletal and developmental anomalies, and, in adolescent patients, primary ovarian failure and sexual infantilism. The physical abnormalities associated with Turner syndrome include a webbed neck, low-set ears, multiple pigmented nevi, micrognathia, epicanthal folds, shield-like chest with microthelia, short metacarpals and metatarsals, an increased carrying angle at the elbows, renal developmental abnormalities, and cardiovascular anomalies (including coarctation of the aorta and aortic stenosis). (In Turner mosaics, patients have more than one sex chromosomal line, with the most common combination being 45/XO, 46/XX; the degree of ovarian dysgenesis varies depending on the ratio of XO to XX germ cells. Patients may present with primary or secondary amenorrhea, may or may not be short, and may have few or many of the physical stigmata of Turner syndrome, depending on the tissue distribution of the XO chromosomal line.)

- Turner 45/XO gonadal dysgenesis: the most common cause of primary amenorrhea.
- Characterized by: fibrous gonadal streaks, female phenotype, short stature, skeletal and developmental anomalies, and, in adolescent patients, primary ovarian failure, sexual infantilism, associated renal developmental abnormalities, and cardiovascular anomalies.
- Turner mosaics: patients have more than one sex chromosomal line. The degree of ovarian dysgenesis varies depending on the ratio of XO to XX germ cells.
- Turner mosaics: patients may present with primary or secondary amenorrhea and may or may not have the physical characteristics of 45/XO.

Anorexia Nervosa

This syndrome is seen almost exclusively in young females and is manifested predominantly by weight loss, amenorrhea, and behavioral disorder. The age at onset is usually younger than 25 years. Weight loss can be extreme and accompanied by a distorted and implacable attitude toward eating and weight. The patients deny their illness and fail to recognize their nutritional needs. Some may manifest unusual hoarding and handling of food; bulimia (excessive food intake) and vomiting are seen in 50% of the patients. Amenorrhea occurs in all young female patients with anorexia nervosa, and in 25% of them, it precedes the weight loss. Other features include bradycardia, hypotension, constipation, impaired temperature regulation (inability to shiver and maintain body temperature in face of hypothermia or hyperthermia), lanugo hair growth, hypercarotenemia, and, in severe cases, dependent edema. Endocrine findings include hypogonadotropism, normal or increased serum levels of GH and low IGF-I, normal serum levels of T_4 and TSH but decreased levels of T_3 and increased reversed T_3 levels, generally increased serum cortisol levels that show normal suppressibility with dexamethasone, decreased 24-hour urinary 17-ketogenic and 17-ketosteroids, and a normal serum level of prolactin. A partial central AVP lack and DI may occur.

- Anorexia nervosa: is seen almost exclusively in young females.
- Predominant manifestations: weight loss, amenorrhea, and behavioral disorder.
- Amenorrhea occurs in almost all patients, and, in 25%, it precedes the weight loss.
- Endocrine findings: hypogonadotropism, normal or increased serum GH, low serum IGF-I, normal serum T_4 and TSH levels, decreased serum T_3 and increased reversed T_3 levels, increased serum cortisol levels (normal suppressibility with dexamethasone), and normal serum level of prolactin. Partial DI may occur.

Androgens in Normal Females

The sources of circulating androgens in adult females are the ovaries, adrenal cortices, and peripheral tissues. Plasma androstenedione is produced by the ovaries (50%) and the adrenals (50%). Plasma testosterone is derived from three sources: the ovaries (25%), adrenals (25%), and conversion of androstenedione in the peripheral tissues (50%). Dehydroepiandrosterone (DHEA) is derived mostly from the adrenals (80%) and, to a small extent, from the ovaries (20%). Dehydroepiandrosterone-sulfate (DHEAS) is derived almost exclusively from the adrenals (95%). The theca-cell system is the source of the ovarian androgens, and it is LH-dependent. The adrenal androgen source is the zona fasciculata/reticularis and is ACTH-dependent.

Plasma testosterone circulates in two forms: free (1%-2%) and bound (98%-99%) components. Testosterone is bound to sex-hormone-binding globulin and albumin. Testosterone is the most potent circulating androgen. It is biotransformed to dihydrotestosterone (DHT) in the pilosebaceous unit through the activity of the enzyme 5α-reductase. DHT is the active androgen in the hair follicles. It is metabolized within the pilosebaceous unit to 3α-androstenediol glucuronide. The other weaker androgens are biotransformed to testosterone or DHT at the androgen target tissues.

In adult females, androgens have several functions: growth of sexual hair, maintenance of libido, and promotion of anabolic functions.

- Circulating androgens in adult females: testosterone, androstenedione, DHEA, and DHEAS.
- Testosterone and androstenedione have an ovarian and adrenal cortical source. DHEAS is almost exclusively (95%) an adrenocortical androgen.

- The ovarian source is the theca-cell system; the adrenocortical source is the zona fasciculata/reticularis.
- Production of androgens is trophic-hormone dependent: ovarian source is LH-dependent; adrenal source is ACTH-dependent.
- Androgens in females are promoters of sexual hair growth, libido, and general anabolic functions.
- In hair follicles, testosterone is converted to dihydrotestosterone via 5α-reductase. Dihydrotestosterone is the active androgen in hair follicles.

Hirsutism and the Hyperandrogenic Syndrome

Hirsutism is defined as androgen-induced excessive hair growth in the androgen-sensitive area of the body of a female. *Virilization* implies the appearance of masculine features in secondary sex characteristics and the sexual organs and results from a more pronounced increase in androgen stimulation. Virilization includes hirsutism, but hirsutism frequently occurs without virilization.

Etiology

An excess of androgens may be from an endogenous or an exogenous source. *Endogenous hyperandrogenicity* results from increased production of androgens by the ovaries and/or the adrenal cortices. From either source, the overproduction may be a consequence of a benign, hyperplastic, trophic hormone-dependent disorder or a neoplastic autonomous disorder. Neoplastic sources include benign or malignant tumors of the adrenal cortex or ovary.

Ovarian LH-dependent disorders include polycystic ovarian syndrome, idiopathic hirsutism, and hyperthecosis. *Adrenocortical ACTH-dependent disorders* include congenital adrenal hyperplasia and ACTH-dependent Cushing disease. Hyperprolactinemia may lead to an ACTH-dependent increase in adrenal androgen production.

Exogenous hyperandrogenicity results from exposure to androgens, anabolic steroids, or to some testosterone-derived progestins. Chronic administration of metyrapone causes increased adrenal androgen production because of selective 11-hydroxylase enzyme block.

Idiopathic hirsutism and polycystic ovarian disease are the commonest causes of the hyperandrogenic syndrome seen in clinical practice. All the other causes are rarely encountered.

- Hyperandrogenicity can be due to an endogenous or an exogenous source of androgens.
- Endogenous sources of androgen production include the ovaries and adrenal cortices. From either source, the etiologic process may be a trophic hormone-dependent hyperplastic process, or an autonomous neoplastic disorder.

- The commonest causes of hyperandrogenicity are idiopathic hirsutism and polycystic ovaries.
- Exogenous hyperandrogenicity may be caused by exposure to androgens or anabolic steroids, some progestins, or metyrapone.

Clinical Features

The clinical features are those of the hyperandrogenic state and its cause. In order of increasing severity, the hyperandrogenic state may present with acne, hirsutism, menstrual and ovulatory disorders, defeminization, and masculinization (temporal hair recession, deepening voice, increased muscle mass, and clitorimegaly).

- Clinical presentations in order of increasing severity: acne, hirsutism, menstrual and ovulatory disorders, defeminization, and masculinization.

Diagnosis

The most important clinical diagnostic clues relate to evaluation of the time at onset, tempo of progression, and severity of the hyperandrogenic state. A benign disorder is suggested by disease onset at puberty and a mild, slowly progressive course. Rapid onset of disease at any age and a severe rapidly progressive course point to a malignant disorder.

1) A detailed drug and family history is important. A positive family history may be seen in familial/racial hirsutism, polycystic ovarian syndrome, and late-onset congenital adrenal hyperplasia. 2) A young woman whose hirsutism is mild and pubertal in onset or who has southern European ancestry, whose menstrual function is normal, and who is free of any underlying significant disorder need not undergo detailed endocrine testing. 3) If the onset of hirsutism is pubertal and associated with menstrual irregularity (oligomenorrhea or amenorrhea) but without virilization, the differential diagnosis includes polycystic ovaries and late-onset congenital adrenal hyperplasia. 4) The serum levels of testosterone and DHEAS are essential for diagnostic laboratory evaluation. Also, a screen for Cushing syndrome (overnight 1-mg dexamethasone suppression test or 24-hour urinary free cortisol) and measurement of serum prolactin are also required. 5) In selected patients and as guided by the clinical history and findings, determining the serum level of 17-hydroxyprogesterone, with or without the cosyntropin test for confirmation of congenital adrenal hyperplasia may be necessary. 6) Also, in selected patients suspected of having neoplasm, pelvic ultrasonography and abdominal CT are indicated. 7) If plasma DHEAS is greater than 7 ng/dL, the differential diagnosis is between adrenal tumor and late-onset congenital adrenal hyperplasia. Proceed with CT of the abdomen; if the findings are negative, proceed with serum 17-hydroxyprogesterone and cosyntropin test. Also, test for dexamethasone suppressibility of DHEAS (see below). 8) Plasma levels of DHEAS that are less than 7 ng/dL exclude adrenal tumor and congenital adrenal hyperplasia. Proceed with measuring serum testosterone; levels greater than 200 ng/dL should raise the suspicion of ovarian tumor; pelvic ultrasonography and CT are required and, if necessary, laparoscopy and exploration. A serum level of testosterone less than 200 ng/dL points to polycystic ovarian syndrome.

- The most important diagnostic clues relate to evaluating the time at onset, tempo of progression, and severity of hyperandrogenic state.
- A benign disorder is suggested by onset at puberty and a mild, slowly progressive course.
- A malignant disorder is suggested by a rapid onset at any age and a severe, rapidly progressive course.
- Serum testosterone and DHEAS: essential for diagnostic laboratory evaluation.
- Ancillary laboratory measurements include that of Cushing syndrome screening test, serum prolactin, and serum 17-hydroxyprogesterone.
- If the plasma level of DHEAS is >7 ng/dL, the differential diagnosis is between adrenal tumor and late-onset congenital adrenal hyperplasia.
- If the plasma level of DHEAS is <7 ng/dL, measure serum testosterone. If the serum testosterone level is >200 ng/dL, suspect ovarian tumor. If the serum testosterone level is <200 ng/dL, polycystic ovarian syndrome.

Selected Hyperandrogenic States

Idiopathic hirsutism—There is a modest increase in androgen production (mostly ovarian), with increased peripheral androgen production and increased sensitivity of the hair follicle. The hyperadrenogenicity is mild and LH-dependent. Also, the onset is at puberty, and the disease has a very slow progression. Menstrual cycles are ovulatory, and the results of pelvic examination are normal. The serum levels of testosterone and DHEAS are normal.

- Idiopathic hirsutism: modest increase in androgen production (mostly ovarian).
- Other features: LH-dependent, onset at puberty, slow progression, menstrual cycles are ovulatory, normal serum levels of testosterone and DHEAS.

Polycystic ovarian syndrome—This is the most common cause of nonvirilizing hyperandrogenicity, but its pathogenesis is poorly understood. Gonadotropin dynamics are abnormal, with loss of the LH surge and increased LH levels. The ovaries are usually enlarged (70% of patients) but may be normal in size and characteristically have multiple cysts and stromal thickening. Hyperandrogenicity is mild to moderate and LH-dependent. In many patients, there is associated obesity and insulin resistence and consequent hyperinsulinism, which further contribute to the androgen excess. The onset of the disorder is at puberty, and its progression is slow and of mild degree. Hirsutism (70% of patients), menstrual abnormality (88%), infertility and anovulation (75%), and obesity (50%) are usually present. The serum level of testosterone is normal or modestly increased (70% of patients) and is nearly always less than 200 ng/mL. DHEAS levels are normal or mildly increased in 25% of patients. Changes seen on pelvic ultrasonography are characteristic (70%); hyperprolactinemia may be present in 25% to 30% of patients. Serum levels of E_2 are normal; estrone levels are increased, and the risk of endometrial hyperplasia is increased.

- Polycystic ovarian syndrome: the most common cause of hyperandrogenicity.
- Hyperandrogenicity: mild to moderate and LH-dependent.
- Features: onset at puberty, slow progression, hirsutism (70% of patients), menstrual abnormality (88%), infertility and anovulation (75%), and obesity (50%).
- Serum level of testosterone: normal or modestly increased (70%); it almost always is <200 ng/mL.
- Serum level of DHEAS: normal or mildly increased.
- Modest degree of hyperprolactinemia occurs in 25%-30% of patients.

Late-onset congenital adrenal hyperplasia—This may be of the "classic" type, with severe enzyme deficiency and neonatal and postnatal presentation. It may also be "nonclassic" or "cryptic," in which the enzyme deficiency is mild and the presentation is pubertal or "late onset." It is inherited as an autosomal recessive trait closely linked to the HLA gene region. Steroidogenic block: may be 21-hydroxylase (most common type), 11-hydroxylase, or 3β-ol-dehydrogenase block. Such steroidogenic blocks lead to accumulation of precursors and shunting of these precursors to the androgenic pathways. All androgen abnormalities are ACTH-dependent, hence dexamethasone suppressible. 21-Hydroxylase deficiency (most common congenital adrenal hyperplasia): increased basal levels of 17-hydroxyprogesterone to greater than 300 ng/dL. If normal, cosyntropin test is indicated; 30 minutes after giving ACTH, a value greater than 1,200 ng/dL is diagnostic.

Virilizing Tumors of the Ovary and Adrenal

These tumors can occur at any age; they produce a hyperandrogenic state that is severe and has a rapid onset and progression. Adrenal tumors characteristically are associated with high levels of DHEAS, whereas ovarian tumors produce high levels of testosterone. Diagnosis requires anatomical delineation: abdominal CT for adrenal tumors and pelvic ultrasonography or CT for ovarian tumors. Rarely, one needs to resort to selective venous sampling for localization.

Endocrine Therapy

Endocrine therapy is temporizing and may need 6 to 12 months to show a clinical effect. The goal is to decrease androgen production or to inhibit the androgen effect of hair follicles.

Oral contraceptives are indicated for the management of idiopathic hirsutism and polycystic ovaries. This therapy suppresses LH, increases SHBG, and inhibits DHT binding to its receptor. It is important to avoid the progestin norgestrel because of its androgenic effect.

Glucocorticoid therapy—The primary role of glucocorticoid therapy is in the management of late-onset congenital adrenal hyperplasia, but it also may be used in polycystic ovaries if DHEAS levels are increased. Dexamethasone (0.25-0.75 mg) or prednisone (5-7.5 mg) is given at bedtime. The well-known risks of exogenous Cushing syndrome and hypothalamic-pituitary-adrenal axis suppression may occur. In congenital adrenal hyperplasia, the efficacy of glucocorticoid therapy can be monitored by measuring the level of 17-hydroxyprogesterone.

Androgen receptor-blockers—Spironolactone, the well-known aldosterone antagonist, is also an androgen-receptor blocker and inhibitor of androgen action. It also decreases androgen production by its effect on steroidogenesis. The usual dose is 50 to 200 mg daily; spironolactone should be used only in conjunction with effective contraception. Cimetidine is an alternate androgen receptor blocker but is less effective than spironolactone. Newer promising approaches include use of flutamide (an androgen receptor blocker) and finasteride (a 5α-reductase blocker). Cyproterone acetate is an antiandrogen that decreases dihydrotestosterone production and action. It also decreases LH release. It is given with topical or oral estrogen and is not available in the U.S.

- Endocrine therapy is temporizing.
- It may need 6-12 months to show an effect.
- Goal: decrease androgen production or inhibit androgen effect on hair follicles.
- Oral contraceptives: management of idiopathic hirsutism and polycystic ovaries.
- Glucocorticoid therapy: primary role in managing late-onset congenital adrenal hyperplasia.
- Spironolactone: blocks androgen receptor and inhibits androgen action.

HYPERLIPIDEMIAS

Hyperlipidemias are important clinical disorders because of the two threats they pose to health: the dominant threat of premature vascular disease and the less frequent threat of acute pancreatitis.

Etiology

Hyperlipidemias may be primary and familial or secondary to other identifiable disorders or to the use of drugs. The basic pathophysiologic derangements are an increase in production and/or a reduction in metabolism and clearance.

- Hyperlipidemias: genetic or acquired disorders that can result from increased production and/or reduced clearance.

Some of the primary hyperlipidemias are outlined in Table 7-2 and the causes of secondary hyperlipidemias are outlined in Table 7-3.

Clinical Features

Ischemic vascular disease—Increased risk of atherogenesis has been associated with the following lipoprotein abnormalities: increased low-density lipoprotein (LDL), increased intermediate-density lipoprotein (IDL), increased Lp(a), and decreased high-density lipoprotein (HDL). Increased HDL is associated with decreased atherogenic risk. Hypertriglyceridemia may be atherogenic in two ways: 1) it may induce alterations in other lipoproteins that might increase the risk of atherogenesis (e.g., it may decrease HDL-cholesterol [HDL-C], increase small density LDL, increase apo B, increase very-low-density lipoprotein [VLDL] remnants and IDL) and 2) it may have a yet unidentified direct atherogenic action.

Pancreatitis—The risk of pancreatitis is conferred by increased triglyceride-rich lipoproteins, the chylomicrons, and VLDL.

Xanthomas—These occur with significant increase in certain lipoproteins: tendon xanthomas with increase in LDL, tuberous and tuboeruptive xanthomas with increase in IDL, eruptive xanthomas with increase in chylomicrons, and planar xanthomas with increase in IDL.

- Clinical presentations: ischemic vascular disease, pancreatitis, or xanthomas.

Diagnosis and Management

The Adult Treatment Panel of the National Cholesterol Education Program (NCEP) has recommended that all adults older than 20 years be evaluated for hypercholesterolemia to identify those at risk for coronary heart disease. Such persons should be identified by total serum cholesterol (TC) and HDL-C levels. If indicated, they should be classified further for treatment based on LDL-cholesterol (LDL-C) levels. Many authorities think that serum triglycerides should be obtained at the initial screening.

Lipid screening tests should be conducted in the free living state and not during an acute illness or hospitalization. Plasma TC does not vary much with meals and can be measured non-fasting. Because plasma triglycerides fluctuate considerably after meals, they must be measured in the fasting state. Determination of plasma HDL-C is recommended as part of the initial evaluation. HDL-C levels cannot be evaluated fully without knowledge of the serum triglyceride levels (plasma triglyceride exchanges into the core regions of HDL and displaces cholesterol esters; the quantity of triglyceride-rich lipoproteins in plasma determines the cholesteryl ester content of HDL; there is an inverse logarithmic dependence of HDL-C on triglycerides). Plasma LDL-C is estimated with the Friedwald equation (LDL-C = Total C- [HDL-C + 5 Triglycerides]). This correlates well with LDL-C obtained by ultracentrifugation as long as the triglyceride level is <400 mg/dL. Ultracentrifugation and the newer immunoseparation methods may be used to assay LDL-C directly.

Lp(a) is believed to be an independent risk factor. Many authorities believe that Lp(a) should be a part of the risk assessment for coronary heart disease only in patients with established coronary heart disease.

- Lipid screening tests should be conducted in the free living state and not during an acute illness or hospitalization.
- Standard lipid tests: total cholesterol, triglycerides, HDL-C, and a calculated LDL-C (Friedwald equation; only useful if triglyceride levels are <400 mg/dL).
- Lp(a) is the only other atherogenic lipid proven to be an independent risk factor.
- The NCEP recommends that all adults older than 20 years have their total cholesterol and HDL-C checked. If indicated, they should be further classified for treatment based on their LDL-C levels.

Assessment of other cardiovascular risks—Risk factors other than hypercholesterolemia include males older than 45 years, females older than 55 years or a female with premature menopause who is not on estrogen replacement therapy, history of definite cerebrovascular or peripheral vascular disease, family history of premature coronary heart disease (definite myocardial infarction or sudden death before age 55 in a parent or a sibling), smoking (currently smokes >10 cigarettes/day), hypertension, diabetes mellitus, and an HDL-C less than 35 mg/dL. Protective factor is HDL-C greater than 60 mg/dL. High risk is defined as a net of two or more risk factors.

- Assessment of the other coronary risk factors is important for assessment of the overall atherogenic risk and planning effective management.

Table 7-2.—Features of Primary Hyperlipidemias

Feature	Familial hypercholesterolemia	Familial combined hyperlipidemia	Familial dysbetalipoproteinemia	Familial hypertriglyceridemia	Severe hypertrigylceridemia of early onset	Severe hypertriglyceridemia of adult onset
Pathophysiology	Defective LDL receptor/or defective apo B-100; impaired catabolism of LDL	Overproduction of hepatic VLDL-apo B-100 but not of VLDL-Tg	Defective or absent apo E: excess of CM-remnants and VLDL in the fasting state	Overproduction of hepatic VLDL-Tg but not of apo B-100	Lipoprotein lipase deficiency Apo C-II deficiency; defect in CM- and VLDL-catabolism	Overproduction of VLDL triglyceride Delayed catabolism of chylomicrons and VLDL
Mode of inheritance	Autosomal codominant	Autosomal dominant	Autosomal recessive	Autosomal dominant	Autosomal recessive	Autosomal recessive
Estimated population frequency	1:500	1:50	1:5,000	1:50	<1:10,000	Rare
Risk of coronary heart disease	+++	++	+	+ in families in which HDL-C is deficient	-	+
Physical findings	Arcus senilis Tendinous xanthomas	Arcus senilis	Arcus senilis Tuboeruptive and palmar xanthomas	None	Lipemia retinalis Eruptive xanthomas	Milky plasma Lipemia retinalis Eruptive xanthomas Pancreatitis
Associated findings		Obesity Glucose intolerance Hyperuricemia HDL deficiency	Obesity Glucose intolerance Hyperuricemia	Obesity Glucose intolerance Hyperuricemia HDL deficiency	HDL deficiency Recurrent abdominal pain Pancreatitis Hepatosplenomegaly	Obesity Glucose intolerance Hyperuricemia HDL deficiency Pancreatitis
Treatment	Diet Niacin and resin Statin and resin Probucol and resin	Diet Drugs singly or in combination with niacin, statin, gemfibrozil, resin	Diet Niacin Gemfibrozil Statin	Diet Niacin Gemfibrozil Abstain from alcohol, estrogen	Diet Fish oil	Diet Control diabetes when present Avoid alcohol, estrogen Gemfibrozil Fish oil

C, cholesterol; CM, chylomicrons; HDL, high-density lipoprotein; LDL, low-density lipoprotein; Tg, triglyceride; VLDL, very-low-density lipoprotein; +++, very high; ++, high; +, moderate; -, no increased risk.

Etiologic diagnosis—After a lipid disorder has been documented, the next step is to exclude secondary causes of hyperlipidemia (Table 7-3). A family history is obtained, and when appropriate, a family screen is conducted.

Recommended assessment plan—1) If the patient has established cardiovascular disease, a known lipid disorder or xanthomas, TC, triglyceride, and HDL-C levels should be measured after an overnight fast. Otherwise, assessment starts with measurement of TC and HDL-C in the fasting or nonfasting state. 2) Patients who have desirable TC (<200 mg/dL) and HDL-C (>50 mg/dL) levels should have their values checked within 5 years. 3) If the patient has a borderline high value for TC (200-239 mg/dL), information about other risk factors for coronary heart disease should be obtained. If the

Table 7-3.—Causes of Secondary Hyperlipidemias

Increased LDL cholesterol	Increased triglycerides	Decreased HDL
Hypothyroidism	Obesity	Hypertriglyceridemia
Dysglobulinemia	Diabetes mellitus	Obesity
Nephrotic syndrome	Hypothyroidism	Diabetes mellitus
Obstructive liver disease	Sedentary life	Cigarette smoking
Progestins	Alcohol	Sedentary life
Anabolic steroids, glucocorticoid therapy	Renal insufficiency	β-Blockers
Anorexia nervosa	Estrogens	Progestins
Acute intermittent porphyria	β-Blockers	Anabolic steroids
	Thiazides, steroids	
	Dysglobulinemias	
	Systemic lupus erythematosus	

patient has a borderline high value of TC (200-239 mg/dL) and a normal HDL-C level in the absence of clinical coronary heart disease or two or more risk factors for this disease, dietary information should be provided and the TC checked within the next year. 4) If the patient has a borderline high value of TC (200-239 mg/dL) and a history of coronary heart disease or two or more risk factors or if the patient has a high risk TC value (>240 mg/dL) or a low HDL-C value (<35 mg/dL), LDL-C levels should be assessed so that an appropriate treatment regimen can be determined. LDL-C is routinely calculated after measuring TC, triglyceride, and HDL-C levels after an overnight fast.

Therapy

The therapeutic goals take into account the presence of coronary heart disease, other atherosclerotic cardiovascular diseases, and other cardiovascular risk factors. The application of the National Cholesterol Education Program Guidelines must be individualized for each patient, considering the presence of such factors as age, the presence of other disease, and the patient's level of motivation and discipline. Treatment of hyperlipidemia in patients with coronary heart disease or other clinical atherosclerotic sequelae is known as "secondary prevention." Treatment in patients without such disorders is termed "primary prevention." Table 7-4 outlines these recommendations.

1) Lowering LDL-C levels in patients with established atherosclerotic disease reduces cardiovascular events and total mortality; therefore, aggressive treatment to lower LDL-C in secondary prevention is clinically indicated and cost-effective. 2) Lowering TC or LDL-C in patients without coronary heart disease reduces cardiovascular events and mortality. Therefore, LDL-C lowering in primary prevention is indicated for high-risk patients. In patients considered to be at low risk,

the emphasis is on dietary and lifestyle modification and less on drug therapy

Treatment modalities include dietary modifications, behavior and lifestyle modification, correction of secondary causes when feasible, and prudent use of antihyperlipidemic drugs.

Diet Therapy (Table 7-5)

General principles. Achieve and maintain normal body weight. Decrease saturated fats and cholesterol intake. If no coronary heart disease, start at American Heart Association (AHA) step I. If coronary heart disease is present, start at step II diet.

Behavior Modification

Weight reduction enhances the cholesterol-lowering effect of low cholesterol/low saturated fat diet, decreases triglycerides, increases HDL-C, and decreases blood pressure and the risk of diabetes mellitus. Smoking cessation increases HDL-C. Regular exercise increases HDL-C. Stress reduction and alcohol restriction often reduce VLDL.

Drug Therapy

Drug therapy for hyperlipidemias is outlined in Table 7-6. General principles—1) The use of drugs is likely to be for lifetime; so institute drug therapy only after vigorous efforts at dietary therapy and after educating patients about the goals of the therapy, the side effects of the drug, and the need for long-term commitment. 2) Recheck lipids and potential side effects of the drug at 4 to 6 weeks and again at 3 months. 3) If the response is adequate, check again in 4 to 6 months; if the response is inadequate, increase the dose. If the response is still inadequate, switch to another drug or use a combination of drugs. 4) Avoid the combination of statins and fibric acid derivatives and possibly statins and niacin because of the increased risk of myositis.

- Drug therapy only after a good attempt at dietary restrictions; more liberal use of drug therapy in patients with established coronary heart disease, because diet alone rarely lowers LDL-C to the desirable range of <100 mg/dL.
- Drug therapy is for lifetime.
- Use drug in progressively larger doses until maximal dose allowed; if still ineffective, try combination drug therapy.
- If at all possible, avoid combinations of statins and fibrates and statins and niacin (increased risk of myositis).

Patients with increased LDL-C: 1) For the younger asymptomatic patient, resins are the drugs of choice. Alternatively, niacin or a combination of resins and niacin can be used. 2) For the patients with severe hypercholesterolemia or coronary heart disease, the elderly, or those who cannot tolerate resins or niacin, statins (reductase inhibitors) should be used; the combination of smaller doses of statin and resin or statin/niacin/resin can be tried. 3) For estrogen-deficient women, estrogen replacement is quite effective in decreasing LDL-C and increasing HDL-C, and its use is associated with a significant decrease in coronary heart disease. Oral estrogens generally should not be given to patients with hypertriglyceridemia, but the use of an estrogen patch or the addition of another antihypertriglyceridemic drug can be considered.

Patients with increased LDL-C and triglycerides: 1) For the younger asymptomatic patients, the drug of choice is niacin.

2) For patients who cannot tolerate this medication and older persons, a statin should be used. Alternatives include gemfibrozil, the combination of resin and niacin, and the combination of resin and gemfibrozil.

Patients with hypertriglyceridemia and normal LDL-C: Clear guidelines for drug therapy are not available. 1) For moderate hypertriglyceridemia, a program of weight reduction, elimination of secondary causes, and lifestyle modifications. 2) If triglycerides are greater than 1,000 mg/dL while the patient is on a restricted diet, steps to reduce the risk of pancreatitis are necessary (stop oral estrogen or alcohol, control diabetes mellitus, and restrict calories and fats). The drug of choice is gemfibrozil, because most patients have diabetes mellitus and niacin worsens the diabetic state. Niacin can be tried in the absence of the diabetic state. Fish oil capsules (1 g) at a dose of 3 to 5 capsules twice daily may be effective.

Patients with low HDL-C: In the absence of heart disease, lifestyle modification (diet and exercise and cessation of smoking) is prescribed, and an attempt is made to discontinue drugs that can lower HDL-C (e.g., β-blockers, androgens). In the presence of coronary artery disease, lowering LDL-C to less than 100 mg/dL with a reductase inhibitor is indicated. Drugs that can increase HDL-C include nicotinic acid, gemfibrozil, and, in postmenopausal women, estrogen replacement therapy.

Patients with increased Lp(a): Exercise may decrease Lp(a). Nicotinic acid and neomycin, singly or in combination, and, in postmenopausal women, estrogen replacement may be effective.

Table 7-4.—Overview of Therapy for Hyperlipidemias

Clinical risk assessment	Initiate diet	Initiate drug therapy	Goal of therapy
No CHD; less than risk factors	>160 mg/dL	>190 mg/dL	<160 mg/dL
No CHD; two or more risk factors	>130 mg/dL	>160 mg/dL	<130 mg/dL
CHD step II AHA diet	>100 mg/dL	>130 mg/dL	<100 mg/dL

AHA, American Heart Association; CHD, coronary heart disease.

Table 7-5.—Dietary Recommendations for Hyperlipidemia (American Heart Association)

	Average U.S. diet	Step I diet	Step II diet
Total fat, %	36	<30	<30
Saturated fat, %	15	<10	<7
Polyunsaturated fat, %	6	<10	<10
Monounsaturated fat, %	15	Up to 15	Up to 15
Cholesterol, mg/dL	400-500	<300	<200

Table 7-6.—Drug Therapy for Hyperlipidemias

Drug	Bile acid sequestrants	Nicotinic acid	Fibric acid derivatives (e.g., gemfibrozil)	HMG-CoA reductase inhibitors (statins)	Probucol
Mechanism of action	Bind bile acids in gut, increase hepatic LDL-catabolism	Decreases VLDL and LDL production	Decrease production and enhance clearance of VLDL	Inhibit the rate-limiting enzyme in cholesterol synthesis, upregulate LDL receptors, increase LDL uptake and catabolism	Lipophylic, incorporated into LDL, increases LDL clearance by nonreceptor pathways
Indications	↑LDL	↑LDL, ↑VLDL, ↑Lp(a)	↑VLDL	↑LDL	↑LDL
Usual dose	8-10 g bid, start with low dose and increase gradually	1 g bid, start with low dose and increase gradually	600 mg bid	Lovastatin: 20-40 mg bid Simvastatin: 10-20 mg qd or bid Pravastatin: 20-40 mg at bedtime Fluvastatin: 20-40 mg qd Atorvastatin: 10-40 mg qd	500 mg bid
LDL-C	↓ 10%-20%	↓ 10%-20%	↓ 0-15%	↓ 15%-40%	↓ 10%-15%
Triglycerides	May ↑	↓ 40%	↓ 35%	↓ 10%-20%	No effect
HDL-C	↑ 5%	↑ 15%-20%	↑ 5%-15%	↑ 5%-10%	May be ↓ by 15%-30%
Lp(a)	No effect	↓ 15%-20%	No effect	No effect	No effect
Patient's tolerance	Relatively poor	Relatively poor	Excellent	Excellent	Excellent
Side effects	Bloating Constipation Interference with absorption of some drugs (take drugs 1 hr before or 4 hr after the resin)	Flushing Pruritus Gastric irritation Hepatotoxicity (especially with slow-release niacin) Hyperglycemia Hyperuricemia	GI side effects Myositis Hepatotoxicity Warfarin interaction	GI side effects Hepatotoxicity Myositis Headaches Insomnia	GI side effects
Contra-indications	Pregnant and lactating women	Liver dysfunction Active peptic ulcer Pregnant and lactating women Caution: in NIDDM not on insulin	Pregnancy and lactation Liver dysfunction Renal dysfunction	Children Pregnant and lactating women Risk of myositis is increased if statin is combined with gemfibrozil or cyclosporine	Patients with low HDL Pregnant and lactating females Children

GI, gastrointestinal; LDL, low-density lipoprotein; NIDDM, noninsulin-dependent diabetes mellitus; VLDL, very-low-density lipoprotein.

THE ENDOCRINE PANCREAS

Diabetes Mellitus

Etiology and Classification

Diabetes mellitus is a metabolic disorder whose basic defect is an absolute or relative lack of insulin. In its complete form, it is manifested by hyperglycemia, accelerated atherosclerosis, microvascular disease (retina and kidney), and neuropathy. It affects about 5% of the population in the U.S.

Type 1 diabetes mellitus (type 1 DM) is characterized by severe absolute insulin deficiency, the patient's dependence on exogenous insulin therapy, and a high predisposition to ketosis. It affects 10% to 20% of the diabetic population, usually appearing in patients younger than 20 years old, but it can occur at any age. Both genetic and environmental factors are involved in its pathogenesis. There is concordance in twins in about 50% of cases, frequent association with certain histocompatibility antigen HLA types, and association with abnormal immune responses, including islet-cell antibodies. The risks of developing type 1 DM in the population at large are 1/500; in siblings, 1/14; in monozygotic twins, 1/3; in offspring of a female with type 1 DM, 1/50; and in the offspring of a male with type 1 DM 1/20. Some patients with type 1 DM may have a remission of up to several months after initial insulin therapy restores the metabolic balance. This "honeymoon" is transient and followed by recurrence of insulin deficiency and symptomatic diabetes mellitus.

- Type 1 DM is characterized by: severe absolute insulin deficiency, patient's dependence on exogenous insulin therapy, and a high predisposition to ketosis. It affects 10%-20% of the diabetic population. Genetic and environmental factors are involved in its pathogenesis.
- Concordance in twins: about 50%. Frequent association with certain histocompatibility antigen HLA types. Association with abnormal immune responses.
- Some patients may have remission of up to several months after initial insulin therapy restores metabolic balance. This "honeymoon" is transient.

Type 2 DM is characterized by partial absolute or relative insulin deficiency (and thus not ketosis-prone) and, in most patients, by insulin resistance at target tissues (the bulk of the insulin resistance is postreceptor in site, particularly at the glycogen synthesis step). Which of these defects is primary is not known, but both defects are required for the expression of type 2 DM. Type 2 DM affects 80% to 90% of the diabetic population and can occur at any age, but it usually appears in older obese patients. Genetic susceptibility is strong (the nature of the genetic influence is not known in most patients), and

twin concordance is almost 100%. Environmental factors such as obesity have a definite role in the development of the disease.

- Type 2 DM is characterized by: partial absolute or relative insulin deficiency, resistance to development of ketosis, and (in most patients) insulin resistance at target tissues. It affects 80%-90% of the diabetic population and usually appears in older obese patients.
- Genetic susceptibility is strong. Twin concordance is almost 100%.
- Environmental factors such as obesity have a definite role in the development of type 2 DM.

Maturity-onset diabetes of the young is clearly linked to mutations in the glucokinase gene located on the short arm of chromosome 7. It is transmitted as an autosomal dominant trait and is expressed as mild hyperglycemia and resistance to ketosis in young persons.

Clinical Features

Type 1 DM usually has a dramatic onset related to abrupt severe insulin deficiency. It usually presents with polyuria, polydipsia, polyphagia with associated weight loss, severe dehydration, ketoacidosis, and, eventually, coma. In very young children, nocturnal enuresis may signal the onset of disease.

Type 2 DM usually has an insidious onset. Initially, the patient may be asymptomatic, and the diagnosis is suggested by the presence of glycosuria or is made by the finding of fasting hyperglycemia. Patients may complain of blurring of vision and myopia, generalized pruritus, and episodes of recurrent infections, carbuncles, furuncles, urinary tract infections, monilial vaginitis in females, and balanitis in males. Occasionally, patients may present with evidence of chronic diabetic complications (neuropathy, nephropathy, or retinopathy), without symptoms relating to glucose intolerance. Polyuria, polydipsia, and polyphagia may develop under certain conditions when the insulin output is stressed (e.g., in pregnancy, with infection, and with the use of certain drugs such as glucocorticoids). Occasionally, patients can present with hyperosmolar nonketotic coma. Some patients may present with transient postprandial hypoglycemia.

- Type 1 DM has a dramatic onset related to abrupt severe insulin deficiency.
- Presentation: polyuria, polydipsia, polyphagia with associated weight loss, severe dehydration, and ketoacidosis.
- Type 2 DM of insidious onset. Initially, patients may be asymptomatic. Episodes of recurrent infections, carbuncles, furuncles, urinary tract infections, monilial vaginitis, or

balanitis. Evidence of chronic diabetic complications. Under certain conditions when insulin output is stressed, polyuria, polydipsia, polyphagia may develop. Patients occasionally present with hyperosmolar nonketotic coma.

Diagnosis

Fasting plasma glucose. Normal fasting plasma glucose is less than 115 mg/dL. In adults (but not pregnant women), values of 140 mg/dL or greater on two or more separate occasions confirm the diagnosis of diabetes mellitus. *The American Diabetes Association has recommended lowering the level for diagnosis from 140 mg/dL to 126 mg/dL (July 1997).* Adults should be tested for diabetes every 3 years beginning at age 45. Persons at risk should undergo earlier or more frequent screening: members of a high-risk ethnic group, obese persons, those with hypertension or HDL cholesterol levels less than 35 mg/dL and/or triglyceride levels greater than 250 mg/dL, and those with first-degree relative with diabetes.

- In adults (not pregnant women): fasting plasma glucose values ≥140 mg/dL on two or more separate occasions confirm the diagnosis of diabetes mellitus.

Oral glucose tolerance test (oral GTT). The main usefulness of this test is to establish or refute the diagnosis of diabetes in the following circumstances: 1) when the fasting plasma glucose values are borderline (between 115 and 139 mg/dL), 2) when the patient presents with symptoms related to diabetes or its known chronic complications and fasting plasma glucose is normal or borderline, and 3) when a diagnosis of diabetes must be made during pregnancy.

Interpretation. A diagnosis of diabetes mellitus is made if on two separate occasions the fasting plasma glucose is 140 mg/dL or greater and the 2-hour value and one additional value between 0.5 and 1.5 hours are 200 mg/dL or greater. A 2-hour plasma glucose value less than 140 mg/dL effectively rules out the diagnosis of diabetes mellitus. A diagnosis of impaired glucose tolerance is made if the fasting plasma glucose is less than 140 mg/dL, the 2-hour value is 140 to 200 mg/dL, and the intervening values are 200 mg/dL or greater. Over time, patients with impaired glucose tolerance may decompensate to frank diabetes, may revert to normal glucose tolerance, or may remain unchanged. They should be reevaluated periodically or if clinical indications develop.

- The main usefulness of the oral glucose tolerance test: when fasting glucose values are borderline, when patient presents with symptoms related to diabetes mellitus or its known chronic complications and fasting plasma glucose is normal or borderline, and when the diagnosis of diabetes mellitus must be made during pregnancy.

- Diabetes mellitus: on two separate occasions the fasting plasma glucose is ≥140 mg/dL and the 2-hour value and one additional value between 0.5 and 1.5 hours are ≥200 mg/dL. A 2-hour plasma glucose value <140 mg/dL effectively rules out the diagnosis of diabetes mellitus.
- Impaired glucose tolerance: the fasting plasma glucose is <140 mg/dL, the 2-hour value is 140-200 mg/dL, and the intervening values are ≥200 mg/dL. Over time, patients with impaired glucose tolerance may decompensate to frank diabetes, revert to normal glucose tolerance, or remain unchanged. They should be reevaluated periodically.

Patients with previous abnormality of glucose tolerance have a history of documented hyperglycemia and have subsequently returned to normal glucose homeostasis. They include those with gestational diabetes and those in whom hyperglycemia developed during the acute phase of myocardial infarction, during serious trauma or sepsis, or during ingestion of diabetogenic drugs. *Patients with potential abnormality of glucose tolerance* have normal glucose tolerance but compared with the general population are at increased risk for development of diabetes. They include monozygotic twins or other first-degree relatives of diabetic patients, obese persons, women who have delivered babies weighing more than 9 pounds, and certain racial/ethnic groups such as Native Americans and African and Hispanic Americans.

Therapy for Type 1 DM

Patients with type 1 DM are severely insulinopenic and are insulin-dependent for survival. Therapy has three critical components, insulin, nutrition plan, and exercise, which need to be balanced on a daily basis. The treatment program must be flexible to allow for changing lifestyles without sacrificing metabolic control. Also, the patient needs to be involved in monitoring the treatment program and in making the necessary adjustments. For most patients, the goal of therapy should be achievement of optimal glycemic control. The Diabetes Control and Complications Trial (DCCT) has demonstrated conclusively that intensive therapy prevents or markedly lessens the risks of chronic microvascular complications of diabetes.

Nutrition

Total calories. Allow maintenance of a reasonable weight and for growth in children and adolescents; do not limit caloric intake if the patient is not overweight.

Nutrient distribution. Protein, 10% to 20%; total fat, less than 30% of total calories; saturated fat, less than 10%; cholesterol, less than 300 mg/day; carbohydrates and monounsaturated fats, 60% to 70% of total calories. The distribution can vary and is individualized on the basis of therapy goals.

- Pay attention to quantity (allow maintenance of reasonable weight; avoid obesity) and quality of food (prudent saturated fat, cholesterol, and salt intake); follow AHA step I diet.

Exercise

Take into consideration the factors that affect the metabolic response to exercise: fitness, duration, and intensity of exercise and the time of exercise in relation to meals and to insulin therapy. Consider steps to be taken to avert hypoglycemia in the face of sporadic unusual activity. Monitor blood glucose before, during, and after exercise to determine efficacy. Moderately severe exercise may deplete glycogen stores and result in sustained food requirement to replace glycogen; hypoglycemia may occur well after exercise (12 hours after jogging). Patients should be careful about planning vigorous exercise in the evening hours.

- Encourage physical activity and take it into consideration in the therapeutic plan.
- Monitor effects of exercise on glycemic control, and adjust insulin and diet accordingly.
- Hypoglycemia may occur several hours after exercise; be prudent about evening exercise.

Insulin Therapy

Consider the patient's endogenous insulin secretion, which components of the insulin secretory profile need to be replaced or supplemented (basal or postprandial insulin secretion), and the time action profiles of the available insulin preparations.

Conventional Insulin Programs

Early after diagnosis of type 1 DM, some insulin reserve is still present and the options available are 1) a twice daily mixture of regular insulin and intermediate-acting insulin, the so-called mixed insulin regimen (NR-O-NR-O) and 2) a morning mixture of regular and intermediate-acting insulin, presupper regular insulin, and bedtime intermediate-acting insulin to minimize nocturnal hypoglycemia and to counteract the dawn phenomenon (NR-O-R-N). Adjust intermediate insulin to control prebreakfast and predinner blood glucose levels; adjust regular insulin to optimize prelunch and prebedtime blood glucose levels.

- Early after diagnosis of type 1 DM, some insulin reserve is still present and the options available are NR-O-NR-O and NR-O-R-N.

Several years after diagnosis, insulin secretion is lost, and these programs become inadequate to meet glycemic control needs, at which time an intensive insulin program is needed. The indication for intensive insulin therapy is to optimize glycemic control by providing basal insulin levels and post-meal bursts of insulin.

Multiple dose insulin program (MDI). 1) Replacement of prandial insulin secretion—Provide preprandial injections of rapid onset, short-acting insulin before each meal, and adjust individually to provide meal insulinemia appropriate to the size of the meal. This program permits total flexibility in meal timing. Regular insulin is given 20 to 30 minutes before a meal; this interval is not needed with the very rapid onset lispro. 2) Replacement of basal insulin secretion—Two options: a) intermediate-acting human insulin (isophane insulin suspension [NPH] or insulin zinc suspension [Lente]) at bedtime plus a small morning dose or b) 1 or 2 injections of human insulin zinc suspension, extended (Ultralente).

Continuous subcutaneous insulin infusion (CSII). This uses an insulin pump that provides a programmed, regular, continuous subcutaneous infusion of insulin. Its advantages are that it replicates 1) basal insulin secretion (may be decreased overnight and increased early morning to counteract the dawn phenomenon), 2) meal-stimulated insulin secretion (the pump is activated 20-30 minutes before meals to provide meal boluses to meet prandial insulin needs), and 3) response of insulin secretion to exercise (with increased physical activity, insulin delivery may be suspended to reduce the risk of exercise-induced hypoglycemia). The disadvantages of CSII are the 1) use of the pump; 2) the use of regular insulin, so any interruption of flow leads to rapid deterioration of control, and 3) infection at catheter site.

- MDI: attempts to mimic the normal insulin secretory profile. Replacement of prandial insulin secretion: preprandial bursts of short-acting insulin. Replacement of the basal insulin secretion: intermediate-acting insulin (p.m. and a.m.) or insulin zinc suspension, extended (Ultralente) (1 or 2 injections/day).
- CSII: attempts to mimic the normal insulin secretory profile. Disadvantages: use of pump; use of regular insulin, so any interruption of flow leads to rapid deterioration of control; and infection at catheter site.

Requirements of an intensive program include a motivated, sophisticated patient capable of careful monitoring (self-monitored blood glucose) 4 times/day and who has knowledge of insulin dose modification. Also required are patient education, surveillance and counselling, patient's awareness of hypoglycemia, and those around the patient being aware of the danger of hypoglycemia and its mode of therapy, including the use of glucagon.

In the absence of motivation, education, or frequent monitoring of blood glucose, one has to resort to the use of the suboptimal conventional insulin programs.

Insulin dosage. The insulin dosage required for meticulous glycemic control in typical patients with type 1 DM who are within 20% of their ideal body weight and in the absence of intercurrent illness or other periods of instability approximates 0.5 to 1.0 U/kg per day. The doses are less during the honeymoon period and may increase significantly during intercurrent illness dosage and the adolescent growth spurt. *Initiation*: about 40% to 50% of the total insulin dosage is used to provide basal insulinemia; the rest is divided among the meals, either empirically proportional to the relative carbohydrate content of the meals or by initially giving approximately 1.0 to 1.2 units of insulin for every 10 g of carbohydrate consumed. *Adjustment*: a plan is provided to enable the patient to alter therapy to achieve individually defined blood glucose targets; actions are guided by self-monitored blood glucose levels and daily records.

Glycemic Goals of Optimal Therapy

1) Blood glucose targets: fasting and premeal, 70 to 105 mg/dL; 1 hour postprandially, 100 to 160 mg/dL; 2 hours postprandially, 80 to 120 mg/dL; bedtime, 100 to 140 mg/dL; and 2:00 to 4:00 a.m., 70 to 105 mg/dL. 2) Glycosylated hemoglobin C, 6% to 7%. 3) Absence of ketonuria. 4) Achievement of these goals without significant side effects. These targets need to be modified in the following circumstances: 1) lower target levels (pregnancy, see below) and 2) higher target levels in patients who are at risk of or from hypoglycemia because of the inability to recognize hypoglycemic symptoms, the inability to recover spontaneously from hypoglycemia, or the presence of ischemic cardiac or cerebrovascular disease.

Assessment and Monitoring

These include glycosylated hemoglobin determination to monitor long-term glycemic control. Self-monitored blood glucose must be done on a daily basis. On most days, it should be 4 times per day before meals and at bedtime. Additional samples should be obtained at 2:00 to 4:00 a.m. once every 1 to 2 weeks and at any time the overnight insulin dosage is to be altered and any time hypoglycemia is suspected. Periodically, postprandial blood samples are also obtained. The patient should keep a careful diary of blood glucose measurements, insulin doses, hypoglycemic episodes, and departures from daily routines. Patient compliance and responsibility for management should be assessed on a regular basis. A random plasma glucose value is used to compare with that obtained by the patient using his or her own monitoring system.

- Monitoring: glycosylated hemoglobin every 2-3 months; self-monitored blood glucose at least 4 times a day; 2:00 - 4:00 a.m. blood sugar every 1-2 weeks; when hypoglycemia

is suspected; periodic postprandial blood sugars. Important to evaluate patient's compliance and responsibility.

Therapy for Type 2 DM

The standard goals of therapy include glycemic control to correct fasting and preprandial hyperglycemia and to minimize postprandial hyperglycemia. The targets are fasting and preprandial plasma glucose levels less than 115 mg/dL, 2-hour postprandial blood glucose less than 140 mg/dL, and a normal or near-normal glycosylated hemoglobin (HbA1 or HbA1c). Another goal is control of other cardiovascular risk factors: to optimize lipid and blood pressure control, to encourage exercise and smoking cessation, and to keep body weight stable and as close to the ideal as possible. Most patients with type 2 DM are obese and lead sedentary lifestyles; therefore, a nutritional plan and promotion of physical activity are the cornerstones of management. In some patients, they may be the only therapeutic intervention required to restore glycemic control.

- Goals: optimal control of type 2 DM and of other cardiovascular risk factors.

Nutrition

Use calorie restriction when appropriate to promote weight reduction. Weight reduction in the obese, even though it may be modest, leads to improvement in insulin resistance, diabetes control, glucose toxicity, and blood pressure and lipid control. A healthy balanced diet includes 1) carbohydrates (45%-60%; encourage dietary fiber consumption and avoidance of excess simple sugars); 2) total fat, less than 30% of calories; low saturated fat, less than 10% of calories (a significant increase in carbohydrate intake may increase the triglyceride levels; monounsaturated fats are increased when there is need to restrict carbohydrates); 3) low cholesterol, less than 300 mg/day; 4) sodium, more than 3,000 mg/dL; 5) proteins, 10% to 20%. Spacing between meals should be adequate: 4 to 5 hours apart. Appropriate modifications of the diet need to be made in the presence of dyslipidemia, hypertension, and renal disease.

- Calorie restriction when appropriate to promote weight reduction; a healthy balanced diet (AHA step I diet); appropriate modifications of the diet need to be made in the presence of dyslipidemia, hypertension, and renal disease.

Exercise

Exercise improves insulin action, facilitates weight loss, and reduces cardiovascular risks (increases HDL-C, decreases VLDL-triglycerides, and increases fibrinolytic activity), and increases sense of well-being. There are limitations to any exercise plan in patients with type 2 DM: 1) preexisting coronary or peripheral vascular disease (preexercise evaluation should include an exercise-stress electrocardiogram in all persons older than 35 years to detect silent ischemic heart disease), 2) proliferative retinopathy, 3) peripheral and autonomic neuropathy, and 4) poor glycemic control. All patients should be encouraged to increase physical activity to a level tolerable to them, to start slowly and build up gradually, and to monitor their glycemic response to exercise.

- A prudent exercise program to encourage weight reduction, cardiovascular fitness, and sense of well-being.
- Remember the limitations: preexisting coronary or peripheral vascular disease (preexercise evaluation should include an exercise-stress electrocardiogram), proliferative retinopathy, peripheral and autonomic neuropathy, poor glycemic control.

Drug Therapy

Oral agents. The oral agents in common use and their use in the management of type 2 DM are outlined in Table 7-7.

Sulfonylureas. The best response occurs early in the disease when endogenous secretory capability is still present. The ideal setup for effectiveness includes fasting plasma level of glucose less than 250 mg/dL, age at onset of type 2 DM older than 40 years, duration of diabetes less than 5 years, normal or excessive weight, and no previous therapy with insulin or insulin dose less than 40 U/day. Use of second-generation sulfonylureas: the second-generation agents (glyburide, glipizide), which are analogues of the first-generation drugs, are nonionically bound to plasma proteins and so are not displaced by other ionically charged drugs such as warfarin and phenylbutazone. Concurrent use of the latter medications does not lead to variation in bioavailability of the second-generation oral antidiabetic agents. *Secondary failures*: remember that transient failures may be due to intercurrent acute medical/surgical illness, failure to adhere to the diet, and weight gain. Side effects uniquely associated with chlorpropamide use include antabuse-like effect and syndrome of inappropriate ADH.

Metformin. Association with lactic acidosis is extremely rare if the specific exclusion criteria for the use of metformin are followed: 1) renal impairment: plasma creatinine values of 1.5 mg/dL or greater for men and 1.4 mg/dL for women, 2) cardiac or respiratory insufficiency that is likely to cause central hypoxia or reduced peripheral perfusion, 3) history of lactic acidosis, 4) severe infection that could lead to reduced tissue perfusion, 5) liver disease (including alcoholic liver disease) as demonstrated by abnormal liver function tests, 6) alcohol abuse with binge drinking sufficient to cause acute hepatic toxicity, and 7) use of intravenous radiographic contrast agents.

The use of *troglitazone (Rezulin)* has been associated with hepatocellular injury, which is usually modest and reversible but can be severe and irreversible. It should not be given to patients with liver disease or those taking bile acid sequestrants. It is recommended that the drug not be used if serum alanine transaminase (ALT) levels are greater than 1.5 times upper limit of normal. Serum ALT should be measured every month of drug use for the first 8 months, then every 2 months for the next 4 months, and periodically thereafter. If serum ALT increases to 3 times or greater the upper limit of normal, the use of troglitazone should be discontinued.

Repaglinide (Prandin) acts on the B cells to increase insulin secretion and has recently been approved by the U.S. Food and Drug Administration for the treatment of type 2 DM, as monotherapy or in combination with metformin. Its clinical efficacy is similar to that of the sulfonylureas. It is given preprandially in a dose of 0.5 to 4 mg before each meal (the dose is skipped if the meal is missed). Its important side effect is hypoglycemia.

- Sulfonylureas: remember the requirements for effective therapy; second-generation drugs are nonionically bound to plasma proteins; transient failures may be due to intercurrent acute medical/surgical illness, failure to adhere to the diet, and weight gain; side effects uniquely associated with chlorpropamide use include antabuse-like effect and SIADH.
- Metformin: association with lactic acidosis is extremely rare if the specific exclusion criteria for the use of metformin are followed.
- Troglitazone: insulin sensitizer; can cause liver dysfunction.
- Repaglinide: increases insulin secretion; is given preprandially; can cause hypoglycemia.

Insulin therapy. This is a second-line therapy for patients with type 2 DM in whom diet and oral agents (monotherapy and combination therapy) have failed. Insulin therapy is commonly used as first-line therapy in patients with type 2 DM who are nonobese, young, or severely hyperglycemic or who are pregnant. It also is used temporarily during severe stress, injury, infection, or surgery. Insulin therapy carries the disadvantage of hypoglycemia and requires vigilance. It should not be used in patients at high risk for hypoglycemia (e.g., alcoholics and poorly compliant patients).

In patients with some degree of meal-stimulated endogenous insulin secretion, one can use one daily dose of intermediate insulin either in the morning, or, to diminish overnight hepatic glucose output, in the evening. This may be supplemented by an oral agent during the day to facilitate meal-stimulated endogenous insulin release. Alternatively, one can use a split-dose of intermediate insulin: in the morning before breakfast and in the evening before dinner, or preferably at

Table 7-7.—Comparison of Common Oral Agents Used to Treat Type 2 Diabetes Mellitus

	Sulfonylurea	Metformin	Acarbose	Troglitazone
Mode of action	Stimulates insulin secretion by β-cell	Enhances insulin effect on the liver and peripheral tissues: decreases neoglucogenesis	An α-glucosidase inhibitor; interferes with digestion of disaccharides and complex carbohydrates Decreases postprandial glycemic excursions	An insulin sensitizer; improves insulin resistance and potentiates the efficacy of insulin therapy
Indications	Mild to moderately severe type 2 DM, monotherapy or in combination with metformin, acarbose, or insulin	Same as sulfonylureas; monotherapy or in combination with sulfonylureas	Type 2 DM with mild fasting hyperglycemia and modest postprandial hyperglycemia particularly in the obese Monotherapy or in combination with sulfonylureas or insulin	Approved only for use in patients with inadequately controlled type 2 DM who are on insulin
Contraindications	Type 1 DM Pregnancy and lactation Hepatic or renal failure Sulfa allergy	Type 1 DM Pregnancy and lactation Renal impairment Conditions associated with propensity to lactic acidosis	As monotherapy in moderately severe type 2 DM Type 1 DM Pregnancy and lactation	Type 1 DM Pregnancy and lactation
Primary failure	20%	Same as sulfonylureas		
Secondary failure	5-10% per year	Same as sulfonylureas		
Side effects and complications	Hypoglycemia Others are rare: gastrointestinal, dermatologic, hematopoietic	Decreased appetite Nausea Abdominal discomfort Diarrhea Lactic acidosis in renal impairment or in conditions with propensity to lactic acidosis	Abdominal fullness, flatulence, and occasional diarrhea Avoid use with metformin: decreases bioavailability of metformin; gastrointestinal side effects may be additive	Liver dysfunction (see text) Long-term effects are unknown May reduce efficacy of oral contraceptives
Advantages	Ease of administration Oral Efficacy in mild to moderate hyperglycemia in type 2 DM	Same as sulfonylureas No hypoglycemia Weight loss Improvement in lipid profile	As monotherapy, no risk of hypoglycemia In combination with sulfonylurea or insulin, may increase the risk of hypoglycemia	Improved control Decrease in insulin dosage

Table 7-7.—Continued

	Sulfonylurea	Metformin	Acarbose	Troglitazone
Agent and dosage	Second generation: glyburide: 1.25-20 mg qd glipizide: 2.5-40 mg qd glipizide-GITS: 5-20 mg qd micronized glyburide: 0.75-12 mg qd Third generation glimepiride: 1-8 mg qd	Metformin: 500-2,500 mg/day	Acarbose: 25-100 mg with each meal	Troglitazone (Rezulin): 200-600 mg once daily

DM, diabetes mellitus.

bedtime. In patients with a more severe insulin deficiency, a multiple dose regimen may be used involving a split/mixed program (e.g., NR-O-NR-O or NR-O-R-N). However, it is important to consider the clinical context of the patient's disease, the patient's motivation and ability to perform self care, and the level of diabetes education.

- In patients with some degree of meal-stimulated endogenous insulin secretion, one can use one daily dose of intermediate insulin, either in the morning or, to diminish overnight hepatic glucose output, in the evening. This may be supplemented by an oral agent during the day. Alternatively, use a split-dose of intermediate insulin.
- In patients with a more severe insulin deficiency, a multiple dose regimen may be used involving a split/mixed program (e.g., NR-O-NR-O or NR-O-R-N).

Combination therapy. The four classes of antidiabetic agents currently available differ in their mechanism of action, raising the possibility that the use of combination therapy can be beneficial in optimizing glycemic control. 1) Combination of sulfonylurea and metformin—when therapy with one agent fails, the addition of the other significantly improves control. Such combination therapy should be considered only after maximizing therapy with the first agent. 2) Acarbose can also be added to sulfonylurea, especially in patients who experience significant postprandial hyperglycemia. In this setting, the acarbose dose can be titrated by following the 1-hour post-prandial plasma glucose levels. 3) The evidence about the efficacy of acarbose-metformin combination therapy is insufficient. 4) The use of sulfonylurea in combination with insulin has produced variable results. In patients with type 2 DM who require large doses of insulin for control, sulfonylurea has been added in an attempt to reduce the insulin requirement; for the

most part, the benefits obtained have been limited. A sequential sulfonylurea-insulin therapy regimen has been tried. A commonly used sequence is the addition of intermediate-acting insulin at bedtime to control nocturnal and fasting hyperglycemia and the continued use of sulfonylurea in the morning to control daytime hyperglycemia. This regimen, termed "BIDS" (bedtime insulin-daytime sulfonylurea) can be used as an intermediate step for patients in whom sulfonylurea therapy has failed before switching to insulin therapy alone. 5) There have been no controlled studies to document the efficacy of metformin-insulin.

- Effective combinations: sulfonylurea and metformin; acarbose and sulfonylurea; troglitazone and insulin; repaglinide and metformin.
- Variable results with sulfonylurea-insulin combinations.
- Untested: acarbose and metformin; metformin and insulin.

Hypoglycemia in Treated Diabetics

Etiology
1) Mismatch of food, exercise, and insulin or sulfonylurea: missed meal, erratic nutrient intake or timing, exercise (glucose needs, increased insulin absorption from exercising limbs), and gastroparesis. 2) Excessive insulin dosage: failure to reduce insulin dosage after periods of increased requirements (after recovery from illness, after pregnancy, during the honeymoon period in the evolution of type 1 DM); unrealistic or inappropriate attempt to maintain normoglycemia, and hypoglycemic unawareness (frequently the result of recurrent hypoglycemia due to attempts to achieve normoglycemia; hypoglycemic unawareness can be reversed when hypoglycemia is prevented for 3 months). 3) Longer duration of diabetes may increase the risk of hypoglycemia for several

reasons: more frequent and larger doses of insulin are necessary to maintain normoglycemia; after several years, type 1 DM patients lose their ability to release glucagon in response to hypoglycemia; after 10 to 15 years, a few patients also begin to lose the ability to secrete epinephrine in response to hypoglycemia (this is a form of autonomic neuropathy and/or resetting of CNS activation points for glucoregulation). With the loss of epinephrine, type 1 DM patients become virtually defenseless against hypoglycemia ("the poor counterregulators") and are at increased risk for developing hypoglycemia with intensive insulin program. 4) Prolonged insulin action: renal failure, circulating insulin antibodies. 5) Decreased neoglucogenesis: alcohol excess, advanced liver disease, loss of counterregulatory hormones (adrenomedullary failure of long-standing diabetes, β-adrenergic blockade, Addison disease, hypopituitarism). 6) Intentional overdosage (factitial or suicidal).

- Etiology: mismatch of food, exercise, and insulin or sulfonylurea; excessive insulin or sulfonylurea dosage; hypoglycemic unawareness; longer duration of diabetes and loss of counterregulatory defenses; prolonged insulin action; decreased neoglucogenesis of various causes (notably alcohol, other endocrinopathies, and drugs); intentional overdosage (factitial or suicidal).

Clinical Features

The symptoms of hypoglycemia are described below. Symptomatic hypoglycemia is classified into mild hypoglycemia (the patient is not impaired), moderately severe hypoglycemia (the patient is still alert and able to seek self-treatment), and severe hypoglycemia (coma, seizure, or sufficient neurologic impairment so that the patient requires the assistance of another person to treat the hypoglycemia). Patients with hypoglycemic unawareness develop severe neuroglycopenic manifestations such as seizures or coma without warning signs. These patients have lost their ability to counterregulate effectively, and they no longer recognize the neurogenic or neuroglycopenic warning symptoms. After a patient experiences one episode of severe hypoglycemia, the risk of a subsequent episode during the next year increases severalfold. All episodes of hypoglycemia have to be treated with vigilance regardless of how trivial the cause may appear to be.

Nocturnal hypoglycemia (predawn phenomenon). More than 50% of all episodes of severe hypoglycemia occur during the night or before breakfast, when patients are asleep and commonly unaware of premonitory symptoms of nocturnal hypoglycemia. Insulin requirements to maintain normoglycemia are 20% to 30% lower in the predawn period than at dawn (the predawn phenomenon). Intermediate-acting insulin given before dinner to lower prebreakfast glucose levels often produces relative hyperinsulinemia at 1:00 to 3:00 a.m. (the waning insulin phenomenon).

- Symptoms are classified into mild, moderate, or severe, depending on the extent of neuroglycopenia and a patient's awareness and ability to institute self-care to correct the hypoglycemia.
- More than 50% of all episodes of severe hypoglycemia occur during the night or before breakfast when patients are asleep.
- After a patient experiences one episode of severe hypoglycemia, the risk of subsequent episodes during the next year increases severalfold.
- All episodes of hypoglycemia have to be treated with vigilance.

Prevention. Education of the patient, family, and roommate is paramount. Education includes hypoglycemic manifestations. Hypoglycemic symptoms can change with time; they become less noticeable. Education also includes need for periodic checks of 1:00 to 3:00 a.m. blood glucose level; need to use glucagon when oral feeding is not possible. Check prebedtime blood sugar: if less than 120 mg/dL, increase the size of bedtime snack, add protein to the carbohydrate content. *Nocturnal hypoglycemia*: increase bedtime snack; modify insulin regimen (reduce predinner intermediate insulin or switch predinner intermediate insulin to bedtime or use predinner insulin zinc suspension, extended [Ultralente] instead of the predinner intermediate insulin).

Unexplained Morning Hyperglycemia in Insulin-Treated Diabetic Patients

Consider the *dawn phenomenon*. This phenomenon refers to the transient state of insulin resistance in the early morning seen mostly in type 1 DM patients. It probably is caused by the nocturnal secretion of GH and increased liver glucose output. Management includes moving intermediate insulin from presuppertime to bedtime. Also consider the waning effect of previous dinnertime intermediate insulin, other factors such as a large evening meal or late snack, and rebound posthypoglycemic hyperglycemia, which is seen very infrequently, in fact, most often, the plasma glucose levels in the morning after nocturnal hypoglycemia are low and remain low for several hours.

- Unexplained morning hyperglycemia: the dawn effect and the waning effect (switch intermediate insulin from predinner to bedtime); rebound posthypoglycemic hyperglycemia is seen very infrequently (decrease the dose of insulin). Differential diagnosis: check 3:00 a.m. blood glucose level.

Acute Complications of Diabetes Mellitus

Diabetic Ketoacidosis

The dominant pathogenetic features of diabetic ketoacidosis are severe insulin deficiency and excess of counterregulatory hormones. The disorder is characterized by hyperglycemia, osmotic diuresis, dehydration, and hyperosmolar state and by lipolysis, ketogenesis, ketonemia, and metabolic acidosis. The patient usually has type 1 DM, and diabetic ketoacidosis may be the initial presentation of the diabetic state.

The *clinical features* are characterized by gradual deterioration (in some patients, over days) and include polyuria, polydipsia, dehydration, anorexia, nausea and vomiting, abdominal pain, tachypnea, obtundation, and coma. The physical findings include clinical evidence of dehydration, decreased mentation, deep and rapid Kussmaul respiration, and acetone breath.

The *precipitating factors* are failure to take insulin or to increase insulin and consume extra fluids during acute illness, infection, other intercurrent illness such as myocardial infarction, pancreatitis, stroke, trauma, or emotional stress.

The *diagnosis* is based on the demonstration of significant hyperglycemia, ketonemia, and metabolic acidosis. Associated biochemical abnormalities include hyponatremia, azotemia, and hyperamylasemia of nonpancreatic origin. Serum levels of potassium, phosphate, and magnesium (despite large body losses) may be normal, increased, or decreased.

Pitfalls: 1) Hyperglycemia may be of only moderate degree (plasma glucose level <500 mg/dL), particularly with pregnancy or alcohol use. 2) Ketoacidosis may be present but undetected by the commonly used nitroprusside tests (Ketostix, Acetest). Such tests react mainly with acetoacetate, less so with acetone, and none at all with β-hydroxybutyrate. The ratio of β-hydroxybutyrate to acetoacetate is usually 3:1. At pH 7.1, it increases to 6:1 and may be greater than 30:1 in the presence of alcohol excess or lactic acidosis (altered redux state).

- Diabetic ketoacidosis: severe insulin deficiency and excess of counterregulatory hormones.
- Characteristics: hyperglycemia, hyperosmolar dehydration, hyperketonemia, and metabolic acidosis; patient usually has type 1 DM. It may be the initial presentation of the disease.
- The clinical features evolve gradually, sometimes over days.
- Abdominal pain is not due to diabetic ketoacidosis if the patient is older than 40 years or (if younger than 40 years) the bicarbonate level is >10 mEq/L.
- Diagnosis: significant hyperglycemia, ketonemia, and metabolic acidosis.
- Ketoacidosis may be present with negative finding on nitroprusside tests (Ketostix, Acetest).

- The diagnostic process is not complete without a thorough search for precipitating factors and assessment of complications.

Therapy

The goals of therapy are to correct the hyperglycemia, hyperketonemia and acidosis, hyperosmolar dehydration, and electrolyte depletion. These goals are achieved by insulin administration, replacement of fluid and electrolytes, treatment of precipitating factors, and avoidance of complications. Metabolic and volume correction have to be initiated rapidly. After improvement is established, one can proceed more cautiously.

1. Insulin therapy. Regular insulin is the mainstay of therapy. Insulin infusion is preferred over subcutaneous or intramuscular insulin regimens because it provides smoother control with less risk of hypoglycemia. Initially, give a priming dose of 10 to 20 units intravenously and then set up an insulin infusion at the rate of 10 U/hr. This provides a plasma level of about 200 mU/mL, adequate to inhibit lipolysis and hepatic glucose production and to maximize glucose uptake.

2. Fluids. The aim is to restore volume and to correct electrolyte and fluid losses and hyperosmolarity. The average fluid deficit in adults is 5 to 8 L. Give 2 L of normal saline in the first hour, 1 L/hr in the second and third hours, and 250 to 500 mL/hr until the vital signs stabilize. Next, switch to 0.45% saline and adjust as needed. As plasma glucose values approach 300 mg/dL, change to 0.45% saline in 5% dextrose in water. Maintain the plasma glucose value between 200 and 250 mg/dL during the first 12 to 24 hours to reverse ketosis, to avoid rapid decrease in osmolarity and cerebral edema, and to avoid hypoglycemia.

3. Electrolytes. Potassium—The potassium deficit is about 300 to 500 mEq. Regardless of the initial serum level of potassium, the total body stores of potassium are low. With therapy and correction of acidosis and hyperglycemia, the serum level of potassium decreases. Potassium should be added to the intravenous fluids as soon as renal perfusion and urine flow are assured. Add 40 mEq of potassium to each liter of intravenous fluid as potassium chloride. Phosphate—Phosphate repletion is indicated in the presence of phosphate levels less than 1 mg/dL. Give phosphate in the dose of 0.08 mM/kg intravenously over 6 hours. (Neutral potassium phosphate, 1 ampule contains 3 mM phosphate and 15 mEq of potassium.) Monitor the serum level of phosphate carefully because of the risk of hypocalcemia, seizures, and death. Bicarbonate—If pH is less than 7.1, give bicarbonate (44 mEq/L) until pH increases to about 7.1.

Avoid excessive bicarbonate because it exacerbates hypokalemia and may result in paradoxical CSF fluid acidosis.

- Goals: to correct hyperglycemia, hyperketonemia and acidosis, hyperosmolar dehydration, and electrolyte depletion.
- Achieve goals by: insulin administration, replacement of fluid and electrolytes, treatment of precipitating factors, and avoidance of complications.

Complications

The major complications of diabetic ketoacidosis result mostly from therapy failures: persistent ketosis/acidosis, hypoglycemia, hypokalemia, paradoxical CSF acidosis, cerebral edema, and metabolic alkalosis can be prevented.

Prognosis

The mortality rate is 5% to 15% (higher among the elderly) and in most patients is due to the associated catastrophic illness such as myocardial infarction, cerebrovascular accident, or sepsis. After successful therapy, the goal is to avoid recurrence by properly managing the diabetic state and by patient education, sick day management, and testing urine ketones when blood glucose greater than 300 mg/dL.

- Main complications result from therapy failures: persistent ketoacidosis, hypoglycemia, hypokalemia, paradoxical CSF acidosis, cerebral edema, metabolic alkalosis.
- Prognosis: 5%-15% mortality; higher rate among the elderly and due to associated catastrophic illness.
- After successful therapy, the goal is to avoid recurrence by properly managing the diabetic state and by patient education.

Hyperglycemic Hyperosmolar Nonketotic Coma

Hyperglycemic hyperosmolar nonketotic coma is characterized by significant hyperglycemia, hyperosmolar dehydration, and the absence of ketoacidosis. Its pathophysiology includes insulin deficiency, osmotic diuresis, dehydration, and decreased renal function; however, enough insulin is available to inhibit excess lipolysis and ketogenesis. It occurs predominantly in type 2 DM, and it is often precipitated by acute illness such as myocardial infarction, pancreatitis, pneumonia or other infections, surgical stress, dialysis, hyperalimentation, and the use of such drugs as glucocorticoids, thiazides, and phenytoin. Hyperglycemic hyperosmolar nonketotic coma may be the first presentation of type 2 DM.

- Characteristics: significant hyperglycemia and dehydration without ketoacidosis.
- Pathophysiology: insulin deficiency, osmotic diuresis, dehy-

dration, and decreased renal function. Enough insulin is available to inhibit excess lipolysis and ketogenesis.
- Occurs predominantly in type 2 DM; it is often precipitated by acute illness or by glucocorticoids, thiazides, or phenytoin. It may be the first presentation of type 2 DM.

Diagnosis

The disorder should be suspected in any diabetic patient presenting with altered sensorium, obtundation or coma, and severe dehydration. Laboratory evaluation reveals significant hyperglycemia (often >600 mg/dL), absence of significant ketonemia, and plasma hyperosmolarity (>320 mOsm/L). Associated findings may include renal insufficiency and lactic acidosis. A search for an underlying etiologic disorder is an integral part of the diagnostic process.

- Suspect the disorder in any diabetic patient with altered sensorium, obtundation/coma, and severe dehydration.
- Laboratory evaluation shows: significant hyperglycemia (often >600 mg/dL), no significant ketonemia, and plasma hyperosmolarity (>320 mOsm/L).
- Associated findings: renal insufficiency and lactic acidosis.
- Search for complications and precipitating disorder.

Therapy

Prompt management is indicated. The objectives are to restore volume and osmolarity and to manage the hyperglycemia. Supportive measures are initiated to manage shock, coma, and, in patients who have been or are receiving steroids, to provide increased dosages appropriate for an acute illness. 1) Initial fluid therapy should be with normal saline to restore vascular volume and tissue perfusion: 1 L normal saline per hour for 2 to 4 hours or longer, followed by 0.45% saline to correct the hyperosmolarity. As the blood glucose level decreases with appropriate insulin therapy, 5% dextrose in water can be added. 2) A dose of 20 units of regular insulin is given intravenously if the plasma glucose level is greater than 600 mg/dL, then insulin infusion is begun. It is important to decrease the plasma glucose gradually to a level between 200 and 300 mg/dL to avoid cerebral edema. Next, stop the infusion and start giving insulin subcutaneously. 3) Electrolyte replacement—Potassium, phosphate, and magnesium replacements are as outlined above for diabetic ketoacidosis. 4) Lactic acidosis usually responds to volume replacement; if the pH is less than 7.1, bicarbonate can be given. 5) Monitoring—The patient's condition has to be monitored closely. Repeated neurologic evaluation is needed because focal deficits or seizures may become apparent during therapy.

The complications include vascular events such as myocardial infarction or cerebrovascular accident, hypoglycemia, cerebral edema, and hypokalemia. Mortality is 50%.

- Objectives: restore volume and osmolarity and manage hyperglycemia.
- Initial fluid therapy: give normal saline to correct volume deficit, then 0.45% saline to correct hyperosmolarity.
- Regular insulin to correct the hyperglycemia; gradually decrease plasma glucose to a level around 200 mg/dL.
- Patient must be monitored closely.
- Complications: vascular events, hypoglycemia, cerebral edema, and hypokalemia.
- Mortality: 50%.

Chronic Sequelae of Diabetes Mellitus

Eye Disease in Diabetes

In type 1 DM, the prevalence of diabetic retinopathy is 50% to 70% by 10 years and higher than 95% by 15 to 20 years; it is rare in those who have had diabetes mellitus for less than 5 years. In type 2 DM, the prevalence is 15% to 20% at the time of diagnosis and 50% by 15 years.

Retina. 1) Background diabetic retinopathy: micro-aneurysms, hard yellow exudates, hemorrhages, retinal edema, and local maculopathy. Management: diabetes control, blood pressure control, focal laser treatment for macular edema. 2) Preproliferative retinopathy: soft white exudates (infarcted nerve fibers), venous beading, intraretinal microvascular abnormalities, areas of capillary closure, and diffuse maculopathy. Management: diabetes control, blood pressure control, grid laser therapy around macula for macular edema. 3) Proliferative retinopathy: neovascular proliferation, glial proliferation, retinal elevation, vitreous hemorrhage. Management: panretinal photocoagulation to decrease stimulus for angiogenesis factors, vitrectomy after repeated vitreous hemorrhage, repair of retinal tears, and blood pressure control.

Iris. Impairment of pupil reaction to light and accommodation; rubeosis iridis and resultant neovascular glaucoma. Therapy: panretinal photocoagulation to decrease stimulus for new vessels; diagnose and treat glaucoma; cryoablation of the ciliary body is a last resort.

Lens. Subcapsular cataract in young patients (posterior pole opacities, rapidly progressive). Therapy: diabetes control; surgical removal. Accelerated typical senile cataract due to polyol accumulation and glycosylation of crystalline proteins; irreversible. Therapy: surgical removal.

Dilated ophthalmic evaluation by an experienced ophthalmologist is critical to identify patients at risk, at least annually from the time of diagnosis in type 2 DM, and 5 years after diagnosis of type 1 DM in postpubertal patients. For pregnant women with type 1 DM, obtain an ophthalmologic consultation in the first trimester and follow closely during pregnancy. No screening is required for women with gestational diabetes.

- Dilated ophthalmic evaluation is critical for all diabetic patients: in type 2 DM, at diagnosis and then annually; for type 1 DM, after puberty and annually beginning 5 years after diagnosis.

The Skin and Diabetes

Diseases include necrobiosis lipoidica diabeticorum, diabetic dermopathy, Dupuytren contractures, and diabetic cheirarthropathy in type 1 DM; also, finger stiffness, periarticular swelling, and waxy thickened skin, resembling scleroderma. Eruptive xanthomas in patients with uncontrolled diabetes due to significant hypertriglyceridemia.

Infections and Diabetes

Increased frequency of cutaneous infections (*Staphylococcus* infections, furuncles, pyoderma, and carbuncles), urinary tract infections (cystitis, pyelonephritis, and papillary necrosis), lung infections (pneumonia), extremity infections (gram-negative and anaerobic infections), and genital tract infections (vulvovaginitis and balanitis). Three unusual conditions have specific relationships with the diabetic syndrome: malignant external otitis, rhinocerebral mucormycosis, and emphysematous cholecystitis.

Macrovascular Disease in Diabetes

Ischemic cardiovascular disease appears earlier and is more extensive in diabetic patients than in the general population. It presents clinically as peripheral vascular disease (with intermittent claudication, gangrene, and impotence), coronary artery disease (with angina and myocardial infarction), and cerebrovascular disease (e.g., stroke).

Coronary artery disease accounts for 70% of deaths in the diabetic population and tends to involve the proximal and distal vessels in the right and left coronary arterial systems. Atypical manifestations may occur; angina may present with epigastric distress, heartburn, and neck or jaw pain; myocardial infarction may be silent (in 15% of patients) because of autonomic neuropathy. It should be suspected in those patients with sudden onset of left ventricular failure. *Cardiomyopathy and heart failure* occur in fewer than 15% of patients in the absence of other identifiable causes and with a normal coronary arterial system on angiography. *Peripheral vascular disease* has a higher frequency of distal involvement, particularly in the lower extremities. Use arteriography with caution and only if the patient is a candidate for vascular surgery; use with caution if the patient has diminished renal function (acute tubular necrosis may develop).

Diabetic foot ulcers result from neuropathy and vascular disease. Abnormal pressure distribution results in callus formation, and ill-fitting shoes cause blisters. Foreign bodies lead to abrasions and punctures. Ulcers are painless and frequently complicated by infection and osteomyelitis. Therapy: prevention or relief of maldistribution of pressure; prompt treatment of infections; correction of vascular insufficiency.

Hyperlipidemia in Diabetics

Abnormalities occur in the three major classes of lipoproteins. 1) In type 1 DM, lipid levels are usually normal if the diabetic state is well controlled and there is no renal impairment. 2) Diabetic ketoacidosis: increased VLDL synthesis by the liver and decreased catabolism of VLDL and chylomicrons because of inhibition of lipoprotein lipase; triglyceride levels may reach very high levels, and eruptive xanthomas may appear. 3) In type 2 DM, triglyceride-rich lipoproteins are increased because of overproduction of VLDL and decreased lipoprotein lipase activity. Both defects are improved with better control of the diabetic state. HDL-C levels are low and levels do improve but usually do not normalize with control of diabetes. LDL-C levels usually are not affected by the diabetic state and may be elevated in the presence of renal failure, genetic diseases, or other associated diseases such as hypothyroidism. Compositional changes in LDL may occur (including glycosylation, increased susceptibility to oxidation, and small dense low-density lipoprotein) and may increase the atherogenicity of LDL-C in patients with diabetes.

Diabetes and Pregnancy

Normal gestational changes in fuel metabolism include 1) fetal siphoning of glucose and neoglucogenic precursors, resulting in a tendency to fasting maternal hypoglycemia and to starvation ketosis, and 2) anti-insulin action of placental hormones (human placental lactogen, estrogen, and progesterone) and increased cortisol secretion. Because of these stresses, gestational diabetes may develop in pregnant women with reduced beta-cell reserve. In those with established diabetes, there is worsening of control. *The well-being of the fetus dictates tight glucose control.* Inadequate control early in pregnancy increases the risk of congenital malformations, and inadequate control in the latter part of pregnancy increases the risk of macrosomia, neonatal hypoglycemia, hypocalcemia, polycythemia, hyperbilirubinemia, and respiratory distress.

- Inadequate control in early pregnancy: increased risk of congenital malformations.
- Inadequate control in latter part of pregnancy: increased risk of macrosomia, neonatal hypoglycemia, hypocalcemia, polycythemia, hyperbilirubinemia, and respiratory distress.

Gestational diabetes complicates 2% to 3% of all pregnancies. All pregnant women should be evaluated at 24 to 28 weeks or, if at high risk, at the first visit. (In July 1997,

the ADA recommended that testing does not need to be performed in women at low risk, i.e., those younger than 25 years, normal body weight, no family history of the disease, and not members of a high-risk ethnic group.) A 50-g oral glucose load is given and the plasma glucose level is measured 1 hour later. A plasma glucose level greater than 140 mg/dL indicates the need for a complete oral glucose tolerance test. In the oral glucose tolerance test during pregnancy, 100 g of glucose is given orally. The diagnostic criteria are those of O'Sullivan and Maher. Two or more of the following plasma glucose values must be met or exceeded: fasting, 105 mg/dL; 1 hour, 190 mg/dL; 2 hours, 165 mg/dL; and 3 hours, 145 mg/dL.

- Early detection and optimal management of diabetes during pregnancy can prevent congenital malformations and decrease neonatal morbidity and mortality.
- Gestational diabetes complicates 2%-3% of all pregnancies.
- Screen all pregnant women at 24-28 weeks; if at high risk, screen at first visit.
- 50-g oral glucose load; 1 hour later, plasma glucose level >140 mg/dL indicates need for complete oral glucose tolerance test.
- Oral glucose tolerance test during pregnancy: give 100 g of glucose orally. Diagnostic criteria of O'Sullivan and Maher.

Therapy

Pregnancy is an absolute indication for consideration of intensive insulin therapy. Optimal glycemic control is essential in pregnancy and before conception to avoid higher risk of fetal anomalies. Pregnant women with type 1 DM and women with type 1 DM who are planning pregnancy require excellent glycemic control to reduce the risk of fetal malformations and maternal and fetal complications. Pregnancy in diabetic women should be planned in advance, and women not attempting to conceive should use effective methods of contraception.

The goals of therapy are to ensure tight control of diabetes, with avoidance of hypoglycemia and fasting ketonemia, and to ensure adequate nutrition and optimal weight gain. Home monitoring for blood glucose and urine ketones is important. Glycemic targets are stringent: fasting, 60 to 90 mg/dL; preprandial, 60 to 105 mg/dL; postprandial 1 hour, 70 to 140 mg/dL; postprandial 2 hours, 60 to 120 mg/dL; bedtime, 60 to 120 mg/dL; and 2:00 to 4:00 a.m., 60 to 100 mg/dL. Treatment should include more frequent self-monitored blood glucose, extra snacks to avoid hypoglycemia, and expectation of a progressive increase in insulin requirement during the course of gestation as a consequence of insulin resistance induced by placental hormones. Regular office visits and monthly glycohemoglobin values are required. In patients with prepregnancy diabetes, insulin requirements may decrease early in pregnancy, but after mid-pregnancy, requirements increase progressively. Immediately post partum, insulin requirements usually return to prepregnancy levels. Timing of the delivery is based on tests of fetal maturity. An uncomplicated pregnancy should be allowed to progress to at least 37 weeks.

- Goals of therapy: ensure tight control of diabetes (avoiding hypoglycemia and fasting ketonemia), ensure adequate nutrition and optimal weight gain, and home monitoring for blood glucose and urine ketones.
- Intensive insulin therapy is essential.
- In patients with prenatal diabetes, insulin requirements may decrease early in pregnancy and increase progressively after mid-pregnancy. Immediately post partum, insulin requirements usually return to prepregnancy levels.
- Timing of delivery: based on tests of fetal maturity.

Women with gestational diabetes who become euglycemic in the postpartum state should be followed up periodically; the risk of developing type 2 DM approaches 60% in 15 years.

- Periodic follow-up of patients with gestational diabetes who become euglycemic post partum.
- Risk of developing type 2 DM is almost 60% at 15 years.

In women with type 1 DM and significant chronic diabetic complications, pregnancy may exacerbate retinopathy. Nephropathy may lead to toxemia, and borderline cardiac status may be decompensated. Patients with well-controlled diabetes and mild and early chronic complications have a good chance for a normal pregnancy, without harm to the mother or the fetus.

HYPOGLYCEMIA IN NONDIABETIC PATIENTS

Etiology

Glucose is an essential metabolic fuel for the brain. Hypoglycemia normally is prevented by a decrease in glucose utilization by extraneural tissues and an increase in hepatic glucose output. The hormonal mediators of this physiologic response are a decrease in insulin secretion and an increase in secretion of counterregulatory hormones. Hypoglycemia may be caused by insulin excess, counterregulatory hormone deficiency, or a liver disorder.

Hypoglycemia may occur in the postabsorptive (fasting) or postprandial state and is classified into either insulin-mediated (insulin levels not suppressed) or noninsulin-mediated (insulin levels suppressed).

- Classifications of hypoglycemia: postabsorptive (fasting) or postprandial; insulin-mediated or noninsulin-mediated.

Insulin-Mediated Hypoglycemia

This may be a consequence of exogenous insulin excess, endogenous insulin excess, or mismatch between insulin and meal-induced glucose excursions, the so-called reactive hypoglycemia. *Exogenous hyperinsulinemia* occurs in insulin-treated diabetics and with surreptitious administration of insulin. *Endogenous hyperinsulinemia* occurs in insulinoma and with therapeutic or surreptitious administration of sulfonylureas, which stimulate insulin secretion by the B cells. Insulin antibodies that bind circulating insulin and prevent its degradation also result in hyperinsulinemia. *Postprandial hypoglycemia* may occur from gastric surgery and some congenital deficiencies of enzymes of carbohydrate metabolism (such as in galactosemia or hereditary fructose intolerance) or it may be idiopathic.

Noninsulin-Mediated Hypoglycemia

This may occur as a consequence of alcohol use (alcohol metabolism impairs neoglucogenesis), deficiency of counterregulatory hormone(s) (primary or secondary cortisol deficiency), or GH deficiency in children (isolated glucagon deficiency has not been documented in adults; isolated epinephrine deficiency does not cause hypoglycemia). It also may occur with the presence of an insulin-like factor such as IGF-II in nonbeta-cell mesenchymal or epithelial tumors or the presence of insulin-receptor antibodies. Other causes are critical organ failure (liver, kidney, or heart failure), sepsis, inanition (mechanism unknown), extensive liver disease, and congenital deficiency of glycogenolytic or neoglucogenic enzymes.

- Insulin-mediated hypoglycemia usually results from insulin excess of endogenous or exogenous source. Rarely, it may be postprandial or reactive.
- Noninsulin-mediated hypoglycemia may occur with alcohol use, loss of counterregulatory hormone(s), presence of insulin-like factor, critical organ failure, or extensive liver disease.

The most common causes of hypoglycemia seen in emergency rooms are drugs (particularly insulin and sulfonylureas), alcohol, and sepsis. All the other causes of hypoglycemia are uncommon. In hospitalized patients, drugs and critical illness (particularly renal failure) are the most common causes of hypoglycemia.

Clinical Features

The clinical manifestations are those related to hypoglycemia and its cause. Hypoglycemic symptoms may be sympathoadrenal activation or neuroglycopenic. Symptoms of sympathoadrenal activation include sweating, palpitation, tremor, nervousness, hunger, faintness, weakness, and sacral and perioral numbness. These symptoms may be blunted or absent in patients receiving β-adrenergic blocking agents. Neuroglycopenic symptoms include headache, diplopia, confusion, inappropriate affect, motor incoordination, and, when hypoglycemia is severe, seizures, coma, and (ultimately) death. These symptoms usually predominate when plasma glucose levels decline slowly and reach lower levels (≤40 mg/dL). The manifestations of hypoglycemia are usually reversible, but permanent brain damage can result from a prolonged severe episode.

Diagnosis

Evaluation of patients for possible hypoglycemia has two diagnostic objectives: to demonstrate that the clinical manifestations are due to hypoglycemia and to identify the underlying cause. 1) The diagnosis of hypoglycemia requires the demonstration of the Whipple triad: the presence of suggestive symptoms, the documentation of a low plasma glucose level (<50 mg/dL in males and <40 mg/dL in females) and prompt relief of symptoms with ingestion or infusion of glucose. 2) The diagnosis of hypoglycemia can be made during the spontaneous occurrence of symptoms or after provocation of symptoms by fasting (in fasting or postabsorptive hypoglycemic state) or by administration of food (in postprandial or reactive hypoglycemic state). 3) It is important to rule out artifactual hypoglycemia. Whole-blood glucose values may be spuriously low in polycythemia vera, leukemia, or thrombocythemia (this occurs when the blood sample is withdrawn for glucose measurement and is not separated promptly, allowing continued glucose utilization by blood cells; measurement of plasma glucose in these conditions should provide an accurate result). 4) The possibility of laboratory error should be excluded by repeated measurements. 5) Remember that blood glucose monitoring devices are neither accurate nor precise in the definition of low glucose levels.

- Document the presence of hypoglycemia: the Whipple triad (symptoms, low blood sugar, relief of symptoms by administration of glucose) in a spontaneous or provoked setting.
- Exclude artifactual hypoglycemia and possibility of laboratory error.
- Do not rely on blood glucose measurements by glucose monitoring devices.

Evaluation of Fasting, With or Without Postprandial, Hypoglycemia

The two critical laboratory determinations are measurement of plasma glucose (to document hypoglycemia) and serum insulin (to categorize its cause). They can be measured during a spontaneous attack, after an overnight fast, or after a provoked attack (during a 72-hour fast). Serum levels of C peptide are checked in blood samples that document hyperinsulinemia.

- Two critical laboratory determinations in evaluating fasting hypoglycemia: measuring plasma glucose (to document hypoglycemia) and serum insulin (to determine whether hypoglycemia is insulin-mediated).

Insulin-Mediated Fasting Hypoglycemia

A normal endocrine pancreas responds to decrease in plasma glucose levels during fasting by suppression of insulin release. During continued fasting in normal persons, plasma glucose and serum insulin levels decline together. Hyperinsulinism is identified by plasma insulin levels greater than 6 mU/mL in association with plasma glucose of less than 50 mg/dL in males and less than 40 mg/dL in females.

- Hyperinsulinism: plasma insulin levels >6 mU/mL in association with plasma glucose of <50 mg/dL in males and <40 mg/dL in females.

If fasting hypoglycemia is insulin-mediated, the next step is to determine the source of the excess insulin. The differentiation between an exogenous and endogenous source is based primarily on serum C-peptide levels. Endogenous insulin is derived from proinsulin by the splitting of the C-peptide connecting link; the B cell secretes insulin and C peptide in equimolar concentrations. Exogenous insulin is purified and free from the C peptide. Hyperinsulinemia with a low C-peptide level (<200 pmol/L) points to an exogenous insulin source, whereas that associated with an appropriately increased C-peptide level (>200 pmol/L) points to an endogenous source (insulinoma, use of oral sulfonylureas, or the very rare presence of insulin-autoantibodies).

- If hyperinsulinism is present, consider an endogenous or exogenous source.
- Endogenous hyperinsulinemia is associated with a parallel increase in C-peptide levels and is seen in insulinoma, surreptitious use of sulfonylureas, or with insulin autoantibodies.
- Exogenous hyperinsulinemia is associated with undetectable C-peptide levels and is seen in surreptitious administration of insulin.

Surreptitious administration of insulin or oral sulfonylureas occurs most commonly in patients who have ready access to these medications (family members of insulin-dependent diabetics or medical/paramedical personnel). *Insulinomas* are rare islet-cell pancreatic tumors occurring at all ages but most frequently in the 4th to 7th decades, with a slight preponderance in females.

The tumors usually are sporadic, solitary, and benign (80%), and less than 10% are multiple or malignant or occur in the setting of MEN I. *Autoantibodies to insulin* occur very rarely in non-diabetic persons and are one cause of autoimmune hypoglycemia. These autoantibodies bind the normally secreted insulin and release it slowly in an unregulated manner; endogenous insulin is suppressed and free C-peptide levels are reduced. However, the total C-peptide levels are high because these same antibodies also bind the secreted proinsulin.

- Surreptitious use of insulin or sulfonylureas: by medical or paramedical personnel or relatives of diabetics.
- Insulinomas: rare tumors of B cells of pancreatic islets; single sporadic benign tumor (80%), multiple tumors (<10%), malignant (<10%), or familial and in the setting of MEN I (<10%).
- Insulin autoantibodies: provoked in an insulin-taking diabetic, in a surreptitious user of insulin, or in autoimmune hypoglycemia.

The diagnosis of insulinoma is based on the demonstration of the Whipple triad and appropriately increased plasma insulin and C-peptide levels in the absence of detectable sulfonylurea in the blood or urine. Additional diagnostic measures that may be helpful in selected patients include the following: 1) C-peptide suppression test, which can help distinguish physiologically controlled pancreatic B-cell islet from autonomous nonsuppressible insulin production in insulinoma. (Suppression is assessed by measuring serum C peptide after administering insulin to produce hypoglycemia.) 2) Provocative agents such as tolbutamide, glucagon, leucine, or calcium elicit more insulin secretion from insulinomas than from normal B cells. 3) Plasma proinsulin levels are increased in most patients with insulinomas. 4) Serum levels of human chorionic gonadotropin (hCG) or its α- or β-subunits are increased in two-thirds of patients with malignant insulinomas but not in those with benign disease.

After the diagnosis of insulinoma has been made, an attempt to localize the tumor is pursued. Ultrasonography, CT, or MRI of the pancreas can delineate tumors larger than 1 or 2 cm. Angiography may be needed to detect smaller tumors. Transhepatic venous sampling after the administration of calcium to stimulate insulin secretion may be helpful. The use of intraoperative ultrasonography has contributed significantly to identification of small tumors.

- In hyperinsulinemic states associated with an appropriate increase in C-peptide levels: the exclusion of surreptitious administration of sulfonylureas points to insulinoma as the cause of the hyperinsulinemic state.
- In selected patients, additional tests may be necessary; the most useful is the C-peptide suppression test.

- High levels of proinsulin or hCG or its subunits raise the suspicion of a malignant insulinoma.

Noninsulin-Mediated Fasting Hypoglycemia

If hyperinsulinism is not present in patients with documented hypoglycemia, the differential diagnosis includes hypopituitarism, hypoadrenalism, liver disease, drug-induced hypoglycemia, and extrapancreatic tumor. If the clinical evidence suggests hypopituitarism or hypoadrenalism, appropriate endocrine tests are in order. Severe liver disease or ingestion of alcohol, drugs, or toxins can generally be distinguished by the medical history, physical examination, and liver function tests. With inborn hepatic enzyme defects, symptoms usually begin in infancy, and the diagnosis depends on the clinical setting and appropriate enzyme assays. The diagnosis of primary liver disease usually is obvious, but remember that if hypoglycemia is noted in a patient with liver cirrhosis, the presence of hepatoma needs to be excluded. The presence of an extrapancreatic tumor that causes hypoglycemia is likely if the clinical findings and specific laboratory tests do not support one of the above conditions, especially if significant wasting or an abdominal mass is present.

- If hyperinsulinism is absent in patients with documented hypoglycemia, the differential diagnosis includes hypopituitarism, hypoadrenalism, liver disease, drug-induced hypoglycemia, and extrapancreatic tumor. The clinical picture and appropriate laboratory studies usually point to the underlying cause.
- For hypoglycemia noted in the course of cirrhosis, exclude hepatoma.
- The presence of extrapancreatic tumor causing hypoglycemia is likely if the clinical findings and specific laboratory tests do not support one of the above conditions, especially in the presence of wasting or an abdominal mass.

Alcohol-induced hypoglycemia is a common cause of fasting hypoglycemia. The symptoms of hypoglycemia often are mistakenly attributed to drunkenness. The plasma glucose level should be determined in all symptomatic patients with a history of significant alcohol intake. Blood alcohol levels may not be increased when a patient with hypoglycemia is examined. Diabetic patients taking insulin or oral agents are especially susceptible to ethanol-induced hypoglycemia.

- Alcohol-induced hypoglycemia is a frequent cause of fasting hypoglycemia.
- Its manifestations often are mistakenly attributed to drunkenness.
- When a patient with alcohol-induced hypoglycemia is examined, blood alcohol levels may not be increased.

- Diabetic patients taking insulin or oral agents are especially susceptible to ethanol-induced hypoglycemia.

Postprandial Hypoglycemia

Postprandial hypoglycemia is due to asynchronous or excessive insulin secretion relative to prandial plasma glucose levels and is characterized by symptomatic hypoglycemia occurring 1 to 5 hours after food ingestion. It can occur in the following clinical settings: 1) a rare hereditary abnormality in children in whom hypoglycemia may follow the ingestion of fructose, galactose, or leucine; 2) in some patients who have impaired glucose tolerance, symptomatic hypoglycemia, or "diabetic" hypoglycemia (hypoglycemia may develop 4-6 hours after glucose ingestion; it is attributed to an excessive and delayed insulin response to a glucose load); and 3) "alimentary" hypoglycemia most often follows gastrectomy, jejunostomy, or vagotomy and pyloroplasty. Symptomatic hypoglycemia in alimentary hypoglycemia occurs earlier (1-2 hours after a glucose meal) than in other forms of postprandial hypoglycemia. The mechanism is believed to be due to the rapid entry of large amounts of glucose into the small bowel, causing a precipitous increase in the plasma glucose level and a dramatic secretion of insulin. Alimentary hypoglycemia may also occur in patients with thyrotoxicosis or rapid gastric emptying of unknown cause.

Contrary to popular belief, idiopathic postprandial syndrome (reactive or functional) is distinctly rare. Some patients may erroneously attribute many types of symptoms to hypoglycemia such as lack of energy, chronic anxiety, lethargy, mental dullness, and similar complaints; an oral glucose tolerance test may provoke these symptoms and show "hypoglycemia." However, it is important to remember that normal subjects may have as low a plasma glucose after an oral glucose load and be asymptomatic, symptoms in these patients are not associated with a low plasma glucose, and persons who have "hypoglycemia" after oral glucose frequently have normal glucose levels after a mixed meal. Diagnosis requires documentation of the Whipple triad after a mixed meal; an oral glucose tolerance test should not be used to make the diagnosis.

- Postprandial hypoglycemia: due to asynchronous or excessive insulin secretion relative to prandial plasma glucose levels. It is characterized by symptomatic hypoglycemia occurring 1-5 hours after food ingestion.
- May occur in the setting of "alimentary hypoglycemia" and in patients with impaired glucose tolerance.
- Idiopathic postprandial syndrome (reactive or functional) is rare. Diagnosis requires documentation of the Whipple triad after a mixed meal; an oral glucose tolerance test should not be used to make the diagnosis.

Therapy

Treatment is directed at the hypoglycemia and the underlying disorder. For the hypoglycemia, it is important to restore and to maintain euglycemia. For mild hypoglycemia in an alert patient, give 20 g oral glucose in the form of glucose tabs, soft drinks, candy, fruit juices, or milk and repeat as necessary. For patients unable to take oral nutrient, give parenteral therapy in the form of intravenous glucose (25 g [50 mL of 50% dextrose in water]) and repeat in 15 to 20 minutes if necessary. If this is not feasible, give glucagon, 1 mg subcutaneously, intramuscularly, or intravenously, to stimulate endogenous glucose production. Recovery from hypoglycemia is usually prompt; rarely, it is delayed for hours or days, presumably because of cerebral edema. Subtle cognitive defects can result from a severe and recurrent hypoglycemic episode, but permanent neurologic deficits are uncommon.

- Treatment: hypoglycemia and the underlying disorder.
- Hypoglycemia: oral or parenteral glucose; glucagon can be given when patient is not able to take oral feedings and when parenteral glucose is not feasible.
- Recovery from hypoglycemia is usually complete and prompt; it sometimes may take hours; permanent deficits are unusual.

Treatment is directed at the underlying cause, such as discontinuation of an offending drug, excision of an offending tumor, or treatment of the causative illness. For insulinoma, management is surgical and consists of excision of the tumor or distal pancreatectomy if the tumor is not localized at exploration (these tumors are evenly distributed in the pancreas). Medical treatment is indicated for patients who are poor surgical risks, who refuse surgery, in whom a tumor is not found at surgery, or who have persistent/recurrent malignant insulinoma. Glucose is given as needed; diazoxide is given to inhibit insulin secretion. Alternatively, phenytoin, propranolol, or verapamil or octreotide can be used. Chemotherapy with streptozocin and fluorouracil can benefit a few patients with malignant insulinoma.

- Treatment of insulinoma: surgical tumor excision or distal pancreatectomy.
- For persistent disease: diazoxide or its alternates; chemotherapy for malignant persistent/recurrent disease.

MULTIPLE ENDOCRINE NEOPLASIA

MEN I

MEN I, or Wermer syndrome, is the association of neoplasms of the parathyroid, endocrine pancreas, and anterior pituitary. It is familial and inherited as an autosomal dominant trait with essentially 100% penetrance. The MEN I locus has been mapped to a specific region on chromosome 11 and the gene has been identified recently and belongs to the category of tumor suppressor genes. Each affected person carries one mutated gene transmitted as an autosomal dominant trait; if the normal copy from the unaffected parent is mutated, the syndrome results.

Primary Hyperparathyroidism

This is the most common manifestation; it shows nearly 100% penetrance by age 40 to 50 years and usually is caused by parathyroid hyperplasia and, occasionally, by single or multiple adenomata. Hypercalcemia is commonly expressed by age 40 and is similar in its presentation and complications to sporadic hyperparathyroidism. Diagnosis is by the presence of hypercalcemia and increased intact PTH. The differential diagnosis includes other familial syndromes associated with hypercalcemia: familial hyperparathyroidism (differentiation is based on family history and long-term observation to determine whether other features of MEN I develop) and familial hypocalciuric hypercalcemia (hypercalcemia is present at birth; hypocalciuria, usually not associated with complications of hypercalcemia). The two options for therapy are removal of 3.5 parathyroids or total parathyroidectomy and transplantation of parathyroid tissue into the forearm; the rate of recurrence of hyperparathyroidism is high.

Islet Cell Neoplasia

This is the second most common neoplasm in MEN I and is probably the most important manifestation because of its malignant potential. Hypersecretory syndromes include hypersecretion of pancreatic polypeptide (75%-85% of patients), gastrin (60%), insulin (25%-35%), VIP (3%-5%), glucagon (5%-10%), and somatostatin (1%-5%). Islet cell tumors may hypersecrete other peptides, including ACTH, CRH, and GHRH. Distinctively, one-third of the tumors are malignant. Diagnosis depends on the clinical recognition of characteristic syndromes, measurement of hormones with or without provocative stimulation, and radiologic techniques. *Gastrinoma* (or *Zollinger-Ellison syndrome*): clinical features of increased gastric acid production, recurrent multiple peptic ulcers, diarrhea, and esophagitis. Diagnosis: increased gastric acid secretion, increased basal gastrin, and an exaggerated gastrin response to secretin or calcium. (For insulinoma, see section above on Hypoglycemia in Nondiabetic Patients.)

Pituitary Tumors

More than 15% of gene carriers have pituitary tumors, which are usually multicentric. The most common tumor is a pro-

lactinoma. Acromegaly in MEN I may be caused by a pituitary GH tumor or an ectopic GHRH tumor. Cushing syndrome in MEN I may be caused by ACTH pituitary tumor or an ectopic ACTH or CRH tumor.

Other Manifestations of MEN I

These include 1) carcinoid tumors, mostly of the foregut, which may produce serotonin, calcitonin, or CRH; 2) thyroid and adrenal adenomas; and 3) subcutaneous or visceral lipomas.

Screening for MEN I

Currently, there is no compelling evidence that early detection decreases mortality and morbidity. If a decision is made to evaluate asymptomatic family members, this is best done with serum levels of calcium (albumin-adjusted or ionized) and intact PTH. Laboratory evaluation and/or imaging studies for pancreatic or pituitary tumors are not indicated in the absence of relevant symptoms. Specific genetic testing for MEN I should be forthcoming now that the responsible gene and its mutations have been identified.

MEN II

MEN II includes two major syndromes: MEN IIA (medullary carcinoma of the thyroid, pheochromocytoma, and primary hyperparathyroidism) and MEN IIB (medullary carcinoma of the thyroid, pheochromocytoma, mucosal neuromas, intestinal ganglioneuromatosis, and marfanoid features). These two familial syndromes are inherited in an autosomal dominant pattern with high penetrance.

MEN IIA

Medullary carcinoma of the thyroid is the most common manifestation (>90% of patients) of MEN IIA; it develops in childhood and usually begins as C-cell hyperplasia. Measurement of calcitonin after provocation with pentagastrin or calcium allows for early diagnosis.

Pheochromocytomas occur in about 50% of patients, and about 50% of the tumors are bilateral. These tumors have an increased incidence of malignancy (20%-40%) and of epinephrine-producing tumors. In the 50% with apparently unilateral disease, unilateral adrenalectomy is followed in about 50% of patients by development of a contralateral tumor in 8 to 10 years.

Hyperparathyroidism develops in 15% to 20% of the patients.

MEN IIA has two subtypes: familial medullary carcinoma of the thyroid and MEN IIA with cutaneous lichen amyloidosis.

MEN IIB

The endocrine manifestations differ from those of MEN IIA in the absence of hyperparathyroidism and in the fact that medullary carcinoma of the thyroid develops earlier in life and appears to be more virulent. The occurrence of hypercalcemia should make one think about osseous metastases. Mucosal true neuromas are the most distinctive features of MEN IIB. They may occur at the tip of the tongue, on the eyelids or lips, and along the gastrointestinal tract. Intestinal neuromas may cause intermittent obstruction or diarrhea.

Genetics of MEN II

The genetic locus is in the pericentromeric region of chromosome 10; abnormal mutation in the *RET* gene is present in 95% to 98% of affected persons. Other chromosomal abnormalities may contribute to progression of the disease.

Screening for MEN II

Medullary carcinoma of the thyroid is potentially fatal, but it can be cured or prevented by early thyroidectomy. This provides the strongest rationale for screening. Screening includes DNA analysis for *RET* mutations; basal and provoked calcitonin; and urinary fractionated catecholamines, metanephrines, and vanillylmandelic acid. Begin screening in early childhood, preferably before age 5 years. Testing for the *RET* proto-oncogene allows endocrine screening tests to be targeted at persons at risk.

Other genetic tumor syndromes do not fit neatly into either the MEN I or MEN II pattern (e.g., mixed syndromes such as familial pheochromocytoma and islet cell tumors).

QUESTIONS

Multiple Choice (choose the one best answer)

1. Fasting hypoglycemia may occur in:
   a. Cushing syndrome
   b. Alcohol intoxication
   c. Primary aldosteronism
   d. Pheochromocytoma
   e. All the above

2. Clinical presentations of primary hypothyroidism may include all of the following *except*:
   a. Shortness of stature and failure of sexual maturation in an adolescent
   b. Amenorrhea-galactorrhea and a sellar mass in a young woman
   c. Hypercholesterolemia
   d. Pericardial effusion
   e. Polycythemia

3. Which of the following statements is *not true* about Graves disease?
   a. It is the most common cause of diffuse goiter associated with hyperthyroidism
   b. It is the only cause of hyperthyroidism that may be associated with chemosis, proptosis, and extraocular muscle dysfunction
   c. It may be associated with other autoimmune disorders such as Addison disease, vitiligo, and pernicious anemia
   d. Typically, it occurs in a triphasic pattern: transient

hyperthyroidism, followed by transient hypothyroidism, and then eventual restoration of euthyroidism
   e. Typical laboratory abnormalities include a high serum level of free thyroxine, suppressed serum TSH, and high radioiodine uptake

4. A high serum level of TSH may be seen in all of the following disorders *except*:
   a. The recovery stage from acute nonthyroidal illness
   b. A patient with pituitary tumor, hyperthyroidism, and high radioiodine uptake
   c. A patient with hyperthyroidism, a high serum level of T_4 and T_3, and a positive family history of generalized resistance to thyroid hormone
   d. A patient with diffuse bosselated goiter, hypothyroidism, and positive antimicrosomal antibodies
   e. An elderly patient with a multinodular goiter, atrial fibrillation, and a high serum level of T_3

5. All the following statements about the symptoms of hypoglycemia are true *except*:
   a. They are absent in artifactual hypoglycemia
   b. They occur in response to rapid or significant decrease in plasma glucose levels
   c. They are nonspecific and are not sufficient alone to diagnose the presence of hypoglycemia
   d. They are preceded by counterregulatory hormone release
   e. They differ between insulin-mediated and noninsulin-mediated hypoglycemia

6. An *increased radioiodine uptake* measured over the thyroid in a hyperthyroid patient is characteristic of:
   a. Toxic multinodular goiter
   b. Painless lymphocytic thyroiditis
   c. Surreptitious ingestion of thyroid hormone(s)
   d. Iodide-induced thyrotoxicosis
   e. Ectopic thyroid tissue producing thyrotoxicosis

7. All the following alterations in thyroid function tests can be seen in *non-thyroidal illness except*:
   a. Low serum triiodothyronine (T$_3$)
   b. Low serum thyroxine (T$_4$)
   c. Low serum sTSH
   d. High serum T$_4$
   e. High serum thyroglobulin

8. All the following statements about insulinoma are true *except*:
   a. Can cause postprandial or postabsorptive hypoglycemia
   b. Hypoglycemia is associated with high serum levels of insulin and low serum levels of C peptide
   c. Clinical features may resemble the hypoglycemia induced by the surreptitious administration of an oral sulfonylurea
   d. The presence of hypoglycemia is confirmed by the presence of suggestive symptoms, the finding of a low plasma level of glucose, and the relief of symptoms by the administration of glucose, the so-called Whipple triad
   e. Liver disease, cortisol deficiency, a large mesenchymal retroperitoneal tumor should also be considered in the differential diagnosis.

9. All the following statements about bromocriptine are true *except*:
   a. It suppresses hyperprolactinemia and restores normal gonadal function in 80% to 90% of the patients with hyperprolactinemia irrespective of the cause
   b. It may cause regression in tumor size in a significant number of patients who harbor a prolactin-producing pituitary tumor
   c. It is temporizing therapy; discontinuation of its use usually leads to the reemergence of hyperprolactinemia
   d. In bromocriptine-treated young women who harbor a macroprolactinoma and who desire fertility, use of the drug is stopped at the earliest sign of pregnancy because there is not risk of tumor growth during pregnancy
   e. In patients who have a nonfunctioning pituitary tumor and hyperprolactinoma due to the "stalk effect," bromocriptine can normalize prolactin levels but will not cause regression in tumor size

10. All the following statements about hypoparathyroidism are true *except*:
    a. It may be associated with hypocalcemia, hyperphosphatemia, increased serum level of immunoreactive parathyroid hormone, and increased serum level of creatinine
    b. It may be associated with other endocrine deficiencies in polyglandular autoimmune disorder (PGA) type I
    c. It may be associated with basal ganglia calcification and parkinsonian features
    d. It is characterized by hypocalcemia, hyperphosphatemia, normal serum levels of creatinine, and low or undetectable serum levels of immunoreactive parathyroid hormone
    e. It most commonly occurs as a result of inadvertent damage to the parathyroid glands during thyroid surgery

11. A 58-year-old man has a blood pressure of 160/100 mm Hg on a routine insurance examination. He is not taking any medications. Serum potassium is 3.2 mEq/L (normal, 3.6-4.8 mEq/L). Primary aldosteronism is suspected, and an appropriate work-up is conducted. Primary aldosteronism is characterized by all the following *except*:
    a. Unprovoked hypokalemia due to increased and inappropriate renal potassium loss
    b. Hypokalemic alkalosis
    c. Increased aldosterone levels in the blood and urine that are not suppressed by saline administration
    d. High renin production that is not suppressed by salt loading
    e. Low plasma renin activity that does not respond to stimulation by volume depletion or upright posture

12. A 61-year-old man with type 2 diabetes mellitus that had been adequately controlled with 10 mg of glyburide per day is brought to the emergency room because of fever and gradual obtundation of 4 days' duration. He is significantly dehydrated and hypotensive. Chest radiography shows evidence of left lower lobe pneumonitis. A random plasma glucose is 960 mg/dL, serum creatinine is 2 mg/dL, and urinalysis shows heavy glycosuria but without ketonuria. Plasma ketones are negative. The physician considers a diagnosis of hyperglycemia hyperosmolar nonketotic state (HHNK). All the following statements about this condition are true *except*:
    a. Insulin deficiency, osmotic diuresis, dehydration, and decreased renal function have a role in the pathogenesis. Enough insulin is present, however, to inhibit excessive lipolysis and ketogenesis
    b. HHNK occurs predominantly in type 2 diabetes mellitus and is usually its first presentation. It is often

precipitated by acute illness or by the use of gluco-corticoids, thiazides, or phenytoin

c. HHNK should be suspected in any diabetic patient who presents with altered sensorium and severe dehydration. The diagnosis is confirmed by finding significant hyperglycemia and plasma hyperosmolality and the absence of significant ketonemia. A search for a precipitating disorder is important

d. The primary objectives of therapy are to restore volume and osmolality (initially by the use of normal saline to correct volume and then by 0.45% saline to correct hyperosmolality) and management of the glycemic disorder with the use of regular insulin

e. Complications are rare, and the disorder does not carry any added morbidity or mortality

13. Secondary causes of diabetes mellitus include all of the following *except*:
    a. Acromegaly
    b. Hemochromatosis
    c. Primary aldosteronism
    d. Hypopituitarism
    e. Pheochromocytoma

14. All the following statements about gestational diabetes are true *except*:
    a. Early detection and management of diabetes can significantly decrease perinatal mortality and morbidity
    b. Screening for glucose intolerance is advisable in all pregnant women and is usually done at 24 to 26 weeks of gestation
    c. The diagnostic criteria for diabetes in the oral glucose tolerance test are the same as those for nonpregnant patients
    d. The risk of gestational diabetes is increased in patients with obesity, advanced maternal age, and an abnormal obstetric history, such as large babies, unexplained stillbirths, and polyhydramnios
    e. Gestational diabetes can recur in subsequent pregnancies; frank type 2 diabetes will develop in 60% of the patients at 15 years

15. All the following statements about insulin-induced hypoglycemia in an 18-year-old man with type 1 diabetes mellitus are true *except*:
    a. Early in the course of the disease, catecholaminergic symptoms typically appear first, particularly if the rate of decrease in the plasma level of glucose is rapid
    b. Neuroglycopenic symptoms predominate when the rate of decrease in plasma glucose is gradual, when the degree of hypoglycemia is severe, or when the patient has hypoglycemia unawareness

c. Intensive insulin therapy and near-normal glycemic control are associated with an increased incidence of hypoglycemia but a decreased risk of the development of microvascular complications

d. Incidence is reduced by heavy exercise and with the use of alcohol

e. Incidence is increased by the occurrence of renal failure or cortisol deficiency

16. All the following statements about Cushing disease are true *except*:
    a. Serum levels of ACTH are normal or modestly increased in most patients
    b. In most patients, the hypercortisol state is not suppressed by the administration of a high dose of dexamethasone (8 mg/day for 2 days)
    c. Most patients harbor an ACTH-producing pituitary tumor, but imaging of the sella with CT or MRI is negative in more than 50% of patients
    d. The clinical and biochemical features may be indistinguishable from those of Cushing syndrome caused by an ectopic ACTH-producing bronchial carcinoid
    e. Petrosal venous sampling with CRH provocative testing shows a central-to-peripheral ACTH gradient greater than 2:1

17. An 18-year-old man presents with failure of sexual maturation. He is eunuchoidal and has bilateral gynecomastia and small firm testes. His sense of smell is normal. The serum level of testosterone is low, and the serum levels of LH and FSH are increased. The most likely diagnosis is:
    a. Kallmann syndrome
    b. Prolactin-producing pituitary tumor
    c. Craniopharyngioma
    d. Klinefelter syndrome
    e. Testicular feminization

18. A 17-year-old woman is referred for the evaluation of primary amenorrhea. She is sexually immature. Laboratory studies document low serum levels of estradiol, LH, and FSH. Diagnostic considerations include all the following *except*:
    a. Craniopharyngioma
    b. Autoimmune oophoritis
    c. Anorexia nervosa
    d. Kallmann syndrome
    e. Prolactin-producing pituitary tumor

19. Functional reversible hypothalamic amenorrhea may occur in association with all the following *except*:
    a. Situational stresses

b. Significant weight changes

c. Hyperprolactinemia of any cause

d. Hyperandrogenic states of ovarian or adrenal origin

e. Postpartum pituitary necrosis

20. Exogenous gonadotropin therapy may restore fertility potential in a hypogonadal male in all of the following disorders *except*:

a. Craniopharyngioma

b. Post-radiation hypopituitarism

c. Post-surgical hypopituitarism

d. Mumps orchitis

e. Congenital isolated hypogonadotropism associated with anosmia

21. Clinical features that suggest an ovarian or adrenal neoplasm as the cause of hyperandrogenic syndrome in a 28-year-old woman include all the following *except*:

a. Abrupt onset of hyperandrogenic features of few months' duration

b. Severe rapidly progressive hyperandrogenicity

c. Serum testosterone and DHEAS may be normal or mildly elevated but always less than 2 times the upper limit of normal

d. Serum testosterone or DHEAS are significantly increased and are non-trophic-hormone dependent

e. The presence of an abdominal or a unilateral pelvic mass

22. All the following statements about estrogen therapy in menopause are true *except*:

a. Oral and transdermal estrogen are equally effective in the management of hot flashes and genitourinary atrophy

b. Increases the risk of endometrial cancer; this increased risk is prevented by supplemental progestin

c. Prevents the rapid phase of bone loss characteristic of menopause

d. Useful in the management of hypercholesterolemia

e. Useful in the management of hypertriglyceridemia

23. Which of the following is typically seen in classic Turner syndrome (45/XO)?

a. Anosmia and hypogonadotropic hypogonadism

b. Precocious isosexual puberty

c. Shortness of stature that responds to therapy with estrogen

d. Fibrous gonadal streaks and hypergonadotropic hypogonadism

e. Female phenotype, absence of sexual hair, short vagina, and absence of female internal genitalia

24. Which of the following statements about Kallmann syndrome is true?

a. Low serum level of testosterone and high serum levels of LH and FSH

b. Panhypopituitarism

c. Azospermia is present

d. Diabetes insipidus, hyperprolactinemia, and the presence of hypothalamic mass on MRI

e. Chromosomal sex is 46,XXY, the gonads are testes, and the phenotype of the internal and external genitalia is male

25. All the following are true about pheochromocytoma *except*:

a. Symptoms may be paroxysmal. In most patients, the paroxysmal symptoms are stereotypic and vary only in frequency and severity

b. Can be asymptomatic and discovered incidentally on abdominal imaging

c. May be familial. Familial pheochromocytoma may be isolated or part of MEN IIA or MEN IIB syndromes

d. Diagnosis can be excluded in a patient with hypertension by the confirmed findings of normal urinary free catecholamines, metanephrines, and vanillylmandelic acid

e. β-Adrenergic blockade is the cornerstone of medical therapy and is instituted as soon as the diagnosis is made to control hypertension, to prevent hypertensive crisis, and to prepare the patient for tumor excision

ANSWERS

1. Answer b.
Alcohol intoxication is a common cause of fasting hypoglycemia because the hepatic metabolism of alcohol inhibits hepatic neoglucogenesis. All the other options are causes of secondary diabetes and are not associated with fasting hypoglycemia.

2. Answer e.
Anemia, and not polycythemia, is commonly seen in association with primary hypothyroidism. The anemia is usually normocytic normochromic and due to a direct effect of the hypothyroid state on erythropoiesis (it will respond only to thyroid hormone replacement). Spontaneous primary hypothyroidism is most often due to Hashimoto thyroiditis; macrocytic anemia may occur and be due to associated pernicious anemia. Microcytic anemia caused by iron deficiency is most often related to menometrorrhagia due to anovulation, which occurs in hypothyroid adult females.

3. Answer d.
Although the hyperthyroid state in Graves disease may fluctuate in intensity, in most patients it is persistent until therapy is instituted. The triphasic pattern is characteristically seen in subacute (granulomatous) or silent (painless) types of thyroiditis.

4. Answer e.
An elderly patient with a multinodular goiter, atrial fibrillation, and high serum levels of T_3 has hyperthyroidism, and, consequently, the serum TSH should be suppressed.

5. Answer e.
The diagnosis of hypoglycemia requires the demonstration of the Whipple triad: suggestive symptoms, documentation of low plasma glucose, and the relief of symptoms by the administration of sugar or glucose. The symptoms of hypoglycemia are the same regardless of the cause.

6. Answer a.
Toxic multinodular goiter is caused by the overproduction of thyroid hormones by the autonomous nodules and is associated with an increased radioiodine uptake. All the other causes of hyperthyroidism mentioned in the question are associated with suppressed radioiodine uptake.

7. Answer e.
Nonthyroidal illness occurs in several forms: the low T_3 form, low T_3/T_4 form, and the low T_3/high T_4 form. In all these forms, serum TSH is either normal or low. Alterations in serum thyroglobulin are not a feature of nonthyroidal illness.

8. Answer b.
In insulinoma, the neoplastic B cell secretes insulin and C peptide in equimolar proportions. In insulinoma, in the face of hypoglycemia, the serum levels of insulin and C peptide are inappropriately increased.

9. Answer d.
Patients with macroprolactinoma in whom pregnancy is induced either by the administration of prolactin-suppressive dopamine-agonist therapy such as bromocriptine or by the use of exogenous gonadotropins have a risk of about 25% to 40% of tumor enlargement during pregnancy. They should be followed up carefully during pregnancy with a monthly visual field examination. When the clinical features suggest tumor expansion, MRI of the head is indicated.

10. Answer a.
The characteristic biochemical features of parathyroid hormone deficiency are hypocalcemia and hyperphosphatemia. The diagnosis of hypoparathyroidism depends on the presence of hypocalcemia, hyperphosphatemia, normal serum level of creatinine, and a very low serum level of PTH.

11. Answer d.
Primary aldosteronism is characterized by autonomous hypersecretion of aldosterone. The consequent enhanced renal reabsorption of sodium and water and the expansion of the extracellular volume lead to suppression of renin by secretion by the juxtaglomerular cells. All the other options are correct.

12. Answer e.
HHNK is a serious disorder. Despite the best therapeutic efforts, it carries a 30% to 50% mortality due primarily to cardiovascular events and to the hazards of therapy such as hypoglycemia, hypokalemia, or cerebral edema. Early diagnosis and prudent therapy are critical

13. Answer d.
Hypopituitarism is associated with the tendency to hypoglycemia because of the loss of the neoglucogenic activity of cortisol. All the other disorders mentioned can cause secondary diabetes.

14. Answer c.
The oral GTT for the diagnosis of gestational diabetes is different from the standard oral GTT in the nonpregnant population in two ways: 100 g of glucose is given, and the diagnostic criteria are those of O'Sullivan and Maher (two or more

of the following plasma glucose values must be met or exceeded: fasting, 105 mg/dL; 1 hour, 190 mg/dL; 2 hours, 165 mg/dL; and 3 hours, 145 mg/dL).

15. Answer d.

The incidence of hypoglycemia in all insulin-taking diabetics is increased by heavy exercise or the use of alcohol.

16. Answer b.

Two-thirds of the patients with Cushing disease show suppressibility of cortisol production during an 8-mg dexamethasone suppression test (either administered in a dose of 2 mg/6 hr for 48 hours or as an 8-mg overnight single dose).

17. Answer d.

Klinefelter syndrome is characterized by primary gonadal failure and, thus, by hypergonadotropic hypogonadism. In testicular feminization, the phenotype is female and the serum testosterone levels are in the normal male range. All other disorders are characterized by central hypogonadotropic hypogonadism.

18. Answer b.

In autoimmune oophoritis, ovarian failure is primary and, thus, the serum LH and FSH levels are characteristically high, that is, the hypoestrogenic state is hypergonadotropic in type. All the other conditions listed are associated with central hypogonadotropic hypogonadism.

19. Answer e.

In central hypogonadotropism, it is important to consider the common causes of functional reversible hypogonadotropism. Postpartum pituitary necrosis is characterized by pituitary infarction, and the ensuing hypopituitarism is characteristically permanent and irreversible.

20. Answer d.

In mumps orchitis, the testicular disorder is primary and irreversible. The seminiferous tubules are damaged and cannot respond to exogenous gonadotropins.

21. Answer c.

The hyperandrogenic state resulting from an ovarian or adrenal neoplasm is characteristically abrupt in onset, rapidly progressive, and severe. It can occur at any age. The serum androgen levels are characteristically increased significantly and are usually at least 2 times higher than normal. The finding of such levels in a hyperandrogenic female should prompt consideration of an underlying ovarian or adrenal neoplasm.

22. Answer e.

The administration of oral estrogens leads to an increase in VLDL production by the liver. In most patients the increase in triglycerides is modest, but in some, particularly those with a genetic predisposition, the increase in triglycerides may be massive and result in increased risk of development of pancreatitis. In general, oral estrogen therapy is contraindicated in patients with familial hypertriglyceridemia or in patients with a significant increase in triglycerides. Susceptible patients who are given oral estrogens should have their triglycerides rechecked in 1 or 2 months after the initiation of therapy.

23. Answer d.

Classic Turner syndrome (karyotype 45X) is characterized endocrinologically by fibrous gonadal streaks, sexual infantilism, and hypergonadotropic hypogonadism.

24. Answer c.

Kallmann syndrome is characterized by the presence of isolated hypogonadotropism (due to absence of GnRH-producing hypothalamic neurons) and anosmia (due to the maldevelopment of the olfactory bulbs).

25. Answer e.

α-Adrenergic blockade is the cornerstone of medical management of pheochromocytoma and is essential for the control of hypertension, prevention of crisis, and restoration of euvolemia. β-Adrenergic blockade alone may aggravate the hypertension because of the blockade of the β-receptor-mediated vasodilatation in the muscular bed. β-Adrenergic blockade should always follow the institution of α-blockade.

NOTES

CHAPTER 8
GASTROENTEROLOGY

Thomas R. Viggiano, M.D.
John J. Poterucha, M.D.

PART I
Thomas R. Viggiano, M.D.

ESOPHAGUS

Esophageal Function

The upper esophageal sphincter (or cricopharyngeus muscle) and the muscle of the proximal one-third of the esophagus are striated muscle under voluntary control. A transition from skeletal to smooth muscle occurs in the mid-esophagus. In the distal one-third of the esophagus, the muscle is smooth muscle that is under involuntary control. The lower esophageal sphincter is a zone of circular muscle located in the distal 2 to 3 cm of the esophagus. To transport food from the mouth through the negative-pressured chest into the positive-pressured abdomen, the esophagus must transport food against a pressure gradient. To prevent reflux of gastric contents, the lower esophagus has a sphincter for unidirectional flow. Normal esophageal motility accomplishes both transport and prevention of reflux.

- The esophagus must transport food against a pressure gradient and prevent reflux of gastric contents.

Normal Motility

After a person swallows, the upper esophageal sphincter relaxes within 0.5 second. A primary peristaltic wave then passes through the body of the esophagus at a rate of 1 to 5 cm/s, generating an intraluminal pressure of 40 to 100 mm Hg. Within 2 seconds after the swallow, the lower esophageal sphincter relaxes and stays relaxed until the wave of peristalsis passes through it. Next, the lower esophageal sphincter contracts again to maintain its resting tone. Two major symptom complexes result if the esophagus is unable to perform its two major functions: dysphagia (transport dysfunction) and reflux (lower esophageal sphincter dysfunction).

- Dysphagia: transport dysfunction.
- Reflux: lower esophageal sphincter dysfunction.

Dysphagia

Dysphagia is the defective transport of food and is usually described as "sticking." Odynophagia is pain on swallowing. The two causes of dysphagia must be distinguished: mechanical (obstructed lumen) and functional (motility disorder). Answers to three questions frequently suggest the diagnosis: 1) what type of food produces the dysphagia, 2) what is the course of the dysphagia, and 3) is there heartburn (Fig. 8-1)? Dysphagia with an intermittent course is caused by a ring, a web, or a motility disorder.

- Be able to distinguish mechanical dysphagia from functional dysphagia.
- Intermittent dysphagia is caused by a ring, a web, or a motility disorder.

Mechanical Cause

Mechanical obstruction occurs if the lumen diameter is less than 12 mm. With mechanical obstruction, the course is progressive; dysphagia for solids is greater than for liquids, and there is associated weight loss.

- Mechanical obstruction: progressive course, weight loss, dysphagia for solids is greater than for liquids.

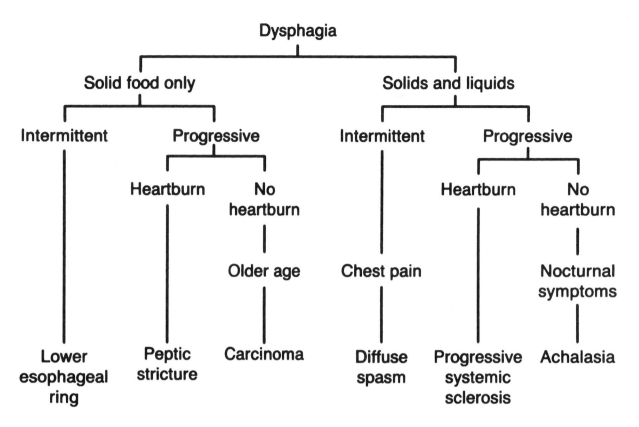

Fig. 8-1. Diagnostic scheme for dysphagia. Obtaining answers to three questions (see text) often yields the most likely diagnosis. (From MKSAP VI: Part 1:44, 1982. American College of Physicians. By permission.)

1. Stricture—Peptic stricture results from prolonged reflux and is usually a short (<2 to 3 cm long) narrowing in the distal esophagus.

- Peptic stricture results from prolonged reflux, usually in the distal esophagus.

Barrett esophagus is characterized by abnormal columnar epithelium in the distal esophagus. It can present as a stricture in the mid-esophagus that may occur with an ulcer. Barrett esophagus is a complication of reflux and, thus, is acquired and not congenital. Normal squamous mucosa is replaced by columnar epithelium, which has an increased risk to develop adenocarcinoma.

- Barrett esophagus: abnormal columnar epithelium in the distal esophagus that is a complication of chronic reflux and predisposed to the development of adenocarcinoma.

Lye stricture—Alkali is more injurious to the esophagus than acid (in postgastrectomy patients, alkaline reflux can produce severe esophagitis). Do not induce vomiting after lye ingestion. Stricture tends to occur at the three physiologic narrowings where the initial passage of the corrosive may have been delayed. Bougienage after 3 or 4 weeks may prevent occurrence of stricture. There is increased incidence of squamous cell cancer.

- Postgastrectomy alkaline reflux can produce severe esophagitis.
- Do not induce vomiting after lye ingestion.
- Lye stricture is associated with an increased incidence of squamous cell cancer.

2. Tumor—Benign. Leiomyoma is the most common benign tumor. It is usually asymptomatic. Be able to recognize the appearance of this tumor on barium swallow fluoroscopy. Perform endoscopy even if classic changes are seen on barium swallow.

Malignant. Recognize the appearance of malignant tumors on barium swallow fluoroscopy. Also, know the conditions that predispose to esophageal squamous cell carcinoma: achalasia, lye stricture, Plummer-Vinson syndrome, human papillomavirus, tylosis, smoking, and alcohol. In the U.S., 20% of the malignant tumors are squamous and 80% are adenocarcinoma. Progressive dysphagia with weight loss is usually seen. Diagnosis is established by endoscopy with biopsy and cytology. *Prognosis:* 5-year survival is only 7% to 15%, 28% have lung metastases, and 25% have liver metastases. The prognosis is poor in U.S. because of late detection of the tumor, but in China, the prognosis is excellent because of screening programs and early detection. *Treatment:* squamous cell carcinoma is more radiosensitive than adenocarcinoma. Surgery is difficult for proximal lesions. Surgery and preoperative irradiation are used for distal one-third lesions. *Palliation:* laser endoscopy, bougienage, stent placement. *Chemotherapy:* no agents are known to be beneficial. Squamous cell carcinoma can produce ectopic parathyroid hormone; thus, hypercalcemia does not mean the tumor is unresectable. Barrett esophagus predisposes to adenocarcinoma of the esophagus.

- Know the radiographic appearance of leiomyoma and esophageal cancer.
- Conditions that predispose to esophageal squamous cell cancer: achalasia, lye stricture, Plummer-Vinson syndrome, human papillomavirus, tylosis, smoking, and alcohol. Barrett esophagus predisposes to adenocarcinoma.
- Esophageal cancers are usually unresectable; palliative treatment.
- 5-Year survival is only 7%-15% in the U.S.

3. Ring—A ring is a mucosal membrane that marks the junction of the esophageal and stomach mucosa. Muscular rings are rare. It presents as intermittent dysphagia for solids or as a sudden obstruction from food bolus (steak house syndrome). Know the radiographic appearance. Treatment is dilatation.

- Ring: intermittent dysphagia and food bolus impaction.
- Know its radiographic appearance.
- Treatment is dilatation.

4. Web—A web is a membrane of squamous mucosa that occurs anywhere in the esophagus. It presents as intermittent dysphagia. Plummer-Vinson syndrome: cervical esophageal web, iron deficiency anemia, and 15% chance of oropharyngeal or esophageal squamous cell cancer.

- Web presents as intermittent dysphagia.
- Plummer-Vinson syndrome: cervical esophageal web, iron deficiency anemia, and 15% chance of oropharyngeal or esophageal squamous cell cancer.
- Intermittent dysphagia is caused by rings, webs, or motility disorders.

Functional Cause

With functional obstruction (motility disorders), there is dysphagia for solids and liquids and an intermittent course;

weight loss may or may not occur. The three important motor abnormalities of the esophagus are achalasia, diffuse esophageal spasm, and scleroderma.

- Functional obstruction: dysphagia for solids and liquids; intermittent course; with or without weight loss.

1. Achalasia—Denervated esophagus (degeneration of Auerbach ganglion cells). Chest radiography shows air-fluid level. Barium swallow fluoroscopy shows dilated esophagus with beak-like tapering. *Motility pattern:* incomplete relaxation of the lower esophageal sphincter; hypertensive lower esophageal sphincter (usually does not have reflux); and aperistalsis in body (most important). Always endoscopically examine patients with achalasia, because cancer of the esophagogastric junction may present with the radiographic appearance and motility pattern of achalasia (pseudoachalasia). A clue would be an older patient with dysphagia and heartburn. Treatment is with pneumatic dilatation and not bougienage. Pneumatic dilatation is as effective as Heller myotomy.

   In Brazil, the parasite *Trypanosoma cruzi* (Chagas disease) produces a neurotoxin that destroys the myenteric plexus. Esophageal dilatation identical to that of achalasia, megacolon, and megaloureter is seen in Chagas disease.

- Achalasia: chest radiograph shows air-fluid level.
- Dilated esophagus with beak-like tapering on barium swallow fluoroscopy.
- Most important motility pattern in achalasia: aperistalsis.
- Always endoscopically examine patients with achalasia.
- Treat achalasia with pneumatic dilatation and not with bougienage.
- Chagas disease has esophageal dysfunction identical to that of achalasia.

2. Diffuse esophageal spasm—Diffuse esophageal spasm usually presents as chest pain but may cause intermittent dysphagia, which is aggravated by stress and hot or cold liquids. Barium swallow fluoroscopy shows a corkscrew esophagus. *Motility:* simultaneous contractions of high amplitude in the body of the esophagus. If the patient is asymptomatic during the test, motility may be normal. The lower esophageal sphincter is hypertensive or has defective relaxation in one-third of patients. Medical treatment (nitrates, anticholinergic agents, nifedipine) has unpredictable results. Surgical treatment is long myotomy.

- Diffuse esophageal spasm usually presents as chest pain.
- It is aggravated by stress and hot or cold liquids.
- Barium swallow fluoroscopy shows corkscrew esophagus.

- Medical treatment has unpredictable results.

3. Scleroderma—Esophageal involvement with scleroderma is associated with Raynaud phenomenon. Barium swallow fluoroscopy shows a common esophagogastric tube. *Motility:* aperistalsis in the body of the esophagus and incompetence of the lower esophageal sphincter, which causes severe reflux.

- Scleroderma: Raynaud phenomenon, aperistalsis, reflux.

Oropharyngeal Dysphagia

Oropharyngeal dysphagia is the result of faulty transfer of a food bolus from the oropharynx to the esophagus caused by structural abnormalities or disorders of either neural regulation or skeletal muscle (Table 8-1). Oropharyngeal dysphagia presents as high esophageal dysphagia associated with coughing, choking, or nasal regurgitation. After recognizing that oropharyngeal dysphagia is present, other associated symptoms may lead to the diagnosis of the underlying illness (e.g., a young person with oropharyngeal dysphagia, central scotoma, and neurologic symptoms has multiple sclerosis).

- Oropharyngeal dysphagia is the result of faulty transfer of a food bolus from the oropharynx to the esophagus caused by structural or neuromuscular disorders.
- It presents as cervical esophageal dysphagia associated with coughing, choking, or nasal regurgitation.

Gastroesophageal Reflux Disease

Reflux

The lower esophageal sphincter is the major barrier to reflux. This sphincter is a 2- to 4-cm-long specialized segment of circular smooth muscle in the terminal esophagus. The pressure of this sphincter varies markedly during the day, but the normal resting pressure is 15 to 30 mm Hg. Swallowing causes the pressure to decrease promptly (within 1 or 2 seconds after the onset of swallowing) and for the sphincter to remain relaxed until the peristaltic wave passes over it. The sphincter then contracts to maintain the increased resting pressure that prevents reflux. Pressure of the lower esophageal sphincter decreases significantly for 2 hours after a meal. Transient relaxations of the lower esophageal sphincter cause some gastroesophageal reflux to occur in everyone during the day but do not cause symptoms or esophagitis. Patients with clinically symptomatic reflux or inflammation show more frequent transient lower esophageal sphincter relaxations of unknown cause and have more frequent and longer lasting episodes of reflux.

- Lower esophageal sphincter pressure decreases for 2 hours after a meal.
- Patients with clinically symptomatic reflux show transient lower esophageal sphincter relaxations.

The degree of tissue damage is the real concern in gastroesophageal reflux disease. Several factors that determine whether reflux esophagitis occurs include 1) frequency of transient relaxations of the lower esophageal sphincter, 2) volume of gastric contents, 3) rate of gastric emptying (if delayed, reflux may develop), 4) potency of refluxate (acid, pepsin, bile), 5) efficiency of esophageal clearance (motility, salivary bicarbonate), and 6) resistance of esophageal tissue to injury and ability to repair.

The evaluation of esophagitis is designed to answer four important questions (Table 8-2): Does the patient have reflux and, if so, how severe? Does the patient have esophagitis and, if so, to what extent? Are the patient's symptoms due to reflux? What is the mechanism of reflux?

Table 8-1.—Causes of Oropharyngeal Dysphagia

Muscular disorders	Neurologic disorders	Structural causes
Amyloidosis	Amyotrophic lateral sclerosis[*]	Cervical osteophytes
Dermatomyositis[*]	Cerebral vascular accident	Cricopharyngeal dysfunction
Hyperthyroidism	Diphtheria	Goiter
Hypothyroidism	Huntington disease[*]	Lymphadenopathy
Myasthenia gravis[*]	Multiple sclerosis[*]	Zenker diverticulum
Myotonia dystrophica[*]	Parkinson disease	
Oculopharyngeal myopathy	Polio	
Stiff-man syndrome	Tabes dorsalis	
	Tetanus	

[*]Know the symptoms of these illnesses.

Table 8-2.—Evaluation of Esophagitis

Question	Tests for reflux (the more sensitive one is listed first)
Is reflux present?	pH probe; isotope scan
Is esophagitis present?	Biopsy; endoscopy
Are symptoms due to reflux?	Acid perfusion (Bernstein test)
Mechanism of reflux?	Motility

Internists should know how to use tests that evaluate reflux in a cost-effective way. In most patients, the medical history is sufficiently typical to warrant a trial of therapy without conducting expensive tests. Testing should be performed in patients with an atypical medical history, refractory symptoms, long-standing reflux, dysphagia, weight loss, or possible complications of esophagitis.

Atypical symptoms of gastroesophageal reflux disease include noncardiac chest pain, asthma, chronic cough, and hoarseness. Reflux is the most common cause of noncardiac chest pain. Asthmatic patients with coexisting reflux should have treatment for reflux, because it may improve control of respiratory symptoms. Reflux should be considered in asthmatic patients with postprandial or nocturnal wheezing. Complications of reflux include ulceration, bleeding, stricture, aspiration, Barrett esophagus, and adenocarcinoma of the esophagus.

- In most patients, the medical history is sufficiently typical to warrant a trial of therapy without tests.
- Testing should be performed in patients with an atypical medical history, refractory symptoms, long-standing reflux, dysphagia, weight loss, or possible complications of esophagitis.
- Atypical symptoms of gastroesophageal reflux: noncardiac chest pain, asthma, chronic cough, and hoarseness.
- Complications of gastroesophageal reflux: ulceration, bleeding, stricture, aspiration, Barrett esophagus, and adenocarcinoma of the esophagus.

Esophageal Tests

1. Barium swallow fluoroscopy—Reflux is found in 60% of patients with esophagitis but also in 25% of control subjects. It is a qualitative test and does not distinguish between "normal" and abnormal reflux. Upper gastrointestinal radiography is used primarily as a screening test to exclude other diagnoses (e.g., ulcer) and to identify complications of reflux (e.g., strictures, ulcers, cancer or mass). Patients with reflux and dysphagia should have barium esophagography first. Radiography may not detect Barrett esophagus.

- Reflux is found in 60% of patients with esophagitis but also in 25% of control subjects.
- Patients with reflux and dysphagia should have barium esophagography first.

2. Esophagoscopy—This is the most definitive test if gross inflammation is present. However, 40% of patients may have symptomatic reflux with no gross inflammation. This is the preferred first test in long-standing cases of reflux to rule out Barrett esophagus. It is also the first test for patients with reflux without dysphagia.

- Esophagoscopy is the test preferred first in long-standing cases of reflux to rule out Barrett esophagus.
- It is the first test for patients with reflux without dysphagia.

3. Esophageal biopsy—In patients with reflux but without gross esophagitis, the basal cell layer and papillae are elongated. Esophagoscopy and biopsy are about 60% sensitive for detecting reflux. Eosinophilia in the biopsy specimen is 100% sensitive for a diagnosis of esophagitis. If Barrett esophagus is found, biopsy specimens should be obtained from along the length of Barrett epithelium as surveillance for dysplasia (premalignant changes) or malignancy.

- Biopsy may detect esophagitis when gross inflammation is not present.
- With Barrett esophagus, it is important to obtain biopsy specimens from along the length of the mucosa as surveillance for dysplasia (premalignant changes) or malignancy.

4. 24-Hour pH monitoring—Monitoring the pH in the distal esophagus of patients during a 24-hour period of normal routine allows a more physiologic evaluation of reflux during daily activities. This test is valuable in patients with atypical symptoms, reflux symptoms refractory to therapy, a nondiagnostic evaluation, or pulmonary symptoms.

- 24-Hour pH monitoring allows a more physiologic evaluation of reflux during daily activities.
- This test is valuable in patients with atypical symptoms.

5. Acid perfusion (Bernstein test)—Saline perfusion for 10 minutes should not cause symptoms; next, switch to 0.1N HCl to determine whether the pain is reproduced. If heartburn and chest pain occur after acid instillation, treat for reflux.

- If heartburn and chest pain occur after acid instillation, treat for reflux.

6. Esophageal manometry—Manometry is reserved for patients with suspected esophageal motility disorders or for preoperative evaluation of surgical candidates.

- Esophageal manometry is reserved for suspected esophageal motility disorders.

Treatment of Reflux

Treatment of gastroesophageal reflux disease is divided into three phases:

Phase 1 therapy—Lifestyle modifications: elevate the head of the bed 6 inches, modify the diet so there is less fat and more protein, three meals a day, no eating for 3 hours before reclining, weight loss if overweight, and avoidance of specific foods (fatty foods, chocolate, alcohol, citrus juices, tomato products, coffee, carminatives). The patient should stop smoking and avoid alcohol. Avoid drugs that decrease lower esophageal sphincter pressure: anticholinergic agents, sedatives, tranquilizers, theophylline, progesterone or progesterone-containing birth control pills, nitrates, β-adrenergic agonists, and calcium channel blockers. Therapy is with antacids or alginic acid 30 minutes after meals and at bedtime.

Phase 2 therapy—Therapy includes drugs that decrease gastric acid output: H_2 blockers, all are equally effective. A dose twice daily (bid) is preferable for treating gastroesophageal reflux disease, for example, cimetidine, 400 mg bid; ranitidine, 150 mg bid; famotidine, 20 mg bid; nizatidine, 150 mg bid. Proton pump inhibitors: omeprazole and lansoprazole are the most effective agents to relieve symptoms and to promote mucosal healing. It is best to treat gross esophagitis for 6 weeks. Long-term use of these agents is safe. Drugs that increase the lower esophageal sphincter pressure and esophageal clearance—cisapride, metoclopramide, bethanechol—have a limited role in treating reflux and often cause side effects.

Phase 3 therapy—This therapy includes antireflux surgery, which is reserved for patients who are refractory to medical therapy or who develop complications. Nissen fundoplication is the preferred operation; fundoplication increases lower esophageal sphincter pressure.

- Phase 1 therapy: modify lifestyle, avoid drugs that decrease lower esophageal sphincter pressure, and use antacids as the first line of treatment.
- Phase 2 therapy: H_2 blockers or omeprazole.
- Phase 3 therapy: antireflux surgery is reserved for patients who are refractory to medical therapy or who develop complications.

Noncardiac Chest Pain

Chest pain is a frightening symptom, and patients are often referred to internists and gastroenterologists when cardiac evaluation does not have positive findings. Internists must understand the limitations of the diagnostic studies used to evaluate noncardiac chest pain. First, significant cardiac disease must be ruled out. Esophageal pain may be due to a motor disorder or esophagitis. Gastroesophageal reflux disease is the most common cause of noncardiac chest pain. Esophageal spasm can closely mimic angina. Esophagogastroduodenoscopy rules out mucosal disease, that is, inflammation, neoplasms, and chemical injury. Perform esophageal motility study to look for motor disorders, for example, esophageal spasm, "nutcracker esophagus." Therapy for noncardiac chest pain includes avoidance of precipitants. Antacids may be beneficial in patients with inflammation. Sublingual nitroglycerin or calcium channel blockers are sometimes helpful in motor disorders, but their efficacy is unproven. If appropriate, reassure the patient that cardiac disease is not present.

- For noncardiac chest pain, rule out significant cardiac disease.
- Gastroesophageal reflux disease is the commonest cause of noncardiac chest pain.
- Esophageal spasm can closely mimic angina.
- Esophagogastroduodenoscopy detects mucosal disease.
- Motility studies detect motility disorders.
- Sublingual nitroglycerin or calcium channel blockers are sometimes helpful.

Infections of the Esophagus

Patients with immunodeficiency disorders (AIDS), diabetes mellitus, malignancies (especially lymphoma and leukemia), or esophageal motility disorders are susceptible to opportunistic infections of the esophagus. These infections present as odynophagia. The most important infections to recognize are *Candida*, herpes, and cytomegalovirus. *Candida infection:* barium radiography shows small nodules in the upper one-third of the esophagus, and endoscopy shows cottage cheese-like plaques. Diagnosis is made by seeing pseudohyphae on KOH preparations. Treatment is with nystatin or clotrimazole for colonization and ketoconazole or fluconazole for esophagitis. Rarely, amphotericin B is used. *Herpes infection:* barium radiography and endoscopy show small discrete ulcers without plaques. Diagnosis is based on finding intranuclear inclusions (Cowdry type A bodies). Treatment is with acyclovir. *Cytomegalovirus infection:* radiography and endoscopy show severe inflammation with large ulcers. Intranuclear inclusions may be seen, but viral cultures are unreliable. Treatment is with ganciclovir or foscarnet (if ganciclovir-resistant).

- Opportunistic infections present as odynophagia in immuno-suppressed patients.

Other Esophageal Problems

Medication-Induced Esophagitis

Medication-induced esophagitis presents as odynophagia or dysphagia and is more likely to occur if there is abnormal motility, stricture, or compression (left atrial enlargement). It is more common in the elderly and is recognized as inflammation in the mid-esophagus, with sparing of the distal esophagus. Medications commonly associated with esophagitis include tetracycline, doxycycline, quinidine, potassium supplements, alendronate (Fosamax), ferrous sulfate, and ascorbic acid.

- Mid-esophageal inflammation is associated with abnormal motility, stricture, or compression and is more common in the elderly.
- Medicines responsible for esophagitis: tetracycline, doxycycline, quinidine, potassium supplements, alendronate, ferrous sulfate, and ascorbic acid.

Mallory-Weiss Syndrome

Mallory-Weiss syndrome is mucosal laceration at the esophagogastric junction. It accounts for about 10% of cases of upper gastrointestinal tract bleeding: 75% of patients have a history of retching or vomiting before bleeding, 72% have diaphragmatic hernias, and 90% stop bleeding. Vasopressin, endoscopic injection, or electrocautery may control bleeding. Surgical treatment for persistent bleeding is rarely necessary.

- Mallory-Weiss syndrome: mucosal laceration at the esophagogastric junction.
- Accounts for about 10% of cases of upper gastrointestinal tract bleeding. Bleeding stops spontaneously in 90%.
- 75% of patients have a history of retching and vomiting before bleeding.

Esophageal Perforation

Esophageal perforation commonly occurs after dilatation in an area of stricture. Spontaneous perforation of the esophagus (Boerhaave syndrome) follows violent retching, often after an alcoholic binge. It also occurs after heavy lifting, defecation, seizures, and forceful labor (childbirth). The most common site of perforation is the left posterior part of the distal esophagus. If pleural fluid is present, it may have an increased concentration of amylase. Zenker diverticulum, cervical osteophytes (difficult intubations), and endoscopy (intubation) are causes of perforation of the cervical esophagus.

- Esophageal perforation commonly occurs after dilatation.
- Boerhaave syndrome follows violent retching, often after an alcoholic binge.

STOMACH AND DUODENUM

Peptic ulcers are defects in the gastric or duodenal mucosa that result from an imbalance between the digestive activity of acid and pepsin in the gastric juice and the host's protective mechanisms to resist mucosal digestion. Recent advances in our understanding of peptic ulcer pathogenesis have caused us to modify our presumption that idiopathic acid hypersecretion is a major etiologic factor. Newer classifications of peptic ulcers categorize ulcers as being associated with three possible etiologic factors: 1) *Helicobacter pylori;* 2) nonsteroidal anti-inflammatory drugs (NSAIDs), including aspirin; or 3) miscellaneous causes. Miscellaneous causes include ulcers due to hypersecretion from gastrinomas (Zollinger-Ellison syndrome), idiopathic hypersecretion, and duodenogastric reflux of gastric mucosal barrier-breaking agents such as bile salts or lysolecithin. Recent reports estimate that fewer than 5% of ulcers are due to miscellaneous causes. Thus, at least 95% of peptic ulcers are due to either *Helicobacter pylori* or NSAIDs.

Helicobacter pylori

The Organism

H. pylori is a gram-negative, spiral-shaped, microaerophilic bacillus that contains 4 to 6 unipolar, sheathed flagella. This fastidious organism resides beneath and within the mucus layer of the gastric mucosa and produces several enzymes such as urease and mucolytic proteases that are important for its survival and its pathogenic effect. After it has been ingested, the organism moves into and through the mucus layer of the stomach. It has been postulated that several virulent factors are needed for successful colonization of the gastric mucosa, including motility, adhesins, proteases, phospholipases, cytokines, cytotoxins, and urease. Urease is thought to protect the organism from the acid environment. After colonization, the organism multiplies in the gastric mucus layer. Defense mechanisms may help control the infection, but unless treated, the organism remains in the gastric mucus layer for life.

H. pylori is a "slow" bacterium that causes persistent gastric infection and chronic inflammation. Ingestion of *H. pylori* can cause acute symptoms. Within weeks to months after infection, a chronic superficial gastritis develops, and after years to decades, chronic atrophic gastritis or gastric malignancy may develop.

Epidemiology

In the U.S., *H. pylori* has an age-related prevalence, occurring in 10% of the general population younger than 30 years and in 60% of those older than 60 years. *H. pylori* is present in 40% to 50% of the general population overall; it is more prevalent in blacks and Hispanics, poorer socioeconomic groups, and institutionalized persons. In developing countries such as India and Saudi Arabia, 50% of the population is infected by age 10, 70% by age 20, and 85% to 95% of the population overall is infected. Evidence of person-to-person transmission includes clustering within families, higher than expected prevalence among institutionalized persons, transmission by endoscopy and biopsy, and a higher prevalence of infection among gastroenterologists. The fecal-oral route of transmission has been postulated, and indeed, *H. pylori* has been isolated from human feces. In the future, detection of the organism in stool may provide a noninvasive approach to the diagnosis of *H. pylori* infection.

Associated Diseases

Active Chronic Gastritis

In patients with active chronic gastritis that is not associated with immunologic mechanisms (type A gastritis—pernicious anemia) or chemical injury (type C gastritis—alcohol, NSAIDs, aspirin, bile salts), *H. pylori* infection (type B gastritis) is universally found. *H. pylori*-induced active chronic gastritis is the most common type of chronic gastritis, and in some patients, it may progress to chronic atrophic gastritis. An important concept is that *H. pylori*-induced gastritis is the basic disease, and the development of duodenal or gastric ulcers or malignancy is a complication of the gastritis.

Duodenal Ulcer

H. pylori is found in 90% to 95% of patients with duodenal ulcers. The most important link between *H. pylori*-induced gastritis and the development of duodenal ulcers is the presence of gastric metaplasia in the duodenal bulb. Some data suggest that the gastric metaplasia must be infected by *H. pylori* to permit the development of duodenitis or duodenal ulcer. If *H. pylori*-positive patients with duodenal ulcer do not receive treatment, most have relapse within 1 year. However, if the infection is eradicated, the rate of relapse approaches zero. *H. pylori* infection causes basal and meal-stimulated gastrin release. Asymptomatic carriers of the bacillus may have a protective mechanism that prevents the hypersecretion of gastric acid. Enhanced gastric acid secretion occurs only in ulcer patients.

Gastric Ulcer

H. pylori is found in about 80% of patients with gastric ulcer. Eradication of *H. pylori* decreases the relapse rate of gastric ulcers. *Adenocarcinoma*—Studies from the U.S. and Great Britain have established a strong association between *H. pylori* infection (serum samples) and the emergence of noncardia gastric adenocarcinoma. It is postulated that *H. pylori* gastritis progresses to atrophic gastritis and, in the presence of other risk factors, gastric adenocarcinoma eventually develops. This appears to be a rare occurrence. A cause-and-effect relationship remains to be established, and further studies are needed to determine the exact role of *H. pylori* in the development of gastric adenocarcinoma. *Primary B-cell lymphoma*—*H. pylori* has also been associated with primary B-cell lymphoma of the stomach. Of 450 patients with *H. pylori*-positive gastritis, 125 (28%) had mucosal lymphoid follicles and 8 (1.8%) had B lymphocytes infiltrating the epithelium, consistent with the development of early lymphoma.

Nonulcer Dyspepsia

Nonulcer dyspepsia is common, affecting about 20% of the people in the U.S. Of those with functional dyspepsia, approximately 50% are infected with *H. pylori*, similar to the prevalence of *H. pylori* in asymptomatic persons. There is no convincing evidence that treatment of *H. pylori*-positive patients with nonulcer dyspepsia results in significant clinical improvement.

Diagnostic Tests for H. pylori Infection

Various diagnostic tests are available for determining whether *H. pylori* infection is present. The choice of which test to use is determined by the clinical setting of the patient and the cost.

Serology

H. pylori produces not only a local immune response but also a systemic immune response. Current detection methods exist for antibodies of the IgG, IgA, and IgM classes. Serologic testing is the most cost-effective, noninvasive way to diagnose primary *H. pylori* infection, but serologic results remain positive over time, which limits the usefulness of this test in follow-up evaluation. The sensitivity is 95%, the specificity is 90% to 95%, and the cost is $40 to $100.

Breath Test

A radiolabeled dose of urea is given orally to a patient. If *H. pylori* is present, the urease splits the urea and radiolabeled CO_2 is exhaled. The advantage of this test is that it is quick, easy to perform, and does not require endoscopy. As the breath test becomes more widely available, it will be the test of choice for follow-up evaluation. The sensitivity is 95% to 98%, the specificity is 95% to 98%, and the cost is $100 to $200.

Biopsy Urease Tests

A biopsy specimen is impregnated into auger that contains urea and a pH indicator. As the urea is split, the pH of the medium changes the color of the auger from yellow to red. This test depends on bacterial urease, and the greater the number of organisms, the more rapid the test turns positive. The sensitivity is 95%, the specificity is 98%, and the cost is $20 (plus the cost of endoscopy to obtain tissue).

Histology

An advantage of histology is being able to examine the underlying inflammatory reaction. *H. pylori* can be demonstrated with Gram stain, hematoxylin and eosin stain, Giemsa stain, and the Warthin-Starry (silver) stain. The sensitivity is 98%, the specificity is 98%, and the cost is $250.

Culture

Culturing *H. pylori* is tedious and expensive and should be reserved for special circumstances, for example, when an antibiotic-resistant organism is suspected or if virulence testing is being done. The sensitivity is 90% to 95%, the specificity 100%, and the cost is $150.

Currently, because many symptomatic patients undergo endoscopy, histologic examination and biopsy urease tests are used most commonly in the initial evaluation. Newer, inexpensive serologic tests that can be performed in minutes are being investigated.

Treatment

The goal of treatment of an *H. pylori*-positive duodenal or gastric ulcer is to heal the ulcer and to eradicate (not suppress) the bacteria. Combination therapy with antisecretory agents and antimicrobial therapy for *H. pylori* is most effective. There is extensive research to determine the simplest and most efficacious agents for combination therapy, and specific recommendations for treatment regimens are constantly changing. The following general principles should guide treatment:

1. All patients with gastric or duodenal ulcer who are infected with *H. pylori* should receive combination therapy.
2. Patients with a well-documented ulcer who are infected with *H. pylori* but who are in remission with maintenance antisecretory therapy should receive combination therapy, then maintenance antisecretory therapy will not be necessary.
3. Maintenance antisecretory therapy is unnecessary except in patients with recurrent *H. pylori*-negative ulcers and in some patients with a previous history of bleeding from an ulcer.
4. Currently, treatment is not recommended for nonulcer dyspepsia and asymptomatic *H. pylori*-infected patients.

Nonsteroidal Anti-Inflammatory Drug-Induced Ulcers

NSAIDs inhibit gastroduodenal prostaglandin synthesis, which results in decreased secretion of mucus and bicarbonate and reduced mucosal blood flow. NSAID-induced ulcers occur more commonly in the stomach than in the duodenum, and they typically are located in the prepyloric area or antrum of the stomach.

The risk of peptic ulcer disease with NSAIDs is dose-dependent. It is important for physicians to understand that the anti-inflammatory properties of NSAIDs predispose to ulceration (prostaglandin inhibition) and there are different dose-response relationships for analgesia and anti-inflammatory properties of NSAIDs. The maximal analgesic effect plateaus well below the effective anti-inflammatory dose. Low doses of aspirin or NSAIDs give pain relief but have little anti-inflammatory activity. The newer NSAIDs have been marketed with more convenient (less frequent) dosing intervals and in dosages that have marked anti-inflammatory activity. Thus, the use of newer NSAIDs may subject the patient to an increased risk for ulcer without providing increased analgesia. In many instances, the use of NSAIDs can be discontinued and simple analgesic therapy with acetaminophen substituted. For patients who require NSAIDs, an attempt should be made to use the lowest possible dose. It is also important for physicians to know that the risk of peptic ulcer disease with NSAID use is maximal in the first month of treatment (ulcers may occur shortly after treatment is begun) and elderly patients and patients with a previous history of peptic ulcer disease are at highest risk.

H_2-receptor antagonists and sucralfate are ineffective in preventing gastric ulcers and for reducing the frequency of NSAID-induced mucosal erosions. Prostaglandin replacement with the synthetic prostaglandin misoprostol decreases the incidence of NSAID-induced gastric ulcers. However, diarrhea develops in many patients, thus limiting the usefulness of misoprostol.

Duodenal Ulcer

H. pylori infection and associated antral gastritis are present in approximately 95% of patients with duodenal ulcer. However, only 10% to 20% of all patients who are infected with *H. pylori* ever develop an ulcer; therefore, other risk factors must be involved. Other risk factors that contribute to duodenal ulceration include 1) NSAIDs, 2) acid hypersecretion, 3) cigarette smoking, 4) cirrhosis, 5) chronic pulmonary disease, and 6) chronic renal disease. There is no evidence that diet, alcohol, corticosteroids, caffeine, or stress increases the risk of duodenal ulceration.

Gastric Ulcer

H. pylori infection and associated antral gastritis are present in 80% of patients with gastric ulcer. Most gastric ulcers occur in areas of gastritis on the lesser curvature of the stomach near the junction of the body and antrum. In patients with gastric ulcer, acid secretion is normal or low; thus, it is believed that gastric ulceration occurs when the gastric mucosal barrier of mucus and bicarbonate is damaged. The risk factors other than *H. pylori* that contribute to gastric ulceration include 1) NSAIDs, 2) bile reflux, and 3) cigarette smoking. Bile reflux may occur from previous gastroduodenal surgery or from abnormal antral motility or pyloric sphincter function. Alcohol can cause gastritis, but there is no evidence that alcohol predisposes to gastric ulceration.

- 95% of duodenal ulcers are caused by *H. pylori* or NSAIDs, including aspirin.
- Risk factors for duodenal ulcers: *H. pylori*, NSAIDs, acid hypersecretion, cigarette smoking, cirrhosis, chronic pulmonary disease, and chronic renal disease.
- Risk factors for gastric ulcers are 1) *H. pylori*, 2) NSAIDs, 3) bile reflux, and 4) cigarette smoking.

Zollinger-Ellison Syndrome

Zollinger-Ellison syndrome is characterized by the triad of peptic ulceration, acid hypersecretion, and diarrhea caused by a gastrin-producing tumor. The tumor is usually located in the pancreas, but it can occur in the wall of the duodenum. Two-thirds of gastrinomas are malignant and can metastasize to regional lymph nodes and the liver. One-fourth of gastrinomas are related to a multiple endocrine neoplasia syndrome (MEN-I) and are associated with pituitary adenoma and hyperparathyroidism.

The most common clinical presentation is duodenal bulb ulceration, although multiple ulcers and postbulbar ulcers occur. The coexistence of duodenal ulcer with diarrhea or duodenal ulcer with hypercalcemia should raise suspicion of Zollinger-Ellison syndrome. A duodenal ulcer that is not related to *H. pylori* infection or to NSAID use should also raise suspicion of Zollinger-Ellison syndrome. Gastrinoma also should be considered in patients with recurrent ulcers, intractable ulcers, a family history of ulcer disease or MEN-I syndrome, or evidence of gastric acid hypersecretion (enlarged rugal folds, dilated duodenum, increased acid output).

The serum level of gastrin should be determined if Zollinger-Ellison syndrome is suspected. Serum levels of gastrin greater than 1,000 pg/mL in patients who produce gastric acid are essentially diagnostic of gastrinoma. Increased serum levels of gastrin may also be seen in atrophic gastritis, pernicious anemia, postvagotomy states, and renal failure, because gastric acid output is low in these conditions. Basal and stimulated gastric acid secretory studies should be performed in all patients who have increased levels of gastrin. The basal acid output is greater than 10 mEq/hr. When the laboratory results are equivocal, a secretin test should be performed. An intravenous bolus of secretin produces an increase in the serum level of gastrin in patients with gastrinoma.

Tumor localization can be difficult. Computed tomographic (CT) scanning detects 50% of tumors and is the procedure of choice for locating a gastrinoma. If the CT findings are normal, selective arteriography will localize 33% of tumors. Combined CT and arteriography localizes 70% to 80% of gastrinomas. Surgical exploration is indicated to locate an isolated tumor in a patient who does not have evidence of metastases or MEN-I syndrome.

Approximately 20% to 25% of gastrinomas can be completely removed surgically. If the tumor cannot be removed, some advocate a parietal cell vagotomy, which helps control acid secretion. Patients who are not candidates for surgery or who have an unresectable tumor can be managed medically by acid suppression and chemotherapy. High-dose, long-term treatment with H_2-receptor blockers or proton pump inhibitors is safe and effective. Chemotherapy with streptozocin and 5-fluorouracil is effective in 50% of patients with metastatic disease.

- Zollinger-Ellison syndrome: peptic ulceration, acid hypersecretion, and diarrhea caused by a gastrin-secreting tumor.
- Rule out Zollinger-Ellison syndrome in patients with *H. pylori* and NSAID-negative duodenal ulcers, duodenal ulcers with diarrhea, duodenal ulcers with hypercalcemia.
- Do not explore surgically if metastatic disease or MEN-I syndrome is present.

Stress Ulcers

Stress ulceration is caused by gastric mucosal ischemia due to an underlying illness. *H. pylori* is not an important pathogenic factor. The underlying conditions for stress ulcers are trauma, sepsis, and serious illness. Most of the hemorrhages occur 3 to 7 days after the traumatic event. Burns, especially those involving more than 35% of the body, may cause ulcers. Central nervous system trauma produces Cushing ulcer, which is seen in 50% to 75% of patients with head injury. This ulcer tends to be deep and to perforate more often than other ulcers.

- Underlying conditions for stress ulcers: trauma, sepsis, serious illness.
- Hemorrhaging occurs 3-7 days after the traumatic event.
- Burns involving >35% of body may produce ulcers.
- Stress ulcers are seen in 50%-75% of patients with head injury (Cushing ulcers).

Prophylaxis against bleeding is to keep pH greater than 4.0. Antacids clearly decrease the incidence of bleeding over that of placebo. H_2-receptor antagonists are equally as effective as antacids and sometimes easier to use. Sucralfate is as effective as antacids and H_2 blockers, according to some studies. Also, sucralfate may decrease nosocomial pneumonia in ventilator-dependent patients, because gastric pH is not lowered (decreased bacterial overgrowth). Prostaglandins may have a role in prophylaxis. Enteral feedings can maintain intragastric pH greater than 3.5. If antacids cannot be used, use H_2 blockers or sucralfate; combination treatment may be helpful.

- Prophylaxis: keep pH >4.0.
- Antacids, H_2-receptor antagonists, and sucralfate decrease incidence of bleeding.
- Sucralfate may decrease nosocomial pneumonia in ventilator-dependent patients.

Medical therapy for bleeding, acute gastric mucosal ulcers: correct the underlying predisposing condition. In general, upper gastrointestinal tract bleeding stops spontaneously about 85% of the time. Some advocate the use of iced saline lavage or intragastric levarterenol. Angiographic therapeutic techniques include intra-arterial vasopressin and transcatheter embolization. Endoscopic techniques are electrocautery (bicap heater probe) and laser photocoagulation. Surgical therapy for bleeding acute gastric mucosal ulcers must be considered when blood requirement is more than 4 to 6 units per 24 to 48 hours. The mortality rate for all forms of surgical therapy is 30% to 40%.

Nonerosive Nonspecific Chronic Gastritis

Chronic gastritis is divided into two types: type A and type B. Type A, or autoimmune, gastritis involves the body and fundus of the stomach. A subset of patients develops atrophic gastritis (inflammation of the gland zone with variable gland loss). Pernicious anemia with hypochlorhydria or achlorhydria and megaloblastic anemia may result. Antiparietal cell antibodies are found in 90% of patients. Intrinsic factor antibodies are seen less commonly. Other autoimmune diseases such as Addison disease and Hashimoto thyroiditis are often present. The serum levels of gastrin are increased. Gastric carcinoid tumors rarely develop. Gastric polyps occur, and intestinal metaplasia may be a precursor to gastric adenocarcinoma.

- Type A gastritis is associated with pernicious anemia and other autoimmune disorders.
- Serum levels of gastrin are increased.
- Type A gastritis is associated with gastric carcinoids, polyps, and adenocarcinoma.

Type B gastritis involves the antrum and is associated with *H. pylori* infection. Serum levels of gastrin are normal. Gastric ulcers and duodenal ulcers occur commonly, and the incidence of gastric adenocarcinoma is increased.

- Type B gastritis is associated with *H. pylori* infection.
- Serum levels of gastrin are normal.
- Type B gastritis is associated with gastric and duodenal ulcers and adenocarcinoma.

Gastric Cancer

In the 1940s, gastric cancer was the most common malignant disease in the U.S. Since then, the decrease in incidence has been dramatic. Japan has the highest mortality rate from gastric cancer. Migration studies show a decrease in incidence among migrants from high-risk areas to low-risk areas and a suggestion of increased risk among persons moving from low-risk to high-risk areas. Environmental factors include diet—increased association with starch, pickled vegetables, salted fish/meat, smoked foods, increased salt consumption, and nitrate and nitrite consumption. Genetic factors include blood group A, because patients with blood group A have two- to threefold greater incidence among relatives. The population at risk are persons older than 50 years. The male:female ratio is as high as 2:1. Also, it is more common in lower socioeconomic groups.

- Dramatic decrease in the incidence of gastric cancer in the U.S. since the 1940s.
- Decreased incidence among migrants from high-risk areas.
- Increased association with starch, pickled vegetables, salted fish/meat, smoked foods, increased salt consumption, and nitrate and nitrite consumption.
- A two- to threefold greater incidence among relatives.

Possible Precancerous Lesions/Situations

1) Chronic atrophic gastritis and intestinal metaplasia are frequently found in patients with gastric cancer; however, both conditions are found frequently in older persons without gastric carcinoma. 2) Chronic benign gastric ulcer rarely progresses to cancer. 3) Pernicious anemia—previous autopsy studies showed a prevalence of 10%. Recent endoscopic screening study of 123 patients with pernicious anemia showed a prevalence of gastric neoplastic lesions of 8.1%. 4) Postgastrectomy minimally increases the risk, but surveillance endoscopy is not necessary.

- Chronic atrophic gastritis is found frequently in patients with gastric cancer.
- Chronic benign gastric ulcer rarely progresses to cancer.
- Pernicious anemia prevalence of 10%.
- Postgastrectomy: minimal increased risk, endoscopy screening not necessary.

Clinical Aspects

Gastric cancer is often asymptomatic, but abdominal discomfort and weight loss are the common presenting complaints. Physical examination is often unrevealing, but up to 30% of patients have an epigastric mass. Perform endoscopy, with multiple (7 or 8) biopsies and CT scanning of abdomen (to identify extragastric extension).

● Abdominal discomfort and weight loss are common presenting complaints.
● 30% of patients have an epigastric mass.
● Perform endoscopy, with multiple (7-8) biopsies.

Treatment and Prognosis

For local disease—Resection often requires total gastrectomy for tumor-free margins. Omentum and spleen (splenic hilus nodes) are often removed in curative resection. For disseminated disease—Surgical treatment is necessary only for palliation. Response to chemotherapy is generally poor. The only consistent factor is extent of disease. Five-year survival is 90% if the tumor is confined to the mucosa and submucosa, 50% if the tumor is through the serosa, and 10% if the tumor involves lymph nodes.

Gastric Polyps

Gastric polyps are rare; 0.5% prevalence in an autopsy series. The two types of polyps are hyperplastic and adenomatous. Hyperplastic polyps are more common and not premalignant. No therapy is needed. Adenomatous polyps are premalignant, especially if larger than 2 cm. They occur most often in achlorhydric stomachs, that is, pernicious anemia, and are usually localized in the antrum. If pedunculated, the polyp can be removed endoscopically.

● Hyperplastic polyps are more common and not premalignant.
● Adenomatous polyps are premalignant, especially if larger than 2 cm.

Gastroduodenal Dysmotility Syndromes

Symptoms of abnormal gastric motility may include nausea, vomiting, bloating, early satiety, dyspepsia, heartburn, anorexia, weight loss, and food avoidance. The specific cause of abnormal gastric motor function is unknown but is believed to be related to autonomic neuropathy. Diabetes mellitus is probably the most common medical cause of symptomatic gastric motor dysfunction. Conditions causing gastroparesis are listed in Table 8-3.

● Nausea, vomiting, bloating, early satiety, dyspepsia, heartburn, anorexia, weight loss, and food avoidance may suggest abnormal gastric motility.

● It is believed to be related to autonomic neuropathy.
● Diabetes mellitus: most common medical cause of symptomatic gastric motor dysfunction.

Treatment—Currently, several prokinetic drugs are available in the U.S. These drugs normalize and/or augment motility, with an accompanying enhancement of movement of luminal contents. Metoclopramide is a dopamine antagonist and a cholinergic agonist that increases the rate and amplitude of antral contractions. It crosses the blood-brain barrier and frequently causes such side effects as drowsiness, athetosis, and prolactin release. Domperidone is a selective dopamine antagonist that works only on peripheral receptors in the gut. It has no cholinergic effects and fewer side effects than metoclopramide. Cisapride facilitates the release of acetylcholine from the myenteric plexus (local cholinergic agonist). It does not antagonize dopamine and has few side effects. Bethanechol is a systemic cholinergic agonist with side effects. It may be useful in low dosage in combination with other agents. Erythromycin stimulates both cholinergic and motilin receptors.

● Metoclopramide is a dopamine antagonist and cholinergic agonist.
● Domperidone is a selective dopamine antagonist.
● Cisapride is a selective cholinergic agonist.
● Erythromycin stimulates both cholinergic and motilin receptors.

SMALL INTESTINE

Diarrhea

Patients use the term "diarrhea" to refer to any increase in the frequency, fluidity, or volume of the stool or any change in its consistency. Normally, stools are generally solid and brown, but these features may vary with diet. Frequency of stools varies among persons from 1 to 3 stools daily to 2 or 3 stools

Table 8-3.—Conditions Causing Gastroparesis

Acute conditions	Chronic conditions
Anticholinergic drugs	Amyloidosis
Hyperglycemia	Diabetes mellitus
Hypokalemia	Gastric dysrhythmias
Morphine	Pseudo-obstruction
Pancreatitis	Scleroderma
Surgery	Vagotomy
Trauma	

weekly. Blood, pus (leukocytes), and oil are not present in normal stools (Table 8-4).

Physicians define diarrhea as an increase in stool weight or volume. Because a stool is 65% to 80% water, stool weight is proportional to stool water. Dietary fiber content influences the water content of the stool and, thus, stool weight can vary according to the diet of a culture. In the U.S., normal daily stool weight is less than 200 g/day and normal stool volume is less than 200 mL/day (compared with <400 g/day and 400 mL/day, respectively, in rural Africa).

It is important to understand normal daily intestinal fluid balance. Each day, 9 or 10 L of isotonic fluid is presented to the proximal small intestine (2 L, diet and 8 L, endogenous secretions). The small bowel absorbs most of the fluid (7-9 L), and the colon absorbs all the 1 or 2 L presented to it each day except for less than 200 mL and forms a soft solid stool. There is considerable reserve, because the maximal absorptive capacity is 12 L/day for the small bowel and 4 to 6 L/day for the colon.

Mechanisms of Diarrhea

Osmotic diarrhea occurs when water-soluble molecules are poorly absorbed, remain in the intestinal lumen, and retain water in the intestine. Osmotic diarrhea follows ingestion of an osmotically active substance and stops with fasting. Stool volume is less than 1 L/day, and the stool has an osmolar gap—stool osmolality is greater than the sum of electrolyte concentrations. Often, stool pH is less than 7.0. Clinical examples of osmotic diarrhea include lactase deficiency, sorbitol foods, saline cathartics, and antacids.

- In osmotic diarrhea, stool volume is <1 L/day.
- Diarrhea stops with fasting.
- Stool has an osmolar gap.
- Causes of osmotic diarrhea: lactase deficiency, sorbitol foods, and antacids.

In secretory diarrhea, fluid and electrolyte transport are abnormal, that is, the intestine secretes rather than absorbs fluid. Stool volume is greater than 1 L/day, and its composition is similar to that of extracellular fluid, so there is no osmolar gap. The diarrhea persists despite fasting and often presents with hypokalemia. Clinical examples of secretory diarrhea include bacterial toxins, hormone-secreting tumors, surreptitious laxative ingestion, bile acid diarrhea, and fatty acid diarrhea.

- In secretory diarrhea, stool volume is >1 L/day.
- There is no osmolar gap.
- Diarrhea persists despite fasting.
- Causes of secretory diarrhea: bacterial toxins, hormone-secreting tumors, surreptitious laxative ingestion, bile acid diarrhea, and fatty acid diarrhea.

In exudative diarrhea, membrane permeability is abnormal, and there is exudation of serum proteins, blood, or mucus into the bowel from sites of inflammation, ulceration, or infiltration. The diarrhea is small volume and may be associated with bloody stools. Examples include invasive bacterial pathogens (*Shigella, Salmonella*, etc.) and inflammatory bowel disease.

- Exudative diarrhea: abnormal membrane permeability.
- Diarrhea is small volume.
- Invasive bacterial pathogens (*Shigella, Salmonella*, etc.) and inflammatory bowel disease.

Motility disorders—Both rapid transit (inadequate time for chyme to contact absorbing surface) and delayed transit (bacterial overgrowth) can cause diarrhea. Rapid transit occurs after gastrectomy and intestinal resection and in hyperthyroidism and carcinoid syndrome. Delayed transit occurs with structural defects (strictures, blind loops, small-bowel diverticuli) or underlying illnesses that cause visceral neuropathy (diabetes) or myopathy (scleroderma), that is, pseudo-obstruction.

- Rapid transit: causes diarrhea because of malabsorption.
- Delayed transit: causes diarrhea because of bacterial overgrowth.

Mixed mechanisms—Many disease processes may have more than one mechanism for causing diarrhea, for example, generalized malabsorption has osmotic and secretory components (fatty acids cause secretion in the colon).

Clinical Approach

It is useful to differentiate small-bowel ("right-sided") diarrhea from colonic ("left-sided") diarrhea (Table 8-5). Right-sided diarrhea is large in volume, with a modest increase in the number of stools. Symptoms attributed to inflammation of the rectosigmoid are absent, and proctoscopic examination findings are normal. Left-sided diarrhea presents as frequent

Table 8-4.—Normal Stool Composition

		Electrolytes, mEq/L	
Weight	<200 g	Na$^+$	40
Percent water	65-80	K$^+$	90
Fat	<7 g	Cl$^-$	15
Nitrogen	<2.5 g	HCO$_3^-$	30

Table 8-5.—Right-Sided and Left-Sided Diarrhea: Contrasts in Clinical Presentation

Right-sided, or small-bowel, diarrhea	Left-sided, or colonic, diarrhea
Reservoir capacity intact	Reservoir capacity decreased
Large stool volume	Small amounts of stool
Modest increase in number	Frequency
No urgency	Urgency
No tenesmus	Tenesmus
No mucus	Mucus
No blood	Blood

small-volume stools with obvious evidence of inflammation, and proctosigmoidoscopic examination usually confirms inflammation. Left-sided diarrhea usually suggests an exudative mechanism, whereas the mechanism for right-sided diarrhea is nonspecific.

Acute Diarrhea

Acute diarrhea is abrupt in onset and usually resolves in several days (3-10 days). It is self-limited, and the cause usually is not found (? viral). No evaluation is necessary unless there are bloody stools and fever or infection is suspected (e.g., travel history, common source outbreak). If these conditions exist, do not treat with antimotility agents. Begin the work-up with stool studies for bacterial pathogens, ova, and parasites and proctosigmoidoscopy. Recognize the common situations that predispose to specific infections (see infectious diarrhea below).

- For acute diarrhea, no evaluation is necessary unless there are bloody stools and fever or infection is suspected.
- Do not administer antimotility agents if there are bloody stools and if fever or infection is suspected.

Chronic Diarrhea

Chronic diarrhea is an initial episode lasting longer than 4 weeks or diarrhea that recurs after the initial episode. The most common cause of chronic diarrhea is irritable bowel syndrome, but always rule out lactase deficiency. Be able to differentiate organic diarrhea from functional diarrhea (Table 8-6).

- The most common cause of chronic diarrhea is irritable bowel syndrome.
- Always rule out lactase deficiency in suspected irritable bowel syndrome.
- Differentiate organic diarrhea from functional diarrhea.

Chronic Watery Diarrhea

The evaluation of chronic watery diarrhea usually requires distinguishing secretory diarrhea from osmotic diarrhea (Table 8-7). This can be done by collecting stools and measuring volume, osmolality, and electrolyte content and observing the patient's response to fasting.

- Evaluation of chronic watery diarrhea requires distinguishing secretory diarrhea from osmotic diarrhea.

Anatomy of Nutrient Absorption

The sites of nutrient, vitamin, and mineral absorption are the following: 1) the duodenum absorbs iron, calcium, magnesium, folate, water-soluble vitamins, and monosaccharides; 2) the jejunum absorbs fatty acids, amino acids, monosaccharides, and water-soluble vitamins; and 3) the ileum absorbs

Table 8-6.—Features Differentiating Organic Diarrhea From Functional Diarrhea

	Organic diarrhea	Functional diarrhea
Weight loss	Often present	Not present
Duration of illness	Variable (weeks to years)	Usually long (>6 months)
Quantity of stool	Variable but usually large (>200 g/24 hr)	Usually small (<200 g/24 hr)
Presence of blood in stool	May be present	Never present (unless from hemorrhoids)
Timing when diarrhea occurs	No special pattern	Usually in the morning but rarely wakes patient
Fever, arthritis, skin lesions	May be present	Not present
Emotional stress	No relation to symptoms	Usually precedes or coincides with symptoms
Cramping abdominal pain	Often	May be present

From Matseshe JW, Phillips SF: Chronic diarrhea: a practical approach. Med Clin North Am 62:141-154, Jan 1978. By permission of WB Saunders Company.

monosaccharides, fatty acids, amino acids, fat-soluble vitamins (A, D, E, K), vitamin B_{12}, and conjugated bile salts.

The distal small bowel can adapt to absorb nutrients. The proximal small bowel cannot adapt to absorb vitamin B_{12} or bile salts. Fat absorption is the most complex process. Dietary fat consists mostly of triglycerides that must be digested by pancreatic lipase to fatty acids and glycerol, which are solubilized by micelles for absorption. The fatty acids and monoglycerides are reesterified by intestinal epithelial cells into chylomicrons that are absorbed into the circulation by lymphatic vessels (Table 8-8). Medium chain triglycerides are absorbed directly into the portal vein and do not require micellar solubilization.

- The distal small bowel can adapt to absorb nutrients.
- The proximal small bowel cannot adapt to absorb vitamin B_{12} or bile salts.

Suspect malabsorption if the medical history suggests steatorrhea or if there is diarrhea with weight loss (especially if intake is adequate), chronic diarrhea of indeterminate nature, or nutritional deficiency (know the symptoms and signs of malabsorption) (Table 8-9).

- Diarrhea with iron deficiency anemia (evaluation for blood loss is negative) = proximal small bowel, e.g., sprue.
- Diarrhea with metabolic bone disease = decreased calcium and protein, thus, proximal small bowel.
- Hypoproteinemia with normal fat absorption suggests "protein-losing enteropathy." If eosinophilia is present, eosinophilic gastroenteritis; if lymphopenia is present, intestinal lymphangiectasia.
- Oil droplets (neutral fat) or muscle fibers (undigested protein) present in stool = pancreatic insufficiency (maldigestion).
- Serum levels of calcium, magnesium, and iron are usually normal in pancreatic insufficiency. Serum levels of albumin may also be normal.
- Howell-Jolly bodies (if there is no history of splenectomy) or dermatitis herpetiformis suggests celiac sprue (small-bowel biopsy is not diagnostic for sprue, but the response to gluten-free diet is).
- Fever, arthralgias, neurologic symptoms = Whipple disease.

Helpful hints in the medical history, physical examination, or laboratory results may suggest the possibility of diarrhea or

Table 8-7.—Typical Findings in Osmotic and Secretory Diarrheas

	Osmotic diarrhea	Secretory diarrhea
Daily stool volume, L	<1	>1
Effect of 48-hr fasting	Diarrhea stops	Diarrhea continues
Fecal fluid analysis		
Osmolality, mOsm	400	290
Na + K x 2,[*] mEq/L	120	280
Solute gap[†]	>100	<50

[*]Multiplied by 2 to account for anions.

[†]Calculated by subtracting ([Na] + [K]) x 2 from osmolality.

From Krejs GJ, Hendler RS, Fordtran JS: Diagnostic and pathophysiologic studies in patients with chronic diarrhea. *In* Secretory Diarrhea. Edited by M Field, JS Fordtran, SG Schultz. Bethesda, MD, American Physiological Society, 1980, pp 141-151. By permission of publisher.

Table 8-8.—Mechanisms of Fat Malabsorption

Alteration	Mechanism	Disease state
Defective digestion	Inadequate lipase	Pancreatic insufficiency
Impaired micelle formation	Duodenal bile salt concentration	Common duct obstruction or cholestasis
Impaired absorption	Small-bowel disease	Sprue and Whipple disease
Impaired chylomicron formation	Impaired β-globulin synthesis	Abetalipoproteinemia
Impaired lymphatic circulation	Lymphatic obstruction	Intestinal lymphangiectasia and lymphoma

malabsorption (Table 8-10). Other hints in the history might include 1) age—youth suggests lactase deficiency, inflammatory bowel disease, or sprue, 2) travel—parasites, toxigenic agents (exposure to contaminated food or water), 3) drugs--laxatives, antacids, antibiotics, colchicine, lactulose, 4) family history—celiac sprue, inflammatory bowel disease, polyposis coli, lactase deficiency.

Medical history: previous surgery (short-bowel syndrome, dumping syndrome, blind loop syndrome, postvagotomy diarrhea, and ileal resection), radiation, systemic disease.

Diseases Causing Diarrhea

Osmotic Diarrhea

Lactase deficiency—Lactose is normally split by lactase into glucose and galactose, which are absorbed in the small bowel. In lactase deficiency, lactose is not absorbed in the small intestine but enters the colon, where it is fermented in the lumen by bacteria to lactic acid. The result is diarrhea of low pH and increased intestinal motility. The most common disaccharidase deficiency is lactase deficiency. "Acquired" lactase deficiency (genetic?) is common in Orientals, blacks, Eskimos, and people from the Middle East. Diarrhea, abdominal cramps, and flatulence occur after ingestion of dairy products. There is improvement with diet. The pH of the stool is less than 6.0. *Lactose tolerance test*— Blood sugar increases less than 20 mg/100 mL after lactose ingestion. Abnormal hydrogen breath test. Jejunal biopsy results are normal (disaccharidase levels are decreased). Lactose intolerance can occur in any clinical setting in which the intestinal mucosa is damaged.

- Lactase deficiency: lactose is not absorbed in the small intestine.

Table 8-9.—Causes of Symptoms in Malabsorption

Extra-gastrointestinal symptom	Result of
Muscle wasting, edema	Decreased protein absorption
Paresthesias, tetany	Decreased vitamin D and calcium absorption
Bone pain	Decreased calcium absorption
Muscle cramps	Weakness, excess potassium loss
Easy bruisability, petechiae	Decreased vitamin K absorption
Hyperkeratosis, night blindness	Decreased vitamin A absorption
Pallor	Decreased vitamin B_{12}, folate, or iron absorption
Glossitis, stomatitis, cheilosis	Decreased vitamin B_{12} or iron absorption
Acrodermatitis	Zinc deficiency

Table 8-10.—Associated Symptoms of Systemic Illnesses Causing Diarrhea

Symptom or sign	Diagnosis to be considered
Arthritis	Ulcerative colitis, Crohn disease, Whipple disease, *Yersinia* infection
Marked weight loss	Malabsorption, inflammatory bowel disease, cancer, thyrotoxicosis
Eosinophilia	Eosinophilic gastroenteritis, parasitic disease
Lymphadenopathy	Lymphoma, Whipple disease
Neuropathy	Diabetic diarrhea, amyloidosis
Postural hypotension	Diabetic diarrhea, Addison disease, idiopathic orthostatic hypotension
Flushing	Malignant carcinoid syndrome
Proteinuria	Amyloidosis
Peptic ulcers	Zollinger-Ellison syndrome
Hyperpigmentation	Whipple disease, celiac disease, Addison disease, pancreatic cholera, eosinophilic gastroenteritis

From Fine KD, Krejs GJ, Fordtran JS: Diarrhea. *In* Gastrointestinal Disease: Pathophysiology Diagnosis Management. Fourth edition. Edited by MH Sleisenger, JS Fordtran. Philadelphia, WB Saunders Company, 1989, pp 290-316. By permission of publisher.

- Diarrhea of low pH and increased intestinal motility.
- The most common disaccharidase deficiency is lactase deficiency.
- Diarrhea, abdominal cramps, flatulence occur after ingestion of dairy products.
- Abnormal hydrogen breath test.
- Patients on a weight reduction diet who drink diet soda or chew sugarless gum may develop osmotic diarrhea from sorbitol.

Secretory Diarrhea

Watery diarrhea, hypokalemia, achlorhydria—WHDA, or Verner-Morrison, syndrome is also called "pancreatic cholera." It is a massive diarrhea (5 L/day) with dehydration and hypokalemia. The patient may have numerous other endocrine tumors (hypercalcemia, hyperglycemia). This diarrhea is associated with a non-beta islet cell tumor of the pancreas. Vasoactive intestinal peptide is the most common mediator, followed by prostaglandin, secretin, and calcitonin. Clinical recognition is by pancreatic scan/angiography and measurement of hormone levels. Treatment is with somatostatin or operation.

- Pancreatic cholera: massive diarrhea, dehydration, hypokalemia.
- Patients may have other multiple endocrine tumors.
- It is associated with a non-beta islet cell tumor of the pancreas.

Carcinoid syndrome—Carcinoid syndrome results from tumors of enterochromaffin cells of neural crest origin; 90% of the tumors are in the terminal ileum. There is episodic facial flushing (lasting up to 10 minutes), watery diarrhea, wheezing, right-sided valvular disease (endocardial fibrosis), and hepatomegaly. If the gut is normal, look for bronchial tumors or gonadal tumors. Dietary tryptophan is converted into serotonin (causes diarrhea, abdominal cramps [intestinal hypermotility], nausea, and vomiting), histamine (responsible for the flushing), and other chemicals (bradykinin, ACTH). Carcinoid syndrome means that hepatic metastases are present. The diagnosis of carcinoid syndrome is made by finding increased urinary levels of 5-hydroxyindoleacetic acid (5-HIAA) and by liver biopsy. This syndrome is not associated with hypertension. Treatment is with octreotide.

Laxative abuse—Of the population over age 60, 15% to 30% take laxatives regularly. This is laxative abuse. With surreptitious laxative ingestion, patients complain of diarrhea but do not admit taking laxatives. In referral centers, this is the commonest cause of watery diarrhea. Proctoscopy reveals melanosis coli. Barium enema shows "cathartic colon," that is, dilated, hypomotile, absent haustra. Laxatives causing melanosis coli include anthracene derivatives (senna, cascara, aloe). Diagnosis: stool phenophthalein. Address underlying emotional problems.

- Proctoscopy reveals melanosis coli.
- Barium enema shows "cathartic colon," i.e., dilated, hypomotile, absent haustra.
- Address underlying emotional problems.

Bile Acid Malabsorption

Bile acid malabsorption is caused by ileal resection or disease. The diarrhea due to bile acid malabsorption may produce two different clinical syndromes, each requiring a different treatment. 1) Limited resection (<100 cm)—Malabsorbed bile acids enter the colon and stimulate secretion. Liver synthesis can compensate, so bile acid concentration in the upper small bowel is greater than the critical micelle concentration. No steatorrhea. Fecal fat is less than 20 g/24 hr. Treat with cholestyramine, which binds bile acids. 2) Extensive resection (>100 cm)—Bile acids are severely malabsorbed, and enterohepatic circulation is interrupted. This limits synthesis, and the liver cannot compensate. Bile acid concentration is decreased in the upper small bowel, micelles cannot be formed, and fat malabsorption results. The malabsorbed fatty acids themselves stimulate secretion in the colon. Treat with low fat diet (<50 g/day) rich in medium chain triglycerides. Cholestyramine would further decrease bile acid concentration and increase steatorrhea.

- Limited resection: treat with cholestyramine.
- Extensive resection: treat with low fat diet rich in medium chain triglycerides.

Bacterial Overgrowth

The proximal small intestine is usually sterile. The major defense mechanisms in the proximal small bowel are gastric acid, normal peristalsis (the most important defense), and intestinal IgA. When defenses are altered, bacterial overgrowth results. The mechanism of steatorrhea is deconjugation of bile acids by bacteria that normally are not present in the proximal intestine. Deconjugation of the bile acids changes the ionization coefficient, and the deconjugated bile acids can be passively absorbed in the proximal small bowel. Normally, conjugated bile acids are actively absorbed distally in the ileum. As a result, the critical micellar concentration is not reached, and mild steatorrhea results from the intraluminal deficiency of bile acids.

- Normal peristalsis is the most important defense in the proximal small bowel.
- Deconjugated bile salts can be absorbed passively.

● Mild steatorrhea results from the intraluminal deficiency of bile acids.

Clinical features of bacterial overgrowth are steatorrhea (10-20 g/day), vitamin B_{12} malabsorption (macrocytic anemia), positive jejunal cultures (>10^5 organisms), increased folate levels due to bacterial production, and abnormal bile acid breath test. Breath test—bile acid breath test—^{14}C-labeled bile acids release $^{14}CO_2$ when deconjugated by bacteria in the gut. This test has low sensitivity (20%-30% false-negative).

Associated conditions—Postoperative (blind loops, enteroenterostomy, gastrojejunocolic fistula), structural (diverticula, strictures, fistulas), motility disorders (scleroderma, pseudo-obstruction), achlorhydria (atrophic gastritis, gastric resections; achlorhydria corrects with antibiotics), and impaired immunity. Two types of the latter are hypogammaglobulinemic sprue (no plasma cells in lamina propria and flat villi on small-bowel biopsy) and nodular lymphoid hyperplasia associated with IgA deficiency—know radiographic appearance—predisposes to *Giardia lamblia* infection.

● Diarrhea, vitamin B_{12} deficiency, and above conditions suggest bacterial overgrowth.

Infectious Diarrheas

The toxigenic and invasive causes of bacterial diarrhea and the associated features are outlined in Tables 8-11 and 8-12.

Staphylococcus aureus—The diarrhea is of rapid onset; it lasts for 24 hours. There is no fever, vomiting, or cramps. The toxin is ingested in egg products, cream, and mayonnaise. Treatment is supportive.

Clostridium perfringens ("church picnic diarrhea")—The toxin is ingested in precooked foods, usually beef and turkey. Heat-stable spores produce toxins. Although the bacteria are killed and the toxin is destroyed, the spores survive. When food is rewarmed, the spores germinate, producing toxin. The diarrhea is worse than the vomiting and is later in onset. It lasts 24 hours. Treatment is supportive.

E. coli ("traveler's diarrhea")—The toxin is ingested in water and salads. It is a plasmid-mediated enterotoxin. Treatment is rehydration with correction of electrolytes and ciprofloxacin, norfloxacin, or trimethoprim-sulfamethoxazole. *E. coli* may be important in nursery epidemic diarrhea.

Vibrio cholerae—The toxin is ingested in water. It is the only toxigenic bacterial diarrhea in which antibiotics clearly shorten the duration of the disease. Treatment is with tetracycline.

Table 8-11.—Causes of Bacterial Diarrhea: Toxigenic

Organism	Onset, hr	Mediated by cyclic Amp	Fever	Intestinal secretion
Staphylococcus aureus	1-6	+	-	+
Clostridium perfringens	8-12	-	±	+
Escherichia coli	12	+	+	+
Vibrio cholerae	12	+	Due to dehydration	++++
Bacillus cereus	1-6	+	-	+

Table 8-12.—Causes of Bacterial Diarrhea: Invasive

Organism	Fever	Bloody diarrhea	Bacteremia	Antibiotic effective
Shigella	+	+	+	+
Salmonella	+	-	-	-
Vibrio parahaemolyticus	+	+	-	+(?)
Escherichia coli	+	-	-	-
Staphylococcus aureus (enterocolitis)	+	+	±	+
Yersinia enterocolitica	+	+	+	?
Campylobacter	+	+	±	+
Vibrio vulnificus	+	+	+	+

Bacillus cereus—The source of the toxin is fried rice in oriental restaurants. One type has rapid onset and resembles *S. aureus* infection; the other type has a slower onset and resembles *C. perfringens* infection. The diagnosis is made by isolating the organism from contaminated food and by the medical history. Treatment is supportive.

Other toxigenic bacteria—*C. botulinum* produces a neurotoxin that is ingested in improperly home-processed vegetables, fruits, and meats. It interferes with the release of acetylcholine from peripheral nerve endings. *C. difficile*—See antibiotic/pseudomembranous colitis.

- Toxigenic bacterial diarrhea: watery, no fecal leukocytes.
- *S. aureus*: rapid onset.
- *C. perfringens*: "church picnic diarrhea," precooked foods, later in onset.
- *E. coli*: "traveler's diarrhea."
- *B. cereus*: fried rice in oriental restaurants.

Bacterial Diarrhea (Invasive)

Shigella—It is often acquired outside the U.S. Bloody diarrhea is characteristic, and fever and bacteremia occur. Diagnosis is based on positive stool and blood cultures. Treatment is with ampicillin. Resistant strains are emerging for which chloramphenicol is an alternative. (Plasmids are responsible for antibiotic deactivation resistance.)

Salmonella (non-*typhi*)—In the U.S., *Salmonella typhimurium* is the most common agent. The toxin is ingested with poultry. Fever is present. The absence of bloody diarrhea is the main characteristic that distinguishes it from *Shigella* infection. Diagnosis is based on positive stool culture. Treatment is supportive. Treat severe symptoms only with ciprofloxacin. Treating mild symptoms with other antibiotics may result in prolonged carrier state.

Vibrio parahaemolyticus—The toxin is ingested with undercooked shellfish. This infection is increasing in frequency in the U.S. (it is common in Japan). Fever and bloody diarrhea are the chief characteristics. Diagnosis is based on positive stool culture. Antibiotics are of questionable value in treating this infection, but erythromycin may be most effective.

E. coli—In the U.S., enteroinvasive *E. coli* is a rare cause of diarrhea. Enteroinvasive *E. coli* involves the colon and presents with fever, bloody diarrhea, and profound toxicity (similar to *Shigella* infection). Enterohemorrhagic *E. coli* (serotype O157:H7) produces a cytotoxin that damages vascular endothelial cells. *E. coli* O157:H7 can cause sporadic or epidemic illness from contaminated meat and raw milk. Enterohemorrhagic *E. coli* infection should be suspected when bloody diarrhea occurs after eating hamburger and when bloody diarrhea is complicated by hemolytic uremic syndrome or thrombotic thrombocytopenic purpura.

S. aureus (enterocolitis)—Diagnosis is based on positive stool culture or Gram stain, which shows predominance of gram-positive cocci and a paucity of other organisms.

- Invasive bacterial diarrhea: fever, bloody stools, and fecal leukocytes.
- *Shigella*: bloody diarrhea.
- *S. typhimurium*: no bloody diarrhea, treat with antibiotics only if blood cultures are positive.
- *V. parahaemolyticus*: undercooked shellfish, bloody diarrhea.
- *E. coli*: bloody stools, abdominal pain but no fever. Follows from eating hamburgers; may cause hemolytic uremic syndrome and thrombotic thrombocytopenic purpura.

"Newer" Enteric Bacterial Pathogens

Yersinia enterocolitica—The spectrum of disease includes acute enteritis and chronic enteritis. Acute enteritis is similar to shigellosis and usually lasts 1 to 3 weeks. It is characterized by fever, diarrhea, leukocytosis, and fecal leukocytes. Chronic enteritis is found especially in children. There is diarrhea, failure to thrive, hypoalbuminemia, and hypokalemia. Other features are acute abdominal pain (mesenteric adenitis), right lower quadrant pain, tenderness, nausea, and vomiting. It mimics appendicitis or Crohn disease. This gram-negative rod is hardy and can survive in cold temperatures. It grows on special medium (cold enriched). It is an invasive pathogen. Fecal-oral transmission in water and milk.

Extraintestinal manifestations are nonsuppurative arthritis and ankylosing spondylitis (in HLA-B27). Skin manifestations are erythema nodosum and multiforme. Thyroid manifestations are Graves disease and Hashimoto disease. Multiple liver abscesses and granulomata are present.

Treatment is with aminoglycosides, trimethoprim-sulfamethoxazole (Bactrim). The bacteria are variably sensitive to tetracycline and chloramphenicol. Beta lactamases are frequently produced. Penicillin resistance is common.

- *Y. enterocolitica* infection: acute abdominal pain (differential diagnosis includes appendicitis and Crohn disease).
- Fecal-oral transmission in water and milk.
- Manifestations include nonsuppurative arthritis and ankylosing spondylitis (in HLA-B27).

Campylobacter jejuni—These are comma-shaped, motile, microaerophilic gram-negative bacilli. Transmission is linked to infected water, unpasteurized milk, poultry, sick dogs, and infected children. The incubation period is 2 to 4 days before invasion of the small bowel. Infection results in the presence of blood and leukocytes in the stool. It may mimic granulomatous or idiopathic ulcerative colitis. It may also mimic small-bowel secretory diarrhea, with explosive, frequent watery diarrhea due to many species that produce a cholera-type toxin. The diarrhea usually lasts 3 to 5 days but may relapse. Antibiotic treatment is with erythromycin when severe, but treatment often is not needed. Postdiarrheal illnesses are hemolytic uremic syndrome and postinfectious arthritis.

- *C. jejuni*: transmission linked to infected water, unpasteurized milk, poultry, sick dogs, and infected children.
- May mimic granulomatous or idiopathic ulcerative colitis.
- Diarrhea: usually lasts 3-5 days but may relapse.

Vibrio vulnificus (noncholera)--The organisms are extremely invasive and produce necrotizing vasculitis, gangrene, and shock. They are routinely isolated from seawater, zooplankton, and shellfish along the Gulf of Mexico and both coasts of the U.S., especially in the summer. Two clinical syndromes are 1) wound infection, cellulitis, fasciitis, or myositis after exposure to seawater or cleaning shellfish and 2) septicemia after ingesting raw shellfish (oysters). Patients at high risk for septicemia include those with liver disease, congestive heart failure, diabetes mellitus, renal failure, immunosuppressive states, or hemochromatosis. Treatment is with tetracycline.

- *V. vulnificus* is extremely invasive, producing necrotizing vasculitis, gangrene, and shock.
- Wound infection, cellulitis, fasciitis, or myositis occurs after exposure to seawater or cleaning shellfish.
- Septicemia occurs after ingesting raw shellfish (oysters).

Aeromonas hydrophilia—Previously, the pathogenicity of the bacteria was questioned. Although the infection is often mistaken for that of *E. coli*, *A. hydrophilia* is now recognized as an increasingly frequent cause of diarrhea after swimming in fresh or salt water. The organism produces several toxins. Treatment is with trimethoprim-sulfamethoxazole and tetracycline.

Malabsorption Due to Diseases of the Small Intestine

Celiac Sprue

Celiac sprue is a gluten-sensitive enteropathy. It presents in children as growth retardation and in adults, as an iron deficiency that is unresponsive to iron given orally. Osteomalacia can be present without steatorrhea if the proximal small bowel is involved. Splenic atrophy and abnormal blood smear with Howell-Jolly bodies may be clues to the diagnosis in 10% to 15% of patients. The skin manifestation is dermatitis herpetiformis. The endomysial antibody test is effective for screening. If the result is positive, then a small-bowel biopsy

should be performed. If the result of the endomysial antibody test is negative, another diagnosis should be considered. Small-bowel biopsy is *not* diagnostic, but response to gluten-free diet is diagnostic. If the patient is unresponsive to the diet, review the diet for inadvertent gluten ingestion. If unresponsive after 10 to 15 years of successful dietary management, rule out lymphoma (especially if there is also abdominal pain).

- Celiac sprue: iron deficiency that is unresponsive to iron given orally; osteomalacia with or without steatorrhea.
- Splenic atrophy and abnormal blood smear with Howell-Jolly bodies may be clues to the diagnosis in 10%-15% of patients.
- Lymphoma is a late complication.

Tropical Sprue

In tropical sprue, diarrhea occurs 2 to 3 months after travel to the tropics. After 6 months, megaloblastic anemia develops because of folate deficiency and possible coexisting vitamin B_{12} deficiency. The infectious agents are *Klebsiella* and *E. coli*. Small-bowel biopsy shows blunted villi similar to those in celiac sprue. Treatment is with tetracycline (250 mg four times daily) and folate with or without vitamin B_{12}.

- Tropical sprue: diarrhea and megaloblastic anemia after travel to the tropics.
- Cause: coliforms bacteria (*Klebsiella* more than *E. coli*).
- Treatment: tetracycline (250 mg 4 times daily) and folate with or without vitamin B_{12}.

Whipple Disease

Whipple disease is a systemic infectious disease involving the central nervous system (CNS), heart, kidneys, and small bowel. It is caused by gram-positive bacilli. Small-bowel biopsy shows periodic-acid Schiff (PAS)-positive granules in the macrophages. Suspect Whipple disease in patients with recurrent arthritis, pigmentation, adenopathy, or CNS symptoms (dementia, myoclonus, ophthalmoplegia, visual disturbances, coma, seizures). Treatment is with trimethoprim-sulfamethoxazole or tetracycline for 1 year.

- Suspect Whipple disease in patients with recurrent arthritis, pigmentation, adenopathy, or CNS symptoms.
- Small-bowel biopsy shows PAS-positive granules in the macrophages.
- Treatment: trimethoprim-sulfamethoxazole or tetracycline for 1 year.

Eosinophilic Gastroenteritis

Patients with eosinophilic gastroenteritis have a history of allergies (asthma, etc.) and food intolerances and episodic symptoms of nausea, vomiting, abdominal pain, and diarrhea.

Laboratory findings include eosinophilia, iron deficiency anemia, and steatorrhea or protein-losing enteropathy. Small-bowel radiographs show coarse folds and filling defects, and biopsy shows infiltration of the eosinophils in the mucosa and, occasionally, absence of villi. Rule out parasitic infection. Treatment with steroids produces a rapid response.

- Mucosal eosinophilic gastroenteritis: allergies, food intolerances, eosinophilia, and episodic intestinal symptoms.
- Rule out parasitic infection.
- Steroids produce a rapid response.

Systemic Mastocytosis

Systemic mastocytosis is a proliferation of mast cells in the skin (urticaria pigmentosa), bones, lymph nodes, and parenchymal organs. Histamine is released, and 50% of patients have gastrointestinal symptoms, that is, diarrhea and peptic ulcer. "Bath pruritus" (itching after hot bath) is a clue to the diagnosis.

- Systemic mastocytosis causes urticaria pigmentosa.
- 50% of patients have gastrointestinal symptoms.
- "Bath pruritus" is a clue to the diagnosis.

Intestinal Lymphangiectasia

Intestinal lymphangiectasia is a disorder due to lymphatic obstruction. Hypoplastic lymphatics cause lymph to leak into the intestine. The clinical features are edema (often unilateral leg edema), chylous peritoneal or pleural effusions, and steatorrhea or protein-losing enteropathy. Laboratory findings include lymphocytopenia (average, 600/mm^3) due to enteric loss. All serum proteins are decreased, including immunoglobulins. Small-bowel radiographs show edematous folds, and small-bowel biopsy shows dilated lacteals and lymphatics in the lamina propria that may contain lipid-laden macrophages. The same biopsy findings are seen in obstruction of mesenteric nodes (lymphoma, Whipple disease, Crohn disease) and obstruction of venous inflow to the heart (constrictive pericarditis, severe right heart failure). Diagnosis is based on abnormal small-bowel biopsy findings and documented enteric protein loss by increased alpha$_1$-antitrypsin levels in the stool. Treatment is with low fat diet and medium chain triglycerides (they enter the portal blood rather than lymphatics). Occasionally, surgical excision of the involved segment is useful if the lesion is localized.

- Intestinal lymphangiectasia: unilateral lymphedema of the leg and chylous peritoneal or pleural effusions.
- Lymphocytopenia is universal.
- Decreased serum proteins.
- Small-bowel biopsy shows dilated lacteals and lymphatics.
- Treatment: low fat diet and medium chain triglycerides.

Amyloidosis

Systemic amyloidosis is characterized by a diffuse deposition of an amorphous eosinophilic extracellular protein polysaccharide complex in the tissue. The major sites of amyloid deposition are blood vessel walls and the mucous membranes and muscle layers of the intestine. Any portion of the gut can be involved. Amyloid damages tissues by infiltration (muscle and nerve infiltration causes motility disorders, malabsorption) and ischemia (obliteration of vessels causes ulceration and bleeding). Intestinal dysmotility can produce diarrhea, constipation, pseudo-obstruction, megacolon, and fecal incontinence. Clinical findings in amyloidosis include macroglossia, hepatomegaly, cardiomegaly, proteinuria, and peripheral neuropathy. Pinch (post-traumatic) purpura or periorbital purpura after proctoscopic examination occurs. *Diagnosis*—Small-bowel radiography shows symmetrical, sharply demarcated thickening of the valvulae conniventes. Fat aspirate confirms the diagnosis in 90% to 95% of patients and rectal biopsy stained with Congo red in 70% to 85%.

Miscellaneous Small-Bowel Disorders

Meckel diverticulum, the persistence of the vitelline duct, is the most frequent developmental abnormality of the gut. It usually is found within 100 cm from the ileocecal valve on the antimesenteric border of the ileum. It contains all layers of the intestinal wall and so is a true diverticulum. The mucosa is usually ileal but may be gastric (pancreatic, intestinal). Complications include obstruction due to intussusception and volvulus around the band fixing the diverticulum to the bowel wall. Benign (leiomyomas) and malignant (carcinoids, leiomyosarcoma) tumors have been found in diverticula. Diverticulitis is uncommon. Incarceration in an indirect inguinal hernia (Littre hernia) and perforation that causes peritonitis may occur. Hemorrhage is the common complication and results from ulceration of the ileal mucosa adjacent to the gastric mucosa. This accounts for 50% of the cases of lower gastrointestinal tract bleeding in children and young adults. Radiography usually is not helpful in making the diagnosis. A nuclear scan (parietal cells concentrate technetium) may show the diverticulum, but false-positive and false-negative results can occur.

- Meckel diverticulum is the most frequent developmental abnormality of the gut.
- It accounts for 50% of the cases of lower gastrointestinal tract bleeding in children and young adults.

Aortoenteric fistula—A history of gastrointestinal tract bleeding in a patient who has had a previous aortic graft demands immediate evaluation to rule out an enteroenteric fistula. If the patient presents with massive bleeding, do not attempt endoscopy or arteriography. Emergency surgery is indicated.

- If a patient presents with massive bleeding, do not attempt endoscopy or arteriography. Emergency surgery is indicated.

Chronic Intestinal Pseudo-Obstruction

Pseudo-obstruction is a syndrome characterized by the clinical findings of mechanical bowel obstruction but without occlusion of the lumen. The two types are primary and secondary. The primary type, also called "idiopathic pseudo-obstruction," is a visceral myopathy or neuropathy. The secondary type is due to an underlying systemic disease or precipitating causes.

Idiopathic (primary) pseudo-obstruction is associated with recurrent attacks of nausea, vomiting, cramping abdominal pain, distension, and constipation, which are of variable intensity and duration. If it is a familial cause, the patient will have a positive family history and the condition will be present at a young age. Esophageal motility is abnormal (achalasia) in most patients. Occasionally, urinary tract motility is abnormal, and diarrhea or steatorrhea results from bacterial overgrowth. Upper gastrointestinal tract and small-bowel radiographs show dilatation of the bowel and slow transit (not mechanical obstruction).

- Idiopathic pseudo-obstruction is due to a familial cause or to sporadic visceral myopathy or neuropathy.
- Recurrent attacks have variable frequency and duration.
- Abnormal esophageal motility occurs in most patients.
- Steatorrhea is caused by bacterial overgrowth.

Secondary pseudo-obstruction is due to underlying systemic disease or precipitating causes. These causes include the following (significant causes to remember are in italics):

1. Diseases involving the intestinal smooth muscle: *amyloidosis*, scleroderma, systemic lupus erythematosus, myotonic dystrophy, and muscular dystrophy.
2. Neurologic diseases: *Parkinson disease*, Hirschsprung disease, Chagas disease, and familial autonomic dysfunction.
3. Endocrine disorders: *myxedema* and hypoparathyroidism.
4. Drugs: *antiparkinsonian medications* (*L-dopa*), phenothiazines, tricyclic antidepressants, ganglionic blockers, clonidine, and narcotics.

Approach to the Patient With Chronic Intestinal Pseudo-Obstruction

First, rule out a mechanical cause for the obstruction. Second, look for an underlying precipitating cause such as metabolic abnormalities, medications, or an underlying associated disease. If a familial idiopathic cause is suspected, assess esophageal motility. Suspect scleroderma if intestinal radiography shows large-mouth diverticula of the small and large intestines. Suspect amyloidosis if the skin shows palpable purpura, and proteinuria and neuropathy are present.

- Secondary pseudo-obstruction is due to an underlying systemic disease or precipitating cause.
- Scleroderma presents as large-mouth diverticula of the intestine.
- Amyloidosis presents with palpable purpura, proteinuria, and neuropathy.

Inflammatory Bowel Disease

"Idiopathic inflammatory bowel disease" refers to two disorders of unknown cause: chronic ulcerative colitis and Crohn disease. Other possible causes of inflammation, especially infection, should be excluded before making the diagnosis of idiopathic inflammatory bowel disease.

Ulcerative colitis is a mucosal inflammation involving only the colon. Crohn disease is a transmural inflammation that can involve the intestine anywhere from the esophagus through the anus. The rectum is involved in about 95% of patients with ulcerative colitis and in only 50% of those with Crohn disease. Ulcerative colitis is a continuous inflammatory process extending from the anal verge to more proximal colon (depending on the extent of the inflammation). Crohn disease is a segmental inflammation in which inflamed areas alternate with virtually normal areas. Ulcerative colitis usually presents as frequent bloody bowel movements with minimal abdominal pain, whereas Crohn disease presents with fewer bowel movements, less bleeding, and, more commonly, abdominal pain. Crohn disease is associated with intestinal fistula and fistula to other organs as well as perianal disease. Ulcerative colitis does not form fistulas; perianal disease is uncommon. Strictures of the intestine are common with Crohn disease but rare in ulcerative colitis (when they are present, they suggest cancer).

- Ulcerative colitis involves only the colon.
- Crohn disease can involve the intestine anywhere from the esophagus through the anus.
- Ulcerative colitis is a continuous process.
- Crohn disease is a segmental inflammation.
- Ulcerative colitis has frequent bloody bowel movements.
- Crohn disease has fewer bowel movements, less bleeding, and more abdominal pain.
- Crohn disease is associated with intestinal fistula, strictures, and perianal disease.

Extraintestinal Manifestations of Inflammatory Bowel Disease

Arthritis occurs in 10% to 20% of patients, usually monarticular or pauciarticular involvement of large joints. Joint symptoms mirror bowel activity: joints flare when colitis flares and joints improve as colitis improves. Also, ankylosing spondylitis (relationship with HLA-B27) and sacroiliitis—which are usually progressive and do not improve when colitis improves—can develop.

- The joint symptoms mirror bowel activity.
- Ankylosing spondylitis and sacroiliitis can develop.

Skin lesions occur in 10% of patients. The three types of lesions are erythema nodosum, pyoderma gangrenosum, and aphthous ulcers of the mouth. All these skin conditions usually improve with treatment of colitis. Severe, refractory skin disease is an indication for surgical treatment.

- The skin lesions are erythema nodosum, pyoderma gangrenosum, and aphthous ulcers of the mouth.

Eye lesions occur in 5% of patients. The lesion is usually episcleritis and/or uveitis. These usually improve with treatment of inflammatory bowel disease.

Liver disease also occurs in 5% of patients. Primary sclerosing cholangitis is more common in chronic ulcerative colitis than in Crohn disease. If the alkaline phosphatase level is increased in a patient with inflammatory bowel disease, the work-up for primary sclerosing cholangitis includes ultrasonography, endoscopic retrograde cholangiopancreatography, and liver biopsy.

- If increased alkaline phosphatase occurs with inflammatory bowel disease, rule out primary sclerosing cholangitis.

Renal stones occur in 5% to 15% of patients. In Crohn disease with malabsorption, calcium oxalate stones occur. In chronic ulcerative colitis, uric acid stones are due to dehydration and loss of bicarbonate in the stool, leading to acidic urine.

Indications for Colonoscopy

Colonoscopy is indicated for evaluating the extent of the disease and for stricture (biopsy) and filling defect (biopsy). It is also indicated for differentiating Crohn colitis from ulcerative colitis when the two are otherwise indistinguishable. Another indication is for monitoring by random mucosal biopsy the development of dysplasia or cancer in patients who have had ulcerative colitis or Crohn colitis for more than 8 years.

- Know the indications for colonoscopy in inflammatory bowel disease.

Toxic Megacolon

In patients with active inflammation, avoid the causes of toxic megacolon, including aerophagia, opiates, anticholinergic agents, hypokalemia, and barium enema.

- In patients with active inflammation, avoid the causes of toxic megacolon.

Treatment of Ulcerative Colitis

Medical—5-Aminosalicylic acid (ASA) (the active agent) is bound to sulfapyridine (vehicle). Colonic bacteria break the bond, releasing 5-ASA. 5-ASA is not absorbed but stays in contact with the mucosa and exerts its anti-inflammatory action. The efficacy of 5-ASA may be related to its ability to inhibit the lipoxygenase pathway of arachidonic acid metabolism or its ability to function as an oxygen free-radical scavenger (further studies are needed). It is effective in acute disease and in maintaining remission. Side effects (male infertility, malaise, nausea, pancreatitis, rashes, headaches, hemolysis, impaired folate absorption, hepatitis, aplastic anemia, and exacerbation of colitis) occur in 30% of patients who take sulfasalazine and are related to the sulfapyridine moiety. 5-ASAs are a group of new drugs that deliver 5-ASA to the intestine in various ways. They eliminate sulfa toxicity but are more expensive than sulfasalazine. Two of these drugs are mesalamine and olsalazine. Mesalamine can be given topically (Rowasa suppositories, Rowasa enema) or orally (Asacol, 5-ASA coated with acrylic polymer that releases 5-ASA in the terminal ileum, and Pentasa, ethyl cellulose coating releases 50% of the 5-ASA in the small bowel). Olsalazine consists of two 5-ASA molecules conjugated with each other. Bacteria break the bond, releasing 5-ASA into the colon.

Aminosalicylates are used for mild to moderately active ulcerative colitis and in Crohn disease. Topical forms are useful in proctitis or left-sided colitis; systemic forms are used for pancolitis. Of the patients who do not tolerate sulfasalazine, 80% to 90% will tolerate oral 5-ASA preparations. Side effects include hair loss, pancreatitis (often in patients who developed pancreatitis while taking sulfasalazine), reversible worsening of underlying renal disease, and exacerbation of colitis.

- Sulfasalazine is effective in acute disease and in maintaining remission.
- Sulfasalazine: side effects occur in 30% of patients.
- Aminosalicylates are equally effective but more expensive; they are useful in 80%-90% of patients intolerant to sulfasalazine.

Corticosteroids—Topical preparations should be used twice daily for patients with active mild-to-moderate disease that is limited to the distal colon. Corticosteroids should be added to the regimen of patients with more proximal disease if sulfasalazine does not control the attacks. Up to 50% of the dose can be absorbed (depending on the preparation used and its vehicle). Oral preparations are indicated in active pancolonic disease of moderate severity in doses of 40 to 60 mg once daily or 20 to 40 mg daily in cases of mild disease that are unresponsive to topical steroids and sulfasalazine. Prednisolone, the active metabolite, is the preferred form of drug in patients with cirrhosis (these patients may not be able to convert inactive prednisone to prednisolone). For patients with a prompt response to oral corticosteroids, the dose may be tapered gradually at a rate not to exceed a 5-mg reduction in the total dose every 3 to 7 days. Intravenous preparations should be used in large doses (prednisolone, 100 mg in divided doses) for up to 10 to 14 days in severely ill patients. At that time, if there is improvement, it should be possible to convert the medication to oral corticosteroids (60-100 mg/day). If there is no improvement, surgical intervention (colectomy) is required. Corticosteroids are not believed to prevent relapse and, therefore, should not be used after the patient has complete remission and is symptom-free.

- Prescribe topical preparations twice daily for patients with active mild-to-moderate disease that is limited to the distal colon.
- Corticosteroids should be added to the regimen of patients with more proximal disease if systemic steroids and sulfasalazine have not controlled the attacks.
- Oral preparations are useful in active pancolonic disease of moderate severity.
- Intravenous preparations are used for severely ill patients.

Total parenteral nutrition does not alter the clinical course of an ongoing attack. Indications for its use include 1) severe dehydration and cachexia with marked fluid and nutrient deficits, 2) excessive diarrhea that has failed to respond to standard therapy for chronic ulcerative colitis, and 3) debilitated patients undergoing colectomy. Opiates (or their synthetic derivatives) and anticholinergic agents are contraindicated in chronic ulcerative colitis because they are ineffective and can contribute to the development of toxic megacolon.

- Total parenteral nutrition does not alter the clinical course of the ongoing attack.
- Use of opiates and anticholinergic agents is contraindicated in chronic ulcerative colitis.

Surgical—Surgical treatment is curative in chronic ulcerative colitis. Indications for colectomy are severe intractable disease, acute life-threatening complications (perforation, hemorrhage, toxic megacolon unresponsive to treatment), symptomatic colonic stricture, and suspected or documented colon cancer. Other indications include intractable moderate-to-severe colitis, refractory uveitis or pyoderma gangrenosum, growth retardation in pediatric patients, cancer prophylaxis, or inability to taper a regimen to low doses of corticosteroid (i.e., <15 mg/day) over a period of 2 to 3 months. Procedures include proctocolectomy with ileoanal anastomosis, Koch pouch, or conventional Brooke ileostomy.

- Surgical treatment is curative in chronic ulcerative colitis.

Treatment of Crohn Disease

Medical—For sulfasalazine, see Treatment of Ulcerative Colitis above. This drug is more effective for colonic disease than for small-bowel disease, although 5-ASA products designed to be released and activated in the small bowel may prove to be effective in the colon. Sulfasalazine does not have an additive effect or a steroid-sparing effect when used with corticosteroids, nor does it maintain remission in Crohn disease as it does in ulcerative colitis. Nothing is effective in the prophylaxis of Crohn disease.

- Sulfasalazine is more effective for colonic disease than for small-bowel disease.
- It does not have an additive effect or sparing effect when used with corticosteroids.
- It does not maintain remission in Crohn disease.

Corticosteroids, see Treatment of Ulcerative Colitis above. The agents that most quickly control an acute exacerbation of Crohn disease are corticosteroids. They are the most useful drugs for treating small-bowel Crohn disease.

In the National Crohn Disease Cooperative Study, azathioprine was not significantly different from placebo with regard to therapeutic response. However, this study has been criticized because azathioprine was given for a short period and its potential beneficial effect may have been missed—4 to 6 months are needed to realize any benefit from immunosuppressive drugs like azathioprine or 6-mercaptopurine.

6-Mercaptopurine, the active metabolite of azathioprine, has a steroid-sparing effect. Its use should be reserved for patients with active disease who are taking steroids when there is need to reduce the corticosteroid dose (or to maintain a given dose in the face of worsening disease activity).

- 6-Mercaptopurine is the active metabolite of azathioprine.
- It has a steroid-sparing effect.

Metronidazole (at a dose of 20 mg/kg) is quite effective for treating perianal disease. Six weeks may be needed for the therapeutic effect to become manifest; unfortunately, recurrences often occur when the drug dose is tapered or discontinued, leading to chronic therapy. It is as effective as sulfasalazine for disease of the colon. If a patient is unresponsive to sulfasalazine, it is worthwhile switching to metronidazole, but not vice versa. It is less effective for small-bowel disease. Side effects include glossitis, metallic taste, vaginal and urethral burning sensation, neutropenia, dark urine, urticaria, disulfiram (Antabuse) effect, and paresthesias.

- Metronidazole is quite effective for perianal disease.
- Recurrences are frequent when the drug dose is tapered or discontinued.
- It is as effective as sulfasalazine for disease of the colon.

Nutrition—Bowel rest per se does not have any role in achieving remission in Crohn disease. However, providing adequate nutritional support does help facilitate remission; any form of nutritional support is acceptable as long as it is adequate in amount. Adequate nutrition can be essential in maintaining growth in children with severe Crohn disease.

Surgical—If Crohn disease is present during exploration for presumed appendicitis, the acute ileitis should be left alone (many of these patients do not develop chronic Crohn disease). An appendectomy can be performed if the cecum and appendix are free of disease. Of the Crohn patients receiving surgical treatment, 70% to 90% require reoperation within 15 years (many within the first 5 years after the initial operation). The anastomotic site is the most likely site for recurrence of disease. Indications for surgical treatment include intractable symptoms, acute life-threatening complications, obstruction, unhealed fistulas that cause complications, abscess formation, and malignancy.

- 70%-90% of Crohn patients operated on require reoperation within 15 years.
- The anastomotic site is the most likely site for disease recurrence.

GASTROINTESTINAL MANIFESTATIONS OF AIDS

Gastrointestinal tract symptoms occur in 30% to 50% of North American and European patients with AIDS and in nearly 90% of patients in developing countries. The most frequent gastrointestinal tract symptom is diarrhea, which is often chronic and associated with weight loss. Dysphagia, odynophagia, abdominal pain, and jaundice are less frequent. Gastrointestinal tract bleeding is rare. The goal of evaluation is to identify treatable causes of infection or symptoms.

- The majority of AIDS patients with diarrhea have one or more identifiable pathogens.
- Some have no identifiable cause despite extensive evaluation. This may represent idiopathic AIDS enteropathy or, as yet, unidentified pathogens.

The gastrointestinal tract in AIDS is predisposed to a spectrum of viral, bacterial, fungal, and protozoan pathogens.

Viral

Cytomegalovirus

Cytomegalovirus is one of the most common and potentially serious opportunistic pathogens. It most commonly affects the colon and esophagus, although the entire gut, liver, biliary tract, and pancreas are susceptible. There is a patchy or diffuse colitis that may progress to ischemic necrosis and perforation. *Symptoms:* watery diarrhea and fever; less commonly, hematochezia and abdominal pain. *Diagnosis:* biopsy specimens show cytomegalic inclusion cells with surrounding inflammation (owl's eye). *Treatment:* ganciclovir, 5 mg per kg twice daily for 14 to 21 days. If resistant, use foscarnet.

Herpes Simplex Virus

The three gastrointestinal tract manifestations of herpes simplex virus infection in patients with AIDS are perianal lesions (chronic cutaneous ulcers), proctitis, and esophagitis. The organs affected are the colon and esophagus. *Symptoms:* perianal lesions are painful; proctitis causes tenesmus, constipation, and inguinal lymphadenopathy; and esophagitis causes odynophagia, with or without dysphagia. *Diagnosis:* cytologic identification of intranuclear (Cowdry type A) inclusions in multinucleated cells. Diagnosis is confirmed by viral cultures. *Treatment:* acyclovir given orally or intravenously.

Adenovirus

Adenovirus recently has been reported to cause diarrhea. The organ affected is the colon. *Symptoms:* watery, nonbloody diarrhea. *Diagnosis:* culture and biopsy. *Treatment:* none.

Bacteria

Mycobacterium avium-intracellulare

Infection of the gut occurs in patients with disseminated disease. The small intestine is affected more commonly than the colon. *Symptoms:* fever, weight loss, diarrhea, abdominal pain, and malabsorption. *Diagnosis:* acid-fast organisms in the stool and tissue confirmed by culture from stool and biopsy specimens. *Treatment:* multiple drug therapy with ethambutol, rifampin, ciprofloxacin, and clarithromycin.

Salmonella (typhimurium and enteritidis)

Treatment is with amoxicillin, trimethoprim-sulfamethoxazole, or ciprofloxacin.

Shigella flexneri

Treatment is with trimethoprim-sulfamethoxazole, ampicillin, or ciprofloxacin.

Campylobacter jejuni

Treatment is with erythromycin or ciprofloxacin.

Salmonella, Shigella flexneri, and *Campylobacter jejuni* have a substantially higher incidence of intestinal infection, bacteremia, and prolonged or recurrent infections in AIDS patients because of antibiotic resistance or compromised immune function or both.

Fungi

Candida albicans

In AIDS patients, *Candida* causes locally invasive mucosal disease in the mouth and esophagus. Disseminated candidiasis is rare because neutrophil function remains relatively intact. The presence of oral candidiasis in persons at risk for AIDS should alert the physician to possible HIV infection. If oral candidiasis is present, endoscopy is required to confirm esophageal involvement. *Symptoms:* odynophagia suggests esophageal involvement. *Diagnosis:* histologic examination shows hyphae, pseudohyphae, or yeast forms. *Treatment:* nystatin, ketoconazole, fluconazole, or amphotericin.

Histoplasma capsulatum

Histoplasma capsulatum is an important opportunistic infection in AIDS patients who reside in endemic areas. Colonic involvement is more common than small bowel involvement. *Symptoms:* diarrhea, weight loss, fever, and abdominal pain. *Diagnosis:* is established by culture. Colonoscopy may show inflammation and ulcerations and histologic examination with Giemsa staining shows intracellular yeast-like *Histoplasma capsulatum* within lamina propria macrophages. *Treatment:* amphotericin or itraconazole.

Protozoa

Cryptosporidium

Cryptosporidium is among the commonest enteric pathogens, occurring in 10% to 20% of patients with AIDS and diarrhea in the U.S. and in 50% of those in developing countries. The organs affected are the small and large intestines and the biliary tree. *Symptoms:* voluminous watery diarrhea, severe abdominal cramps, weight loss, anorexia, malaise, and low-grade fever. Biliary tract obstruction has been reported. *Diagnosis:* microscopic identification of organisms in stool specimens with modified acid-fast staining or specific *Cryptosporidium* stains. Organisms may also be identified in biopsy specimens or in duodenal fluid aspirates. *Treatment:* paromomycin reduces the diarrhea.

Isospora belli

Isospora belli is the more common cause of diarrhea in developing countries. It resembles *Cryptosporidium* oocysts. The small intestine is affected primarily, but the organisms can be identified throughout the gut and in other organs. *Symptoms:* watery diarrhea, cramping abdominal pain, weight loss, anorexia, malaise, and fever. *Diagnosis:* oval oocysts in stool seen with modified Kinyoun acid-fast stain. Biopsy specimen from small intestine may show organisms in the lumen or within cytoplasmic vacuoles in enterocytes. *Isospora belli* oocysts contain two sporoblasts and differ from *Cryptosporidium* oocysts, which are small, round, and contain four sporozoites. *Treatment:* trimethoprim-sulfamethoxazole.

Microsporidia (Enterocytozoon bieneuisi)

Microsporidia are emerging as an important pathogen; the organisms have been identified in up to 33% of AIDS patients with diarrhea. The organ affected is the small intestine. *Symptoms:* watery diarrhea with gradual weight loss but no fever and no anorexia. *Diagnosis:* based on electron microscopic identification of round-to-oval meront (proliferative) and sporont (spore-forming) stages of Microsporidia in the villous but not crypt epithelial cells of the duodenum and jejunum. There are reports of positive stool specimens with Giemsa staining. *Treatment:* none known.

Entamoeba histolytica

Treatment is with metronidazole.

Giardia lamblia

Treatment is with metronidazole.

Blastocystis hominis

Because there is no evidence that *Blastocystis hominis* is pathogenic, it does not need to be treated.

The rates of symptomatic infection with *Entamoeba histolytica, Giardia lamblia,* and *Blastocystis hominis* are not significantly higher than in non-HIV patients. *Entamoeba histolytica* is a nonpathogenic commensal in most patients with AIDS. Giardiasis may require prolonged treatment, as in other immunocompetent persons.

DIAGNOSTIC EVALUATION OF PATIENTS WITH AIDS WHO HAVE DIARRHEA

Initial studies include 1) examination for stool leukocytes; 2) stool cultures for *Salmonella* species, *Shigella flexneri*, and *Campylobacter jejuni* (at least three specimens); 3) stool examination for ova and parasites (using saline, iodine, trichrome, and acid-fast preparations), and 4) stool assay for *Clostridium difficile* toxin. Additional studies include 1) gastroscopy to inspect tissue, aspirate luminal material, and obtain biopsy specimens; 2) examining duodenal aspirate for parasites and culture; 3) duodenal biopsy specimens cultured for cytomegalovirus and mycobacteria; 4) colonoscopy to inspect tissue and obtain biopsy specimens; 5) biopsy specimens cultured for cytomegalovirus, adenovirus, mycobacteria, and herpes simplex virus; 6) biopsy specimens stained with hematoxylin-eosin for protozoa and viral inclusion cells, with methenamine silver or Giemsa stain for fungi, and with Fite for mycobacteria.

If the initial studies and the additional studies listed above do not yield a diagnosis, then there is controversy about further evaluation. Most experts advocate empiric treatment with loperamide (Imodium). Others recommend that biopsy specimens from the duodenum be examined with electron microscopy for Microsporidia or from the colon for adenovirus. I favor empiric treatment with loperamide, because there is no treatment for either Microsporidia or adenovirus.

COLON

Pseudomembranous Enterocolitis

This is a necrotizing inflammatory disease of the intestines characterized by the formation of a membrane-like collection of exudate overlying a degenerating mucosa. Associated conditions are colon obstruction, uremia, ischemia, intestinal surgery, and all antibiotics (except vancomycin).

Antibiotic Colitis

The symptoms of antibiotic colitis are fever, abdominal pain, and diarrhea (mucus and blood), which usually occur 1 to 6 weeks after antibiotic therapy. Sigmoidoscopy shows pseudomembranes and friability. Biopsy reveals inflammation and microulceration with exudation. The condition usually remits, but it recurs in 15% of cases. Complications include perforation and megacolon. *Pathogenesis:* the antibiotic alters colonic flora so there is overgrowth of *Clostridium difficile*. The toxin produced by *C. difficile* is cytotoxic, causing necrosis of the epithelium and exudation (pseudomembranes). *Diagnosis:* toxin assay is positive in 98% of cases, and cultures are positive in about 75%. Radiography reveals pseudomembranes. Proctoscopic findings may be normal or show classic pseudomembranes. *Treatment:* discontinue use of antibiotics and provide general supportive care (fluids, etc.). Avoid use of antimotility agents. If no response, metronidazole, 250 mg three times daily, is 80% effective and inexpensive. Vancomycin, 125 mg four times daily, is also 80% effective but very expensive. If the patient is very ill, cholestyramine binds toxin. For first recurrence, the same antibiotic can be used or the drug can be switched. For multiple recurrences, add cholestyramine and prolong the course of treatment with antibiotics.

- Antibiotic colitis: symptoms include fever, abdominal pain, diarrhea 1-6 weeks after antibiotic therapy.
- Toxin assay is positive in 98% of patients.
- Culture is positive in 75%.
- Metronidazole is the initial treatment.
- 15% have recurrence.

Radiation Colitis

Radiation injury usually affects both the colon and the small bowel. Endothelial cells of small submucosal arterioles are very radiosensitive and respond to large doses of radiation by swelling, proliferating, and undergoing fibrinoid degeneration. The result is an obliterative endarteritis. Disease spectrum— 1) *Acute disease* occurs during or immediately after radiation; the mucosa fails to regenerate, and there is friability, hyperemia, and edema. 2) *Subacute disease* occurs 2 to 12 months after radiation. Obliterative endarteritis produces progressive inflammation and ulceration. 3) *Chronic disease* consists of fistulas, abscesses, strictures, and bleeding from intestinal mucosal vessels. Predisposing factors include 1) other diseases that produce microvascular insufficiency, for example, hypertension, diabetes mellitus, atherosclerosis, and heart failure, because they accelerate the development of vascular occlusion; 2) total radiation dose of 40 to 50 Gy; 3) previous chemotherapy; 4) adhesions; 5) previous surgery and pelvic inflammatory disease; and 6) age, the elderly are more susceptible. Radiography of acute disease shows fine serrations of the bowel, and of chronic disease, stricture of the rectum. Endoscopy shows atrophic mucosa with telangiectatic vessels. *Treatment:* endoscopic coagulation is effective.

- Radiation colitis involves both the colon and the small bowel.
- The endothelial cells of the small submucosal arterioles are very radiosensitive.
- The result is obliterative endarteritis.
- Predisposing factors: hypertension, diabetes mellitus, atherosclerosis, chemotherapy, and >40 Gy of radiation.
- The rectum is involved most commonly.

Ischemia

Review of Vascular Anatomy

The celiac trunk supplies the stomach and duodenum. The superior mesenteric artery supplies the jejunum, ileum, and right colon. The inferior mesenteric artery supplies the left colon and rectum.

Acute Ischemia

The symptoms of acute ischemia are sudden severe abdominal pain, vomiting, and diarrhea (with or without blood). Early in the course of ischemia, physical examination findings are normal, but later findings indicate peritonitis. Risk factors include severe atherosclerosis, congestive heart failure, atrial fibrillation (source of emboli), hypotension, and oral contraceptives. There are several syndromes.

1. Acute mesenteric ischemia is due to obstruction of the superior mesenteric artery in 80% of cases. Most (95%) emboli lodge in this artery because of laminar flow, vessel caliber, and the angle it takes off from the aorta. The clue to search for emboli is atrial fibrillation. This syndrome results in a loss of small bowel and produces short-bowel syndrome. Radiography shows ileus, small-bowel obstruction, and, later, gas in the portal vein. The treatment is embolectomy

2. Ischemic colitis is due to poor perfusion. It commonly involves areas of the colon between adjacent arteries, that is, "watershed areas," such as the splenic flexure and rectosigmoid. This syndrome presents with abdominal pain and rectal bleeding. *Radiography:* thumbprinting of watershed areas is characteristic on radiography. *Treatment:* supportive and, if the condition deteriorates, surgical resection.

3. Nonocclusive ischemia is due to poor tissue perfusion caused by inadequate cardiac output. It can involve both the small and the large bowel. Its distribution does not conform to an area supplied by a major vessel. It occurs in patients with cardiac failure or anoxia or who are in shock. It is questioned whether digitalis causes mesenteric vasoconstriction.

- Acute superior mesenteric artery syndrome is usually due to emboli.
- Ischemic colitis: diagnosis is based on radiographic finding of thumbprinting of watershed areas.

Chronic Ischemic Colitis

Chronic ischemic colitis is uncommon. Symptoms include postprandial pain and fear of eating (weight loss). At least two of three major splanchnic vessels must be occluded. It is associated with hypertension, diabetes mellitus, and atherosclerosis. Abdominal bruit is a clue to the diagnosis.

Angiography is diagnostic in about 50% of cases and shows a stenotic area in two of three major vessels. Treatment is with surgical revascularization.

Occlusion of the superior mesenteric vein accounts for approximately 10% of the cases of bowel ischemia. Risk factors include hypercoagulable states such as polycythemia vera, liver disease, pancreatic cancer, intra-abdominal abscess, and portal hypertension. It presents as abdominal pain that gradually becomes severe. Diagnosis is based on angiographic findings. Treatment is surgical.

- Chronic ischemic colitis is associated with hypertension, diabetes mellitus, and atherosclerosis.
- Mesenteric venous thrombosis occurs with hypercoagulable states.

Amebic Colitis

The colon is the usual site of the disease initially. Symptoms vary from none to explosive bloody diarrhea with fever, tenesmus, and abdominal cramps. Proctoscopy shows discrete ulcers with undermined edges and normal adjacent mucosa. If an exudate is present, swab and make wet mount preparations for trophozoites. Indirect hemagglutination is useful for invasive disease. Radiography shows concentric narrowing of the cecum in 90% of cases. Treat with metronidazole (Flagyl). *Entamoeba histolytica* is the only pathogenic ameba in humans.

- The colon is the initial site of disease.
- Proctoscopy shows discrete ulcers with undermined edges.
- Radiography shows concentric narrowing of the cecum in 90% of cases.
- *Entamoeba histolytica* is the only pathogenic ameba in humans.

Tuberculosis

Tuberculosis presents as diarrhea, a change in bowel habits, and rectal bleeding. The ileocecal area is the most commonly involved site. Radiography shows a contracted cecum and ascending colon and ulceration. Proctoscopy reveals deep and superficial ulcers. The rectum may be spared. A hypertrophic ulcerating mass may be seen. Biopsy samples stained with Ziehl-Neelsen stain are positive for acid-fast bacilli. All cases are associated with pulmonary or miliary tuberculosis.

- Tuberculosis is associated with diarrhea, change in bowel habits, and rectal bleeding.
- The ileocecal area is commonly involved.
- Deep and superficial ulcers are characteristic findings.
- All cases are associated with pulmonary or miliary tuberculosis.

Streptococcus bovis endocarditis is associated with colon disease (diverticulosis or cancer). The colon should be evaluated.

Irritable Bowel Syndrome

The term "irritable bowel syndrome" is used for symptoms that are presumed to arise from the small and large intestines. Irritable bowel syndrome refers to a well-recognized complex of symptoms arising from interactions of the intestine, the psyche, and, possibly, luminal factors. Most patients have abdominal pain that is relieved with defecation or associated with a change in the frequency or consistency of the stool. Other associated symptoms include abdominal bloating and passage of excessive mucus with the stool.

Patients with irritable bowel syndrome usually have a long duration of symptoms, symptoms associated with situations of stress and no weight loss, no intestinal bleeding, and no associated organic symptoms (arthritis, fever, etc.). Irritable bowel syndrome is a diagnosis of exclusion: the diagnosis is confirmed by an appropriate medical evaluation that does not reveal any organic illness. Always ask if the patient's symptoms are related to ingestion of dairy foods, because lactase deficiency must be ruled out. Patients who have upper abdominal discomfort and bloating may require an ultrasonographic examination of the abdomen and esophagogastroduodenoscopy. Patients with lower abdominal discomfort or with a change in stool habits may require stool studies, proctoscopic examination, and colon radiography or colonoscopy.

The treatment of irritable bowel syndrome is reassurance, stress reduction, high fiber diet, or the use of fiber supplements. The use of antispasmodics to control abdominal pain or antimotility agents to control diarrhea should be reserved for patients who do not have a response to a high fiber diet.

Nontoxic Megacolon (Pseudo-Obstruction)

Acute pseudo-obstruction of the colon occurs postoperatively (nonabdominal operations) and with spinal cord injury, sepsis, uremia, electrolyte imbalance, and drugs (narcotics, anticholinergics, and psychotropic agents). When the cecum is larger than 13 or 14 cm in diameter, the risk of perforation increases. Obstruction should be ruled out with Hypaque enema. Treatment includes placement of a nasogastric tube, discontinuation of drug therapy, correction of metabolic abnormalities, and, if needed, colonoscopic decompression or cecostomy.

Chronic pseudo-obstruction of the colon is seen in disorders that cause generalized intestinal pseudo-obstruction.

Congenital Megacolon

Congenital megacolon (Hirschsprung disease) occurs in 1 of 5,000 births. There is increased incidence with Down syndrome. Congenital megacolon usually becomes manifest in infancy; however, it can present in adulthood. There is a variable length of aganglionic segment from the rectum to the proximal colon (usually confined to the rectum or rectosigmoid). The diagnosis is usually made at birth because of meconium ileus or obstipation. If the diagnosis is made in an adult, the patient has a history of chronic constipation. Colon radiographs show a characteristically narrowed distal segment and a dilated proximal colon. Rectal biopsy shows aganglionosis. Anorectal manometry shows loss of the anorectal reflex. *Treatment:* sphincter-saving operations.

- Congenital megacolon: increased incidence with Down syndrome.
- In adults, chronic constipation.
- Colon radiographs show characteristically narrowed distal segment and dilated proximal colon.
- Rectal biopsy shows aganglionosis.
- Motility: absent and rectal inhibitory reflex.

Lower Gastrointestinal Tract Bleeding

The evaluation of rectal bleeding should begin with the digital examination, anoscopy, and proctosigmoidoscopy. If a definitive diagnosis cannot be made, next perform a barium enema or arteriography, depending on the nature of the bleeding. The inability to cleanse the colon appropriately during active bleeding makes the barium enema difficult to perform and interpret. Some advocate the use of nuclear scanning if the activity of the bleeding is uncertain. With active bleeding, angiography is the diagnostic procedure of choice. It is also indicated for patients with recurrent episodes of rectal bleeding who have had normal results on previous standard tests, that is, barium enema or colonoscopy. Colonoscopy is not useful if lower gastrointestinal tract bleeding is torrential, but it may be of some benefit if there is a slower rate of bleeding. Colonoscopy is valuable for evaluating patients with unexplained rectal bleeding and persistently positive findings on tests for occult blood in the stool.

- Initial evaluation of rectal bleeding: digital examination, anoscopy, and proctosigmoidoscopy.
- If activity of bleeding is uncertain, try bleeding scan.
- Colonoscopy is not useful if there is torrential lower gastrointestinal tract bleeding.
- Angiography is the procedure of choice for active bleeding.

The important causes of lower gastrointestinal tract bleeding are the following:

- Angiodysplasia—it usually involves the right colon and small bowel and may respond to endoscopic treatment.
- Diverticular disease—there usually is bleeding without other symptoms.

- Inflammatory bowel disease (colitis)—5% of patients present with this.
- Ischemic colitis—painful and bloody diarrhea.
- Cancer—rarely causes significant bleeding.
- Meckel diverticulum—the commonest cause of lower gastrointestinal tract bleeding in young patients. It is usually painless.
- Hemorrhoids—are usually present as rectal outlet bleeding.

Evaluation of lower gastrointestinal tract bleeding—Stabilize the patient, perform proctoscopy to rule out rectal outlet bleeding, and obtain nasogastric tube aspirate or use esophagogastroduodenoscopy to rule out upper gastrointestinal tract bleeding. Radionuclide-tagged red blood cell scan may help determine if bleeding is occurring, but it may not precisely localize the bleeding site. If there is active bleeding, perform angiography. If bleeding stops or occurs at a slow rate, perform colonoscopy. If the patient is young, perform a Meckel scan.

Treatment—If angiography localizes the bleeding site, vasopressin, infusion, or embolization may be useful. If the bleeding is found by colonoscopy, epinephrine injection, electrocoagulation, or laser coagulation may be useful. If bleeding is massive or if significant bleeding continues, surgical management is needed.

Diverticular Disease of the Colon

Definitions

Diverticula are acquired herniations of the mucosa and submucosa through the muscular layers of the colonic wall. *Diverticulosis* is the mere presence of uninflamed diverticula of the colon. *Diverticulitis* is the inflammation of one or more diverticula. The diagnosis and management of the complications of diverticular disease are outlined in Table 8-13.

Diverticulitis

Microperforation or macroperforation of the diverticulum with subsequent peridiverticular inflammation is necessary to produce diverticulitis. The severity of the clinical symptoms depends on the extent of the inflammation. Free perforation is infrequent (diverticula are invested by longitudinal muscle and mesentery). Local perforations may dissect along the colon wall and form intramural fistulas. The clinical presentation is left lower quadrant pain, fever, abdominal distension, constipation, and, occasionally, a palpable tender mass. Treatment includes resting the bowel or using a low fiber diet and antibiotics and obtaining an early surgical consultation. Indications for surgical treatment during the acute phase include the development of generalized peritonitis, an enlarging

Table 8-13.—Diagnosis and Management of Complications of Diverticular Disease

Complication	Symptoms	Findings	Treatment
Diverticulitis	Pain, fever, and constipation or diarrhea (or both)	Palpable tender colon, leukocytosis	Liquid diet, with or without antibiotics or elective surgery
Pericolic abscess	Pain, fever (with or without tenderness), or pus in stools	Tender mass, guarding leukocytosis, soft tissue mass on abdominal films or ultrasonography	Nothing by mouth, intravenous fluids, antibiotics, early surgical treatment with colostomy
Fistula	Depends on site: dysuria, pneumaturia, fecal discharge on skin or vagina	Depends on site: fistulogram, methylene blue	Antibiotics, clear liquids, colostomy, and, later, resection
Perforation	Sudden severe pain, fever	Septic patient, leukocytosis, free air	Antibiotics, nothing by mouth, intravenous fluids, immediate surgical treatment
Liver abscess	Right upper quadrant pain, fever, weight loss	Tender liver, tender bowel or mass, leukocytosis, alkaline phosphatase, lumbosacral scan (filling defect)	Antibiotics, surgical drainage, operation for bowel disease
Bleeding	Bright red or maroon blood, or clots	Blood on rectal exam, sigmoidoscopy, colonoscopy, angiography	Conservative: blood transfusion if needed, with or without operation

inflammatory mass, fistula formation, colonic obstruction, inability to rule out a carcinoma in an area of stricture, or recurrent episodes of diverticulitis.

- Diverticulitis: the clinical symptoms depend on the extent of inflammation.
- Free perforation is infrequent.
- Clinical presentation: left lower quadrant pain, fever, abdominal distension, constipation, and, occasionally, a palpable tender mass.
- Treatment: rest bowel, give antibiotics, and obtain a surgical consultation.

Angiodysplasia

Angiodysplasia is a common and increasingly recognized cause of lower gastrointestinal tract bleeding in elderly patients. Acquired vascular ectasias are believed to be associated with aging. Angiodysplasia is associated with cardiac disease, especially aortic stenosis. It usually involves the cecum and the ascending colon. There are no associated skin or visceral lesions. The ectasias appear to be due to the chronic, partial, intermittent, and low-grade obstruction of submucosal veins where they penetrate the colon. Obstruction is from muscle contraction and distention of the cecum. Colon radiography is of no diagnostic value. Angiography localizes the extent of involvement. Colonoscopy may show lesions. Apply cautery.

- Acquired vascular ectasias are associated with aging.
- Angiodysplasia is associated with cardiac disease, especially aortic stenosis.
- It usually involves the cecum and ascending colon.
- Colonoscopy may show lesions. Apply cautery.

Colon Polyps

Types of epithelial polyps include 1) hyperplastic polyps—metaplastic, completely differentiated glandular elements; they are benign. 2) Hamartomatous polyps—a mixture of normal tissues; they are benign. 3) Inflammatory polyps—an epithelial inflammatory reaction; they are benign. 4) Adenomatous polyps—failure of differentiation of glandular elements. Adenomatous polyps are the only neoplastic (premalignant) polyp. The three types of adenomatous polyps are tubular adenoma, mixed (tubulovillous) adenoma, and villous adenoma (syndrome of hypokalemia, profuse mucus). The risk of cancer in any adenomatous polyp depends on two features: size greater than 1 cm and presence of villous elements. If a polyp is found on flexible sigmoidoscopy and biopsy shows hyperplastic polyp, no further work-up is needed. If biopsy shows adenomatous polyp, perform colonoscopy to look for additional polyps and to perform polypectomy.

- Adenomatous polyps are the only neoplastic (premalignant) polyp; there are three types.
- The risk of cancer in any adenomatous polyp depends on: size >1 cm and presence of villous elements.
- If biopsy shows adenomatous polyp, perform colonoscopy.

Hereditary Polyposis Syndromes

Only those polyposis syndromes associated with adenomatous polyps have risk of cancer.

Familial polyposis: adenomatous polyps of the colon. More than 95% of the patients develop colorectal carcinoma. There are no extra-abdominal manifestations except for bilateral congenital hypertrophy of the retinal pigment epithelium. Diagnosis is based on family history and documentation of adenomatous polyps. Screening of all family members is indicated, and colectomy is indicated before malignancy develops.

- More than 95% of patients with familial polyposis develop colorectal carcinoma.
- There are no extra-abdominal manifestations except for bilateral congenital hypertrophy of the retinal pigment epithelium.
- Colectomy is indicated before malignancy develops.

Gardner syndrome: adenomatous polyps involving the colon, although the terminal ileum and proximal small bowel are rarely involved. More than 95% of patients develop colorectal cancer. Extraintestinal manifestations include congenital hypertrophy of the retinal pigment epithelium; osteomas of the mandible, skull, and long bones; supernumerary teeth; soft tissue tumors; thyroid and adrenal tumors; and epidermoid and sebaceous cysts. Screening of family members is indicated, and colectomy should be performed before malignancy develops.

- More than 95% of patients with Gardner syndrome develop colorectal cancer.
- There are extraintestinal manifestations.
- Screening of family members is indicated.

Turcot-Despres syndrome: adenomatous polyps of the colon associated with malignant gliomas and other brain tumors. Autosomal recessive inheritance.

Polyposis Syndromes Not Associated With Risk of Cancer

Peutz-Jeghers syndrome: hamartomas of the small intestine and less commonly of the stomach and colon. Pigmented lesions of the mouth, hands, and feet are associated with ovarian sex cord tumors and tumors of the proximal small bowel.

- Peutz-Jeghers syndrome: hamartomas of the small intestine.
- Pigmented lesions of the mouth, hands, and feet are associated with ovarian sex cord and proximal small bowel tumors.

Juvenile polyposis: hyperplastic polyps involving the colon and, less commonly, the small intestine and stomach. It presents as gastrointestinal tract bleeding or intussusception with obstruction.

- Only adenomatous polyps are premalignant.
- Perform colectomy for diffuse polyposis only if they are adenomatous.
- Screen family of patients with heritable polyposis syndromes only if the polyps are adenomatous.
- All the above syndromes are autosomal dominant except Turcot-Despres syndrome.

Colorectal Cancer

Epidemiology

Epidemiology is important in etiologic theories. Colorectal carcinoma is the second most common cancer in the U.S. There are 100,000 new cases and 60,000 deaths annually. Six percent of Americans eventually develop colon cancer. The mortality rate has not decreased since the 1930s. The incidence varies widely among different populations; it is highest in "westernized" countries. Compared with past rates, rates for cancer of the right colon and sigmoid colon have increased but decreased for the rectum: cecum/ascending colon, 25%; sigmoid, 25%; rectum, 20%; transverse colon, 12%; rectosigmoid, 10%; and descending colon, 6%.

- Colorectal cancer is the second most common cancer in the U.S.
- Rates for cancer of the right colon and sigmoid colon have increased.

Etiology

The role of the environment as a cause of colorectal cancer is supported by regional differences and migrant studies of incidence. Diet—A high fat diet increases the risk and may enhance the cholesterol/bile acid content of bile which is converted by colonic bacteria to compounds that may promote tumors. A high fiber diet is protective. Increased stool bulk may dilute carcinogens/promoters and decrease exposure by decreasing transit time. Fiber components may bind carcinogens or decrease bacterial enzymes that form toxic compounds. Charbroiled meat/fish and fried foods contain possible mutagens. Antioxidants (vitamins A and C), selenium, vitamin E, yellow-green vegetables, and calcium may protect against cancer.

- High fat diet increases the risk of colorectal cancer.
- High fiber diet has a protective effect.
- Charbroiled meat/fish and fried foods contain possible mutagens.

Genetic Factors

Certain oncogenes amplify or alter gene products in colon cancer cells. Aneuploidy is characteristic of more aggressive tumors. The carbohydrate structure of colonic mucus is altered in colon cancer. Cell-cell interaction possibly has a role in cancer development. Also, genetic predisposition has a role in many colon cancer patients. Familial adenomatous polyposis syndromes are autosomal dominant. Most colon cancers arise in adenomatous polyps. Hereditary nonpolyposis colon cancer (HNPCC or Lynch syndrome) is an autosomal dominant disease that may account for up to 5% of colon cancers. Genetic susceptibility in the general population also has a role, for example, a threefold increased risk of colorectal cancer in first-degree relatives of patients with sporadic colorectal cancer.

- Aneuploidy is characteristic of more aggressive tumors.
- Genetic predisposition to cancer exists in many colon cancer patients.
- Familial adenomatous polyposis is autosomal dominant.
- There is a threefold increased risk of colorectal cancer in first-degree relatives of patients with sporadic colorectal cancer.

Risk Factors for Colorectal Cancer

The risk factors for colorectal cancer include the following: 1) age older than 40 years—the risk increases sharply at age 40, doubles each decade until age 60, and peaks at age 80. 2) Personal history of adenoma or colon cancer—the risk increases with the number of adenomas; 2% to 6% patients with colon cancer have synchronous colon cancer and 1.1% to 4.7% have metachronous cancers. 3) Family history of colon cancer. 4) Inflammatory bowel disease—dysplasia precedes cancer. Cancer rate begins to increase after 7 years of chronic ulcerative colitis and increases 10% per decade of disease. After 25 years, the risk is 30%. The risk is greatest for universal colitis. The risk is delayed a decade in left-sided colitis and is negligible in ulcerative proctitis. Cancer risk is *not* related to severity of the first attack, disease activity, or age at onset. Cancer arising in chronic ulcerative colitis has a prognosis similar to that of other colon cancers. The rate of colon cancer is also increased 4 to 20 times in Crohn colitis or ileocolitis. 5) A personal history of female genital or breast cancer carries a twofold increased risk of colon cancer.

- Colorectal cancer risk factor: age > 40 years.
- Risk increases with the number of adenomas.

- 2%-6% of patients with colon cancer have synchronous colon cancer and 1.1%-4.7% have metachronous cancers.
- Cancer rate begins to increase after 7 years of chronic ulcerative colitis.
- After 25 years, the risk is 30%.
- The risk is greatest for universal colitis.
- Crohn colitis: the rate of colon cancer is increased (4x-20x).

Pathology and Prognostic Indicators

Cancer arises in the epithelium and invades transmurally to penetrate the bowel wall and then enters the regional lymphatics to reach distant nodes. Hematogenous spread is via the portal vein to the liver.

Surgical-pathologic stage of primary tumor—The depth of invasion and the extent of regional lymph node involvement are important in determining prognosis.

Modified Dukes classification (Astler-Coller, 1954): A—mucosa, submucosa (80% 5-year survival); B1—into, not through, the muscularis propria without nodal involvement (65%); B2—through the bowel wall without regional nodal involvement (43%); C1—B1 with regional nodes involved (53%); C2—B2 with regional nodes involved (15%); and D—distant metastases (5%-10%).

The extent of regional node involvement and prognosis: 1 to 4 nodes, 35% recur and more than 4 nodes, 61% recur.

Other pathologic features and prognosis include 1) ulcerating/infiltrating tumor is worse than exophytic/polypoid tumor; 2) poorly differentiated histologic features are worse than highly differentiated ones; 3) venous/lymphatic invasion has a poor prognosis, as does aneuploidy.

Clinical features and prognosis—A high preoperative level of carcinoembryonic antigen is associated with a high recurrence rate and a shorter time before recurrence occurs. Poor prognosis if present with obstruction/perforation. Prognosis is worse in younger than in older patients.

- The depth of invasion and the extent of regional lymph node involvement are important in determining prognosis.
- High preoperative level of carcinoembryonic antigen is associated with high recurrence and a shorter time before recurrence.
- Poor prognosis if present with obstruction/perforation.
- The prognosis is worse in younger than in older patients.

Diagnosis

The clinical presentation is that of a slow growth pattern. Disease may be present for 5 years before symptoms appear. The symptoms depend on the location of the disease. A proximal colon tumor may present with symptoms of anemia, abdominal discomfort, or a mass. The left colon is narrower, and patients may present with obstructive symptoms, change in bowel habits, and rectal bleeding.

If cancer is suspected, perform an air-contrast barium enema and flexible sigmoidoscopy or colonoscopy. If cancer is detected with an air-contrast barium enema or flexible sigmoidoscopy, colonoscopy is needed to rule out synchronous lesions.

Metastatic survey includes physical examination, evaluation of liver-associated enzymes, and chest radiography. Image the liver if levels of liver-associated enzymes are abnormal. The preoperative level of carcinoembryonic antigen is helpful in prognosis and follow-up.

- Proximal colon disease: presenting symptoms may be anemia, abdominal discomfort, or mass.
- Left colon disease: obstructive symptoms, change in bowel habits, and rectal bleeding.
- Preoperative level of carcinoembryonic antigen is helpful in prognosis and follow-up.

Treatment

For most cases, surgical resection is the treatment of choice. This includes wide resection of the involved segment (5-cm margins), with removal of lymphatic drainage. In rectal carcinoma, a low anterior resection is performed if an adequate distal margin of at least 2 cm can be achieved; this rectal sphincter-saving operation does not make the prognosis worse in comparison with abdominal perineal resection. The tumor may require resection to prevent obstruction or bleeding even if distant metastases are present.

- For most cases, surgical resection is the treatment of choice.

Postoperative Management—No Apparent Metastases

Repeat colonoscopy in 6 to 12 months and then every 3 years if the findings are negative. Annually test for occult blood in stool.

Adjuvant chemotherapy—5-Fluorouracil and levamisole decrease recurrence by 41% and mortality by 33% in colonic stage C; they may be beneficial for stage B2. Radiotherapy plus 5-fluorouracil decreases the recurrence rate in rectal cancer stages B2 and C, but it is not clear if there is any survival advantage.

- Repeat colonoscopy in 6-12 months and then every 3 years if the findings are negative.
- Annual testing for occult blood in stool.
- 5-Fluorouracil and levamisole decrease recurrence by 41% and mortality by 33% in colonic stage C.

Prevention of Colorectal Carcinoma

Primary prevention—The steps to be taken in primary prevention are not known, although epidemiologic data indicate that a high fiber, low fat diet is reasonable. Secondary prevention—Identify and eradicate premalignant lesions and detect cancer while it is still curable. Screening includes occult blood screening and sigmoidoscopy. With occult blood screening, earlier stage lesions are detected, but this has not decreased mortality. The Hemoccult test has a 20% to 30% positive predictive value for adenomas and 5% to 10% for carcinomas. With sigmoidoscopy, earlier stage lesions are detected, and the removal of adenomas results in a lower than expected incidence of rectosigmoid cancers, but none show decreased mortality. Flexible sigmoidoscopy detects 2 to 3 times more neoplasms than rigid proctoscopy.

Recommendations for screening—1) For average risk (i.e., anyone not in the high-risk group): annual rectal examination after age 40; annual occult blood test after age 50; sigmoidoscopy after age 50 (every 3-5 years after negative findings on two examinations 1 year apart). 2) For previous adenoma or carcinoma: annual occult blood testing; colonoscopy every year until normal x2, then every 3 years. 3) For familial adenomatous polyposis: annual sigmoidoscopy beginning at puberty until polyposis is diagnosed, then colectomy. 4) For hereditary nonpolyposis cancer syndromes: colonoscopy at age 20, then annual Hemoccult test and colonoscopy every 3 years. 5) For first-degree relative with colorectal cancer: annual occult blood test and periodic sigmoidoscopy beginning at age 40. 6) For a woman with breast/genital cancer: annual occult blood test and periodic sigmoidoscopy. 7) For ulcerative colitis: annual colonoscopy and multiple biopsies starting after 7 years of universal chronic ulcerative colitis or after 15 years of left-sided chronic ulcerative colitis; dysplasia indicates the need for more frequent endoscopic follow-up and may lead to colectomy.

- Earlier stage lesions can be detected, but early detection has not been shown to decrease mortality.
- Flexible sigmoidoscopy detects 2x-3x more neoplasms than rigid proctoscopy.

PANCREAS

Embryology

The pancreas develops in the 4th week of gestation as a ventral and dorsal outpouching or bud from the duodenum. Each bud has its own duct. As the duodenum rotates, the buds appose and join, and the ducts anastomose. Pancreas divisum results from the failure of the ducts of the dorsal and ventral pancreas to fuse. It is controversial whether this may predispose to acute or recurrent pancreatitis. In annular pancreas, part of the ventral pancreas encircles the duodenum (usually the second part, proximal to the ampulla) and causes obstruction.

- Pancreas divisum: failure of dorsal and ventral pancreas to fuse. Might predispose to acute pancreatitis. Be able to recognize this condition on radiographs.
- Annular pancreas: part of the ventral pancreas encircles the duodenum (usually the second part, proximal to the ampulla) and causes obstruction. Be able to recognize this on radiographs.

Classification of Pancreatitis

Acute—reversible inflammation. 1) Interstitial pancreatitis accounts for 80% of cases. Perfusion of the pancreas is intact. It is less severe, with less than 1% mortality. 2) Necrotizing pancreatitis accounts for 20% of cases. It is more severe, with 10% mortality if sterile and 30% if infected.

Chronic—irreversible (i.e., structural disease, with endocrine or exocrine insufficiency). It is documented by pancreatic calcifications on abdominal radiography, by ductal abnormalities on endoscopic retrograde cholangiopancreatography (ERCP), by scarring on pancreatic biopsy, or by endocrine insufficiency (diabetes mellitus) or exocrine insufficiency (malabsorption).

- Acute interstitial pancreatitis: perfusion is intact, mortality is <1%.
- Acute necrotizing pancreatitis: perfusion is compromised, mortality is 10% if sterile and 30% if infected.
- Chronic pancreatitis is documented by pancreatic calcifications, ductal abnormalities, endocrine insufficiency (diabetes), and exocrine insufficiency (malabsorption).

Acute Pancreatitis

In acute pancreatitis, activation of pancreatic enzymes causes autodigestion of the gland. Clinical features are abdominal pain, nausea and vomiting ("too sick to eat"), ileus, peritoneal signs, hypotension, and abdominal mass.

Etiologic Factors

Alcohol is the most common cause and gallstones the second most common cause. The third most common cause is idiopathic (approximately 10%). The following drugs cause pancreatitis: azathioprine, 6-mercaptopurine, L-asparaginase, hydrochlorothiazide diuretics, sulfonamides, sulfasalazine, tetracycline, furosemide, estrogens, valproic acid, pentamidine (both parenteral and aerosolized), and the antiretroviral drug dideoxyinosine (ddI). Know these drugs.

The evidence that the following drugs may also cause pancreatitis is less convincing and not definite: corticosteroids, NSAIDs, methyldopa, procainamide, chlorthalidone, ethacrynic acid, phenformin, nitrofurantoin, enalapril, erythromycin, metronidazole, nonsulfa-linked aminosalicylate derivates (such as 5-aminosalicylic acid and interleukin-2).

Other causes—Hypertriglyceridemia may cause pancreatitis if the triglyceride level is usually greater than 1,000. Look for types I, IV, and V hyperlipoproteinemia and for associated oral contraceptive use. Hypertriglyceridemia may mask hyperamylasemia. Hypercalcemia may also cause pancreatitis; look for underlying multiple myeloma, hyperparathyroidism, or metastatic carcinoma. In immunocompetent patients, mumps and coxsackievirus cause acute pancreatitis. In AIDS patients, acute pancreatitis has been reported with cytomegalovirus infection. Ductus divisum, or incomplete fusion of the dorsal and ventral pancreatic ducts, may predispose to acute pancreatitis in some people, although this is a controversial matter.

- In nonalcoholic patients with acute pancreatitis, review all medications, check lipid levels and calcium levels, and rule out gallstones.
- Know which medications definitely cause acute pancreatitis.

Clinical Presentation

Pain may be mild to severe; it is usually sudden in onset and persistent. The pain typically is located in the upper abdomen, with radiation to the back. Relief may be obtained by bending forward or sitting up. Exacerbation of the pain is common with ingestion of food or alcohol. The absence of pain is a poor prognostic feature, because these patients usually present with shock.

Fever, if present, is low grade, rarely exceeding 101°F in the absence of complications.

Volume depletion—Most patients are hypovolemic because fluid accumulates in the abdomen.

Jaundice—Patients with pancreatitis may have a mild increase in total bilirubin, but they are not usually clinically jaundiced. When jaundice is present, it usually represents obstruction of the common bile duct by stones, compression by pseudocyst, or inflamed pancreatic tissue.

Dyspnea—A wide range of pulmonary manifestations may be seen. In more than half of all cases of acute pancreatitis, some degree of hypoxemia is present. This is usually from pulmonary shunting. Patients often have atelectasis and may develop pleural effusions.

- Fever >101°F suggests infection.

Diagnosis of Acute Pancreatitis

Serum amylase—An increase in the serum level of amylase is the most useful test for acute pancreatitis. The level of amylase increases 2 or 3 hours after an attack and remains elevated for 3 or 4 days. The magnitude of the elevation does not correlate with the clinical severity of the attack. Serum amylase levels may be normal in some (<10%) patients because of alcohol or hypertriglyceridemia. Persistent elevation suggests

a complication, for example, pseudocyst, abscess, or ascites. Serum amylase is cleared by the kidney. The urine amylase level remains elevated after the serum amylase level returns to normal. Isoenzyme identification may aid in distinguishing between salivary (nonpancreatic) and pancreatic sources. Serum lipase may help distinguish between pancreatic hyperamylasemia and an ectopic source (lung, ovarian, or esophageal carcinoma). Lipase levels are also increased longer than amylase levels after acute pancreatitis.

Nonpancreatic hyperamylasemia—Parotitis; renal failure; macroamylasemia; intestinal obstruction, infarction, perforation; ruptured ectopic pregnancy; diabetic ketoacidosis; drugs (such as morphine); burns; pregnancy; and neoplasms (lung, ovary, esophagus).

- If presentation for pancreatitis is classic but amylase value is normal, repeat amylase test, check urine amylase and serum lipase levels, and scan the abdomen.
- Persistent hyperamylasemia suggests a complication.
- If amylase is mildly elevated and there is a history of vomiting but no signs of obstruction, perform esophagogastroduodenoscopy to rule out a penetrating ulcer.

Physical findings include the following: 1) Vital signs—tachycardia and orthostasis. 2) Skin—fat necrosis and xanthelasmas. Grey Turner sign (flank discoloration) or Cullen sign (periumbilical discoloration) suggests retroperitoneal hemorrhage. 3) Abdomen—it often is less impressive than the amount of pain the patient is having.

- Be able to recognize metastatic fat necrosis.
- Grey Turner sign and Cullen sign suggest retroperitoneal hemorrhage.

Laboratory findings: 1) Chest radiography—An isolated left pleural effusion strongly suggests pancreatitis. Infiltrates may represent aspiration pneumonia or adult respiratory distress syndrome. 2) Abdominal flat plate—Look for sentinel loop (dilated loop of bowel over pancreatic area) and colon cutoff sign (abrupt cutoff of gas in the transverse colon). Pancreatic calcifications indicate chronic pancreatitis. 3) Ultrasonography is the procedure of choice in acute pancreatitis, although in the presence of ileus, air in the bowel may obscure visualization of the pancreas. Ultrasonographic examination gives information about the pancreas and is the best method for delineating stones. However, it is not a good method for use in obese patients. 4) CT scanning is the next step when visualization of the pancreas is poor with ultrasonography. It gives the same information as ultrasonography, is slightly less sensitive in picking up stones and texture abnormalities, involves radiation, and is more expensive. CT scanning is indicated in critically ill patients to rule out necrotizing pancreatitis and is the better imaging choice in obese patients. 5) ERCP has no role in the diagnosis of acute pancreatitis and should be avoided because it may cause infection. When acute pancreatitis is associated with jaundice and cholangitis, endoscopic papillotomy is indicated.

- An isolated left pleural effusion on chest radiography is strongly suggestive of acute pancreatitis.
- On an abdominal flat plate, be able to recognize the sentinel loop sign, colon cutoff sign, and pancreatic calcifications.
- Ultrasonographic examination is the procedure of choice in patients with mild acute pancreatitis, in thin patients, and to rule out gallstones.
- CT scanning is indicated in seriously ill patients to rule out necrotizing pancreatitis and in obese patients.
- ERCP has no role in the diagnosis of acute pancreatitis.

Treatment

Supportive care is the backbone of treatment, with monitoring for and treatment of complications when they occur. *Fluids*—Restore and maintain intravascular volume; this usually can be accomplished with crystalloids and peripheral intravenous catheters. Monitor blood pressure, pulse, urine output, daily intake and output, and weight. Eliminate medications that may cause pancreatitis. Use of a nasogastric tube does not shorten the course or severity of pancreatitis, but it should be used in case of ileus or severe nausea and vomiting. *Analgesics*—Meperidine (Demerol), 75 to 125 mg given intramuscularly every 3 or 4 hours, is preferred, especially over morphine, because it causes less sphincter of Oddi spasm. The efficacy of antisecretory drugs such as H_2-blockers, anticholinergic agents, somatostatin, or glucagon has not been documented. Total parenteral nutrition is unnecessary in most cases of pancreatitis. Peritoneal dialysis does not change the overall mortality, although it may decrease early mortality in severe pancreatitis.

- Supportive care is the backbone of treatment.
- Eliminate medications that may cause pancreatitis.
- Nasogastric tube does not shorten the course or severity of pancreatitis.
- Meperidine (Demerol) is preferred because it causes less sphincter of Oddi spasm.

Complications

A local complication is phlegmon, a mass of inflamed pancreatic tissue. It may resolve. Pseudocysts, a fluid collection within a nonepithelial-lined cavity, should be expected if there is persistent pain and persistent hyperamylasemia. In 50% to 80% of cases, this resolves within 6 weeks without intervention. Pancreatic abscess usually develops 2 to 4 weeks after the acute episode and presents as fever (>101°F), persistent abdominal pain, and persistent hyperamylasemia. If a pancreatic abscess is not drained surgically, the mortality rate is virtually 100%. Give antibiotics that are effective for gram-negative and anaerobic organisms. Jaundice is due to common bile duct obstruction. Pancreatic ascites results from disruption of the pancreatic duct or a leaking pseudocyst.

- A local complication of pancreatitis should be suspected if fever, persistent pain, or persistent hyperamylasemia occurs.

A systemic complication is respiratory distress syndrome, a well-recognized complication of acute pancreatitis. Circulating lecithinase probably splits fatty acids off lecithin, producing a faulty surfactant. Pleural effusions occur in approximately 20% of patients with acute pancreatitis. If aspirated, a high amylase content is found. Fat necrosis may be due to increased levels of serum lipase.

- Adult respiratory distress syndrome is a complication of acute pancreatitis.
- Pleural effusions occur in approximately 20% of patients with acute pancreatitis and have a high amylase content.

Assessment of Severity

Most patients with acute pancreatitis recover without any sequelae. The overall mortality rate of acute pancreatitis is 5% to 10%, and death is due most often to hypovolemia and shock, respiratory failure, pancreatic abscess, or systemic sepsis. The Ranson criteria are reliable for predicting mortality in acute pancreatitis (Table 8-14). Mortality: fewer than 3 signs, 1%; 3 or 4 signs, 15%; 5 or 6 signs, 40%; and 7 or more signs, 100%.

- Most patients with acute pancreatitis recover without any sequelae.

Chronic Pancreatitis

Chronic use of alcohol (at least 10 years of heavy consumption) is the most common cause of chronic pancreatitis. Gallstones and hyperlipidemia usually do not cause chronic pancreatitis.

Hereditary pancreatitis is caused by a mutation in the cationic trypsinogen gene, which is inherited as an autosomal dominant trait with variable penetrance. Onset is before age 20, although 20% of patients may present later than this. It is marked by recurring abdominal pain, positive family history, and pancreatic calcifications. It may increase the risk of pancreatic cancer.

Trauma with pancreatic ductal disruption causes chronic pancreatitis. Protein calorie malnutrition is the commonest cause of chronic pancreatitis in Third World countries.

- Chronic pancreatitis is commonly caused by alcohol but seldom by gallstones or hyperlipidemia.
- Hereditary pancreatitis is seen in young people with a positive family history and pancreatic calcifications.
- Protein calorie malnutrition is the commonest cause of chronic pancreatitis in Third World countries.

Triad of Chronic Pancreatitis

The triad consists of pancreatic calcifications, steatorrhea, and diabetes mellitus. Pancreatic calcifications—Diffuse calcification is due to heredity, alcohol, or malnutrition. Local calcification is due to trauma, islet cell tumor, or hypercalcemia. By the time steatorrhea occurs, 90% of the gland has been destroyed and lipase output has decreased by 90%.

- Chronic pancreatitis presents as abdominal pain, pancreatic calcification, steatorrhea, and diabetes mellitus.

Laboratory Diagnosis

Amylase and lipase levels may be normal. Stool fat may be normal. If malabsorption is present, then stool fat is more than 10 g per 24 hours on a 48- to 72-hour stool collection while the patient is on a 100-g fat diet.

Pancreatic function tests—Cholecystokinin (CCK)/secretin stimulation, secretin given intravenously and submaximal CCK, with aspiration of duodenal contents and marker.

Bentiromide test—Para-aminobenzoic acid (PABA)

Table 8-14.—Ranson Criteria

Admission	48 hours
Age >55 yr	pO$_2$ <60 mm Hg
Leukocyte count >15,000	Hematocrit decrease >10%
Glucose >200	Albumin <3.2
Aspartate aminotransferase >250	Blood urea nitrogen increase >5 mg/dL
Lactate dehydrogenase >350	Calcium <8 mg/dL
	Estimated fluid sequestration >4 L

Modified from Ranson JHC: Acute pancreatitis: surgical management. *In* The Exocrine Pancreas: Biology, Pathobiology, and Diseases. Edited by VLW Go, JD Gardner, FP Brooks, E Lebenthal, EP DiMagno, GA Scheele. New York, Raven Press, 1986, pp 503-511. By permission of publisher.

conjugated with *N*-benzoyl tyrosine (bentiromide) is given orally. If chymotrypsin activity is adequate, the molecule is cleaved and PABA is absorbed and excreted in the urine. This test requires a normal small intestine (normal D-xylose test) and is useful only in severe steatorrhea.

CT scans show calcifications, irregular pancreatic contour, dilated duct system, or pseudocysts.

ERCP reveals protein plugs, segmental duct dilatation, and alternating stenosis and dilatation with obliteration of branches of the main duct.

- Amylase and lipase levels may be normal, but evidence for structural disease or endocrine or exocrine insufficiency is present.
- 90% of the gland must be damaged for steatorrhea to occur.

Pain

The mechanism of the pain is not clearly defined; it may be due to ductular obstruction. One-third to one-half of patients have a reduction in pain after 5 years. The possibility of coexistent disease such as peptic ulcer should be considered. Abstinence from alcohol may relieve the pain. Analgesics, aspirin, or acetaminophen is used occasionally with the addition of codeine (narcotic addiction is a frequent complicating factor). Celiac plexus blocks relieve pain for 3 to 6 months, but long-term efficacy is disappointing. A trial of pancreatic enzyme replacement for 1 or 2 months should be tried. Women with idiopathic chronic pancreatitis are most likely to respond. Surgery should be considered only after conservative measures have failed. Patients with a dilated pancreatic duct may have a favorable response to a longitudinal pancreatojejunostomy (Puestow procedure).

- Abstinence from alcohol may relieve pain.
- Narcotic addiction is a frequent complicating factor.
- A 1- or 2-month trial of pancreatic enzyme replacement is worthwhile. Women are more likely to have a response.
- Surgical treatment: only after conservative measures have failed.

Malabsorption

Patients have malabsorption not only of fat but also of essential fatty acids and fat-soluble vitamins. The goal of enzyme replacement is to maintain body weight. Diarrhea will not resolve. Enteric-coated or microsphere enzymes are designed to be released at an alkaline pH, thus avoiding degradation by stomach acid. Their advantage is that they contain larger amounts of lipase. The disadvantages are that they are expensive and bioavailability is not always predictable.

Pancreatic Cancer

Pancreatic carcinoma is more common in men than in women. It usually presents between the ages of 60 and 80 years. The 5-year survival rate is less than 2%. Risk factors include diabetes mellitus, chronic pancreatitis, hereditary pancreatitis, carcinogens, benzidine, cigarette smoking, and high fat diet. Pancreatic carcinoma usually presents late in the course of the disease. Patients may have a vague prodrome of malaise, anorexia, and weight loss. Symptoms may be overlooked until the development of pain or jaundice.

- Courvoisier sign: painless jaundice with a palpable gallbladder suggests pancreatic cancer.
- Trousseau sign: recurrent migratory thrombophlebitis is associated with pancreatic cancer.
- Recent-onset diabetes and nonbacterial (thrombotic) "marantic" endocarditis.

Routine laboratory blood analysis has limited usefulness. Patients may have increased levels of liver enzymes, amylase, and lipase or anemia, although this is variable. Tumor markers are also nonspecific. Abdominal ultrasonography and CT are both approximately 80% sensitive in localizing pancreatic masses. Either imaging method may be used in conjunction with fine-needle aspiration or biopsy to make a tissue diagnosis. ERCP and endoscopic ultrasonography (EUS) are used if the abdominal ultrasonographic or CT results are inconclusive. Both ERCP and EUS have a sensitivity greater than 90%. ERCP also allows aspiration of pancreatic secretions for cytologic analysis. The "double duct" sign is a classic presentation, with obstruction of both the pancreatic and the bile ducts. Biopsy specimens from suspicious lymph nodes may be taken at EUS.

- Abdominal ultrasonography and CT are 80% sensitive in localizing pancreatic masses.
- ERCP and EUS have a sensitivity >90%.

Surgical treatment is the only hope for cure; however, most lesions are nonresectable. The criteria for resectability are a tumor smaller than 2 cm, absence of lymph node invasion, and absence of metastasis. Survival is the same for total pancreatectomy and the Whipple procedure: 3-year survival, 33%; 5-year survival, 1%; and operative mortality, 5%.

Radiation therapy may have a role as a radiosensitizer in unresectable cancer. However, survival is unchanged. The results of chemotherapy have also been disappointing, and studies have not consistently shown improved survival.

Cystic Fibrosis

Because patients with cystic fibrosis are living longer, internists should know the common intestinal complications of this disease. Exocrine pancreatic insufficiency (malabsorption) is the common (85%-90%) and most important complication. Endocrine pancreatic insufficiency (diabetes) occurs in 20% to 30% of the patients. Rectal prolapse occurs in 20%, and a distal small-bowel obstruction from thick secretions occurs in 15% to 20%. Focal biliary cirrhosis develops in 20%.

- Pancreatic insufficiency occurs in 85%-90%.

Pancreatic Endocrine Tumors

Zollinger-Ellison syndrome is a non-beta-cell islet tumor of the pancreas that produces gastrin, causing gastric acid hypersecretion. This results in peptic ulcer disease (see section on Stomach and Duodenum).

Insulinoma is the most common islet cell tumor—a beta-cell islet tumor that produces insulin, which causes hypoglycemia. The diagnosis is based on finding increased fasting plasma levels of insulin and hypoglycemia. CT, endoscopic ultrasonography, or arteriography may be useful in localizing the tumor.

Glucagonoma is an alpha-cell islet tumor that produces glucagon. It presents with diabetes, weight loss, and a classic skin rash (migratory necrolytic erythema). The diagnosis is based on finding increased glucagon levels and failure of blood glucose to increase after the injection of glucagon.

Pancreatic cholera is a pancreatic tumor that produces vasoactive intestinal polypeptide (VIP), which causes watery diarrhea (see Secretory Diarrhea).

Somatostatinoma is a delta-cell islet tumor that produces somatostatin, which inhibits insulin, gastrin, and pancreatic enzyme secretion. The result is diabetes mellitus and diarrhea. The diagnosis is based on finding increased plasma levels of somatostatin.

Octreotide is useful in treating pancreatic endocrine tumors except for somatostatinomas. Octreotide prevents the release of hormone and antagonizes target organ effects.

- Zollinger-Ellison syndrome: non-beta-cell islet tumor of the pancreas.
- Insulinoma: commonest islet cell tumor.
- Pancreatic cholera: pancreatic tumor that produces VIP, which causes secretory diarrhea.
- Octreotide prevents hormone release and antagonizes hormone effects.

PART II
John J. Poterucha, M.D.

INTERPRETATION OF ABNORMAL LIVER TESTS

The frequent use of automated blood tests has increased the recognition of abnormal liver tests. Because these abnormalities usually indicate liver injury and are not true markers of liver function, the term "liver function tests" should be avoided. More specific markers of liver function are direct bilirubin, the serum albumin, and the prothrombin time (PT).

The evaluation of patients with abnormal liver tests hinges on many clinical factors, including the chief complaints of the patient, patient age, risk factors for liver disease, personal or family history of liver disease, medications, and physical examination findings. Because of these multiple factors, designing a standard algorithm for the evaluation of liver test abnormalities is difficult and often inefficient. Nevertheless, with some basic information, a health care provider should be able to evaluate liver test abnormalities in an efficient, cost-effective manner.

COMMONLY USED LIVER TESTS

Aminotransferases (ALT, AST)

The aminotransferases are found in hepatocytes and are markers of liver cell injury, or hepatocellular disease. Hepatocellular injury causes these enzymes to "leak" out of the liver cells, and increased levels of these enzymes are seen in the serum within a few hours after liver injury. The aminotransferases consist of alanine aminotransferase (ALT), also known as "serum glutamate pyruvate transaminase" (SGPT), and aspartate aminotransferase (AST), also known as "serum glutamate oxaloacetate transaminase" (SGOT). ALT is relatively specific for liver injury, whereas AST is found not only in hepatocytes but also in skeletal and cardiac muscle and other organs. Because some automated blood tests assay only for AST, it is useful to determine the serum level of ALT before embarking on an evaluation for liver disease.

Alkaline Phosphatase

Alkaline phosphatase is found on the hepatocyte membrane that borders the bile canaliculi (the smallest branches of the bile ducts). Because alkaline phosphatase is also found in bone and placenta, an isolated increase in the level of the enzyme should prompt further testing to determine whether the increase is from the liver or other tissues. Determination of alkaline phosphatase isoenzymes is one method of doing this. Another is the determination of γ-glutamyl transpeptidase (γ-glutamyltransferase) (GGT). GGT is an enzyme of intrahepatic biliary canaliculi that is more sensitive to biliary obstruction than alkaline phosphatase. Other than to confirm the hepatic origin of an increased level of alkaline phosphatase, GGT has little role in the diagnosis of diseases of the liver because its synthesis can be induced by many medications, thus reducing its specificity for *clinically significant* liver disease.

Bilirubin

Bilirubin is the water-insoluble product of heme metabolism that is taken up by the hepatocyte and conjugated with glucuronic acid to form monoglucuronides and diglucuronides. Conjugation makes bilirubin water soluble, allowing it to be excreted in bile. When bilirubin is measured in the serum, there are direct and indirect fractions. Diseases characterized by overproduction of bilirubin, such as hemolysis or resorption of a hematoma, are characterized by hyperbilirubinemia that is less than 20% conjugated. Hepatocyte dysfunction or bile flow impairment produces hyperbilirubinemia that is usually more than 50% conjugated. Because conjugated bilirubin is water soluble and may be excreted in the urine, patients with liver disease and hyperbilirubinemia have dark urine. In these patients, the stools are lighter in color because of the absence of bilirubin pigments.

Prothrombin Time and Albumin

PT and the serum level of albumin are true markers of liver synthetic function. Abnormalities of PT and albumin imply severe liver disease and should prompt an immediate workup. PT is a measure of the activity of factors II, V, VII, and X, all of which are synthesized in the liver. These factors are also dependent on vitamin K for synthesis, so deficiencies of vitamin K produce abnormalities of PT. Vitamin K deficiency can result from the use of antibiotics during a period of prolonged fasting, small-bowel mucosal disorders such as celiac disease, and severe cholestasis, with an inability to absorb fat-soluble vitamins. True hepatocellular dysfunction is characterized by an inability to synthesize clotting factors even when the stores of vitamin K are adequate. A simple way to distinguish vitamin K deficiency from liver dysfunction in a patient with a prolonged PT is to administer vitamin K. A 10-mg dose of oral vitamin K for 3 days or 10 mg of subcutaneous vitamin K will normalize PT in a vitamin K-deficient patient but will have no effect on PT in a patient with decreased liver synthetic function.

Albumin has a half-life of 21 days; thus, decreased serum levels due to liver dysfunction do not occur acutely. However, the serum level of albumin can decrease relatively quickly in a severe systemic illness such as bacteremia. This rapid decrease likely is due to cytokine release, with accelerated metabolism of albumin. A chronic decrease of albumin in a patient without overt liver disease should prompt a search for albumin in the urine.

HEPATOCELLULAR DISORDERS

Diseases that primarily affect hepatocytes are termed "hepatocellular disorders" and are characterized predominantly by increases in aminotransferases. The disorders are best considered as "acute" (generally < 3 months) or "chronic." Acute hepatitis may be accompanied by malaise, anorexia, abdominal pain, and jaundice. Common causes of acute hepatitis are listed in Table 8-15.

Diseases that produce a sustained (> 3 months) increase in aminotransferase levels are in the category of "chronic hepatitis." The increase (usually two- to fivefold) in aminotransferases is more modest than that in acute hepatitis. Patients may be asymptomatic but occasionally complain of fatigue and right upper quadrant pain. The differential diagnosis of chronic hepatitis is relatively lengthy; the more important and common disorders are listed in Table 8-16.

CHOLESTATIC DISORDERS

The diseases that predominantly affect the biliary system are called "cholestatic diseases." They can affect the microscopic ducts (e.g., primary biliary cirrhosis), large bile ducts (e.g., pancreatic cancer causing common bile duct obstruction), or both (e.g., primary sclerosing cholangitis). In general, the predominant abnormality in these disorders involves alkaline phosphatase. Although diseases that cause an increase in bilirubin are often referred to as "cholestatic," it is important to remember that severe hepatocellular injury, as in acute hepatitis, also produces hyperbilirubinemia because of hepatocellular dysfunction. The common causes of cholestasis are listed in Table 8-17.

JAUNDICE

The evaluation of a patient with jaundice is an important diagnostic skill. Jaundice is visibly evident hyperbilirubinemia and occurs when the bilirubin concentration is greater than 2.5 mg/dL. As mentioned above, it is important to note whether the bilirubin increase is predominantly conjugated or unconjugated. A common disorder that produces unconjugated hyperbilirubinemia is Gilbert syndrome. Total bilirubin is

Table 8-15.—Common Causes of Acute Hepatitis

Disease	Clinical clue	Diagnostic test
Hepatitis A	Exposure history	IgM anti-HAV
Hepatitis B	Risk factors	HBsAg, IgM anti-HBc
Drug-induced	Compatible medication/timing	Improvement after withdrawal from agent
Alcoholic hepatitis	History of alcohol excess, AST:ALT >2	Liver biopsy, improvement with abstinence
Ischemic hepatitis	History of severe hypotension	Rapid improvement of aminotransferase levels
Acute duct obstruction	Abdominal pain, fever	Cholangiography

ALT, alanine aminotransferase; AST, aspartate aminotransferase; HAV, hepatitis A virus; HBc, hepatitis B core; HBsAg, hepatitis B surface antigen.

Table 8-16.—Common Causes of Chronic Hepatitis

Disease	Clinical clue	Diagnostic test
Hepatitis C	Risk factors	Anti-HCV
Hepatitis B	Risk factors	HBsAg
Nonalcoholic steato-hepatitis	Obesity, diabetes, hyperlipidemia	Ultrasonography, liver biopsy
Hemochromatosis	Arthritis, diabetes mellitus, family history	Iron studies, gene test, liver biopsy
Alcoholic liver disease	History, AST:ALT >2	Liver biopsy
Autoimmune hepatitis	ALT 200-1,500, usually female, other autoimmune disease	Antinuclear or anti-smooth muscle antibody, liver biopsy

ALT, alanine aminotransferase; AST, aspartate aminotransferase; HBsAg, hepatitis B surface antigen; HCV, hepatitis C virus.

generally less than 3.0 mg/dL, whereas direct bilirubin is 0.3 mg/dL or less. Bilirubin concentration is generally higher in the fasting state or when the patient is ill. A presumptive diagnosis of Gilbert syndrome can be made in an otherwise well patient with unconjugated hyperbilirubinemia and normal levels of hemoglobin (to exclude hemolysis) and normal liver enzymes (to exclude liver disease).

Direct hyperbilirubinemia is more common in a patient with jaundice. These patients can be categorized as those with nonobstructive conditions and those with obstruction. Abdominal pain, fever, or a palpable gallbladder (or a combination of these) suggests obstruction. Risk factors for viral hepatitis, a bilirubin concentration greater than 15 mg/dL, and persistently high aminotransferase levels suggest that the jaundice is due to hepatocellular dysfunction. A sensitive, specific, and noninvasive test to exclude obstructive causes of cholestasis is hepatic ultrasonography. Diseases characterized by large bile duct obstruction generally show intrahepatic bile duct dilatation, especially if the bilirubin concentration is greater than 10 mg/dL and the patient has had jaundice for more than 2 weeks. Acute large bile duct obstruction, usually from a stone, may produce markedly increased aminotransferase levels. If the clinical suspicion for bile duct obstruction is still strong despite negative ultrasonographic results, endoscopic retrograde cholangiography should be considered.

ALGORITHMS FOR PATIENTS WITH ABNORMAL LIVER TESTS

Algorithms for the management of patients with abnormal liver tests are at best guidelines and at worst misleading. Always remember that the patient's clinical presentation should be considered in interpreting (or not interpreting) abnormal liver tests. In general, patients with abnormal liver tests that are less that twice the normal value can be followed unless the patient is symptomatic or the albumin level, PT, or bilirubin concentration is abnormal. Persistent abnormalities should also be evaluated. Algorithms for the management of patients with increased levels of ALT or alkaline phosphatase are shown in Figures 8-2 and 8-3, respectively.

SPECIFIC LIVER DISEASES

Viral Hepatitis

Hepatitis A

Hepatitis A virus (HAV) is a small RNA virus that accounts for 20% to 25% of cases of acute hepatitis in developed countries. The disease generally is transmitted by the fecal-oral route and has an incubation period of 15 to 50 days. Spread is more common in overcrowded areas with poor hygiene and poor sanitation. Hepatitis caused by HAV is generally mild, especially in children who often have a subclinical or nonicteric illness. Infected adults are more ill and usually develop jaundice. The prognosis is excellent. Rarely, HAV may cause fulminant hepatitis. Chronic liver disease does not develop from HAV. Serum IgM anti-HAV is present during an acute illness, generally persists for 2 to 6 months, and is followed by IgG anti-HAV, which offers immunity from further infection. Immune serum globulin should be given for household contacts of infected patients. When a common source of foodborne infection is identified, serum globulin should be given to those exposed. A hepatitis A vaccine has been developed and approved for use in the U.S. Persons traveling abroad and patients with chronic liver disease are good candidates for hepatitis A vaccine.

- HAV is transmitted by the fecal-oral route.
- The incubation period is 15-50 days.
- The prognosis is excellent.
- Chronic liver disease does not develop.
- IgM anti-HAV is present during the acute illness.
- Give immune serum globulin for household contacts.

Hepatitis B

Hepatitis B virus (HBV) is a DNA virus with a surface and a core. The core consists of a core antigen and "e" antigen. The disease is transmitted parenterally or by sexual contact. In high prevalence areas, for example, certain areas of Asia, infants may acquire infection from the mother during childbirth. High-risk groups in the U.S. include injection drug users,

Table 8-17.—Common Causes of Cholestasis

Disease	Clinical clue	Diagnostic test
Primary biliary cirrhosis	Middle-aged woman	Antimitochondrial antibody
Primary sclerosing cholangitis	Association with ulcerative colitis	Cholangiography (ERCP)
Large bile duct obstruction	Jaundice and pain are common	Ultrasonography, ERCP
Drug-induced	Compatible medication/timing	Improvement after withdrawal of the agent
Intrahepatic mass lesion	History of malignancy	Ultrasonography, computed tomography

ERCP, endoscopic retrograde cholangiopancreatography.

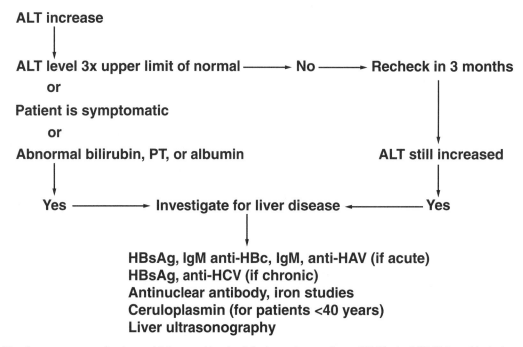

Fig. 8-2. Algorithm for management of patients with increased levels of alanine aminotransferase (ALT). Anti-HAV, hepatitis A virus antibody; anti-HBc, hepatitis B core antibody; anti-HCV, hepatitis C virus antibody; HBsAg, hepatitis B surface antigen; PT, prothrombin time.

persons with multiple sexual contacts, and health care workers. The clinical course of HBV infection varies. Most infections in adults are subclinical, and even when symptomatic, the disease resolves within 6 months. During acute hepatitis, symptoms (when present) are generally more severe than those of HAV. Jaundice rarely lasts longer than 4 weeks. Some patients may have preicteric symptoms of "serum sickness," including arthralgias and urticaria. These symptoms may be related to immune complexes, which can also lead to polyarteritis and glomerulonephritis.

- HBV is transmitted parenterally or by sexual contact.
- Infants may acquire infection from mothers.
- High-risk groups: injection drug users, persons with multiple sexual contacts, and health care workers.
- Most infections in adults are subclinical.
- Jaundice rarely lasts >4 weeks.

HBV is not directly cytopathic, and acute hepatocellular necrosis is due to a host immune response to viral-infected cells. This inflammatory response accounts for the symptoms of acute hepatitis B. Thus, patients with symptomatic HBV are more likely to "clear" the virus than those with subclinical infection. For example, patients with fulminant hepatitis B who recover rarely develop chronic hepatitis B. Viral markers in the blood during a self-limited infection with HBV are shown in Figure 8-4.

- Host immune response causes hepatocellular necrosis and accounts for HBV symptoms.
- Patients who recover from fulminant hepatitis B rarely develop chronic hepatitis B.

Note that IgM hepatitis B core antibody (anti-HBc) is nearly always present during acute hepatitis B. Some patients with acute hepatitis B, particularly those with fulminant hepatitis B, may lack hepatitis B surface antigen (HBsAg). HBV-DNA and hepatitis B e antigen (HBeAg) correlate with ongoing viral replication and indicate high infectivity. Patients with hepatitis B mutants may have high HBV-DNA levels but lack HBeAg. Commonly encountered serologic patterns of HBV are shown in Table 8-18.

Ten percent of patients acquiring HBV as adults and 90% of those infected as neonates do not clear HBsAg from the serum within 6 months and, thus, become chronically infected. Chronicity is more common in patients with a defect of the immune system. Patients with chronic hepatitis B but normal findings on liver tests and histologic examination of the liver are called "carriers" and have a good prognosis. Chronic liver inflammation due to HBV may lead to cirrhosis and liver failure. Spontaneous conversion from an HBeAg-positive state to HBeAg-negativity is accompanied by an increase in the level of aminotransferases. Patients with chronic HBV liver disease, particularly if cirrhosis is present, are at high risk for the development of hepatocellular carcinoma and, every

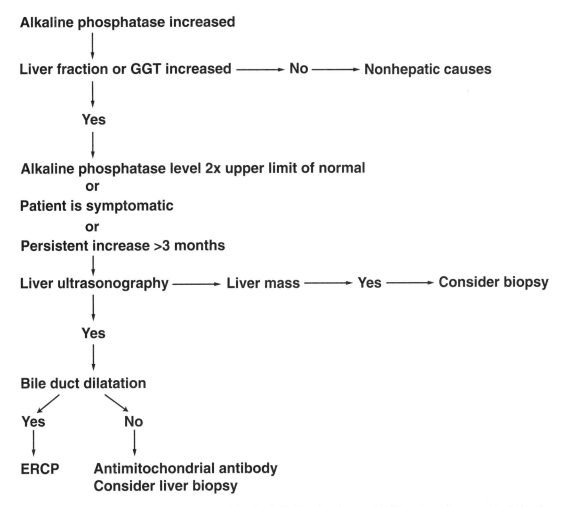

Fig. 8-3. Algorithm for management of patients with increased levels of alkaline phosphatase. ERCP, endoscopic retrograde cholangiopancreatography; GGT, γ-glutamyl transpeptidase.

6 to 12 months, liver ultrasonography should be performed and the alpha-fetoprotein level determined.

- IgM anti-HBc is nearly always present during acute hepatitis B.
- HBV-DNA and HBeAg correlate with ongoing viral replication and indicate infectivity.
- 10% of patients acquiring HBV as adults and 90% of those infected as neonates do not clear HBsAg.
- Most chronic carriers of HBsAg have essentially a normal liver histologically and a good prognosis.
- Chronic hepatitis due to HBV may lead to cirrhosis.
- Patients with HBV-induced cirrhosis are at high risk for development of hepatocellular carcinoma.

Patients with chronic hepatitis B and active viral replication are potential candidates for therapy. Interferon-alfa results in a 30% to 40% response rate as measured by loss of HBeAg and HBV-DNA. A few patients will also clear HBsAg. Patients more likely to respond to interferon include those with a relatively recent diagnosis of chronic hepatitis B, high serum levels of aminotransferases, active hepatitis without evidence of cirrhosis on biopsy, and low serum levels of HBV-DNA. Patients with HBV who have a response to interferon may have a transient increase in aminotransferase levels after about 8 weeks of treatment. Lamivudine, an oral nucleoside analog, lowers HBV-DNA levels and may be useful for patients with chronic hepatitis B, particularly if they have symptoms. Lamivudine decreases HBV-DNA levels in nearly all patients, and 20% have seroconversion to antibodies to hepatitis B e (anti-HBe). Lamivudine-resistant mutations occur in 30% of patients who have received treatment for 1 year, but the mutations are less virulent than the wild-type strain.

Hepatitis D

The delta agent is a small RNA particle that requires the presence of HBsAg to cause infection. Hepatitis D virus (HDV) infection can occur simultaneously with acute HBV

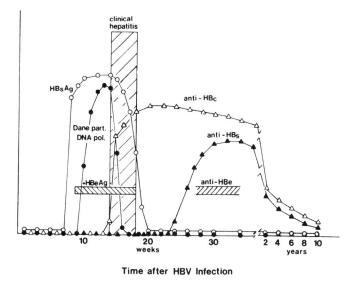

Time after HBV Infection

Fig. 8-4. Viral markers in blood during self-limited hepatitis B virus infection. Anti-HBc, hepatitis B core antibody; anti-HBe, hepatitis B e antibody; anti-HBs, hepatitis B surface antibody; HBeAg, hepatitis B e antigen; HBsAg, hepatitis B surface antigen. (From Robinson WS: Biology of human hepatitis viruses. *In* Hepatology: A Textbook of Liver Disease. Vol 2. Second edition. Edited by D Zakim, TD Boyer. Philadelphia, WB Saunders Company, 1990, pp 890-945. By permission of publisher.)

(coinfection) or may infect a chronic HBsAg carrier (superinfection). HDV is strongly associated with injection drug abuse in the U.S. Infection with HDV should be considered only in patients with HBsAg and is diagnosed by anti-HDV seroconversion. Acute delta hepatitis is self-limited but may cause fulminant hepatitis. Like HBV, HDV recurs in a transplanted liver.

- Delta agent requires the presence of HBsAg to cause infection.
- HDV is strongly associated with injection drug abuse.
- HDV infection occurs only in patients with HBsAg.
- Diagnosed by anti-HDV seroconversion.
- HBV and HDV recur in transplanted liver.

Hepatitis C

Hepatitis C virus (HCV), an RNA virus, is the most common chronic blood-borne infection in the United States. Although the number of new cases of hepatitis C infection is decreasing, the propensity of the virus to cause chronic infection will result in an increasing number of deaths. HCV has a role in 40% of all cases of chronic liver disease and is the leading indication for liver transplantation. Hepatitis C is a parenterally transmitted virus. The most common risk factor is illicit drug use. Persons with a history of transfusion of blood products before 1990 (when routine testing of blood products for HCV was introduced) are also at significant risk

for infection with HCV. Sexual transmission of HCV occurs but seems to be inefficient, and only about 2% of long-term spouses of chronic hepatitis C patients have serologic evidence of hepatitis C infection. The risk of transmission of hepatitis C to health care workers by percutaneous (needlestick) exposure is also low, probably around 2%. For a health care worker who has a needlestick exposure from a patient with hepatitis C, baseline testing for anti-HCV and ALT is recommended. Follow-up testing can be with HCV RNA at 4 to 6 weeks and/or anti-HCV and ALT at 4 to 6 months. Prophylactic immune globulin or anti-hepatitis C therapy is not recommended.

Antibodies to HCV (anti-HCV) indicate exposure to the virus and are not protective. The presence of anti-HCV can indicate either current infection or a previous infection with subsequent clearance. The presence of anti-HCV in a patient with an abnormal ALT and risk factors for hepatitis C acquisition is strongly suggestive of current HCV infection. The initial test for anti-HCV is done by enzyme-linked immunoassay (EIA). This test is very sensitive (few false-negative results) but the specificity is variable. If the anti-HCV by EIA is negative, it is extremely unlikely that the patient has hepatitis C. The specificity of EIA is improved with the addition of the recombinant immunoblot assay (RIBA) for anti-HCV. A guide to interpretation of anti-HCV tests is given in Table 8-19.

The reference standard for the diagnosis of hepatitis C infection is the presence of HCV RNA as determined by polymerase chain reaction (PCR). Quantitative HCV RNA tests are also available. These assays can measure the amount of HCV RNA present but are not as sensitive as HCV RNA determination by PCR. Levels do not correlate with disease severity, and the major use of quantitative assays is to stratify the response to therapy.

- Hepatitis C is a parenterally transmitted virus and a common cause of chronic hepatitis.
- Common modes of transmission are illicit drug use and transfusion of blood products before 1990.
- Anti-HCV indicates exposure to the virus.
- HCV RNA by PRA is the reference standard for diagnosis.

Infection with HCV rarely presents as acute hepatitis. About 85% of persons acquiring hepatitis C develop a chronic infection, and subsequent spontaneous loss of the virus is rare. Consequently, most patients with hepatitis C present with chronic hepatitis with mild to moderate increases in ALT. Some patients have fatigue and/or vague right upper quadrant pain. Patients may also come to medical attention because of complications of end-stage liver disease or, rarely, extrahepatic complications such as cryoglobulinemia or porphyria cutanea tarda. Up to 30% of patients chronically infected with

Table 8-18.—Common Serologic Patterns of Hepatitis B Virus

HBsAg	Anti-HBs	Anti-HBc	HBeAg	Anti-HBe	Interpretation
+	-	IgM	+	-	Acute HBV infection, high infectivity
+	-	IgG	+	-	Chronic HBV infection, high infectivity
+	-	IgG	-	+	Late-acute or chronic HBV infection, low infectivity or
+	+	+	±	±	HBsAg of one subtype and heterotypic anti-HBs (common)
					Process of seroconversion from HBsAg to anti-HBs (rare)
-	-	IgM	±	±	Acute HBV infection Anti-HBc window
-	-	IgG	-	±	Low-level HBsAg carrier or Remote past infection
-	+	IgG	-	±	Recovery from HBV infection
-	+	-	-	-	Immunization with HBsAg (after vaccination) or Remote past infection

Anti-, antibody; HBc, hepatitis B core; HBcAg, HBc antigen; HBe, hepatitis B e; HBeAg, HBe antigen; HBs, hepatitis B surface; HBsAg, HBs antigen; HBV, hepatitis B virus.

From Dienstag JL, Wands JR, Isselbacher KJ: Acute hepatitis. *In* Harrison's Principles of Internal Medicine. Twelfth edition. Edited by JD Wilson, E Braunwald, KJ Isselbacher, RG Petersdorf, JB Martin, AS Fauci, RK Root. New York, McGraw-Hill, 1991, pp 1322-1337. By permission of publisher.

Table 8-19.—Interpretation of Anti-HCV Results

Anti-HCV by EIA	Anti-HCV by RIBA	Interpretation
Positive	Negative	False-positive EIA, patient does not have true antibody
Positive	Positive	Patient has antibody*
Positive	Indeterminate	Uncertain antibody status

EIA, enzyme-linked immunoassay; HCV, hepatitis C virus; RIBA, recombinant immunoblot assay.

*Remember that anti-HCV does not necessarily indicate current hepatitis C infection (see text).

HCV have a persistently normal ALT. Because the majority of patients with hepatitis C are asymptomatic, treatment is aimed at preventing future complications of the disease. About 20% to 30% of patients with chronic hepatitis C develop cirrhosis over a 10- to 20-year period. Patients with cirrhosis due to HCV generally have had disease for longer than 20 years.

Currently, interferon alpha in combination with ribavirin is the standard of care for patients with hepatitis C who are deemed candidates for treatment. This combination given for 6 to 12 months results in a sustained clearance of HCV RNA from the serum in 38% to 43% of patients. On the basis of the natural history of hepatitis C and the response to therapy, an algorithm for patients without any contraindication to treatment can be proposed (Fig. 8-5). These guidelines apply generally to the large percentage of the patients with hepatitis C who are asymptomatic or have nonspecific symptoms such as fatigue.

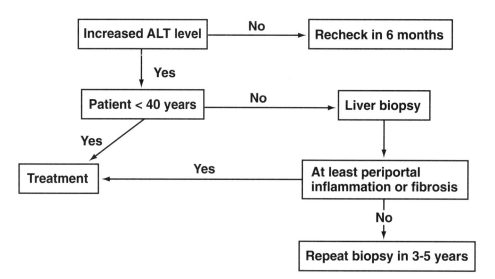

Fig. 8-5. Treatment algorithm for patients with hepatitis C virus infection who have no contraindication to therapy. ALT, alanine aminotransferase.

Therapy should be offered to patients who have extrahepatic manifestations of hepatitis C, such as vasculitis related to cryoglobulinemia.

Patients who are not treatment candidates should be evaluated annually with routine liver tests. Patients with cirrhosis are at increased risk for hepatocellular carcinoma, particularly if there is a history of alcohol excess. The risk of hepatocellular carcinoma complicating hepatitis C with cirrhosis is 1.4% to 4% per year. Screening with alpha-fetoprotein and liver ultrasonography every 6 to 12 months is advised for patients with the tumor who are candidates for treatment with modalities such as liver transplantation or percutaneous ablation. Patients with HCV and decompensated cirrhosis should be considered for liver transplantation.

- Symptomatic, clinically recognized acute hepatitis C is unusual.
- 85% of patients acquiring hepatitis C remain chronically infected.
- 20%-30% of patients develop cirrhosis over 20 years.
- The combination of interferon alpha and ribavirin results in sustained clearance of HCV RNA in about 40% of patients.
- Patients with cirrhosis due to hepatitis C are at increased risk for hepatocellular carcinoma, particularly if there is also a history of alcohol excess.

Hepatitis E

Hepatitis E virus (HEV) is an enterically transmitted RNA virus. It can cause acute hepatitis in patients from endemic areas (India, Pakistan, Mexico, and Southeast Asia) and in travelers returning from these regions. Clinically, hepatitis E resembles hepatitis A. A notable exception is the high risk of fulminant hepatitis E in women who acquire the infection during the third trimester of pregnancy. Chronic hepatitis E does not occur. Hepatitis A, B, C, and E are compared in Table 8-20.

- HEV is an enterically transmitted RNA virus.
- It resembles hepatitis A.
- There is a high risk of fulminant hepatitis E in women who acquire the infection during the third trimester of pregnancy.

Miscellaneous

Epstein-Barr virus, cytomegalovirus, and herpes viruses can all cause acute viral hepatitis, which is most serious in immunocompromised patients.

Autoimmune Hepatitis

"Autoimmune hepatitis" (AH) was previously called "autoimmune *chronic* active hepatitis" because the diagnosis required 3 to 6 months of abnormal liver enzymes. However, AH can present as acute hepatitis. AH affects patients at any age, mainly females. The onset is usually insidious, and initial liver biopsy may show cirrhosis.

By definition, patients with AH should have no history of drug-related hepatitis, HBV, HCV, or Wilson disease. Immunoserologic markers, including antinuclear antibody (ANA), smooth muscle antibody, soluble liver antigen antibodies, or antibodies to liver/kidney microsomal (LKM) antigens, are usually seen and may help separate patients into certain groups. There is an association with certain HLA types. Associated conditions include Hashimoto thyroiditis, Coombs-

Table 8-20.—Comparison of Hepatitis A, B, C, and E

Feature	Hepatitis A	Hepatitis B*	Hepatitis C	Hepatitis E
Incubation, days	15-45 (mean, 30)	30-180 (mean, 60-90)	14-160 (mean, 80)	14-60 (mean, 40)
Onset	Acute	Often insidious	Insidious	Acute
Age preference	Children, young adults	Any age	Any age	Young adults
Transmission				
Fecal-oral	+++	-	-	+++
Sexual	±	++	+	±
Percutaneous	Unusual	+++	+++	-
Severity	Mild	Often severe	Variable	Mild
Prognosis	Generally good	Worse with age, debility	Variable	Good
Chronicity	None	Occasional (5%-10%)	Frequent	None
Prophylaxis	Ig	Hepatitis B immune globulin, HBV vaccine	None	?

*Concomitant delta hepatitis is similar to hepatitis B, but more severe outcomes are favored.
From Dienstag JL, Wands JR, Isselbacher KJ: Acute hepatitis. *In* Harrison's Principles of Internal Medicine. Twelfth edition. Edited by JD Wilson, E Braunwald, KJ Isselbacher, RG Petersdorf, JB Martin, AS Fauci, RK Root. New York, McGraw-Hill, 1991, pp 1322-1337. By permission of publisher. Information on hepatitis C is data from Seeff LB: Diagnosis, therapy, and prognosis of viral hepatitis. *In* Hepatology: A Textbook of Liver Disease. Third edition. Edited by D Zakim, TD Boyer. Philadelphia, WB Saunders Company, 1996, pp 1067-1145.

positive hemolytic anemia, diabetes mellitus, and glomerulonephritis. Marked increases in the serum levels of gamma globulin are common, and the aminotransferase levels are generally 4 to 10 times normal. Corticosteroids (30-60 mg/day) produce improvement in 60% to 80% of patients. Changes in results of liver tests and gamma globulin are often dramatic. Azathioprine can be added to allow the use of lower doses of prednisone. The prednisone dose should be reduced to control symptoms and to maintain the serum level of aminotransferases below five times normal. Even after an excellent response to corticosteroids, relapse often occurs and the control of AH often requires maintenance therapy. Although corticosteroids do not seem to prevent progression to cirrhosis, they improve survival in patients with severe disease.

- The onset of AH is usually insidious.
- There should be no history of drug-related hepatitis, HBV, HCV, or Wilson disease.
- Immunoserologic markers are often seen.
- Marked increases in serum levels of gamma globulin are common.
- 60%-80% of patients have improvement with corticosteroids.
- Changes in results of liver tests and gamma globulin are often dramatic.
- The control of AH often requires maintenance therapy.

Alcoholic Liver Disease

Alcoholic Hepatitis

Alcoholic hepatitis is characterized histologically by fatty change, degeneration and necrosis of hepatocytes (with or without Mallory bodies), and inflammatory infiltrate of neutrophils. Almost all patients have increased intralobular connective tissue, and they may have cirrhosis. Clinically, patients may be asymptomatic or jaundiced and critically ill. Common symptoms include anorexia, nausea, vomiting, abdominal pain, and weight loss. The most common sign is hepatomegaly, which may be accompanied by ascites, jaundice, fever, splenomegaly, and encephalopathy. AST is increased in 80% to 90% of cases, but it is almost always less than 400 U/L. Aminotransferase levels greater than 400 U/L are not a feature of alcoholic liver disease and a search for other causes (e.g., ingestion of acetaminophen) should be pursued. The AST:ALT ratio is frequently greater than 2. Leukocytosis is seen, particularly in severely ill patients.

- Alcoholic hepatitis is characterized by fatty change, degeneration and necrosis of hepatocytes (with or without Mallory bodies), and inflammatory infiltrate of neutrophils.
- Common symptoms are anorexia, nausea, vomiting, abdominal pain, and weight loss.
- Common signs are hepatomegaly, ascites, jaundice, fever, splenomegaly, and encephalopathy.

- AST is increased (almost always <400 U/L) in 80%-90% of cases.
- AST:ALT is frequently >2.
- Leukocytosis occurs in severely ill patients.

Poor prognostic markers include encephalopathy, spider angiomata, ascites, renal failure, prolonged PT, and a bilirubin concentration greater than 20 mg/dL. Many patients have progression to cirrhosis, particularly if alcohol intake is not curtailed. Corticosteroids may be beneficial as an acute treatment of alcoholic hepatitis, particularly in patients with severe disease characterized by encephalopathy and a markedly prolonged PT.

- Poor prognostic markers: encephalopathy, spider angiomata, ascites, renal failure, prolonged PT, and bilirubin >20 mg/dL.
- Corticosteroids may be beneficial in severe disease.

Alcoholic Cirrhosis

Cirrhosis is defined histologically by fibrosis with nodular parenchymal regeneration. Typically, the cirrhosis of alcoholics is micronodular. Only 60% of patients with alcoholic cirrhosis have signs or symptoms of liver disease. Most patients with cirrhosis have no history of alcoholic hepatitis. Women are more predisposed to cirrhosis from alcoholism; this may be related to gastric mucosal levels of alcohol dehydrogenase. Liver enzymes may be relatively normal in cirrhosis without alcoholic hepatitis. Concomitant HCV infection is common in patients with alcoholic liver disease. The prognosis of alcoholic cirrhosis depends on whether patients continue to drink and whether there are symptoms (jaundice, ascites, gastrointestinal bleeding) of chronic liver disease. The 5-year survival for patients without ascites, jaundice, or hematemesis and who abstain is 89%, and for those with symptoms and who continue to drink, it is 34%. Liver transplantation is an option for patients with end-stage alcoholic liver disease as long as they have abstained from alcohol for 6 months or longer.

- Cirrhosis of alcoholics is micronodular.
- Only 60% of patients with alcoholic cirrhosis have signs or symptoms of liver disease.
- Women are more predisposed to cirrhosis from alcoholism.
- Liver enzymes may be relatively normal.
- 5-Year survival for patients without ascites, jaundice, or hematemesis and who abstain is 89%.
- 5-Year survival for those with symptoms and who continue to drink is 34%.
- Liver transplantation is an option.

Nonalcoholic Steatohepatitis

Nonalcoholic steatohepatitis (NASH) is a common cause of abnormal liver tests. About 60% of patients with NASH are obese or have hyperlipidemia or diabetes mellitus. The aminotransferase levels are usually abnormal, and the alkaline phosphatase level is increased in about one-third of patients. By definition, all patients have fatty change and inflammation on histologic examination of the liver, and some have fibrosis and even cirrhosis. The pathogenesis of NASH is uncertain, and the effect of weight loss and control of hyperlipidemia and hyperglycemia is variable. From 20% to 30% of patients with NASH have progression to cirrhosis.

Chronic Cholestatic Liver Diseases

Primary Biliary Cirrhosis

Primary biliary cirrhosis is a chronic, progressive, cholestatic liver disease that primarily affects middle-aged women. Its cause is unknown but appears to involve an immunologic disturbance resulting in small bile duct destruction. Many patients are identified because of asymptomatic increase of alkaline phosphatase. Common early symptoms are pruritus and fatigue. Patients also may have symptoms due to Hashimoto thyroiditis or sicca complex. Biochemical features include increased alkaline phosphatase and IgM levels. Later, bilirubin concentration increases, the serum level of albumin decreases, and PT is prolonged. Steatorrhea may occur because of progressive cholestasis. Fat-soluble vitamin deficiencies and metabolic bone disease are common.

- Primary biliary cirrhosis primarily affects middle-aged women.
- Common early symptoms: pruritus and fatigue.
- Alkaline phosphatase and IgM levels increase.
- Fat-soluble vitamin deficiencies and metabolic bone disease are common.

Circulating antimitochondrial antibodies (AMA) occur in 90% to 95% of patients. The classic histologic lesion is granulomatous infiltration of septal bile ducts. Recently, ursodeoxycholic acid has been shown to be beneficial in patients with primary biliary cirrhosis by delaying the need for liver transplantation. Cholestyramine may be helpful for pruritus. Fat-soluble vitamin deficiencies should be treated. Cyclosporine, colchicine, and methotrexate are suggested as treatments to arrest disease progression, but the data about them are not conclusive.

- AMA occur in 90%-95% of patients.
- Classic histologic lesion: granulomatous infiltration of septal bile ducts.
- Treatment: ursodeoxycholic acid.

Primary Sclerosing Cholangitis

Primary sclerosing cholangitis (PSC) is a chronic cholestatic liver disease characterized by obliterative inflammatory fibrosis of extra- and intrahepatic bile ducts. An immune mechanism has been implicated. Patients may have an asymptomatic increase in alkaline phosphatase or progressive fatigue, pruritus, and jaundice. Bacterial cholangitis is uncommon unless biliary tract surgery or instrumentation has been performed previously. Cholangiography establishes the diagnosis of PSC, showing short strictures of bile ducts with intervening segments of normal or slightly dilated ducts, producing a beaded appearance. This cholangiographic appearance can be mimicked by that of acquired immunodeficiency syndrome (AIDS) cholangiopathy (due to cytomegalovirus or cryptosporidium) and ischemic cholangiopathy after intra-arterial infusion of fluorodeoxyuridine.

- PSC: obliterative inflammatory fibrosis of extra- and intrahepatic bile ducts.
- An immune mechanism is implicated.
- An asymptomatic increase in alkaline phosphatase.
- Bacterial cholangitis is uncommon.
- Cholangiography establishes the diagnosis.
- AIDS cholangiopathy mimics the cholangiographic appearance of PSC.

The most commonly associated disease accompanying PSC is chronic ulcerative colitis. Ulcerative colitis occurs in 70% of patients with PSC and may antedate, accompany, or even follow the diagnosis of PSC. Proctocolectomy performed for ulcerative colitis has no effect on the development of PSC. Patients with PSC are at higher risk for bile duct cancer; its development may be indicated by rapid clinical deterioration, with jaundice, weight loss, and abdominal pain. Treatment for PSC is generally supportive. Percutaneous or endoscopic balloon dilatation of bile duct strictures may offer palliation, especially in patients with recurrent cholangitis. Many patients have progressive liver disease and require liver transplantation.

- Ulcerative colitis occurs in 70% of patients with PSC.
- Proctocolectomy has no effect on the development of PSC.
- PSC patients are at higher risk for bile duct cancer.
- Treatment for PSC is generally supportive.
- Many patients require liver transplantation.

Hereditary Liver Diseases

Genetic Hemochromatosis

Hemochromatosis is a genetically transmitted disorder of iron metabolism characterized by iron overload. The basic defect may be inappropriately high absorption of iron from the gastrointestinal tract. The gene for genetic hemochromatosis has been identified and termed *HFE*. Genetic hemochromatosis is transmitted in an autosomal recessive manner. In the general population, the heterozygote frequency is 10%. Only homozygotes manifest progressive iron accumulation.

- Genetic hemochromatosis is a disorder of iron metabolism.
- Characteristic: high absorption of iron from the gastrointestinal tract.
- Autosomal recessive transmission.
- Only homozygotes have progressive iron accumulation.

Patients usually present with end-stage disease. The peak incidence is between the ages of 40 and 60 years. Iron overload is manifested more often and earlier in men than women, because women are somewhat protected by menstrual losses of iron. Clinical features include arthropathy, hepatomegaly, skin pigmentation, diabetes mellitus, cardiac dysfunction, and hypogonadism. Routine liver biochemistry studies generally show little disturbance. The serum level of iron is increased, and transferrin saturation is greater than 60%. Serum levels of ferritin are high, and levels greater than 1,000 suggest hemochromatosis. Increased iron and ferritin levels also occur in other liver diseases, particularly alcoholic cirrhosis. Testing for mutations in the *HFE* gene and liver biopsy with quantitation of hepatic iron concentration are standard methods for diagnosing hemochromatosis. Generally, hepatic iron levels in hemochromatosis are greater than 10,000 $\mu g/g$ dry weight.

- Patients usually present with end-stage disease.
- Iron overload is more common in men.
- Clinical features: arthropathy, hepatomegaly, skin pigmentation, diabetes mellitus, cardiac dysfunction, and hypogonadism.
- Serum levels of ferritin are high.
- Standard tests for making the diagnosis: genetic testing and liver biopsy with hepatic iron concentration.

Hemochromatosis is treated with removal of iron by repeated phlebotomies. The standard recommendation is to remove 500 mL per week to the point of mild anemia. A maintenance program of 4 to 8 phlebotomies per year is required. When initiated in the precirrhotic stage, removal of iron can render the liver normal and may improve cardiac function and diabetes mellitus. Treatment does not reverse arthropathy or hypogonadism, nor does it eliminate the increased risk (30%) of hepatocellular carcinoma if cirrhosis has already developed. All first-degree relatives of patients should be evaluated for evidence of iron overload.

- Hemochromatosis is treated with repeated phlebotomies.
- Iron removal can render the liver normal.

- Treatment does not reverse arthropathy, hypogonadism, or eliminate increased risk of hepatocellular carcinoma.
- First-degree relatives should be screened.

Wilson Disease

Wilson disease is an autosomal recessive disorder characterized by increased amounts of copper in tissues. The basic defect involves an inability to prepare copper for biliary excretion. The liver is chiefly involved in children, but neuropsychiatric manifestations are prominent in older patients. The Kayser-Fleischer ring is a brownish pigmented ring at the periphery of the cornea. It is not invariably present and is more frequent in patients with neurologic manifestations. Hepatic forms of Wilson disease include fulminant hepatitis (often accompanied by hemolysis and renal failure), chronic hepatitis, and insidiously developed cirrhosis. The development of hepatocellular carcinoma is rare. Neurologic signs include tremor, rigidity, altered speech, and changes in personality. Fanconi syndrome and premature arthritis may occur.

- Wilson disease: an autosomal recessive disorder characterized by increased copper in tissues.
- Basic defect: inability to prepare copper for biliary excretion.
- Kayser-Fleischer ring: brownish pigmented ring at the periphery of the cornea.
- Hepatocellular carcinoma is rare.
- Neurologic signs: tremor, rigidity, altered speech, and changes in personality.

Evidence of hemolysis (total bilirubin increased out of proportion to direct bilirubin), low or normal level of alkaline phosphatase, and a low serum level of uric acid (due to Fanconi syndrome) suggest Wilson disease. The diagnosis is established on the basis of a low level of ceruloplasmin and an increased urinary concentration of copper. Ceruloplasmin levels can be misleading—they can be increased by estrogen or biliary obstruction and decreased by liver failure of any cause. High concentrations of copper in the liver are found in Wilson disease; similarly high values can also occur in cholestatic syndromes. Penicillamine chelates and increases the urinary excretion of copper. Trientine is an alternative to penicillamine. Zinc inhibits gastrointestinal tract absorption of copper and can be used as adjunctive therapy. All siblings of patients should be evaluated for copper. Liver transplantation corrects the metabolic defect of Wilson disease.

- Diagnosis: low ceruloplasmin and increased urinary concentration of copper.
- High concentrations of liver copper: Wilson disease and cholestatic syndromes.
- Treatment: trientine or penicillamine

- Liver transplantation corrects the metabolic defect.

Alpha₁-Antitrypsin Deficiency

Alpha$_1$-antitrypsin is synthesized in the liver. The gene is on chromosome 14. M is the common normal allele, and Z and S are frequent abnormal alleles. Intrahepatic accumulation of alpha$_1$-antitrypsin in the ZZ phenotype causes liver disease; however, disease occurs in only 10% to 20% of ZZ patients. During the first 6 months of life, the patients often have a history of cholestatic jaundice that resolves. In later childhood or adulthood, cirrhosis may develop. The prevalence of cirrhosis in patients with the MZ phenotype is increased, but the risk is small. Hepatocellular carcinoma can complicate alpha$_1$-antitrypsin deficiency, especially in males. The diagnosis of alpha$_1$-antitrypsin deficiency is made by determining the alpha$_1$-antitrypsin phenotype. The serum levels of alpha$_1$-antitrypsin may vary and be unreliable. Liver transplantation corrects the metabolic defect and changes the recipient's phenotype to that of the donor.

- Intrahepatic accumulation of alpha$_1$-antitrypsin causes liver disease.
- During the first 6 months of life, cholestatic jaundice resolves.
- Hepatocellular carcinoma can complicate alpha$_1$-antitrypsin deficiency, especially in males.
- The diagnosis is made by determining the alpha$_1$-antitrypsin phenotype.
- Liver transplantation corrects the metabolic defect.

Fulminant Hepatic Failure

Fulminant hepatic failure is defined as hepatic failure with encephalopathy developing less than 8 weeks after the onset of jaundice in patients with no history of liver disease. Its common causes are listed in Table 8-21. Poor prognostic markers include a drug-induced cause (other than acetaminophen), older age, grade 3 or 4 encephalopathy, acidosis, and PT greater than 3.5 INR. Treatment is supportive, and steroids offer no benefit. Patients should be transferred to a medical center where liver transplantation is available.

- Fulminant hepatic failure: hepatic failure with encephalopathy developing <8 weeks after the onset of jaundice and in patients with no history of liver disease.
- Poor prognostic markers: drug-induced (not acetaminophen), older age, grade 3 or 4 encephalopathy, PT >3.5 INR.
- Steroids offer no benefit.

Drug-Induced Liver Disease

Drugs cause toxic effects in the liver in many ways, often mimicking naturally occurring liver disease. Most drug-induced

Table 8-21.—Common Causes of Fulminant Hepatic Failure

Infective
    Hepatitis virus A, B, C(?), D, E
    Herpes simplex
Drug reactions and toxins
    Halothane
    Isoniazid-rifampicin
    Antidepressants
    Nonsteroidal anti-inflammatory drugs
    Valproic acid
    Acetaminophen overdose
    Mushroom poisoning
    Herbal remedies
Ischemic
    Ischemic hepatitis ("shock" liver)
    Acute Budd-Chiari syndrome
Metabolic
    Wilson disease
    Fatty liver of pregnancy
    Reye syndrome
Miscellaneous (rare)
    Massive malignant infiltration
    Severe bacterial infection

From Sherlock S, Dooley J: Diseases of the Liver and Biliary System. Ninth edition. Oxford, Blackwell Scientific Publications, 1993, p 102. By permission of publisher.

liver disorders are idiosyncratic and not dose-related; 2% of the cases of jaundice in hospitalized patients and 25% of the cases of fulminant hepatitis are drug-induced. Consequently, all drugs that have been used by a patient with liver disease must be identified.

Acetaminophen toxicity may occur at relatively low doses in alcoholics, because alcohol induces hepatic microsomal P450 enzymes, which metabolize acetaminophen to its toxic metabolite. Disulfiram can also cause fulminant hepatitis. Amoxicillin/clavulinic acid causes severe cholestatic hepatitis, and valproic acid, tetracycline, and zidovudine can cause severe steatosis. Amiodarone may cause hepatotoxicity, whose histologic features can mimic those of alcoholic liver disease. Methotrexate in a total dose of more than 2 g can cause hepatic fibrosis; some physicians advocate annual liver biopsies in patients receiving long-term methotrexate treatment for psoriasis or rheumatoid arthritis. Intravenous cocaine can cause massive necrosis and death, probably because of ischemia. Trovafloxacin and troglitazone are newer agents that have been associated with acute hepatitis.

- Most drug-induced liver disorders are idiosyncratic, not dose-related.
- 2% of cases of jaundice (hospitalized patients) and 25% of cases of fulminant hepatitis are drug-induced.
- Identify all drugs that have been used by a patient with liver disease.
- In alcoholics, acetaminophen toxicity may occur at relatively low doses.
- Amoxicillin/clavulinic acid causes severe cholestatic hepatitis.
- Amiodarone may cause hepatotoxicity.
- A total dose of methotrexate >2 g can cause hepatic fibrosis.
- Intravenous cocaine can cause massive necrosis.

Liver Tumors

Hepatocellular Carcinoma

The risk of hepatocellular carcinoma is increased in cirrhosis of nearly any cause but particularly if due to HBV, HCV, hemochromatosis, or alcoholic liver disease. Alpha-fetoprotein is increased in only 50% of patients with hepatocellular carcinoma. Common metastatic sites are lymph nodes, lung, bone, and brain. Paraneoplastic syndromes include gynecomastia, hypercalcemia, hypoglycemia, polycythemia, and clubbing. Liver transplantation is an option for selected patients, particularly those with cirrhosis. Percutaneous alcohol ablation may be useful for small tumors.

- The risk of hepatocellular carcinoma is increased in cirrhosis of nearly any cause.
- Alpha-fetoprotein is increased in 50% of patients with hepatocellular carcinoma.
- Common metastatic sites: lymph nodes, lung, bone, and brain.
- Paraneoplastic syndromes: gynecomastia, hypercalcemia, hypoglycemia, polycythemia, and clubbing.
- Liver transplantation: an option for selected patients.

Cholangiocarcinoma

The incidence of cholangiocarcinoma is increased in patients with PSC, *Opisthorchis* infection, and a history of choledochal cysts. Cholangiocarcinoma can be difficult to diagnose, especially in patients with PSC. For most patients, surgical resection is the treatment of choice, although resection is not possible in many patients.

Adenoma

Adenomas are associated with the use of oral contraceptives. Patients can present with acute right upper quadrant pain and hemodynamic compromise because of bleeding.

Cavernous Hemangioma

Cavernous hemangioma is the most common benign tumor of the liver. CT scan with contrast agent is often diagnostic.

Metastases

Metastases are more common than primary tumors of the liver. Frequent primary sites are the colon, stomach, breast, lung, and pancreas. Surgical resection of isolated colon cancer metastases has limited effect on long-term survival.

Complications of End-Stage Liver Disease

Ascites

The pathogenesis of ascites is disputed but probably involves a combination of decreased effective circulatory blood volume (underfill theory) and inappropriate renal sodium retention with expansion of plasma volume (overfill theory). The initial event may be vasodilatation. Patients with ascites generally have a low urinary concentration of sodium. The treatment of ascites involves sodium restriction, diuretics, and (occasionally) fluid restriction. Generally, spironolactone (100-200 mg/day) is used initially, although a low dose of furosemide (20-40 mg) is often added. The goal is to increase urinary sodium and to allow the loss of 1 L of ascitic fluid (1 kg weight) per day. Paracentesis is indicated for diagnostic purposes and should be done therapeutically in patients with tense ascites or with respiratory compromise from abdominal distention. Large-volume or even total paracentesis in combination with 6 g of albumin per liter of ascitic fluid removed is safe and well tolerated.

- The pathogenesis of ascites probably involves a combination of decreased effective circulatory blood volume and inappropriate renal sodium retention with expansion of plasma volume.
- Patients generally have a low urinary concentration of sodium.
- Treatment: sodium restriction, diuretics.
- Large-volume paracentesis is safe and well tolerated.

Pleural effusion occurs in 6% of patients with cirrhosis and is right-sided in 67%. Edema usually follows ascites and is related to hypoalbuminemia and possibly increased pressure on the inferior vena cava by the intra-abdominal fluid. The sudden onset of ascites should raise the possibility of hepatic venous outflow obstruction (Budd-Chiari syndrome). Tests most useful for determining the cause of ascites are measurements of total protein and the serum-ascitic fluid albumin gradient [albumin (serum) minus albumin (ascites)]. An albumin gradient greater than 1.1 g/dL almost always indicates portal hypertension. Ascites secondary to portal hypertension induced by congestive heart failure can be distinguished from cirrhotic ascites because congestive heart failure usually has an ascitic fluid protein greater than 2.5. Exudative ascites from cancer or tuberculosis generally has an ascitic fluid protein greater than 2.5 and an albumin gradient less than 1.1 (Table 8-22).

Refractory ascites is uncommon. Most physicians advocate therapeutic paracentesis as needed. Peritoneovenous shunts are complicated by disseminated intravascular coagulation and shunt malfunction and, in comparison with diuretics and paracentesis, do not improve survival. Transjugular intrahepatic portosystemic shunts (TIPS) are effective in some patients with refractory ascites.

- Pleural effusion occurs in 6% of patients with cirrhosis and is right-sided in 67%.
- The sudden onset of ascites raises the possibility of hepatic venous outflow obstruction (Budd-Chiari syndrome).
- An albumin gradient >1.1 g/dL almost always indicates portal hypertension.
- Peritoneovenous shunts do not improve survival.

Spontaneous Bacterial Peritonitis

Spontaneous bacterial peritonitis occurs in 10% to 20% of cirrhotic patients with ascites. It is defined as a bacterial infection of ascitic fluid without any intra-abdominal source of infection. Fever, abdominal pain, and abdominal tenderness are classic symptoms; however, many patients have few or no symptoms. Spontaneous bacterial peritonitis should be suspected in any patient with cirrhotic ascites. For all patients, diagnostic paracentesis is advisable as an initial step. Coagulopathy and thrombocytopenia should not prohibit performing diagnostic paracentesis. A cell count and culture of ascitic fluid should be performed on all patients. Bedside inoculation of blood culture bottles with ascitic fluid increases the diagnostic yield. Spontaneous bacterial peritonitis is more common in patients with large-volume ascites and those with

Table 8-22.—Use of Single Measurements to Determine the Cause of Ascites

	Serum-ascites albumin gradient, g/dL	Ascites protein, g/dL
Cirrhosis	>1.1	<2.5
Congestive heart failure	>1.1	>2.5
Malignancy	<1.1	>2.5

a low ascitic fluid protein (<1.5 g). Also, blood from all patients with spontaneous bacterial peritonitis should be cultured, because almost 50% of these cultures will be positive. Variants of spontaneous bacterial peritonitis are listed in Table 8-23.

Spontaneous bacterial peritonitis and culture-negative neutrocytic ascites should be treated with a third-generation cephalosporin. The response to antibiotics should be assessed by repeat paracentesis 48 hours after the initiation of therapy. The polymorphonuclear count should decrease by 50% and cultures should be sterile. The hospital mortality rate of spontaneous bacterial peritonitis is 50% to 70%, and even if a patient survives hospitalization, the 1-year mortality rate is 60% to 80%. A polymicrobial infection of ascitic fluid should prompt a search for an intra-abdominal focus of infection; spontaneous bacterial peritonitis nearly always involves one organism. The presence of bacterascites is thought to be due to contamination, and repeat paracentesis is advised.

- Spontaneous bacterial peritonitis occurs in 10% to 20% of cirrhotic patients with ascites.
- Classic symptoms: fever, abdominal pain, and abdominal tenderness.

- Many patients have few or no symptoms.
- Bedside inoculation of blood culture bottles with ascites increases the diagnostic yield.
- Spontaneous bacterial peritonitis is more common in cases of large-volume ascites and in patients with low ascitic fluid protein (<1.5 g).
- Spontaneous bacterial peritonitis nearly always involves only one organism.

Hepatorenal Syndrome

Hepatorenal syndrome, or functional renal failure, consists of renal failure with normal tubular function in patients with portal hypertension. The differential diagnosis is given in Table 8-24. Hepatorenal syndrome is difficult to distinguish from prerenal azotemia; thus, a brief trial of colloid expansion may be needed. Hepatorenal syndrome is often precipitated by vigorous diuretic therapy. Treatment is supportive, although TIPS has been useful in a few patients. After liver transplantation is performed, kidney function returns to normal.

- Hepatorenal syndrome: renal failure with normal tubular function in a cirrhotic patient.

Table 8-23.—Variants of Spontaneous Bacterial Peritonitis

	Ascitic fluid poly-morphonuclear cells, no. cells/mL	Ascitic fluid cultures
Spontaneous bacterial peritonitis	>250	Positive
Culture-negative neutrocytic ascites	>250	Negative
Bacterascites	<250	Positive

Table 8-24.—Differential Diagnosis for Hepatorenal Syndrome

	Prerenal azotemia	Hepatorenal syndrome	Acute renal failure
Urinary sodium concentration, mEq/L	<10	<10	>30
Urine-to-plasma creatinine ratio	>30:1	>30:1	<20:1
Urinary osmolality	At least 100 mOsm > plasma osmolality	At least 100 mOsm > plasma osmolality	Equal to plasma osmolality
Urinary sediment	Normal	Unremarkable	Casts, debris

From Epstein M: Functional renal abnormalities in cirrhosis: pathophysiology and management. *In* Hepatology: A Textbook of Liver Disease. Vol 2. Second edition. Edited by D Zakim, TD Boyer. Philadelphia, WB Saunders Company, 1990, pp 493-512. By permission of publisher.

- It is difficult to distinguish from prerenal azotemia.
- It is often precipitated by vigorous diuretic therapy.
- After liver transplantation, kidney function returns to normal.

Portal Systemic Encephalopathy

Portal systemic encephalopathy is a reversible decrease in the level of consciousness in patients with severe liver disease. Disturbed consciousness, personality change, intellectual deterioration, and slowed speech are common manifestations. The electroencephalogram is often abnormal, and patients often have asterixis (flapping tremor). The grading system commonly used for portal systemic encephalopathy is given in Table 8-25.

The sudden development of portal systemic encephalopathy in patients with stable cirrhosis should prompt a search for bleeding, infection, or electrolyte disturbances; however, simple precipitating events may include increased dietary protein or constipation. Serum or arterial levels of ammonia are usually increased. Treatment consists of dietary protein restriction and lactulose. Lactulose has a laxative effect to decrease the nitrogenous compounds presented to the liver. Oral neomycin can be used as an adjunct to lactulose.

- Portal systemic encephalopathy: reversible decrease in the level of consciousness in patients with severe liver disease.
- The electroencephalogram is often abnormal.
- Patients often have asterixis, or flapping tremor.
- Sudden development of portal systemic encephalopathy: look for bleeding, infection, or electrolyte disturbances.
- Treatment: dietary protein restriction and lactulose.

Variceal Hemorrhage

Esophageal varices are collateral vessels that develop because of portal hypertension. Varices can also occur in other parts of the gut. Most cirrhotic patients with varices do not hemorrhage, but a first hemorrhage has a 10% to 30% mortality. Bleeding is generally massive. Early endoscopy is indicated for diagnosis and treatment. Endoscopic therapy consists of sclerotherapy or band ligation. Octreotide decreases portal venous pressure and may help stop the hemorrhage. Isolated gastric varices without esophageal varices can occur with sinistral (left-sided) portal hypertension due to splenic vein thrombosis.

- Esophageal varices are collateral vessels that develop because of portal hypertension.
- Most cirrhotic patients with varices do not hemorrhage.
- First hemorrhage: 10%-30% mortality.
- Bleeding is generally massive.
- Early endoscopy is indicated for diagnosis and treatment.

Recurrent bleeding occurs in 80% to 100% of patients within 2 years. Propranolol or nadolol given orally can help prevent rebleeding, although most physicians advocate endoscopic variceal ligation until the varices have been obliterated. Patients with refractory bleeding are candidates for shunting. Surgical shunts have a high rate of mortality and morbidity and are complicated by portal systemic encephalopathy. TIPS is effective in controlling bleeding and has the advantage of avoiding an operation. The incidence of portal systemic encephalopa-

Table 8-25.—Grading System for Portal Systemic Encephalopathy

Grade of encephalopathy	Level of consciousness	Neurologic abnormalities	EEG abnormalities
0	Normal	None	None
1	Trivial lack of awareness	Slight tremor Uncoordination	Symmetric slowing (5-6 cps)
	Personality change Day-night reversal	Asterixis	Triphasic waves
2	Lethargic Inappropriate behavior	Asterixis Abnormal reflexes	Symmetric slowing Triphasic waves
3	Asleep but arousable Confused when awake	Asterixis Abnormal reflexes	Symmetric slowing Triphasic waves
4	Unarousable	Babinski response Decerebrate posture Pupillary responses preserved	Very slow (2-3 cps) delta activity

cps, cycles per second; EEG, electroencephalogram.
From Schafer DF, Jones EA: Hepatic encephalopathy. *In* Hepatology: A Textbook of Liver Disease. Vol 1. Second edition. Edited by D Zakim, TD Boyer. Philadelphia, WB Saunders Company, 1990, pp 447-460. By permission of publisher.

thy after TIPS is 10% to 40%, but it usually can be controlled with medical therapy.

- Rebleeding occurs in 80%-100% of patients.
- Patients with refractory bleeding are candidates for shunting.
- The incidence of portal systemic encephalopathy after transjugular intrahepatic portal systemic shunting is 10%-40%.

Biliary Tract Disease

Gallstones and Cholecystitis

Gallstones can be cholesterol or pigment. Cholesterol gallstones occur when bile is supersaturated with cholesterol relative to bile salts. Excessive cholesterol secretion (females, obesity, exogenous estrogens) or deficient bile acid secretion (bile acid sequestrant therapy) can lead to cholesterol gallstones. Pigment stones can occur with hemolysis or cirrhosis, but usually there is no identifying cause. Ultrasonography is 90% to 97% sensitive for detecting gallstones. Cholecystitis may be suggested by gallbladder contraction, marked distention, surrounding fluid, or wall thickening. Ultrasonography also offers the opportunity to detect dilated bile ducts. If radionuclide biliary scanning is performed during an episode of pain, it is helpful in diagnosing cystic duct obstruction with cholecystitis. Positive test results are marked by nonvisualization of the gallbladder despite biliary excretion of radioisotope.

- Cholesterol gallstones occur when bile is supersaturated with cholesterol.
- Pigment stones can occur with hemolysis or cirrhosis.
- Ultrasonography is 90%-97% sensitive for detecting gallstones.
- Radionuclide biliary scanning helps diagnose cystic duct obstruction with cholecystitis.

Asymptomatic gallstones require no therapy, even in high-risk patients. Patients with episodes of biliary colic or acute cholecystitis should have cholecystectomy. Laparoscopic cholecystectomy is the procedure of choice. High surgical risk patients can undergo percutaneous cholecystostomy as a temporary measure. Stone dissolution with ursodeoxycholic acid should be used for only small CT-radiolucent cholesterol stones. This treatment needs to be given for 6 to 24 months.

- Asymptomatic gallstones require no therapy.
- Procedure of choice: laparoscopic cholecystectomy.
- Use ursodeoxycholic acid for only small CT-radiolucent cholesterol stones.

Bile Duct Stones

Most bile duct stones originate in the gallbladder, although a few patients have primary duct stones. CT and ultrasonography are relatively insensitive for common bile duct stones, and diagnosis generally requires cholangiography usually accomplished via endoscopic retrograde cholangiopancreatography (ERCP). Patients can have minimal or no symptoms due to common bile duct stone or they can have life-threatening cholangitis with abdominal pain, fever, and jaundice. Common bile duct stones should be removed. This can be done in 90% of patients with ERCP. The urgency of the procedure depends on the clinical presentation. Patients with minimal symptoms can have elective ERCP, but those with cholangitis and fever unresponsive to antibiotics should have urgent endoscopic treatment. Patients with gallbladder stones who have a sphincterotomy and clearance of their duct stones have only a 10% chance of having further problems with their gallbladder stones.

- Most bile duct stones originate in the gallbladder.
- Diagnosis of common bile duct stones usually requires cholangiography.
- Common bile duct stones should be removed.
- Urgent endoscopic treatment is needed if cholangitis and fever are unresponsive to antibiotics.

Benign Biliary Tract Strictures

Most benign biliary strictures are iatrogenic. They were especially common in the early days of laparoscopic cholecystectomy. Such strictures are usually treated surgically.

Malignant Biliary Obstruction

Malignant biliary obstruction is usually due to carcinoma of the head of the pancreas, bile duct cancer, or metastatic cancer to hilar nodes. If the disease is unresectable, palliative endoscopic or percutaneous stenting is as effective as surgical bypass. One exception is impending duodenal obstruction, at which time operation offers the opportunity for bypass of both biliary and duodenal obstruction. A major complication of stenting is occlusion of the stents, which occurs in 1 to 6 months.

- The usual causes of malignant biliary obstruction: carcinoma of the head of the pancreas, bile duct cancer, and metastatic cancer to hilar nodes.
- Palliative endoscopic or percutaneous stenting is as effective as surgical bypass.
- The major complication of stenting: occlusion of the stents.

Gallbladder Carcinoma

Gallbladder carcinoma has a strong association with calcified (porcelain) gallbladder. For this reason, cholecystectomy is advised in patients with porcelain gallbladder.

Sphincter of Oddi Dysfunction

Sphincter of Oddi dysfunction is a poorly defined entity characterized by right upper quadrant pain without any structural cause. Patients with typical biliary-type pain, increased values on liver tests during the pain, a dilated common bile duct, and delayed drainage of contrast after cholangiography often have improvement after sphincterotomy. Patients without all these criteria generally have a poor response to sphincterotomy.

QUESTIONS

Multiple Choice (choose the one best answer)

1. You are asked to evaluate a 54-year-old man because of difficulty swallowing. For 6 months, he has had increasing difficulty swallowing solids, especially meats, and he has lost 10 pounds. Otherwise, he has been in excellent health and has no other complaints. He has smoked 1 pack of cigarettes daily for 30 years and has taken medications for chronic heartburn for 20 years. Upper gastrointestinal radiography shows narrowing of the esophageal lumen in the mid esophagus, with a small ulcer present. Which of the following is the most likely explanation of these findings?
   a. Achalasia
   b. Diffuse esophageal spasm
   c. Esophageal ring
   d. Barrett esophagus
   e. Nonspecific esophageal motility disorder

2. You are called to the emergency department to evaluate a 27-year-old woman. Four hours ago while eating turkey, she felt something "stick" in the lower chest. She has been unable to vomit and has attempted to swallow water but has not been able to swallow anything. Over the last 2 years, she has had multiple episodes of solid food sticking in the lower chest but was able to "throw up" and the episodes resolved. She denies heartburn and weight loss and is otherwise healthy. Physical examination findings are normal. Which of the following is the most likely explanation of her findings?
   a. Achalasia
   b. Diffuse esophageal spasm
   c. Lower esophageal ring
   d. Peptic stricture
   e. Nonspecific esophageal motility disorder

3. A 37-year-old woman has difficulty swallowing. Over the last 4 years, she has had several episodes of food sticking in the lower esophagus, which were relieved by drinking water. For the last 6 months, she has had difficulty swallowing both solids and liquids and has lost 10 pounds. Upper gastrointestinal radiography shows a smooth beak-like tapering of the distal esophagus and dilatation of the proximal esophagus. Esophagogastroduodenoscopic results are normal. Which of the following is the most likely explanation of her symptoms?
   a. Peptic stricture
   b. Lower esophageal ring
   c. Achalasia
   d. Diffuse esophageal spasm
   e. Nonspecific motility disorder

4. A 49-year-old executive is referred for evaluation of chest pain for 4 months. He describes several episodes of a deep substernal chest pain lasting 30 to 60 minutes, then resolving spontaneously. He exercises regularly and denies exertional chest pain. A cardiology evaluation, including resting and exercise electrocardiograms and coronary angiography, is normal. Results of esophagogastroduodenoscopy with biopsy of the lower esophagus are also normal. His father died of heart disease, and he is very worried about this pain. Which of the following is the next best step in the evaluation of this patient?
   a. Upper gastrointestinal radiography
   b. Computed tomography of the chest
   c. Magnetic resonance imaging of the chest
   d. Bernstein test (acid profusion test)
   e. Esophageal motility study

5. A 39-year-old woman complains of coughing and choking with swallowing and sticking of food in the neck. On occasion, she has had regurgitation of swallowed liquids

into her nose. All the following conditions could explain her symptoms *except*:

a. Achalasia
b. Zenker diverticulum
c. Myasthenia gravis
d. Multiple sclerosis
e. Amyotrophic lateral sclerosis

6. A 27-year-old man with acquired immunodeficiency syndrome has odynophagia for 1 week. Probable causes of his symptoms include all of the following *except*:

a. *Candida*
b. Herpes
c. Cytomegalovirus
d. Bullous pemphigoid

7. A 77-year-old woman, who is taking multiple medications, developed odynophagia 3 days ago. She denies heartburn but has noticed some dysphagia for solids, which is relieved by drinking liquids. Upper gastrointestinal radiography shows inflammation in the mid esophagus, with sparing of the distal esophagus. All the following medications may explain these findings *except*:

a. Potassium supplements
b. Tetracycline
c. Nonsteroidal anti-inflammatory drugs
d. Calcium channel blockers
e. Ascorbic acid

8. A 39-year-old man comes to the free clinic with abdominal discomfort and frequent indigestion. He is a migrant worker, and his eating habits are irregular. He has had two previous upper gastrointestinal radiographic studies, which have demonstrated duodenal ulcers. He denies taking nonsteroidal anti-inflammatory drugs and aspirin, and he does not drink alcohol. A rapid serologic test for *Helicobacter pylori* is positive. Which of the following is the most appropriate next step in his management?

a. Refer for esophagogastroduodenoscopy
b. Perform esophagogastroduodenoscopy and obtain biopsies for *Helicobacter pylori*
c. Determine the serum level of gastrin
d. Treat with antisecretory agents
e. Treat with antibiotics and antisecretory agents

9. A 44-year-old woman has chronic indigestion. She had a duodenal ulcer documented by endoscopy several years ago. She has continued to have dyspepsia and recently has developed diarrhea. She denies taking nonsteroidal anti-inflammatory drugs, aspirin, and alcohol. Her father and brother have had surgery for ulcers. Physical examination

findings are normal. Laboratory evaluation, including complete blood count, and chemistry profiles are normal *except* for calcium of 10.8 mg/dL. A rapid serologic test for *Helicobacter pylori* is negative. Which of the following is the most likely explanation for her symptoms?

a. Nonulcer dyspepsia
b. Gastroesophageal reflux
c. Peptic ulcer disease due to alcohol
d. Peptic ulcer disease due to *Helicobacter pylori* infection
e. Zollinger-Ellison syndrome

10. A 70-year-old man has progressive dysphagia for solids and a 20-pound weight loss over 2 months. He has no previous history of heartburn. Esophagogastroduodenoscopy shows an ulcerated narrowing in the mid esophagus, and biopsy findings are consistent with squamous cell carcinoma. All the following clinical conditions could predispose to esophageal squamous cell carcinoma *except*:

a. Alcohol ingestion
b. Smoking
c. Gastroesophageal reflux disease
d. Achalasia
e. Human papilloma virus

11. A 43-year-old business executive has had diarrhea for 3 days. She has just returned from a business trip to Mexico and noticed her first loose stool on the flight home. She has been having 6 to 7 loose watery stools daily with no blood. She denies fever but has lost 2 pounds. She is in excellent health otherwise and takes no medication. It is inconvenient for her to have such frequent stools. Physical examination findings are normal. Which of the following is the most appropriate course of action at this time?

a. Metronidazole 250 mg t.i.d.
b. Amoxicillin 250 mg q.i.d.
c. Ciprofloxacin 500 mg t.i.d.
d. Stools for culture and sensitivity, ova and parasites, and *Clostridium difficile* toxin assay
e. Advise that she force fluids, and offer her an antimotility agent

12. A 26-year-old woman is evaluated for diarrhea of 1 month. She has had 3 or 4 loose watery, nonbloody stools daily for 1 month. She denies fever and has not been traveling or camping. She has lost 8 pounds intentionally by strictly adhering to a diet over the last month. She has been drinking a lot of diet soda and chewing sugarless gum. Physical examination findings are normal. She appears well hydrated and has no orthostatic blood pressure or pulse changes. Laboratory report: her stools are loose and brown. No

fecal leukocytes are present. Which of the following is the most likely explanation of her symptoms?

a. Secretory diarrhea from a toxigenic bacteria
b. Secretory diarrhea from a hormone-producing tumor
c. Osmotic diarrhea from lactase deficiency
d. Osmotic diarrhea from sorbitol ingestion
e. Diarrhea from a bacterial pathogen

13. A 54-year-old executive is evaluated for diarrhea of 3 months. He has been having 2 or 3 loose brown stools daily for 3 months. He denies fever, weight loss, and has never observed blood in his stools. He denies travel other than a fishing trip to remote areas of Canada. He is otherwise in excellent health. Physical examination findings are normal. Which of the following is the most appropriate course of action at this time?

a. Advise him to drink fluids, and offer an antimotility agent
b. Obtain stool for culture and sensitivity, ova, and parasites
c. Amoxicillin 250 mg q.i.d.
d. Ciprofloxacin 500 mg t.i.d.
e. Metronidazole 250 mg t.i.d.

14. A 22-year-old medical student comes to the emergency room, passing bright red blood per rectum. He is in excellent health; however, he has had 2 previous episodes of blood per rectum at ages 16 and 19 years. Previous evaluations, including stool studies and colonoscopy, have not disclosed a bleeding source. He has been told he had hemorrhoidal bleeding. Physical examination findings are normal. Rectal examination shows bloody red liquid stools. No hemorrhoids are found. Which of the following is the most likely explanation of his symptoms?

a. Crohn disease involving the terminal ileum
b. Juvenile polyps
c. Meckel diverticulum
d. Ulcerative colitis
e. Aortoenteric fistula

15. A 34-year-old schoolteacher is referred for edema for 2 years. He first noticed swelling of his left leg, but for the last 3 months both legs have "become swollen" and the edema has increased. He has also noticed dyspnea on exertion for 1 month. Physical examination reveals 4+ pitting edema of both legs. Examination of the chest reveals dullness and decreased breath sounds at both bases. A complete blood count shows 4,000 leukocytes, 65% segmented neutrophils, 3% eosinophils, 3% band forms, 1% basophils, 5% lymphocytes, and 7% monocytes. Total

protein is 4.0 g/dL; albumin, 2.5 g/dL; globulin, 2.3 g/dL. Urinalysis is normal, with no urine protein. Which of the following is the most likely explanation of these findings?

a. Bacterial overgrowth of small intestine
b. Crohn disease
c. Abetalipoproteinemia
d. Idiopathic cyclic edema
e. Intestinal lymphangiectasia

16. An 18-year-old college freshman comes to the outpatient clinic with nausea, abdominal pain, and diarrhea for 3 to 4 weeks. Her symptoms follow meals; however, she has not been able to identify specific foods that cause worse symptoms. She denies fever and has not been traveling or camping. She is allergic to pollens, dusts, and mold but has had no recent symptoms of allergic rhinitis, and she is not taking any medications. She acknowledges that the demands of school and playing on the basketball team have been stressful. Physical examination findings are normal. The complete blood count is normal, leukocyte count is 9,600, with 60% segmented neutrophils, 4% band forms, 15% eosinophils, and 24% lymphocytes. Stools for ova and parasites and culture and sensitivity are negative. Which of the following is the most likely explanation of her symptoms?

a. Irritable bowel syndrome
b. Infection with *Giardia lamblia*
c. Infection with *Entamoeba histolytica*
d. Eosinophilic gastroenteritis
e. Chronic pancreatitis

17. A 40-year-old woman has osteomalacia and an iron deficiency anemia. Stool studies are negative for occult blood and show a stool fat of 20 g/24 h. She has had no previous surgery. In addition to hypochromic microcytic red blood cells, a peripheral blood smear shows Howell-Jolly bodies. The most likely explanation for this woman's condition is:

a. Whipple disease
b. Intestinal lymphangiectasia
c. Tropical sprue
d. Celiac sprue
e. Bacterial overgrowth

18. A 70-year-old man complains of diarrhea and 4 episodes of arthritis over the last 3 months. His family thinks he is becoming more forgetful. On examination, he appears hyperpigmented and has generalized lymphadenopathy. Stool fat is 20 g/24 hr. Small bowel biopsy shows PAS-positive granules in macrophages in the lamina propria of the small intestine. The most likely cause of this

patient's condition is:

a. Tropic sprue
b. Intestinal lymphangiectasia
c. Abetalipoproteinemia
d. Whipple disease
e. *Vibrio vulnificus* infection

19. All the following enteric pathogens have been found with increased frequency in AIDS *except*:

a. *Cytomegalovirus*
b. *Mycobacterium avium-intracellulare*
c. *Cryptosporidium*
d. *Giardia lamblia*
e. *Salmonella*

20. A 50-year-old man has diarrhea and 10-pound weight loss for 3 months. He has not traveled. Physical examination reveals a large tongue with furrowed edges, a systolic murmur along the left sternal border that increases with inspiration, hepatomegaly, and diminished vibratory sensation in both feet. Complete blood count and chemistry screening profile are normal, and urinalysis shows 4+ proteinuria. Which of the following is the most likely explanation for these findings?

a. Celiac sprue
b. Whipple disease
c. Progressive systemic sclerosis
d. Amyloidosis
e. Intestinal lymphangiectasia

21. A 64-year-old woman has left lower quadrant abdominal pain and constipation. On physical examination, her temperature is 38.3°C (101°F) and a tender left lower quadrant abdominal mass is palpable. Laboratory studies include a normal abdominal radiograph and a complete blood count showing 15,000 leukocytes, with a left shift. The most appropriate management would include:

a. Obtain stool cultures, blood cultures, and perform flexible sigmoidoscopy
b. Obtain stool cultures and schedule a return visit in 2 days for review of the culture report
c. Obtain stool cultures, begin oral antibiotics, and instruct the patient to schedule a return appointment if her symptoms do not improve
d. Admit to the hospital, allow nothing by mouth, begin treatment with intravenous sulfides and antibiotics, and obtain a surgical consultation
e. Emergency surgery

22. A 65-year-old woman has recurrent red rectal bleeding. Physical examination findings are normal *except* for aortic stenosis. A flexible sigmoidoscopy to 30 cm is normal. Colon radiography is normal, and upper GI endoscopy is normal. What is the most appropriate next step of her diagnostic evaluation?

a. Radionuclide bleeding scan
b. Angiography
c. Colonoscopy
d. Small-bowel radiography
e. Small-bowel endoscopy

23. A 75-year-old woman has lower abdominal pain and bloody diarrhea. Proctoscopic examination to 30 cm is normal, and colon radiography shows "thumb-printing" of the splenic flexure. Risk factors for the development of her condition include all the following *except*:

a. Hypertension
b. Diabetes mellitus
c. Diverticulosis
d. Atherosclerosis

24. A 64-year-old man comes to the outpatient clinic with fever, abdominal pain, and diarrhea of 2 days. He was dismissed from the hospital 3 weeks ago after a 4-day admission for treatment of pyelonephritis. Two days ago he developed 3 or 4 loose watery brown stools with a small amount of blood and mucus. He then noticed mild cramping in the left lower quadrant and a temperature of 99.6°F. There is mild tenderness over the left lower quadrant. Laboratory examination includes normal findings on urinalysis, complete blood count, and abdominal radiography. Sigmoidoscopy shows discrete areas of well-demarcated white exudate-like material. Which of the following is the next best step in this patient's management?

a. Stool for ova and parasites
b. Stool for culture and sensitivity
c. Stool for *Clostridium difficile* toxin assay
d. Colonoscopy with biopsy
e. Colon radiography

25. A 62-year-old man comes to the emergency room with abdominal pain, vomiting, and diarrhea of 12 hours' duration. He describes the sudden onset 12 hours ago of a mid-abdominal pain that has increased in severity. He passed 3 stools; the last stool 1 hour ago was bloody. He vomited shortly after arrival in the emergency room. He has a medical history of stable class II angina and a history of nephrolithiasis but is otherwise healthy. Physical examination reveals a man who is in obvious distress because of abdominal pain. His vital signs are normal *except* for an irregular pulse with a rate of 126/min. Complete blood count, urinalysis, electrolytes, and creatinine are normal.

Chest radiographic findings are normal. Electrocardiogram shows atrial fibrillation with no evidence for acute ischemia. Abdominal radiography shows a small distended loop of small intestine in mid abdomen. Serum amylase is 196. Which of the following is the most likely explanation of these findings?

a. Acute pancreatitis
b. Acute cholecystitis
c. Acute ileus
d. Acute mesenteric ischemia
e. Nephrolithiasis

26. A 55-year-old man has diarrhea and weight loss of 4 months' duration. He describes his stool as pale, light-colored, with oil droplets. He has lost 26 pounds. His appetite has been good. He denies recent abdominal pain. He takes no medication, does not smoke, and drinks alcohol "socially." Physical examination findings are normal. Laboratory evaluation includes normal electrolytes and creatinine; blood glucose is 150; albumin, 2.8; serum amylase, 114. Which of the following is the most likely explanation for these findings?

a. Pancreatic ductal adenocarcinoma
b. Acute pancreatitis secondary to alcohol
c. Acute pancreatitis secondary to gallstones
d. Chronic pancreatitis secondary to alcohol
e. Chronic pancreatitis secondary to gallstones

27. A 52-year-old man comes to your office because his family has thought he looked "yellow" for several weeks. He denies abdominal pain and has no history of liver disease and is currently not taking any medication. Physical examination reveals scleral icterus and jaundice. Abdominal examination shows a nontender palpable gallbladder. Laboratory evaluation includes a total bilirubin of 7, direct bilirubin 4, amylase 115. Complete blood count, electrolytes, and creatinine are normal. Ultrasonography of the abdomen shows dilated intrahepatic ducts and an enlarged gallbladder. Which of the following is the most likely explanation for these findings?

a. Acute cholecystitis
b. Choledocholithiasis (common duct stone)
c. Acute pancreatitis
d. Chronic pancreatitis
e. Pancreatic cancer

28. A 49-year-old pharmacist has chronic diarrhea. For 10 years, he has had episodes of loose stool. He denies weight loss and intestinal bleeding, and he has had some normal bowel movements and episodic constipation. He denies

any travel and has no specific food intolerances. He had been evaluated in the past and was given no explanation for his problem. The most likely explanation of these findings is:

a. Diverticulosis of the colon
b. Ulcerative colitis
c. Hirschsprung disease
d. Granulomatous colitis
e. Irritable bowel syndrome

29. A 23-year-old medical student is asymptomatic but comes to your office because of a family history of colon cancer. His father died at age 46 years of colon cancer. He is the oldest of 5 children. Colonoscopic examination reveals several hundred small polyps distributed throughout the colon, and biopsy reveals benign tubular adenomas with moderate dysplasia. All the following are indicated in this patient's management *except*:

a. Screening upper gastrointestinal endoscopy
b. Screening of siblings
c. Genetic counseling
d. Treatment with sulindac and follow-up colonoscopy annually
e. Surgical consultation for proctocolectomy

30. All the following patients are at high risk for colorectal cancer and should be screened aggressively for colorectal cancer *except*:

a. A 36-year-old man with previous adenomatous polyps
b. A 35-year-old man with Peutz-Jeghers syndrome
c. A 40-year-old woman whose mother died of colon cancer at age 60
d. A 50-year-old woman with a history of breast cancer
e. A 50-year-old woman with a history of female genital cancer

31. A 35-year-old man has an increased serum level of aminotransferase. He is asymptomatic and has no significant medical history, although 15 years ago he used intravenous drugs. Physical examination results were unremarkable. Laboratory test results were notable for an alanine aminotransferase level of 94 U/L. He was found to be anti-HBs-, IgG anti-HBc-, and anti-HCV- positive. Which of the following is most correct?

a. This patient will likely be HBsAg-positive
b. Intravenous drug use is a risk factor for hepatitis C but not hepatitis B
c. He will likely be HCV-RNA-positive
d. His liver disease should not be treated because he is asymptomatic
e. The patient should receive hepatitis B vaccination

32. A 45-year-old day-care employee has a 2-week history of fatigue, anorexia, and jaundice. She denies abdominal pain and has no significant medical history, and the only medication she takes is an oral contraceptive. Physical examination results are notable for jaundice without stigmata of chronic liver disease. Laboratory findings included: alanine aminotransferase (ALT), 1,469 U/L; alkaline phosphatase, 2-fold increase; total bilirubin, 17.5 mg/dL; direct bilirubin, 12 mg/dL; and prothombin time, 1.3 International Normalized Ratio (INR). Which of the following is most correct?
   a. Ultrasonography of the liver will likely show dilated bile ducts
   b. Even if ultrasonographic results are negative, ERCP should be performed
   c. Oral contraceptives commonly cause acute hepatitis
   d. Laboratory findings are consistent with alcoholic hepatitis
   e. IgM anti-HAV will likely be positive

33. A 34-year-old man has a 3-month history of a painful rash on the lower extremities. It has not improved with topical corticosteroid therapy. Otherwise, he feels well. His medical history is notable for a bleeding ulcer 10 years ago that required blood transfusions. Physical examination results are notable for a purpuric rash on both lower extremities. Because laboratory tests demonstrated a 2-fold increase in alanine aminotransferase (ALT), hepatitis serologic studies were performed and the patient was found to be anti-HCV-positive. Which of the following is most correct?
   a. The patient should be tested for cryoglobulins
   b. Oral corticosteroid treatment should be given
   c. Interferon will not improve the rash
   d. Renal arteriography would likely demonstrate the characteristic changes of polyarteritis nodosa
   e. Rheumatoid factor will likely be absent

34. A 54-year-old woman has complained of pruritus for 6 months. Otherwise, she feels well. She has been taking pravastatin for 3 months for hypercholesterolemia. Examination results are notable for xanthelasma. Laboratory findings: alkaline phosphatase, 4-fold increase; alanine aminotransferase (ALT), 1.5 times increase; total bilirubin, 2.3 mg/dL; direct bilirubin, 1.2 mg/dL; and cholesterol, 344. Which of the following is most correct?
   a. Pravastatin is the likely cause of the abnormal liver tests
   b. An antinuclear antibody should be performed
   c. Antimitochondrial antibody would likely be present
   d. This condition has a strong association with ulcerative colitis

   e. The patient likely has nonalcoholic steatohepatitis due to the hypercholesterolemia

35. An 18-year-old woman is seen because she has a 2-week history of jaundice and has been lethargic for 24 hours. She has no significant medical history and she denies medications or illegal drugs. Examination findings are notable for jaundice, lethargy, and asterixis. Laboratory findings: alanine aminotransferase (ALT), 182 U/L; alkaline phosphatase, 54 U/L; total bilirubin, 33 mg/dL; direct bilirubin, 10 mg/dL; prothrombin time, 2.3 International Normalized Ratio; and hemoglobin, 8.3 g/dL. Which one of the following is most correct?
   a. A 24-hour urine sample should be collected for copper
   b. The history is consistent with ischemic hepatitis
   c. IgM anti-HAV is likely to be positive
   d. This disease is characterized by positive assays for antinuclear and anti-smooth muscle antibodies
   e. Liver biopsy will demonstrate globules that stain positive with periodic acid-Schiff

36. A 74-year-old woman has a 2-week history of headache and shoulder and hip stiffness. She was previously healthy, and her examination results are normal. Laboratory findings: hemoglobin, 10.7 g/dL with a normal mean corpuscular volume (MCV); alkaline phosphatase, 3-fold increase; alanine aminotransferase (ALT), 1.5 times increase; and erythrocyte sedimentation rate, 104 mm/h. Antimitochondrial antibody, liver ultrasonography, and computed tomography of the head are normal. Which of the following is most correct?
   a. ERCP should be performed
   b. A liver biopsy is needed to make a definitive diagnosis
   c. This disorder responds well to corticosteroids
   d. Ursodiol should be administered
   e. Hepatitis serologic studies should be performed

37. A 55-year-old man has pain in the finger joints. A grandfather and older brother died of hepatocellular carcinoma. Physical examination results are notable for hyperpigmentation, enlargement and deformity of the painful joints, hepatomegaly, and small testes. Laboratory findings: alanine aminotransferase (ALT), 1.5 times increase; and glucose, 153 mg/dL. Which of the following is most correct?
   a. This disease is transmitted in an autosomal dominant manner
   b. Determining the serum level of ceruloplasmin should be the next test

c. The patient has Addison disease

d. Serum iron studies should be performed

e. This disorder is usually treated with chelation therapy

38. A 44-year-old woman has had jaundice and epigastric pain for 24 hours. Examination findings: obese, uncomfortable, temperature 38.9°C, jaundice, and mild epigastric tenderness. Laboratory findings: leukocyte count, 14.4 x 10^9/L with left shift; total bilirubin, 8.4 mg/dL; direct bilirubin, 4.8 mg/dL; alanine aminotransferase (ALT), 543 U/L; alkaline phosphatase, 1.5 times increase; and amylase, 441 U/L. Ultrasonography showed gallbladder stones and normal-sized bile ducts. The distal common bile duct and pancreas were not well seen. After 24 hours of mezlocillin therapy, she was afebrile, the ALT was 82 U/L, and bilirubin was 7.8/4.3 mg/dL. Which of the following is most correct?

a. Computed tomography of the abdomen with fine cuts of the pancreas should be performed

b. The history is compatible with ischemic hepatitis

c. IgM anti-HAV is likely to be positive

d. IgM anti-HBc is likely to be positive

e. The patient has cholangitis due to choledocholithiasis

39. A 60-year-old woman has fatigue and jaundice of 3 weeks duration. For years, she has known of mildly abnormal liver tests that have not been investigated further. Physical examination findings notable for a relatively well-appearing patient with mild jaundice, multiple spider angiomata, and mild splenomegaly. Laboratory findings: alanine aminotransferase (ALT), 1,206 U/L; total bilirubin, 4.3 mg/dL; direct bilirubin, 2.6 mg/dL; prothrombin time, 1.3 International Normalized Ratio; platelets, 83 x 10^9/L, and an increased gamma globulin. Alkaline phosphatase, hemoglobin concentration, leukocyte count, iron saturation,

HbsAg, anti-HCV, and anti-HAV are negative or normal. Liver ultrasonography shows a coarsened echotexture of the liver consistent with chronic parenchymal disease, mild splenomegaly, and no ascites. Which of the following is most correct?

a. The patient should have splenectomy for diagnosis and treatment

b. The serum level of ceruloplasmin should be determined

c. Antinuclear antibody will likely be present

d. This clinical picture is consistent with acute alcoholic hepatitis superimposed on alcoholic cirrhosis

e. ERCP should be done to investigate the jaundice

40. A 50-year-old alcoholic man has a 5-day history of jaundice and lethargy. He is not able to give a coherent history, but his "significant other" states that he had recently had an upper respiratory infection for which he had been taking an unknown "over-the-counter" medication. Examination findings: lethargic but arousable, disoriented, asterixis, fetor hepaticus, spider angiomata, and splenomegaly. Laboratory findings: alanine aminotransferase (ALT), 853 U/L; aspartate aminotransferase (AST), 749 U/L; total bilirubin, 12.5 mg/dL; direct bilirubin, 7.9 mg/dL; prothrombin time, 1.6 International Normalized Ratio; platelets, 78 x 10^9/L; and ammonia, 189 N/dL. Which of the following is most correct?

a. The clinical picture is consistent with alcoholic hepatitis

b. The clinical picture is consistent with acetaminophen hepatotoxicity

c. Alcoholic patients are rarely coinfected with hepatitis C

d. Hepatitis C commonly causes clinically recognized acute hepatitis

e. Liver biopsy would not show steatosis

ANSWERS

1. Answer d.

This patient has progressive dysphagia for solids with chronic heartburn. History suggests a mechanical narrowing or stricture that is most likely secondary to gastroesophageal reflux. The chronicity of symptoms suggests that Barrett esophagus may be a complication, and the presence of a stricture and an ulcer in the mid esophagus strongly suggests that Barrett esophagus is present. Esophageal rings occur in the distal esophagus and usually cause intermittent dysphagia or food bolus impaction. Motility disorders, such as achalasia, diffuse esophageal spasm, or nonspecific motility disorders, usually present as intermittent dysphagia for solids and liquids, and upper gastrointestinal radiography does not show a stricture.

2. Answer c.

The history of intermittent dysphagia and a sudden food bolus impaction strongly suggest a lower esophageal ring. Intermittent dysphagia may also be caused by an esophageal web or a motility disorder. However, food bolus impactions that do not pass after drinking liquids are unusual in these conditions.

3. Answer c.

Intermittent dysphagia for solids that has progressed to dysphagia for both solids and liquids suggests a chronic motility disorder. The smooth beak-like tapering on an upper gastrointestinal radiograph is classic for achalasia. Sometimes achalasia may not be appreciated on an endoscopic examination. A motility study would confirm the diagnosis.

4. Answer e.

This man presents with noncardiac chest pain. The most common cause of noncardiac chest pain is esophageal reflux; however, reflux has been ruled out by the normal findings on endoscopy and biopsy of the lower esophagus. The second most likely cause of noncardiac chest pain is diffuse esophageal spasm and that is the most likely diagnosis in this case. An esophageal motility study is indicated.

5. Answer a.

Cervical esophageal dysphagia associated with coughing, choking, or nasal regurgitation that occurs with the act of swallowing suggests oropharyngeal dysphagia. Oropharyngeal dysphagia may be caused by neurologic, muscular, or structural disorders of the swallowing mechanism. Myasthenia gravis, multiple sclerosis, and amyotrophic lateral sclerosis can cause oropharyngeal dysphagia. Structural causes include Zenker diverticulum, cervical lymphadenopathy, goiter, cricopharyngeal dysfunction, and cervical osteophytes. Achalasia is denervation of the lower esophageal sphincter, and this can cause dysphagia that is localized to the mid or lower chest and is not associated with coughing, choking, or nasal regurgitation. Also, achalasia does not cause cervical dysphagia or dysphagia related to the act of swallowing.

6. Answer d.

Odynophagia, or pain on swallowing, is caused by inflammation, spasm, or distention of the esophagus. In an immunocompromised patient, odynophagia suggests the presence of infection with an opportunistic agent. *Candida*, herpes, and *Cytomegalovirus* are common causes of odynophagia in immunodeficient patients. Bullous pemphigoid can cause odynophagia but is not seen in immunodeficient patients.

7. Answer d.

This patient presents with medication-induced esophagitis. Medications commonly associated with esophagitis include tetracycline, doxycycline, nonsteroidal anti-inflammatory drugs, quinidine, potassium supplements, ferrous sulfate, and ascorbic acid.

8. Answer e.

This man has 2 previously documented duodenal ulcers, is infected with *Helicobacter pylori*, and has never been treated with antibiotics and antisecretory agents. No further evaluation for *Helicobacter pylori* or active ulcer disease is necessary. This patient should be treated and followed to determine if symptoms have resolved. A serum gastrin study should be performed when hypersecretion is suspected or when peptic ulcer disease is not associated with *Helicobacter pylori* infection, or when nonsteroidal anti-inflammatory drugs, aspirin, or alcohol has been ingested. Treatment with antisecretory agents will relieve symptoms but will not prevent recurrence.

9. Answer e.

The history of a previously documented ulcer in a person who is not infected with *Helicobacter pylori* and not taking aspirin, alcohol, or nonsteroidal anti-inflammatory drugs should raise suspicion for a possible hypersecretory syndrome. The family history and increased serum level of calcium also suggest hypersecretory syndrome secondary to multiple endocrine neoplasia. Given this unusual clinical scenario, Zollinger-Ellison syndrome is the most likely diagnosis.

10. Answer c.

The clinical conditions that predispose to squamous cell carcinoma of the esophagus include achalasia, lye stricture, Plummer-Vinson syndrome, human papilloma virus, smoking, alcohol ingestion, and a rare genetic condition called "tylosis." Gastroesophageal reflux disease predisposes to Barrett esophagus and the development of adenocarcinoma of the esophagus.

11. Answer e.

This woman has acute diarrhea related to traveling in Mexico. The most likely cause of the diarrhea is infection with toxigenic *E. coli*. At this point, she needs only to ensure that she is well hydrated because the infection most likely is self-limited. Because she has no fever and no blood in the stool, it would be acceptable to offer her an antimotility agent to minimize the inconvenience of frequent stools.

12. Answer d.

The diarrhea stopped with fasting, suggesting that an osmotic mechanism is the cause of the diarrhea. The woman has been dieting and ingesting diet soft drinks and chewing gum, which contain sorbitol. The most likely explanation of the symptoms is osmotic diarrhea related to sorbitol ingestion.

13. Answer b.

Chronic diarrhea is diarrhea that lasts longer than 1 month or diarrhea that recurs. Stool studies are the first step in the evaluation of chronic diarrhea. The history of traveling suggests an infectious diarrhea. These symptoms would not be uncommon for *Giardiasis*. It is appropriate to evaluate the stool for culture and parasites.

14. Answer c.

Meckel diverticulum is the most common cause of bleeding in the lower gastrointestinal tract in young adults. This is the third episode of bleeding for this young person, whose previous intestinal evaluations have been negative. However, the studies that were performed would not detect Meckel diverticulum. A nuclear scan is indicated to rule out Meckel diverticulum.

15. Answer e.

This man has edema, exertional dyspnea, and clinical evidence for bilateral pleural effusions. All the serum protein levels are low, but there is no loss of protein into urine. These findings are consistent with a protein-losing enteropathy. A protein-losing enteropathy with lymphocytopenia strongly suggests intestinal lymphangiectasia.

16. Answer d.

This young woman has nausea, abdominal pain, and diarrhea following the ingestion of food. The history of previous allergies and the presence of eosinophilia suggest eosinophilic gastroenteritis. Protozoa, such as *Entamoeba histolytica*, do not cause eosinophilia, and stool cultures and the parasite study are normal.

17. Answer d.

This young woman has malabsorption, iron deficiency anemia, and metabolic bowel disease. Malabsorption is usually due to a small intestinal or pancreatic cause. Iron and calcium are absorbed in the proximal small intestine, and this history suggests a disorder that occurs in the proximal small intestine (which is supplied by the celiac artery). These findings in combination with the presence of Howell-Jolly bodies in a patient who has not had a splenectomy strongly suggest celiac sprue as the cause of malabsorption.

18. Answer d.

The presence of malabsorption, central nervous system symptoms, arthritis, hyperpigmentation, and lymphadenopathy strongly suggests Whipple disease. The small bowel biopsy findings confirm the diagnosis of Whipple disease.

19. Answer d.

The rates of symptomatic infection with *Giardia lamblia*, *Blastocystis hominis*, and *Entamoeba histolytica* are not significantly higher in HIV-positive patients than in those without HIV infection.

20. Answer d.

Systemic amyloidosis can involve any portion of the intestine. Amyloid is deposited in the blood vessels and mucus membranes of the intestine and can cause malabsorption, motility disorders, or ischemia, with intestinal ulceration and bleeding. Clinical findings include macroglossia, hepatomegaly, cardiomegaly, peripheral neuropathy, and proteinuria. The diagnosis can be confirmed with a fat aspirate.

21. Answer d.

Acute diverticulitis is a clinical diagnosis that can be made in elderly patients who present with left lower quadrant abdominal pain, fever, and left lower quadrant abdominal tenderness with or without a palpable mass. This patient has significant fever and leukocytosis. The most appropriate course of action would be to rest the intestine and begin treatment with intravenous fluids and antibiotics. A surgical consultation should be obtained to help with the management of the present illness and because the patient is young and will most likely have recurrent diverticulitis and ultimately require surgical management.

22. Answer c.

The most likely explanation for recurrent red rectal bleeding in an older person who does not have diverticulitis is angiodysplasia of the colon. The best test to detect angiodysplasia is colonoscopy. Colonoscopy also offers therapeutic potential if the vascular malformations are localized and amenable to endoscopic coagulation.

23. Answer c.

This elderly woman with lower abdominal pain, bloody

diarrhea, and "thumb-printing" of the colon at the splenic flexure has ischemic colitis. Chronic intestinal ischemia usually occurs in patients with significant arteriosclerotic vascular disease. Risk factors for the development of atherosclerosis are hypertension and diabetes mellitus. Diverticulosis occurs in elderly patients but does not increase the risk for ischemic colitis.

24. Answer c.

This patient has diarrhea, mild abdominal pain, and fever. After an illness that required antibiotics for management, there is no evidence for recurrent urinary tract infection, and proctoscopic examination strongly suggests pseudomembranous colitis. Antibiotic-related pseudomembranous colitis is most often caused by *Clostridium difficile*, and the most sensitive test to document antibiotic-related pseudomembranous colitis is a toxin assay of a stool sample.

25. Answer d.

Ischemia should be considered as a cause of abdominal pain when the pain begins suddenly and is followed by other symptoms of gastrointestinal dysfunction. Ischemia should also be considered in patients with underlying arterial sclerotic vascular disease. The sudden onset of abdominal pain in a patient who is in atrial fibrillation should raise suspicion for an embolic event. The mild ileus and low increase in serum amylase are not consistent with acute pancreatitis, acute hepatobiliary disease, or ileus. The most likely explanation for this patient's findings is acute mesenteric ischemia from an embolic event.

26. Answer d.

This patient has evidence of malabsorption, that is, diarrhea with pale stools and weight loss. The presence of oil droplets implies the ingested fat in the form of triglycerides has not been broken down by pancreatic lipase, thus strongly suggesting pancreatic insufficiency due to chronic pancreatitis. Gallstones rarely or never cause chronic pancreatitis but are a common cause of acute pancreatitis. This man, who admits drinking "socially," most likely has chronic pancreatitis with pancreatic insufficiency due to alcohol ingestion.

27. Answer e.

Painless jaundice with a palpable nontender gallbladder is Courvoisier sign and strongly suggests pancreatic cancer. Acute cholecystitis, choledocholithiasis, and acute pancreatitis usually present with abdominal pain. It is unusual for chronic pancreatitis to present without abdominal pain, and it is also unusual for chronic pancreatitis to present with jaundice. Although chronic pancreatitis could explain these findings, pancreatic cancer more commonly presents this way.

28. Answer e.

The history of long-standing alternating diarrhea, constipation, and normal bowel movements suggests irritable bowel syndrome. In this syndrome, there usually is no weight loss, no intestinal bleeding, and no symptoms to suggest other systemic disease. Always rule out lactase deficiency, and remember that irritable bowel syndrome is a diagnosis of exclusion, that is, the diagnosis is confirmed by an appropriate medical evaluation that is negative.

29. Answer d.

This patient has familial adenomatous polyposis, which carries virtually a 100% risk for colon cancer. The presence of dysplasia suggests that this patient is at high risk for malignancy. Total proctocolectomy should be performed. Familial adenomatous polyposis is an autosomal dominant condition, so siblings should be evaluated, and the family should have genetic counseling. Because there is a small risk of coexistent polyps in the duodenum, upper endoscopy should be performed. Although there are reports of sulindac retarding the growth of polyps, it would be inappropriate to use sulindac in this high-risk situation.

30. Answer b.

Peutz-Jeghers syndrome consists of hamartomas or nonmalignant polyps usually involving the small intestine. The syndrome also includes pigmented lesions of the mouth, hands, and feet, and there is an uncommon association with ovarian sex cord tumors and proximal small-bowel tumors. The high-risk conditions for colorectal cancer include a previous history of adenomas or carcinoma, familial adenomatous polyposis, history of colon cancer in a first-degree relative, women with breast or genital cancer, patients with ulcerative colitis for more than 7 years, and families with hereditary nonpolyposis cancer syndrome. Patients with all of these high-risk conditions should have aggressive screening for colorectal cancer.

31. Answer c.

This man has symptoms and biochemical markers consistent with chronic hepatitis. Patients who have risk factors for hepatitis C, increased aminotransferase levels, and antibodies to hepatitis C are nearly always HCV-RNA-positive, indicating an ongoing infection with hepatitis C. The fact that he is asymptomatic should not preclude him from being considered for treatment. Intravenous drug use is not only a risk factor for hepatitis C but also for hepatitis B. The patient's hepatitis B serologic studies are consistent with a previous HBV infection with resolution and immunity. The HBsAg will be negative, and there is no need for hepatitis B vaccination.

32. Answer e.

This patient has symptoms and biochemical markers consistent with acute hepatitis. She has a marked increase in aminotransferase levels, only a modest increase in the alkaline phosphatase, and an increased bilirubin concentration. Day-care employees are at significant risk for hepatitis A, and the diagnostic test of choice would be the IgM anti-HAV. Because this is a nonobstructive cause of jaundice, ultrasonography likely will not show dilated bile ducts, and there is no need for ERCP. Of note, in somebody with acute jaundice, ultrasonography of the liver may not detect dilated bile ducts even if the jaundice is obstructive and, therefore, if the clinical suspicion is high, ERCP would be reasonable. Because our clinical suspicion for obstructive jaundice is not high in this case, ERCP should not be performed. When oral contraceptives cause liver test abnormalities, cholestasis is more common than hepatitis. It is rare for alcoholic hepatitis to result in an ALT level greater than 400; therefore, that diagnosis is not likely.

33. Answer a.

This patient has abnormal aminotransferase levels, hepatitis C antibody, and lower extremity rash consistent with a vasculitis. This is a characterized scenario of vasculitis due to cryoglobulinemia associated with hepatitis C. Generally, these patients have a good response to interferon, which is considered the treatment of choice for cryoglobulinemia associated with hepatitis C. Oral corticosteroids are sometimes given if interferon fails. Patients who have cryoglobulinemia generally do not demonstrate the changes of polyarteritis nodosa and, therefore, renal arteriography would not be useful. Patients with hepatitis C-associated cryglobulinemia usually have rheumatoid factor present.

34. Answer c.

This patient has biochemical markers and symptoms consistent with cholestasis. Patients with chronic cholestatic liver diseases often have hypercholesterolemia, because of deficient biliary secretion of cholesterol. She also has pruritus, which likely is due to retention of bile acids. A middle-aged woman with a chronic cholestatic condition is very suggestive of primary biliary cirrhosis, and antimitochondrial antibody testing will likely be positive. Pravastatin can cause abnormal liver tests, although there are usually mild aminotransferase increases rather than an increase in alkaline phosphatase. This patient's symptoms of cholestasis started before the administration of pravastatin. An antinuclear antibody would be performed if one suspected autoimmune hepatitis, which would present with predominantly an increase in aminotransferase. Primary sclerosing cholangitis, another cholestatic liver disease, is strongly associated with ulcerative colitis.

Nonalcoholic steatohepatitis is more often characterized by increased aminotransferase levels.

35. Answer a.

This patient has a clinical syndrome of fulminant hepatic failure. This is defined as hepatic failure with encephalopathy developing within 8 weeks after the onset of jaundice in a patient with no history of liver disease. Some relatively unusual things in her laboratory tests are that the aminotransferase levels are relatively low, alkaline phosphatase is low, hyperbilirubinemia is predominantly indirect, and hemoglobin concentration is low. The constellation of these features is suggestive of Wilson disease with hemolysis. This diagnosis should be considered in any young patient who presents with liver failure. Patients can also have neurologic manifestations and Kayser-Fleischer rings, although these findings are less common in patients presenting with acute liver failure. The best test for fulminant Wilson disease is a 24-hour urine copper analysis, and this should be markedly increased (>250 μg/24 hr). Treatment of Wilson disease is chelation of copper with either penicillamine or trientine, although patients presenting acutely usually need liver transplantation. Acute hepatitis A could present similarly, although one would expect the aminotransferase levels to be more increased. Ischemic hepatitis generally occurs in patients with documented hypotension, and it is characterized by marked transient elevations of aminotransferases. Autoimmune hepatitis can occasionally present acutely but should have a more marked increase in aminotransferases. A liver biopsy specimen demonstrating globules that stain positive with PAS is suggestive of alpha$_1$-antitrypsin deficiency, which does not present as an acute hepatitis *except* in the neonatal period.

36. Answer c.

This patient has a systemic illness characterized by headache, joint stiffness, normocytic anemia, and a markedly increased erythrocyte sedimentation rate. She also has mildly cholestatic liver tests. Any infectious or inflammatory state can lead to mildly abnormal liver tests, and this patient's clinical history would be consistent with temporal arteritis with associated polymyalgia rheumatica. This patient should respond well to corticosteroid treatment. The procedure of choice for this patient would be temporal artery biopsy. There is no need for ERCP, given the low clinical suspicion that she has an obstructive process. Liver biopsy could be considered but is a poor way to try to diagnose systemic vasculitis. Urosodiol can be useful for cholestatic liver disease, but it only has proved useful for primary biliary cirrhosis, which is unlikely given the systemic complaints and negative antimitochondrial antibody. Hepatitis serologic studies are not necessary, because of the low clinical suspicion for acute or chronic hepatitis.

37. Answer d.

This man presents with joint complaints involving the hands. He has hyperpigmentation, hepatomegaly, small testes, mild increase in aminotransferases, increased glucose levels, and a family history of hepatocellular carcinoma. All these findings are consistent with a diagnosis of genetic hemochromatosis. This is a disorder of iron overload that is transmitted in an autosomal recessive manner. It is common, occurring in about 1/300 persons of Northern European origin. Patients can have involvement not only of the liver but also of the pancreas, heart, joints, and pituitary gland. Early diagnosis is essential, because treatment in the presymptomatic phase can allow the patient to have a normal life span. Treatment can also be helpful in reversing cardiac disease, although it does not seem to help arthritis or the increased risk of hepatocellular carcinoma. Patients with genetic hemochromatosis have an iron saturation greater than 50% (usually >80%) and an increased ferritin level. A gene test is available and can be helpful in diagnosis. Wilson disease would be unlikely to present in this age group and, therefore, a ceruloplasmin test would not be helpful. Addison disease could account for the hyperpigmentation but would not explain the other findings. Genetic hemochromatosis typically is not treated with chelation therapy because phlebotomy is simpler and effective.

38. Answer e.

This 44-year-old woman has the typical findings of cholangitis. She has abdominal pain, fever, and jaundice. In addition, she has a mild increase in the amylase level, suggesting that there may be an associated pancreatitis. A unifying cause for the cholangitis and pancreatitis would be a distal common bile duct stone. Patients who have a common bile duct stone can initially have marked aminotransferase increases that are quite transient. Also remember that patients who have acute jaundice will not always have dilated bile ducts and if the clinical suspicion remains high, as it should be in this case, ERCP should be performed. Computed tomography of the abdomen with fine cuts of the pancreas would be indicated if one suspected pancreatic carcinoma. Painless jaundice would be more characteristic of pancreatic cancer. Ischemic hepatitis can produce marked transient increases in aminotransferase levels but usually does so in a patient who has a history of hypotension. Acute hepatitis A and B obviously cause increased aminotransferase levels but should not cause this degree of abdominal pain or fever and aminotransferase elevations should be more prolonged than seen in this patient.

39. Answer c.

This woman presents with what appears to be acute hepatitis, but she also has features of chronic liver disease, including spider angiomata and mild splenomegaly with hypersplenism, suggesting portal hypertension. She has an increase in gamma globulin, and this clinical history in a woman is most consistent with autoimmune hepatitis. It is important to remember that even though autoimmune hepatitis is a chronic condition, it can present acutely. Such patients generally have positive assays for anti-smooth muscle and/or antinuclear antibodies. It is best to avoid splenectomy in patients with portal hypertension unless they have marked thrombocytopenia with bleeding. Wilson disease would be rare in a 60-year-old woman. Acute alcoholic hepatitis produces aminotransferase increases but nearly always <400 U/L. There is no need for ERCP because there is no suspicion of an obstructive cause of the patient's jaundice. Hepatitis B and C are largely excluded on the basis of negative hepatitis B surface antigen and anti-HCV.

40. Answer b.

This alcoholic man has jaundice and lethargy. He has a relatively marked increase in aminotransferase levels, evidence of synthetic dysfunction, and a low platelet count, which would be consistent with hypersplenism and portal hypertension. This is suggestive of another case of acute liver disease superimposed on chronic liver disease. Aminotransferase increases in alcoholic hepatitis are generally <400 IU/mL. In addition, patients with alcoholic hepatitis generally have an AST:ALT ratio >2. This particular patient likely has acetaminophen hepatotoxicity on top of chronic alcoholic liver disease. Alcoholics are more likely to develop acetaminophen hepatotoxicity, even with doses of acetaminophen that are not usually considered toxic. Alcoholic persons not only have an accelerated P450 metabolism of acetaminophen, favoring the formation of a toxic metabolite, but they may also be deficient in glutathione because of chronic liver disease, which makes them less likely able to conjugate the toxic metabolite adequately. In patients with acute acetaminophen hepatotoxicity, *N*-acetylcysteine should be given. Alcoholic patients are commonly infected with hepatitis C, although hepatitis C is a rare cause of acute hepatitis. In this alcoholic man with evidence of chronic liver disease and who is actively drinking, liver biopsy is likely to show steatosis in addition to Mallory hyalin.

NOTES

CHAPTER 9

GENERAL INTERNAL MEDICINE

Scott C. Litin, M.D.

INTERPRETATION OF DIAGNOSTIC TESTS

Diagnostic test assessment takes into account two sets of characteristics: those pertaining to the test itself (sensitivity and specificity) and the pretest likelihood that the disease is present in the person being tested (prevalence of disease in a population). When a diagnostic test is applied to a population at risk for the abnormal condition, patients in the studied population can be assigned to one of four groups (Table 9-1):

True-positive = disease present, abnormal test result.
False-positive = disease absent, abnormal test result.
False-negative = disease present, normal test result.
True-negative = disease absent, normal test result.

When data are displayed in a 2-by-2 table, the following test characteristics can be defined (Table 9-1):

1. Sensitivity
   Positive in disease (PID).
   True positivity rate—proportion of patients with the target disorder who have positive test result.
   2-by-2 table definition = $a/(a+c)$.
   "SN out"—a test with 100% **s**ensitivity if **n**egative rules **out** the disorder.
   Screening tests attempt to maximize sensitivity to avoid missing a person with the disease.
   Characteristic of test—not affected by population characteristics.
2. Specificity
   Negative in health (NIH).
   True negativity rate—proportion of patients without the target disorder who have a negative test result.
   2-by-2 table definition = $d/(b+d)$.
   "SP in"—a test with 100% **s**pecificity if **p**ositive rules **in** the disorder.
   Confirmatory tests used in follow-up of screening try to maximize specificity to avoid incorrectly labeling a healthy person as having disease.

Characteristic of test—not affected by population characteristics.
3. Positive predictive value
   When a patient's illness is evaluated by interpreting a diagnostic test, the 2-by-2 table is read horizontally, not vertically. Thus, in judging the value of a diagnostic test, it is not essential to know its sensitivity and specificity but whether a patient with positive test results has the disease, that is, how well the test results predict a disease compared with the reference standard for that disease. Thus, the horizontal properties of the diagnostic test are of primary interest. Among all patients with a positive diagnostic test result, $(a+b)$, in what proportion, $a/(a+b)$, has the diagnosis been correctly predicted or ruled in? This proportion is the positive predictive value (PPV).

- PPV is the proportion of patients who test positive who have the disease.
- This provides information most useful in clinical practice.
- PPV is affected by the prevalence of the disease in the population.
- 2-by-2 table definition, PPV = $a/(a+b)$.

4. Negative predictive value
   It is also important to know the percentage of patients with a negative test result, $(c+d)$, who actually do not have the disease. This proportion, $d/(c+d)$, is the negative predictive value (NPV).

- NPV is the proportion of patients who test negative and have no disease; it is prevalence-dependent.
- 2-by-2 table definition, NPV = $d/(c+d)$.

5. Prevalence
   The PPV and NPV of a diagnostic test depend on the proportion of persons with the disease among the entire group of persons to whom the test is applied. This proportion, $(a+c)/(a+b+c+d)$, is the prevalence.

Table 9-1.--2-By-2 Table

		Target disorder		
		Present	Absent	
Diagnostic test result	Positive	True + a	False + b	a+b
	Negative	c False -	d True -	c+d
		a+c	b+d	a+b+c+d

Prevalence = (a+c)/(a+b+c+d)

Test characteristics

    Sensitivity = a/(a+c)

    Specificity = d/(b+d)

Frequency-dependent properties

    PPV = a/(a+b)

    NPV = d/(c+d)

How to Construct a 2-By-2 Table

The sensitivity, specificity, and predictive values of normal and abnormal test results can be calculated with even a limited amount of information. For example, suppose a new diagnostic test gives abnormal results in 90% of patients who have the disease and normal results in 95% of patients who are disease-free, and furthermore, the prevalence of the disease in the population to which the test is applied is 10%. This provides the following information:

    Sensitivity = 90%

    Specificity = 95%

    Prevalence = 10%

This test is now ready to be applied to a group of patients by filling in a 2-by-2 table (Table 9-2). The calculation is easier if the test is applied to a large number of patients, for example, 1,000, and a+b+c+d = 1,000.

Because the prevalence of the disease is 10%, 100 patients have the disease (0.1 x 1,000 = 100, or a+c = 100). Of the patients, 90%, or 900, are disease-free (0.9 x 1,000 = 900, or b+d = 900).

Because the sensitivity of the test is 90%, of the 100 patients with disease, 90% have a positive test result (a = 0.9 x 100 = 90) and 10% have a negative result (c = 0.1 x 100 = 10).

Specificity of 95% means that of the 900 patients who are disease-free, 95% have a negative test result (d = 0.95 x 900 = 855) and 5% have a positive test result (b = 0.05 x 900 = 45).

The 2-by-2 table (Table 9-2) shows that 135 patients (a+b) have an abnormal test result; however, only 90 of these 135 patients actually have the disease. Therefore, the PPV of an abnormal test is a/(a+b) = 90/135 = 66.7%, that is, only two-thirds of all patients with positive test results will actually have the

disease. Similarly, one can determine that 865 patients (c+d) have a negative test result: 855 of these 865 patients are disease-free. Therefore, the NPV of the test is d/(c+d) = 855/865 = 98.8%.

Clinicians should be able to perform these simple calculations. Clinical decision-making by internists is more likely to depend on the PPV and NPV of test results for a given population than on the sensitivity or specificity of the test.

For example, if the prevalence of the disease in the clinician's population is 2% instead of 10%, the PPV and NPV can be recalculated. The PPV of abnormal test results falls to 26.9%, quite different from the 66.7% above, although the sensitivity and specificity of the test (90% and 95%, respectively) have not changed (Table 9-3).

- An important factor in interpreting a patient's abnormal test result is knowledge of the prevalence of the disease in the population being tested.
- High-risk populations (high prevalence of disease) tend to improve the PPV of an abnormal test result.
- Low-risk populations (screening tests) make the NPV of a normal test result look impressive.

Table 9-2.--2-By-2 Table for Test With 90% Sensitivity, 95% Specificity, and 10% Prevalence

		Disease present	Disease absent	
Diagnostic test result	Positive	90 a	45 b	135 a+b
	Negative	c 10	d 855	c+d 865
		a+c	b+d	a+b+c+d
	Total	100	900	1,000

Prevalence = (a+c)/(a+b+c+d) = 100/1,000 = 10%

Test characteristics

    Sensitivity = a/(a+c) = 90/100 = 90%

    Specificity = d/(b+d) = 855/900 = 95%

Frequency-dependent properties

    PPV = a/(a+b) = 90/135 = 66.7%

    NPV = d/(c+d) = 855/865 = 98.8%

Likelihood ratio (LR) for a positive test result:

    LR+ = Sensitivity/(1-Specificity) = 90%/5% = 18

Likelihood ratio for a negative test result:

    LR- = (1-Sensitivity)/Specificity = 10%/95% = 0.11

Pretest Odds = Prevalence/(1-Prevalence) = 10%/90% = 0.11

Post-Test Odds = Pretest Odds x Likelihood Ratio

Post-Test Probability = Post-Test Odds/(Post-Test Odds + 1)

Table 9-3.--2-By-2 Table for Test With 90% Sensitivity, 95% Specificity, and 2% Prevalence

Test result		Disease present	Disease absent	
	Positive	18 a	49 b	67 a+b
	Negative	c 2	d 931	c+d 933
		a+c	b+d	a+b+c+d
Total		20	980	1,000

Prevalence = (a+c)/(a+b+c+d) = 20/1,000 = 2%

Test characteristics

Sensitivity = a/(a+c) = 18/20 = 90%

Specificity = d/(b+d) = 931/980 = 95%

Frequency-dependent properties

PPV = a/(a+b) = 18/67 = 26.9%

NPV = d/(c+d) = 931/933 = 99.8%

Use of Odds and Likelihood Ratios

Some physicians prefer interpreting diagnostic test results by using the likelihood ratio, a factor by which a pretest probability is altered by a test result. When using likelihood ratios, it is necessary to think in terms of "odds ratios" instead of the more commonly used "probability percentages." Recall that probability compares a portion of the affected population with the entire population and is expressed as a percentage. However, odds compares a portion of the affected population with the unaffected population and is expressed as a ratio. For example, if a condition were seen in 50% of the population, the probability of having that condition would be 50/100, or 50%. The odds ratio of having that condition would be 50 (with condition)/50 (without condition), or an odds ratio equal to 1.

Probability and odds can be converted somewhat interchangeably by the following formulas:

$$\text{Probability} = \frac{\text{Odds}}{1 + \text{Odds}}$$

(in the example above, 0.50 = 1/1+1)

$$\text{Odds} = \frac{\text{Probability}}{1 - \text{Probability}}$$

(in the example above, 1 = 0.50/1-0.50)

The likelihood ratio of either a positive or a negative test result can be determined if the odds ratio form of pretest esti-

mation of disease likelihood is used. These formulas are provided in Table 9-2. Using the same numbers as in the Table 9-2 example, one could determine that the likelihood ratio for a positive test result in this scenario would be 18. The pretest odds of having the condition would be 0.11. The post-test odds for a positive test could be determined by multiplying the pretest odds (0.11) by the likelihood ratio (18): 0.11 x 18 = 1.98. This can be converted to post-test probability by placing the numbers in the formula:

$$\frac{\text{Post-Test Odds}}{(\text{Post-Test Odds} + 1)} = \frac{1.98}{2.98} = 66.4\%$$

This is nearly identical to the previously determined positive predictive value.

PREOPERATIVE MEDICAL EVALUATION

The Art of Medical Consultation

This section is concerned with advice given by an internist to a surgeon in assessing preoperative risk in managing perioperative problems (J Gen Intern Med 2:257-269, 1987). Guidelines for the internist to optimize compliance with the advice are listed below:

1. Limit the number of recommendations to five or fewer.
2. Focus on crucial recommendations and avoid diluting management plan with trivial suggestions.
3. Be specific, especially regarding drug dosages. Recommend not only which drug to use, but specify dose and frequency of administration.
4. Advice about therapy (i.e., initiating or discontinuing drug therapy) is heeded more often than diagnostic suggestions (i.e., ordering tests).
5. Labor-intensive advice that requires the surgeon to do something (look at a blood smear, perform a procedure, etc.) is poorly heeded. If such tasks must be performed, the medical consultant should do them personally.
6. Oral communication with the surgeon usually enhances compliance.
7. Follow-up visits and notes further improve compliance.

Successfully communicating one's assessment and plan is an art. A three-step approach–diagnosis/treatment/prognosis–is often helpful.

1. Diagnosis–the internist creates a problem list that is a table of contents for anyone involved in the care of patient. It is particularly useful to anesthesiologists and surgeons.
2. Treatment–the internist offers recommendations that will diminish the surgical risks associated with the patient's problem. The emphasis is on therapeutics aimed only at diminishing surgical risk.

3. Prognosis–the internist states the surgical and anesthetic risk for each problem (often available in published literature). When this information is lacking, the internist has to substitute personal judgment.
4. The internist should comment on the cumulative risk for a patient with multiple medical problems, such as cardiac, pulmonary, and liver disease. The risk in such patients may become prohibitive.

- Diagnosis–a problem list.
- Treatment–recommendations only for decreasing surgical risk.
- Prognosis–surgical and anesthetic risk for each problem.
- Internist should comment on cumulative risk for patient with multiple medical problems.

Risks of Anesthesia and the Operation

Operative deaths are uncommon because of the many technical advances made in recent years in surgery and anesthesia. The risk of dying in the perioperative period (i.e., intraoperatively or within 48 hours postoperatively) is about 0.3% when all operations are considered. In major surgical procedures, the mortality risk is still less than 1% in patients younger than 65 years, but it increases to about 5% for those between 65 and 80 years old. Deaths occur in three periods: anesthetic induction (10%), intraoperatively (35%), and in the first 48 hours postoperatively (55%). Postoperative mortality between 48 hours and 6 weeks is usually due to pneumonia, sepsis, cardiac arrest, pulmonary embolus, or renal failure. The American Society of Anesthesiologists (ASA) has published a classification scheme to aid clinicians (Table 9-4). This classification is subjective, and many physicians favor a systematic assessment as opposed to a global impression. However, ASA class IV and V patients have roughly 100 times the mortality of class I patients for a surgical procedure. Also, an emergency procedure roughly doubles the risk in any ASA classification of patients.

- The risk of dying in the perioperative period is 0.3% of all operations.
- Three periods in which deaths (%) occur: anesthetic induction (10%), intraoperatively (35%), and within 48 hours postoperatively (55%).

Many physicians have mistakenly assumed that spinal anesthesia is safer than general anesthesia in high-risk patients. From a cardiopulmonary standpoint, this is not true. Spinal anesthesia may be associated with wide fluctuations in blood pressure, anxiety, and less control of the airway and ventilation. Thus, it is inappropriate for the internist to write, "patient too ill for general anesthesia; okay if done under spinal." The final decision about the type of anesthesia is the responsibility of the anesthesiologist.

- From a cardiopulmonary point of view, spinal anesthesia is not safer than general anesthesia.
- Spinal anesthesia may be associated with wide fluctuations in blood pressure.
- The final decision about the type of anesthesia is the responsibility of the anesthesiologist.

The type of operation performed is an important determinant of morbidity and mortality (Table 9-5). Procedures associated with low risk (reported cardiac risk generally <1%) include breast surgery, eye surgery, dilatation and curettage, herniorrhaphy, superficial procedures, and endoscopic procedures. Certain other procedures are associated with high perioperative risk (reported cardiac risk often >5%), including emergent operations (particularly in the elderly), aortic and other major vascular procedures, peripheral vascular surgery, craniotomy, and cardiac operations. Other operations would be considered intermediate risk (reported cardiac risk generally <5%), including carotid endarterectomy, orthopedic surgery (as well as head and neck operations), and interperitoneal, intrathoracic, and prostate operations.

Table 9-4.--American Society of Anesthesiologists Classification of Anesthetic Mortality Within 48 Hours Postoperatively

Class	Physical status	48-Hour mortality
I	Normal healthy person <80 years old	0.07%
II	Mild systemic disease	0.24%
III	Severe but not incapacitating systemic disease	1.4%
IV	Incapacitating systemic disease that is a constant threat to life	7.5%
V	Moribund patient not expected to survive 24 hours, regardless of surgery	8.1%
E	Suffix added to any class indicating emergency procedure, e.g., IE, IIE, IIIE	Doubles risk

Table 9-5.--Cardiac Risk* Stratification for Noncardiac Surgical Procedures

Risk	Procedure
High	
Reported cardiac risk often >5%	Emergent major operations, particularly in the elderly
	Aortic and other major vascular
	Peripheral vascular
	Anticipated prolonged surgical procedures associated with large fluid shifts and/or blood loss
Intermediate	
Reported cardiac risk generally <5%	Carotid endarterectomy
	Head and neck
	Intraperitoneal and intrathoracic
	Orthopedic
	Prostate
Low†	
Reported cardiac risk generally <1%	Endoscopic procedures
	Superficial procedure
	Cataract
	Breast

*Combined incidence of cardiac death and nonfatal myocardial infarction.

†Do not generally require further preoperative cardiac testing.

From Report of the American College of Cardiology/American Heart Association Task Force on Practice Guidelines (Committee on Perioperative Cardiovascular Evaluation for Noncardiac Surgery): Guidelines for perioperative cardiovascular evaluation for noncardiac surgery. J Am Coll Cardiol 27:910-948, 1996. By permission of American Heart Association and American College of Cardiology.

However, the importance of associated disease in determining surgical risk may outweigh the nature of the procedure or the type of anesthesia used in predicting outcome. The following sections discuss risk assessment and management strategies grouped by organ system.

Pulmonary Risks and Management

Pulmonary complications (hypoventilation, atelectasis, and pneumonia) occur in about one-third of patients postoperatively and account for 50% of overall perioperative mortality. Patients at definite risk for pulmonary complications include smokers, patients with chronic obstructive pulmonary disease, obesity, thoracic surgery, and upper abdominal surgery. Patients with probable increased risk include those older than 70 years whose duration of anesthesia is longer than 2 hours or who currently have respiratory infection.

- Pulmonary complications account for 50% of overall perioperative mortality.

Preoperative pulmonary function testing should be part of the evaluation of high-risk patients. The interpretation of these tests regarding risk assessment is controversial. However,

most authors agree that the simple spirometric measurement of forced expiratory volume in 1 second (FEV_1) is probably as good a predictor as any of surgical risk. If the FEV_1 is greater than 2 L, the patient can safely undergo the surgical procedure. If the FEV_1 is between 1 and 2 L, the risk of postoperative pulmonary complications is increased. An FEV_1 less than 1 L is indicative of a high risk of postoperative pulmonary complication.

- FEV_1 is a good predictor of surgical risk.
- FEV_1 >2 L, patient can safely undergo procedure.
- FEV_1 <1 L, high risk of postoperative pulmonary complication.

Several measures have been advocated to decrease the pulmonary risks. Preoperative measures to decrease pulmonary risk include instruction in respiratory maneuvers, cessation of cigarette smoking, use of bronchodilators, antibiotic treatment of chronic bronchitis, and chest physiotherapy. Postoperative measures include chest physiotherapy and inspiratory maneuvers, minimization of postoperative narcotic analgesia, and early mobilization of elderly patients.

Cardiac Risks and Management

Each year about 1 out of 10 U.S. citizens undergoes a noncardiac operation. Because of the increasing prevalence of surgical procedures in the elderly, about one-third of all noncardiac surgical patients are at risk for cardiac morbidity or mortality after taking into account the prevalence of coronary artery disease or the high-risk status in this population. Patients with known or suspected cardiac disease are commonly referred to a general internist or cardiologist for assessment before a noncardiac procedure is performed. Several questions are posed during these consultations:

1. How can the high-risk patient be identified?

2. What selective testing needs to be performed (if any) to further define risk?

3. What intervention or perioperative management is appropriate to decrease cardiac-related morbidity and mortality during noncardiac surgical procedures?

A risk-factor index, the Goldman index, was devised through a prospective analysis of patients older than 40 years undergoing noncardiac general surgery in an attempt to allow clinicians to estimate cardiac risk after clinical assessment (N Engl J Med 297:845-850, 1977). This scale has been validated prospectively and has formed the framework of preoperative cardiac evaluation (Tables 9-6 and 9-7).

Table 9-6.--The Goldman Cardiac Risk-Index for Noncardiac Surgery

Clinical variable	Point assessment
History	
Age >70 years	5
Recent myocardial infarction (≤6 mo)	10
Physical examination	
Ventricular gallop or jugular venous pressure ≥12 cm H_2O	11
Significant valvular aortic stenosis	3
Electrocardiogram	
Rhythm other than sinus or atrial ectopy on preoperative tracing	7
More than 5/min ectopic ventricular beats on any tracing preoperatively	7
Poor general medical condition (any of the following)	
Po_2 <60 mm Hg or Pco_2 >50 mm Hg	
Serum potassium <3.0 meq/L or bicarbonate <20 meq/L	
Blood urea nitrogen >50 mg/dL or creatinine >3.0 mg/dL	3
Chronic liver disease	
Noncardiac debilitation	
Surgical procedure	
Intraperitoneal, intrathoracic, aortic	3
Emergency	4
Maximum score	53

Modified from Goldman L, Caldera DL, Nussman SR et al: Multifactorial index of cardiac risk in noncardiac surgical procedures. N Engl J Med 297:845-850, 1977.

Table 9-7.--Cardiac Complications Stratified by the Goldman Risk Index

Risk-index class	Point score	No or minimal complications, %	Severe complications, %	Cardiac death, %
I	0-5	99	0.6	0.2
II	6-12	96	3	1
III	13-25	86	11	3
IV	≥26	49	12	39

Modified from Goldman L, Caldera DL, Nussman SR et al: Multifactorial index of cardiac risk in noncardiac surgical procedures. N Engl J Med 297:845-850, 1977.

More recently, the American College of Cardiology/American Heart Association Task Force (ACC/AHA) reported their guidelines to instruct physicians in the perioperative cardiovascular evaluation of patients for noncardiac surgical procedures (J Am Coll Cardiol 27:910-948, 1996). These guidelines go further than the Goldman index in presenting the framework for determining which patients are candidates for cardiac testing. The physician must consider several interacting variables and give them appropriate weight. Because there are no adequate controlled or randomized clinical trials to define this process, a collection of outcome data and expert opinion formed the basis of the algorithmic approach shown in Figure 9-1.

Myocardial infarction (MI) is the most feared perioperative complication. Of perioperative MIs, 50% are fatal and 60% are not accompanied by anginal pain. The risk of perioperative MI peaks 24 to 48 hours postoperatively. Patients with recent MIs are at greatest risk for perioperative MIs. The risk of perioperative MI without cardiac disease = 0.2%. According to retrospective studies, the risk of perioperative MI in patients with recent MI (<3 months) = 27%; if the MI occurred 3 to 6 months ago, 11%; and if the MI was more than 6 months ago, 5%. With hemodynamic catheters and aggressive intensive care management, the perioperative MI rate of patients with recent MI could be markedly decreased (MI <3 months = 5.7%; MI 4 to 6 months = 2.3%). Traditional teaching has suggested delaying nonemergent surgery for at least 6 months after MI. However, it has more recently become possible to risk-stratify MI patients during convalescence (Fig. 9-1). If a recent stress test has shown no residual myocardium at risk, the likelihood of reinfarction after noncardiac surgery would be low. Thus, if clinically indicated, it may be possible to perform surgery in selected post-MI patients 4 to 6 weeks after the infarction.

- Of perioperative MIs, 50% are fatal and 60% are silent.
- The risk of perioperative MI peaks 24 to 48 hours postoperatively.
- Patients with recent MI are at greatest risk for perioperative MI, but this rate can be decreased with hemodynamic catheters and aggressive intensive care management.
- Standard recommendation—delay nonemergent surgery for at least 6 months after MI.

Monitoring for Perioperative Myocardial Ischemia

In high-risk patients undergoing noncardiac operations, early postoperative myocardial ischemia is an important correlate of adverse cardiac outcomes. Patient subgroups who are at high risk for postoperative ischemia and who might benefit most from intensive Holter monitoring in the post-operative period can be identified preoperatively: left ventricular hypertrophy, coronary artery disease (CAD), diabetes mellitus, hypertension, and digoxin use. By identifying high-risk patients and monitoring them postoperatively with real-time monitors with alarms triggered by ST-segment depression, ischemia could be identified instantaneously so rapid intervention could potentially prevent clinical ischemia events. However, this hypothesis is as yet unstudied and unproven, and these interventions, if performed in all at-risk patients, would drive up costs tremendously! For patients at increased risk for perioperative MI, the ACC/AHA guidelines recommend electrocardiography (ECG) preoperatively, immediately postoperatively, and daily for the first 2 days after surgery.

- Early postoperative myocardial ischemia is an important correlate of adverse cardiac outcome in high-risk noncardiac surgical patients.

Valvular Heart Disease

Patients with valvular heart disease present specific risks in noncardiac surgery. Significant aortic stenosis is associated with a "fixed" cardiac output that cannot increase in response to surgical stress. Although such patients have minimal risk with local anesthesia, spinal anesthesia increases the risk because of the frequent induction of vasodilatation, which can cause cardiovascular collapse. Although general anesthesia can be performed with acceptable risks in selected hemodynamically monitored patients with severe aortic stenosis, conventional wisdom is to repair the valve preoperatively (when possible) in patients with critical aortic stenosis.

- Significant aortic stenosis is associated with a "fixed" cardiac output that cannot increase with surgical stress.
- Although selected patients with severe aortic stenosis can tolerate general anesthesia, the valve should be repaired preoperatively when possible in those with critical aortic stenosis.

When mitral or aortic valve regurgitation is present, the status of left ventricular function is of primary importance. Patients with regurgitant valvular disease and preserved left ventricular function tolerate vasodilatation well.

- Patients with valvular regurgitation and preserved left ventricular function tolerate vasodilatation well.
- Patients with valvular heart disease should receive endocarditis prophylaxis in accordance with the standard recommendations of the American Heart Association.

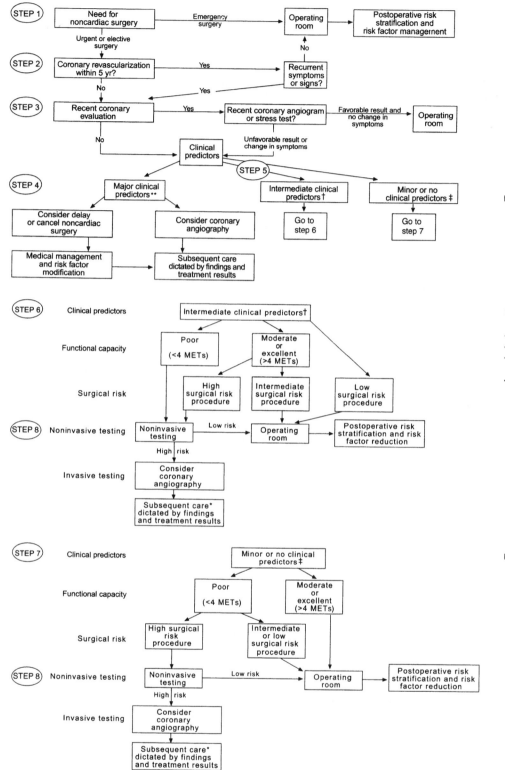

Fig. 9-1. Stepwise approach to preoperative cardiac assessment. >4 METs: the ability to climb a flight of stairs or walk up a hill. The ability to walk on level ground at 4 miles/hr or run a short distance. The ability to do heavy housework, e.g., scrubbing floors or lifting or moving heavy furniture. High, intermediate, and low risk surgical procedures are defined in Table 9-5. *Subsequent care may include cancellation or delay of surgery, coronary revascularization followed by noncardiac surgery, or intensified care. CHF, congestive heart failure; ECG, electrocardiogram; METs, metabolic equivalents; MI, myocardial infarction. (From Report of the American College of Cardiology/American Heart Association Task Force on Practice Guidelines [Committee on Perioperative Cardiovascular Evaluation for Noncardiac Surgery]: Guidelines for perioperative cardiovascular evaluation for noncardiac surgery. J Am Coll Cardiol 27:910-948, 1996. By permission of American Heart Association and American College of Cardiology.)

Anticoagulation Issues in Patients With Mechanical Prosthetic Heart Valves Undergoing Noncardiac Operations

No randomized controlled trials have been conducted on anticoagulation in noncardiac surgical patients with mechanical heart valves. However, the following suggestions are offered.

1. Consult with the surgeon to determine whether the intensity of anticoagulation needs to be altered. Procedures such as dental extractions, cataract removal, and other minor operations often can be performed safely with minimal or no decrease in the intensity of anticoagulation.

2. Many factors must be considered when determining a risk-to-benefit assessment of continuous anticoagulation in patients with mechanical prosthetic cardiac valves. Mitral prosthetic valves are more thrombogenic than aortic prostheses, regardless of what type of valve has been used. In general, the older caged-ball valves (Starr-Edwards) are more thrombogenic than bileaflet valves (St. Jude Medical), and *bioprosthetic valves* are the least thrombogenic. Associated factors such as atrial fibrillation, severely impaired left ventricular function, or history of previous thromboembolism also increase the risk of thromboembolism.

3. After a risk-to-benefit assessment has been completed, one of the following strategies can be chosen: a) discontinue warfarin therapy for several days before the procedure to allow the International Normalized Ratio (INR) to decrease to less than 1.5 (a level at which it is considered safe to perform surgery) in an outpatient setting; b) decrease the dose of warfarin (outpatient setting) to maintain the intensity of anticoagulation in a lower or subtherapeutic range during the procedure (discuss this with the surgeon); c) discontinue warfarin therapy and institute heparin therapy coverage (inpatient setting)–administration of heparin can be discontinued 4 hours before the operation and reinstituted, in conjunction with oral anticoagulant therapy, postoperatively, when it is considered safe; or d) discontinue warfarin therapy and institute coverage with low-molecular-weight heparin (outpatient setting)–discontinuing the heparin an adequate number of hours before the operation and then postoperatively, when it is considered safe, reinstituting heparin therapy in conjunction with oral anticoagulant therapy.

In many situations, strategy a or b can be undertaken safely at considerable cost advantage (because of the need for fewer hospitalization days or heparin-related costs) without appreciable increase in risk to the patient. Preoperative heparin therapy during warfarin withdrawal is recommended for those situations in which the risk of operative bleeding with anticoagulant therapy and the risk of thromboembolism without anticoagulant therapy are high (for example, major surgical procedure in a patient with mitral valve prosthesis, cardiomyopathy, and previous thromboembolism). Reinstitution of anticoagulation as early as safely possible is appropriate for all three of the strategies mentioned above.

- Teeth extractions, cataract operations, and other minor procedures usually can be performed safely with therapeutic levels of anticoagulation.
- Prosthetic valves in the mitral position are more thrombogenic than aortic prostheses.
- Older caged-ball valves are more thrombogenic than bileaflet valves.
- Bioprosthetic valves are least thrombogenic.
- Anticoagulation in patients with mechanical prosthetic cardiac valves substantially decreases the incidence of thromboemboli but never eliminates it entirely.

Congestive Heart Failure

Patients with congestive heart failure (CHF) have an incidence of perioperative pulmonary edema ranging from 3% (New York Heart Association class I) to 25% (class IV). Patients with a history of CHF but no preoperative evidence of this disorder have a 6% incidence of perioperative pulmonary edema. Although preoperative CHF is the greatest risk factor for development of pulmonary edema, 50% of those who develop this complication have no history of CHF. Most patients who develop CHF perioperatively do so in the first hour after termination of anesthesia. CHF should be aggressively treated preoperatively, and the therapy for chronic compensated CHF should be maintained in the perioperative period.

- Incidence of perioperative pulmonary edema is from 3% to 25% in patients with CHF.
- The greatest preoperative risk for developing pulmonary edema is CHF.
- If CHF develops perioperatively, it usually does so in the first hour after anesthesia is terminated.
- Treat CHF aggressively preoperatively, and in the perioperative period, maintain therapy for chronic compensated CHF.

Hypertension

Ideally, patients should have well-controlled hypertension (i.e., ≤140/90 mm Hg) for several months preoperatively to minimize lability of intraoperative blood pressure as well as postoperative and neurologic complications. However, studies have shown that when hypertension is stable and diastolic blood pressure is 110 mm Hg or less, no benefit is derived from postponing elective procedures to achieve better control.

If diastolic blood pressure is greater than 110 mm Hg, it should be stabilized preoperatively to diminish risk. Although systolic blood pressure is less well studied, most medical consultants suggest the systolic blood pressure be controlled to less than 180 mm Hg before the induction of anesthesia for elective procedures. In the perioperative period, antihypertensive agents should be continued. Parenteral agents should be substituted for oral medications in patients who are unable to take pills by mouth or nasogastric tube.

- If diastolic blood pressure is >110 mm Hg, it should be stabilized preoperatively.

Hematologic Risk and Management

Patients with poorly controlled polycythemia vera have a high surgical morbidity and mortality because of an excess of thromboembolic events and decrease in oxygen transport due to high blood viscosity. In polycythemia vera, phlebotomy should be performed to decrease the hematocrit to less than 45% before elective operations. Platelet counts less than 50,000/mm^3 or greater than 1,000,000/mm^3 should be evaluated with bleeding times and corrected preoperatively. A platelet count of 50,000/mm^3 usually provides adequate hemostasis for most surgical procedures. If the count is less than 20,000/mm^3, spontaneous bleeding is common. A bleeding time, activated partial thromboplastin time (APTT), and prothrombin time (PT) should be determined preoperatively only if the medical history and physical examination results indicate increased bleeding risk, such as previous bleeding with major or minor surgery, easy bruising, or a family history of bleeding disorder.

- Patients with poorly controlled polycythemia vera have high surgical morbidity and mortality because of thromboembolic events and high blood viscosity.
- In polycythemia vera, perform phlebotomy to decrease hematocrit to <45% before elective operation.
- Platelet count of 50,000/mm^3 usually provides adequate hemostasis for most operations.
- Preoperatively determine bleeding time, APTT, and PT only if medical history and physical examination finding indicate increased bleeding risk.

Liver Risks and Management

Patients with chronic liver disease, particularly those with progressive hepatic failure, possess a high operative risk. Preoperatively, the internist should concentrate on correcting electrolyte abnormalities and abnormal clotting variables, reducing ascites, treating encephalopathy, and improving the patient's nutritional status.

Endocrinologic Risks and Management

Patients who are thyrotoxic are at high risk for surgical complications, such as arrhythmias, high output CHF, and death. Thyroid storm occurs in 20% to 30% of these patients. Thus, elective surgery should be postponed and treatment (antithyroid drugs or radioiodine) should be given for at least 3 months until the patient is euthyroid. If an operation is emergent, a patient who is thyrotoxic should be pretreated with propranolol, propylthiouracil, potassium iodide, and hydrocortisone. The hypothyroid patient can undergo surgical procedures at very low risk. Severely myxedematous patients should receive thyroxine replacement therapy, careful monitoring, and supportive therapy, including free water restriction and diuretics.

- Thyrotoxic patients are at high risk for surgical complications.
- This condition should be treated for 3 months or until patient is euthyroid before any elective operation is performed.
- In case of an emergency operation, pretreat with propranolol, propylthiouracil, potassium iodide, and hydrocortisone.

Patients with diabetes mellitus have a greater risk of surgical complications due to underlying cardiovascular and cerebrovascular disease. It is preferable to have the patient in moderate diabetic control preoperatively to diminish the risk of infection. Remember that the patient may not be able to recognize the signs and symptoms of hypoglycemia in the perioperative period. Thus, oral hypoglycemic agents are withheld and the insulin dose is cut in half on the day of the operation. Metformin, a nonsulfonylurea oral hypoglycemic agent, is discontinued before surgery to avoid possibly inducing lactic acidosis in situations where renal function may fluctuate unpredictably. The serum glucose level should be maintained in the 150 to 250 mg/dL range in the perioperative period.

- In cases of diabetes mellitus, there is greater risk of surgical complications because of underlying cardiovascular and cerebrovascular disease.
- Withhold oral hypoglycemic agents, cut insulin dose in half on the day of the operation, and maintain the serum glucose level at 150 to 200 mg/dL in the perioperative period.

To be on the safe side, adequate preoperative and perioperative corticosteroid replacement prep should be given to any patient who has received suppressive doses of corticosteroids for 2 weeks or more during the past year.

Nutrition

Perioperatively, malnourished patients have increased complications related to wound infection, pneumonia, respiratory insufficiency, and adversely affected cellular and humoral immune function. In nutritional assessment, clinical judgment of malnutrition is as accurate as objective measurements. Thus, detailed laboratory measurements of albumin and other substances are not usually necessary. There is some rationale in giving preoperative nutritional supplementation to malnourished patients, and continuing support through the perioperative period.

Thromboembolism Prophylaxis

Although all surgical patients are at some risk for venous thromboembolic disease, certain patients form a high-risk subset, including elderly patients, patients undergoing prolonged anesthesia or operation, patients with previous venous thromboembolic disease, patients with hereditary disorders of thrombosis, or those with prolonged immobilization or paralysis, malignancy, obesity, varicosities, or estrogen use. Reasonable guidelines for thromboembolism prophylaxis in surgical patients to decrease the overall risk of deep vein thrombosis or pulmonary embolism are given in Table 9-8.

Perioperative Antibiotic Prophylaxis

Antibiotics are given perioperatively to prevent infection of normal sterile tissues by direct contamination during the surgical procedure. The risk of wound infection depends largely on the type of operation. "Clean" operations are ones in which the gastrointestinal, genitourinary, and respiratory tracts are not entered and there is no surrounding inflammation. Previously, antibiotic prophylaxis was not required for this type of procedure because the risk of infection was only about 5%, as opposed to a much higher risk in other procedures, which required prophylactic treatment with antibiotics to prevent wound infection (clean-contaminated, contaminated, and dirty operations). However, antibiotic prophylaxis is now recommended for simple clean procedures such as inguinal hernia repair and breast surgery. A short course of prophylactic therapy (one dose of antibiotic preoperatively and no more than one dose postoperatively) is as effective as longer regimens and is less likely to be associated with toxicity or development of resistant organisms in clear or clean-contaminated operations. Technically, the antibiotics used in dirty or contaminated procedures are for treatment of established infection rather than for prophylaxis and are often continued for 5 to 10 days postoperatively.

Preoperative Laboratory Tests

Few laboratory tests should be ordered solely because an operation is planned. In the absence of symptoms, signs, or risk factors for a disease, results of routinely ordered tests are usually normal, and when abnormal, they are usually ignored. Authors looking at specific preoperative tests have suggested that chest radiography, ECG, PT, APTT, and bleeding time are not justified as "routine" preoperative tests in young healthy persons. In the cost-containment climate of modern medical practice, tests should be performed for specific clinical indications and not because a patient is being seen in the outpatient clinic, hospital, or operating room (Table 9-9).

Because ECG abnormalities increase with age and certain abnormalities are related to major perioperative morbidity, most medical consultants suggest a routine ECG in all patients older than 50 years before elective operations. Although the relationship between chest radiographic findings and perioperative morbidity is not well-defined, elderly patients frequently need postoperative chest radiographs performed because of pulmonary complications, and a baseline preoperative radiograph is helpful in patients older than 60 years.

- Chest radiography, ECG, PT, APTT, and bleeding time are not "routine" preoperative tests in young healthy persons.
- Tests should be performed for specific clinical indications.

Geriatric Surgical Patients

The number of surgical procedures performed on elderly patients has steadily increased. Elderly patients comprise 15% of the population but account for one-third of all surgical procedures, one-half of all emergency surgical procedures, and three-fourths of overall surgical mortality. Age is an independent risk factor for perioperative cardiovascular morbidity. Most elderly patients have at least one associated chronic medical illness. This and the pathophysiologic effects of aging on the cardiovascular and pulmonary systems probably explain why geriatric patients have a higher perioperative mortality rate than younger patients. Intervention aimed at meticulously looking for and treating perioperative complications (anemia, infection, pneumonia) leads to improved outcomes (less postoperative delirium, fewer hospital days, etc.) in geriatric patients.

- Elderly patients account for one-third of all surgical procedures.
- Age is an independent risk factor for perioperative cardiovascular morbidity.
- Geriatric patients have a much higher prevalence of CAD.
- Geriatric patients have a higher perioperative mortality rate.

Perioperative Medication Management

The internist tailors perioperative drug therapy to individual circumstances with particular attention to three factors:

1. Have the indications and doses for the specific drug been clearly defined?
2. What are the likely anesthetic and surgical interactions and complications?
3. Is a clinically important withdrawal syndrome likely, and how can it be managed safely?

Table 9-8.--Prevention of Venous Thromboembolism

Patient Characteristics	Recommended Therapy
Low-risk general surgery patients	Early ambulation
Moderate-risk general surgery patients	LDUH, LMWH, IPC, or ES
Higher risk general surgery patients	LDUH, or higher-dosage LMWH
Higher risk general surgery patients prone to wound complications, e.g., hematomas and infection	IPC is an alternative
Very high-risk general surgery patients with multiple risk factors	LDUH or LMWH, combined with IPC
Selected very high-risk general surgery patients	Perioperative warfarin (goal INR 2.5; range, 2.0 to 3.0)
Patients undergoing total hip replacement surgery[*]	LMWH, started 12 to 24 hr after surgery; or warfarin, started before or immediately after surgery (goal INR 2.5; range, 2.0 to 3.0); or adjusted-dose heparin, started preoperatively; possible adjuvant use of ES or IPC[†]
Patients undergoing total knee replacement surgery[*]	LMWH, warfarin, or IPC
Patients undergoing hip fracture surgery	LMWH, or warfarin (goal INR 2.5; range, 2.0 to 3.0) started preoperatively or immediately after surgery
High-risk patients undergoing orthopedic surgery	IVC filter placement, only if other forms of anticoagulant-based prophylaxis are not feasible, because of active bleeding; this should rarely be necessary
Patients undergoing intracranial neurosurgery	IPC with or without ES: LMWH and LDUH may be acceptable alternatives; consider IPC or EC, with LMWH or LDUH, for high-risk patients
Patients with acute spinal cord injury	LMWH; although ES and IPC appear ineffective when used alone, ES and IPC may have benefit when used with LMWH, or if anticoagulants are contraindicated; during rehabilitation, consider continuation of LMWH or conversion to full-dose oral anticoagulation
Trauma patients with an identifiable risk factor for thromboembolism	LMWH, as soon as considered safe; consider initial prophylaxis with IPC if administration of LMWH will be delayed or is contraindicated; in high-risk patients with suboptimal prophylaxis, consider screening with duplex ultrasonography, or filter placement in the IVC
Patients with MI	LDUH or full-dose anticoagulation; IPC and possibly ES may be useful when heparin is contraindicated
Patients with ischemic stroke and lower-extremity paralysis	LDUH or LMWH; IPC with ES also is probably effective
General medical patients with clinical risk factors for venous thromboembolism, particularly those with CHF or chest infections	LDUH or LMWH
Patients with long-term indwelling central vein catheters	Warfarin (1 mg/day), or LMWH daily to prevent axillary-subclavian venous thrombosis
Patients having spinal puncture or epidural catheters placed for regional anesthesia or analgesia	LMWH should be used with caution

[*]Optimal duration of prophylaxis is uncertain; 7 to 10 days is recommended with LMWH or warfarin; 29 to 35 days with LMWH may offer additional protection.
[†]LDUH, aspirin, dextran, and IPC reduce the overall incidence of venous thromboembolism but are less effective.
CHF, congestive heart failure; ES, elastic stockings; LDUH, low-dose unfractionated heparin; INR, International Normalized Ratio; IPC, intermittent pneumatic compression; IVC, inferior vena cava; LMWH, low-molecular-weight heparin; MI, myocardial infarction.
From Clagett GP, Anderson FA Jr, Geerts W et al: Prevention of venous thromboembolism, Chest 114(suppl):7-8, 1998.

Table 9-9.--Indications for Standard Preoperative Tests in Nonemergency Situations

Test	Indications
Hematocrit	All women; men >60 years old; anticipated blood loss
Electrolytes	Patients >60 years or with renal disease or diabetes, or who take diuretics, steroids, bowel preparations
Prothrombin and partial thromboplastin times, platelet count	Patients with liver disease, bleeding, or malignancy, or who take anticoagulants
Electrocardiography	Patients >50 years or with cardiovascular disease, lung disease, peripheral vascular disease, or diabetes
Chest radiography	Patients >60 years or with pulmonary or cardiovascular disease or acute pulmonary symptoms

Modified from MKSAP X: Part A, Book 3, 1994. American College of Physicians. By permission.

Most drugs used in managing chronic medical conditions can and should be continued through the perioperative period. Often, patients can receive medications with sips of water on the morning of the operation and resume oral medications or parenteral substitution later in the day. Should particular questions occur about the continuation of a specific drug, communicate with the anesthesiologist.

● Most drugs for chronic medical conditions should continue to be used through the perioperative period.

CURRENT CONCEPTS IN ANTICOAGULATION THERAPY

INR

What Is Its Significance?

INR was developed to standardize reporting of the PT assay test results. Standardization was necessary because of the variability in the responsiveness of the different thromboplastins used as reagents throughout the world. The International Sensitivity Index (ISI) is the value representative of the responsiveness of a given thromboplastin to the reduction of vitamin K-dependent coagulation factors. The variations in ISI between different thromboplastins are due to differences in their manufacture and source and in the method of preparation. A more responsive thromboplastin produces less rapid stimulation of coagulation factors, producing a greater prolongation of the PT for a given reduction in clotting factors. A less responsive thromboplastin activates residual clotting factors more rapidly and results in a less prolonged PT, despite a comparable decrease in clotting factors. Therefore, with use of a more responsive thromboplastin, a lower dose of warfarin is required to maintain the PT at a desired ratio than the dose required with a less

responsive thromboplastin—that is, an acceptable PT ratio using a very responsive thromboplastin might give a false sense of security in a patient who is actually at risk for clotting. If a less responsive thromboplastin were used, that same ratio might give a false sense of security in a patient who is actually at risk for major bleeding. The INR is simply an exponential mathematical transformation of PT (usually reported in seconds) into a "corrected" ratio value.

● INR standardizes reporting of PT assay test results.

How Can the INR be Calculated?

The INR is calculated from the patient's PT ratio, which is a simple calculation, and the ISI, which is more complicated. The ISI is calculated by the manufacturer of the thromboplastin or by the laboratory performing the test. The formula is

$$INR = \left(\frac{Patient\ PT}{Mean\ Control\ PT} \right)^{ISI}$$

How Does the INR Help in Clinical Practice?

The ISI of most thromboplastins used in the U.S. varies from 1.0 to 2.8. Because there is no "typical" North American thromboplastin, the earlier habit of using PT ratios has inadvertently left many patients at risk because of over or under anticoagulation. The use of the INR offers several advantages, as listed below:

● Smooth regulation of anticoagulant therapy.
● Benefit to patients who travel, because there is consistency among laboratories using different types of thromboplastin.
● Standardization of anticoagulant therapy in clinical trials and scientific publications.
● Potentially decreased risk of bleeding or thrombotic complications associated with oral anticoagulant therapy.

What Are Recommended INR Therapeutic Ranges for Oral Anticoagulant Therapy?

The recommended INR therapeutic ranges are summarized in Table 9-10. In short, an INR of 2.0 to 3.0 is used for most indications except for those few high-risk conditions (e.g., mechanical prosthetic heart valves) in which a slightly higher INR is suggested.

Antithrombotic Therapy for Venous Thromboembolic Disease

Guidelines for anticoagulation in patients with venous thromboembolic disease are summarized in Table 9-11.

Table 9-10.--Recommended Therapeutic Range for Oral Anticoagulant Therapy

Indication	INR
Prophylaxis of venous thrombosis (high-risk surgery)	2.0-3.0
Treatment of venous thrombosis	2.0-3.0
Treatment of pulmonary embolism	2.0-3.0
Prevention of systemic embolism	
Tissue heart valves[*]	2.0-3.0
Acute myocardial infarction (to prevent systemic embolism)[†]	2.0-3.0
Valvular heart disease	2.0-3.0
Atrial fibrillation	2.0-3.0
Antiphospholipid-antibody syndrome (secondary prevention)	2.5-3.5
Mechanical prosthetic heart valves	
AVR and no risk factors[‡]	
Bileaflet valve	2.0-3.0
Other disk valve or Starr-Edwards	2.5-3.5
AVR and risk factor[§]	2.5-3.5
MVR[§]	2.5-3.5

AVR, aortic valve replacement; INR, International Normalized Ratio; MVR, mitral valve replacement.

[*]Treatment usually for 3 months unless other risk factors continue.

[†]If oral anticoagulant therapy is elected to prevent recurrent myocardial infarction, an INR of 2.5 to 3.5 is recommended, consistent with Food and Drug Administration recommendations.

[‡]Risk factors: atrial fibrillation, left ventricular dysfunction, previous thromboembolism, hypercoagulable state.

[§]Consider addition of ASA 80 to 100 mg once daily to decrease embolic risk.

Modified from Litin SC, Gastineau DA: Current concepts in anticoagulant therapy. Mayo Clin Proc 70:266-272, 1995 and data from Bonow RO, Carabello B, de Leon AC Jr et al: ACC/AHA guidelines for the management of patients with valvular heart disease: executive summary. A report of the American College of Cardiology/American Heart Association Task Force on Practice Guidelines (Committee on Management of Patients With Valvular Heart Disease). Circulation 98:1949-1984, 1998.

Anticoagulation in Prosthetic Heart Valves

What Are the Recommendations for Anticoagulation in Patients With Mechanical Prosthetic Heart Valves?

It is strongly recommended that all patients with mechanical prosthetic heart valves receive warfarin. Levels of warfarin that prolong INR to 2.5 to 3.5 are recommended. Levels of warfarin producing an INR less than 1.8 have a high risk of thromboembolic events, and levels that increase INR to more than 4.5 have a high risk of excessive bleeding. In high-risk patients, aspirin (80 to 100 mg/day) in addition to warfarin further decreases risk of thromboembolism without increasing the risk of major bleeding, although minor bleeding is increased.

- All patients with mechanical prosthetic heart valves should receive warfarin.
- Use warfarin levels that prolong INR to 2.5 to 3.5.
- Warfarin levels that 1) decrease INR <1.8 have high risk of thromboembolic events or 2) increase INR >4.5 have high risk of excessive bleeding.
- A low dose of aspirin plus warfarin may have additive benefit without causing major bleeding (increases minor bleeding).

What Is Recommended if a Patient With a Prosthetic Heart Valve Has a Systemic Embolism Despite Adequate Therapy With Warfarin (INR 2.5 to 3.5)?

Such patients may also respond to a slight increase in the warfarin dose, thus increasing the INR to 3.5 to 4.5. In addition to the warfarin, one could add aspirin (80 to 100 mg/day).

- No regimen ever eliminates the risk of systemic embolization or the risk of bleeding!

What Are the Recommendations for Anticoagulation in Patients With Bioprosthetic Heart Valves?

It is recommended that all patients with bioprosthetic valves in the mitral position receive warfarin therapy (INR, 2.0 to 3.0) for the first 3 months. Anticoagulant therapy of patients with bioprosthetic valves in the aortic position who are in sinus rhythm is also reasonable during the first 3 months. Certain patients with bioprosthetic valves have underlying conditions (i.e., atrial fibrillation, left atrial thrombus) that require long-term warfarin therapy to prevent systemic emboli. Among patients with bioprosthetic heart valves who are in sinus rhythm, long-term therapy with aspirin (325 mg daily) may offer protection against thromboembolism and appears reasonable for patients without contraindication.

- Patients with bioprosthetic valves receive warfarin therapy (INR, 2.0 to 3.0) for 3 months.

Table 9-11. --Guidelines for Anticoagulation in Adults With Venous Thromboembolic Disease

Deep venous thrombosis or pulmonary embolus	Guidelines for anticoagulation
Suspected	Obtain baseline APTT, PT, CBC Check for contraindication to heparin therapy Give unfractionated heparin, 5,000 U IV and order imaging study
Confirmed	Rebolus with heparin, 80 U/kg IV and start maintenance infusion at 18 U/kg per hour[*] or use appropriate regimen of subcutaneous fixed-dose low-molecular-weight heparin Start warfarin therapy on first day at 5 mg and then administer warfarin daily at estimated maintenance dose Discontinue low-molecular-weight or unfractionated heparin when it has been administered jointly with warfarin for at least 4 or 5 days and the INR ≥2.0 for 2 consecutive days Anticoagulate with warfarin for at least 3 months at an INR of 2.0 to 3.0 (longer treatment should be given to patients with ongoing risk factors or recurrent thrombosis)

APTT, activated partial thromboplastin time; CBC, complete blood count; PT, prothrombin time.
[*]If unfractionated heparin is used, check APTT at 6 hours to keep APTT between 1.5 and 2.5 times control (blood heparin level, 0.2 to 0.4 U/mL by protamine sulfate or 0.3 to 0.6 U/mL by an amidolytic anti-Xa assay) and check platelet count daily.

- Patients with bioprosthetic valves who have atrial fibrillation or left atrial thrombus require long-term warfarin therapy to prevent systemic emboli.
- Long-term therapy with aspirin may protect patients with bioprosthetic heart valves who are in sinus rhythm against thromboembolism.

Hemorrhagic Complications of Anticoagulation

When the Anticoagulant Effect of Warfarin Needs to Be Reversed, What Is the Best Way to Do This?

The anticoagulant effect of warfarin can be reversed by stopping treatment, administering vitamin K, or, in urgent situations with significant bleeding, replacing vitamin K-dependent coagulation factors with fresh frozen plasma. When warfarin therapy is discontinued, no significant effect is seen on the INR for 2 days or more because of the half-life of warfarin (36 to 42 hours) and the delay before newly synthesized functional coagulation factors replace dysfunctional coagulation factors.

Administering vitamin K lowers the INR more rapidly, depending on the dosage of vitamin K and severity of the anticoagulant effect. When high doses of vitamin K are used, reversal is rapid and seen by about 6 hours. The disadvantage is that patients often remain resistant to warfarin for up to a week, making continued warfarin treatment difficult. This problem can be overcome by using much lower dosages of vitamin K given orally, subcutaneously, or by slow intravenous infusion.

- Anticoagulant effect of warfarin can be reversed by stopping treatment, giving vitamin K, or replacing vitamin K-dependent coagulation factors with fresh frozen plasma.
- Replacement of vitamin K-dependent coagulation factors with fresh frozen plasma produces an immediate effect and is the treatment of choice in cases of life-threatening bleeding or serious warfarin overdosages.

Are There Certain Patient Characteristics That Increase the Risk of Hemorrhagic Complications of Anticoagulant Treatment?

A strong relationship between intensity of anticoagulant therapy and risk of bleeding has been reported in patients receiving treatment for deep venous thrombosis and prosthetic heart valves. The concurrent use of drugs that interfere with hemostasis and produce gastric erosions (aspirin, nonsteroidal anti-inflammatory drugs) increases the risk of serious upper gastrointestinal tract bleeding. Other drugs such as trimethoprim-sulfamethoxazole and disulfiram inhibit the clearance of warfarin, thus potentiating its effect. Instead of memorizing the long list of drugs that may interact with warfarin, physicians should consider any medication a source of potential interaction until proved otherwise. Several comorbid disease states associated with increased bleeding during warfarin therapy are treated hypertension, renal insufficiency, hepatic insufficiency, and cerebrovascular disease.

- The relationship between the intensity of anticoagulant therapy and the risk of bleeding is strong.
- Concurrent use of drugs that interfere with hemostasis and produce gastric erosions increases the risk of serious upper gastrointestinal tract bleeding.
- Trimethoprim-sulfamethoxazole and disulfiram inhibit the clearance of warfarin, potentiating its effect.

COMMON CLINICAL PROBLEMS IN GENERAL INTERNAL MEDICINE

Treatment of Hyperlipidemia

Case

A 55-year-old man with stable class II angina is referred for consideration of drug treatment for hyperlipidemia. He is otherwise healthy. He quit smoking cigarettes 2 years previously and has no other known risk factors for CAD. He has closely followed the advice of a dietitian for the past 6 months, but his cholesterol levels have shown no significant decrease. His most recent values are: total cholesterol, 240 mg/dL; high-density lipoprotein cholesterol (HDL-C), 35 mg/dL; and triglycerides, 75 mg/dL.

Discussion

Evidence has shown that lowering increased low-density lipoprotein cholesterol (LDL-C) levels is associated with both primary and secondary prevention of coronary events. Moreover, several angiographic trials have shown consistent decreases in progression and increases in regression of atherosclerotic plaques followed up for several years.

The second report of the National Cholesterol Education Program defined high-risk status as definite CAD and/or atherosclerotic disease or two of the following risk factors:

1. Positive risk factors
- Male ≥45 years old.
- Female ≥55 years old or premature menopause without estrogen replacement.
- Family history of CAD (definite MI or sudden death before 55 years of age in father or other first-degree male relative or before 65 years of age in mother or other first-degree female relative).
- Current cigarette smoker.
- Hypertension (blood pressure ≥140/90 mm Hg or taking antihypertension medications).
- Low HDL-C (<35 mg/dL).
- Diabetes mellitus.
2. Negative risk factor
- High HDL-C ≥60 mg/dL (if HDL-C level is ≥60 mg/dL, subtract one risk factor).

LDL-C is used to monitor patients with hypercholesterolemia and is calculated from the following formula:

$$LDL\text{-}C = (\text{Total Cholesterol}) - (\text{HDL Cholesterol}) - (\text{Triglycerides}/5)$$

In this patient, LDL-C = (240) - (35) - (75/5) = 190 mg/dL.

Secondary causes of hyperlipidemia should be ruled out in all patients. Secondary causes of hyperlipidemia may be caused by diseases (hypothyroidism, diabetes, nephrotic syndrome, renal failure, obstructive liver disease), drugs (corticosteroids, progestins, thiazides, β-blockers), or diet (alcohol abuse, increased saturated fats).

- Rule out secondary causes of hyperlipidemia in all patients.

After secondary causes are ruled out, the next line of treatment involves weight reduction in overweight patients, increased physical activity, and dietary therapy (Table 9-12). Both weight reduction and exercise not only promote lowering of cholesterol levels but have other benefits, such as decreasing triglycerides, increasing HDL-C, decreasing blood pressure, and decreasing the risk of diabetes mellitus.

Dietary therapy to decrease elevated serum levels of cholesterol is initiated in patients without CAD or risk factors if LDL-C is 160 mg/dL or greater, for patients without CAD but at least two risk factors if LDL-C is 130 mg/dL or greater, and for patients with CAD if LDL-C is greater than 100 mg/dL. Generally, a minimum of 6 months of intensive dietary therapy and counseling should be carried out in primary prevention before initiating drug therapy; shorter periods can be considered in patients with severe increases of LDL-C (220 mg/dL) or known CAD. If drug therapy is initiated, it should be added to dietary therapy and not substituted for it. Drug treatment should be considered in patients without CAD and with fewer than two risk factors if LDL-C is 190 mg/dL or greater, without CAD but with two or more risk factors if LDL-C is 160 mg/dL or greater, or with CAD if LDL-C is 130 mg/dL or greater (Table 9-12).

- If at least 6 months of dietary therapy fail to lower cholesterol to goal level, consider drug therapy.

If hypolipidemic drugs are used, the choice of drug depends on the mechanism of action, side-effect profile, efficacy, and cost. The following discussion considers the most common classes of drugs used in the treatment of hyperlipidemia.

Bile acid sequestrants (e.g., cholestyramine and colestipol)— Clinical trials have documented their benefit and safety. Their mechanism of action involves removing plasma LDL by depleting the bile acid pool, which causes an increase in hepatic LDL receptors. These drugs are often used alone (in patients

Table 9-12.--Treatment Decisions Based on Low-Density Lipoprotein Cholesterol Level

Patient category	Initiation level	LDL goal
Dietary therapy		
Without CAD and with fewer than two risk factors	≥ 160 mg/dL	< 160 mg/dL
Without CAD and with two or more risk factors	≥ 130 mg/dL	< 130 mg/dL
With CAD	> 100 mg/dL	≤ 100 mg/dL
Drug treatment		
Without CAD and with fewer than two risk factors	≥ 190 mg/dL	< 160 mg/dL
Without CAD and with two or more risk factors	≥ 160 mg/dL	< 130 mg/dL
With CAD	≥ 130 mg/dL	≤ 100 mg/dL

CAD, coronary artery disease; LDL, low-density lipoprotein.
From Expert Panel on Detection, Evaluation, and Treatment of High Blood Cholesterol in Adults: Summary of the second report of the National Cholesterol Education Program (NCEP) Expert Panel on Detection, Evaluation, and Treatment of High Blood Cholesterol in Adults (Adult Treatment Panel II). JAMA 269:3015-3023, 1993.

with mild increases in LDL-C levels) or in combination with other drugs (in patients with greater increases in LDL-C levels). Side effects include gastrointestinal symptoms, binding of other concurrently administered drugs, constipation, and increased triglyceride levels, especially in patients who begin with increased levels.

Nicotonic acid (niacin)—This agent is effective in decreasing total cholesterol and triglyceride levels as well as increasing HDL-C levels. Side effects are common and, thus, limit the use of this drug in many patients. Side effects can include flushing, nausea, abdominal discomfort, and skin itching. Increased levels of plasma glucose, uric acid, and hepatic enzymes may also occur. Slow-release preparations reduce the side effect of flushing, but the incidence of liver dysfunction increases significantly, especially with higher doses. Small doses of aspirin taken before the niacin may block flushing.

The HMG-CoA reductase inhibitors, or "statins" (e.g., lovastatin, pravastatin, simvastatin, atorvastatin, cerivastatin, and fluvastatin)—These drugs are highly effective in decreasing LDL-C by blocking hepatic cholesterol synthesis, which causes an increase in LDL liver receptors. They have few side effects, although myalgias, myopathy, and increase in hepatic enzymes may occur. Myopathy can increase with concurrent use of cyclosporine, niacin, erythromycin, and fibrates (fibric acid derivatives). Long-term safety remains to be demonstrated; therefore, these drugs should be used with caution in young men and premenopausal women. At least one primary prevention study has shown decreased mortality risks with the use of statins. In large secondary prevention trials, statin drugs have been shown to reduce total mortality, cardiac mortality, and the incidence of stroke. They are attractive choices for treatment of severe forms of hypercholesterolemia.

Fibrates (e.g., gemfibrozil, fenofibrate)—These are the drugs of choice for decreasing isolated increased levels of triglycerides. In some patients, these drugs slightly lower LDL-C and raise HDL-C levels. Fenofibrate is more effective in lowering LDL-C than gemfibrozil. Side effects are rare and mostly related to the gastrointestinal tract. These drugs may also increase the risk of gallstones. Therapeutically, they are most useful for disorders of hypertriglyceridemia, especially in patients with diabetes mellitus.

All the above-mentioned drugs have the potential to interact with warfarin (bile acid sequestrants can bind the drug, thus decreasing the INR, and the other hypolipidemic drugs may potentiate warfarin, thus increasing the INR). Therefore, when they are used in anticoagulated patients, close monitoring is indicated.

In general, the following drugs alone or sometimes in combination are recommended.

1. For patients with increased levels of LDL-C: bile acid sequestrants, HMG-CoA reductase inhibitors, and nicotinic acid.
2. For patients with increased levels of LDL-C and triglycerides: nicotinic acid, fibrates, and HMG-CoA reductase inhibitors.
3. For patients with isolated hypertriglyceridemia if treatment is indicated: fibrates and nicotinic acid.
4. Estrogen replacement in postmenopausal women is potential alternative or adjunct to drug therapy in those with increased levels of LDL-C.

Drug therapy for hyperlipidemia must be individualized. In general, a positive effect is gained and fewer side effects experienced by starting therapy with low doses of medication and increasing the dose slowly, if necessary. No studies have supported or condemned the use of drug therapy in the elderly.

Tobacco Abuse

Case

A 60-year-old woman comes to your office for her annual mammogram, breast examination, and pelvic examination. You note from the preexamination questionnaire that she is a current smoker and has smoked one pack per day for 30 years. Examination of the lungs reveals scattered rhonchi and wheezes with a prolonged expiratory phase. You broach the subject of smoking cessation with the patient, but she quickly and defensively counters with a number of statements. She states that after 30 years of smoking "the damage is done" and there is no sense in quitting. She also fears gaining weight after quitting and says that when she did try to quit several years ago, she quickly became so nervous and edgy that she could not sleep and was unpleasant to be around. How might you devise a plan to deal effectively with this patient's tobacco abuse problem?

Discussion

Tobacco use is the leading cause of preventable premature death in the U.S. In addition to being the causative factor for nearly 90% of all cases of lung cancer, smoking is associated with cancer of the oral cavity, larynx, esophagus, stomach, pancreas, uterine cervix, and genitourinary tract. However, among ex-smokers abstinent for 15 years or longer, the incidence of lung cancer is reduced to the rates seen in nonsmokers.

Smokers are 2 to 6 times as likely to have an MI as non-smokers, and 20% of all deaths due to cardiovascular disease are attributable to smoking. After several years of abstinence, the cardiovascular risk of ex-smokers is not significantly different from that of those who have never smoked.

Compared with smokers, ex-smokers have less phlegm production and wheezing, greater FEV_1 and vital capacity, better immune function, and lower mortality from pulmonary infections, bronchitis, and emphysema. Although some lung damage is irreversible, ex-smokers have significant improvement in their pulmonary function during the first year of cessation. After that, the decline in lung function stabilizes at a nonsmoker's rate. Smokers continue to show a decline in lung function at twice the rate of ex-smokers.

Often, one of the most compelling arguments for a patient to stop smoking is that it harms others. It is estimated that more than 50,000 people die annually in the U. S. from medical complications of passive smoking. Most of these deaths are from accelerated heart disease, although the number of lung cancer deaths is also significant. Studies have estimated that nonsmoking spouses of smokers have an all-cancer risk about 1.5 times that of nonsmoking spouses of nonsmokers.

The National Cancer Institute advises physicians to use an easy-to-remember four-step approach in counseling their patients in smoking cessation.

1. **Ask** about smoking at every opportunity.
   The physician should question patients about smoking at any new encounter, inquiring not only if they smoke, but how much they smoke. It is also helpful to ask whether they have ever tried to stop smoking and if so, what happened.

2. **Advise** all smokers to stop.
   Fewer than two-thirds of physicians report advising their patients to stop smoking, and only two-thirds of patients report receiving smoking cessation advice from their physician. This counsel can often be an influential message to patients. The physician should state the advice clearly; for example, "As your physician, I must advise you to stop smoking now." It helps to personalize the "quit smoking" message by referring to other illnesses the patient has, family history, passive smoking issues, etc.

3. **Assist** the patient in stopping to smoke.
   Set a quit date with the patient. Try to do it within 4 weeks, acknowledging with the patient that the time never is ideal. Provide self-help materials. Recommend or prescribe nicotine gum, nicotine patches, intranasal nicotine spray, nicotine inhaler, or bupropion, especially for any patient who smokes more than 10 cigarettes daily and is motivated to attempt a smoking cessation. Consider signing a stop-smoking contract with the patient. Finally, if the patient is not willing to quit at this time, provide motivating literature and bring the topic up again at the next visit.

4. **Arrange** follow-up visits.
   Set up a follow-up visit within 1 or 2 weeks after the quit date. Counseling programs and behavioral therapy programs can be effective in smoking cessation. A transdermal nicotine patch together with behavioral therapy results in significantly higher cessation rates than transdermal nicotine alone. If during follow-up visits you discover the patient has relapsed, advise them that this is not uncommon. Encourage the patient to try again immediately.

Pharmacologic therapy to aid in smoking cessation should be recommended to most patients. In clinical trials, smoking cessation rates at 6 to 12 months are more than doubled among those using active therapy, compared with placebo treatment. Two categories of pharmacologic smoking cessation treatment are available: nicotine replacement therapy and nonnicotine therapy. Nicotine replacement therapy is available in several forms. A transdermal nicotine patch releases nicotine at a steady rate for 16 to 24 hours and is associated with higher patient compliance because of its once-a-day dosing schedule. Nicotine gum, nicotine nasal spray, and nicotine inhaler are immediate-release forms of nicotine replacement and are effective in smoking cessation treatment but must be used several times each day. These forms of nicotine replacement have the advantage of allowing patients to use them in response to smoking urges. Bupropion is the only nonnicotine therapy currently available with proven efficacy for smoking cessation. Bupropion should not be used if the patient has any significant seizure risk; otherwise, it is appropriate for any smoker who is motivated to stop smoking. Bupropion may have the added advantage of attenuating postcessation weight gain.

Several other important concerns that patients have can be addressed and answered. For those worrying about weight gain with smoking cessation, it is useful to let them know that although the majority of patients do gain weight, the average weight gain is about 3 kg, and this can be anticipated and dealt with effectively. For patients who have noted difficulties with nervousness and poor sleep after smoking cessation, advise them that these symptoms are related to nicotine withdrawal and usually resolve after 2 or 3 weeks. Nicotine replacement therapies can often help control these symptoms. Some patients notice an increase in coughing after they stop smoking. This can be explained as a temporary response caused by an increase in the lung's ability to remove phlegm and, thus, represents recovery of the lung's own defense mechanisms. After cessation has been achieved, the patient should be advised to refrain from having even an occasional cigarette, because nicotine addiction seems to be triggered quickly in most ex-smokers.

Acute Low Back Pain

Case

A 55-year-old man comes to your office with a 3-day history of severe low back pain in the lumbosacral area. He recalls no specific trauma, and the review of systems is negative for fever, weight loss, or other constitutional symptoms. He does not complain of numbness, tingling, or weakness in his legs, and he has no bladder or bowel symptoms. He works in a factory, and his job requires some minor lifting and bending. Make a diagnostic assessment, therapeutic plan, and suggestions about levels of activity.

Discussion

In December 1994, the Agency for Health Care Policy and Research published clinical practice guidelines relating to adult patients with acute low back problems. The following discussion focuses on suggestions from these Guidelines.

Acute low back problems are one of the most common reasons for patients to visit a physician's office. Acute low back problems are defined as activity intolerance due to lower back or back-related leg symptoms of less than 3 months' duration. It is important to know that 90% of patients with acute low back problems have a spontaneous recovery and return to previous levels of activity within 1 month. On the initial assessment of such a patient, a focused medical history and physical examination should be performed so that a potentially dangerous underlying condition is not overlooked. Based on this evaluation, low back symptoms can be classified into one of three working categories:

1. *Potentially serious spinal conditions*—This category includes tumor, infection, fracture, or major neurologic disorder. One would look for "red flags" in the history or examination that would point to these conditions, that is, a history of trauma (fracture) or cancer (spinal epidural metastases), risk factors for spinal infection and/or fever/chills (infection), saddle anesthesia or bladder and bowel dysfunction (cauda equina syndrome).

2. *Sciatica*—This category includes back-related lower limb symptoms suggestive of lumbosacral nerve root compromise. Sciatica would be further suggested by a positive straight leg raise, as defined by pain below the knee at less than 70° of leg elevation, aggravated by dorsiflexion of the ankle. Crossover pain (i.e., eliciting pain in the leg with sciatica by straight raising of the unaffected leg) is an even stronger indication of nerve root compression. Correlative findings on sensory examination, specific muscle strength loss, and reflex changes can be used to further diagnose sciatica and to localize the nerve root suspected to be involved.

3. *Nonspecific back symptoms*—This category includes low back pain without signs or symptoms of a serious underlying condition or nerve root compression.

The patient in the case example appears to have nonspecific back discomfort. After this diagnosis is made, the physician could educate the patient about this problem, reassuring him that the evaluation results do not suggest a dangerous problem and that a rapid recovery can be expected. Should the patient not recover within a month, a more extensive evaluation may be needed, including radiography and special studies.

In the interim, the physician must address the need for symptom control measures. This can include oral medications. The safest effective medication for acute low back problems appears to be acetaminophen, which has a low side-effect profile. Nonsteroidal anti-inflammatory drugs can be used, but the disadvantages are cost and side-effect profile (gastrointestinal tract irritation/ulceration, etc.). Muscle relaxants seem to be no more effective than nonsteroidal anti-inflammatory drugs in treating low back symptoms and even a combination of relaxants and nonsteroidal anti-inflammatory drugs has not demonstrated benefit. They also can produce significant drowsiness. Opioids appear no more effective than safer analgesics and should be avoided if possible. If opioids are chosen, they should be used for only a short time and the patient must be warned of the potential side effects of drowsiness, cloudy mentation, and constipation and the potential for dependency.

Physical methods are often used in the treatment of acute back problems; however, most of these methods, including traction, massage, ultrasound, and trigger point injections, have not been proven effective in patients with symptoms. Some have suggested that spinal manipulation is safe and might be effective for appropriate patients who have acute low back symptoms but no radiculopathy.

Activity alteration is a balance between avoiding undue back irritation and preventing debility due to inactivity. Most patients do not require bed rest. In fact, it has been suggested that patients with acute low back pain who continue ordinary activities within the limits permitted by the pain recover more rapidly than those treated with bed rest or back-mobilizing exercises. If bed rest is used, it should be used for only 2 or 3 days, because prolonged bed rest has a potential debilitating effect and its efficacy in treatment is unproven. Bed rest

generally is reserved for patients with severe limitations due to sciatica. Certain postures and activities can increase stress on the back and aggravate the symptoms. Patients must be taught to minimize the stress of lifting by keeping the object being lifted close to the body at the level of the naval. Lifting with the legs as opposed to the back must be emphasized. Prolonged sitting can sometimes aggravate problems, and patients should be encouraged to change their position frequently. Until the patient returns to normal activity, aerobic conditioning may be recommended to help avoid debilitation from inactivity. When requested, it may be appropriate for the physician to offer specific instructions about activity at work for patients with acute limitations due to low back symptoms. The physician should make it clear to both the patient and the employer that even moderately heavy unassisted lifting may aggravate back symptoms and that any restrictions are intended to allow for spontaneous recovery or for time to build activity tolerance through exercise.

QUESTIONS

Multiple Choice (choose the one best answer)

1. A 70-year-old woman has been at partial bed rest for a week because of a sprained knee. She presents to your urgent care center complaining of right-sided pleuritic chest pain. Her temperature is 37.5°C. She is comfortable at rest but somewhat dyspneic with exertion. She complains of a dry cough and her chest radiograph shows a small amount of atelectasis in the right base. You consider the diagnosis of pulmonary embolism and estimate her chance of having this diagnosis is 50% (prevalence in this patient). You also know that the fibrin degradation product, D-dimer, measured by ELISA assay can be a helpful test in this clinical situation. You know that with a cutoff of 500 µg/L for the D-dimer test, diagnostic sensitivity of this test for pulmonary embolism is 99% and its specificity is 40%. If the D-dimer test is positive (>500), what is the chance that this patient has a pulmonary embolus?
   a. 38%
   b. 62%
   c. 99%
   d. 98%
   e. 40%

2. Using the same clinical scenario, if the D-dimer test is negative (<500), what is the chance that the patient has no pulmonary embolism?
   a. 38%
   b. 62%
   c. 99%
   d. 98%
   e. 40%

3. A 75-year-old woman is referred for a preoperative evaluation. She has a left mammographic abnormality, and she and the surgeon have decided on mastectomy if the biopsy specimen shows malignancy. Because of a previous stroke, she has mild residual left hemiparesis. She is wheelchair-bound and uses a walker. Her only medication is atenolol, 50 mg daily. Her blood pressure is 160/80 mm Hg, pulse is 60, with occasional extrasystoles; heart and lung examination findings are otherwise unremarkable. No abnormality is found on chest radiography. Electrocardiography does not show any acute change but premature ventricular contractions in a quadrigeminy pattern. Which of the following statements is correct?
   a. Her β-blocker should be withheld before surgery
   b. She should have a dipyridamole thallium scan to assess cardiac risk before surgery

c. She should have echocardiography to assess cardiac risk before surgery

d. It is all right to proceed to surgery without further cardiac testing

e. She should have a treadmill exercise test to assess risk before surgery

4. A 70-year-old diabetic man with arteriosclerosis obliterans is to have aortobifemoral bypass surgery. You perform a preoperative evaluation and are asked to comment specifically on the need for additional preoperative testing. He is not very active because of his severe claudication at 100 feet. He golfs but uses a motorized cart. Chest radiographic and electrocardiographic findings are unremarkable. Which of the following statements is correct?

a. He should have a dipyridamole thallium study for further risk stratification

b. He should have a treadmill exercise test for further risk stratification

c. He should have echocardiography for further risk stratification

d. He should proceed to coronary angiography for further risk stratification

e. He needs no further testing and may proceed directly to surgery

5. You are consulted to give management advice for a 30-year-old woman who presents with an unprovoked left popliteal deep vein thrombosis. Her family history is negative for venous thromboembolism. She has a history of systemic lupus erythematosus and takes prednisone, 10 mg daily, because of previous glomerulonephritis (now stable) and arthritis. She has one child but has had two miscarriages. An APTT test performed before starting anticoagulation in this patient was prolonged, but her PT was normal. Which statement is most likely to be correct?

a. Because her APTT is increased already, heparin should be withheld and warfarin treatment initiated

b. The patient should be encouraged to use oral contraceptives to prevent pregnancy during the time she is anticoagulated

c. Her history suggests she will need heparin and then anticoagulation with warfarin at an INR of 2.5 to 3.5, perhaps indefinitely

d. History suggests that she will need anticoagulation with heparin and then warfarin at an INR of 2.0 to 3.0 for 3 months

e. Because of the clot in her popliteal vein she would not be at risk for embolization and, thus, would not need anticoagulation at this time

6. A frail 80-year-old man who weighs 48 kg is admitted for a first episode of deep vein thrombosis of the right deep femoral veins. Three weeks earlier, he had right total knee arthroplasty and walks with crutches. He is otherwise healthy. Which statement is correct?

a. A vena caval filter should be placed to decrease the risk of pulmonary embolism because anticoagulants would be too risky in this early postoperative situation

b. If unfractionated heparin is used for treatment, the goal APTT should be kept at 2.5 to 3.5 times control

c. The estimated dose of warfarin for this man would be 10 mg daily

d. Because this deep vein thrombosis was unprovoked, at least 6 months of anticoagulation treatment is indicated

e. Heparin could be discontinued after being given in conjunction with warfarin for 5 days if the INR is greater than or equal to 2.0 for at least 2 days

7. On two separate occasions a 45-year-old man has been found to be hyperlipidemic, with a total cholesterol of 270 mg/dL, triglycerides 150 mg/dL, and high-density lipoprotein cholesterol 40 mg/dL. He has no symptoms of coronary artery disease, is not a smoker, is not diabetic, and is not hypertensive. His 50-year-old brother recently had a myocardial infarction, prompting the patient to seek your advice. Which statement is incorrect?

a. He should have sTSH checked

b. His low-density lipoprotein cholesterol is 180 mg/dL

c. He does meet the NCEP definition of high-risk status

d. His low-density lipoprotein goal should be less than 130 mg/dL

e. If drug therapy were initiated, nicotinic acid would be a reasonable choice

8. A 58-year-old insulin-dependent diabetic man comes for an evaluation. He has a history of treated hypertension, gout, and peripheral vascular disease. His fasting plasma glucose is 190 and his glycosylated hemoglobin is 10%. His total cholesterol is 260 mg/dL, triglycerides 190 mg/dL, and high-density lipoprotein cholesterol 30 mg/dL. He had similar blood test values 6 weeks ago. Which advice is least appropriate for this patient?

a. He should be referred to a dietitian

b. He should begin a fibrate drug

c. He should begin taking nicotinic acid

d. He should begin taking an HMG-CoA reductase inhibitor

e. He should be referred to a diabetic specialist

9. The following statements about a patient's tobacco use are true *except*:

a. It can be harmful to others through passive smoking

b. Cancer of the genitourinary tract and cervix is increased in smokers

c. The majority of physicians do not do an effective job in advising and assisting patients through smoking cessation

d. The rates of smoking cessation using transdermal nicotine products are improved when combined with a behavioral therapy program

e. Weight gain occurs in most patients who quit smoking and averages 15 pounds

10. A 42-year-old laborer has had acute low back pain since lifting a heavy box 2 days ago at work. He denies fever, significant trauma, cancer, or other "red flags" in his history. On examination, a paraspinal spasm is found in the left low lumbar region. He is unable to flex his back more than 45° without pain in the back. Straight leg raising at 30° also causes pain in the back. Muscle strength in his legs is normal, and reflexes are intact. The most appropriate management option at this point is:

a. Reassure him that the evaluation does not suggest a serious problem or require further testing and rapid recovery should be expected

b. Suggest that he be excused from work for 1 week of bed rest

c. A plain film of the lumbar spine should be ordered

d. A muscle relaxant and codeine should be prescribed for symptom relief

e. Magnetic resonance imaging of the lumbar spine should be performed

ANSWERS

1. Answer b.

This is an example of a 2-by-2 table that needs to be constructed to answer the question. The question is related to the positive predictive value of D-dimer test in a patient with a 50% prevalence of disease. The answer is a/a+b or 495/795, approximately 62%.

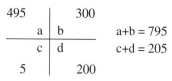

2. Answer d.

The negative predictive value in the same patient with a D-dimer test that is negative would be d/c+d or 200/205, approximately 98%.

3. Answer d.

This patient has minor clinical predictors, and even though she has poor functional capacity, she is to have a low-risk surgical procedure. Therefore, according to the ACC/AHA stepwise approach, she should proceed to surgery without any further cardiovascular testing.

4. Answer a.

This patient has intermediate clinical predictors (diabetes mellitus) and poor functional capacity. He is to undergo a high-risk surgical procedure. It is most appropriate to proceed with noninvasive testing in this patient. He would be unable to perform a treadmill exercise test. Echocardiography alone would not give valuable risk stratification information. There would be no indication at this time for coronary angiography, unless perhaps the noninvasive testing placed him in a high-risk category. Therefore, a dipyridamole thallium study would be appropriate.

5. Answer c.

The clinical scenario described is classic for a patient with antiphospholipid antibodies (lupus anticoagulant). She has an elevated APTT without heparin treatment, has had previous miscarriages, has lupus, and now has an unprovoked venous thrombosis. These patients require anticoagulation with an INR of 2.5 to 3.5, perhaps indefinitely. Her elevated APTT without heparin treatment does not protect her in this situation, and it would be appropriate to use heparin while initiating warfarin therapy. Oral contraceptives are relatively contraindicated in patients with lupus and idiopathic thromboses. The popliteal vein is in the deep venous system, and she is at risk for embolization and needs anticoagulation.

6. Answer e.

The patient is not at high risk for bleeding and, therefore, should be anticoagulated without a vena caval filter. The goal APTT with unfractionated heparin should be 1.5 to 2.5 times control. The estimated daily dose of warfarin for an elderly man of his size would be 5 mg or less per day. A deep vein thrombosis shortly after knee surgery is not considered idiopathic or unprovoked.

7. Answer b.

All the listed statements are correct *except* b. His low-density lipoprotein cholesterol would be calculated in the following manner: total cholesterol minus high-density lipoprotein cholesterol minus triglycerides/5; or 270 - 40 - 150/5 = 200.

8. Answer c.

This patient has insulin-dependent diabetes and gout. Therefore, nicotinic acid would be an inappropriate choice for lipid-lowering therapy, because it is associated with increasing both glucose and uric acid levels. The other options are all reasonable.

9. Answer e.

Although weight gain is seen in most patients who quit smoking, the average increase is only 3 kg. All the other statements are correct.

10. Answer a.

This patient has acute nonspecific back pain. He should be reassured at this point; no further testing is indicated. If analgesics were prescribed, simple ones such as acetaminophen would be reasonable as an initial therapy. There is no evidence that bed rest will help him get better or return to work any sooner. However, his work activity may well need to be modified in the short term so that he does not continue to aggravate his discomfort. Ideally, heavy lifting and so forth could be modified until recovery. For acute nonspecific back pain without "red flags" in the history or examination, there is no role for a lumbar spine film or magnetic resonance imaging.

NOTES

CHAPTER 10

GENETICS

Virginia V. Michels, M.D.

Genetic factors play a role in the development of many types of human disease. Genetic determinants may be single gene defects, mitochondrial mutations, chromosome abnormalities, or multifactorial.

CHROMOSOME ABNORMALITIES

Approximately a sixth of all birth defects and cases of congenitally determined mental retardation are due to chromosome abnormalities. Chromosome abnormalities occur in about 1 in 180 live births. One-third of these abnormalities involve an abnormal number (aneuploidy) of non-sex chromosomes (autosomes). Factors known to result in a higher-than-average risk for having a child with autosomal aneuploidy are maternal age 35 years or older and having previously had an affected child. Prenatal diagnosis by karyotyping of fetal cells obtained by amniocentesis or chorionic villus sampling can be offered to pregnant women who are at increased risk.

- Chromosome abnormalities occur in 1 in 180 live births.
- Risk factors for autosomal aneuploidy: maternal age ≥35 years and having had an affected child.

Down Syndrome

The most common autosomal aneuploidy syndrome in term infants is Down syndrome (incidence, 1 in 880). The most serious consequence of Down syndrome is mild-to-moderate mental retardation (average IQ, about 50). Forty percent of patients with Down syndrome have a congenital heart defect, most frequently ventricular septal defect or atrioventricular canal defect, although other congenital heart defects may occur. Thyroid disease is frequent, and Alzheimer's disease develops at a relatively early age in many. A few patients have hypoplasia of the odontoid, which is important to diagnose before participation in certain sports. Males with Down syndrome are usually sterile, but affected

females are fertile and have a very high risk of having an affected child. Most persons with Down syndrome have trisomy 21 as a result of a new mutation nondisjunctional event; in these cases, the risk to the parents of having another affected child is 1% to 2% or higher, depending on maternal age. In 3% of persons with Down syndrome, a translocation chromosome abnormality is present, in which the extra chromosome 21 is attached to another chromosome, most commonly 14 (Fig. 10-1). These translocation chromosomes may be inherited in an *unbalanced* form from a parent carrying a *balanced* form of the translocation; these parents have a 5% to 15% risk of having another affected child. For identification of these high-risk families, chromosome analysis should be done on all patients with Down syndrome. Even if the parents have completed their childbearing, the karyotype of the affected individual should be determined so that other relatives (e.g., adult siblings) can be counseled. The same principles are presumed to be true for other autosomal aneuploidy syndromes.

- Most common autosomal aneuploidy syndrome in term infants is Down syndrome.
- Most serious consequence of Down syndrome is mild-to-moderate mental retardation.
- Most frequent heart defect in Down syndrome is ventricular septal defect or atrioventricular canal defect.
- Males with Down syndrome are usually sterile, but females are fertile.
- Most persons with Down syndrome have trisomy 21.

Sex Chromosome Aneuploidy Syndromes

Approximately 35% of chromosome abnormalities in live-born infants involve sex chromosome aneuploidy. These infants may have an additional X or Y chromosome or be lacking one. Patients with 47,XXX or 47,XYY karyotypes usually have no major birth defects or mental retardation, although the mean IQ may be 90 rather than 100. Patients with 47,XYY

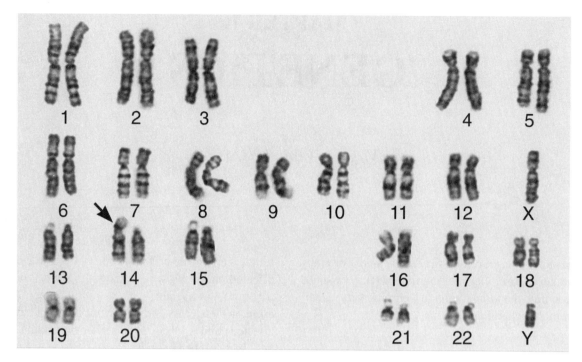

Fig. 10-1. Karyotype 46,XY,-14,+t(14;21)(p11;q11) from patient with Down syndrome. Extra chromosome 21 material is translocated to a chromosome 14. Result is robertsonian translocation. (Karyotype courtesy of G. Dewald, Ph.D.)

usually are detected incidentally. Patients with a 47,XXY karyotype (Klinefelter syndrome) have small testes, infertility, and a tall eunuchoid body habitus. Patients with a 45,X karyotype (Turner syndrome) or its variants—one structurally abnormal X, such as 46,X,i(X)q (Fig. 10-2)—or mosaicism for an X or Y chromosome—such as 45,X/46,XX—usually are mentally normal. Streak gonads are usually present. Patients have a risk of approximately 30% for a congenital heart defect. Bicuspid aortic valve with or without coarctation of the aorta is particularly common. Short stature, webbed neck, increased number of pigmented nevi, failure to develop secondary sexual characteristics, short 4th or 5th metacarpals or metatarsals, renal malformations, and increased risk for thyroid disease are also variably present. Ordinarily, parents of patients with sex chromosome aneuploidy are not at increased risk for having another affected child, and these parents do not routinely need chromosome analyses.

- 47,XXY karyotype (Klinefelter syndrome): small testes, infertility, tall eunuchoid body habitus.
- 45,X karyotype (Turner syndrome): short stature, lack of secondary sex characteristics, usually mentally normal, 30% risk of congenital heart defect, commonly bicuspid aortic valve.
- Other possible features of 45,X karyotype: webbed neck, increased number of pigmented nevi, short 4th or 5th metatarsals or metacarpals.

Other Chromosome Abnormalities

Thirty-four percent of chromosome abnormalities involve structural changes such as deletions, duplications, inversions, or translocations. The translocations may be balanced (no net loss or gain of genetic material) or unbalanced. People with balanced translocations are usually phenotypically normal and healthy but may be at increased risk for miscarriages or their children may have birth defects. Patients with net loss or gain of genetic material by any of the mechanisms listed above have phenotypic abnormalities that usually include mental retardation and frequently other major or minor birth defects. Parents of all patients with a structural chromosome abnormality should have chromosome analyses to determine whether they are carriers of a balanced translocation.

- Parents of all patients with a structural chromosome abnormality should have chromosome analyses.

Fragile X-Linked Mental Retardation

The fragile X-linked mental retardation syndrome occurs in about 1 in 1,000 males. This unusual chromosome abnormality is characterized by a visible fragile site on the long arm of an X chromosome at band q27 when the lymphocytes are cultured in media deficient in folic acid (Fig. 10-3). The fragile site is never observed in all cells, and the frequency may be as low as 4%. Some carrier females do not express the fragile site cytogenetically.

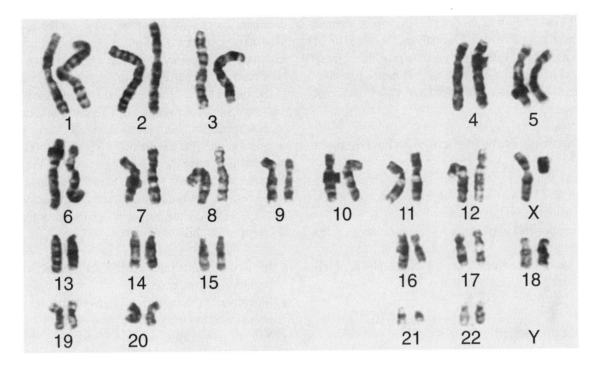

Fig. 10-2. Karyotype 46,X,r(X) from patient with Turner syndrome. (Karyotype courtesy of G. Dewald, Ph.D.)

Affected males may be physically normal or have a long, thin face with prominent jaw, large simplified ears, and enlarged testes. The degree of mental retardation ranges from mild to profound. An occasional male is clinically normal and is referred to as a "transmitting" male. Initially puzzling aspects of this syndrome included the observations that transmitting males had daughters who, although obligate carriers, rarely showed signs of the disease. However, these daughters could have typically affected sons. Carrier females may be phenotypically normal or mildly retarded and dysmorphic; occasionally they are moderately or severely retarded. This now can be explained by the discovery of a DNA trinucleotide repeat (CGG) that is more likely to expand and thereby become more abnormal during transmission through a female. Direct DNA

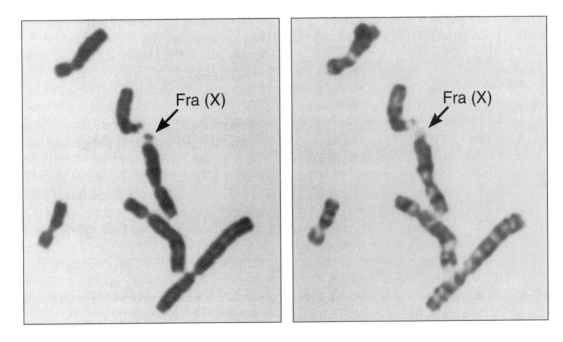

Fig. 10-3. Chromosome analysis from patient with fragile X syndrome. Fragile site is visible on long arm of X chromosome at band q27 when lymphocytes are cultured in media deficient in folic acid. (Photograph courtesy of G. Dewald, Ph.D.)

analysis of the size of the trinucleotide repeat is a more accurate method than standard cytogenetic analysis for detection of carrier females. Males with repeat expansion to 200 or more (referred to as a full mutation) are generally mentally retarded. Females with repeats of this size have a 50% chance of mental subnormality.

- Fragile X: fragile site on long arm of X chromosome at band q27.
- Males with fragile X: may be physically normal or have long, thin face, prominent jaw, large ears, enlarged testes, mild to profound mental retardation.
- Carrier females: phenotypically normal or mildly retarded and dysmorphic.
- To detect carrier females: direct DNA analysis of trinucleotide repeat is most accurate.

PATTERNS OF INHERITANCE

Autosomal Dominant

In autosomal dominant inheritance, the responsible gene is located on one of the autosomes and the gene overrides its homologue in terms of clinical effect. Therefore, one copy of the gene is sufficient for the trait to be expressed or for the disease to be present, and heterozygotes have the disease. There is a 50% chance that any child born to an affected person will inherit the abnormal gene.

- Autosomal dominant inheritance: responsible gene is located on autosome and overrides its homologue.
- 50% chance that child of affected person will inherit abnormal gene.

The severity of the disease caused by the abnormal gene may be uniform for some conditions, such as achondroplasia, but the severity may be variable for other conditions, such as neurofibromatosis and Marfan syndrome. This difference of severity is referred to as "variable expression." In contrast, the term "incomplete penetrance" means that some persons who have inherited the gene show no signs of it. Obviously, the clinical decision regarding whether a person has signs of the gene defect depends on the thoroughness of the examination and the sensitivity of the investigative techniques. For example, many families with hypertrophic cardiomyopathy were thought to include members with incomplete penetrance until asymptomatic relatives were examined with echocardiography. Although transmission of a disease through members of either sex through multiple generations of a family strongly suggests autosomal dominant inheritance, it is important to remember that autosomal dominant diseases can occur without a positive family history. This can occur because of incomplete penetrance, incorrect assignment of paternity, new mutation, or somatic mosaicism. New mutation events represent changes in the genetic material of the individual egg or sperm that gives rise to the fetus. Although the risk for siblings of a person whose disease arose by new mutation is not increased over that of the general population, the risk for the offspring still is 50%. Somatic mosaicism refers to the possibility that one of the parents has the gene defect in only some cells, including the reproductive cells (germinal mosaicism), such that the person has no or few signs of the disease but potentially can transmit the disease to one or more children.

- In autosomal dominant inheritance, disease severity may be uniform or variable.
- Incomplete penetrance: no signs of abnormal gene in a person who has inherited it.
- Somatic mosaicism: person has gene defect in only some cells.

Some of the diseases with autosomal dominant inheritance are listed in Table 10-1 and summarized on the following pages.

Ehlers-Danlos Syndromes

Type I

There may be up to 15 forms of Ehlers-Danlos syndrome. Type I, or gravis type, was the first described and serves as a prototype for discussion of this group of genetically heterogeneous disorders. The syndrome is inherited as an autosomal dominant condition. The basic defect in type I disease has just recently been defined for some cases, and it is a defect in the α-1 chain of type V collagen. Whether this disorder will prove to be genetically heterogeneous at the locus level remains unknown. The disorder is characterized by velvety textured, hyperextensible, fragile skin that splits easily and heals poorly, resulting in wide, thin scars. Many tissues are friable, which is an important consideration when surgical procedures are considered. Even fetal membranes are affected and frequently rupture before term, resulting in premature birth. "Molluscoid pseudotumors" are areas of sagging, wrinkled, redundant skin that may develop over the knee and elbow joints. Small fat or mucin-containing spherules may be present in the subcutaneous tissue and may be calcified. The joints are hyperextensible and prone to dislocations. Pes planus, scoliosis, degenerative arthritis, visceral diverticulosis, and spontaneous pneumothorax may occur.

- Ehlers-Danlos type I is an autosomal dominant condition.
- Features: velvety textured, hyperextensible, fragile skin.

Table 10-1.--Diseases With Autosomal Dominant Inheritance

Achondroplasia
Amyloidosis (many types)
Ehlers-Danlos syndrome, types I, II, III, VIII, some type IV, VI, and VII
Huntington disease
Hypertrophic cardiomyopathy
LEOPARD syndrome
Low-density lipoprotein (LDL) receptor deficiency (hypercholesterolemia)
Marfan syndrome
Multiple endocrine neoplasia, types I, IIa, and IIb
Myotonic dystrophy
Neurofibromatosis, types 1 and 2
Noonan syndrome[*]
Osler-Weber-Rendu disease (hereditary hemorrhagic telangiectasia)
Osteogenesis imperfecta, types I and IV, most type II
Polycystic kidney disease (some forms are autosomal recessive)
Porphyria (several types)
Pseudoxanthoma elasticum (some forms are autosomal recessive)
Spherocytosis
Tuberous sclerosis
Von Hippel-Lindau disease
Von Willebrand disease

[*]Most cases are sporadic, but there is good evidence that they have new mutation autosomal dominant disease.

- Joints are hyperextensible and prone to dislocation.
- Associated conditions: pes planus, scoliosis, degenerative arthritis, visceral diverticulosis, spontaneous pneumothorax.

Involvement of small blood vessels results in easy bruisability. Mitral valve prolapse may occur in 50% of patients. Dilatation of the aortic root or pulmonary artery and prolapse of the tricuspid valve may occur. Vascular rupture is relatively rare.

- Ehlers-Danlos type I: mitral valve prolapse in 50%.
- Vascular rupture is uncommon.

Type II

Ehlers-Danlos syndrome type II, or mitis type, is similar to type I but milder; it also is inherited as an autosomal dominant disorder. A significant number of patients have mitral valve prolapse. It is uncertain whether all cases of this disorder result from a mutation at the same locus as for type I, but at least some families have an α-1 chain of type V collagen.

- Ehlers-Danlos type II is milder than type I.

Type III

The joint hypermobility of Ehlers-Danlos syndrome type III, or benign familial hypermobility syndrome, is similar to that in type I and may result in joint dislocations. However, skin hyperextensibility and scarring are minimal or absent. There is a wide range of expression both within and between families. Families with the mildest manifestations merge with the general population in terms of normal variation in joint mobility. It is an autosomal dominant or multifactorial disorder.

- In Ehlers-Danlos type III, joint hypermobility is similar to that in type I.
- Skin hyperextensibility and scarring are minimal or absent.

Type IV

Ehlers-Danlos syndrome type IV, or vascular type, may be genetically heterogeneous with both autosomal dominant and, perhaps less commonly, autosomal recessive forms. It is usually due to deficiency of type III collagen synthesis or secretion in skin, aorta, uterus, and intestine. This is the most severe form of Ehlers-Danlos syndrome and is characterized by rupture of large arteries, the colon, or the gravid uterus. Angiography and other invasive procedures may precipitate vascular or organ rupture and should be done only after careful consideration of the risk:benefit ratio. Mitral valve prolapse frequently is present. In some patients the skin is extremely thin, allowing visualization of the underlying venous network (Fig. 10-4). Despite this, there is a tendency to form keloid scars and contractures. In contrast to other forms of Ehlers-Danlos syndrome, the skin and connective tissues may not be hyperextensible. Occasional complications include spontaneous pneumothorax and severe periodontal disease. This defect is expressed in cultured skin fibroblasts, so prenatal diagnosis theoretically is possible. Although it has been suggested that type III collagen also is deficient in some patients with congenital cerebral aneurysms or acquired abdominal aortic aneurysms who do not have classic Ehlers-Danlos syndrome, demonstrable defects occur in only a very small proportion of patients.

- Ehlers-Danlos type IV has autosomal dominant and possibly autosomal recessive forms.
- It is due to deficiency of type III collagen synthesis.
- Angiography and other invasive procedures may precipitate vascular or organ rupture.
- Mitral valve prolapse is frequently present.
- Occasional complications: spontaneous pneumothorax and severe periodontal disease.

Type V

Ehlers-Danlos syndrome type V is an X-linked recessive disease. The molecular defect is unknown. Clinically, it is

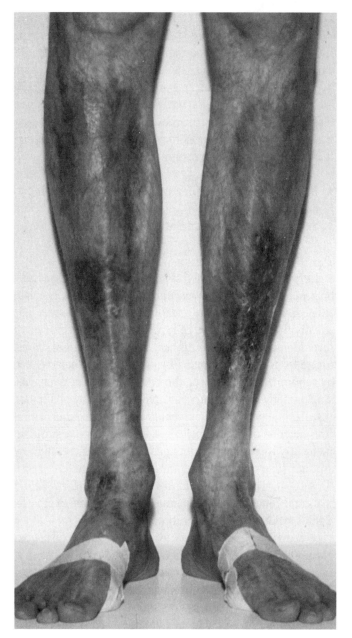

Fig. 10-4. Thin, prematurely aged-appearing skin in young man with Ehlers-Danlos syndrome type IV.

aortic rupture, and gastrointestinal hemorrhage also can occur. Prenatal diagnosis is possible only in families with a documented biochemical defect.

- Ehlers-Danlos type VI is called ocular type.
- Blindness from retinal detachment is a complication.
- Some cases are autosomal recessive.
- Scoliosis, joint dislocations, aortic rupture, and gastrointestinal hemorrhage can occur.

Type VII

Ehlers-Danlos syndrome type VII, or arthrochalasis multiplex congenita, is characterized by extreme joint laxity and dislocations. Some patients might have defective conversion of procollagen to collagen, which is an autosomal recessive defect. However, more commonly, others have structural abnormalities of half their α-2 chains of type I collagen which interfere with the enzymatic conversion of procollagen to collagen. This is an autosomal dominant condition that sometimes arises as a new mutation.

- Ehlers-Danlos type VII usually is autosomal dominant.

Type VIII

Ehlers-Danlos syndrome type VIII is similar to types I and II but includes particularly severe periodontal disease. It is an autosomal dominant disorder, and the basic defect is unknown.

- Ehlers-Danlos type VIII is autosomal dominant.

There is marked clinical and genetic heterogeneity in all the Ehlers-Danlos syndromes that have been chemically defined.

Hypertrophic Cardiomyopathy

Isolated hypertrophic cardiomyopathy frequently is inherited as an autosomal dominant disorder. Penetrance ranges from more than 60% to 100% in different families when relatives are studied with electrocardiography and echocardiography. Investigation of first-degree relatives is necessary. Even if parents are normal by echocardiography, the possibility of new mutation cannot be excluded, and children born to an affected parent must be considered to be at risk and should be evaluated. The possibility of an autosomal dominant disorder can never be excluded on the basis of a negative family history.

- Isolated hypertrophic cardiomyopathy is autosomal dominant.
- Investigation of first-degree relatives is necessary.
- Children of affected parents are at risk.

As with any autosomal dominant disorder, the risk of passing

similar to Ehlers-Danlos type II. Mitral and tricuspid valve prolapse or insufficiency may be present.

- Ehlers-Danlos type V is X-linked recessive disease.

Type VI

Ehlers-Danlos syndrome type VI is called the ocular type because blindness from retinal detachment or ocular rupture is a serious complication. In some cases the disease is due to an autosomal recessively inherited deficiency of procollagen lysyl hydroxylase. Severe scoliosis, recurrent joint dislocations, the abnormal gene to each child is 50%. The course of the disease may be variable, even within a family; therefore, the age at onset cannot be predicted precisely. It is not rare to study a child who presents with symptoms and to discover, after family investigations, that an asymptomatic parent is affected.

- In hypertrophic cardiomyopathy, the risk of passing the gene to each child is 50%.
- Course of disease is variable.
- Age at onset cannot be predicted.

Hypertrophic cardiomyopathy with or without outflow obstruction has been observed within single families. This is compelling evidence that they are different manifestations of the same disease.

Less than 30% of families with hypertrophic cardiomyopathy have a defect in the β cardiac myosin heavy-chain gene on chromosome 14q. However, other families have not shown linkage to this locus, a finding demonstrating genetic heterogeneity. Other gene defects that may cause hypertrophic cardiomyopathy include cardiac troponin T, troponin I, α-tropomyosin, myosin-binding protein C, ventricular myosin essential light chain, ventricular myosin-regulating light chain, and possibly others that remain unidentified.

- Less than 30% of families with hypertrophic cardiomyopathy have defect in β cardiac myosin heavy-chain gene.

Marfan Syndrome

The Marfan syndrome is relatively common; its incidence is 1 in 20,000. It is an autosomal dominant disorder with extremely variable expression, and approximately 20% of cases arise by new mutation. There are no well-documented instances of nonpenetrance.

- Marfan syndrome is relatively common—1 in 20,000.
- It is an autosomal dominant disorder.
- About 20% of cases arise by new mutation.

The disease involves the musculoskeletal, cardiovascular, and ocular systems. Skeletal abnormalities include tall stature, a low upper:lower segment ratio because limbs are relatively long compared with the trunk, scoliosis or kyphosis, and pectus deformities. These features result from overgrowth of the tubular bones. Increased joint laxity and hyperextensibility are common, but occasionally patients have limited extension of fingers and elbows. The face may be long and the palate highly arched. This "marfanoid habitus" may be present in patients with other disorders such as other connective tissue dysplasias, mucosal neuroma syndrome (multiple endocrine neoplasia type IIb), Stickler syndrome, and homocystinuria.

The characteristic body habitus is never sufficient evidence for making the diagnosis of Marfan syndrome in the absence of other characteristic features or a well-documented family history of Marfan syndrome.

- Marfan syndrome involves the musculoskeletal, cardiovascular, and ocular systems.
- Skeletal abnormalities: tall stature, low upper:lower segment ratio, scoliosis or kyphosis, pectus deformities.
- Increased joint laxity and hyperextensibility are common.

The ocular abnormalities associated with Marfan syndrome may include subluxation of the lenses, myopia, and retinal detachment. As the most specific ocular feature, dislocation of the lenses is very helpful in making the diagnosis of Marfan syndrome, although ectopia lentis also can occur in other disorders such as homocystinuria and Weill-Marchesani syndrome. Dislocations occur in 50% to 80% of patients; the lens frequently is displaced upward, but this is not always the case. Gross dislocations may be evident without the aid of special equipment, but lesser degrees of dislocation may be evident only by slit-lamp examination. Therefore, all patients suspected of having Marfan syndrome must have a complete ophthalmologic evaluation, including slit-lamp examination. Patients with Marfan syndrome should have frequent ophthalmologic examinations to permit early detection of complications such as retinal detachment or glaucoma.

- Ocular abnormalities of Marfan syndrome: subluxation of lenses, myopia, retinal detachment.
- Dislocation of lenses is helpful for diagnosis; ectopia lentis can occur in homocystinuria and Weill-Marchesani syndrome.
- Dislocations occur in 50%-80% of cases.
- All patients must have ophthalmologic evaluation.

The life expectancy of patients with Marfan syndrome is shortened because of cardiovascular disease. The most common manifestation is mitral valve prolapse with or without mitral regurgitation. Dilatation of the ascending aorta is the next most common cardiovascular disorder; it may lead to aortic regurgitation, aortic rupture, or dissecting aneurysm. Although less than 70% of patients have evidence of cardiovascular disease on physical examination, more than 80% have abnormalities detected by echocardiography.

- Life expectancy in Marfan syndrome is shortened by cardiovascular disease.
- Most common cardiovascular manifestations are mitral valve prolapse and dilatation of ascending aorta.
- More than 80% of patients have abnormalities found on echocardiography.

Mitral valve prolapse in patients with Marfan syndrome initially may involve only the posterior leaflet; it may be late systolic or pansystolic and often is progressive. Prophylactic antibiotic therapy for bacterial endocarditis is warranted. The prevalence of mitral valve prolapse is similar in males and females. In one retrospective series of 166 patients who had had echocardiography before age 22 years, 8 patients died as a result of mitral valve regurgitation and the complication developed in an additional 15 patients. Mitral insufficiency may be present in infants with Marfan syndrome. Acute onset of severe mitral regurgitation due to rupture of chordae tendineae may occur even in childhood. Mitral valve prolapse in a patient with a "marfanoid" body habitus is not a sufficient basis for the diagnosis of Marfan syndrome in the absence of a positive family history of Marfan syndrome or other characteristic findings. Patients with some forms of Ehlers-Danlos syndrome and nonspecific connective tissue dysplasias can have a similar body habitus, joint laxity, and mitral valve prolapse.

- Mitral valve prolapse in Marfan syndrome is progressive.
- Prophylactic antibiotic for bacterial endocarditis is warranted.

In two series, aortic abnormalities were found in 60% to 90% of patients with Marfan syndrome. In children and adults, the diameter of the aortic root usually is abnormal in proportion to body surface area. Aortic dilatation is progressive, with symmetric involvement in the region of the sinus of Valsalva and sinotubular ridge. The maximal aortic root diameter is several centimeters superior to the level of aortic leaflet insertion. A greater degree of aortic root dilatation is positively correlated with aortic regurgitation and dissection. Progression of aortic root dilatation may be due to the strain of left ventricular ejection, and β-adrenergic blockers may protect against progressive dilatation. In a controlled study, patients with aortic root dilatation who were given propranolol to decrease left ventricular inotropy by 30% had a significantly lesser degree of dilatation and less morbidity.

- Aortic abnormalities occur in 60%-90% of cases of Marfan syndrome.
- Aortic dilatation is progressive.

Although surgical risks are increased in patients with Marfan syndrome because of tissue friability, surgical treatment frequently is successful for mitral and aortic regurgitation and for aortic dissection. In one series of 41 patients who had a total of 79 operations for aneurysms or valvular insufficiencies, the early mortality rate was 3%; 62% survived at least 15 years. This study spanned 16 years, and 7 of the 11 late deaths may have been prevented by surgical techniques that now are available.

- Surgical risks are increased in Marfan syndrome.
- Surgical treatment is often successful for mitral and aortic regurgitation and aortic dissection.

Patients with Marfan syndrome are prone to traumatic aortic rupture, so contact sports and strenuous exercise should be avoided. The risk of cardiovascular complications during pregnancy poses a special problem for women with Marfan syndrome. Acute aortic dissection may occur before, during, or after labor. A retrospective review of one series of patients suggested that the risk of maternal death was "low in patients with minimal preexisting vascular disease" but the risk may be "significant" in those with moderate degrees of aortic root dilatation. Therefore, aortic root diameter must be considered when counseling women who are considering childbearing. Some physicians advise women with aortic root dilatation not to become pregnant. Those who decide to become pregnant should receive care appropriate for high-risk obstetric patients and careful echocardiographic monitoring.

- Patients with Marfan syndrome should avoid contact sports and strenuous exercise (risk of aortic rupture).
- In pregnant women with Marfan syndrome, aortic dissection may occur before, during, or after labor.
- Some physicians advise women with aortic root dilatation not to become pregnant.

Additional features sometimes associated with Marfan syndrome include decreased amounts of subcutaneous tissue, skin striae, inguinal hernias, pneumothorax, and degenerative joint disease.

In addition to physical examination, the diagnostic evaluation of patients suspected of having Marfan syndrome should include chest radiography, ophthalmologic examination (including slit-lamp evaluation of the lenses), and echocardiography. A thorough family history should be obtained. For patients with a well-documented family history of Marfan syndrome, characteristic involvement of the skeletal, cardiovascular, or ocular organ systems may be sufficient for the diagnosis to be made. However, in patients without a positive family history, the patient must have the characteristic body habitus and either aortic root dilatation or ectopia lentis. In those with ectopia lentis, homocystinuria must be excluded. In patients with the characteristic body habitus and mitral valve prolapse but without aortic root dilatation, the diagnosis cannot be made definitely. If skin hyperextensibility, poor skin and wound healing, or atrophic skin scarring is present, the patient probably has a form of Ehlers-Danlos syndrome. If no other abnormality is present, it may be impossible to exclude the diagnosis of Marfan syndrome, and subsequent evaluations are warranted.

● Diagnostic evaluation for Marfan syndrome includes chest radiography, ophthalmologic evaluation, and echocardiography.

First-degree relatives should be evaluated even if they have no obvious stigmata of Marfan syndrome. Families have been observed in which a child presented with obvious phenotypic features of Marfan syndrome and a parent was found to be affected only after echocardiography revealed aortic dilatation or slit-lamp examination revealed ectopia lentis.

The basic cause of Marfan syndrome is a defect in fibrillin; the gene encoding fibrillin is on chromosome 15q15-21. This discovery potentially makes presymptomatic and prenatal diagnosis possible in families known to have the disease, and in the near future it also may allow for diagnostic testing in patients with equivocal signs of the disease.

● Cause of Marfan syndrome is a defect in fibrillin.

Myotonic Dystrophy

Myotonic dystrophy, the most common form of muscular dystrophy in adults, has an incidence of approximately 1 per 8,000 to 20,000. The inheritance pattern is autosomal dominant with extremely variable expression. Although average age at onset is in the second to third decade of life, the disease may be evident at birth or first be noticed in the seventh decade. The disease is characterized by myotonia, muscle atrophy and weakness, ptosis of the eyelids, and expressionless facies resulting from particularly severe involvement of facial and temporal muscles. Rate of progression of the disease is variable, but disability is usually severe within 15 to 20 years after onset. Associated abnormalities may include premature frontal baldness, testicular atrophy or menstrual irregularities, gastrointestinal symptoms related to smooth muscle involvement, and cardiac disease. Distinctive refractile posterior subcapsular cataracts often are evident by slit-lamp examination. Although glucose intolerance is common, overt diabetes mellitus occurs in only about 6% of patients.

● Myotonic dystrophy is most common form of muscular dystrophy in adults.
● Incidence is 1 in 8,000-20,000.
● Autosomal dominant inheritance with extremely variable expression.
● Age at onset is usually second to third decade of life.
● Characteristics: myotonia, muscle atrophy and weakness, ptosis of eyelids, expressionless facies.
● Disability is severe within 15-20 years after onset.
● Associated abnormalities: premature frontal baldness, testicular atrophy or menstrual irregularities, gastrointestinal symptoms, cardiac disease.
● Diabetes mellitus occurs in 6% of patients.

The diagnosis is based on clinical findings and a typical electromyographic pattern characterized by prolonged rhythmic discharges. The gene for myotonic dystrophy is located on chromosome 19 at band q13, and genetic counseling is warranted for the patient and family. First-degree relatives should be investigated. The risk for children born to an affected parent is 50%. The molecular basis of most cases of myotonic dystrophy is expansion of a CTG trinucleotide repeat sequence in a gene encoding a protein kinase. Thus, direct DNA-based diagnosis of the disease is possible in most cases. The size of the DNA repeat expansion tends to increase during transmission from one generation to the next. This increasing size correlates with worsening disease severity in subsequent generations, a phenomenon known as "anticipation." Affected females also need to be aware of the additional risk of having an affected infant with severe, sometimes fatal, hypotonia and mental deficiency. This infantile form of the disease rarely occurs when the father is the affected parent.

● Diagnosis of myotonic dystrophy is based on clinical and electromyographic findings or DNA analysis.
● Genetic counseling is warranted for patients and family members with myotonic dystrophy.
● First-degree relatives should be investigated.

Cardiac disease is present in approximately two-thirds of patients with myotonic dystrophy, and sudden death may occur. There is prolongation of the P-R or QRS interval, and there are changes in the T wave and ST segment. Intra-atrial and His-Purkinje conduction may be prolonged, and heart block may require implantation of a pacemaker. There seems to be degeneration of the conducting tissue before other cardiac muscle is involved. If general anesthesia is required, caution must be taken. Many affected patients have central and alveolar hypoventilation resulting in a serious risk of postanesthetic respiratory depression, which can occur several hours after the patient seems to be alert and stable.

● Cardiac disease occurs in 2 of 3 patients with myotonic dystrophy, and sudden death may occur.
● Many patients have central and alveolar hypoventilation.

Neurofibromatosis

Type 1

Neurofibromatosis type 1 is an autosomal dominant disorder with an incidence of approximately 1 in 3,000 to 4,000. Approximately 50% of patients have the disease because of a new mutation. The disorder has markedly variable expression but very high penetrance. The diagnosis is based on two or more of the following clinical criteria: six or more café-au-lait macules of 1.5 cm or more in diameter (in a child, five or more that are 0.5 cm), axillary or inguinal freckling, two or more Lisch nodules of the iris, two or more neurofibromas or one plexiform neurofibroma, a definitely positive family history, or one of these and one of the uncommon characteristic manifestations such as orbital or sphenoid wing dysplasia, optic or other central nervous system glioma, renal artery dysplasia with or without abdominal aorta coarctation, or tibial pseudofracture. Additional, less specific signs of the disease may include pheochromocytoma and scoliosis. Fewer than 10% of patients develop malignancy, often neurofibrosarcoma. Patients should have, at minimum, an annual physical examination, including blood pressure check and thorough neurologic assessment. The gene has been identified and is a GTPase-activating protein involved in the *ras* signaling process. The gene is very large, and multiple different mutations have been identified; there is no evidence for non-allelic heterogeneity. Because of the multitude of different mutations, DNA-based testing for direct diagnosis is difficult. Linkage analysis can be used for presymptomatic or prenatal diagnosis in informative families (see Linkage Analysis, page 397).

- Neurofibromatosis type 1 is autosomal dominant.
- Incidence is 1 in 3,000-4,000.
- Disorder has markedly variable expression but very high penetrance.
- Fewer than 10% of patients develop malignancy (often neurofibrosarcoma).
- Multiple different mutations have been identified.

Type 2

Neurofibromatosis type 2 is an autosomal dominant disorder that is genetically distinct from neurofibromatosis type 1. It is characterized by bilateral vestibular schwannomas (commonly referred to as "acoustic neuroma" in the past) or a family history of neurofibromatosis type 2 with a unilateral vestibular schwannoma, or two of the following: menginoma, glioma, neurofibroma, schwannoma, or posterior subcapsular lenticular opacities. Café-au-lait macules may or may not be present. The gene has been identified and is localized to the long arm of chromosome 22. It has been referred to as either "merlin" or "schwannomin." In addition to occurring in the germline of neurofibromatosis type 2 patients, acquired mutations in this gene occur in some sporadic meningiomas and schwannomas. DNA-based diagnosis is available by linkage analysis in some familial cases or by direct mutation analysis in some patients. Patients should have, at minimum, an annual physicial examination with thorough neurologic assessment, monitoring of hearing, and magnetic resonance imaging of the head. Magnetic resonance imaging of the spine should be done in patients with newly diagnosed disease or patients with symptoms referable to the spinal cord.

- Neurofibromatosis type 2 is autosomal dominant.
- Characteristics: vestibular schwannomas, sometimes nervous system gliomas, subcapsular cataracts, café-au-lait macules.

Osteogenesis Imperfecta

Historically, osteogenesis imperfecta has been divided into four types. Type I is the most common form of osteogenesis imperfecta tarda, and type IV tends to be more severe. Osteogenesis imperfecta congenita includes types II and III. Type II is lethal in the perinatal period, whereas type III may be compatible with prolonged survival with extreme crippling and short stature. The disease is characterized by multiple bone fractures, and some patients have opalescent teeth, blue sclerae, and child- or adult-onset hearing loss. Some patients have increased bruisability. The clinical expression is extremely variable between and within families. Multiple defects in the genes encoding the α-1 and α-2 chains of type I collagen have been reported, and thus the disease is extremely heterogeneous at the DNA level.

Types I and IV, most type II, and some type III osteogenesis imperfecta cases are autosomal dominant. Mitral valve prolapse is increased in frequency but infrequently progresses to significant regurgitation. The mean aortic root diameter is slightly but significantly increased, and aortic regurgitation occurs in 1% to 2% of patients.

Tuberous Sclerosis

Tuberous sclerosis is an autosomal dominant disorder with variable expression and high penetrance. Approximately 50% of cases arise by new mutation. It is characterized by cortical or retinal tubers, seizures, mental retardation in less than 50%, depigmented "ash leaf" macules, facial angiofibromas, dental pits, subungual or periungual fibromas, shagreen patches, and renal cysts or angiomyolipomas. Cardiac rhabdomyomas are more frequent in the fetus and infant and often resolve with age. Pulmonary fibrosis resulting in a "honeycomb" appearance by radiography or computed tomography is more frequent in young women and tends to progress rapidly. Central nervous system astrocytomas may occur. There is non-allelic heterogeneity, with one gene defect that causes tuberous sclerosis on chromosome 9 and another on chromosome 16. The gene on chromosome 9 is referred to as hamartin; that on chromosome 16 is called tuberin. Both act as tumor suppressor genes.

- Tuberous sclerosis is autosomal dominant and has high penetrance.

- About 50% of cases arise by new mutation.
- Characteristics: cortical or retinal tubers, seizures, mental retardation in <50%, "ash leaf" macules, angiofibromas, subungual or periungual fibromas, shagreen patches, renal cysts or angiomyolipomas.

Von Hippel-Lindau Disease

Von Hippel-Lindau disease is characterized by retinal, spinal cord, and cerebellar hemangioblastomas, cysts of the kidneys, pancreas, and epididymis, and renal cysts and cancers. Other manifestations include hemangioblastomas of the medulla oblongata, cysts and hemangiomas of other visceral organs, pancreatic cancer, and pheochromocytomas.

- Characteristics of von Hippel-Lindau disease: retinal, spinal cord, and cerebellar hemangioblastomas; cysts of kidneys, pancreas, and epididymis.

Retinal hemangioblastomas often are the earliest manifestation of von Hippel-Lindau disease. The mean age at diagnosis is 21 to 28 years, but they can occur as early as 4 years. Initially, the lesion appears as a small red dot that may enlarge at a variable rate to appear as a gray disk or globular, red tumor. The lesions leak, and localized retinal detachment is frequent. Large lesions may be obscured by exudate or gliosis, or they may calcify. Multiple or bilateral lesions occur in 20% to 58% of patients, and 16% to 36% of those with retinal lesions have diminished vision.

- Retinal hemangioblastomas may be earliest manifestation of von Hippel-Lindau disease.

Hemangioblastomas of the central nervous system in von Hippel-Lindau disease are benign, and associated morbidity is due to space-occupying effects. They occur most frequently in the cerebellum and spinal cord but also can be in the medulla oblongata and rarely in the cerebrum. The average age at onset of symptoms is 30 years. Recently, tumors of the endolymphatic sac have been recognized as a component of von Hippel-Lindau disease.

- Hemangioblastomas of central nervous system in von Hippel-Lindau disease are benign tumors with morbid effects.

Renal cysts, hemangiomas, and benign adenomas are usually asymptomatic. Rarely, cysts are so extensive as to mimic polycystic kidney disease and cause renal failure. The cysts vary in size from a few millimeters to more than 2 cm; they are bilateral in 60% and frequently multiple. Renal clear cell cancers are bilateral or multiple in 40% to 87% of cases.

They are the leading cause of death, which occurs at a mean age of 44 years.

- Renal cysts, hemangiomas, and benign adenomas are usually asymptomatic in von Hippel-Lindau disease.
- Renal cancer is a major cause of death.

Most pancreatic cysts are asymptomatic. They rarely lead to diabetes mellitus or steatorrhea. Pancreatic cystadenocarcinoma or islet cell tumors also can occur.

Adrenal cysts, adenomas, and cortical hyperplasia are asymptomatic. Pheochromocytomas are bilateral in 17% to 34% of patients, and the average age at diagnosis is 25 to 34 years. Pheochromocytomas tend to cluster within certain families, particularly those with missense mutations as opposed to those mutations that lead to a truncated gene product.

- Pheochromocytomas of von Hippel-Lindau disease cluster within certain families.

Many male patients with von Hippel-Lindau disease have benign, asymptomatic epididymal lesions, although occasionally fertility is impaired. An epididymal cyst in a relative at risk is not sufficient by itself to diagnose von Hippel-Lindau disease.

Inheritance is autosomal dominant, and the risk for any child born to an affected person is 50%. Expression is variable, and penetrance is high in thoroughly evaluated families. Males and females are affected equally.

- Von Hippel-Lindau disease is autosomal dominant.

Patients with a hemangioblastoma should have a review of the family history, magnetic resonance imaging with gadolinium of the head and upper spine, ophthalmologic examination, and computed tomography or ultrasonography of the abdomen. Patients with bilateral epididymal cysts or polycystic pancreas should also be screened, and it should be considered in patients with pheochromocytomas, polycystic kidneys, or renal cancer. Patients with von Hippel-Lindau disease need annual physical and ophthalmologic examinations, peripheral blood cell count, urinalysis, computed tomography or magnetic resonance imaging of the head, and computed tomography or ultrasonography of the abdomen. Evaluation of urinary catecholamines is reasonable, particularly if the patient is hypertensive or has a family history of pheochromocytoma. Patients should have genetic counseling, and first-degree relatives should have physical and ophthalmologic examinations beginning at age 2 to 4 years, imaging of the head and spine at 11 years, and imaging of the abdomen at 18 years. It is unknown at what age one can safely discontinue screening for at-risk members. The gene that causes von Hippel-Lindau disease is localized to chromosome 3p25-26. The normal gene acts as a tumor suppressor. Presymptomatic and prenatal diagnosis by use of linked DNA markers is available in some families. DNA diagnosis by direct mutation analysis is possible for many patients. Acquired mutations in this gene also have been found in sporadic renal cell carcinomas.

Autosomal Recessive

Autosomal recessive disease occurs because of abnormal genes that are located on the autosomes. However, one copy of the abnormal gene is not sufficient to cause disease, and heterozygotes (carriers) are not clinically different from the general population. When two persons who are heterozygotes for a given gene defect mate, the children are at 25% risk of inheriting the abnormal gene from both parents and, thus, of having the disease.

- Autosomal recessive inheritance: abnormal genes are located on autosomes, but one copy of gene is not sufficient to cause disease.
- Heterozygotes (carriers) are not clinically different from the general population.

Because the heterozygous state may be transmitted silently through many generations before the chance mating of two heterozygotes occurs, it is not surprising that there rarely is a family history of the disease in previous generations. The occurrence of multiple affected siblings within a family suggests autosomal recessive inheritance; however, because of the small average family size in this country, many autosomal recessive diseases seem to occur as isolated cases.

The risk for the children of a person who has an autosomal recessive disease depends on the frequency of the abnormal gene in the population. Except for common diseases such as cystic fibrosis or sickle cell anemia, the risk is usually small, provided that this person does not marry a relative or a person who has a family history of the same disease.

Many diseases that are caused by an identified metabolic defect, such as homocystinuria, are autosomal recessive diseases due to an enzyme deficiency. When the enzymatic defect is established, carrier testing and prenatal diagnosis sometimes are possible.

Some of the diseases with autosomal recessive inheritance are listed in Table 10-2 and summarized on the following pages.

Friedreich Ataxia

This is an autosomal recessive disorder. The first sign of the disease is ataxic gait. The mean age at onset is approximately 12 years. Dysarthria, hypotonic muscle weakness, loss of vibration and position senses, and loss of deep tendon reflexes

develop subsequently. In some patients, diabetes mellitus, nystagmus, optic atrophy, dementia, respiratory dysfunction due to kyphoscoliosis, and decreased sensory nerve conduction velocities also develop. Since detection of the gene defect, many atypical cases have been recognized, such as with preservation of deep tendon reflexes.

- Friedreich ataxia is autosomal recessive.
- First sign of disease is ataxic gait.
- Mean age at onset is 12 years.
- Dysarthria, hypotonic muscle weakness, loss of vibration and position senses, and loss of deep tendon reflexes develop subsequently.

In one series, 60 of 82 patients with Friedreich ataxia had clinical evidence of cardiac dysfunction 4 months to 4 years before death, and 56% died of heart failure. The mean age at death was 36.6 years. Cardiac arrhythmias, particularly atrial fibrillation, were common and occurred in 50% of fatal cases. At autopsy, most cases had marked thickening of the left ventricle with extensive interstitial fibrosis and focal degeneration of muscle fibers. Muscle fibers were hypertrophied and many had large nuclei. The cardiomyopathy may be of the hypertrophic type with subaortic stenosis.

- Cardiac arrhythmias occur in 50% of fatal cases of Friedreich ataxia.

The risk for a sibling being affected is 25%. The gene has been localized to chromosome 9q12-21.1 by genetic linkage

Table 10-2.--Diseases With Autosomal Recessive Inheritance

Alkaptonuria
α_1-Antitrypsin deficiency
Cystic fibrosis
Familial Mediterranean fever
Friedreich ataxia
Gaucher disease
Glycogen storage disease, types I, II, III, IV, V, VII
Hemochromatosis
Homocystinuria
Oculocutaneous albinism
Phenylketonuria
Pseudoxanthoma elasticum (some forms are autosomal dominant)
Refsum disease
Sickle-cell disease
Tay-Sachs disease
α- and β-Thalassemia
Wilson disease

studies of affected families. The gene involved has been named frataxin, and the mechanism of mutation is most frequently expansion of GAA trinucleotide repeat. This potentially allows for prenatal or presymptomatic diagnosis of cases in which one affected child already has been diagnosed.

- Risk of Friedreich ataxia in sibling of affected person is 25%.

Gaucher Disease

Gaucher disease is an autosomal recessive disorder due to deficiency of the enzyme glucocerebrosidase, which results in lipid storage in the spleen, liver, bone marrow, and other organs. Type 1 (non-neuronopathic) disease is most frequent in Ashkenazi Jews (carrier frequency, 1 in 10). The disease may be asymptomatic at any age or present in childhood or adulthood with splenomegaly, hepatosplenomegaly, thrombocytopenia, anemia, degenerative bone disease, or pulmonary disease. Type 2 (infantile, neuronopathic) has no ethnic predisposition, and type 3 (juvenile form) has intermediate clinical signs. The first sign of neurologic involvement in types 2 and 3 is supranuclear ophthalmoplegia.

- Gaucher disease is autosomal recessive.
- Disease is due to deficiency of the enzyme glucocerebrosidase.
- Type 1 is most frequent in Ashkenazi Jews.
- Type 2 has no ethnic predisposition.
- First sign of neurologic involvement in types 2 and 3 is supranuclear ophthalmoplegia.

Enzyme replacement is effective treatment for non-neuronopathic forms of the disease, but it is not yet known whether it is effective for patients with neurologic involvement.

- Enzyme replacement therapy is effective for non-neuronopathic Gaucher disease.

Glycogen Storage Diseases

Glycogen storage disease type I is due to deficiency of the enzyme glucose-6-phosphatase. It is characterized by hypoglycemia, hypercholesterolemia, hyperuricemia, lactic acidosis, short stature, hepatomegaly, and delayed onset of puberty. Adults with this disease may develop malignant hepatomas, premature coronary disease, pancreatitis, gout, and renal disease.

- Glycogen storage disease type I is due to deficiency of the enzyme glucose-6-phosphatase.
- Characteristics: hypoglycemia, hypercholesterolemia, hyperuricemia, lactic acidosis, short stature, hepatomegaly, delayed puberty.

Glycogen storage disease type II (Pompe disease) is an autosomal recessive disorder due to deficiency of the lysosomal enzyme α-1,4-glucosidase (acid maltase). The infantile form is characterized by hypotonia, macroglossia, and progressive cardiomyopathy resulting in death within the first year of life. The electrocardiogram is characterized by high-voltage QRS complexes in all leads and a short PR interval. Cardiac catheterization frequently reveals biventricular hypertrophy with left outflow tract obstruction. The myocardium is different histologically from the myocardium in isolated hypertrophic cardiomyopathy. There is evidence of glycogen storage with vacuolation of heart muscle. Histologic examination of tissues such as liver and kidney may reveal engorged lysosomes, but in muscle the lysosomes may have ruptured and cytoplasmic glycogen is seen. The diagnosis can be confirmed by determination of α-1,4-glucosidase activity in skeletal muscle or cultured fibroblasts. Prenatal diagnosis through enzyme analysis of amniotic fluid cells is possible.

- Glycogen storage disease type II is autosomal recessive.
- Disease is due to deficiency of the enzyme α-1,4-glucosidase.
- Characteristics of infantile form: hypotonia, macroglossia, progressive cardiomyopathy.

Juvenile and adult forms of glycogen storage disease type II also exist. The presenting characteristic is skeletal muscle weakness, and cardiac involvement usually is absent or minimal. At least one patient had a cardiac arrhythmia that required implantation of a ventricular pacemaker, but her echocardiogram showed no cardiomegaly.

- Characteristics of juvenile and adult forms of glycogen storage disease: skeletal muscle weakness, minimal or absent cardiac involvement.

Glycogen storage disease type III is due to an autosomal recessively inherited deficiency of amylo-1,6-glucosidase (debrancher) activity. The enzyme is deficient in liver, and in some patients also in skeletal muscle, cultured skin fibroblasts, and leukocytes. Clinically, the disorder is characterized by hepatomegaly and growth retardation that resolves at puberty. There may be hypoglycemia and hyperlipidemia. Skeletal muscle weakness may develop in adult life. Cardiomyopathy, when present, may be life-threatening and mimic hypertrophic cardiomyopathy. Histologic evaluation of cardiac tissue reveals increased intracellular glycogen with no disarray of myofibers or myofibrils. Deficiency of the enzyme has been documented in cardiac muscle from one patient.

- Glycogen storage disease type III is autosomal recessive.

- Disease is due to deficiency of amylo-1,6-glucosidase activity.
- Characteristics: hepatomegaly, growth retardation that resolves at puberty.

Hemochromatosis

Clinical features of the disease may be gray-brown skin pigmentation, cardiomyopathy, hepatomegaly with fibrosis or cirrhosis, diabetes mellitus, hypogonadism, and bone demineralization. The disease is due to tissue damage by iron overload, although the extent of iron overload in an organ does not always correspond to the severity of tissue damage. Biochemical abnormalities include increased serum iron and ferritin levels, increased transferrin saturation, and increased urinary iron excretion, especially in response to deferoxamine administration. Hemochromatosis is inherited as an autosomal recessive condition. Recently, a major histocompatibility complex class I-like gene, named HFE, has been identified as being mutated in patients with hereditary hemochromatosis.

- Features of hemochromatosis: gray-brown skin pigmentation, cardiomyopathy, hepatomegaly, diabetes mellitus, hypogonadism, bone demineralization.
- Disease is due to tissue damage by iron overload.
- Disease is autosomal recessive.

The risk for siblings of an affected patient is 25%, and therefore all should be screened for biochemical evidence of the disease or undergo molecular genetic testing. Patients with iron overload should have phlebotomy until the excess iron is removed, regardless of whether clinical signs of the disease are present. The risk for children of affected individuals is relatively low (approximately 1 in 20) but is not negligible because of the relatively high gene frequency in the general population. Therefore, older children should be screened to determine whether they are at risk for the disease.

- Siblings of patients with hemochromatosis have risk of 25% for the disease.
- Children of patients with hemochromatosis need to be screened.

Heart disease occurs in 15% to 20% of patients with clinically evident hemochromatosis, and the earliest signs may be electrocardiographic changes characterized by decreased QRS amplitude and T-wave flattening or inversion. Later, congestive heart failure and arrhythmias may occur. The heart condition sometimes resolves after phlebotomy.

- Heart disease occurs in 15%-20% of patients with hemochromatosis.

Homocystinuria

The classic form of homocystinuria is due to autosomal recessively inherited deficiency of cystathionine β-synthase. The gene is expressed in skin fibroblasts and amniocytes, so prenatal diagnosis by determination of enzyme activity in amniocytes is feasible.

- Homocystinuria is autosomal recessive disease.
- Disease is due to deficiency of cystathionine β-synthase.

The incidence of the disease is approximately 1 per 200,000. Clinically, it is characterized by tall stature with a low upper segment:lower segment ratio, pectus deformities, scoliosis, genu valgum, pes planus, and a highly arched palate. Lens dislocation is progressive, and the direction of displacement is usually, but not always, downward. Myopia, retinal detachment, secondary glaucoma, fair hair and skin, cutaneous flushing, and hernias may be present. Approximately 50% of patients are mentally retarded, but this is variable even within a sibship. The electroencephalogram may be abnormal, and some patients have seizures, focal neurologic signs, and hemiatrophy of the brain. Acute psychiatric disturbances or schizophrenic behavior may occur. Osteoporosis with a tendency to fractures and "codfish"-shaped, collapsed vertebrae may be evident radiographically. None of the features are present consistently in all patients, and some affected individuals appear normal.

- Incidence of homocystinuria is about 1 per 200,000.
- Clinical features: tall stature, pectus deformities, scoliosis, genu valgum, pes planus, highly arched palate.
- Lens dislocation is progressive.
- About 50% of patients are mentally retarded.
- Acute psychiatric disturbances or schizophrenic behavior may occur.
- Osteoporosis and "codfish"-shaped, collapsed vertebrae may be seen on radiographs.

Cardiovascular abnormalities include arterial or venous thrombosis, angina pectoris, coronary occlusions at a young age, renal artery narrowing resulting in hypertension and renal atrophy, cerebrovascular accidents, thrombophlebitis, and pulmonary emboli. Dilatation of the pulmonary artery and left atrial endocardial fibroelastosis have been reported. Thrombi are particularly likely to occur after operation, venipuncture, or catheterization.

- Cardiovascular abnormalities of homocystinuria: arterial or venous thrombosis, angina pectoris, coronary occlusions at young age.
- Thrombi are likely after operation, venipuncture, catheterization.

Histologic examination of the arteries reveals marked fibrous thickening of the intima. Aortic intimal fibrosis may be severe enough to mimic coarctation. Medial changes consist of thrombosis and dilatation with widely spaced, frayed muscle fibers. The elastic fibers of the large arteries may be fragmented, and dilatation of the ascending aorta has been observed. No consistent platelet defect has been noted.

The disease sometimes may be diagnosed by positive results of urinary nitroprusside test and confirmed by quantitative urinary homocystine determination. Levels of plasma homocysteine and its precursor, methionine, are increased. Testing of the plasma homocysteine level is the most sensitive, with levels more than 200 µmol/L. This should not be confused with the lesser increases that occur in hyperhomocysteinemia. The goal of treatment is to lower the plasma homocysteine level, which seems to result in slower progression and fewer symptoms of the disease; 50% of patients respond to pyridoxine therapy (25-1,000 mg/day). Supplemental folate also should be given because patients who are potentially capable of responding to pyridoxine may not do so in the presence of folate deficiency. A low-protein, low-methionine diet can be useful, but adults find it difficult to comply with this. For infants, a low-methionine formula is available. Betaine also has been reported to be of benefit in decreasing plasma homocysteine levels.

- In homocystinuria, levels of plasma homocysteine and its precursor, methionine, are increased.
- Goal of treatment: lower plasma homocysteine level.

A rare form of homocystinuria is due to deficiency of *N*-methyltetrahydrofolate-homocysteine methyltransferase. Affected patients have additional neurologic symptoms, and the plasma methionine levels may be normal. Patients with homocystinuria due to abnormal cobalamin metabolism also have normal plasma methionine levels and may have methylmalonic aciduria and megaloblastic anemia.

Mild hyperhomocysteinemia, sometimes associated with polymorphisms in methylenetetrahydrofolate reductase, is believed to be a risk factor for atherosclerosis but is a different condition.

Pseudoxanthoma Elasticum

There are two hereditary forms of pseudoxanthoma elasticum: autosomal dominant and autosomal recessive. Both forms are characterized by yellowish skin papules, especially on the neck and flexural areas, angioid streaks and choroiditis of the retina, and vascular complications, including angina pectoris, claudication, calcification of peripheral arteries, and renal vascular hypertension. In one series of patients, 50% had angina pectoris, 14% had calcification of peripheral arteries, and 18% had intermittent claudication. The age at onset of

complications is variable, and they may occur in early adolescence. Endocardial thickening may result in deformity of the valves, and the conduction system also may be involved, resulting in arrhythmias. Histologically, the arteries show fragmented elastic fibers with granular deposits in place of amorphous elastin. The basic defect is not known.

- Two hereditary forms of pseudoxanthoma elasticum: autosomal dominant and autosomal recessive.
- Characteristics: yellowish skin papules, angioid streaks and choroiditis of retina, vascular complications.

Refsum Disease

Refsum disease is an autosomal recessive neurodegenerative disease characterized by cerebellar ataxia, hypertrophic polyneuropathy, and retinitis pigmentosa. Deafness, ichthyosis, and cardiac conduction defects are frequently present. Onset of the disorder may be in infancy or middle age, and the course is progressive. Cerebrospinal fluid protein concentration is increased, and phytanic acid accumulates in serum and organs. Hypertrophic interstitial neuritis and degenerative changes of nuclei and fiber tracts are observed histologically in the brain stem. The electrocardiogram is characterized by a prolonged PQ interval and ST-segment and T-wave changes. Impaired atrioventricular conduction, bundle branch block, and sudden death from cardiac arrhythmia may occur. Myocardial fibrosis has been reported.

- Refsum disease is autosomal recessive.
- Characteristics: cerebellar ataxia, hypertrophic polyneuropathy, retinitis pigmentosa.
- Frequently present: deafness, ichthyosis, cardiac conduction defects.

Phytanic acid is a fatty acid present in dairy products and fat from grazing animals. Patients with Refsum disease are deficient in the catabolic enzyme phytanic acid α-hydroxylase, which results in accumulation of ingested phytanic acid in fatty deposits in the involved organ systems. The enzyme deficiency is expressed in cultured skin fibroblasts, and prenatal diagnosis is possible.

- Patients with Refsum disease are deficient in phytanic acid α-hydroxylase.

Dietary restriction of phytanic acid results in clinical improvement and stabilization of the disease. Electrocardiographic changes sometimes resolve after treatment. Plasmapheresis removes phytanic acid from the body and may allow liberalization of the diet; it can be extremely valuable in the management of acutely ill patients.

Tay-Sachs Disease

Tay-Sachs disease is an autosomal recessive disease due to deficiency of hexosaminidase A. The classic infantile form of the disease is rapidly fatal and is due to storage of ganglioside GM_2 in neural tissue. It is particularly common in people of Ashkenazi Jewish ancestry; the carrier frequency is 1 in 30. Therefore, screening for carriers by determination of enzyme activity in serum (or leukocytes, particularly in pregnant women, in whom the serum level is unreliable) is recommended in this population. Prenatal diagnosis is available when both the mother and the father are carriers.

- Tay-Sachs disease is autosomal recessive.
- Disease is due to deficiency of hexosaminidase A.

Rare juvenile and adult forms of the disease exist and may present with ataxia, upper motor neuron disease, or other neurologic disorders. These late-onset variants have less of an ethnic predisposition.

X-Linked Recessive

X-linked recessive diseases are caused by abnormal genes located on the X chromosome. Female heterozygotes, who have one abnormal gene on one X chromosome and one normal gene on the other X chromosome, usually are clinically normal. Exceptions may occur because of the phenomenon of lyonization, in which one X chromosome is inactivated at random early in fetal life; if the normal gene is inactivated in a critical number of cells, the woman may have symptoms or clinical signs of the disease. However, the disease usually is less severe than in males. The likelihood of clinical signs of the disease developing in a female varies by disease. For example, it is rare for female carriers of hemophilia VIII to have severe bleeding problems, but it is relatively common for carriers of ornithine carbamoyltransferase (ornithine transcarbamoylase) deficiency to have intermittent symptoms.

- X-linked recessive diseases are caused by abnormal genes on X chromosome.
- Development of clinical signs of disease in female varies by disease.

Males who inherit the abnormal gene have no corresponding genetic loci on the Y chromosome and therefore are referred to as "hemizygotes." Any male child born to a heterozygous female is at 50% risk for having the disease; female children are at 50% risk for inheriting the gene and being carriers. All the daughters of affected males are carriers, and all the sons are unaffected (i.e., male-to-male transmission cannot occur).

- Males with abnormal gene are called "hemizygotes."
- Male child of heterozygous female has 50% risk of disease.
- Female child is at 50% risk of inheriting the gene.

X-linked recessive diseases also may arise by new mutation affecting either the mother or the afflicted son. Genetic counseling is difficult in these situations because if the mother represents the new mutation the risk for her future male children is 50%. However, if the child represents the new mutation, there is no significant risk for siblings of that child. New advances in DNA-based diagnosis have resulted in opportunities for carrier detection for some diseases, which circumvent problems created by lyonization.

Some of the conditions with X-linked recessive inheritance are listed in Table 10-3 and summarized on the following pages.

Duchenne and Becker Muscular Dystrophies

Duchenne muscular dystrophy is one of the most common types of muscular dystrophy; its incidence is approximately 1 in 3,500 newborn males. It is an X-linked recessive disease, and approximately a third of the cases arise by new mutation. Progressive skeletal weakness beginning at 2 to 5 years of age, with death in the late teens or 20s, is characteristic. The diagnosis is made on the basis of clinical findings and markedly increased creatine kinase levels. The muscle biopsy findings are relatively nonspecific. Becker muscular dystrophy has later onset.

- Incidence of Duchenne muscular dystrophy is 1 in 3,500 newborn males.
- Duchenne muscular dystrophy is X-linked recessive.
- Skeletal weakness at 2- 5 years of age is characteristic.

The genetic defect that results in both Duchenne and Becker muscular dystrophies involves the dystrophin gene

Table 10-3.--X-Linked Recessive Conditions

Adrenoleukodystrophy ("X-linked" form)
Chronic granulomatous disease (many cases; autosomal recessive forms are less common)
Color blindness
Duchenne and Becker muscular dystrophies
Fabry disease
Glucose-6-phosphate dehydrogenase deficiency
Hemophilia A and B
Ocular albinism
Rickets, hypophosphatemic
Testicular feminization

located on chromosome X at band p2l. Approximately two-thirds of patients have a submicroscopic partial gene deletion, and the rest have undetected deletions, duplications, or other abnormalities. The dystrophin gene is very large, consisting of at least 60 exons and l,800 kilobases. The entire gene has been cloned. The protein product of this gene, dystrophin, is a rod-shaped cytoskeletal protein that is predominantly localized to the surface membrane of striated muscle cells. Identification of the molecular defect has resulted in improved ability to determine carrier status in female relatives by DNA analysis. This is a significant improvement over carrier testing by measurement of creatine kinase levels, because levels are increased in only 70% of obligate carriers. DNA analysis also can be used for prenatal diagnosis. All mothers, sisters, and children of patients with Duchenne or Becker muscular dystrophy should have genetic counseling.

- Mothers, sisters, and children of patients with Duchenne or Becker muscular dystrophy need genetic counseling.

The heart disease in patients with Duchenne muscular dystrophy is characterized by significant changes in systolic time intervals suggestive of compromised left ventricular function. There are histologic changes characterized by multifocal dystrophic areas with fibrosis and loss of myofilaments. These changes are most marked in the posterobasal segment and contiguous lateral and inferior walls of the left ventricle. Some families with dystrophin defects have dilated cardiomyopathy without significant skeletal muscle weakness.

- Heart disease in Duchenne muscular dystrophy involves changes in systolic time intervals.

Fabry Disease

Fabry disease is a lysosomal storage disease due to deficiency of α-galactosidase A. The inheritance pattern is X-linked recessive, although females may have less severe signs of the disease than males. Glycosphingolipids accumulate in the endothelium, perithelium, and smooth muscle of blood vessels. There is less accumulation in ganglion cells, myocardial cells, reticuloendothelial cells, and connective tissue cells.

- Fabry disease is due to deficiency of α-galactosidase A.
- Disease is X-linked recessive.
- Females may have less severe signs than males.

The first signs of the disease may be telangiectatic angiokeratomas of the skin and mucous membranes. Acroparesthesias and episodes of severe burning pain in the palms and soles with proximal radiation also may occur in childhood and adolescence. Whorl-shaped corneal opacities and cataracts

develop. In adulthood, cardiovascular and renal diseases are the major causes of morbidity and mortality. Cardiac problems, including ischemia, infarction, congestive heart failure, mitral insufficiency, and aortic stenosis, may result from progressive glycosphingolipid infiltration. Systemic hypertension due to infiltration of renal parenchymal vessels may aggravate the cardiac disease. Electrocardiography may show signs of left ventricular hypertrophy, ST-segment changes, and T-wave inversion. Occasionally, patients have arrhythmias and a short P-R interval.

- First signs of Fabry disease may be telangiectatic angiokeratomas of skin and mucous membranes.
- Acroparesthesias may occur in childhood and adolescence.
- Whorl-shaped corneal opacities and cataracts develop.
- In adults, cardiovascular and renal diseases develop.

The interventricular septum and posterior left ventricular wall may be thickened. Cardiomegaly, especially involving the left atrium and ventricle, is observed. The right atrium and ventricle may be dilated. Myocardial cells show extensive glycosphingolipid deposited around the nucleus and between myofibrils. Endothelial cells and smooth muscle cells are hypertrophied. The mitral valve frequently is thickened and has normal or thick papillary muscles; the tricuspid valve may be involved, but the aortic and pulmonary valves usually are normal. Lipid-filled cells are seen within the fibrous tissue of involved valves.

Neurologic signs result from small-vessel involvement in the brain. The most frequent cause of death is renal failure.

Dilantin and carbamazepine are useful for treating the pain. Renal transplantation can prolong life. The gene has been cloned, and prenatal diagnosis is possible.

MITOCHONDRIAL MUTATIONS

Mitochondria each contain several circular copies of their own genetic material, mitochondrial DNA. This mitochondrial DNA is approximately 16,000 base pairs in length and encodes for transfer-RNAs and several proteins involved in the mitochondrial respiratory chain. Many mitochondrial enzymes, including some others of the respiratory chain complex, are encoded by nuclear DNA and transported into the mitochondria. Mitochondrial DNA mutations cause Leber's optic atrophy and the multisystem syndromes of multiple episodes of lactic acidosis and stroke (MELAS), myoclonic epilepsy with ragged red fibers (MERRF), and neuropathy, ataxia, and retinitis pigmentosa (NARP). Many cases of Kearns-Sayre syndrome (cardiomyopathy and ophthalmoplegia) are due to mitochondrial mutations. Mitochondrial disorders can arise as new mutations or be maternally inherited; only the egg contributes mitochondria to the zygote, the sperm does not. Mitochondrial mutations may be homoplasmic (present in all mitochondrial DNA) or heteroplasmic (present in only some of the mitochondrial DNA).

- Mitochondrial DNA mutations cause Leber's optic atrophy and multisystem syndromes.
- Many cases of Kearns-Sayre syndrome are due to mitochondrial mutations.
- Only the egg contributes mitochondria to the zygote, the sperm does not.

MULTIFACTORIAL CAUSATION

Multifactorial means that the disease or trait is determined by the interaction of environmental influences and a polygenic (many gene) predisposition. Human conditions that may have multifactorial causation include many common birth defects—such as congenital heart defects, cleft lip and palate, and neural tube defects—and many common diseases—such as diabetes mellitus, asthma, hypertension, and coronary artery atherosclerosis.

- Multifactorial causation: disease or trait is due to environmental influences and polygenic predisposition.
- Birth defects that may have multifactorial causation: congenital heart defects, cleft lip and palate, neural tube defects.
- Diseases that may have multifactorial causation: diabetes mellitus, asthma, hypertension, coronary artery atherosclerosis.

The multifactorial model predicts that there will be a tendency for familial aggregation of the condition but without a strict mendelian pattern of inheritance. Familial aggregation also can be due to common environmental factors, so familial aggregation by itself is not sufficient to prove multifactorial causation.

Because familial aggregation exists for multifactorial disorders, it is implicit that the occurrence risk will be increased for members of an affected family over that of the general population. As expected, the risk is highest for first-degree relatives (parents, siblings, children), who have half of their genes in common. The risk is less for second-degree relatives (grandparents, aunts, uncles, grandchildren, nephews, nieces), who share one-quarter of their genes. The risk decreases exponentially thereafter; third-degree relatives (great-grandparents, cousins, great-grandchildren) share only one-eighth of their genes. Empiric (observed) risk figures for some well-studied multifactorial disorders fit well with the predicted risks.

The genetic liability in multifactorial causation is due to the cumulative effect of many genes, each having a small effect, rather than to the effect of one major gene. These genes create a liability that presumably is continuously distributed within the population. If the genetic liability is strong enough, under an unfortunate set of environmental circumstances the disorder will occur.

- Genetic liability in multifactorial causation is due to cumulative effect of many genes.

For many multifactorial conditions, there is a difference in predilection between males and females which could result directly from genetic differences or from different internal (e.g., hormonal) or external environmental factors. Furthermore, if a member of the less commonly affected sex has the condition, his or her genetic liability was probably greater and therefore the risk for his or her relatives is greater. Similarly, if a person has a more severe form of the disease, the risk for relatives is higher. For disorders in which disease frequency increases with age, earlier onset sometimes implies a greater risk for relatives. Finally, the greater the number of affected individuals within the family, the higher risk for other relatives. There also are racial differences in the frequency of many disorders of multifactorial causation.

When the inheritance pattern of any disease is being determined, the possibility of genetic heterogeneity always must be considered. For example, there are both autosomal dominant and multifactorial causes of atrial septal defect which may be indistinguishable clinically. Failure to recognize that different genetic diseases can cause the same or similar clinical entities can result in confusion when determining risks.

Table 10-4 lists some conditions of multifactorial causation.

PRESYMPTOMATIC AND PRENATAL DIAGNOSIS OF GENETIC DISEASE BY DNA ANALYSIS

Presymptomatic and prenatal diagnosis of genetic diseases utilizing peripheral blood specimens or specimens obtained by amniocentesis or chorionic villus sampling has become a routine part of clinical practice because of the identification of the basic genetic defect underlying numerous mendelian conditions and the capability for direct DNA diagnosis. In addition, even when the causative genetic defect has not yet been identified, knowledge of its chromosome localization may allow for diagnosis by linkage analysis. Because individual genes are too small to be seen microscopically, standard chromosome analysis generally is not helpful even when the gene has been localized to a specific chromosome region.

The DNA-based laboratory procedures used for diagnosis, the limitations of the tests, and the importance of an accurate clinical diagnosis and family history are described below. A discussion of the prenatal diagnosis of Duchenne muscular dystro-

Table 10-4 .--Conditions of Multifactorial Causation

Atherosclerosis
Atopic disease or allergy
Cancer
Cardiac defects (congenital)
Cleft lip or palate
Diabetes mellitus
Hypertension
Neural tube defects
Schizophrenia

phy (DMD) provides an excellent example of these issues. Although the following examples describe prenatal diagnosis, the same principles apply to presymptomatic diagnosis.

Importance of an Accurate Clinical Diagnosis and Family History

The importance of a correct diagnosis in the index patient when diagnosis by DNA analysis is being contemplated cannot be overemphasized. This criterion is in contrast to many instances of genetic diagnosis by chromosome analysis in which the cytogeneticist usually can be relied on to note most abnormalities (fragile X and subtle deletions are examples of exceptions) regardless of the exact indication for the study. This approach is possible because the procedure of chromosome analysis involves examination of all 46 chromosomes in a given cell to look for gross structural changes. In contrast, it is impossible to systematically examine each of a person's 100,000 genes to detect all abnormalities.

● It is impossible to systematically examine each of a person's 100,000 genes.

The laboratory's process of detection of even one abnormal gene must be directed by the precise clinical diagnosis. The DNA-based assays are specific for the disease being studied, and abnormalities elsewhere in the genome will not be detected. Thus, if the incorrect assay is chosen because of an incorrect clinical diagnosis, the disease-causing mutation will not be detected. For example, if a pregnant woman's brother and uncle are believed to have DMD but the correct diagnosis is X-linked Emery-Dreifuss muscular dystrophy, the wrong DNA analysis will be performed and may result in an erroneous prediction as to whether the fetus is affected. It is the responsibility of the physician to obtain medical records or to arrange for one of the affected relatives to be examined to confirm the reported diagnosis, and the physician may want the assistance of a medical geneticist or other specialist in this process.

In addition to confirmation of the diagnosis, an accurate family pedigree is necessary. It is important to know whether the index patient represents a sporadic case or whether other family members also are affected. This information must be considered in the determination of whether DNA diagnosis is possible and in the interpretation of the results of DNA analysis. In sporadic cases, diagnosis by linkage analysis (see below), which is based on tracking the mutation through the family, may be impossible.

● Accurate family pedigree is necessary for diagnosis.

In these sporadic cases, diagnosis often can be established only for diseases for which direct DNA diagnosis is possible. In contrast, in families with multiple affected members, direct DNA diagnosis is the first diagnostic choice when possible, followed by linkage analysis if the mutation cannot be directly identified. For other diseases, linkage studies are the only option. For example, in DMD, approximately 60% of patients have a deletion identifiable by techniques in routine use for clinical testing. If a deletion is detected in a sporadic patient with DMD, it usually is possible to determine whether the mother is a carrier and, if so, direct DNA diagnosis can be applied for her male fetuses. If a deletion cannot be detected in a sporadic patient with DMD, then specific prenatal diagnosis is not possible for the mother's future children, although exclusion of a disease may still be possible by use of linked markers. The mother of a sporadic patient with DMD has a prior risk for being a carrier of approximately 2 in 3, and the options include fetal sex determination followed by termination of all male fetuses, although at least 2 of 3 would be expected to be unaffected, or termination of fetuses that inherited the same markers as the index patient, in which at least 1 of 3 would be unaffected.

● In families with multiple affected members, direct DNA diagnosis is first diagnostic choice.

Alternatively, if there are multiple affected family members with DMD, the issue of new mutation is not a concern. If a deletion is detected in these multiplex families, this is the simplest approach for testing male fetuses of carrier women within the family. However, if a deletion is not detected, then blood specimens can be collected from multiple family members for linkage analysis (Fig. 10-5).

Linkage Analysis

Linkage analysis for prenatal diagnosis is based on the biologic fact that individual units of genetic material (genes) are situated in linear order on one of the 24 types of chromosomes (22 autosomes plus the X and Y chromosomes). The word "alleles" refers to the different forms of genetic material at the same gene locus, for example, the A and B alleles at the ABO blood group locus. Genes located on different chromosomes segregate independently, so there is a 50% chance that an individual egg or sperm will contain the same or different alleles encoded within these two chromosomal loci (Fig. 10-6).

● "Alleles" are different forms of genetic material at the same gene locus.

Genes located on the same chromosome are *syntenic*. During the pairing of homologous chromosomes during meiosis, crossovers can occur between genes even if they are located on the same chromosome. The average number of crossovers per chromosome per meiosis is two. Genes located far apart on the same chromosome are more likely to be separated by crossovers than are genes located close together. If the genes are so far apart that they are separated by crossovers at least 50% of the time, then these genes are not linked even though they are syntenic, and they exhibit random segregation (Fig. 10-7).

● Genes located on same chromosome are *syntenic*.

Of course, linkage is not an all-or-none phenomenon. There is the potential for crossover to occur between any two gene loci, and this could happen in 20% of meioses, 2% of

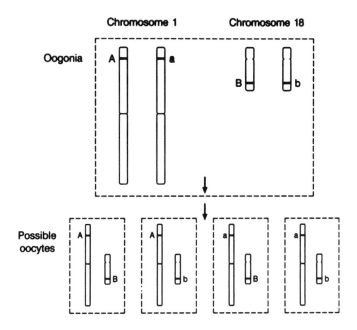

Fig. 10-6. Random segregation of gene locus on chromosome 1 in relation to gene locus on chromosome 18. There is a 50% chance that allele A will segregate with allele B or allele b. These loci are not syntenic and do not demonstrate linkage.

meioses, or 0.2% of meioses, for example, depending on the "distance" between them. Although physical distance is correlated with the likelihood of crossover, other factors such as location of the genes adjacent to the chromosome centromere and sex of the individual also influence the likelihood of crossover. Therefore, a measure of the functional likelihood of crossover, a centimorgan (cM), is used to describe the observed recombination rate. Thus, if crossovers occur in 10% of meioses, the loci are said to be 10 cM apart. On average, 1 cM corresponds to approximately 1,000 kilobases of DNA. The degree of linkage of specific genes must be generated from clinical observations in numerous families.

For tests used in clinical practice, it is important to know the frequency of crossovers occurring between the disease gene and the marker gene, because this is one factor that limits the accuracy of the test. If the disease gene and the marker gene are 2 cM apart, it is important for the patient to know that the accuracy will be less than 98%. The use of flanking markers, that is, markers on both sides of the gene, if available, can help circumvent the problem of undetected crossovers. Although known genes sometimes are used for markers, more commonly DNA segments of unknown function are used for markers. These "anonymous" DNA segments, like genes themselves, can be highly variable in their nucleotide sequence. These normal variations are located extensively throughout the genome and can be recognized by one of many different kinds of bacterial enzymes that cut

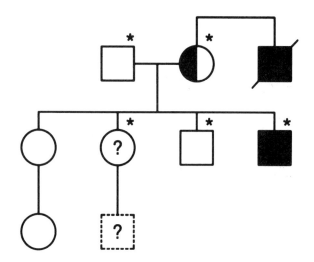

Fig. 10-5. Sample pedigree of family with males with Duchenne muscular dystrophy (shaded symbols). Carrier females are shown with half-shaded symbols. Members for whom blood was requested for DNA linkage analysis are marked with an asterisk. Squares, males; circles, females; line through square indicates that person is deceased; dashed-line square indicates male fetus. Note that blood for DNA from pregnant woman's father and unaffected brother is helpful for DNA linkage studies. Most laboratories offering these tests assist the referring physician in determining which family members need testing.

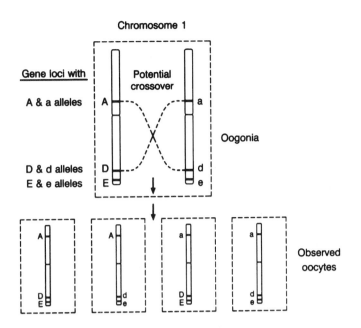

Fig. 10-7. Three gene loci on chromosome 1. Locus with allele A and allele a is located at sufficient distance from loci with alleles D/d and E/e that random segregation occurs. However, loci with alleles D/d and E/e always show D and E together or d and e together (not drawn to scale). Loci for D/d and E/e do not show random segregation and thus are linked.

DNA at specified sites. DNA polymorphisms located within the gene of interest are less likely to show recombination with the mutation site than those located adjacent to the gene (Fig. 10-8).

● The accuracy of linkage-based diagnosis is variable from one disease to another, depending on how tightly the disease gene and marker DNA are linked.

The size of the DNA fragments generated by these cutting enzymes varies among individuals because of normal variations in our DNA sequences. These different-sized fragments are referred to as restriction fragment length polymorphisms. These can be separated by size by electrophoresis on a gel. Once separated by size, the DNA fragments can be transferred to a nylon membrane as part of the procedure known as Southern blot analysis.

Southern Blot Procedure

After a patient's DNA has been extracted from peripheral blood lymphocytes, subjected to enzyme cutting, and electrophoresed to separate different sizes of DNA fragments, a radioactive probe for the disease gene or for the marker DNA segments is applied and hybridizes to the complementary DNA sequences of interest. The fragments then can be visualized on x-ray film. An example of linkage analysis by Southern blotting in a family with DMD is shown in Figure 10-9.

In addition to linkage analysis, Southern blotting can be used in some cases for direct detection of deletion or duplication types of mutations, or for single-base mutations if the enzyme restriction site is directly altered by the mutation. An example of direct detection of a deletion in a patient with DMD is shown in Figure 10-10.

Polymerase Chain Reaction

Another method of DNA diagnosis that has had great impact on clinical practice is the polymerase chain reaction (PCR). The PCR involves replication of a specific, relatively small segment of DNA in an exponential fashion, so that up to a billion copies are produced. One uses known DNA sequences from within the area of interest, and these known DNA sequences allow creation of synthetic oligonucleotides that serve as primers to hybridize with the patient's DNA sequence to initiate the amplification process (Fig. 10-11).

The multiple copies of the DNA segment that are produced by the PCR then can be identified by various techniques, including direct visualization after gel electrophoresis. This allows detection of mutations in the patient's DNA. For example, the PCR can be used for detection of mutations in

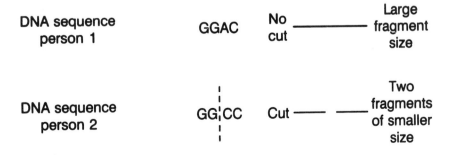

Fig. 10-8. Bacterial restriction enzyme *HAE* III. There are hundreds of types of bacterial enzymes that recognize and cleave specific DNA sequences. Appropriate enzyme that provides most information for DNA markers near disease gene of interest will be selected by the laboratory performing the test. Resulting fragments of differing sizes in different persons are restriction fragment-length polymorphisms.

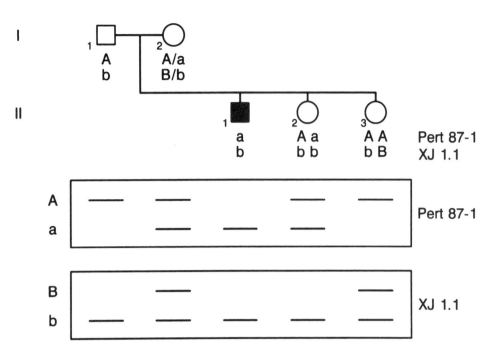

Fig. 10-9. Representation of a family segregating for Duchenne muscular dystrophy and data for two probes that detect restriction fragment-length polymorphism, Pert 87-1 and XJ 1.1. Bottom half of figure represents Southern blot analysis of these two probes with arbitrary designation of alleles A/a for Pert 87-1 and B/b for XJ 1.1. Square, normal male; circle, female; shaded symbol, affected individual. Sister II.3 of affected male II.1 inherited Ab haplotype from her father and AB haplotype from her mother. Because her brother has ab haplotype, it can be predicted that she is not a carrier and her fetus is not at increased risk. Although sister II.2 did inherit the ab haplotype, it cannot be determined with certainty that she is a carrier because it is not known whether the mutation arose in brother or whether mother is a carrier. Sister II.2 could elect prenatal diagnosis, with the realization that males who inherit the ab haplotype might be affected or unaffected, whereas those who inherit the Ab haplotype would most likely be unaffected.

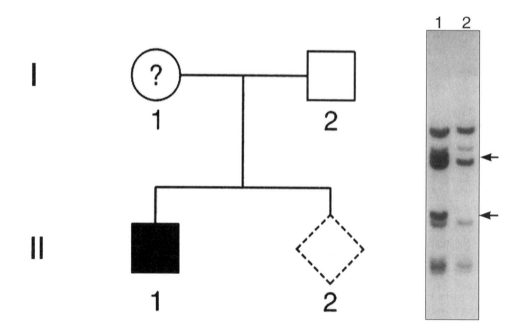

Fig. 10-10. Mother (I.1) of this patient (II.1) with sporadic Duchenne muscular dystrophy wanted to know whether she was a carrier or whether a new mutation had occurred in her son, because of her concern for the risk for future children. Southern blot analysis detected a deletion in her son (II.1) (lane 2 as compared to control in lane 1). By densitometry, the mother seemed to have less than the expected amount of DNA (not shown) corresponding to her son's deletion. Thus, she was diagnosed as being a carrier for the dystrophy and can be offered specific prenatal diagnosis. If no deletion had been detectable (by various methods), then her carrier status could not have been determined.

specific regions of the dystrophin gene for the diagnosis of DMD and other diseases.

Diseases Amenable to DNA Diagnosis

The number of diseases diagnosable by DNA analysis is increasing as additional disease genes are localized or identified and cloned. Humans are believed to have approximately 100,000 genes; currently, approximately 6,000 genes have been mapped. Some diseases for which DNA diagnosis is available are listed in Tables 10-5 through 10-7, but these lists will change rapidly and are not meant to be all-inclusive.

Furthermore, when diagnosis is based on linkage, some families may not have the necessary number of family members available to allow for informative DNA analysis. Other families may have a sufficient number of family members who are willing to participate but the DNA markers in common usage to study their specific gene defect may not be informative in a particular family. An example of this problem is shown in Figure 10-12.

Thus, the physician who encounters a clinical situation for the first time which may be amenable to DNA-based diagnosis should discuss the testing procedure and its limitations with the laboratory personnel or a geneticist familiar with the details of the specific disease testing before a detailed discussion of the prenatal diagnosis with the patient. Ideally, these discussions should take place before a woman becomes pregnant. For example, if a woman provides a family history of a brother with DMD and she is deciding whether to have a child, it would be prudent to confirm the diagnosis and get a detailed family history to determine whether prenatal diagnosis seems feasible rather than simply stating that prenatal diagnosis is possible.

Table 10-5.--Some Autosomal Dominant Diseases Diagnosable by DNA Analysis

Amyloidosis, some forms
Familial adenomatous polyposis coli
Familial hypercholesterolemia (low-density lipoprotein receptor defects)
Huntington disease
Marfan syndrome
Multiple endocrine neoplasia, types I, II, and IIb
Myotonic dystrophy
Neurofibromatosis, types 1 and 2
Osteogenesis imperfecta, some forms
Polycystic kidney disease
Spinocerebellar ataxia, types I and III
Retinoblastoma
Von Hippel-Lindau disease
Von Willebrand disease

Table 10-6.--Some Autosomal Recessive Diseases Diagnosable by DNA Analysis

α_1-Antitrypsin deficiency
Congenital adrenal hyperplasia (21-hydroxylase deficiency)
Cystic fibrosis
Gaucher disease
Hemochromatosis
Phenylketonuria
Sickle-cell disease
Spinal muscular atrophy
Tay-Sachs disease
α- and β-Thalassemia

This woman would be in a difficult situation if she became pregnant while assuming that prenatal diagnosis was possible only to find out later that prenatal diagnosis was not possible because her brother was a sporadic case or is deceased and she has no detectable deletion. Parenthetically, deletions can be much more difficult to detect in a woman heterozygous for an X-linked disease than in a hemizygous affected male.

- DNA-based diagnoses cannot be used for all families, even when DNA tests for a specific disease are available.

An example of an X-linked disease has been used throughout this discussion, but the same general principles apply to autosomal dominant and recessive diseases. Prenatal diagnoses of cystic fibrosis, sickle-cell disease, and the thalassemias are particularly important because of their high frequency. Virtually all cases of sickle-cell disease and most cases of thalassemia can be diagnosed by direct DNA analysis with the PCR without the need for linkage analysis. Direct DNA analysis with the PCR of the phenylalanine 508 mutation, which accounts for approximately 70% of cystic fibrosis mutations, is possible;

Table 10-7.--Some X-Linked Diseases Diagnosable by DNA Analysis

Alport syndrome (X-linked form)
Duchenne and Becker muscular dystrophies
Fragile X-linked mental retardation
Hemophilia A and B
Kennedy spinobulbar atrophy
Lesch-Nyhan syndrome
Ornithine transcarbamoylase deficiency
Wiskott-Aldrich syndrome
X-linked ichthyosis
X-linked lymphoproliferative disease

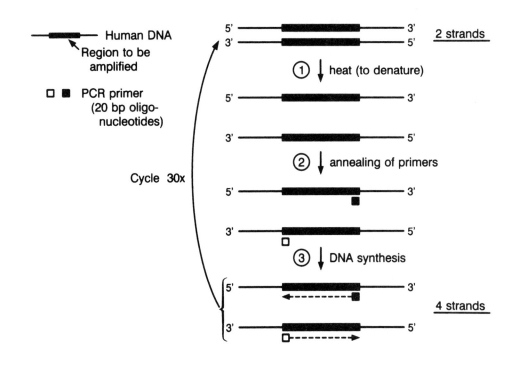

Fig. 10-11. PCR is used to make multiple copies of short segment of DNA of interest. DNA from patient is denatured to single-stranded DNA in the presence of oligonucleotide primers. DNA sequences of these primers are made to specification to anneal with DNA sequences on both sides of DNA segment of interest. DNA between these primers is then synthesized, and entire process can be repeated automatically.

however, the remaining 30% of mutations are so diverse that more extensive gene testing or linkage analysis is necessary.

Occasionally, linkage analysis can be applied even if the affected family member is deceased or represents a sporadic case. If multiple alleles are analyzed that flank the site of the gene defect, it may be possible to deduce the marker genotype of the deceased person by studying other family members.

Another potential pitfall in prenatal diagnosis by DNA analysis is genetic heterogeneity. For example, most patients with autosomal dominant polycystic kidney disease have a gene defect linked to markers on chromosome 16. However, up to 10% of families have a phenotypically similar disease due to a different, nonallelic genetic mutation that does not show linkage to these markers. Thus, in the minority of families linkage cannot be performed for presymptomatic or prenatal diagnosis; if the family is not recognized to be one of the "unlinked" families, an erroneous diagnosis may be made. There are numerous other examples of this type of genetic heterogeneity, including retinitis pigmentosa, spinocerebellar ataxias, and Charcot-Marie-Tooth disease.

It is anticipated that the rapid advances made in molecular genetics in the past several years will accelerate as the genetic bases of additional diseases are identified and newer techniques for molecular diagnosis become available.

● Genetic heterogeneity can confound DNA linkage studies.

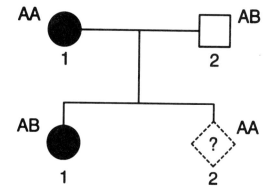

Fig. 10-12. Mother (I.1) and first child (II.1) are affected by autosomal dominant disease. Marker alleles linked to this disease are shown next to each person's symbol. Because mother's genotype is AA, it cannot be determined whether the fetus inherited the chromosome with the A marker and the disease gene or the other A marker without the disease gene. This family is said to be noninformative.

GLOSSARY

Autosome: Chromosome other than sex chromosome.

Chromosome: Long strands of double-stranded DNA that encode genes and that are associated with a protein framework. Normal human has 46 chromosomes per cell.

Deletion: Structural abnormality in which part of a chromosome is missing.

Duplication: Structural abnormality in which an extra copy of part of a chromosome is present.

Gene: A portion of DNA molecule that codes for a specific RNA or protein product.

Hemizygote: A person who has a gene form on one chromosome but no homologous chromosome with a corresponding gene site. The term usually refers to males because they have only one X chromosome.

Heterozygote: A person who has different gene forms at a given site on two homologous chromosomes.

Homozygote: A person who has the same gene forms at a given site on two homologous chromosomes.

Inversion: Structural abnormality characterized by reversal of a segment within the chromosome.

Karyotype: The chromosome complement of an individual person.

Linkage (genetic linkage): Physical proximity of two gene loci on the same chromosome such that segregation is nonrandom.

Phenotype: The observable biochemical or physical characteristics of an individual as determined by genetic material and environment.

Proband: The index patient.

Recurrence: Occurrence of another case of a specific condition in the same family.

Translocation: Structural abnormality characterized by transfer of a piece of one chromosome to another chromosome.

QUESTIONS

Multiple Choice (choose the one best answer)

1. An 18-year-old woman with short stature presents with primary amenorrhea. To evaluate for possible Turner syndrome, the most appropriate genetic test is:
   a. Peripheral blood karyotype
   b. Peripheral blood fluorescent in situ hybridization (FISH)
   c. Bone marrow karyotype
   d. Skin fibroblast FISH
   e. Ovarian biopsy FISH

2. A 27-year-old man is apparently healthy *except* for a history of ectopia lentis. The family history is negative for sudden death. An appropriate investigation includes:
   a. Karyotype
   b. Echocardiography only if murmur is present
   c. Echocardiography regardless of murmur
   d. DNA analysis
   e. Echocardiography only if arterial pulse pressure is widened

3. Hereditary hemochromatosis is diagnosed in a 50-year-old man with diabetes mellitus and cirrhosis. The genetic risk to his sisters for homozygosity is:
   a. 100%
   b. 75%
   c. 50%
   d. 25%
   e. 0%

4. A healthy 20-year-old woman is planning a family and informs you that her sister has a congenital heart defect and Down syndrome due to trisomy 21. Your patient should have:
   a. Peripheral blood chromosome analysis
   b. Amniotic fluid chromosome analysis when pregnant
   c. Echocardiography
   d. No special studies related to her history
   e. Echocardiography and peripheral blood chromosome analysis

5. A patient with myotonic dystrophy is experiencing spells of "light-headedness." The most likely cause is:
   a. Orthostatic hypotension
   b. Seizures
   c. Psychosomatic
   d. Allergic reaction
   e. Atrioventicular block

6. Renal cysts are diagnosed in a 40-year-old man with a history of cerebellar hemangioblastoma. His father was blind and died at age 30 of renal failure. The most likely diagnosis is:
   a. Tuberous sclerosis
   b. Neurofibromatosis
   c. von Hippel-Lindau disease
   d. Multiple endocrine neoplasia
   e. Polycystic kidney disease

7. A woman is concerned about her 10-year-old son, who has intermittent pain in his feet and unexplained fevers. Her brother has Fabry disease but she was told as a teenager that she was unaffected. The most likely explanation is:
   a. She and her son both have Fabry disease
   b. She is a carrier and her son has Fabry disease
   c. Her son has Fabry disease but the gene skipped a generation
   d. Anticipation resulted in Fabry disease in her son
   e. Her son has Fabry disease inherited from his father

8. Mitochondrial inheritance is characterized by:
   a. Transmission through females only to sons
   b. Transmission through males only to daughters
   c. Transmission through females to sons or daughters
   d. Transmission through males to sons or daughters
   e. Transmission through males only to sons

9. A boy, his uncle, and a male maternal first cousin all have mental retardation. Fragile X studies were normal by chromosome and DNA analysis. One can conclude:
   a. The males are each mentally retarded for a different reason
   b. An autosomal recessive gene defect is most likely
   c. An autosomal dominant gene defect is most likely
   d. An X-linked recessive gene defect is most likely
   e. Fragile X syndrome is most likely

10. A 30-year-old man has a mother and brother with neurofibromatosis type 1. He has one café-au-lait macule and wonders whether he is affected. Linkage with an intragenic marker shows:
    a. The study is uninformative
    b. The man is affected
    c. The man is partially affected (incomplete penetrance)
    d. The study shows non-paternity
    e. The man is unaffected

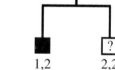

ANSWERS

1. Answer a.

Peripheral blood karyotyping should be performed rather than the FISH procedure because FISH could miss a partially deleted X or a partially deleted Y chromosome that would have significant implications for management. There is no need to do bone marrow, skin, or ovarian studies.

2. Answer c.

Ectopia lentis is one of the major features of Marfan syndrome. Echocardiography is recommended regardless of whether or not a murmur is present because a dilated aorta would still warrant monitoring and would confirm the diagnosis but would not necessarily be associated with aortic insufficiency or murmur. A karyotype would not be at all useful because patients with this single gene disorder do not have a cytogenetically visible abnormality. DNA analysis is not the criterion for diagnosis because not all fibrillin mutations can be detected through DNA analysis and some patients who have fibrillin defects may not have Marfan syndrome.

3. Answer d.

Hemochromatosis is an autosomal recessive disorder and often is asymptomatic, whereas significant iron overload is accumulating. Therefore, the risk for a sibling is 1 in 4, or 25%.

4. Answer d.

Trisomy 21 implies that there are three separate number 21 chromosomes in the patient with Down syndrome. This is not a familial condition, and one would not expect healthy relatives to have any chromosome abnormality. One can presume that the heart defect in the sister is directly related to the Down syndrome. Therefore, no special investigations need to be performed for the healthy sister.

5. Answer e.

Although any of the conditions could cause "light-headedness," a particularly frequent association with myotonic dystrophy is symptomatic atrioventricular block.

6. Answer c.

The answer to this question relates to knowledge of the association of renal cysts, cerebellar hemangioblastoma, and blindness due to retinal angiomas, which are characteristic of von Hippel-Lindau disease. Tuberous sclerosis can be associated with renal cysts; usually the hamartomas of the retina are asymptomatic and it is not associated with cerebellar hemangioblastomas. Neurofibromatosis is not associated with renal cysts or cerebellar hemangioblastoma, but blindness could occur from an optic glioma. Multiple endocrine neoplasia is not associated with any of these findings. Polycystic kidney disease is not associated with cerebellar hemangioblastomas or blindness.

7. Answer b.

Fabry disease is an X-linked disorder. Sometimes female carriers (heterozygotes) can have some symptoms. However, the case as described here indicates that only her son has symptoms. Therefore, she must be a carrier and one would not say that she has Fabry disease. Genes do not "skip" generations, only clinical symptoms can "skip," but there is no need to invoke this because asymptomatic carrier status is very common with X-linked conditions. There is no evidence for anticipation or expansion of trinucleotide repeats in Fabry disease. A son cannot inherit an X-linked disorder from the father. The likely explanation for the woman being told she was not a carrier years ago was the lack of sensitivity of enzyme testing, and DNA testing has only recently become available.

8. Answer c.

Mitochondria are only passed in eggs, not in sperm; thus, only females can transmit the disorder. The sex of the child is irrelevant.

9. Answer d.

There are many causes of X-linked mental retardation. DNA analysis is extremely sensitive for making this diagnosis. It would be a remarkable coincidence for all these individuals to have mental retardation for different reasons. The autosomal recessive pattern would not fit because one would not expect an uncle and cousin to be affected. An autosomal dominant pattern is unlikely because the case does not suggest that the parents of these boys are affected. Therefore, an X-linked recessive gene defect of some type is most likely, although the specific gene cannot be specified.

10. Answer e.

This case presents markers linked to the neurofibromatosis type 1 gene. The assignment of a haplotype as 1 or 2 is arbitrary. The affected individual shown by the solid symbols in the pedigree has type 1 and type 2 haplotypes. Because the father has only a type 2 haplotype and the mother is also affected, the neurofibromatosis gene must be traveling with the type 1 haplotype. The sibling in question has only type 2 haplotypes and therefore must have inherited the opposite allele from his affected mother and can be predicted to be unaffected.

NOTES

CHAPTER 11

GERIATRICS

Darryl S. Chutka, M.D.

DEMOGRAPHICS

The age at which a person becomes elderly is not fixed. People age at different rates and the chronologic age often does not match the physiologic age. The process of aging begins when one is born, and from that time on, a combination of anatomical and physiologic changes occurs that results in the changes of aging. In addition to these changes, various disease states often occur, producing additional changes in the person. Most organs have the necessary reserve capacity to handle the changes due to normal aging and many disease states. However, with aging, most organs lose some of their organ reserve capacity, thus subjecting persons to many of the common problems seen in aged persons, such as adverse drug reactions, bone fracture, urinary incontinence, and so on.

The demographics of aging suggest that with time those older than 65 years will represent a larger proportion of our population. Currently, the elderly represent about 12% of the U.S. population. If current trends continue, this number is expected to double during the next 40 years. The most rapid increase in the elderly population is expected between the years 2010 and 2030, the years those born between 1945 and 1965 ("baby boomers") reach the age of 65. The elderly can be divided into three groups: the "young-old" (65-75 years), "middle-old" (75-85 years), and "old-old" (>85 years). The "old-old" are growing faster than other segments of the population. The significance of this relates to the greater likelihood of health problems for this segment of the population and the greater expense generated for the care of the "old-old." The estimated growth of the population of women is twice that of men. The poorest segments of the population include the "old-old," elderly widows, and elderly with little formal education. Social security is the primary source of income for approximately one-third of the elderly.

Two important terms to understand are "life expectancy" and "life span." Life expectancy has increased as our culture has progressed through time. This increase is not thought to be due to improved technology, better medications or other factors, which would directly benefit the elderly, but rather from improved nutrition, sanitation, and immunizations. Much of the increase in life expectancy is due to the reduction in premature mortality in children and young adults and not to a decrease in mortality of the elderly. Although life expectancy has shown an increase with time, life span has remained fixed at approximately 100 to 110 years. More people are living closer to the end of their life span, and fewer are dying prematurely. This is known as the "rectangularization of the survival curve."

The sex ratio (M:F) decreases with advancing age. Of the group of people older than 65 years, there are approximately 75 men for every 100 women. Among those older than 85 years, there are only 50 men for every 100 women. A relatively small percentage, only 5% of those older than 65 years reside in a nursing home; however, with advancing age, this percentage increases (20% of those >85 years). Over two-thirds of the elderly live in a family setting with their spouse or children.

- People >65 years currently represent about 12% of the U.S. population.
- Life expectancy has increased primarily because of improved nutrition, sanitation, and immunizations.
- Life expectancy has increased with time; life span has not.
- The "old-old" (>85 years) is the fastest growing segment of the population.
- Only 5% of those >65 years live in a nursing home.

HEALTH CARE FINANCING

The cost of health care for the elderly is substantial. It is estimated that the elderly account for 36% of U.S. health care costs. Those older than 65 years have four times the number of physician visits and four to five times the length of hospital stays as those younger than 65 years. Most of the health care cost for the elderly is for hospital care (40%). The costs for physician visits (20%) and long-term care (20%) are also significant. Financing long-term care can be particularly difficult for the elderly. Many assume Medicare will provide coverage when in fact it covers very little (2%). Half of all long-term care financing is private pay by individual patients. Medicaid, a medical assistance program, provides 40% for those demonstrating financial need. Long-term care insurance provides only 5% of the cost.

- The elderly account for 36% of U.S. health care costs.
- The elderly have four times the number of physician visits and four to five times the length of hospital stays.
- Most of the financing for long-term care is by private pay. Medicare provides coverage for only 2%.

REHABILITATION/ASSISTIVE DEVICES

Rehabilitation is important to many elderly and may be either restorative (improve a loss in function) or maintenance (prevent loss of function currently present). The importance of improving or maintaining one's functional status cannot be overstated because functional status often determines whether a person can safely live independently in the community or requires nursing home placement. Currently, a significant number of nursing home admissions are for rehabilitation, with the expectation that the person will eventually leave the facility and return home after some recently lost function is regained. This is common after prolonged hospitalizations or hospitalizations for various orthopedic procedures. The need for rehabilitative services can be determined by reviewing one's ability to perform activities of daily living (ADLs), which include dressing, eating, bathing, toileting, transferring, and ambulation.

Often assistive devices are prescribed to assist a person in gaining functional status in one or more ADLs. These devices often allow many to live independently and delay or prevent institutionalization. Before an assistive device is recommended, several factors need to be considered. Patients need to accept that they have an impairment, the assistive device will help them, and the device is something they are willing to use. Also, the assistive device must be fitted properly, affordable, and relatively easy to use.

Walkers and canes are useful for elderly patients with sensory impairments, problems maintaining balance, or weakness/pain of the lower extremities. Canes can support up to 25% of body weight and are most useful for those with balance difficulties or *unilateral* leg weakness or pain. The cane should be fitted to the proper length, so that the elbow is flexed at a 20° to 30° angle. Walkers are useful for persons who have a balance problem or weakness that is greater than can be managed effectively with a cane. Walkers also are useful

for persons with *bilateral* lower extremity weakness and can support up to 50% of body weight, depending on the type of walker. Patients with Parkinson disease often have a tendency to fall backward and usually do best with walkers that have wheels on the front. Persons with significant upper extremity weakness often do best with four-wheeled walkers, because they may be unable to lift the walker as they ambulate. Wheelchairs are commonly prescribed for the elderly, for both short-term and long-term use. It is extremely important for the wheelchair to be fitted properly to the patient by a trained therapist. Both the height and width of the chair need to be carefully assessed. An improperly sized wheelchair can contribute to pressure sores, deep venous thrombosis, falls, and serious injury.

- Assistive devices are important in maintaining independence and mobility.
- Canes benefit those with unilateral disabilities of the lower extremities or sensory impairments and can support up to 25% of one's body weight.
- Walkers benefit those with bilateral lower extremity weakness or pain and can support up to 50% of one's body weight.

FALLS

Falls are a common cause of morbidity and an important contribution to mortality in the elderly. They increase in frequency with advancing age, because the likelihood of injury also increases. It is estimated that three-fourths of all deaths related to falls occur in those older than 65 years. The increased frequency of falls in the elderly reflects multiple age-related changes, including a reduction in strength due to a loss of muscle mass, decreased visual and hearing acuity, decreased proprioception, and slowed reaction time. These changes can result in an alteration of gait and decreased balance in an elderly person.

An accident, usually related to hazards in the environment (throw rugs, slippery floors, lack of grab bars in bathtubs, and inadequate lighting), is the most common cause of falls among the elderly living independently. Most of these falls occur while the person is performing typical daily activities such as walking or changing position (e.g., sitting to standing). Most falls (70%) occur in the person's home. A significant percentage (10%) occur on stairs, more commonly while the person is descending the stairs. Falls that occur in nursing homes are more likely due to medical problems such as gait abnormalities, balance problems, weakness, and confusion and are less likely to be caused by an environmental hazard. The common risk factors for falls include weakness of the legs (stroke or neuropathy), gait instability (Parkinson disease), balance disorder (vertigo or orthostatism), cognitive impairment (dementia), and the use of multiple medications. Medications that may contribute to falls include antihypertensive agents, diuretics, tricyclic antidepressants (which may produce orthostatic hypotension), sedative/hypnotics, ethanol, and neuroleptics (which may impair balance).

- An accident, usually related to hazards in the environment, is the most common cause of falls in the elderly living independently.
- Falls that occur in a nursing home are more likely due to medical problems.
- The common risk factors for falls include weakness of the legs, gait instability, balance disorder, cognitive impairment, and the use of multiple medications.

Evaluation of Falls

A thorough medical history is the most important component of the assessment of a fall. If the reason for the fall is not known after the patient's history has been taken, it is unlikely that the cause will be found on physical examination or laboratory testing. The history should include the patient's perception of the cause of the fall, any warning symptoms the patient experienced before the fall, and any associated symptoms that occurred with the fall. The patient should also be questioned about how he or she felt immediately after the fall. Loss of consciousness may suggest a cardiac or neurologic event (arrhythmia, seizure, or cerebrovascular event).

The physical examination should include a neurologic examination testing gait, balance, sensory impairment, and extremity strength. Any sensory impairment should be noted. Because falls may be associated with acute illnesses, patients should be assessed for infections, myocardial infarction, and gastrointestinal hemorrhage. Orthostatic hypotension, although common among the elderly, may also indicate a medication effect or hypovolemia from hemorrhage or dehydration.

- A thorough medical history is the most important component of the assessment of a fall.
- The physical examination should include a neurologic examination testing gait, balance, sensory impairment, and extremity strength.

Prevention and Treatment of Falls

The goal of the assessment of a fall is to reduce the likelihood of additional falls. The treatment plan is based on the findings of the assessment. However, more than one factor is often identified as contributing to falls. Potential interventions for the prevention of falls may include the following:

- Reduction in environmental hazards (provide adequate lighting, remove obstacles from floors, eliminate slippery floors, use appropriate footwear, eliminate side rails).
- Physical therapy (improve gait, balance, and strength).
- Assistive devices (improve gait and balance).
- Review of the medication program (avoid drug-drug interactions, eliminate potentially offending drugs).
- Treat medical problems that may contribute to falls (cataract extraction, Parkinson disease, postural hypotension).

SYNCOPE

"Syncope" is defined as a transient loss of consciousness with loss of postural tone. It becomes more common with advancing age and has many causes. Although the cause of the syncopal spell itself is usually benign, several serious consequences can result from the fall, including bone fracture and subdural hematoma. Regardless of the cause of syncope, the underlying mechanism is inadequate cerebral blood perfusion. It is estimated that as many as one-third of the cases of syncope have a cardiac cause. These include valvular heart disease (aortic stenosis, mitral regurgitation, and mitral stenosis), hypertrophic cardiomyopathy, myocardial infarction, and cardiac arrhythmias (tachyarrhythmias, bradyarrhythmias). An orthostatic decrease in blood pressure is also common in the elderly, because of changes in baroreceptor function. In addition, several disease states can be associated with orthostatic hypotension, including peripheral neuropathy, Parkinson disease, and Shy-Drager syndrome. Also, various medications can produce hypotension, including antihypertensive agents, tricyclic antidepressants, neuroleptics, and diuretics. Although vasovagal syncope is more common in younger persons, it can occur in the elderly. Carotid sinus hypersensitivity, an exaggerated hypotensive reflex that occurs in response to carotid sinus massage, can also be a cause of syncope. Other exaggerated cardiovascular reflexes that can result in syncope include micturition, defecation, and coughing. Seizures, hypoxemia (pulmonary embolism, respiratory failure), severe hypoglycemia, and anemia can also produce syncope.

The medical history is the most important part of the evaluation of syncope. The physical examination should focus on the signs related to cardiovascular or neurologic disease. Orthostatic blood pressure should be measured and carotid massage performed. Findings from the history and physical examination should guide the selection of tests to be performed. Tests that may be of value are electrocardiography and, occasionally, ambulatory cardiac monitoring when a cardiac arrhythmia is suspected. Rarely, electrophysiologic studies should be considered. When neurologic abnormalities are found on examination, an imaging study (computerized tomography [CT] or magnetic resonance imaging [MRI]) of the head may yield important information. Electroencephalography (EEG) is useful when a seizure disorder is thought to cause syncope.

Laboratory blood tests do not commonly give the diagnosis for syncope; however, several of these tests may be helpful in certain circumstances. A blood count and electrolyte and creatinine determinations can give information about volume status. Determining cardiac enzymes may be useful when a recent myocardial infarction is suspected. Echocardiography should be performed if there is evidence of structural cardiac disease.

● Cardiovascular disease is a common cause of syncope in the elderly and includes valvular disease, arrhythmias, and hypotension.

● The medical history is the most important part of a syncope evaluation.

VISION CHANGES

A combination of anatomical and physiologic changes related to aging and various disease states common in the elderly frequently cause decreased vision. Vision loss increases with advancing age, and more than one-quarter of those older than 85 years report significant visual impairment. More than 90% of the elderly wear eyeglasses. It is estimated that at least 25% of nursing home residents are legally blind. The most common eye problem in the elderly is presbyopia, difficulty with close focus. Presbyopia is the result of decreased lens flexibility, which occurs with aging. Cataracts are also more common with advancing age; they begin forming early in life, but the progression varies from person to person. Cataracts can be classified as nuclear, cortical, and subcortical. Although cataracts are usually bilateral, one eye may be affected more than the other. Cataract surgery with intraocular lens implantation is effective in restoring visual acuity. The decision about the surgical treatment of cataracts should be individualized and based on the patient's disability.

Glaucoma is the most common cause of blindness worldwide and is characterized by increased intraocular pressure and associated optic nerve damage. The two major types of glaucoma are open-angle and angle-closure. Open-angle glaucoma is more common. Chronic open-angle glaucoma produces a slow progressive loss of peripheral vision that often is not appreciated by the patient until a significant amount of vision is lost. Glaucoma is more common among black Americans than whites and is the most common cause of blindness in black Americans. Funduscopic examination shows atrophy and cupping of the optic disk. Visual field testing reveals typical field defects. A small number of patients with funduscopic or visual field changes of glaucoma have normal intraocular tension. If the physician routinely checks for glaucoma, it can be diagnosed and treated effectively before significant visual loss occurs. The decision to treat glaucoma is not based only on the degree of increased ocular tension.

Treatment is started when there is evidence of visual loss or physical evidence of ocular damage, such as cupping of the optic disks.

There are several options for the treatment of glaucoma, including surgery and medication. Medications are effective in reducing the production of aqueous humor or in increasing its outflow. Pilocarpine causes pupillary constriction and opens the trabecular meshwork, resulting in increased flow of aqueous humor. β-Blockers such as timolol decrease the production of aqueous humor, as do carbonic anhydrase inhibitors. Epinephrine decreases the production of aqueous humor and increases its flow. The goal of surgical treatment is to increase the flow of aqueous humor. Laser trabeculectomy is occasionally performed for open-angle glaucoma and is usually successful in increasing the outflow of aqueous humor.

Acute angle-closure glaucoma is less common than chronic open-angle glaucoma and represents about 5% of glaucoma cases. It often presents after pupillary dilation. It results from the obstruction of aqueous humor as it flows from the anterior chamber of the eye through Schlemm canal. This obstruction abruptly increases intraocular pressure. Patients with acute angle-closure glaucoma present with symptoms of intense eye pain, blurred vision with halos around lights, headache, and nausea. Physical examination reveals a slightly dilated pupil unresponsive to light. Urgent treatment is necessary to prevent permanent loss of vision.

Macular degeneration is the most significant disease of the retina in the elderly. It is associated with the gradual and progressive loss of central vision, while peripheral vision is spared. Although it initially tends to develop in one eye, it eventually becomes bilateral in many patients. Macular degeneration is associated with aging, tobacco use, and possibly with hypertension. It results in atrophy of the pigmented retinal epithelium. Impaired function of the photoreceptors eventually occurs, resulting in the characteristic loss of central vision and sparing of peripheral vision. The breakdown of the epithelium results in the deposition of drusen. The pathologic changes of macular degeneration generally can be seen on funduscopic examination. Laser treatment can be beneficial in some types of macular degeneration; however, most cases are managed with devices used to assist vision, such as increased lighting and magnifying lenses.

● Chronic open-angle glaucoma is more common than angle-closure glaucoma.

● Symptoms of open-angle glaucoma are slowly progressive and consist of loss of the peripheral field of vision.

● Symptoms of angle-closure glaucoma are abrupt in onset and consist of eye pain, headache, nausea, and vomiting.

● Macular degeneration is a disease of the retina and results in the loss of central vision.

HEARING CHANGES

Hearing loss in the elderly is commonly due to a central auditory processing disorder, which causes difficulty with speech perception. The ability to discriminate speech is worse than predicted for the amount of pure tone lost. The prevalence of hearing loss, especially of high frequencies (presbycusis), increases significantly among persons older than 65 years, approaching 50% in those older than 80. Noise-induced hearing loss produces a similar high-frequency hearing loss. Elderly patients with a high-frequency loss usually have the most difficulty with appreciating consonant sounds.

Causes of conductive hearing loss include cerumen impaction, perforation of the tympanic membrane, cholesteatoma, Paget disease, and otosclerosis. Hearing aids may benefit many elderly with hearing loss and many improvements have been made in these devices. Some models of hearing aids are able to select the optimal frequency amplification for the specific environment, others can be programmed to amplify the specific frequencies that the patient has lost. A less complex version amplifies the higher frequencies, the frequencies most commonly lost with aging. Hearing aids are most beneficial when used in an environment with minimal background noise, for example, a one-on-one conversation in a quiet room. They are least helpful when used in crowds with extensive background noise.

- Hearing loss due to a central auditory processing disorder causes difficulty with speech perception worse than predicted for the amount of pure tone lost.
- The elderly tend to have greater difficulty appreciating consonants than vowels.
- Chronic exposure to loud noise can produce a high-frequency hearing loss.

RHEUMATOLOGIC PROBLEMS

Rheumatologic problems are among the commonest complaints of the elderly. These diseases tend to be chronic and often accumulate with time. Although most of these diseases are not life-threatening, they commonly cause an alteration in lifestyle and lead to significant disability. Osteoarthritis is extremely common among the elderly and is present to some degree in more than 80% of them. It produces joint symptoms that vary with time and degree of activity. Osteoarthritis usually can be differentiated from rheumatoid arthritis by the medical history and physical examination findings. Osteoarthritis tends not to produce systemic symptoms, which are common in rheumatoid arthritis. Joint inflammation occurs in osteoarthritis, but it is more pronounced in rheumatoid arthritis. Although disease activity varies, acute worsening of a specific joint should make one suspicious of a superimposed crystalline arthritis (gout or pseudogout) or septic arthritis, which occasionally are found in patients with underlying chronic joint disease.

- Osteoarthritis is the commonest rheumatologic disease among the elderly.
- Acute joint symptoms in patients with osteoarthritis or rheumatoid arthritis may represent crystalline or septic arthritis.

Osteoarthritis

Osteoarthritis has a predilection for the hands (distal and proximal interphalangeal joints, first carpometacarpal joint of the thumb), knees, hips, and feet (first tarsometatarsal joint), with relative sparing of the elbow, wrist, metacarpophalangeal joints, and ankle. Osteoarthritis has a typical radiographic appearance that includes asymmetrical narrowing of the joint space, presence of osteophytes, subchondral sclerosis, and cystic changes in the bone. Systemic symptoms do not occur. Joint pain is common with joint use and weight-bearing activity. Rest usually provides relief from the pain. The treatment of osteoarthritis includes adequate rest, local heat, and exercise to strengthen periarticular muscles, occasionally the injection of corticosteroid into the joint space when inflammation is present, and analgesics. Because only joint inflammation is rarely significant in osteoarthritis, an analgesic such as acetaminophen should be tried initially for pain relief. Nonsteroidal anti-inflammatory drugs (NSAIDs) can be quite effective; however, they carry a risk of significant adverse effects, especially when taken chronically.

- Osteoarthritis produces asymmetric narrowing of the joint space.
- Osteoarthritis has a predilection for the hands, hips, knees, and feet.

Rheumatoid Arthritis

Rheumatoid arthritis is often found in elderly patients, most commonly as a chronic disease that was acquired earlier in life. It can also develop later in life and has two presentations. As in younger persons, it may present with symmetrical distal joint inflammation, positive rheumatoid factor, and a tendency to progress with time. The second presentation is common in the elderly and consists of the acute onset of proximal joint pain and stiffness, which can be very similar to polymyalgia rheumatica. Rheumatoid factor is often negative and rheumatoid nodules are often absent. In contrast to osteoarthritis, patients with rheumatoid arthritis have systemic symptoms. Extra-articular manifestations are occasionally present with rheumatoid arthritis and include potential involvement of the skin (rheumatoid nodules), lung (fibrosis, rheumatoid nodules, pleural effusions), blood vessels (vasculitis), nervous system (mononeuritis multiplex), and hematologic system (Felty syndrome). Sjögren syndrome (splenomegaly, leukopenia) also occasionally accompanies rheumatoid arthritis. Radiographs of joints involved with rheumatoid arthritis characteristically show symmetrical narrowing of the joint space. The diagnosis usually is made by demonstrating inflammatory, symmetrical arthritis on physical examination. Laboratory tests can often be misleading in the elderly. Testing for rheumatoid factor is often negative in many elderly patients with rheumatoid arthritis; however, the test can be false positive in many elderly patients who do not have the disease, although usually at a low titer. Elderly patients with rheumatoid arthritis receive the same therapeutic agents as younger patients: NSAIDs, chloroquine, methotrexate, gold, and low doses (5 to 7.5 µg/day) of corticosteroids.

- Approximately 10% of the cases of rheumatoid arthritis develop in persons >65 years.
- Radiographs of rheumatoid arthritis show symmetrical narrowing of the joint space.
- Elderly patients with rheumatoid arthritis often have negative results on testing for rheumatoid factor, and others without rheumatoid arthritis can have false-positive results.

Crystalline Arthropathy

Crystalline arthropathy is common in the elderly population. Whereas gout tends to be more common in men and to involve more distal joints (especially the great toe), pseudogout is more common in women and tends to involve more proximal joints (especially the knee).

Gout is usually a monoarticular arthritis caused by intra-articular deposition of uric acid crystals. It is associated with hyperuricemia, which may be produced by thiazide diuretics. Gouty attacks may be precipitated by stressful events such as surgery, severe illnesses, or trauma. Although gout usually is diagnosed on the basis of the medical history and physical examination, the diagnosis is confirmed by microscopic evaluation of the synovial fluid from an affected joint. Urate crystals are long and needle-shaped. They are negatively birefringent with polarizing microscopy. Treatment for an acute attack of gout includes the use of NSAIDs. Colchicine, orally or intravenously, may be given to patients who should not receive NSAIDs. In some circumstances, intra-articular or systemic corticosteroids may be necessary. Long-term suppressive therapy usually is not initiated until several acute episodes of gout have occurred. Suppressive therapy may include allopurinol or probenecid daily or low doses of oral colchicine. Treatment of asymptomatic hyperuricemia is rarely necessary, although it is initiated in patients with uric acid renal

stones or, occasionally, when starting chemotherapy for various hematologic malignancies.

- Gout is a monoarticular arthritis; it is more common in men.
- Gout is associated with hyperuricemia, which may be produced by thiazides.
- Urate crystals are long, needlelike, and negatively birefringent with polarizing microscopy.
- Initial treatment of an acute attack of gout is with NSAID.

Pseudogout (calcium pyrophosphate deposition disease) is usually a monoarticular arthritis that most frequently involves the knee or wrist. As with gout, an acute attack can occur with a stressful event such as surgery, trauma, or illness. Radiographs of joints with pseudogout often show linear articular calcification, although approximately 25% of the elderly have articular calcification with no clinical evidence of the disease. Calcium pyrophosphate crystals are rectangular and exhibit positive birefringence with polarizing microscopy. An acute attack is treated with NSAIDs or with corticosteroids injected into the affected joints. Daily therapy with a low dose of colchicine may decrease the frequency of acute attacks.

- Pseudogout is a monoarticular arthritis and commonly involves the knee.
- Calcium pyrophosphate crystals are rectangular and positively birefringent with polarizing microscopy.
- An acute attack of pseudogout is treated with NSAIDs or intra-articular steroid.

Polymyalgia Rheumatica and Temporal Arteritis

Polymyalgia rheumatica and temporal arteritis occur more commonly in women than in men and in persons older than 50 years. Patients with polymyalgia rheumatica describe stiffness, aching, and weakness of proximal muscles (shoulders, hips), especially in the morning. This is thought to be due to synovitis of the shoulder and/or hip joint. The clinical presentation of polymyalgia rheumatica may be very similar to that of rheumatoid arthritis in the elderly. Patients may also complain of nonspecific malaise, fatigue, low-grade fever, and anorexia with weight loss. Although patients commonly describe weakness, muscle strength is normal when tested. The diagnosis is usually suspected from the classic history obtained from the patient; no specific laboratory test is diagnostic for the disease. Patients usually have an increased erythrocyte sedimentation rate and, occasionally, mild anemia. The levels of muscle enzymes (creatine kinase and aspartate aminotransferase) are not increased. The response to treatment is very characteristic and often can be used to support the diagnosis. Treatment with low doses of oral corticosteroids (prednisone, 15-20 mg/day) produces a dramatic improvement in symptoms, often within 24 hours. After treatment has been initiated, the corticosteroid dose can be gradually tapered, using the patient's clinical response and erythrocyte sedimentation rate as indicators of disease activity.

- Polymyalgia rheumatica is more common in women.
- Although patients commonly complain of weakness, muscle strength is normal.
- Laboratory findings include an increased erythrocyte sedimentation rate and, occasionally, mild anemia.
- The response to treatment with oral corticosteroids is dramatic.

Temporal arteritis develops in about 15% of patients with polymyalgia rheumatica. Pathologically, there is inflammation of medium-sized arteries, which arise from the aortic arch. Systemic symptoms include low-grade fever and fatigue; anorexia with weight loss is also common. A majority of patients have a unilateral or bilateral headache, usually in the temporal area. Many patients also have scalp tenderness and jaw claudication due to facial artery involvement with disease. Loss of vision, including unilateral or bilateral visual blurring, visual field loss, diplopia, or blindness caused by ischemic optic neuritis, may occur and is the most worrisome symptom. As with polymyalgia rheumatica, temporal arteritis is usually suspected on the basis of the patient's description of the symptoms. Few findings are documented on physical examination. Some patients have tender, swollen, or pulseless temporal arteries. Rarely, bruits may be heard over medium-sized arteries involved with disease. Although no diagnostic laboratory test is specific for temporal arteritis, almost all patients have a significantly increased erythrocyte sedimentation rate, often greater than 100 mm/hr. Mild anemia may also be present. After temporal arteritis is suspected, the diagnosis should be confirmed with temporal artery biopsy. A 4- to 5-cm piece of temporal artery should be obtained, initially on the side of the patient's symptoms. If the pathologic findings are negative, a similar biopsy should be performed on the contralateral side. The inflammatory changes in the artery may be spotty or confined to a small portion of the artery, occasionally causing difficulty in confirming the diagnosis pathologically. Temporal artery biopsy should not be performed routinely in those with polymyalgia rheumatica without symptoms of temporal arteritis. Treatment consists of high doses of steroids (prednisone, 60 mg/day) and may be started before the biopsy sample is obtained, assuming the biopsy is to be performed within 48 hours. The prednisone dose should be tapered by assessing the patient's clinical response to treatment and measuring the erythrocyte sedimentation rate.

- Temporal arteritis develops in about 15% of patients with polymyalgia rheumatica.

- Patients with polymyalgia rheumatica should not have temporal artery biopsies unless they have symptoms of temporal arteritis.
- Temporal arteritis commonly presents with a unilateral or bilateral headache.
- Loss of vision is the most worrisome symptom.
- The erythrocyte sedimentation rate is usually increased.
- Treatment with high-dose corticosteroids should be initiated when the disease is suspected and can be started before temporal artery biopsy.

THYROID DISEASE

Thyroid disease becomes more common with advancing age. Most elderly patients with hyperthyroidism present with typical findings; however, a small but significant proportion have atypical symptoms. Some elderly develop anorexia with weight loss, altered stool frequency (either diarrhea or constipation), or cardiovascular abnormalities, including hypertension, increased angina, myocardial ischemia, congestive heart failure, and atrial fibrillation. Other symptoms that may develop include apathy, depression, tremor, and myopathy. Decline in bone density is also accelerated with hyperthyroidism. Ophthalmopathy, lid lag, tachycardia, and increased perspiration are relatively more uncommon in the elderly than in younger patients. The development of a goiter with hyperthyroidism is noted in only about 60% of the elderly. The commonest cause of hyperthyroidism in the elderly is Graves disease. Radioiodine therapy is the safest and most economical treatment for hyperthyroidism in elderly patients.

- Hyperthyroidism associated with goiter is uncommon in the elderly.
- Graves disease is the commonest form of hyperthyroidism in the elderly.

The diagnosis of hypothyroidism in elderly patients is usually made by finding low levels of total serum thyroxine (T_4) and/or an increased sTSH on laboratory testing of asymptomatic patients. The common symptoms of hypothyroidism are vague (constipation, cold intolerance, dry skin) and often attributed to the many "symptoms of aging." Almost all the patients have hypothyroidism due to primary thyroid failure rather than to pituitary or hypothalamic insufficiency. The commonest cause of hypothyroidism in the elderly is Hashimoto thyroiditis. Treatment of hypothyroidism should begin with a low dose of thyroid supplement (25-50 μg/day), which is increased by 25 μg every 3 to 4 weeks. Patients with coronary artery disease should receive an even lower starting dose and more gradual dose increments because a too rapid thyroid replacement can precipitate cardiac ischemia. It takes approximately 6 to 8 weeks for a given dose of thyroid supplement to equilibrate; therefore, the sTSH should not be checked before this time to assess whether the dose of thyroid supplement is correct. Thyroid hormone requirements decrease with advancing age, and most elderly require 75 to 100 µg/day; however, some require as little as 50 µg/day. Subclinical hypothyroidism can be found in approximately 15% of the elderly. These patients are clinically euthyroid and have a low-normal total (serum) T_4 level and a slightly elevated sTSH level. Whether to treat these patients is a matter of controversy. Most physicians choose to observe and follow these patients unless symptoms of hypothyroidism develop or the sTSH level continues to increase.

- Hypothyroidism is often difficult to detect in the elderly.
- Most cases of hypothyroidism are due to primary thyroid failure rather than to pituitary or hypothalamic disease.
- Hashimoto thyroiditis is the commonest cause of hypothyroidism in the elderly.
- Very low starting doses and very gradual dose increments should be prescribed in hypothyroid patients with coronary artery disease.

Euthyroid sick syndrome is common in elderly hospitalized patients. Patients are clinically euthyroid, but with low serum levels of T_3 and T_4, and a low-normal level of sTSH. Laboratory values tend to return to normal after the patient has recovered from the illness. The syndrome may be caused by a decreased amount of thyroid-binding protein and a substance that inhibits T_4 binding.

SEXUAL FUNCTION AND SEXUALITY

Multiple physical and social changes occur with aging that can result in changes in the desire and capacity of an older person for sexual activity. Although there is evidence that interest in sexuality is retained well into older ages, for several reasons the frequency of sexual activity tends to be reduced with aging. Whereas this is true for the elderly population in general, there is great variability in sexual interest and activity from one elderly person to another. One of the most important factors that may determine whether a person is sexually active is the availability of a partner who is capable of sexual activity. The setting in which the elderly live can also have a role in whether a person is sexually active. Many elderly live in an environment in which sexual activity is difficult or not condoned, for example, in a nursing home or in the home of their children. Because privacy may not be possible in these settings, intimacy is unlikely to occur.

Little is known about the influence sexual hormones have in libido for either the male or female. Although it is not thought that estrogen or progestin have a role in sexual desire in females, evidence suggests that androgens increase sexual interest. Lack of estrogen can produce reduced vaginal lubrication and mucosal atrophy, which can cause dyspareunia. Painful conditions such as osteoarthritis may also have a role in diminishing desire for sexual activity. Erectile dysfunction increases in frequency with advancing age and is the most common reason for a man to reduce his degree of sexual activity. It may be related to psychosocial as well as to physical factors. An erection is a result of a combination of neurologic and vascular activity. The brain sends impulses that produce relaxation of the arterial smooth muscle and sinuses corpus cavernosum, which results in increased blood flow in the cavernosal sinus. The distended sinuses compress and reduce the venous drainage of the penis, resulting in erection. The rigidity of the penis is due to an increase in arterial inflow and a decrease in venous outflow. Aging tends to produce both a slowing of vascular filling and an increase in venous drainage.

With age, testosterone levels tend to decrease in males. This age-related change does not appear to be related to erectile dysfunction; however, it may produce a reduced interest in sexual activity. Many cases of erectile dysfunction are associated with complications of atherosclerotic disease such as coronary artery disease, peripheral arterial disease, and stroke. Hypertension and antihypertensive medications have also been associated with erectile dysfunction. Diabetes mellitus is associated with a high incidence of erectile dysfunction, which may be secondary to the vascular and/or neurologic complications of diabetes.

The evaluation of a patient with erectile dysfunction begins with a medical history. The patient's libido should be determined, as should the frequency and quality of erections. Hypogonadism should be suspected when a marked reduction in libido has occurred. This may also be caused by depression. The medications that are taken and the amount of alcohol use also need to be reviewed carefully. Medications that have been associated with erectile dysfunction include antihypertensive agents, phenothiazines, antidepressants, H_2-receptor antagonists, digoxin, and clofibrate. Symptoms of medical problems such as diabetes mellitus, peripheral neuropathy, peripheral arterial disease, hypertension, thyroid disease (both hypo- and hyperthyroidism) and uremia should be sought. The physical examination should concentrate on findings that would suggest the presence of hypogonadism, peripheral arterial disease, or peripheral neuropathy. Appropriate laboratory tests should include sTSH, fasting blood glucose, and total and bioavailable testosterone. When hypogonadism is suspected, luteinizing hormone (LH) and prolactin levels should be determined. Nocturnal penile tumescence testing is considered unreliable and does not reliably distinguish between psychogenic and organic causes. A duplex scan of the penile arteries can be useful to assess blood flow to the penis. This test can be performed before and after vasodilator therapy and can predict the response to vasodilator therapy.

Treatment for erectile dysfunction includes both mechanical and pharmacologic therapies. Appropriate treatment for specific medical disorders that can be associated with erectile dysfunction should be started. Patients with hypogonadism should be given androgens. Androgens alone should not be expected to reverse erectile dysfunction. Vacuum devices are safe and relatively effective for any cause of erectile dysfunction. Intracorporeal injection of prostaglandin E_1 is also effective in producing a sustained erection. Patients tend to lose their enthusiasm for injections with time, probably because of the relatively invasive nature of the treatment. Sildenafil (Viagra) has been the first of several oral medications approved for the treatment of erectile dysfunction. It is effective in up to 70% of patients regardless of the underlying cause. It inhibits the breakdown of cyclic guanosine monophosphate and improves blood flow to the penis. Because of the potential for hypotension, it is contraindicated for persons receiving nitrate therapy.

- The availability of a partner is one of the most important factors influencing whether an elderly person is sexually active.
- The age-related reduction in testosterone levels in men does not appear to be related to erectile dysfunction; however, it may produce reduced libido.
- Erectile dysfunction may be due to various medications, complications of diabetes mellitus, arterial insufficiency, neuropathy, or thyroid disease.
- Nocturnal penile tumescence is not a reliable test for evaluating erectile dysfunction.

DEMENTIA

Dementia is an acquired cognitive impairment that affects all spheres of the intellect. It is a gradually progressive disorder and becomes more common with increasing age. Approximately 10% to 20% of the population older than 65 years have some degree of dementia. The number increases with age and has been reported to be as high as 50% among those older than 90 years. Dementia involves considerably more than the loss of memory. Other cognitive functions that are affected include judgment, abstract thinking, attention, ability to learn new material, and eventually, the recognition and production of speech. Personality changes frequently accompany dementia. The commonest form of irreversible dementia is Alzheimer disease (50%-70%), followed by vascular dementia (15%-25%). In the recent past, the prevalence of reversible dementias was thought to be as high as 30%.

Currently, it is believed that in most patients with some reversibility in cognitive impairment, the improvement is only transient and most of the patients eventually develop irreversible dementia. The prevalence of truly reversible dementia is quite low, from 1% to 2%. The most common causes of dementia with potential reversibility are depression (pseudodementia), selected drugs, metabolic disorders (hypothyroidism, hyperthyroidism, hyperparathyroidism), toxic agents (heavy metals, pesticides, alcohol, various organic solvents), nutritional deficiencies (vitamin B_{12}, niacin, thiamine), normal-pressure hydrocephalus, subdural hematoma, central nervous system (CNS) tumors, and CNS infections (neurosyphilis, chronic fungal or bacterial meningitis, human immunodeficiency virus [HIV]).

- From 10%-20% of persons older than 65 years have some form of dementia (50% of those older than 90 years).
- The most common cause of cognitive impairment with a potential for being reversed is depression.
- The commonest cause of irreversible dementia is Alzheimer disease.

The diagnosis of Alzheimer disease cannot be confirmed until postmortem examination: no laboratory test, including CT or MRI of the head, is specific for the disease. The diagnosis is made primarily on the basis of the history, usually from family members, and a determination of the cognitive status of the patient. The accuracy of clinicians in diagnosing Alzheimer disease is as high as 95%. Alzheimer disease is a gradually progressive impairment of cognition. Eventually, behavioral problems develop in many patients, including the tendency to wander and to develop paranoia, agitation, delusions, or hallucinations (or a combination of these). Typically, patients with Alzheimer disease have little insight into the disease process and are often brought to the physician by a family member. Pathologically, the CNS findings include neuronal plaques, which represent extracellular deposits of protein containing amyloid, and neurofibrillary tangles, which are intracellular protein, bound to microtubules. Neuronal plaques and neurofibrillary tangles are also found in nondemented persons but in much smaller amounts. Alzheimer disease is associated with a reduced amount of CNS neurotransmitters. Acetylcholine deficiency is especially prominent, as is a reduction in choline acetyltransferase activity.

The evaluation of a demented patient establishes the existence and degree of cognitive impairment, ruling out reversible dementias. Baseline cognitive tests are performed to follow future deterioration. This evaluation consists of a medical history and physical examination (including neurologic examination) and general laboratory tests. Accepted laboratory tests include a complete blood count; electrolyte panel; liver function;

serum levels of creatinine, glucose, and vitamin B_{12}; thyroid function; syphilis serology; chest radiography; and electrocardiography (ECG). Although some form of brain imaging study (CT or MRI) is usually performed, there are arguments for and against this practice. An imaging study is done to rule out various types of potentially reversible CNS lesions such as mass lesions, normal pressure hydrocephalus, or previous strokes and not to check for cerebral atrophy. In patients who have had dementia for an extended period, have no focal findings on neurologic examination, no history of head trauma, and no headache, an imaging study may not be cost-effective. A formal psychometric evaluation is useful to help establish an early diagnosis as well as to follow the progressive decline of the patient's condition. EEG and lumbar puncture are performed only in unusual circumstances and are rarely necessary.

Until recently, the treatment of Alzheimer disease has been limited to controlling abnormal behavior (agitation, delusions, hallucinations, paranoia) with various neuroleptic drugs (sedative-hypnotics and major tranquilizers). None of the neuroleptic medications commonly used improve cognitive function, and very often, they worsen memory and orientation. Major tranquilizers may also cause movement disorders (tardive dyskinesia) and can contribute to falls. The recent availability of tacrine and donepezil, acetylcholinesterase inhibitors, has given clinicians the first true option for treating Alzheimer disease. Acetylcholinesterase inhibitors can transiently delay cognitive decline and should be considered in patients who have mild to moderate dementia. The high prevalence of hepatic toxicity associated with tacrine is not seen with donepezil. Evidence suggests that estrogen therapy, vitamin E, selegiline, and NSAIDs decreased the likelihood of developing Alzheimer disease.

- No laboratory test is specific for diagnosis of Alzheimer disease.
- Evaluation is important for ruling out reversible dementias.
- Medications commonly used in the management of dementia (major tranquilizers, sedative/hypnotics) do not improve memory or orientation.
- Acetylcholinesterase inhibitors can transiently stop the cognitive decline in early-to-moderate dementia.

In addition to Alzheimer disease, several other types of dementia exist. Vascular dementia is common and can be difficult to differentiate from Alzheimer disease. The patient usually demonstrates a stepwise progression consistent with the multiple ischemic infarcts, often with focal neurologic deficits also produced by the ischemic CNS events. Several types of vascular dementias are possible, including cortical multiinfarct, subcortical multiinfarct, and small-vessel ischemia with demyelination (Binswanger disease). Dementia associated with Parkinson disease is another type of dementia. Up to 40% of patients with Parkinson disease develop dementia, many indistinguishable from those with Alzheimer disease. These patients have the typical features of Parkinson disease, that is, resting tremor, rigidity, and bradykinesia in addition to the intellectual impairments of the dementia. In some cases, effective treatment of Parkinson disease with dopamine improves cognitive status. In those with more severe dementia, treatment of the parkinsonian symptoms does not affect cognitive status. Pick disease is an uncommon cause of dementia, with an early age of onset, usually in the fifth or sixth decade. Pick disease is characterized by prominent changes in personality and behavior, with less prominent disturbance of memory. Pathologically, the frontal and temporal lobes of the brain are involved, which can be recognized with CNS imaging. Swollen neurons known as "balloon cells" and argentophilic inclusion bodies are seen microscopically. Creutzfeldt-Jakob disease is an uncommon cause of dementia that has an earlier onset than Alzheimer disease, usually in the sixth decade. The progression of the disease is rapid, eventually producing a vegetative state and the development of myoclonic jerks and seizures. Most patients die within 1 year after disease onset. The cause is thought to be infectious and due to an unidentified slow virus. Huntington disease is autosomal dominant and has early onset of symptoms (usually in the fourth or fifth decade). Eventually, choreiform movements develop. Acquired immunodeficiency syndrome (AIDS) dementia affects up to 50% of people with AIDS and is uncommon in the elderly population.

- Several forms of vascular dementia exist. Dementia due to multiple CNS infarcts is characterized by a stepwise progression.
- Dementia associated with Parkinson disease may improve with treatment of the disease.
- Pick disease is associated with behavioral and personality changes.
- Creutzfeldt-Jakob disease is associated with early onset dementia, with rapid progression and development of myoclonic jerks.

Delirium is an acute confusional disorder frequently mistaken for dementia. It is associated with a decreased level of consciousness, hallucinations, and delusions. Its several causes include 1) many common medical illnesses (urinary tract infection, sepsis, pneumonia) in patients with limited organ reserve function or organ failure; 2) drugs, including sedative-hypnotics, anticholinergic agents, NSAIDs, β-blockers, and antipsychotic agents; 3) metabolic disturbances, such as hyper- or hypoglycemia and hypercalcemia; 4) hypoxia; and 5) hypotension. It is important to differentiate delirium from dementia because of the potential for reversibility of cognitive impairment associated with delirium. Patients with delirium frequently have a preexisting mild (often unrecognized) dementia.

CARDIOVASCULAR CHANGES

It is difficult to know whether the cardiovascular physiologic changes seen in the elderly are due to the normal aging process or to cardiovascular disease. Most likely, the changes are due to a combination of aging, lifestyle, and disease. At rest, the cardiovascular system has relatively few changes. However, like most other organ systems, the reserve capacity of the heart is reduced under conditions of stress and significant changes become apparent. Some of the cardiac changes are a result of lesions in the blood vessels. With age, arterial walls thicken because of intimal thickening. The collagen content increases and results in increased arterial wall stiffness. This produces an increase in peripheral vascular resistance, an increase in pulse wave transmission, and an increase in systolic blood pressure. As a result, the thickness of the left ventricular wall increases. Although there is a decrease in overall number of myocytes with age, the size of individual myocytes increases.

At rest, there is no age-related change in cardiac index or left ventricular ejection fraction. Resting cardiac contractility also remains unchanged. Although the resting heart rate is slightly decreased, this is balanced by a mildly increased stroke volume. Cardiac contractility and left ventricular ejection fraction remain unchanged. There is a reduction in the rate of early diastolic filling and slight increase in left atrial size. In the elderly, the left atrial contraction becomes increasingly important in left ventricular filling. This increase becomes apparent when elderly patients develop atrial fibrillation and lose the atrial contribution to ventricular filling. It results in a significant decrease in the left ventricular ejection fraction and may produce findings of congestive heart failure.

With exercise, the physiologic changes become more pronounced. The maximal heart rate decreases, as does the cardiac index and left ventricular ejection fraction. Cardiac contractility also decreases. Both the end-diastolic and the end-systolic volumes increase. There is an increased plasma level of catecholamines (epinephrine and norepinephrine), with reduced β-adrenergic responsiveness.

- Age-related vascular changes include an increase in peripheral vascular resistance, an increase in pulse wave transmission, and an increase in systolic blood pressure.
- Age-related cardiac changes at rest include a slight reduction in the resting heart rate and a mildly increased stroke volume.
- Age-related cardiac changes with exercise include a reduction in maximal heart rate, cardiac contractility, cardiac index, and left ventricular ejection fraction.
- There is an age-related reduction in β-adrenergic responsiveness and an increased level of circulating catecholamines.

PREOPERATIVE ASSESSMENT OF THE ELDERLY

Elderly patients commonly undergo anesthesia and surgery, and age alone should not be a contraindication for a surgical procedure. Most elderly have some increased risk of perioperative complications as a result of a combination of normal physiologic changes of aging and, more importantly, various disease states. Most perioperative deaths are due to cardiac or respiratory complications. It can be difficult to determine preoperatively if an elderly patient has marked cardiac or respiratory disease. The high prevalence of inactivity in the elderly commonly masks the presence of coronary or pulmonary disease, because symptoms may be present only with exercise. Usually, an older patient who is active, without symptoms, at low risk for cardiorespiratory disease, and scheduled for a nonvascular operation does not require further testing. However, asymptomatic patients who are inactive and have several risk factors for cardiorespiratory disease may benefit from noninvasive cardiac and/or pulmonary testing.

The patient's medications should be reviewed preoperatively. Because of the increased risk of postoperative bleeding, aspirin should be discontinued at least 1 week before the operation. NSAIDs can also increase the risk of bleeding and should be discontinued preoperatively. Because of a shorter antiplatelet effect, NSAIDs may be used up to 48 hours before the operation. Because of the risk of hypoglycemia, oral hypoglycemic medications should not be given the morning of the operation. The blood level of glucose can be managed by the administration of regular insulin if needed. Other medications that the patient takes daily should be given the morning of the operation. Cardiovascular medications, especially β-blockers and clonidine, should not be discontinued abruptly. If corticosteroids have been taken recently in doses capable of suppressing adrenal function, corticosteroids should be given preoperatively.

In addition to the questions typically asked of younger patients in a preoperative assessment, functional ability and cognitive status should be assessed in the elderly. A Mini-Mental State Examination is an adequate screening test for cognitive impairment. Patients with cognitive impairment preoperatively are at increased risk for postoperative delirium. They also may have difficulty completing a physical therapy program.

- Although most elderly have an increased risk of anesthesia and surgery, age alone should not be a factor in deciding whether an operation should be performed.

- Most perioperative deaths among the elderly are due to cardiac or respiratory complications.
- Usually, an older patient who is active, without symptoms, and at low risk for cardiorespiratory disease does not require further testing for a nonvascular operation.
- Aspirin and NSAIDs should be discontinued preoperatively to decrease the likelihood of perioperative bleeding.

PREVENTIVE GERIATRICS

In many disease states, there is evidence to recommend continuing screening tests with advanced aging. In other areas, data about whether screening in the elderly is beneficial is insufficient. In these situations, clinical judgment (taking into account the patient's functional status) is important in deciding whether certain screening tests should be performed. Before a screening test is indicated, several basic principles must hold true:

1. The incidence of the disease is high enough to warrant performing screening tests.
2. There must be a period during which the disease is present but the patient is asymptomatic and the disease can be diagnosed with a screening test.
3. Effective treatment for the disease is available.
4. Early treatment of the disease has a better outcome than it would if the diagnosis is made after symptoms develop.
5. The screening test has a reasonable sensitivity and specificity and is relatively inexpensive and safe.

Cardiovascular Disease

- The benefits of lowering cholesterol have not been clearly demonstrated in the elderly; most authorities do not recommend routine lipid screening in the asymptomatic elderly population. For the elderly with an established diagnosis of coronary artery disease or with multiple risk factors, clinical judgment should be used in determining the benefits of checking lipid values.
- The risks of hypertension as well as the benefits of treatment have been shown to extend to the elderly, and it is recommended that screening for hypertension be performed in the elderly.
- Routine screening for carotid artery disease in the elderly is not recommended; however the recommendations of the U.S. Preventive Services Task Force recommend carotid auscultation in symptomatic elderly persons or those with multiple risk factors for cardiovascular or cerebrovascular disease.
- Routine screening with a resting or exercise ECG is not recommended for elderly patients.

Malignancy

- Because breast cancer continues to increase in incidence with age, continued annual screening with mammography

is recommended. In patients older than 75 years, clinical judgment should be used. If appropriate, it is reasonable to continue mammography as long as the patient's life expectancy exceeds 5 years.
- Although colon cancer is common among the elderly, screening recommendations require clinical judgment. Tests with an acceptable sensitivity and specificity (colonoscopy and barium enema) are difficult for many elderly and have some associated risks. Simple tests such as digital rectal examination or fecal occult blood tests have a low sensitivity and specificity. Despite this, the American Cancer Society recommends annual fecal occult blood testing with flexible sigmoidoscopy every 5 years. For those at increased risk for colorectal cancer, colonoscopy should be performed periodically.
- If cervical Papanicolau smears have been performed appropriately at younger ages and the results have been negative, performing the smears may be discontinued at age 65.
- Although prostate cancer is very common in males, screening tests are controversial. Clinical judgment is advised by the U.S. Preventive Task Force in performing any screening prostate examination. The American Cancer Society recommends performing a digital rectal examination and prostate-specific antigen yearly. It has not been documented that screening for prostate cancer has resulted in reduced mortality.
- There are no recommended screening tests for lung cancer, for either smokers or nonsmokers. Neither routine screening with chest radiography or sputum cytology has shown any reduction in mortality.
- There are no recommended tests for early detection of ovarian cancer.

PULMONARY CHANGES

Pulmonary function declines with advancing age, likely because of a combination of normal anatomical and physiologic changes of aging, injury from exposure to various environmental toxins (tobacco and air pollution), and disease states that affect the lung. Changes in the shape of the thorax contribute to changes in pulmonary physiology. The apical-to-base length of the lungs decreases as the anterior-to-posterior length increases with age. The bronchioles and alveolar ducts increase in diameter, decreasing alveolar surface area. The aged lungs also have reduced compliance because of decreased lung elasticity. These anatomical and physiologic changes result in reduced air flow rates, decreased efficiency of air exchange, and alterations in lung volumes. Changes that occur with aging in pulmonary physiology include a decrease in mucociliary clearance, vital capacity, 1-second forced expiratory volume (FEV_1), maximal breathing capacity, and diffusing capacity (DLCO). The lung residual volume and alveolar-arterial oxygen gradient (AaO$_2$) increase with age. Aging has no effect on total lung capacity.

- Pulmonary function declines with age because of a combination of changes due to aging, environmental exposure, and disease.
- Changes in lung shape contribute to changes in pulmonary physiology.
- Changes in pulmonary physiology include a reduction in vital capacity, FEV$_1$, maximal breathing capacity, and DLCO and an increase in residual volume and AaO$_2$ gradient.

RESPIRATORY DISEASE

Pneumonia is one of the top 10 causes of death among the elderly and is the cause of death in 15% of nursing home residents. The bacterial organisms that cause pneumonia change with advancing age. Elderly patients have an increased number of gram-negative bacteria as part of their normal oral flora. They also have an increased likelihood of aspirating oral secretions, which contributes to the increased incidence of pneumonia caused by gram-negative and anaerobic bacteria. The likely cause of a pneumonia depends on the setting in which the patient acquired the infection. Overall, *Streptococcus pneumoniae* is the commonest etiologic organism. *Haemophilus influenzae*, other gram-negative bacteria, and anaerobes are common among the elderly in nursing homes and hospitals. Organisms such as *Legionella, Chlamydia,* and *Moraxella catarrhalis* are also seen occasionally in the elderly. Treatment for pneumonia should reflect the most likely etiologic agent. Recently, a large percentage of *S. pneumoniae* organisms have become penicillin-resistant. Appropriate empirical treatment for pneumonia acquired by an elderly patient in an outpatient setting would be a second-generation cephalosporin. An extended spectrum macrolide (clarithromycin or azithromycin) would also be acceptable. For hospital-acquired pneumonia, additional coverage is needed for gram-negative and atypical bacteria. Acceptable treatment includes a third-generation cephalosporin with erythromycin given intravenously. An extended spectrum quinolone could also be used. Although nursing home-acquired pneumonia can be quite serious, if the patient's condition is not toxic and appears stable, the pneumonia can be treated in the nursing home if the patient is observed closely. Generally, a third-generation cephalosporin given intramuscularly or an extended spectrum quinolone is the treatment of choice for these patients.

- Pneumonia is among the top 10 causes of death among the elderly.
- Elderly patients have a greater number of gram-negative bacteria as part of their normal oral flora.
- Aspiration is more likely to occur in elderly persons.
- Treatment must reflect the likely causal organisms.

Tuberculosis, after declining in frequency for many years, is increasing in frequency. The number of reported cases has increased 20% over the past 10 years. Tuberculosis is more common with advancing age, with the elderly having two to four times the case rate of those younger than 65 years. Persons residing in nursing homes have from two to six times the case rate of the general population. Most cases of tuberculosis in the elderly are due to reactivation of a previous infection rather than being newly acquired disease. It is thought that about 4% of patients with a positive tuberculin skin test (PPD) eventually develop active tuberculosis. Tuberculosis is suspected on the basis of clinical findings, which can be subtle and include fatigue, anorexia with weight loss, and cough. Chest radiographic findings may also help in suspecting the disease. Confirmation of the disease requires evaluation of sputum and gastric washings for the presence of the acid-fast organisms. Cultures may take up to 6 weeks to become positive. An increasing number of multidrug-resistant *Mycobacterium tuberculosis* is being found; however, these organisms are not commonly seen in the elderly because most cases are due to reactivation of the disease acquired many years ago.

Without symptoms, the PPD is the best test available to determine the possibility of tuberculosis. Intermediate strength tuberculin (5 TU) is administered intradermally and the degree of induration (not erythema) is determined.

On admission to a nursing home, the patient should be administered a two-stage PPD. The first skin test should be interpreted 7 days after it is administered. The second test is administered on the seventh day if the patient has less than 10 mm of induration. The second test is interpreted 2 days after it is applied. Up to 15% of additional patients with a positive reaction are identified with this method. If the PPD is positive, chest radiography should be performed. If the findings are negative and the patient is asymptomatic, no treatment should be initiated unless it can be shown that the patient has had conversion to a positive PPD within the last 2 years. If the chest radiographic findings are abnormal, sputum and gastric washings should be obtained and cultured.

Chemoprophylaxis for persons older than 35 years consists of isoniazid for 6 to 12 months. It is indicated if the PPD is positive and the patient 1) has had conversion to a positive PPD within the last 2 years, 2) is an intravenous drug user, 3) has a coexisting medical problem (e.g., silicosis, such malignancies as leukemia or lymphoma, chronic renal failure, or diabetes mellitus) or is HIV positive, 4) has recently had rapid weight loss, 5) is immunocompromised (including patients taking corticosteroids), 6) has been in a household with and/or in close contact with a tuberculosis patient, or 7) has abnormal chest radiographic findings.

Elderly patients with proven tuberculosis should start receiving treatment with more than two antituberculin drugs until the results of sensitivity testing are known. If the tuberculosis organism is not a resistant strain, the patient may receive treatment with two drugs, usually isoniazid and rifampin. Isoniazid-induced hepatotoxicity is common with advancing age and develops in up to 5% of those older than 65. The baseline level of aspartate aminotransferase should be determined and checked periodically in elderly patients taking isoniazid. Elderly patients taking isoniazid should also receive vitamin B_6 (pyridoxine) supplements (10 to 25 mg/day) to prevent peripheral neuropathy.

- Tuberculosis is increasing in frequency.
- Most tuberculosis in the elderly is due to reactivation of disease rather than to new infection.
- Patients admitted to a nursing home should have a two-stage PPD test.
- Isoniazid can produce liver toxicity in the elderly, and liver function tests should be monitored.
- Elderly patients taking isoniazid should receive pyridoxine to prevent peripheral neuropathy.

IMMUNIZATIONS

Pneumococcal pneumonia vaccine is effective against 23 of the strains of *S. pneumoniae*, which account for 80% of the strains that commonly cause pneumonia. Because of decreasing effectiveness, revaccination should be considered after 6 years in those who received their initial vaccination before age 65. The influenza vaccine is changed on a yearly basis, depending on the prevalent strain. It should be given in the late autumn, and it should be given annually to high-risk persons, persons older than 65 years, and those in frequent close contact with the elderly. After receiving the vaccine, it takes about 2 to 3 weeks to develop immunity to influenza. Any of the elderly who are unvaccinated during an influenza epidemic should be given amantadine or rimantadine.

- Reimmunization of pneumococcal vaccine is advised after 6 to 7 years.
- The influenza vaccine should be administered to the elderly once yearly in the autumn.

OSTEOPOROSIS

Osteoporosis and its complications are extremely common among the elderly. Osteoporosis results in a loss of bone density, with a normal bone-to-mineral ratio. Hip, wrist, and vertebral compression fractures are common causes of morbidity and mortality. Peak bone density is achieved at about age 30, with men having a greater bone density than women at all ages. After age 30, bone density gradually decreases. In females, loss of estrogen, either because of surgery (bilateral oophorectomy) or menopause, causes a more rapid decrease in bone density.

No simple laboratory tests are available that can confirm the diagnosis of osteoporosis. The diagnosis is usually made clinically. The following help to establish the diagnosis: 1) presence of multiple risk factors, including advanced age, female gender, caucasian race, low calcium intake through much of one's lifetime, thin build, a history of steroid or tobacco use, history of previous fracture (especially vertebral), Northern European ancestry, prolonged inactivity, and positive family history for osteoporosis; 2) ruling out secondary causes (glucocorticoid excess, hypogonadism, hyperthyroidism, hyperparathyroidism, osteomalacia, myeloma); 3) physical examination findings (loss of height, increased thoracic kyphosis); and 4) radiographic findings of osteopenia or vertebral compression fractures. Bone density can be measured by several techniques, the most common of which is dual X-ray absorptiometry. Bone density may be determined for one of several reasons: to assess the risk of fracture, to check the progression of disease, and to evaluate the response to treatment.

Previously, the treatment of osteoporosis was disappointing and was aimed at prevention. Currently, several therapeutic options are available that can provide effective treatment for established osteoporosis. Premenopausal women require 1,000 mg/day of elemental calcium, and postmenopausal women, 1,500 mg/day. The initial treatment for osteoporosis in postmenopausal women should be adequate calcium intake, weight-bearing exercise, adequate vitamin D (600-800 IU/day), and hormonal replacement therapy. Hormonal therapy is most effective when initiated at or shortly after menopause. Progestin should be used with estrogen to prevent the increased risk of endometrial cancer seen with unopposed estrogen use. Both cyclic and continuous hormonal therapy are effective in treating osteoporosis. Progestin is not necessary for those who have had a hysterectomy. In addition to showing a reduction in bone loss after menopause, there is evidence that starting hormonal treatment in women with osteoporosis decreases the rate of hip and vertebral fracture. Alendronate, a bisphosphonate, also increases bone density and decreases the rate of hip and vertebral fractures. Compliance with this medication can be a problem. Alendronate is poorly absorbed and binds to food and calcium and, thus, must be taken with tap water before food is ingested. The medication has also been associated with esophagitis, and to minimize this, the patient must remain upright for at least 30 minutes after taking the medication. Calcitonin increases vertebral bone density, but more data are needed to know whether it decreases the risk of hip fracture. Calcitonin appears to have an analgesic effect and may be useful in patients with painful osteoporotic vertebral compression fracture. Raloxifene is a selective estrogen receptor modulator that reduces bone resorption. Although it has estrogen-like effects on bone, it acts as an estrogen antagonist in the breast and uterus. It can cause a modest increase in bone mineral density in the hip and spine. Fluoride increases bone density in most women; however, the fracture rate may increase because of an increase in bone fragility. More recent studies with lower doses of fluoride have had encouraging results. Currently, fluoride has not been approved by the FDA for the treatment of osteoporosis.

- Osteoporosis is common with advancing age as bone density decreases.
- Hip and vertebral compression fractures are common causes of morbidity and mortality.
- No simple laboratory tests are available to confirm the diagnosis of osteoporosis.

OSTEOMALACIA

Osteomalacia is the result of defective bone mineralization and is most commonly caused by a deficiency of vitamin D. It may be due to inadequate intake of vitamin D, lack of exposure to the sun, malabsorption, chronic liver disease, or chronic renal disease (resulting in inadequate conversion of 25-hydroxyvitamin D to 1,25-dihydroxyvitamin D). Radiographically, the bone appears osteopenic and can resemble osteoporosis. Unlike osteoporosis, several abnormal laboratory findings are associated with osteomalacia, including decreased levels of calcium, phosphorus, 1,25-dihydroxyvitamin D_3, and increased levels of alkaline phosphatase. Defective bone mineralization may also be caused by very low levels of phosphate. This can be due to excessive use of aluminum-containing antacids, tumor effect, or renal tubule disorders.

- Osteomalacia can resemble osteoporosis and is due to inadequate vitamin D resulting from various mechanisms.
- Unlike osteoporosis, osteomalacia has laboratory abnormalities that include low serum levels of serum calcium and phosphorus and an increased level of alkaline phosphatase.

PRESSURE ULCERS

Seventy percent of pressure ulcers occur in persons older than 70 years. Approximately 60% of pressure ulcers develop during hospitalization, 18% in nursing homes, and the rest at home. They are especially common among the elderly in intensive care units. The most important risk factor for the development of a pressure ulcer is immobility. Nutritional deficiencies, age-related changes in skin, and urinary incontinence are also contributing risk factors. Most pressure ulcers occur below the waist. The common sites include the sacrum, greater trochanter, ischial tuberosity, calcaneous, and lateral malleolus of the ankle. Four factors are thought to be important in the development of pressure ulcers: pressure, shearing force, friction, and moisture. When the persistent pressure of skin overlying a bony prominence exceeds the capillary pressure, the blood supply to the tissues is impaired. After approximately 2 hours, tissue ischemia can occur and skin ulceration can result. This is the basis for rotating patients at least every 2 hours when they are incapable of turning themselves. Friction and shearing forces have a role when the patient is dragged across a bed or chair. This has the effect of causing angulation and occlusion of subcutaneous blood vessels and producing ischemia of the underlying tissue. Chronic skin moisture produces tissue maceration and promotes skin breakdown. This tends to magnify skin damage.

Pressure ulcers can be classified into one of four stages (I through IV).

- Stage I: Nonblanchable erythema of intact skin. There may be associated edema.
- Stage II: Partial-thickness skin loss involving the epidermis or dermis or both. The ulcer is superficial and may present as an abrasion, a blister, or a shallow crater.
- Stage III: Full-thickness skin loss with damage or necrosis of subcutaneous tissue. The damage may extend to the fascia. The ulcer is a deep crater.
- Stage IV: Full-thickness skin loss with extensive destruction, tissue necrosis, or involvement of muscle, bone, or tendons. Sinus tracts may be present.

Pressure ulcers tend to be understaged because the underlying tissue damage often is not immediately apparent.

The most important component of the treatment of pressure ulcers is prevention. Preventive strategies include repositioning patients at least every 2 hours to minimize tissue ischemia over sites at risk. Several commercial devices are available to help reduce contact pressure. The use of pressure-reducing mattresses can decrease the pressure over a given area of tissue. Minimizing head elevation and lifting the patient instead of dragging will prevent friction and shearing force. Keeping the patient as dry as possible when incontinent and keeping the skin moisturized helps maintain skin integrity.

After a pressure ulcer has developed, the basic strategy for its treatment includes the following:
- Relieving pressure over the ulcer.

- Debridement of nonviable tissue.
- Optimizing the wound environment (preventing wound maceration and avoiding friction and shearing forces) to promote the formation of granulation tissue.
- Management of other conditions (malnutrition or infection when present) that may delay wound healing.

Stages II, III and IV pressure ulcers should be debrided of necrotic tissue when present. Stage II ulcers can be debrided mechanically with wet-to-wet (saline) gauze dressings changed every 6 hours. Several enzymatic debriding agents are also available and effective. Surgical debridement may also be useful, especially for deeper ulcers (stages III and IV). This should be done with caution in patients with lower extremity ulcers and arterial disease. Water debridement (whirlpool) is useful for larger ulcers. A moist wound environment is optimal for wound healing. Heat lamps dry the ulcer and should not be used. Several products are available to help maintain a moist wound environment, including semipermeable polyurethane films and foams, hydrocolloid dressings, and hydrophilic polymer gels. Topical iodine-povidone, hydrogen peroxide, and acetic acid compounds can impair wound healing and should not be used on pressure ulcers. Infection commonly complicates the healing pressure ulcers. Infected ulcers require the use of systemic antibiotics. Topical antibiotics have little penetration into deeper tissue and can promote the development of resistant bacteria. Culturing the surface of an ulcer does not accurately represent the bacteria involved in an infected ulcer; all skin ulcers develop surface bacterial colonization. An accurate determination of the bacteria involved requires deep tissue cultures.

An ulcer that does not heal should alert the physician to the presence of osteomyelitis. Bone radiographs and bone scans are often made in patients with suspected osteomyelitis but have a rather high incidence of false-negative and false-positive results. MRI is an effective diagnostic test when osteomyelitis is suspected; however, bone biopsy with culture is the best confirmatory test.

Platelet-derived growth factor is occasionally useful in stimulating the healing of pressure ulcers. For large or very deep ulcers, surgical treatment may be necessary. The use of skin grafts or rotation flaps using neighboring subcutaneous tissue and muscle may be the best option for these patients.

URINARY INCONTINENCE

Urinary incontinence is common among the elderly, affecting at least 15% of those living independently and about 50% of those in institutions. It causes numerous medical, social, and economic complications and is a common reason for nursing home placement. Complications of incontinence include urinary tract infection, skin breakdown, social isolation, and depression. Understanding urinary incontinence requires a knowledge of urinary tract anatomy and the physiology of micturition. Failure to appreciate this information can result in an inaccurate diagnosis and ineffective treatment.

Anatomy

The detrusor muscle consists of three muscular layers. Its functions include urine storage (relaxed detrusor) and urine emptying (detrusor contraction). Both sympathetic and parasympathetic nerves innervate the detrusor muscle. Stimulation of the sympathetic nerves results in relaxation of the detrusor muscle and stimulation of the parasympathetic nerves produces contraction of the detrusor muscle. The internal sphincter is a smooth muscle under involuntary (sympathetic innervation) control. Sympathetic stimulation produces increased internal sphincter tone. The external sphincter is striated muscle under voluntary (pudendal innervation) control. It contracts in response to transient increases in intra-abdominal pressure (cough, sneeze, etc.). The external sphincter rapidly fatigues and has little role in maintaining continence.

Stretch receptors in the detrusor wall send information to the central nervous system. The spinal cord transmits sensory (ascending) signals to the brain and motor (descending) signals to the bladder. The brain causes stimulation of the sympathetic nerves when urine storage is desired (detrusor relaxation and internal sphincter contraction) and stimulation of the parasympathetic nerves when bladder emptying is desired (detrusor contraction). With parasympathetic nerve stimulation, the internal sphincter relaxes with inhibition of the sympathetic nerves.

- The urinary bladder receives both a sympathetic and a parasympathetic innervation, relaxing and filling with sympathetic stimulation and contracting and emptying with parasympathetic stimulation.
- The internal urinary sphincter contracts with sympathetic stimulation, promoting bladder filling, and relaxes with bladder emptying as a result of sympathetic inhibition.

Effects of Age

Changes in the urinary system that occur with age do not cause urinary incontinence: incontinence is not a normal result of aging. However, the changes that occur can contribute to the problem of incontinence. These changes include a smaller bladder capacity, early contractions of the detrusor muscle, decreased ability to suppress detrusor muscle contractions and postpone urination, and increased nocturnal urine production.

Medications Affecting Urination and Continence

Medications that can affect urination and continence include

1) potent diuretics, which cause brisk filling of the bladder; 2) anticholinergic agents that can impair detrusor muscle contraction; 3) sedative-hypnotics that may cause confusion; 4) narcotics that impair detrusor muscle contraction; 5) α-adrenergic agonists that increase internal sphincter tone; 6) α-adrenergic antagonists that decrease internal sphincter tone; and 7) calcium channel blockers that decrease detrusor muscle tone.

Established Incontinence

Patients are more likely to have reversible incontinence if the incontinence is of recent onset. Although established incontinence is more difficult to treat, it can be managed with significant benefit to the patient. Overactivity of the detrusor muscle (urge incontinence) is a common cause of established incontinence, accounting for 40% to 70% of cases. It causes early detrusor contractions at low bladder volumes. Symptoms include urinary frequency and urgency, with losses of small-to-moderate urine volumes. Nocturia often occurs. Detrusor overactivity is seen with CNS disease (mass lesions, Parkinson disease, stroke) or bladder irritation (infection, benign prostatic hyperplasia, fecal impaction, atrophic urethritis).

Overflow incontinence is uncommon. It is seen with urinary outflow obstruction (benign prostatic hyperplasia, prostate cancer, pelvic tumor) or detrusor underactivity/hypotonic bladder (autonomic neuropathy). Symptoms are low urine flow and frequent urinary dribbling.

Outlet incompetence (stress incontinence) is common in women and rare in men (unless sphincter damage has occurred). It is caused by pelvic floor muscle laxity and lack of bladder support, resulting in small losses of urine with transient increases in intra-abdominal pressure (cough, sneeze, etc.).

Functional incontinence is the inability of normally continent patients to reach toilet facilities in time. Often, it is due to various medications (e.g., potent diuretics) and some limitation of mobility (restraints or hemiparesis).

- Detrusor overactivity is common in the elderly, accounting for 40%-70% of cases of urinary incontinence.
- Detrusor overactivity may be seen with CNS disease or disorders that cause bladder irritation.
- Overflow obstruction is uncommon. It is seen with urinary outflow obstruction or a hypotonic detrusor muscle.
- Outlet incompetence is common in women and rare in men.

Evaluation of Incontinence

The evaluation of urinary incontinence includes a thorough medical history, physical examination, and several simple laboratory tests. The history is most important and should include the amount of urine lost, precipitating factors, whether symptoms of obstruction exist, and the patient's functional status. Also, symptoms of neurologic disease, associated disease states, menstrual status and parity, and the medications used should be documented.

Physical examination of the abdomen should evaluate bladder distention and possible abdominal masses. In examining the pelvis, check for uterine, bladder, or rectal prolapse; atrophic vaginitis; and pelvic masses. The rectal examination should document any masses, fecal impaction, sphincter tone, and prostate enlargement or nodules. A neurologic examination should be performed to search for disease of the CNS or the spinal, autonomic, or peripheral nerves.

Laboratory tests should include 1) urinalysis and urine culture to check for infection, pyuria, and hematuria; 2) blood urea nitrogen and creatinine determination to assess renal function; 3) calcium and glucose measurements to assess polyuric states; 4) occasionally, intravenous pyelography and/or renal ultrasonography to check for hydronephrosis, which may occur with chronic bladder outlet obstruction; and 5) postvoid residual bladder volume to estimate the degree of bladder emptying. Urodynamics usually are not necessary to establish the diagnosis of incontinence. Occasionally, the urodynamic test results do not fit the clinical picture. Urodynamic studies are indicated when patients have medically confusing histories or more than one type of urinary incontinence. Cystometry measures bladder volume and pressure and can be used to detect uninhibited detrusor muscle contractions, lack of bladder contractions, and bladder sensation. Voiding cystourethrography measures the urethrovesical angle and residual urine volume. Uroflow measures urinary flow rate, and electromyography evaluates the external sphincter and detects detrusor-sphincter dyssynergia.

- Most cases of urinary incontinence can be diagnosed by the medical history and physical examination findings.
- Common laboratory tests that may help in the diagnosis include urinalysis, urine culture, blood urea nitrogen, creatinine, serum calcium, and blood glucose.
- A postvoid residual bladder volume may be helpful in determining the degree of bladder emptying.
- Urodynamic studies are not usually necessary to establish the diagnosis of urinary incontinence.

Treatment of Incontinence

The treatment of detrusor overactivity is aimed at suppressing the early detrusor contractions. Behavioral training is often successful, including scheduled toileting and prompted voiding. Medications that inhibit parasympathetic stimulation of the bladder muscle are also effective. Drugs with anticholinergic activity that are used include oxybutynin, flavoxate, imipramine and tolterodine. Calcium channel blockers used as smooth muscle relaxants may also be successful, although they have not been approved for the treatment of urinary incontinence. Topical estrogen therapy is effective in some women when atrophic urethritis is the cause of early detrusor contractions.

The treatment of overflow incontinence is aimed at providing complete bladder drainage from a bladder that either is not contracting adequately or has significant outflow obstruction. In treating a hypotonic bladder, medications that increase the tone of the detrusor muscle can be tried, including the cholinergic agonist bethanechol. This is often effective for short-term use, as in postoperative patients with a transient hypotonic bladder; however, adverse effects are common in the elderly and limit its long-term use. Treatment of obstruction includes operation (transurethral resection of the prostate) and use of α-adrenergic antagonists (prazosin, terazosin, or doxazosin), which decrease the tone of the internal sphincter. An external (condom) urinary catheter is of little benefit, because it does not drain the bladder. An indwelling catheter or intermittent catheterization is occasionally necessary.

The treatment of outlet incompetence is aimed at surgically restoring the normal posterior urethrovesical angle of 90° to 100°. Increasing the tone of the internal sphincter with α-adrenergic agonists (pseudoephedrine, phenylpropanolamine, and imipramine) may be of limited short-term benefit. Hormonal (topical estrogen) therapy helps restore the mucosa of the urethra, increasing its resistance. Pelvic floor (Kegel) exercises are also useful, although they must be performed for several months before any benefit is recognized.

Urologic Consultation

In most elderly patients, the diagnosis of urinary incontinence can be established without the need for evaluation by a urologist. The following conditions indicate the need for urologic evaluation: high postvoid residual urine volume, outflow obstruction, significant uterine or bladder prolapse, abnormal findings on prostate examination, recurrent urinary tract infections, hematuria, unknown diagnosis, or failure to improve with treatment.

Use of Urinary Catheters

External (condom) catheters have a slight risk of infection, and problems with penile skin breakdown limit long-term use. They also have minimal benefit in overflow incontinence. Intermittent catheterization has a small risk (from 1%-20% depending on patient setting) of infection with each catheter insertion. It is very useful for temporary incontinence, as in postoperative patients with a transient hypotonic bladder. Postvoid residual volumes should be used as a guide in determining the frequency of catheterization. Intermittent catheterization is of limited use in the management of chronic incontinence in nursing home patients because of catheter expense and in those living independently if they

have limited manual dexterity or poor vision. Essentially all patients with indwelling catheters eventually develop significant bacteriuria. The chronic use of suppressive antibiotics is not recommended because it does not prevent long-term suppression of bacteriuria and results in infections caused by resistant organisms. Antibiotic treatment should be reserved for symptomatic infections only, although it may be difficult to determine when a symptomatic urinary tract infection is present in a catheterized elderly patient.

URINARY TRACT INFECTIONS

Urinary tract infections become more common with advancing age and cause a wide spectrum of disease. Urinary tract infection is the most common infection in nursing home residents and the most common cause of sepsis in the elderly. It may also produce the syndrome of asymptomatic bacteriuria. Incomplete emptying of the bladder, which is commonly found in the elderly (cystocele, benign prostatic hyperplasia), as well as urinary instrumentation and chronic catheterization all predispose the elderly to urinary tract infection. The elderly have various bacterial organisms that produce urinary tract infections. *Escherichia coli*, the most common organism that causes urinary tract infections in the younger population, causes about only half of these infections in the elderly. Other gram-negative organisms such as *Enterococcus* sp, *Proteus* sp, *Klebsiella* sp, and *Pseudomonas* sp are common in the elderly. Because of the varieties of organisms, urine culture should be performed when evaluating an elderly patient with a urinary tract infection. Treatment may be started with typical antibiotics (e.g., trimethoprim/sulfamethoxazole, amoxicillin, cephalosporins) pending the results of urine culture. Those who have potential for resistant organisms or have had an indwelling urinary catheter should receive an antibiotic with a wider spectrum of coverage, such as a quinolone.

Asymptomatic bacteriuria becomes more common with age and has been associated with increased mortality; however, the mortality appears to be unrelated to the bacteriuria and is likely a marker for increased severity of illness and debility. Asymptomatic bacteriuria should not be treated unless there is a history of chronic urinary obstruction.

Patients with chronic indwelling catheters will eventually develop bacteriuria, and these bacterial organisms change with time. Routine surveillance cultures should not be performed in these patients, and the bacteriuria should not be treated unless the patient is symptomatic. In patients who have had urinary catheters removed, the bacteriuria should be treated if the urine remains bacteriuric for more than 48 hours. In many cases, the bacteriuria will resolve with removal of the urinary catheter alone.

● The elderly have a wider array of bacteria causing urinary tract infections than younger persons; therefore, urine cultures should be performed in elderly patients with a urinary tract infection.

- Asymptomatic bacteriuria does not lead to increased morbidity and mortality as a result of infection and should not be routinely treated.
- Patients with chronic indwelling catheters eventually develop bacteriuria. Surveillance cultures should not be done, and the bacteriuria should not be treated unless the patient becomes symptomatic.

USE OF MEDICATIONS IN THE ELDERLY

More than 30% of all prescriptions are written for persons older than 65 years. Medications are a common cause of iatrogenic disease in the elderly and are handled differently in the elderly because of various changes in pharmacokinetics and pharmacodynamics. The overall results are 1) a longer duration of activity of many drugs, 2) lower doses needed to achieve desired therapeutic effects, 3) more frequent adverse drug effects or drug-drug interactions, and 4) greater likelihood of drug toxicity.

- More than 30% of all prescriptions are written for persons older than 65 years.
- Changes occur in pharmacokinetics and pharmacodynamics in the elderly.

Pharmacokinetics includes drug absorption, distribution, metabolism, and elimination. There are age-related changes that have an effect on each of these variables, affecting some more than others. Age-related changes that could have an effect on drug absorption include a decreased blood supply to the small bowel, villous atrophy resulting in a reduced surface area for the absorption of drugs, and decreased gastric acidity. There is little evidence that there is a significant reduction in drug absorption with advancing age. Drug distribution has a major role in altered pharmacokinetics and changes significantly with age resulting from alterations in the various volumes of distribution in the elderly. These changes include an increase in adipose tissue, a reduction in total body water and lean body mass, and for many, a change in levels of plasma protein. The result of increased adipose tissue is an increase in the volume of distribution for lipid-soluble drugs, which can result in an increase in drug half-life. The decrease in body water creates a smaller volume of distribution for water-soluble drugs, potentially leading to a higher than expected drug concentration. A reduction in plasma protein (e.g., albumin) results in less protein-bound (inactive) acidic drugs and a greater amount of free (active) drug. α_1-Acid glycoproteins are acute phase reactants and increase in patients with significant inflammation. This can produce an increase in basic drug (lidocaine, propranolol) protein-binding and less free drug.

Drug metabolism occurs primarily in the liver. With advanced age, the ability of the liver to metabolize drugs decreases because of various factors, including a decrease in the number of functioning hepatocytes, reduced hepatic blood flow, and reduced hepatic enzymatic activity. Phase I metabolism involves the oxidation or reduction of a drug by the cytochrome P450 system. This type of metabolism produces active metabolites and slows with age. Phase II metabolism involves acetylation and produces inactive metabolites. It shows no changes with advancing age. It is extremely difficult to predict a patient's ability to metabolize a specific drug because there is no simple test to perform.

Drug elimination refers primarily to the ability of the renal system to excrete drugs from the circulation. In general, there is a reduction in renal function with age, with both a decreased renal plasma flow and glomerular filtration rate (up to 30%) although the variability among elderly persons is great. The serum level of creatinine is not a good measure of renal function in the elderly and tends to underestimate the degree of renal insufficiency. Creatinine is a product of muscle breakdown. Because there is decreased lean body mass with advancing age, less creatinine is produced. Thus, it is possible to have a normal serum level of creatinine in an elderly patient who has as much as a 30% reduction in renal function. A more accurate estimate of renal function is the following:

$$\text{Creatinine Clearance} = \frac{(140 - \text{Age}) \times \text{Weight (kg)}}{72 \times \text{Creatinine}} (\times 0.85 \text{ for Women})$$

Pharmacodynamic changes also occur with aging and have an effect on the action of medications. The term "pharmacodynamics" refers to drug sensitivity, which can change with age. These changes may reflect an alteration of receptor number or receptor sensitivity to drug or an altered receptor response to a drug. Less is known about altered pharmacodynamics than about pharmacokinetics; however, the pharmacodynamic changes for several drugs have been identified. There is a reduced responsiveness of β-adrenergic drugs (e.g., less tachycardia with isoproterenol, less bradycardia with β-blockers), increased sedation with benzodiazepines, greater analgesia with opiates, and greater anticoagulant activity with warfarin.

Adverse drug effects are common in the elderly and frequently cause serious complications. Elderly patients often have limited organ reserve function and are unable to respond as younger persons can to an adverse effect. Drug-drug effects tend to occur more commonly in the elderly. The likelihood of a drug-drug effect is related to the number of medications taken.

As a result of altered pharmacokinetics and pharmacodynamics with aging, medications need to be used carefully in the elderly, avoiding polypharmacy whenever possible and watching for evidence of adverse drug effects and drug-drug interactions, both of which increase in frequency with age.

- Pharmacokinetics include drug absorption, distribution, metabolism, and elimination.
- Alteration in drug absorption is the least important alteration

in pharmacokinetics.
- Drug distribution includes an increase in adipose tissue, decrease in body water, and, in many, a change in plasma protein.
- Drug metabolism and clearance tend to decrease with age but are difficult to predict.

QUESTIONS

Multiple Choice (choose the one best answer)

1. A 72-year-old woman complains of urinary incontinence. She describes the sensation of an urgent need to void. However, because of her arthritic knees, she often is unable to reach the toilet before she loses urine. These urinary symptoms have been present for several years but have gotten progressively worse, and she is now afraid to go out in public. The patient also describes some loss of urine with coughing or sneezing, but these symptoms have been present for about 15 years and have remained relatively stable with time. She does not describe dysuria or hematuria. Her medications include isosorbide, metoprolol, and a stool softener. Her medical history is significant for hypertension, a previous myocardial infarction, and deep venous thrombosis. Which of the following is the most appropriate first step in the management of this patient's urinary incontinence?
   a. Referral to a urologist for cystoscopy and urodynamic studies
   b. Trial of oral conjugated equine estrogen
   c. Trial of imipramine
   d. Instruct patient in Kegel exercises and timed voidings
   e. Referral to a gynecologic surgeon for bladder suspension surgery

2. You receive a call from a nursing home about a 78-year-old resident who has dementia, hypertension, and diabetes mellitus. The nurse reports increased agitation and confusion over the past several days. The resident has been verbally and physically abusive to others, occasionally striking out at the caregivers. Medications currently taken by the resident include glyburide, furosemide, and enalapril. What is most appropriate in the evaluation and management of this patient?

   a. Trial of lorazepam 0.5 mg twice daily
   b. Trial of a selective serotonin reuptake inhibitor (SSRI) antidepressant for probable depression
   c. Computed tomography of the head
   d. Assess the patient for an acute medical problem
   e. Trial of haloperiodol 0.5 mg twice daily and as needed for extreme agitation

3. A 69-year-old man is evaluated for a recent spell involving loss of consciousness that occurred 1 week ago. The spell occurred while he was standing. The patient had been ill with gastroenteritis and had poor oral intake at the time. He thinks he was unconscious for 1 to 2 minutes, although the fall was not witnessed. He recalled no loss of urine with the fall and states that he felt normal when he regained consciousness. After the spell, he was able to stand and walk to his bed. The patient described a chronic history of infrequent palpitations consisting of an occasional "skipped beat." The patient's medications include furosemide, potassium, digoxin, and lisinopril, which he takes for congestive heart failure. A recent echocardiogram revealed left ventricular ejection fraction of 28%. On physical examination, a faint right carotid bruit was found. Cardiac examination revealed a normal sinus rhythm with a grade 2/6 holosystolic murmur heard at the cardiac apex. The lungs were clear, and there was no evidence of pedal edema. The cause of this patient's fall is most likely to be determined by:
   a. Electrocardiography
   b. The medical history
   c. 24-Hour Holter monitoring
   d. Electroencephalography
   e. Echocardiography

4. A 68-year-old woman complains of progressive generalized weakness for the past 3 months. The patient has a

history of depression and describes loss of appetite and early morning awakening. She has had a weight loss of 20 pounds over the past 6 months. She describes no ambition and feels she becomes exhausted with minimal exertion. She describes a 2-month history of loose stools and pains in her knees, which she attributes to her "arthritis." Physical examination reveals an irregularly irregular cardiac rhythm at 105 beats/min. No other abnormalities are found. Laboratory values include hemoglobin, 10.1; leukocytes, 7,800, with a normal differential; and mild thrombocytopenia of 98,000. The erythrocyte sedimentation rate is 12 mm/hr. Serum calcium is slightly elevated at 10.7. The most likely cause of this patient's symptoms is:

a. An underlying malignancy
b. Polymyalgia rheumatica
c. Temporal arteritis
d. Hyperthyroidism
e. Depression

5. An 82-year-old man is about to be admitted to a nursing home after the recent death of his wife. He feels well and describes no specific symptoms of illness. He has hypertension, diabetes mellitus, and mild renal insufficiency and takes the following medications: thiazide, 25 mg once daily, and glyburide, 10 mg once daily. Physical examination revealed no significant abnormalities. Before entering the nursing home, the patient is told he needs to be tested for tuberculosis. To his knowledge, he has never had a tuberculin skin test (PPD). Which of the following statements is true?

a. The patient should receive a PPD, and if negative, he should receive a second PPD in 2 weeks
b. If the initial PPD is negative, no further testing is needed
c. If the PPD is positive, the patient should receive 9 months of isoniazid
d. If this patient is given isoniazid, renal function (serum Cr) should be followed closely
e. A positive PPD would warrant starting treatment with a four-drug regimen because of multidrug resistant strains of tuberculosis

6. A 84-year-old woman returns to the nursing home after 1-week hospitalization for pneumonia. On examination, she is found to have a 2- by 3-cm stage II sacral pressure sore. Which of the following statements about this patient is true?

a. The tissue damage involves full-thickness skin loss with damage to the subcutaneous tissue
b. The surface of the ulcer should be cultured for bacteria

to determine if an antibiotic will be useful in treatment
c. This ulcer will heal fastest with a heat lamp keeping the ulcer dry
d. This ulcer should not be debrided if the patient has peripheral arterial disease
e. If the wound is thought to be infected, systemic antibiotics are more effective than topical antibiotics

7. A 78-year-old man is admitted to the nursing home after hospitalization for a hip fracture resulting from a fall. The patient developed urinary retention postoperatively, and an indwelling urinary catheter was inserted. He was admitted to the nursing home with the indwelling urinary catheter. The patient has a history of mild obstructive urinary symptoms from BPH; however, he never had a problem with urinary retention preoperatively. Which of the following statements about this patient is true?

a. Catheter removal followed by prompted voiding and intermittent catheterization checking postvoid residual volumes will likely result in restoration of normal bladder function
b. Fluid restriction and clamping the catheter for 4 hours, 4 times a day is the best way for this patient to regain normal bladder function
c. If the catheter will be required for more than 2 months, treatment should be started with suppressive antibiotic to prevent bacteriuria
d. The indwelling catheter should be replaced with an external (condom) catheter because it has a lower risk of the eventual development of bacteriuria
e. Removing the catheter and starting oxybutinin will help the patient regain normal bladder function

7. A 68-year-old woman is brought to the clinic for evaluation of increased forgetfulness, confusion, and decreased ability to manage her household. She is taking no medications, and physical examination reveals no focal neurologic abnormalities. A mental status exam (MMSE) is performed and suggests mild cognitive impairment. Laboratory tests, including computed tomography of the head, reveal no specific abnormalities. The diagnosis is early Alzheimer disease. The family requests a medication to help their mother. Which of the following medications has *not* been suggested to have benefit in slowing the progression of Alzheimer disease or its symptoms?

a. Vitamin E
b. Nonsteroidal anti-inflammatory drugs
c. Tacrine
d. Estrogen
e. Vitamin B_{12}

9. A 67-year-old man has a very painful, swollen, red left great toe of 2 days' duration. He has never had a similar episode. He has a history of coronary artery disease, moderate renal insufficiency, and hypertension. He has a past history of peptic ulcer disease. His current medications include isosorbide, hydrochlorothiazide, potassium chloride, and atenolol. On examination, the patient has a very tender swollen left great toe. Joint arthrocentesis reveals negatively birefringent needle-like crystals. Which of the following is true about this patient's problem?
   a. He should be treated with an intra-articular injection of steroid
   b. He should be treated with a nonsteroidal anti-inflammatory drug
   c. He should start receiving allopurinol
   d. A daily low dose of aspirin would likely reduce the uric acid level
   e. It is likely that this patient produces an excess of uric acid

10. A 66-year-old man comes to the Outpatient Clinic complaining of difficulty with urination. He describes symptoms of difficulty starting urination, stream hesitancy, and some postvoid dribbling. He has had nocturia 4 times over the past 6 months. He also describes urinary urgency. He denies any dysuria. His medical problems include hypertension, coronary artery disease, and degenerative joint disease. His medications include atenolol, isosorbide, and diltiazem. He also takes amitriptyline for insomnia. The residual urine volume is 100 mL. What is the first treatment that should be initiated for this patient?
   a. Discontinue diltiazem and start doxazocin for the treatment of hypertension
   b. Refer the patient to a urologist for consideration of transurethral resection of the prostate
   c. Start treatment with oxybutynin
   d. Discontinue amitriptyline
   e. Insert an indwelling urinary catheter

ANSWERS

1. Answer d.

The patient describes a combination of urge and stress urinary incontinence. The mechanism for each of these is different. Urge incontinence reflects early contraction of the detrusor muscle, whereas stress incontinence usually implies decreased tone of the internal urinary sphincter. All responses may be of help to this patient; however, one should try the least invasive and safest treatment first. The symptoms are straightforward, and it is doubtful that a urologic investigation would add significant information for management. Although it is possible that hormonal therapy may help both the urge and stress incontinence, there is some risk in giving it to a patient with a previous thrombotic episode. Imipramine may also help both types of incontinence; however, its anticholinergic effects can be expected to worsen the patient's constipation. It is possible that bladder suspension surgery may help urinary stress incontinence; it is not known whether the patient has pathologic changes that warrant surgical treatment. Nonpharmacologic therapy (Kegel exercises, bladder training) should be attempted first in the elderly with urinary incontinence. When properly used, it is effective for both urge and stress incontinence. It is also safe and simple for patients to perform.

2. Answer d.

The recent development of increased confusion and agitation in a patient with dementia may be due to several reasons. One of the common reasons is the development of an acute medical illness. An assessment should be performed to look for evidence of an acute medical problem such as infection (urinary, respiratory), a cardiac event (myocardial infarction, arrhythmia), electrolyte abnormality, dehydration, or drug toxicity. Although computed tomography may show a central nervous system lesion (e.g., stroke or subdural hematoma) that could result in behavior problems, a medical evaluation should be completed first to look for more common conditions that can produce a change in behavior. Psychotropic medications should not be the first form of management of behavioral problems, because many of these problems have a reversible cause.

3. Answer b.

The most important part of the patient evaluation for a spell involving loss of consciousness is the medical history. The physical examination and laboratory tests should be used to confirm the diagnosis suspected from the history. This patient described a gastroenteritis, and, although not specifically stated, one could suspect he had vomiting and/or diarrhea combined with poor oral intake. When this is combined with his chronic use of diuretics, it could result in volume loss. There is no suggestion of a cardiac arrhythmia; the description of the patient's palpitations sounds benign. Although unwitnessed, there is no good evidence for a seizure. Although aortic stenosis can be associated with syncope, the murmur described in the physical examination is more consistent with mitral regurgitation.

4. Answer d.

The patient shows features of apathetic hyperthyroidism, including weight loss, diarrhea, mild anemia, and thrombocytopenia. This is not an uncommon presentation for hyperthyroidism in the elderly. Elderly patients with atrial fibrillation should always be evaluated for hyperthyroidism. Polymyalgia rheumatica and temporal arteritis are less likely because the erythrocyte sedimentation rate is not increased and the symptoms are not typical. Although this patient likely has depression, this does not account for all the symptoms described. An underlying malignancy is possible, although apathetic hyperthyroidism would explain all the patient's symptoms.

5. Answer a.

Patients entering nursing homes require a two-stage PPD. If the initial PPD is negative, a second should be administered in approximately 2 weeks. With this technique, there is a greater likelihood of the second PPD turning positive if there has been a previous exposure to tuberculosis. A positive PPD does not automatically warrant treatment with antituberculin drug(s). Further evaluation should be performed. Isoniazid tends to cause hepatoxicity, especially in the elderly; it is not nephrotoxic.

6. Answer e.

Pressure sores are common in the frail elderly; most of them develop during a hospitalization. Pressure sores can be classified into one of four stages, depending on their depth of tissue damage. A stage II pressure sore is partial thickness skin loss involving the epidermis, dermis, or both. A stage III pressure sore is full-thickness skin loss with involvement of the subcutaneous tissue. Cultures taken of the surface of the ulceration will not accurately reflect the bacteria involved in an infected ulcer. Culturing of deep tissue is required. Pressure ulcers heal fastest in a moist environment, not dry. Nonviable, necrotic tissue should be debrided in a sacral pressure sore. It may be dangerous to debride distal extremity ulcers in patients with advanced peripheral arterial disease because of poor extremity circulation. This generally is not the case for a sacral ulcer. Topical antibiotics do not penetrate very well into the tissue, and systemic antibiotics are more effective when dealing with an infected pressure sore.

7. Answer a.

Elderly patients who have a surgical procedure will occasionally develop urinary retention postoperatively. Usually those who have no previous history of urinary retention preoperatively eventually regain normal bladder function with proper bladder retraining. Prompted voiding is an effective technique to help restore normal bladder function in such patients, who will require intermittent bladder catheterization, with the frequency of catheterization guided by residual urine volumes. Clamping the catheter will not promote a return of bladder contractile function. It will result in bladder distention and stretching of the detrusor muscle, further impairing its contractile function. The aim of treatment should promote bladder drainage with intermittent catheterization, using the postvoid residual urine volume as an indication for the frequency of catheterization. Antibiotics should not be used in patients with indwelling catheters to prevent bacteriuria. Bacteriuria will still develop; however, the bacteria will be resistant to the antibiotic. Bacteriuria is less likely to develop with an external catheter than with an indwelling urinary catheter; however, an external catheter is not helpful in a patient with urinary retention, because the difficulty is getting the urine out of the bladder. Temporary use of cholinergic agonists may be of limited use in patients with an atonic bladder postoperatively. Oxybutinin is an anticholinergic medication that further inhibits contraction of the bladder.

8. Answer e.

Several classes of medications have shown some indication of slowing the progression of Alzheimer disease or the symptoms of cognitive impairment. Antioxidants such as vitamin E have been shown to delay the progression of the neurodegenerative changes. The mechanism of action may be the prevention of damage by free radicals in the brain. Also, evidence suggests that selegiline can inhibit the progression of Alzheimer disease, possibly due to antioxidant activity. Changes of inflammation are seen in the brains of those with Alzheimer disease, and NSAIDs may slow the progression of the disease through anti-inflammatory effects. The acetylcholinesterase inhibitors such as tacrine and donepezil inhibit the degradation of the neurotransmitter acetylcholine. Acetylcholinesterase inhibitors maximize the acetylcholine that is still present. Although the disease continues to progress, the symptoms of cognitive decline may stabilize temporarily. Estrogen may also slow the progression of the disease, but its mechanism of action is not known. It appears to increase cerebral perfusion. Although vitamin

B$_{12}$ deficiency can produce cognitive impairment (and is thought to represent one of the reversible dementias), giving vitamin B$_{12}$ to a patient with Alzheimer disease does not slow the progression of disease.

9. Answer a.

This patient likely is having an acute gouty episode. This diagnosis should be suspected because of the classic location of symptoms, use of a thiazide diuretic, and the description of urate crystals under a polarizing microscope. The use of an NSAID is appropriate therapy for most people with this condition; however, in this patient, it carries an increased risk because of the patient's renal insufficiency and history of peptic ulcer disease. Allopurinol treatment should not be started during an acute episode of gout and generally is not started after a patient's first episode. Low-dose aspirin can produce an increase in uric acid level, and high-dose aspirin can decrease the level. Most patients with gout (90%) have underexcretion of uric acid; overproduction of uric acid is unusual. The best treatment option among those listed is an intra-articular injection of steroid.

10. Answer d.

The patient has an obstructive uropathy, most likely due to benign prostatic hypertrophy. The best initial treatment is to discontinue amitryptyline, because it is not an essential medication. It has anticholinergic activity and can decrease the contraction of the destrusor muscle, contributing to urinary retention, especially in elderly men. Diltiazem can also produce urinary retention through its smooth muscle relaxing activity, and its discontinuation may also need to be considered if symptoms persist. Oxybutynin has anticholinergic activity and may help the symptoms of urinary urgency; however, the urinary retention would likely worsen. An indwelling urinary catheter should not be the first treatment attempted in this patient unless the patient is unable to pass any urine.

CHAPTER 12

HEMATOLOGY

Thomas M. Habermann, M.D.

ANEMIAS

Evaluation of Anemias

The causes of anemia are complex. The World Health Organization defined the lower limit of normal for venous hemoglobin concentration in males older than 14 years living at sea level as 13 g/dL and in nonpregnant females, 12 g/dL. An organized approach to the anemias is essential. Because the initial evaluation of anemia after the history and physical examination begins with the complete blood count (CBC), one way to classify anemia is by the mean corpuscular volume (MCV): microcytic, macrocytic, and normocytic anemia.

CBC is the most commonly ordered blood test. The measured values of the CBC include the total counts for red blood cells (RBCs), platelets, and white blood cells (WBCs) and the volumes of RBCs, platelets, WBCs, and hemoglobin. The calculated values include the hematocrit, MCV, mean corpuscular hemoglobin, mean corpuscular hemoglobin concentration, and red cell distribution width. These values help to differentiate thalassemia from iron deficiency anemia.

In the initial clinical evaluation, anemia can be assessed in different ways. The breakdown of anemias into microcytic, normocytic, and macrocytic is the most useful clinical model, because this information is routinely available from the initial automated CBC. The most common anemias are the microcytic anemias (Tables 12-1 and 12-2).

The differential diagnosis of hypochromic microcytic anemias includes iron deficiency, thalassemic syndromes, anemia of chronic disease, sideroblastic anemias, hemoglobin E, unstable hemoglobins, and lead poisoning. Vitamin B_6 deficiency may cause a microcytic anemia. The causes of iron deficiency include blood loss, increased requirements (as in pregnancy), and decreased absorption (partial gastrectomy and malabsorption syndromes). Disorders associated with blood loss include gastrointestinal (ulcers, malignancy, telangiectasia, hiatal hernia, and long-distance runner's anemia), respiratory (malignancy, pulmonary hemosiderosis), menstruation, phlebotomy (blood donor, diagnostic phlebotomy, polycythemia rubra vera, and self-inflicted), trauma, and surgery.

In a nonreferral practice, iron deficiency anemia is the cause of up to 90% of all hypochromic-microcytic anemias (Plate 12-1). Of the remaining 10%, the thalassemic syndromes are more common than the other rare forms of the hypochromic-microcytic anemias. However, the incidence and prevalence of anemia of chronic disease is variable, depending on whether the setting is inpatient or outpatient and whether a community-based or a referral center. The CBC and other laboratory values provide further information for differentiating these entities (Table 12-2). These studies often provide the major clues to the type of anemia. Blood loss should be considered in the differential diagnosis of any patient with anemia. The evaluation of stool for blood loss is essential in the initial

Table 12-1.—Differentiation of Microcytic Anemias on Basis of Blood Values

	Type of anemia	
	Thalassemia	Iron-deficiency
RBC count	>5.0 x 10^{12}/L	<5.0 x 10^{12}/L
Red cell distribution width	<16	>16
MCV-RBC-(5 x Hb)-3.4	Negative	Positive

Hb, hemoglobin; MCV, mean corpuscular volume; RBC, red blood cell.

Table 12-2.—Comparison of Hypochromic-Microcytic Anemias

Disease state	MCV	Red blood cells	% transferrin saturation	Ferritin, μg/L	Marrow iron
Iron deficiency anemia	Decreased	Decreased	<15	Low	Absent
Anemia of chronic disease	Normal or decreased	Decreased	<15 or normal	Normal or increased	Normal or increased
Thalassemia minor	Decreased	Usually increased	Normal	Normal or increased	Normal

MCV, mean corpuscular volume.
Modified from Savage RA: Cost-effective laboratory diagnosis of microcytic anemias of complex origin. ASCP check sample H84-10(H-153). By permission of American Society of Clinical Pathologists.

work-up and may also provide clues to a combined anemia. A laboratory approach to microcytic anemias is outlined in Figures 12-1 and 12-2. The serum ferritin test is the most useful initial test in documenting iron deficiency, but the values obtained may be increased in the presence of iron deficiency and coexistent inflammatory states, liver disease, hepatocellular carcinoma, and malignancy.

Confusing problems in iron deficiency include patient compliance with iron treatment, wrong dosage schedules, wrong treatment (enteric-coated iron preparations), diminished absorption (previous surgery and mucosal disease of the small bowel), competitive interference with antacids, blood loss in excess of treatment, other causes of anemia, and physician impatience with response. Oral replacement treatment is the treatment of choice in iron deficiency. Ferrous sulfate three times a day at a dose of 325 mg orally 1 hour before or 2 hours after meals is the initial treatment. The CBC should be rechecked 4 weeks after starting iron therapy. Correction of the anemia would be anticipated in 6 weeks. Another 6 months of treatment is necessary to replenish bone marrow reserves.

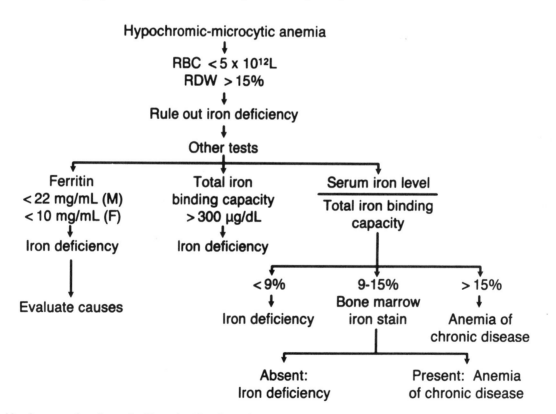

Fig. 12-1. Algorithm for approach to diagnosis of hypochromic-microcytic anemias with normal or decreased red blood cell (RBC) counts. RDW, red cell distribution width. (Modified from Savage RA: Cost-effective laboratory diagnosis of microcytic anemias of complex origin. ASCP check sample H84-10(H-153). By permission of American Society of Clinical Pathologists.)

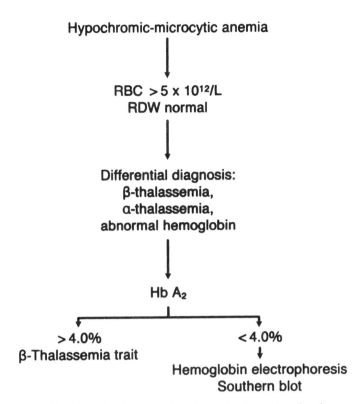

Fig. 12-2. Algorithm for approach to diagnosis of hypochromic-microcytic anemias with an increased total red blood cell (RBC) count. Hb, hemoglobin; RDW, red cell distribution width. (Modified from Savage RA: Cost-effective laboratory diagnosis of microcytic anemias of complex origin. ASCP check sample H84-10(H-153). By permission of American Society of Clinical Pathologists.)

Thalassemia is the most common single gene disorder in the world. β-Thalassemia results when β-globulin chains are decreased (heterozygous) or absent (homozygous), resulting in an excess of α-globulin chains in the RBCs. β-Thalassemia minor patients have a mild anemia and significant microcytosis. β-Thalassemia can be identified by simple screening methods (Tables 12-1 and 12-2 and Fig. 12-2). α-Thalassemia patients have a low normal MVC, with a normal hemoglobin concentration. Genetic counseling is indicated when a diagnosis of α- or β-thalassemia is established.

The differential diagnosis of the macrocytic anemias includes vitamin B_{12} deficiency, folate deficiency, chemotherapy agents, myelodysplasia, liver disease, alcohol abuse, hypothyroidism, cold agglutinin disease, smoking, and hemolysis. A laboratory approach to macrocytic anemias is outlined in Figure 12-3. The pathophysiology of drug-induced macrocytosis includes marrow toxicity with interference with folate metabolism (alcohol), marrow toxicity with other drugs (zidovudine), altered folate metabolism with anticonvulsants (phenytoin, primidone, and phenobarbital), and altered folate metabolism from other drugs (oral contraceptives, triamterene, sulfasalazine, and sulfamethoxazole). Chemotherapy drugs that inhibit purine and pyrimidine synthesis (azathioprine and 5-fluorouracil), deoxyribonucleotide synthesis (hydroxyurea and cytarabine [cytosine arabinoside]), and dihydrofolate reductase inhibitors (methotrexate) are common causes of macrocytosis.

Patients with achlorhydria of any cause do not absorb vitamin B_{12}, because hydrochloric acid is required to free vitamin B_{12} from food. A normal functioning pancreas is required. The causes of vitamin B_{12} deficiency are many and include pernicious anemia, total or partial gastrectomy, ileal resection, bacterial overgrowth syndromes, achlorhydria, and chronic pancreatitis.

The symptoms and signs of vitamin B_{12} deficiency include paresthesias, gait disturbance, mental status changes ("B_{12} maddness"), vibratory/position sense impairment (dorsal column "dropout"), and the absence of ankle reflexes and extensor plantar responses. The MCV is elevated, and Howell-Jolly bodies are typically present, as are hypersegmented neutrophils. A serum level of vitamin B_{12} less than 200 pg/mL is suggestive of the diagnosis of a vitamin B_{12} deficiency. Vitamin B_{12} levels of 100 to 200 pg/mL are not diagnostic of a deficiency state. Urinary methylmalonic acid is increased in vitamin B_{12} deficiency. A low intrinsic factor antibody confirms the diagnosis of pernicious anemia. The serum level of vitamin B_{12} may rarely be normal in pernicious anemia. Serum gastrin levels are high in pernicious anemia. The Schilling test may be required after these tests. The Schilling test confirms a defect in intestinal absorption. In part I, radiolabeled vitamin B_{12} is administered orally, nonradioactive vitamin B_{12} is administered intramuscularly within 1 to 2 hours, and the urine and serum levels are measured. Normal urinary excretion rates after a flushing dose of nonradioactive vitamin B_{12} in the first 24 to 72 hours are greater than 7%. Low urine radioactivity with normal renal function means decreased absorption. The differential diagnosis of an abnormality in part I includes pernicious anemia, small-bowel disease interfering with absorption, and bacterial competition for vitamin B_{12}. True-negative results in part I of the Schilling test include dietary deficiency and cobalamin-binding-protein abnormalities, and false-negative results occur in food-bound malabsorption due to achlorhydria. In part II of the Schilling test, intrinsic factor is added. Patients with pernicious anemia now have normal results. In part II of the Schilling test, false-positive results occur in cases attributable to mucosal megaloblastosis. Antibiotics are given in part III of the Schilling test, and the differential diagnosis of a positive result includes ileal malabsorption and defective intrinsic factor in the test. A negative test result in this stage of the test occurs in the blind loop syndrome secondary to bacterial competition for vitamin B_{12}. The treatment of pernicious anemia is vitamin B_{12}, 1,000 μg intramuscularly for 5 days, followed by 500 to 1,000 μg

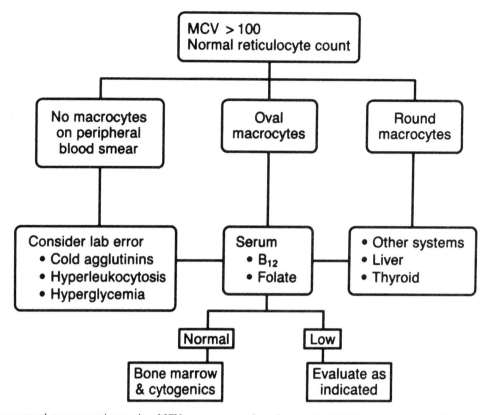

Fig. 12-3. Laboratory approach to macrocytic anemias. MCV, mean corpuscular volume. (Modified from Colon-Otero G, Menke D, Hook CC: A practical approach to the differential diagnosis and evaluation of the adult patient with macrocytic anemia. Med Clin North Am 76:581-597, May 1992. By permission of WB Saunders Company.)

intramuscularly every month. Alternatively, vitamin B_{12} may be given orally at a dose of 500 to 1,000 µg/day.

Megaloblastic anemia due to folate deficiency takes 3 months to develop in contrast to 3 years in vitamin B_{12} deficiency, because of the low storage levels of folic acid in tissues and the relatively high dietary requirement. This anemia is indistinguishable from vitamin B_{12} deficiency morphologically. Folate is absorbed in the proximal small bowel. Deficiency states are associated with increased requirements (pregnancy and hemolytic anemia), poor intake (alcoholics), diseases of the small intestine (sprue), and interference with the recycling of folate from liver stores to tissue (alcohol). The possibility of concomitant vitamin B_{12} and iron deficiency (sprue) should be considered in suboptimal responses to replacement therapy.

The normochromic-normocytic group of disorders present the greatest challenge in differential diagnosis. The differential diagnosis of the normochromic-normocytic anemias includes stem cell dysfunction (aplastic anemia and red cell aplasia), marrow replacement (tumor and fibrosis), renal disease, hemolysis, acute hemorrhage, mixed nutritional deficiency, myelodysplasia, chemotherapy, anemia of acute disease, anemia of chronic disease characterized by a low total iron-binding capacity (acute infections, chronic infections, neoplasia, rheumatoid arthritis, polymyalgia rheumatica, etc.), and erythropoietin deficiency. The anemia of renal failure and liver disease are important in this differential diagnosis. The anemia of renal disease may be related to decreased erythropoietin or shortened RBC survival. It is important to obtain a reticulocyte count to exclude hemolysis early on in the evaluation in patients with normochromic-normocytic anemias. It is essential to exclude blood loss from the gastrointestinal tract that may be acute and not manifested by a microcytic blood picture.

Erythropoietin

Erythropoietin is a glycoprotein that acts through specific receptors on RBC precursors. It is produced primarily in the kidneys, although a small amount is produced in the liver. There are no preformed stores. It is constitutive, constantly present in plasma. The gene is located on chromosome 7. Recombinant human erythropoietin is identical to native erythropoietin. There is an inverse relationship between the circulating concentration of erythropoietin and the hemoglobin or hematocrit value. Regulation is linked to an oxygen sensor, not to peripheral catabolism. Erythropoietin production increases with hypoxia. The serum levels of erythropoietin are not influenced by age or sex. The higher hemoglobin value in men seems to be due to androgenic steroids. The toxicity profile is low. Hypertension may develop or progress in renal dialysis patients.

The serum levels of erythropoietin are low, never absent, in chronic renal failure, polycythemia rubra vera, rheumatoid arthritis, and human immunodeficiency virus (HIV) infection. Zidovudine can increase the serum erythropoietin value. High erythropoietin levels are present in marrow hypofunction (pure red cell aplasia), deficiency states (iron deficiency), tumor, autonomous production (hepatocellular carcinoma), and high altitude.

Anemias of malignancy and the use of neoplastic agents may respond to erythropoietin, particularly multiple myeloma, lymphoma, and solid tumors. It is also useful after bone marrow transplantation. Erythropoietin has been used with efficacious results in the autologous blood donor setting, especially in women and in persons who donate more than 4 units. Approved indications are end-stage renal disease, the anemia of HIV infections, the anemia of malignancy, and the anemias caused by neoplastic agents.

- Erythropoietin: a glycoprotein produced in kidney; production increases with hypoxia.
- Its level is low in renal failure, polycythemia rubra vera, rheumatoid arthritis, and HIV infection.
- Its level is high in pure red cell aplasia, iron deficiency, tumors, and high altitude.
- Indications include end-stage renal disease, the anemia of HIV, and the anemias of malignancy and neoplastic agents.

In evaluating patients with erythrocytosis, a normal or low erythropoietin value associated with an increased RBC mass does not prove autonomous erythropoiesis.

Patients must have adequate iron stores to respond to erythropoietin. If erythropoietin is given to healthy individuals, the hematocrit can increase dramatically. As the hematocrit increases above 60%, the viscosity of the blood rapidly increases. Myocardial infarction or strokes may occur with the misuse of erythropoietin. Doping with erythropoietin for sporting events has been associated with cerebral vascular events secondary to significant increases in the hematocrit.

Hemolytic Anemia

In the initial evaluation of suspected hemolysis, it is essential to determine the presence of hemolytic anemia as manifested by laboratory evidence of an increased rate of erythropoiesis and laboratory evidence of increased RBC destruction. The evidence of increased erythropoiesis includes an elevated reticulocyte count, and the evidence of increased destruction includes an elevated indirect bilirubin and lactate dehydrogenase (LDH) in the initial screening tests. Avoiding this step results in ordering unnecessary laboratory tests. If these tests suggest hemolytic anemia, specific causes should be sought. Hemolytic anemias may be Coombs-negative or Coombs-positive.

The initial evaluation includes a history and physical examination, CBC, morphology, and reticulocyte count. Conditions found during the work-up that can be mistaken for hemolysis include hemorrhage, recovery from deficiency states, metastatic carcinoma, and myoglobinuria. Studies of a family's hematologic history are important. The differential diagnosis of hemolytic anemia is outlined in Figure 12-4.

Inheritance Patterns

Membrane defects and unstable hemoglobin diseases are autosomal dominant. Most enzymopathies are autosomal recessive. However, the most common enzymopathy, glucose-6-phosphate dehydrogenase deficiency, is sex-linked, as is phosphoglycerate kinase deficiency.

- Membrane defects and unstable hemoglobin diseases are autosomal dominant.
- Most enzymopathies are autosomal recessive.
- Glucose-6-phosphate dehydrogenase deficiency is sex-linked.

Laboratory Findings

The bilirubin value is usually 1 to 5 μg/dL and almost exclusively unconjugated or indirect. The direct bilirubin should be less than 15% of total if the bilirubin value is greater than 4 μg/dL. The haptoglobin concentration is usually low, with no compensatory increased rate of synthesis, and the lactate dehydrogenase level is increased. The CBC abnormalities in autoimmune hemolytic anemia include anemia, thrombocytosis, or thrombocytopenia. The presence of autoimmune hemolytic anemia and autoimmune thrombocytopenia is called Evans syndrome. The reticulocyte value is usually persistently increased, reflecting an enhanced bone marrow response.

Peripheral Smear (Differential Diagnosis)

Spherocytes (Plate 12-2) are associated with hereditary spherocytosis, alcohol (Zieve syndrome) burns, *Clostridium* infections, autoimmune hemolytic anemia, and hypophosphatemia. Basophilic stippling occurs in lead poisoning, β-thalassemia, and arsenic poisoning. Hypochromia occurs in thalassemia and lead poisoning. Target cells are present in thalassemia, hemoglobin C and E, obstructive jaundice, hepatitis, lecithin-cholesterol-acyltransferase deficiency, and the splenectomy state (Plate 12-3). Agglutination is present in cold agglutinin disease (Plate 12-4). Stomatocytes are associated with acute alcoholism and are also found as

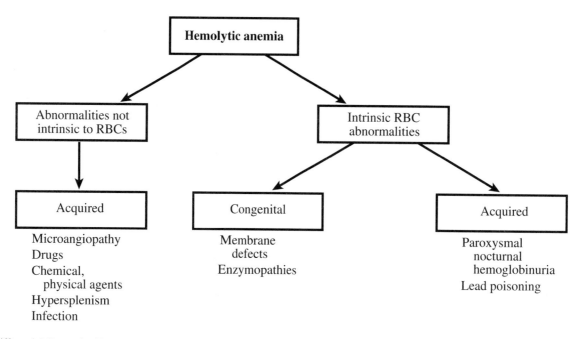

Fig. 12-4. Differential diagnosis of hemolytic anemia. RBC, red blood cell.

an artifact. Spur cells (acanthocytes) (Plate 12-5) are present in chronic liver disease, abetalipoproteinemia, malabsorption, and anorexia nervosa. Burr cells (echinocytes) are present in uremia. Heinz bodies are present in glucose-6-phosphate dehydrogenase deficiency. Howell-Jolly bodies (secondary to fragmentation of the nucleus) indicate hyposplenism and megaloblastic anemia.

Schistocytes: Microangiopathic Hemolytic Anemia

In microangiopathic hemolytic anemia, the RBCs are fragmented and deformed in the peripheral blood (Plate 12-6). The fragmentation is caused by fibrin deposits in small blood vessels leading to mechanical hemolysis. The results of the Coombs test are negative. Patients with microangiopathic hemolytic anemia are often thrombocytopenic.

Microangiopathic hemolytic anemia is associated with thrombotic thrombocytopenic purpura, hemolytic uremic syndrome, malignant hypertension, pulmonary hypertension, acute glomerulonephritis, acute renal failure, renal allograft rejection, HELLP syndrome (hemolysis, elevated liver function tests, and low platelet count), preeclampsia, eclampsia, disseminated intravascular coagulopathy, collagen vascular diseases, scleroderma, systemic lupus erythematosus, Wegener syndrome, periarteritis nodosa, carcinomatosis, small gastric carcinomas, hemangiomas, Kasabach-Merritt syndrome, viral infections (HIV), bacterial infections, drugs (mitomycin C, quinine, ticlopidine, and cyclosporine), acute radiation nephropathy, and post-bone marrow transplantation (total body irradiation, and allogeneic greater than autologous).

Differential Diagnosis of Intravascular Hemolysis

The differential diagnosis includes transfusion reactions from ABO antibodies, microangiopathic hemolytic anemia, paroxysmal nocturnal hemoglobinuria, paroxysmal cold hemoglobinuria, autoimmune hemolytic anemia (uncommon), cold agglutinin syndrome, immune complex drug-induced hemolytic anemia, infections (including falciparum malaria and clostridial sepsis), and glucose-6-phosphate dehydrogenase deficiency.

- Most hemolysis is extravascular.

In intravascular hemolysis, hemoglobin is released into the plasma. It combines rapidly with haptoglobin, which transports it to the liver. When haptoglobin is depleted, hemoglobinemia results, and plasma turns pink-red in color at concentrations of 50 to 100 mg/dL.

Hemoglobinuria occurs when the plasma hemoglobin is less than 25 mg/100 mL. The urine may become pink, red, brown, or black. Other causes of red urine include beets, phenazopyridine (Pyridium), porphyrinuria, and myoglobinuria. Hemosiderinuria is the result of desquamation of renal tubular cells.

Coombs-Positive Hemolytic Anemia

Positive results with a direct Coombs test indicate the presence of C3 and/or IgG on the surface of the patient's RBCs. The three most common causes of Coombs-positive hemolytic anemias are idiopathic, drugs, and malignancy. Malignancies that may be associated with Coombs-positive hemolytic anemia are many and include chronic lymphocytic leukemia, non-Hodgkin lymphoma, and ovarian carcinoma. The Coombs test gives positive results in 8% to 15% of all hospitalized patients, and studies reveal no cause in 95% of these patients. Hemolytic transfusion reactions and drug-related etiologies are important causes of a positive Coombs reaction.

- Coombs test: detects the presence of C3 and/or IgG on RBCs.
- The cause of positive findings on Coombs test is unknown in 95% of hospitalized patients.
- Transfusion-related and drug-related etiologies are important causes of a positive Coombs reaction.

Drug-Induced Hemolytic Anemia (Mechanisms)

Autoantibody mechanism (methyldopa)—This is dose-related, and about 0.3% to 0.8% of patients develop hemolysis. Hemolysis occurs in 18 weeks to 4 years after ingestion of the drug. The direct Coombs test becomes positive in 3 to 6 months and is IgG in high titer. There is no anamnestic response to rechallenge. Discontinuation of use of the drug usually leads to a rapid reversal in hemolysis. The mechanism of action is related to an altered cellular immune system, with a block in the activation of suppressor T cells. Methyldopa induces the formation of anti-Rh antibodies. Other drugs with a similar mechanism known to cause autoimmune hemolytic anemia include procainamide, ibuprofen, and cimetidine.

Drug-adsorption (hapten) immunohemolytic anemia (penicillin)—This complication requires high doses of drug for more than 7 days. The onset is subacute at 7 to 10 days. A high titer of penicillin antibody is always present in the serum. A positive Coombs test develops in 3% of patients and is related to dose in that at 2 million units per day 30% of patients are positive and at 10 million units per day, 100% of patients are positive. A penicillin allergy is not necessarily present. Drug-absorption hemolytic anemia may be fatal if not detected early. Other drugs, including cephalosporins, tetracycline, quinidine, tolmetin, and cisplatin, may cause autoimmune hemolytic anemia by the same mechanism.

Immune-complex mechanism (innocent bystander) (stibophen)—An antidrug antibody forms first and reacts with the drug to form an immune complex. The antidrug antibody complex is then absorbed on the RBCs. The cell-bound complex may activate complement, causing intravascular hemolysis. The Coombs test is positive because of the presence of complement on the RBC surface. Clinically, a small quantity of drug is sufficient to cause autoimmune hemolytic anemia if there is previous exposure. Acute intravascular hemolysis with hemoglobinemia and hemoglobinuria is the usual clinical course. Drugs implicated in this type of autoimmune hemolytic anemia include quinidine, quinine, phenacetin, acetaminophen,

aminosalicylate (PAS), isoniazid (INH), streptomycin, rifampin, methadone, probenecid, insulin, sulfonylureas, hydralazine, hydrochlorothiazide, sulfa drugs, triamterene, and melphalan. Immune hemolytic anemia and renal failure are seen in patients taking captopril, hydrochlorothiazide, rifampin, dipyrone, and mitomycin C.

- Autoantibody mechanism: methyldopa.
- Drug-adsorption mechanism: penicillin.
- Immune-complex mechanism: stibophen, quinine, and quinidine.
- Some drugs produce autoimmune hemolytic anemia by more than one mechanism.

The treatment of warm autoimmune hemolytic anemia includes the following. The first general principle is to treat the underlying disease and to discontinue the use of drugs that have been implicated in hemolysis. If the patient is clinically stable, do not transfuse blood. Avoid transfusion in patients with autoimmune hemolytic anemia. If the patient is symptomatic and studies show improvement in symptoms if the hemoglobin is greater than 8 g/dL, transfuse with packed RBCs only if angina, cardiac decompensation, or neurologic symptoms (e.g., lethargy, weakness, confusion, or obtundation) are present. If transfusion is required, then transfuse with the most compatible RBCs by crossmatch with type-specific ABO and Rh blood. The major risk of transfusion is the formation of autoantibodies to foreign RBC antigens.

If steroids are given, the dose of prednisone should be 60 to 80 mg/day. Most patients have a response in 7 days. If the patient has a relapse during tapering of the drug, return to the previous dose. Splenectomy is required in about 60% of cases. Immunosuppressive drugs such as cyclophosphamide (60 mg/m^2 per day) or azathioprine (80 mg/m^2 per day) are the next line of therapy.

Cold Agglutinin Syndrome (Primary Cold Agglutinin Disease)

Cold agglutinin syndrome is characterized by the presence of agglutination, hemolytic anemia, a positive Coombs test, chronic anemia, and a "monotonous" prognosis. Autoantibodies are maximally reactive at low temperatures. The degree of hemolysis depends on the thermal amplitude: the higher the titer, the more likely to bind complement. The clinical signs and symptoms are related to small vessel occlusion and include acrocyanosis of the ears, tip of the nose, toes, and fingers. Hepatosplenomegaly is uncommon. Skin color is dusky blue and then turns normal or blanches. All digits may be affected equally. This should be differentiated from Raynaud phenomenon, in which one or two fingers turn white to blue to red.

The peripheral blood smear shows agglutination of RBCs that disappears if prepared at 37°C (Plate 12-4). Agglutinated RBCs clump together. In rouleaux, the cells stack up on one another (Plate 12-7). The anemia is mild to moderate, and the Coombs test is positive. The cold agglutinin titer is greater than 1:1,000. Therapy includes avoidance of the cold. Corticoteroids are less effective in cold than in warm autoimmune hemolytic anemia. Splenectomy is generally ineffective. Some patients may respond to immunosuppressive drugs such as cyclophosphamide or chlorambucil. Plasma exchange is not very effective but should be considered if the patient is acutely ill, because IgM is intravascular.

- Cold agglutinin syndrome: agglutination and hemolytic anemia.
- Acrocyanosis of the ears, tip of the nose, toes, fingers; differentiate from Raynaud phenomenon.
- Positive Coombs test response and cold agglutinin titer >1:1,000.

Immunology of Cold Agglutinins

An IgM antibody exhibits a reversible thermal-dependent equilibrium reaction with the I or i antigen which is related to the ABO on RBCs and is favored at lower temperatures. A monoclonal kappa protein is seen in cold agglutinin syndrome, chronic lymphocytic leukemia, multiple myeloma, lymphoma, and Waldenström macroglobulinemia. In secondary diseases, there is a polyclonal light chain reaction with a high thermal cold agglutinin of anti-I specificity (*Mycoplasma pneumoniae*) or anti-i specificity (infectious mononucleosis, cytomegalovirus, and lymphoma).

Mycoplasma pneumoniae (anti-I)—In patients with *Mycoplasma pneumoniae*, 50% have cold agglutinins greater than 1:64, most have splenomegaly, and acrocyanosis is unusual. The course of this complication generally resolves in 2 or 3 weeks, but fatalities have been reported. Treatment includes keeping the patient warm and treating the infection with tetracycline or erythromycin.

Infectious mononucleosis (anti-i)—Of patients with infectious mononucleosis, 40% to 50% have cold agglutinins and 3% have autoimmune hemolytic anemia. The onset occurs by 13 days in 67% of patients. The duration of hemolysis is less than 1 month in 75% of patients and 1 to 2 months in 25%. Hepatosplenomegaly is present in 71% of patients. Steroids are of distinct value in treating this disorder, as may be splenectomy.

Paroxysmal Cold Hemoglobinuria (Complement-Mediated Lysis)

Paroxysmal cold hemoglobinuria is the least common cause of autoimmune hemolytic anemia. Results of the Donath-Landsteiner test are positive. This condition can be idiopathic or secondary. The secondary causes include syphilis (congenital and late), mononucleosis, mycoplasma, chickenpox, mumps, and measles. Measles is the most common secondary cause. Clinical manifestations include shaking chills, fever, malaise, abdominal pain, back pain, and leg pain. There is rapid and severe anemia. The prognosis is good. This condition resolves after the infection clears. Treatment includes protection from the cold, treatment of the underlying disease, and possibly a short course of steroids.

Coombs-Negative Hemolytic Anemias

The differential diagnosis includes the enzymopathies (glucose-6-phosphate dehydrogenase deficiency and pyruvate kinase deficiency), paroxysmal nocturnal hemoglobinuria, hereditary spherocytosis, and thrombotic thrombocytopenic purpura.

Glucose-6-Phosphate Dehydrogenase Deficiency

This is the most common RBC enzyme deficiency. The glucose-6-phosphate dehydrogenase deficiency causes decreased glutathione, which is an antioxidant. It is inherited on the X chromosome and is sex-linked. All enzymopathies are autosomal recessive except glucose-6-phosphate dehydrogenase and phosphoglycerate kinase deficiencies, which are sex-linked. In males, it is present in 12% of U.S. blacks, 20% to 32% of Greeks, and 0.4% of Italians. In females, one X chromosome is inactivated, and the gene is present on both, so the activity ranges from 0% to 100% with a mosaic population. Glucose-6-phosphate dehydrogenase deficiency confers some protection against falciparum malaria. Protection extends to both males and heterozygous females. This selective advantage has been attributed to the inhibition of parasite growth and replication through the mechanism of increased oxidant stress.

The oxidation of hemoglobin leads to the formation of methemoglobin, and sulfhemoglobin may be a product, with precipitation, condensation, and attachment of the denatured portion to the inside of the membrane-forming Heinz bodies. The normal enzyme has a half-life of 62 days, but reticulocytes have a half-life of 124 days and aged cells have a half-life of 31 days. Therefore, in an acute hemolytic state, the glucose-6-phosphate level may be within normal limits. There is individual variability to oxidant stress. It is not possible to stimulate the enzyme with methylene blue or ascorbic acid to counteract the formation of methemoglobin; these drugs may actually exacerbate the anemia.

In the steady state, there is no anemia or RBC defect. There is an increased risk of hemolysis in patients with concurrent renal or hepatic disease, viral and bacterial infections, diabetic acidosis, and low levels of blood glucose. Even a mild infection can produce hemolytic anemia, and this is more common than drug provocation. The organisms commonly associated with this complication are *Salmonella*, *Escherichia coli*, pneumococcus, *Rickettsia*, and viral hepatitis. Favism is seen only in whites and not in blacks.

Drugs commonly causing hemolytic anemia in glucose-6-phosphate dehydrogenase deficiency include antimalarial agents (primaquine and chloroquine), dapsone, sulfonamides (sulfanilamide, sulfamethoxazole, sulfapyridine, and sulfasalazine), nitrofurantoin, diazoxide, and nitrites (which are derived from nitrates from nitroglycerin, fertilizer-contaminating home wells, and amyl nitrite).

Abnormal laboratory findings include intravascular hemolysis, methemoglobinemia, and methemalbuminenia (highly specific for intravascular hemolysis). The presence of Heinz bodies on supravital staining is a good screening test, but the absence of these bodies does not rule out the diagnosis. Reticulocytosis rarely masks the deficiency in whites but it may in blacks and heterozygous females. The glucose-6-phosphate dehydrogenase assay is the definitive test. Treatment includes treating the underlying infection and withdrawing use of the offending drug.

- Glucose-6-phosphate dehydrogenase deficiency: the most common RBC enzyme deficiency; inherited on the X chromosome.
- Falciparum malaria provides some protection.
- Half-life: normal, 62 days; reticulocytes, 124 days; and aged cells, 31 days.
- No anemia or RBC defect occurs in the steady state.
- Important to look for cause, particularly drugs.
- Infection is more common than drug provocation.
- Heinz bodies seen on supravital staining of the peripheral blood is a good screening test.
- Treat underlying infections and withdraw the use of offending drugs.

Other Enzymopathies

About 35 distinct enzymopathies have been identified, and most of them are accepted as an etiologic basis for RBC dysfunction. Two deficiency states comprise the largest number: glucose-6-phosphate dehydrogenase and pyruvate kinase. With the exception of glucose-6-phosphate dehydrogenase deficiency, potentially symptomatic enzymopathies are uncommon. Treatment is supportive and empirical. Other clinically significant enzymopathies include unstable hemoglobins, glucose phosphate isomerase, pyrimidine 5'-nucleotidase, and triose phosphate isomerase deficiencies. In data on a referral population, only 35% of patients who were referred for an enzyme deficiency work-up had an identifiable enzyme deficiency.

Paroxysmal Nocturnal Hemoglobinuria

Paroxysmal nocturnal hemoglobinuria is an acquired clonal chronic hematologic stem cell disorder. Patients with this condition have a median survival of 10 years. It is a clonal disorder in which blood cells are unusually sensitive to activated complement and are lysed. Lysis is complement-mediated. Hemolysis occurs at night because this is when people become more acidotic. The disorder is characterized by abnormal pluripotent stem cells, reticulocytopenia, leukopenia, or thrombocytopenia due to lysis by complement. Normal and abnormal cells occur simultaneously in most patients.

A distinct class of membrane proteins is selectively deleted from the plasma membranes of maturing cells. The abnormal cells in paroxysmal nocturnal hemoglobinuria lack glycosylphosphatidylinositol-linked proteins in erythroid, granulocytic, megakaryocytic, and, in some cases, lymphoid cells. Flow cytometric studies can detect the presence or absence of these GPI-linked proteins, which include CD14, CD16, CD24, CD55, and CD59. This disease involves deficiencies in the surface molecules that normally regulate activation of C3B and C5 to C9 in the complement cascade. There is a decrease in a membrane protein (decay-accelerating factor) and homologous restriction factor that regulates the alternate complement pathway on normal blood cells. Also, the activity of RBC acetylcholinesterase is decreased.

Clinically, paroxysmal nocturnal hemoglobinuria is characterized by a chronic hemolytic anemia with hemoglobinuria and hemoglobinemia (intravascular hemolysis). Venous thrombosis of the portal system, brain, and extremities is associated with 50% of the deaths in paroxysmal nocturnal hemoglobinuria. Episodes of severe pain may occur in the abdomen and back in conjunction with painful or difficult swallowing.

Complications include acute nonlymphocytic leukemia in 5% to 10% of patients (paroxysmal nocturnal hemoglobinuria clone disappears), aplastic anemia (association of aplastic anemia, splenomegaly, and relative reticulocytosis suggests diagnosis), and venous thrombosis (Budd-Chiari syndrome is the major cause of death). Budd-Chiari syndrome is manifested by abdominal pain, tender hepatomegaly, nausea, vomiting, fever, and increased levels of lactate dehydrogenase, serum glutamic-oxaloacetic transaminase, gamma-glutamyltransferase, and conjugated bilirubin. Hepatic ultrasonography and venography are important in making the diagnosis. Treatment includes emergent heparinization, a long-term course of anticoagulation, and fibrinolytic therapy.

Diagnosis—The sucrose hemolysis test can give false-positive results but is a good inexpensive screening test. The Ham test (acid hemolysis test) is a confirmatory test. The most useful assay is flow cytometry to establish the absence of the GPI-linked antigens.

Treatment—Iron therapy: a burst of erythropoiesis can be seen if the patient is iron deficient; however, in most patients, iron may be given safely. Androgen therapy stimulates bone marrow and is of most benefit if the bone marrow is hypoplastic. Prednisone (alternate-day therapy, 15-40 mg) may inhibit activation of complement by the alternate pathway. Prednisone is of no benefit if the bone marrow is hypoplastic or there is mild hemolysis. Discontinue treatment with steroids if no effect occurs in 6 weeks. Transfusions: initially, transfuse with packed RBCs. If complicated by hemolysis, washed or frozen RBCs should be given. A hemolytic crisis may be initiated by infections. Treatment may include steroids, transfusion, and hydration to prevent renal failure. For venous thrombosis, the treatment of choice is heparin, which may activate alternate pathway of complement. Painful episodes are managed with narcotics and rehydration. Bone marrow transplantation is indicated in severe aplastic anemia. Antithymocyte globulin is effective in the management of paroxysmal nocturnal hemoglobinuria.

- Paroxysmal nocturnal hemoglobinuria: a chronic disease caused by an unidentifiable RBC defect.
- Venous thrombosis is associated with 50% of deaths.
- Intravascular hemolysis with hemoglobinuria and hemoglobinemia.
- Leukemia occurs in 5%-10%; aplastic anemia.
- Diagnosis: Ham test, sucrose hemolysis test, and flow cytometry studies.

Hereditary Spherocytosis

Hereditary spherocytosis is most commonly an autosomal dominant disorder in which splenomegaly is invariably present. It is caused by an underlying defect in the RBC membrane cytoskeleton caused by a partial deficiency in one or more of the components called spectrin and band 4.1. Osmotic fragility of RBCs is increased. The incubated osmotic fragility test is almost always abnormal and is the most reliable diagnostic test. The clinical features include jaundice, splenomegaly, negative results with Coombs test, spherocytes, and increased osmotic fragility. Gallstones are present in 43% to 85% of patients. Treatment is splenectomy, which invariably causes cessation of hemolysis. It should be performed after the first decade of life.

- Hereditary spherocytosis: autosomal dominant (75%) as well as autosomal recessive or sporadic.
- Splenomegaly occurs in most patients; cholelithiasis in 55%-75% after the 5th decade.
- Other features: negative results with Coombs test and increased osmotic fragility.
- Treatment: splenectomy after age 5 years in patients with

moderate or severe hemolysis. Asymptomatic adult patients with a hemoglobin value more than 11 g/dL and reticulocyte count less than 6% may be observed.

Idiopathic Thrombotic Thrombocytopenic Purpura

Thrombotic thrombocytopenic purpura is a syndrome rather than a disease. Classically, it is characterized by the pentad of anemia, thrombocytopenia, neurologic signs, fever, and renal abnormalities. Thrombocytopenia and microangiopathy are sufficient to establish the diagnosis. The anemia is normochromic-normocytic, with microangiopathic hemolytic features (Plate 12-6). The Coombs test gives negative results. The results of coagulation studies are normal or only mildly abnormal, in contrast to disseminated intravascular coagulopathy. The cause of this syndrome is unknown in more than 90% of patients. It is related to pregnancy and the use of oral contraceptives.

Clinically, thrombocytopenia is associated with bleeding in 96% of cases—petechiae and purpura, retinal bleeding, hematuria, gingival bleeding, melena, menorrhagia, hematemesis, and hemoptysis. Neurologic signs consist of remittent and frequent changes, including headache, coma, mental changes, paresis, seizure/coma, aphasia, syncope, visual symptoms, dysarthria, vertigo, agitation, confusion, and delirium. Renal abnormalities include a creatinine level greater than 1.5 in less than 20% of cases. Azotemia is an unfavorable prognostic sign. An abnormal urinary sediment with proteinuria, hematuria, pyuria, or casts was present in 82% of patients in one series.

The pathologic findings are characterized by widespread intraluminal hyaline vascular occlusions with platelet aggregates and fibrin, with no inflammatory changes in terminal arterioles or capillaries in virtually any organ. The preferred biopsy site is the bone marrow. Other sites to consider for biopsy are the gingiva, skin, petechial spot, muscle, and lymph nodes. von Willebrand factor (vWF) is believed to participate in the platelet agglutination and thrombus formation. Large multimers of vWF appear to be the aggregating agents of thrombotic thrombocytopenic purpura. In those patients with a single acute episode of thrombotic thrombocytopenic purpura, there is little if any plasma vWF-cleaving protease activity and an IgG antibody probably accounts for the lack of protease activity.

Without treatment, more than 90% of patients die of multiorgan failure. With treatment, 70% to 80% of patients survive the disease with little or no sequelae. The treatment of choice is plasmapheresis with the replacement with fresh frozen plasma or the supernatant fraction from cryoprecipitate preparations (plasma exchange). Other ancillary treatments used at different centers include dipyridamole (400-600 mg/day), aspirin (with a dose from 300 mg twice a week to 600-1,200 mg/day), and prednisone (dose of 60 mg/kg per day). The overall response rate to therapy is 80% to 90%. The projected 10-year risk of relapse in the Canadian Apheresis Group Trial is 36%.

- Thrombotic thrombocytopenic purpura: the pentad of anemia, fever, thrombocytopenia, neurologic signs, and renal abnormalities.
- Its cause is unknown; exclude oral contraceptives and pregnancy as etiologic factors.
- Features: Coombs test gives negative results, microangiopathy, normal prothrombin time, normal activated partial thromboplastin time, and normal fibrinogen.
- There is a relationship with pregnancy and the use of oral contraceptives.
- The treatment of choice is plasmapheresis, with the replacement of fresh frozen plasma.

Adult Hemolytic Uremic Syndrome

Adult hemolytic uremic syndrome is characterized by microangiopathic hemolytic anemia (anemia and thrombocytopenia) with a creatinine level greater than 3 mg/dL. Fever and neurologic signs are not part of this syndrome. The pathologic findings are similar to those in thrombotic thrombocytopenic purpura but are limited to only the kidneys. It is often preceded by an acute infective process. There is a much higher morbidity and mortality rate in adults, and adult hemolytic uremic syndrome is best managed as thrombotic thrombocytopenic purpura is in adults. This may be associated with *E. coli* O 157:H7 diarrhea. The management of the hemolytic-uremic syndrome is supportive in this situation. Dialysis may be necessary. The efficacy of plasmapheresis and plasma exchange has not been proved.

Sickle Cell Anemia

Sickle cell anemia is the most common heritable hematologic disease affecting humans. The gene for the beta chain must be inherited from both parents. It occurs in black Africans and rarely in whites. About 8% of blacks carry the sickle cell gene, with the disease occurring in 1/625 of them. There is a selective advantage from *Plasmodium falciparum* malaria, with preferential sickling of only the parasitized cells. Sickle cell anemia is an example of a balanced polymorphism (a common mutation) that provides a selective advantage but also has the potential to produce a disease state. In the heterozygous state, there is protection against malaria. In the homozygous state, sickle cell anemia is a serious life-shortening disease. Hemoglobin S is different from hemoglobin A in the substitution of valine for glutamic acid at the sixth position, resulting in abnormalities in polymerization (or gelation) of deoxygenation that leads to distortion of shape (sickling). The end result of the polymerization is a permanently altered membrane protein. Two-thirds of the RBCs are removed by extravascular mechanisms.

Sickling is inhibited by hemoglobin F. Hemoglobin F is a very potent inhibitor of polymerization. Polymerization leads to sickling. Sickling is promoted by low oxygen tension, low pH, high cellular concentration of hemoglobins, loss of cell water, hemoglobin D, and HbO-ARAB.

Symptoms are not present until the patient is older than 6 months. Vaso-occlusive disease develops between the ages of 12 months and 6 years. Acute crises are due to recurrent obstruction of the microcirculation by intravascular sickling. Laboratory testing is not helpful. Atypical symptoms should suggest pneumonia, pulmonary infarct, acute pyelonephritis, or cholecystitis.

Bone and joint crises are manifested by bone and joint symptoms, which include gnawing pain and swelling of the elbows and knees. Radiographs may show bone infarcts and periostitis, but these do not appear until symptoms subside. Infarcts and periostitis may be documented with bone scans. Abdominal crises are secondary to small infarcts of mesentery and abdominal viscera with symptoms of 4 or 5 days' duration. This is a nonsurgical problem if bowel sounds are present.

The Cooperative Study of Sickle Cell Disease reported that the incidence of hemorrhagic stroke was highest among patients 20 to 29 years old, with a mortality rate of 26% in the first 2 weeks, with no deaths after infarctive strokes. Transient ischemic attack (TIA) was a strong risk factor for infarctive stroke. Angiographic procedures should not be performed unless the patient has been prepared with RBCs. The therapy for these crises is immediate exchange transfusion. In a randomized study of chronic transfusion, therapy reduced the risk of recurrence of a cerebrovascular event and chronic transfusion therapy is indicated for this complication to maintain hemoglobin S greater than 30%, because the risk of recurrent episodes is greater than 50%. Multivariate analysis found that low steady-state hemoglobin concentration and high leukocyte concentration were not factors for hemorrhagic stroke.

In pulmonary crises, acute chest syndrome accounts for 20% of deaths. Clinical aspects include fever, chest pain, tachypnea, increased WBC count, and pulmonary infarcts. Age makes a difference in cause. In children, infected segments enhance local sickling, so sickling is a secondary phenomenon. The causative organisms include pneumococcus, *Mycoplasma*, *Haemophilus*, *Salmonella*, and *E. coli*. In adults, sickling tends to be a primary event, with no signs of infection.

Aplastic crises usually follow a febrile illness, with disappearance of reticulocytes and normoblasts. They last 5 to 10 days. Hemolytic crises may occur in patients with concomitant glucose-6-phosphate dehydrogenase deficiency, hereditary spherocytosis, and mycoplasmal pneumonia.

Infectious crises are the most frequent cause of death of patients younger than 5 years. The organisms include *Streptococcus pneumoniae* of the blood and spinal fluid (70% of patients). Normally, 80% of the cases of meningitis are caused by *Haemophilus influenzae* in this age group. At ages older than 5 years, gram-negative bacteria predominate, with osteomyelitis caused by *Salmonella*, *Staphylococcus*, and pneumococcus. The causes of infections/infectious crises include decreased IgM, defective alternate pathway, deficiency phagocytosis-promoting peptide tuftsin, and impaired splenic function. The challenge with *Streptococcus pneumoniae* is not followed by appropriate opsonin production.

Chronic manifestations—There is a progressive lag in growth and development after the first decade of life and a chronic destruction of bone and joints, with ischemia and infarction of the spongiosa. The vertebrae become fish-mouthed. Avascular necrosis is common in multiple joints. Ocular manifestations include stasis and occlusion of small vessels that is nonproliferative or proliferative. They may require laser photocoagulation. Cardiovascular manifestations include cardiomegaly, flow murmurs, and a pansystolic murmur with click that mimics mitral regurgitation. Restrictive lung disease may develop. Hepatobiliary manifestations include hepatomegaly with the pathologic features of distended sinusoids, periportal fibrosis, and hemosiderin pigment. Marked hyperbilirubinemia may be due to hepatitis, intrahepatic sickling, choledocholithiasis, or coexistent glucose-6-phosphate dehydrogenase deficiency. There is an increased incidence of pigmented gallstones in 30% to 60% of adults, with symptoms in 10% to 15%. Renal manifestations include papillary necrosis, hyposthenuria by age 6 to 12 months (disruption of countercurrent multiplier system, nocturia, enuresis), hematuria (ulcer in renal pelvis, urate stones), nephrotic syndrome secondary to focal segmental glomerulonephropathy, tubular damage secondary to small infarcts, and priapism. Leg ulcers may occur.

In pregnancy, there is no increase in disease manifestations, but there is an increase in maternal mortality of 20% and fetal mortality of 20%. Early complications of pregnancy include thrombophlebitis, pyelonephritis, and hematuria. Late complications include major infarcts of the lung, kidney, and brain; toxemia; congestive heart failure; and postpartum endometritis.

Laboratory findings include anemia (range, 5.5-9.5 g/dL), sickled cells, cigar cells, ovalocytes, targets, basophilic stippling, polychromatophilia, reticulocytes (8%-12%), and hyposplenia with Howell-Jolly bodies. A persistent increase in the WBC count of 12,000 to 15,000 is characteristic. On hemoglobin electrophoresis, hemoglobin S moves more slowly than hemoglobin A.

The primary treatment is prevention. Infection, fever, dehydration, acidosis, hypoxemia, cold, and high altitude should be avoided. Acetaminophen is indicated for fever because aspirin contributes to an acid load. A temperature higher than 105°F means infection, and infection is uncommon if the temperature is lower than 102°F. Prophylactic use of penicillin is beneficial. Vaccines, including pneumococcal, influenza A, and *Haemophilus*, are indicated, as is folate supplementation, especially in pregnancy. Iron chelation is recommended if the transfusion requirement is high. Splenectomy is recommended for those children who survive the initial splenic sequestration crisis. This is the only indication for splenectomy. Blood transfusion and exchange transfusion are the most effective means of treatment available. The hemoglobin S cells should be decreased to less than 30%. These modalities are especially indicated for the following: history of cerebral vascular accidents, progressive retinopathy, renal or cardiac decompensation preoperatively, and pregnancy (at 30-34 weeks, maintain hemoglobin >10 g/dL). Short-term transfusion therapy is indicated in acute chest syndrome. Other indications for transfusion are priapism, protracted hematuria, and chronic skin ulcers. In vaso-occlusive crises, the cornerstone of treatment includes fluids and correction of urinary sodium losses. Other important considerations are treatment of infections: penicillin in children and coverage for *Staphylococcus* in adults. Analgesics are essential. Blood transfusions do not modify the course. Prenatal diagnosis may be made by analysis of amniotic fluid or chorionic villi biopsy, which is preferred to fetal blood sampling. New approaches that inhibit potassium and water loss from SS RBCs include low-dose clotrimazole and magnesium. In the Multicenter Study of Hydroxyurea in Sickle Cell Anemia, which was a double-blinded, placebo-controlled trial, hydroxyurea decreased the frequency of painful vaso-occlusive crises by about 50%. In patients with severe recurrent episodes, the frequency of the acute chest syndrome was decreased and patients required fewer transfusions. Hydroxyurea increases fetal hemoglobin. Side effects include readily reversible myelosuppression. In addition, hydroxyurea causes slight neutropenia and decreases the reticulocyte count, which may contribute to the efficacy of the drug.

Hematopoietic stem cell transplantation with marrow or umbilical cord blood from HLA-identical siblings have demonstrated that sickle cell disease can be cured. The Cooperative Study of Sickle Cell Disease reported in a prospective analysis that 50% of patients with sickle cell anemia survived beyond the fifth decade. Few patients survive into their 60s. Symptomatic patients had the highest early mortality. A high level of fetal hemoglobin predicted improved survival in young patients. Acute chest syndrome, renal failure, seizures, a baseline WBC count greater than 15×10^9/L, and a low level of fetal hemoglobin were associated with the risk of early death in patients 20 years or older. In adults, 78% of patients died during an acute sickle cell crisis. Acute pain and chest syndrome was the most common cause of death, and stroke was the next most common cause. This was followed by infection (*E. coli*, *Staphylococcus aureus*, HIV, tuberculosis, malaria, pneumococcus, and hepatitis). In children younger than 5 years, the cause of infection is almost universally pneumococcal sepsis.

Sickle cell trait occurs in 8% of American blacks. There is no anemia, RBC abnormalities, increased risk of infections, or increased mortality; 35% to 45% of hemoglobin is hemoglobin S. Associations with sickle cell trait include hematuria, splenic infarction at high altitude (higher than 10,000 feet), hyposthenuria, bacteriuria, pyelonephritis in pregnancy, and reduced mortality from *Plasmodium falciparum* infection.

In hemoglobin SC disease, patients have only hemoglobin S and C, with an absence of hemoglobin A and normal or increased levels of hemoglobin F. Patients with sickle cell hemoglobin C survive longer than those with sickle cell anemia. The sickle cell hemoglobin C disorder is less severe than sickle cell disease with four exceptions: proliferative retinopathy, retinal detachment, aseptic necrosis of the head of the femur, and acute chest syndrome secondary to fat emboli in the final months of pregnancy. There is mild anemia; in 10% of patients, the hemoglobin is less than 10 g/dL. Sickle cells are rare on the peripheral blood smear, and 50% of the cells in the peripheral blood are target cells. The spleen remains functional.

Hemoglobin S/β-thalassemia is less severe than sickle cell disease. Both affect the beta chain. The spleen remains functional, but retinopathy is more common. The protective effect of α-thalassemia is due largely to improvement in hemoglobin concentration.

- Hydroxyurea decreases the frequency of painful vaso-occlusive crises by 50%.
- Acute chest syndrome, renal failure, seizures, a baseline WBC count >15,000/mL, and a low level of fetal hemoglobin are associated with a risk of early death in adults.
- Death is associated with acute pain and chest syndrome, stroke, and infection.
- Patients with sickle cell hemoglobin C survive longer than those with sickle cell anemia.
- High WBC counts are a risk factor for severe pain, acute chest syndrome, and mortality from a hemorrhagic cerebrovascular event.
- The best method of prenatal diagnosis is to sample either from the amniotic sac or chorionic villi and to test for an abnormal endonuclease cleavage pattern.

MALIGNANCIES

Chronic Lymphocytic Leukemia

Chronic lymphocytic leukemia is a lymphoproliferative disorder of mature lymphocytes (Plate 12-8). The clinical diagnosis requires an absolute lymphocytosis of greater than 5,000 mature-appearing lymphocytes per microliter. It is the commonest form of leukemia in patients 60 years and older in the Western world, accounting for 30% of all leukemias at any one time, and 90% of patients are older than 50. It is more common in men. It is rare in Asia.

Chronic lymphocytic leukemia is more of an accumulative than a proliferative disorder of long-lived immunologically incompetent cells. B-CLL is the only major adult leukemia that is not associated with exposure to ionizing radiation, drugs, or chemicals. The two staging classifications are outlined in Tables 12-3 and 12-4.

Predictors of decreased survival include advanced stage, response to initial treatment, WBC count greater than 50,000/mL, cytogenetic abnormalities, increased beta$_2$-microglobulin levels, diffuse bone marrow pattern, and lymphocyte doubling time (unfavorable if <12 months).

The clinical course is chronic in 60% of patients. Complications include recurrent infection; 50% of patients have hypogammaglobulinemia. Fever in chronic lymphocytic leukemia is secondary to infection and not to chronic lymphocytic leukemia. The exception is Richter syndrome. Autoimmune and immunodeficiency complications include autoimmune hemolytic anemia (in 10% of patients), immune-mediated thrombocytopenia (in <5%), that is IgG-mediated and treated with steroids, pure RBC aplasia, hypogammaglobulinemia, impaired delayed-type hypersensitivity, increased susceptibility to micro-organisms, and second malignancies.

- In chronic lymphocytic leukemia, fever is not related to disease but infection, except in Richter syndrome.
- Hypogammaglobulinemia occurs in 50% of patients with recurrent infection.
- Autoimmune hemolytic anemia occurs in 10%.
- Thrombocytopenia occurs in <5%.
- Prophylactic intravenous gamma globulin is indicated for gamma globulin levels <0.3 g/dL with or without previous infection.

The major hematologic malignancy associated with chronic lymphocytic leukemia includes Richter syndrome, which is chronic lymphocytic leukemia that has transformed into diffuse large cell lymphoma and is characterized by fevers, massive asymmetrical adenopathy, splenomegaly, and a poor outcome. Chronic lymphocytic leukemia is associated with increased incidence of solid tumors of the lung and skin (basal cell, squamous cell). Patients may develop secondary drug-induced acute nonlymphocytic leukemia. Infectious complications include *Staphylococcus aureus*, pneumococci, *Pseudomonas*, *Klebsiella*, *Pneumocystis*, cytomegalovirus, *Candida*, herpes simplex, and herpes zoster.

Table 12-3. —Staging: Rai Classification

Stage	Characteristics	No. patients	Median survival time, mo	No. patients[*]	Median survival time, mo
0	Peripheral (>15 x 10^9/L) lymphocytosis, bone marrow lymphocytosis (>40%)	22	>150	79	129
I	Lymphocytosis, lymphadenopathy	29	101	154	74.4
II	Lymphocytosis, splenomegaly	39	71	203	58.2
III	Lymphocytosis, anemia with hemoglobin <11, excluding AIHA	21	19	127	28.1
IV	Lymphocytosis, thrombocytopenia	14	19	105	19.3

[*]Six combined series.

AIHA, autoimmune hemolytic anemia.

Data from Rai KR, Sawitsky A, Cronkite EP, Chanana AD, Levy RN, Pasternack BS: Clinical staging of chronic lymphocytic leukemia. Blood 46:219-234, 1975.

Table 12-4. —Classification of International Workshop on Chronic Lymphocytic Leukemia

Clinical stage	Features
A	No anemia or thrombocytopenia and fewer than three areas of lymphoid enlargement. (Spleen, liver, and lymph nodes in cervical, axillary, and inguinal regions.) A(0), A(I), or A(II).
B	No anemia or thrombocytopenia with three or more involved areas. B(I) or B(II).
C	Anemia (<10 g/dL) and/or thrombocytopenia regardless of the number of areas of lymphoid enlargement. C(III) or C(IV).

From International Workshop on CLL: Chronic lymphocytic leukaemia: proposals for a revised prognostic staging system. Br J Haematol 48:365-367, 1981. By permission of Blackwell Scientific Publications.

Laboratory findings: The diagnosis includes blood lymphocytosis greater than 5,000, mature-appearing lymphocytes (<55% prolymphocytes), and a characteristic phenotype (CD19+, CD20+, CD23+, coexpression of the T-cell marker CD5+, and faint monoclonal light chain restriction). The neoplastic cells usually express high levels of bcl-2 protein, rendering the cells resistant to programmed cell death (apoptosis). Chromosomal abnormalities are found in more than 50% of patients. Two nonrandom chromosomal abnormalities may be associated with chronic lymphocytic leukemia: trisomy 12 and 13Q14 deletions. To date, there is no evidence of pure clonal remissions or cure with treatment. The median survival time of all patients is 5 years from the onset of treatment.

The standard practice in chronic lymphocytic leukemia is to withhold treatment until there is active or progressive disease. A French study compared treatment with no treatment in early stage disease, and there was no difference in survival. In contrast, survival in patients with advanced stage disease is better if the chronic lymphocytic leukemia responds to treatment, with a median response duration of 4 years versus 1 year in nonresponders. Chlorambucil with or without prednisone versus fludarabine is the initial treatment of choice. In a large randomized trial, the complete remission rate and median remission duration with chlorambucil was 3%, and with fludarabine, it was 27%, with a higher median response duration and progression-free survival. To date, there is not a survival advantage in patients treated with fludarabine. Fludarabine may be the initial choice for patients who clinically need a rapid and sustained remission. Prednisone alone may be indicated in isolated immune-related anemia and thrombocytopenia. Fludarabine is the treatment of choice for chronic lymphocytic leukemia in patients who have a relapse after chlorambucil. Fludarabine induces an overall response rate of 32% to 60% in previously treated patients and approximately 80% in previously untreated patients with a median response duration of 33 months. The major toxic effect of fludarabine is myelosuppression and immunosuppression, which predisposes to opportunistic infections secondary to a quantitative suppression in T-helper (CD4) lymphocytes. A large randomized trial has demonstrated the usefulness of recombinant erythropoietin in increasing hemoglobin levels in anemic patients with chronic lymphocytic leukemia. Splenectomy may be indicated in patients with refractory immune anemia and thrombocytopenia, massive splenomegaly, and hypersplenism. Another option is to include systemic chemotherapy with CAP (cyclophosphamide, doxorubicin [Adriamycin], and prednisone). With each relapse, the disease becomes more resistant to treatment.

Treatment guidelines—Rai classification:
Stage 0—No treatment.
Stage I and stage II—The NCI-Working Group recommended treatment if active disease was present and included the presence of disease-related symptoms (weight loss ≥10% in 6 months, fatigue, performance score of 2 or more, fevers without overt infection, or night sweats); massively enlarged nodes or spleen; progressive or rapid rate of increase in the peripheral blood lymphocyte count (<12 months); autoimmune anemia or thrombocytopenia; and repeated infections with or without hypogammaglobulinemia.
Stage III and stage IV—Short median life expectancy, invariably symptomatic. Treat all patients to alleviate symptoms and to improve life expectancy.

Treatment guidelines—International Workshop classification:
Stage A—Observe.
Stage B—Some patients will need treatment, as outlined in stages I and II indications above.
Stage C—Treat all patients.

- Observe stage 0 or stage A patients.
- Treat all patients with Rai stages III and IV disease and International Workshop stage C.
- The optimal treatment of choice is chlorambucil with or without prednisone or fludarabine.
- Fludarabine is the treatment of choice for patients who have relapse after treatment with chlorambucil and/or prednisone.

Patients who have relapse may be followed without therapy until they experience disease-related symptoms or progressive disease, with deterioration of blood cell counts, discomfort from lymphadenopathy or hepatosplenomegaly, recurrent infections, or associated autoimmune disorders.

Hairy Cell Leukemia

Hairy cell leukemia is characterized by an insidious onset of cytopenias without constitutional symptoms. At some time during the course of the disease, 90% of patients have splenomegaly. The hairy cell cytoplasmic projections are "hairy" with multiple, thin, or blunt projections (Plate 12-9). The cells contain tartrate-resistant acid phosphatase (positive TRAP stain). Most are B-cell in nature and clonal, as demonstrated by light- and heavy-chain immunoglobulin gene rearrangements. Hairy cell leukemia accounts for less than 2% of all cases of leukemias. The cause is not known.

- Hairy cell leukemia: cytopenias.
- Splenomegaly is common.
- Hairy cells have cytoplasmic projections.
- B-cell in nature and clonal.
- Constitutes <2% of all cases of leukemias.

Clinical characteristics—The symptoms are related to cytopenias, infections, and splenomegaly.

Laboratory findings reveal anemia, thrombocytopenia, neutropenia, and pancytopenia. More than 75% of patients have anemia, thrombocytopenia, and neutropenia. The bone marrow yields a dry tap on bone marrow aspiration; biopsy specimens are hypercellular with diffuse infiltration. Hairy cells may or may not be seen in the peripheral blood.

- Cytopenias in 75% of patients with hairy cell leukemia.
- Bone marrow: dry tap.
- Hairy cells may not be seen in peripheral blood smear.
- Infection is related to granulocytopenia and impaired cell-mediated immunity.

Complications—Infection is the major cause of death. Infection should be considered when a previously stable patient develops new symptoms. Fever is not a manifestation of the disease but indicates an underlying infection. Localized pyogenic infections are more common, for example, bacterial pneumonia, urinary tract infections, and infections of the skin. Impaired cell-mediated immunity predisposes patients to other infections. The incidence of atypical mycobacterial infections is increased. There is a higher incidence of viral infections, fungal infections, parasitic diseases, toxoplasmosis, histoplasmosis, coccidiosis, and pneumocystis. Bleeding and vasculitis (skin, joint, erythema nodosum) are other complications.

- Hairy cell leukemia: Infection is the major cause of death.
- Fever denotes infection.
- Atypical mycobacterial infections.

Treatment—Observation may be indicated for patients who are asymptomatic with very mild cytopenias. Indications for intervention include significant cytopenia, serious or recurrent infections associated with neutropenia, bleeding secondary to thrombocytopenia, splenic infarction, vasculitis, and increasing number of hairy cells. 2-Chlorodeoxyadenosine produces complete remission in 85% to 88% of patients after a single 7-day continuous, intravenous infusion. Other treatments include interferon alfa-2a or 2b recombinant, which produces a 13% complete remission after 18 months of subcutaneous treatments and a partial remission rate of 66%. 2'-Deoxycoformycin produces complete remission rates in 75% of patients, with a relapse rate of 10%. Splenectomy only improves peripheral blood cell counts and has no effect on the bone marrow. The only indications for splenectomy are a very large spleen and patchy bone marrow involvement in a young patient, splenic infarct, and profound life-threatening bleeding secondary to thrombocytopenia.

- 2-Chlorodeoxyadenosine is the treatment of choice in hairy cell leukemia.
- Other treatments include 2'-deoxycoformycin, interferon alfa-2a or 2b recombinant, and splenectomy.

Lymphadenopathy

The differential diagnosis of lymphadenopathy is very broad. The differential diagnosis of lymphadenopathy and fever with or without splenomegaly includes the following:

Infections—Infectious mononucleosis, Epstein-Barr virus, cytomegalovirus, toxoplasmosis, syphilis, subacute bacterial endocarditis, sarcoidosis, *Salmonella*, tuberculosis, and acquired immunodeficiency syndrome (AIDS).

Malignancies—Hodgkin disease, non-Hodgkin lymphoma, angioimmunoblastic lymphadenopathy, mixed essential cryoglobulinemia, systemic mastocytosis, chronic lymphocytic leukemia, myelofibrosis, Waldenström macroglobulinemia, and multiple myeloma.

Other disorders—Systemic lupus erythematosus and rheumatoid arthritis. Kawasaki disease, Whipple disease, serum sickness, and Kaposi sarcoma.

Infectious Mononucleosis

The outcomes of infectious mononucleosis include acute infectious mononucleosis, asymptomatic primary infection, symptomatic chronic infection, chronic infectious mononucleosis syndrome, malignant lymphoproliferative disorders, hypogammaglobulinemia, and death (200/10 years). Ninety percent of patients have fever of 38°C to 39°C for 10 to 14 days and 70% to 90% of patients develop a sore throat, with an exudative tonsillitis in 30% to 50%. Lymphadenopathy is present in 80% to 90%, splenomegaly in 50% to 60%, hepatomegaly in 10% to 15%, and rash in 5% to 15%. From 50% to 90% of patients are asymptomatic carriers. Laboratory abnormalities include leukocytosis in 70% of patients, lymphocytosis in 50% (variant lymphocytosis and transient increase in suppressor T cells) (Plate 12-10), mild thrombocytopenia in 50%, and increased liver function tests in 80% to 90%. Complications of infectious mononucleosis include fulminant infections in immunodeficient hosts, severe tonsillar hypertrophy, splenic rupture, upper airway obstruction, neurologic (Guillain-Barré syndrome), myocarditis, and bleeding secondary to thrombocytopenia. Malignant diseases associated with Epstein-Barr viral infections include Burkitt lymphoma, nasopharyngeal carcinoma, post-transplantation lymphoproliferative disorders, HIV-related non-Hodgkin lymphoma, and Hodgkin disease. Hematologic complications include autoimmune hemolytic anemia and autoimmune thrombocytopenic purpura.

Hodgkin Disease

With therapy, 75% of cases of Hodgkin disease are cured. Untreated, the 5-year survival rate is less than 5%. Since 1973, Hodgkin disease has ranked second in decreased survival rates in the U.S. There is a bimodal curve in the age at presentation, with the first peak at a median age of about 25 years. Hodgkin disease usually presents as a locally limited disease that progresses in an orderly manner. The typical finding at presentation is lymph node enlargement, but virtually any organ or tissue may be involved (lung, bone marrow, liver, and bone). Less common presentations include pruritus, cytopenias, abnormal liver function tests, and jaundice (extrahepatic biliary obstruction, autoimmune hemolytic anemia, or, rarely, intrahepatic cholestasis). Patients with Hodgkin disease have impaired cell-mediated immunity and are predisposed to herpes zoster and cytomegalovirus infections. A low hemoglobin concentration and a low serum level of albumin are the two most important prognostic factors.

The diagnosis of Hodgkin disease is pathologically based on the presence of Reed-Sternberg (RS) cells, which typically have two or more nuclei with prominent nucleoli that give the cells the appearance of owl's eyes (Plate 12-11).

Disease stage is the principal factor in selecting treatment (Tables 12-5 and 12-6). In the U.S., up to 50% of patients have mediastinal disease on CT scan of the chest that may not be detectable on a standing posterior-anterior chest radiograph. Lymphangiography complements the CT scan and is used infrequently. Special nonroutine procedures include formal staging laparotomy, magnetic resonance imaging, gallium scan, bone scan, and liver/spleen scan.

Before treatment is started, male patients should be advised to store sperm if they intend to have children, and female patients are advised not to become pregnant for 2 years after therapy because 75% of the relapses occur during this period.

Radiotherapy is a consideration in the management of Hodgkin disease emergencies, including acute superior vena cava syndrome, airway obstruction, pericardial tamponade, and epidural spinal cord compression.

Currently, the preferred treatment for pathologic stage I or IIA Hodgkin disease is radiation therapy, at a dose of 35 to 44 Gy, to a mantle (fields extending to include all nodes above the diaphragm) and upper abdominal field. The corresponding rates of freedom from progression and survival at 14 years are 93% and 83%. The treatment of choice in stages IIIA, IIIB, IVA, and IVB is combination chemotherapy (Table 12-7). Although somewhat controversial, stages IB and IIB are also treated with combination chemotherapy. Chemotherapy is also used in the setting of infradiaphragmatic disease. Currently, the standard chemotherapy regimen is ABVD (doxorubicin [Adriamycin], bleomycin, vinblastine, and dacarbazine). The cure rates are up to 65% for patients with advanced disease. There is less sterility and secondary leukemia than with MOPP chemotherapy.

Relapse patterns are relatively predictable in Hodgkin disease. After radiation, relapse occurs in the first 2 years and usually involves nonirradiated sites adjacent to the treated fields. Relapse after chemotherapy occurs at bulky disease sites. Patients who have relapse after radiation therapy have about a 66% chance of cure with salvage chemotherapy. Those who have relapse after chemotherapy currently are offered autologous stem cell or bone marrow transplantation. In one study, comparing autologous bone marrow transplantation with conventional chemotherapy for recurrent or refractory disease, the 3-year event-free survival was 53% for the transplantation group and 10% for the chemotherapy group.

Late complications of Hodgkin disease are significant. The risks include infertility, amenorrhea, pneumococcal sepsis in 7% of patients following splenectomy, hypothyroidism, thyroid carcinoma, avascular necrosis, cardiomyopathy secondary to doxorubicin or radiation therapy, radiation pneumonitis, pulmonary fibrosis, and secondary cancers. The secondary cancers include acute nonlymphocytic leukemia, myelodysplastic syndromes, non-Hodgkin lymphoma, and solid tumors. ABVD is less leukemogenic than MOPP. Patients at highest risk are those who have received multiple courses of chemotherapy. The risk of non-Hodgkin lymphoma is 4% at 10 years. Radiation therapy increases the risk of solid tumors. After 15 years, the risk of secondary solid tumors is 13%; these tumors include cancers of the stomach, breast, lung, thyroid, skin, and head and neck.

- Polymerase chain reaction detects Epstein-Barr virus in 60%-80% of cases of Hodgkin disease.

Table 12-5.—The Cotswolds Staging Classification of Hodgkin Disease

Classification	Description
Stage I	Involvement of a single lymph node region or lymphoid structure
Stage II	Involvement of two or more lymph node regions on the same side of the diaphragm (the mediastinum is considered a single site, whereas hilar lymph nodes are considered bilaterally)
Stage III	Involvement of lymph node regions or structures on both sides of the diaphragm
Stage III-1	With or without involvement of splenic, hilar, celiac, or portal nodes
Stage III-2	With involvement of para-aortic, iliac, and mesenteric nodes
Stage IV	Involvement of one or more extranodal sites in addition to a site for which the designation "E" has been used
	Designations applicable to any disease stage
A	No symptoms
B	Fever (temperature >38°C), drenching night sweats, unexplained loss of >10% of body weight within the preceding 6 months
X	Bulky disease (a widening of the mediastinum by more than 1/3 or the presence of a nodal mass with a maximal dimension >10 cm)
E	Involvement of a single extranodal site that is contiguous or proximal to the known nodal site
CS	Clinical stage
PS	Pathologic stage (as determined by laparotomy)

From Lister TA, Crowther D: Staging for Hodgkin's disease. Semin Oncol 17:696-703, 1990. By permission of WB Saunders Company.

Table 12-6.—Staging Procedures for Hodgkin Disease

History and examination: identification of B symptoms

Imaging procedures: plain chest radiography, computed tomography of the thorax, computed tomographic scan of the abdomen and pelvis, and bipedal lymphangiography

Hematologic procedures: full blood cell count with differential, determination of erythrocyte sedimentation rate, and bilateral bone marrow aspiration and biopsy

Biochemical procedures: tests of liver function and measurement of serum albumin, lactate dehydrogenase, and calcium

Special procedures: laparotomy, ultrasonographic scanning, magnetic resonance imaging, gallium scanning, technetium bone scanning, and liver-spleen scanning

Staging laparotomies: performed only if radiation therapy is the desired treatment, so is not indicated in clinical stage IIIB to IVB patients; the detection of intra-abdominal disease would alter the choice of therapy. Patients should not have adverse features for relapse, such as a large mediastinal mass. The risk of abdominal involvement in females younger than 35 years with nodular sclerosing Hodgkin disease and high cervical neck nodes is low

Modified from Lister TA, Crowther D: Staging for Hodgkin's disease. Semin Oncol 17:696-703, 1990. By permission of WB Saunders Company.

- Disease stage is the principal factor in selecting treatment for patients with Hodgkin disease.
- The treatment of choice for patients who are not part of a clinical trial and who have pathologic stage IA or IIA disease above the diaphragm without a bulky mediastinal mass and <5 nodules in the spleen: mantle field radiation, with radiation fields extending to include the para-aortic regions.
- 66% of patients who have relapse after radiation therapy are in long-term remission after chemotherapy.
- The treatment of choice for patients with pathologic stage

IIB, IIIA2, IIIB, or IV disease: chemotherapy two cycles beyond a complete remission.

- Autologous bone marrow or peripheral blood stem-cell transplantation is indicated after first relapse from any front-line chemotherapy for Hodgkin disease.
- Complications of survival include acute nonlymphocytic leukemia, solid tumors, and cardiomyopathy.

Non-Hodgkin Lymphoma

Non-Hodgkin lymphomas are clinically, pathologically, cytogenetically, and immunologically a diverse group of lymphoproliferative disorders. The prognosis depends on the histologic subtype, stage, and other clinical and laboratory features. The Working Formulation for Clinical Usage, which groups non-Hodgkin lymphomas by natural history and response to therapy, had been the most widely used scheme in the U.S. (Table 12-8). This schema was based on morphologic patterns only. These morphologic patterns have characteristically associated cytogenetic abnormalities and oncogene associations. The most recent classification is the Revised European-American Lymphoma (REAL) Classification (Table 12-9). The REAL Classification subtracted some entities (follicular subsets and large cell subsets), added some new entities (mantle cell, mucosa-associated lymphoid tissue [MALT], monocytoid B cell, and anaplastic large cell), and recognized peripheral T-cell non-Hodgkin lymphomas and new subsets (intestinal T-cell).

The low-grade non-Hodgkin lymphomas, which include the follicular histologic features, are a group of lymphoproliferative disorders that are not curable (unless pathologic stage I disease), most commonly present with advanced stage III and IV disease, are very treatable with simple programs, occur in older patients, and have a long survival (median, 8 years). The paradox of the non-Hodgkin lymphomas is that the low-grade non-Hodgkin lymphomas are not curable, but patients live for a long time even after relapse. In contrast, the intermediate and high-grade lymphomas are potentially curable, but the length of survival is short if the patient does not go into

Table 12-7.—Initial Treatment of Hodgkin Disease

Stage	Type	Response
IA	Radiation therapy (mantle and para-aortic)	93% freedom from progression
IIA	Radiation, extended field (mantle and para-aortic)	82% freedom from progression
IIIA1	Radiation	
IIIA2, IIIB, IV	Chemotherapy	65% of patients receiving ABVD or MOPP/ABVD were alive and disease-free at 5 years

ABVD, doxorubicin, bleomycin, vinblastine, and dacarbazine; MOPP, nitrogen mustard, vincristine, procarbazine, and prednisone.

Table 12-8.—Non-Hodgkin Lymphomas

Classification	
Low grade	Malignant lymphoma: small lymphocytic
	Malignant lymphoma: follicular, predominantly small cleaved cell
	Malignant lymphoma: follicular, mixed small cleaved and large cell
Intermediate grade	Malignant lymphoma: follicular, predominantly large cell
	Malignant lymphoma: diffuse, small cleaved cell
	Malignant lymphoma: diffuse, mixed small and large cell
	Malignant lymphoma: diffuse large cell
High grade	Malignant lymphoma: large cell immunoblastic
	Malignant lymphoma: lymphoblastic
	Malignant lymphoma: small noncleaved cell
Miscellaneous	Composite malignant lymphoma
	Mycosis fungoides
	Extramedullary plasmacytoma
	Unclassified
	Other

Modified from The Non-Hodgkin's Lymphoma Pathologic Classification Project: National Cancer Institute sponsored study of classification of non-Hodgkin's lymphoma: summary and description of a working formulation for clinical usage. Cancer 49:2112-2135, 1982. By permission of Wiley-Liss.

remission. Patients may progress to a more aggressive lymphoma, with a risk that ranges from 10% to 70% in reported series, depending on frequency of new biopsies at the time of progression, follow-up duration, and post-mortem data.

Because the low-grade non-Hodgkin lymphomas are not curable, the most reliable end points are progression-free survival and overall survival. Achievement of a complete remission is not a viable end point in low-grade lymphomas. In addition, immunoglobulin κ/λ light chain restriction studies in peripheral blood and bone marrow with flow cytometry demonstrate malignant cells in peripheral blood after treatment in patients who have been deemed to be in remission, and polymerase chain reaction studies have demonstrated persistent abnormal cell populations in patients believed to be in complete remission.

Most patients with low-grade non-Hodgkin lymphoma have stage III or IV disease, which is not curable with standard treatment regimens. Observation is the initial treatment of choice in asymptomatic patients. The Stanford group reported on 83 patients with advanced disease who were not treated initially and had an actuarially predicted survival of 82% at 5 years and 73% at 10 years. At median follow-up of 50 months, 51 of the 83 patients (61%) required therapy at a median interval of 3 years from the time of diagnosis. Spontaneous regression was observed in 19 patients, partial remission in 13, and complete remission in 6. Treatment with more aggressive regimens has not improved survival. In a randomized trial in selected asymptomatic patients who were randomized to ProMACE-MOPP plus total lymphoid irradiation or to observation, there was no survival difference between the two groups.

For those patients with symptoms, bulky disease, or progressive disease, options with the goal of achieving complete remission include oral chlorambucil taken daily, intravenous CVP (cyclophosphamide, vincristine, and prednisone), CVP with total lymphoid irradiation, or CHOP (cyclophosphamide, doxorubicin, vincristine, and prednisone). CVP or chlorambucil is considered the standard treatment of choice. New treatments include fludarabine and the incorporation of interferon. Anti-CD20, a chimeric human anti-mouse antibody, has been approved for patients who have had relapse.

Gastric MALT lymphomas have clonal gene rearrangements and are associated with *Helicobacter pylori* infections. This is the first malignant lymphoproliferative disorder to respond to an antimicrobial approach. Up to 70% of patients respond to a regimen such as amoxicillin, metronidazole, and omeprazole.

In patients with the histologic features of intermediate-grade non-Hodgkin lymphoma, diffuse large cell lymphoma, anthracycline chemotherapy regimens are the hallmark of therapy, with complete remission rates of 60% to 80% for stage II to IV disease, with the long-term disease-free survival as predicted by the International Index. The intergroup trial in the U.S. compared CHOP (cyclophosphamide, doxorubicin, vincristine, and prednisone), m-BACOD (methotrexate, bleomycin, doxorubicin, cyclophosphamide, vincristine, and dexamethasone), ProMACE-CytaBOM (cyclophosphamide, doxorubicin, etoposide, prednisone, cytarabine, bleomycin, vincristine, methotrexate, and leucovorin), and MACOP-B (methotrexate, doxorubicin, cyclophosphamide, vincristine, bleomycin, and prednisone) and found no statistically significant difference in the 3-year disease-free survival. The mortality rates were higher in m-BACOD and MACOP-B. Trials are now under way comparing standard treatment with the incorporation of autologous bone marrow transplantation as primary treatment. Currently, CHOP is the reference standard of treatment for intermediate-grade non-Hodgkin lymphoma. The long-term complete remission rates are 30% to 86%.

Table 12-9.—Lymphoid Neoplasms Recognized by the International Lymphoma Study Group

---

B-cell neoplasms

I. Precursor B-cell neoplasm: precursor B-lymphoblastic leukemia/lymphoma

II. Peripheral B-cell neoplasms
  1. B-cell chronic lymphocytic leukemia/prolymphocytic leukemia/small lymphocytic lymphoma
  2. Lymphoplasmacytoid lymphoma/immunocytoma
  3. Mantle cell lymphoma
  4. Follicle center lymphoma, follicular
     Provisional cytologic grades: I (small cell), II (mixed small and large cell), III (large cell)
     Provisional subtype: diffuse, predominantly small cell type
  5. Marginal zone B-cell lymphoma
     Extranodal (MALT-type with or without monocytoid B cells)
  6. Provisional entity: Splenic marginal zone lymphoma (with or without villous lymphocytes)
  7. Hairy-cell leukemia
  8. Plasmacytoma/plasma cell myeloma
  9. Diffuse large B-cell lymphoma*
  10. Burkitt lymphoma
  11. Provisional entity: high-grade B-cell lymphoma, Burkitt-like*

T-cell and putative natural killer-cell neoplasms

I. Precursor T-cell neoplasm: precursor T-lymphoblastic lymphoma/leukemia

II. Peripheral T-cell and natural killer-cell neoplasms
  1. T-cell chronic lymphocytic leukemia/prolymphocytic leukemia
  2. Large granular lymphocytic leukemia (LGL)
     T-cell type
     NK-cell type
  3. Mycosis fungoides/Sézary syndrome
  4. Peripheral T-cell lymphomas, unspecified*
     Provisional cytologic categories: medium-sized cell, mixed medium and large cell, large cell, lymphoepithelioid cell
     Provisional subtype: hepatosplenic $\gamma\delta$ T-cell lymphoma
     Provisional subtype: subcutaneous panniculitic T-cell lymphoma
  5. Angioimmunoblastic T-cell lymphoma (AILD)
  6. Angiocentric lymphoma
  7. Intestinal T-cell lymphoma (with or without enteropathy associated)
  8. Adult T-cell lymphoma/leukemia (ATL/L)
  9. Anaplastic large-cell lymphoma (ALCL), CD30+, T and null-cell types
  10. Provisional entity: anaplastic large-cell lymphoma, Hodgkin-like

Hodgkin disease

I. Lymphocyte predominance

II. Nodular sclerosis

III. Mixed cellularity

IV. Lymphocyte depletion

V. Provisional entity: lymphocyte-rich classic Hodgkin disease

---

*These categories are thought likely to include more than one disease entity.

MALT, mucosa-associated lymphoid tissue.

From Harris NL, Jaffe ES, Stein H, Banks PM, Chan JKC, Cleary ML, Delsol G, De Wolf-Peeters C, Falini B, Gatter KC, Grogan TM, Isaacson PG, Knowles DM, Mason DY, Muller-Hermelink HK, Pileri SA, Piris MA, Ralfkiaer E, Warnké RA: A revised European-American classification of lymphoid neoplasms: a proposal from the International Lymphoma Study Group. Blood 84:1361-1392, 1994. By permission of American Society of Hematology.

In nonrandomized studies of patients with relapse who received very high doses of therapy and autologous bone marrow transplant, the overall cure rates have been reported to be 20%. In patients who had relapse after complete remission and who are sensitive to retreatment with standard chemotherapy regimens, the reported cure rates are 35% to 40%. An international study, the PARMA study, randomized patients who were initially in complete remission but subsequently in first or second relapse to DHAP (cis-platinum, cytosine arabinoside, and dexamethasone) chemotherapy or high-dose therapy followed by autologous bone marrow transplantation. Autologous bone marrow transplantion increased the event-free survival and the overall survival. Autologous bone marrow transplantation is considered the standard treatment of intermediate-grade and high-grade non-Hodgkin lymphoma in sensitive relapse. Currently, the role of autologous bone marrow transplantation as part of the initial management of the non-Hodgkin lymphomas is being evaluated in randomized studies.

Prognostic factors are important in lymphoma. The International Index is based on clinical pretreatment characteristics and the relative risk of death. Clinical features that were associated with survival included age ($\leq$60 versus >60 years), LDH (normal or greater), performance status (0,1 versus 2-4), stage (I/II versus III/IV), and extranodal involvement ($\leq$1 site versus >1 site). Patients were divided into different risk groups based on the number of risk factors, with predicted 5-year survivals in the low-risk group (with zero or one factor) of 73%; in the low-intermediate group (with two factors), 51%; in the high-intermediate group (with three factors), 43%; and in the high group (with four or five factors), 26%.

- Non-Hodgkin lymphomas are diverse.
- The Working Formulation for Clinical Usage was the most commonly used classification scheme.
- The REAL Classification is now the most commonly used classification scheme.
- The Ann Arbor Staging System has traditionally been used in lymphoma.
- Currently, the most predictive pretreatment characteristics for the risk of death are age, LDH, performance status, stage, and extranodal involvement (the International Prognostic Factor Index).
- Exceptions to the standard management programs in non-Hodgkin lymphoma include MALT, primary bone, isolated gastric, central nervous system, testicular, bowel, orbital, pulmonary, and cutaneous T- and B-cell lymphomas.
- Most patients with low-grade lymphoma are not curable but have a long survival time.
- Of patients with the histologic features of diffuse large cell advanced intermediate-grade non-Hodgkin lymphoma,

30%-40% are cured of their disease with anthracycline regimens. CHOP chemotherapy is the standard treatment of choice.
- Patients with HIV-related lymphoproliferative disorders with a CD4 count <200/mL response poorly to standard treatment.
- Low-grade lymphomas may transform into intermediate-grade and high-grade lymphomas.
- Lymphoblastic lymphoma and Burkitt lymphoma have a higher risk of central nervous system involvement and tumor lysis syndrome.
- Death rates in non-Hodgkin lymphoma have increased since 1973.

Monoclonal Gammopathies

The differential diagnosis of monoclonal gammopathies includes monoclonal gammopathies of undetermined significance (MGUS) and malignant monoclonal gammopathies. The malignant gammopathies include multiple myeloma (IgG, IgA, IgD, IgE, and free light chains): overt multiple myeloma, smoldering multiple myeloma, plasma cell leukemia, nonsecretory myeloma, osteosclerotic myeloma, plasmacytoma (solitary plasmacytoma of bone, extramedullary plasmacytoma), malignant lymphoproliferative diseases (Waldenström [primary] macroglobulinemia, malignant lymphoma), heavy chain diseases, and amyloidosis (primary, with myeloma).

Monoclonal Gammopathies of Undetermined Significance

In MGUS, the M-protein level is less than 3 g/dL in the serum, and there are less than 10% plasma cells in the bone marrow. The serum level of creatinine is normal, and either a small amount of M protein or no M protein occurs in the urine. The serum level of calcium is normal. There is no anemia and no osteolytic bone lesions. MGUS may be a precursor to multiple myeloma. Twenty-three percent of the patients may have progression to a malignant monoclonal gammopathy. Population-based studies have demonstrated that 1% of adults older than 50 and 3% of those older than 70 years have a monoclonal protein in the serum. Of monoclonal gammopathies, 60% are IgG, 20% are IgM, 10% are IgA, and 7% are free light chains. In most patients, serum protein electrophoresis should be followed initially at 6 months and then at 12-month intervals indefinitely if there is no progression or symptoms. Patients with MGUS should be observed. Unnecessary treatment can lead to the development of a myelodysplastic syndrome or acute leukemia.

- MGUS is the most common dysproteinemia.
- M-protein is $\leq$3 g/dL; <10% plasma cells in the bone marrow; normal hemoglobin, creatinine, and calcium.

- Asymptomatic.
- Stable M-protein measurements.
- Patients are observed safely with no chemotherapy.

Multiple Myeloma

Multiple myeloma is a result of the insidious accumulation in the marrow of neoplastic plasma cells that produce homogeneous immunoglobulin in the serum (85%) and/or in the urine. Osteoclast-activating activity due to exaggerated expression of specific cytokine results in osteolytic bone lesions. Interleukin-6 may be involved in the pathogenesis of myeloma. The median age of multiple myeloma is 65, and it is more common in males and African-Americans. In multiple myeloma, 10% or more plasma cells are found in the bone marrow (Plate 12-12). At least one of the following must be present: M protein in the serum greater than 3 g/dL, M protein in the urine, lytic bone lesions. Anemia, hypercalcemia, or increased creatinine level are present in variable numbers of patients.

Clinical features include bone pain (66% of patients), renal insufficiency (50%), hypercalcemia (30%), and weakness, fatigue, and spinal cord compression (5%). These patients are characteristically at higher risk for infections with encapsulated gram-positive organisms such as *Streptococcus pneumoniae*. The incidence of gram-negative infections and herpes zoster is also increased. The CBC resembles that of normochromic-normocytic anemia. Radiographs show punched-out lytic lesions, osteoporosis, and fractures.

A beta$_2$-microglobulin greater than 2.7 μg/mL and the bone marrow plasma cell labeling index of 0.8% or greater are adverse prognostic factors. If low, the median survival is 6 years. Patients with smoldering myeloma (M protein >3 g/dL, more than 10% plasma cells in the bone marrow, no lytic bone lesions, and no other manifestations of myeloma) should be observed.

Because multiple myeloma is not curable, treatment may be delayed until evidence of progression develops, the patient becomes symptomatic, or treatment is necessary to prevent imminent complications. The median overall survival in multiple myeloma is about 30 months. The standard treatment for patients older than 70 years is melphalan and prednisone given for 7 days every 6 weeks, with a 50% to 60% objective response rate. High-dose dexamethasone in combination with continuous infusion of vincristine and doxorubicin (VAD) is an effective regimen in the management of patients younger than 70 years that does not share the toxic effects of melphalan on stem cells. Palliative radiotherapy in a dose of 20 to 30 Gy is effective in the management of disabling focal pain. Current comparative trials are evaluating the roles of high-dose cyclophosphamide, autologous bone marrow or stem cell transplantation, or allogeneic bone marrow transplantation. The complete remission rates to autologous transplantation are 40%. Most patients have relapse. Fifty percent of patients have a response to erythropoietin. Studies have demonstrated that interferon alfa-2a or 2b recombinant is capable of prolonging the duration of remission in comparison with patients who have received no maintenance, but overall survival differences have not been demonstrated. Bisphosphonate therapy, such as pamidronate, delays the onset of skeleton-related events, reduces bone pain, and modestly extends survival. There is a potential survival benefit with autologous marrow or peripheral stem cell transplantation in patients with relapse.

- Plasma cells: <10% in monoclonal gammopathies of undetermined significance; >10% in myeloma.
- Serum M protein: <3 g/dL in monoclonal gammopathies of undetermined significance; usually >3 g/dL in myeloma.
- Multiple myeloma: usually has a urine M protein.
- Myeloma: bone pain (66% of patients), renal dysfunction (50%), hypercalcemia (30%), spinal cord compression (5%).
- Myeloma: punched-out lytic bone lesions, pneumococcal infection.
- Multiple myeloma patients are at increased risk for infections due to encapsulated organisms, which include *Streptococcus penumoniae*.
- Patients with good-risk disease including a plasma cell labelling index of 0.8% or less or beta$_2$-microglobulin of 2.7 μg/mL or less have a longer overall survival.

Solitary Plasmacytomas

Solitary plasmacytomas may occur without other evidence of multiple myeloma. These extramedullary lesions are potentially curable with radiation therapy.

- Severe back pain may be a manifestation of spinal cord compression, requiring immediate magnetic resonance imaging or computed tomography with dexamethasone, radiation therapy, and possible surgical decompression.

Waldenström Macroglobulinemia

Waldenström macroglobulinemia is characterized by an increase in the IgM paraprotein greater than 3.0 g/dL, lymphadenopathy, anemia, or hepatosplenomegaly. Retinal "sausage" formation may be present. In 20% to 40% of patients, bone marrow involvement with well-differentiated plasmacytoid lymphocytes occurs. Bence Jones proteinuria may be present in 80% of patients. Hyperviscosity syndrome occurs in 15% of patients. Other problems include cryoglobulinemia, sensorimotor peripheral neuropathy, cold agglutinin hemolytic anemia, and renal disease (nephrotic syndrome).

Many patients have only an IgM monoclonal gammopathy of undetermined significance, with no signs or symptoms, and should be monitored without initial treatment.

Hyperviscosity syndrome is characterized by fatigue, dizziness, blurred vision, bleeding from mucous membranes, sausage-shaped retinal veins, and papilledema. The plasma volume is expanded with an increase in serum viscosity. Because 80% of IgM is intravascular, plasmapheresis with albumin and saline replacement is the initial treatment of choice followed by chemotherapy. The disorder most commonly has been treated with chlorambucil (8 mg/m^2) and prednisone (40 mg/m^2 for 10 days at 6-week intervals); 60% of patients respond, with a median survival of 5 years. 2-Chlorodeoxyadenosine or fludarabine is the treatment of choice for patients who have not responded to chlorambucil and prednisone. These are also being evaluated in newly diagnosed patients.

- IgM paraprotein >3.0 g/dL.
- Hyperviscosity syndrome.
- Treatment of choice is chlorambucil, 2-chlorodeoxyadenosine, or fludarabine.

Amyloidosis

Amyloidosis is a group of diseases with extracellular deposition of pathologic insoluble fibrillar proteins, which stain with Congo red, in organs and tissues. The amyloid fibrils in primary amyloidosis are fragments of the variable portions of the immunoglobulin light chains. Patients with amyloidosis present with fatigue, weight loss, hepatomegaly, macroglossia, renal insufficiency, proteinuria, nephrotic syndrome, congestive heart failure, orthostatic hypotension, carpal tunnel syndrome, and peripheral neuropathy. Amyloidosis is classified as primary (90% of patients in U.S.), secondary (chronic infections, autoimmune disease), familial, associated with aging, localized (skin, bladder, etc.), amyloidosis of endocrine glands with medullary carcinoma, and amyloidosis with multiple endocrine neoplasia type II. The most common system involved in patients with primary amyloidosis is the kidney, followed by congestive heart failure secondary to an infiltrative cardiomyopathy (25%), carpal tunnel (20%), peripheral neuropathy, and orthostatic hypotension.

The diagnosis usually is first established by finding a monoclonal protein in the serum or urine. Bone marrow plasma cells are usually less than 20%, and there are no lytic bone lesions. Initial biopsies should include fat aspiration of the abdominal wall (80% positive), rectum (75%), or bone marrow (56%). Nearly 90% of patients with primary systemic amyloidosis have a detectable M protein in the serum or urine, which is lambda in two-thirds. This is the most important screening test when the diagnosis is expected. The bone marrow usually has plasma cells that have a clonal predominance of a light chain isotype. Four of 10 patients present with nephrotic syndrome, 1 in 6 with right-sided congestive heart failure that worsens with calcium channel blockers, and about 1 in 7 with a sensorimotor peripheral neuropathy. Unexplained hypercholesterolemia may be a manifestation of the nephrotic syndrome. The electrocardiogram may show low voltage or pattern of myocardial infarction. The echocardiogram is abnormal in 60% of patients with concentrically thickened ventricles. The neuropathy is progressive, painful, symmetrical, and demyelinating. Peripheral neuropathy is often associated with autonomic failure, as manifested by diarrhea, pseudo-obstruction, or orthostatic syncope. About 50% of patients with amyloid neuropathy have carpal tunnel syndrome. Other symptoms and signs include fatigue, weight loss, change in voice, macroglossia, submandibular swelling, and post-proctoscopic purpura. Acquired inhibitors for thrombin and factor X deficiency may occur.

The median survival of all patients with primary amyloidosis is 13 months: for those with overt congestive heart failure, less than 6 months; with nephrotic syndrome, 27 months; and with peripheral neuropathy, 42 months. The use of oral chemotherapy produces superior results to colchicine.

Treatment with melphalan and prednisone has a response rate of 18%. Treatment with high-dose intravenous melphalan with autologous blood stem cell support results in remission of both the plasma cell dyscrasia and clinical signs and symptoms in 50% to 65% of patients treated. Pathologic characteristics—Primary amyloidosis consists of the variable region of immunoglobulin light chains; secondary amyloidosis consists of protein A.

Acute Leukemias

The cause of acute leukemia is unknown in most cases, but there are many associations, including idiopathic aplastic anemia, paroxysmal nocturnal hemoglobinuria, myeloproliferative disorders, preleukemic syndromes, radiation, benzene, cytotoxic chemotherapy, Down syndrome, Fanconi syndrome, and ataxia-telangiectasia. The classic syndrome of patients who have been exposed to alkylating agents (melphalan, cyclophosphamide, chlorambucil) is pancytopenia in 10 to 36 months, with the chromosome abnormalities of monosomy 5 and 7. It is refractory to standard treatment regimens.

- Alkylating agents should be used in benign diseases, only with consideration of the risk of development of acute myelogenous leukemia, non-Hodgkin lymphoma, bladder cancer, and other solid tumors.
- Recently described secondary leukemias are those related to topoisomerase II inhibitor agents (etoposide).
- High incidence of neoplasms in Down syndrome, Fanconi syndrome, and ataxia-telangiectasia.

Acute Nonlymphocytic Leukemia (Acute Myelogenous Leukemia)

The median age of patients with acute nonlymphocytic leukemia (Plate 12-13) is 65 years. Fifty percent of patients have symptoms for more than 3 months. Good prognostic signs include age younger than 40 years; chromosome abnormalities of t(8,21), t(15,17), inversion 16, or normal chromosomes; and obtaining complete remission with one cycle of induction chemotherapy. Poor prognostic signs include age older than 40 years; preleukemic phase; the chromosome abnormalities of monosomy 5, monosomy 7, t(9,22), trisomy 8, 11q-, and complex cytogenetic patterns; and poor general physical condition or underlying health problems.

For patients who present with extreme leukocytosis (WBC $>100 \times 10^9/L$) with acute leukemia, the initial complication of most concern is cerebral hemorrhage. Emergency treatment includes hydration, alkalinization of urine, allopurinol (600 mg), hydroxyurea (6-8 g orally), cranial irradiation (4-6 Gy), and leukapheresis followed by the treatment of the specific type of leukemia.

- Acute nonlymphocytic leukemia: median age of patients is 65 years; 50% have symptoms >3 months.
- Good prognosis in patients <40 years old, chromosomal abnormalities t(8,21), t(15,17), inv16, or normal chromosomes, and obtaining complete remission with one cycle of induction chemotherapy.

Therapy—Platelet and red blood cell transfusions are required throughout the course of the treatment. Early empiric broad-spectrum antibiotic coverage for fevers is essential.

Induction chemotherapy cytarabine (cytosine arabinoside) with or without an anthracycline agent (daunorubicin or idarubicin). The complete remission rate is 70% to 75% in patients 60 years or younger and 35% to 50% for those older than 60 years, with the potential for cure in 20% of patients. Despite substantial recent advances, most patients with acute myelogenous leukemia eventually have relapse and most do so within 1 year. Of patients who have relapse after induction and consolidation therapy, 30% to 50% achieve a second remission. Remission rates are higher with idarubicin.

Trans-retinoic acid (ATRA)—M3 acute myelogenous leukemia (promyelocytic acute nonlymphocytic leukemia) (Plate 12-14) with a t(5,17) translocation. In a randomized trial by the Eastern Cooperative Oncology Group, trans-retinoic acid (ATRA, All-trans-retinoic acid) resulted in a 67% complete remission rate and more than 70% of patients who received ATRA at any time during treatment were free of relapse at 2.5 years versus 20% who never received ATRA therapy. These patients then need to be treated with cytarabine or a daunorubicin-type program. After remission is achieved, disease-free

survival is excellent, with 76% of patients surviving 6 years as compared with 12% in other acute nonlymphocytic leukemia studies. This is the first malignancy in which a chromosomal alteration has served as the target for induction chemotherapy. Ongoing studies are evaluating the postremission treatments of chemotherapy, autologous bone marrow transplantation, and allogeneic transplantation. The results are controversial but do not suggest a difference in randomized trials.

There are three types of postremission therapy. Maintenance therapy uses low doses of chemotherapy, which avoids severe bone marrow suppression. Consolidation therapy uses regimens similar to those used for induction therapy. Intensification therapy uses more intensive therapy than that used during remission induction. Postremission therapy includes chemotherapy and autologous and allogeneic transplantation. Low-dose combination Ara-C and 6-thioguanine are superior to no further treatment in prolonging disease-free survival after achievement of complete remission. High-dose cytarabine improves remission duration in patients younger than 60 years as compared with conventional-dose cytarabine with or without 6-thioguanine.

The following generalizations may be made about allogeneic bone marrow transplantation in acute nonlymphocytic leukemia. Generally, after 2 years of complete remission, the risk of relapse is lower. Transplantation in cases of relapse is age-dependent: patients younger than 30 years have a better prognosis than those older than 30. Allogeneic bone marrow transplantation in early relapse or in second remission is almost as efficacious as transplantation in first complete remission. Recommendations—If the patient is younger than 55 years, consider bone marrow transplant in first remission of HLA match with poor prognostic factors, including poor-risk cytogenetics and antecedent hematologic disease. In those patients without poor risk factors and not on study, perform transplantation in early relapse or second remission. Results—Currently, the disease-free survival at 5 years for patients undergoing allogeneic transplantation in first remission is 50%; in first relapse, 30%; and in second remission, 28%. Early results of autologous transplantation are encouraging.

Acute Lymphoblastic Leukemia

Acute lymphoblastic leukemia (Plate 12-15) is most common in children, with complete remission rates greater than 90% and with long-term disease-free survival of 60% to 70%. In adults, this leukemia is less common, with remission rates of up to 75%; however, most patients will have relapse. Of adult acute lymphocytic leukemia, 80% of cases are B cell in origin, 20% have T-cell markers, and 1% or 2% express surface immunoglobulin. Most B-cell leukemias express CD10, the common ALL antigen (cALLa). Early pre-B-acute lymphocytic leukemia patients are cALLa negative. Early pre-B acute lymphocytic leukemia is also known as "null acute lymphocytic leukemia." Clinical presentation—One-third of patients present with bleeding, and 25% have symptoms for more than 3 months. Bone pain, lymphadenopathy, splenomegaly, and hepatomegaly are more common in acute lymphoblastic leukemia than in acute nonlymphocytic leukemia. Splenomegaly, lymphadenopathy, and hepatomegaly occur in three-fourths of the patients (compared with one-half of patients with acute myelogenous leukemia).

Prognostic factors—The best prognosis is in children 3 to 10 years old. After the age of 20, survival time continues to decrease with increasing age and shorter complete remission durations. Poor prognostic factors include age, WBC count greater than 30×10^9/L, null cell phenotype, specific chromosome abnormalities, and achievement of remission after more than 4 weeks of intensive chemotherapy. Chromosomal abnormalities—80% to 90% of adults have chromosome abnormalities. Normal chromosomes have the best prognosis. The poorest prognosis is associated with t(9,22); t(4,11); t(8,14); and t(1,19). These patients have lower complete remission rates, shorter remission duration, and very poor survival. Also, t(9,22) has less than 15% survival at 5 years and is present in 25% of adults but in only 2% to 3% of children. Chromosome abnormalities are independent of age, WBC count, and immunophenotype.

Induction therapy consists of the following: the three agents commonly used include vincristine, prednisone, and anthracyclines along with one or more of the following: L-asparaginase, cytarabine, methotrexate, or cyclophosphamide. The complete remission rate is 70% to 90%. The addition of L-asparaginase, cytarabine, or cyclophosphamide may improve remission duration.

Intensification/postinduction therapy is commonly used. Long-term relapse-free survival of 10% to 42% in adults. The use of allogeneic bone marrow transplant in first complete remission results in a 21% to 71% disease-free survival at 2 to 10 years, with relapse rates of 10% to 40%. Trials are under way for evaluating autologous bone marrow transplants and matched unrelated transplants.

In relapse, allogeneic or autologous bone marrow transplants are of benefit in patients who achieve a second complete remission. After a second complete remission and then allogeneic transplant, the disease-free survival ranges from 26% to 54% at various time periods. At second complete remission and then autologous transplant, the disease-free survival ranges from 23% to 31% at various periods of time.

Recent results of unrelated allogeneic donor transplants reveal a 45% leukemia-free survival for patients in first remission, but there are significant logistical and age restrictions. Trials are under way evaluating autologous transplantation.

Indications for bone marrow transplantation include high-risk cytogenetic abnormalities in first remission and patients in second or subsequent remission.

Myelodysplastic Syndromes

Myelodysplastic disorders are characterized by dysplastic bone marrow hyperplasia associated with variable degrees of peripheral blood cytopenias with or without chromosome changes. They are typically heterogeneous and biologically diverse. Myelodysplastic syndromes, as classified by the French-American-British Group (with median survival time), are refractory anemia (26 months), refractory anemia with ringed sideroblasts (34 months), refractory anemia with excess blasts (9 months), refractory anemia with excess blasts in transformation (5 months), and chronic myelomonocytic leukemia (12 months). These disorders present with anemia and other cytopenias. These patients have been reported to have clonal karyotypic abnormalities, predominantly deletions as opposed to acute myelogenous leukemia, which has balanced translocations. Del(5q), del(20q), and –y are the only abnormalities that confer a favorable prognosis, and these patients frequently present with an anemia that requires transfusions. The most life-threatening complication is transformation to acute leukemia. This occurs in 12% of patients with refractory anemia, 8% with refractory anemia with ringed sideroblasts, 44% with refractory anemia with excess blasts, 14% with chronic myelomonocytic leukemia, and 60% with refractory anemia with excess blasts in transition. A significant proportion of patients die of cytopenic complications, most commonly leukopenia. The standard of care in most patients with this disorder is supportive, with RBC transfusions, erythropoietin, and antibiotics for infection. Patients younger than 55 years should be considered for allogeneic bone marrow transplantation if the patient has an HLA match and is younger than 55. New treatment approaches include 5-azacytidine and antithymocyte globulin.

Myeloproliferative Disorders

The myeloproliferative disorders include polycythemia rubra vera, agnogenic myeloid metaplasia, essential thrombocythemia, and chronic granulocytic leukemia. These are clonal processes with a multipotent stem origin that are clinically characterized by peripheral blood and bone marrow proliferation. Their characteristic features are given in Table 12-10. The myeloproliferative disorders are interrelated: polycythemia rubra vera converts to agnogenic myeloid metaplasia in 10% of cases. Essential thrombocythemia converts to agnogenic myeloid metaplasia in 5% of cases. Acute myelogenous leukemia is a complication of polycythemia rubra vera (10% of cases), essential thrombocythemia (>15%), agnogenic myeloid metaplasia (10%-20%), and chronic myelogenous

Table 12-10.—Characteristic Features of Chronic Myeloproliferative Disorders

Characteristic	Polycythemia rubra vera	Agnogenic myeloid metaplasia	Primary thrombocythemia	Chronic granulocytic leukemia
Increased red cell mass	Yes	No	No	No
Myelofibrosis	Later	Yes	Rare	Later
Thrombocytosis	Variable	Variable	Yes	Variable
bcr-abl Oncogene	No	No	No	Yes

From Petitt RM, Silverstein MN: Current clinical management of primary thrombocythemia. Contemp Intern Med Jan 1991, pp 46-52. By permission of Aegean Communications.

leukemia (70%-90%). In each of these disorders, there is a decrease in overall survival of patients compared with age-matched controls. There is also a risk of thrombosis and hemorrhagic complications, especially in polycythemia rubra vera and essential thrombocythemia.

- The myeloproliferative disorders are polycythemia rubra vera, agnogenic myeloid metaplasia, essential thrombocythemia, and chronic granulocytic leukemia.
- Myeloproliferative disorders are interrelated.

Chronic Myelogenous Leukemia (Chronic Granulocytic Leukemia)

Chronic myelogenous leukemia constitutes 20% of all leukemias and is characterized by an acquired defect of clonal origin at the pluripotential cell level. There is a pool of granulocyte precursors with the capacity for normal maturation (Plate 12-16). The Philadelphia chromosome, t(9,22), is the hallmark of this disease in 95% of cases. The translocation results in the fusion of RNA and a protein, a chimeric *bcr-abl*, which can be demonstrated with fluorescence in-situ hybridization (FISH). The hyperproliferation of the *bcr-abl* clone results in production of an upregulated tyrosine kinase. There is expansion of the myeloid compartment and suppression of normal hematopoiesis. New chromosomal abnormalities appear and reappear. The diseases are preleukemic and terminate in a maturation block or blast crisis. Different cell types can be seen, including myeloblasts (50%-60% of patients), megakaryoblasts (15%), B lymphoblasts, erythroblasts (10%), monoblasts, myelomonocytic blasts, and basophilic blasts.

Before the advent of allogeneic bone marrow transplantation and interferon alfa-2a or 2b recombinant, the median survival was 3.5 years after diagnosis. Prognostic factors are different in multiple series. In one study, a good prognosis (61-month median survival versus 34 months) was associated with a spleen size of 0 to 6 cm and 0% to 10% circulating blasts. A poor prognosis was associated with an age older than 45 years and a platelet count greater than 700 x 10^9/L. The

presence of chromosome abnormalities other than t(9,22) is an adverse prognostic factor. The chronic phase is characterized by fewer than 10% blasts in blood and bone marrow and is typically of 2 to 3 years' duration.

Symptoms include malaise, dyspnea, anorexia, fever, night sweats, weight loss, abdominal fullness, easy bruising, bleeding, gout, priapism, and hypermetabolism. Splenomegaly is present in 85% of patients.

Laboratory findings are characterized by the following: Leukocytosis with fewer than 10% blasts in the chronic phase of disease and WBC count of 100,000 are common. Granulocytes in all stages of maturation are present on peripheral blood smear, with basophilia and eosinophilia. The number of platelets is increased, with large bizarre forms present on peripheral blood smears. The hemoglobin concentration ranges from 9 to 12 g/dL. The leukocyte alkaline phosphatase score is low or absent. The differential diagnosis of a low or absent leukocyte alkaline phosphatase score includes paroxysmal nocturnal hemoglobinuria, infectious mononucleosis, and aplastic anemia. The vitamin B_{12} level is increased because of increased transcobalamin I. Other findings include pseudohyperkalemia, pseudohypoglycemia, and false-positive increase in acid phosphatase in the serum. The bone marrow is hyperplastic, with myelofibrosis in 10% to 40% of patients.

- Chronic myelogenous leukemia: acquired defect of clonal origin.
- Philadelphia chromosome, t(9,22), is the hallmark of the disease.
- Increased WBC count; granulocytes in all stages of maturation.
- Bone marrow shows hyperplasia; myelofibrosis in 10%-40% of patients.
- The leukocyte alkaline phosphatase score is low or absent in chronic myelogenous leukemia, paroxysmal nocturnal hemoglobinuria, infectious mononucleosis, and aplastic anemia.
- Increased vitamin B_{12}; increased acid phosphatase.

Treatment—Conventional chemotherapy has not appreciably prolonged survival. There is little evidence that any patient has been cured with conventional therapy, including hydroxyurea and multiagent regimens. The three agents used in the initial treatment of chronic myelogenous leukemia are hydroxyurea, busulfan, and interferon alfa-2a or 2b recombinant. Hydroxyurea was used more commonly, with response rates of 85% to 90%. One study demonstrated that both overall and post-transplant survival are inferior for patients treated with busulfan as compared with hydroxyurea. Hydroxyurea is the treatment of choice for high blast counts and leukostasis lesions, and it is safe in thrombocytopenia. Moreover, it has fewer side effects than busulfan. Recovery from leukopenia or thrombocytopenia after an overshoot is more rapid than with busulfan. Continued maintenance therapy is necessary. Megaloblastic RBCs appear in the peripheral blood. Hydroxyurea should be used in all patients who are considered candidates for bone marrow transplantation, because of the risk of interstitial pneumonitis and veno-occlusive disease with busulfan. The dose of busulfan must be reduced by 50% at a WBC count of 20,000, and its use must be stopped when the WBC count reaches 10,000 to 12,000. Other side effects of busulfan include thrombocytopenia, leukopenia, prolonged bone marrow myelosuppression, increased skin pigmentation, pulmonary toxicity, amenorrhea, germinal cell atrophy, fetal malformations, veno-occlusive disease of liver, and a wasting syndrome.

Interferon alfa-2a or 2b recombinant suppresses the Philadelphia chromosome. Hematologic responses are 40% to 80%, with cytogenetic remissions in the range of 10% to 40%. The median survival is more than 60 months. Prospective randomized trials have demonstrated an improvement in survival and duration of remission in patients treated with interferon alfa-2a or 2b recombinant in comparison with hydroxyurea. The addition of cytarabine to interferon has been reported to improve survival and cytogenetic responses.

The treatment of "blast crisis" includes allopurinol, fluids, hydroxyurea, cranial radiation, and leukocyte apheresis.

- Accelerated phase at 30-36 months; the chronic phase converts to an accelerated or blast phase (75%), which is characterized by blast counts >20%; increase in anemia, thrombocytopenia, basophilia, and leukocyte alkaline phosphatase score; splenomegaly; lymphadenopathy; bone pain; cerebral hemorrhage; fever; headache; and myelofibrosis. Cytogenetic abnormalities precede condition by 6 months.
- If treated with busulfan or hydroxyurea, 10%-15% of patients die in the first year and about 26% per year thereafter.
- Toxicity of busulfan: prolonged myelosuppression, pulmonary toxicity, veno-occlusive disease of the liver.

- Interferon alfa-2a or 2b recombinant suppresses the Philadelphia chromosome and improves survival.
- Intensive treatment with induction chemotherapy in patients with chronic granulocytic leukemia does not postpone or prevent blast crisis or appreciably improve survival.

The only curative regimen to date is high-dose chemotherapy with total body irradiation followed by transplantation of allogeneic bone marrow from HLA-compatible siblings. Allogeneic bone marrow transplantation should be performed in the chronic phase, within the first 12 months in young patients who have an HLA-identical match or an identical twin. Hematologic relapse occurs in 10% to 20% of patients receiving a transplant in the chronic phase. The long-term disease-free survival rates are 40% to 60%.

- Currently, the only curative regimen is HLA-compatible allogeneic bone marrow transplantation.

Because only 15% of all new cases of chronic myelogenous leukemia have an HLA sibling donor, studies are evaluating HLA-matched unrelated volunteer donor bone marrow transplantation protocols and autologous bone marrow transplantation studies. Autologous bone marrow transplantation can improve survival, but there is no evidence of cure.

Agnogenic Myeloid Metaplasia

Splenomegaly occurs in 100% of the patients and is the hallmark of agnogenic myeloid metaplasia. Other features are leukoerythroblastic peripheral blood smear (96% of patients), teardrop cells, and hypocellular marrow (85%) (Plate 12-17). The basic event is the fibroblastic proliferation in bone marrow. Anemia may be caused by expanded plasma volume, ineffective erythropoiesis, blood loss, or hemolysis.

The bone marrow reveals panhyperplasia with modest fibrosis to osteosclerosis. The spleen is pathologically characterized by extramedullary hematopoiesis in the sinusoids of red pulp. Hepatomegaly may occur in 70% of patients because of engorgement by blood, extramedullary hematopoiesis, or hemosiderosis.

- The median survival approaches 5 years.
- Agnogenic myeloid metaplasia: splenomegaly is its hallmark.
- Leukoerythroblastic peripheral blood smear in 96% of patients.
- Teardrop cells.
- Basic event: fibroblastic proliferation of bone marrow.

Treatment—Observe the 20% of asymptomatic patients (80% will remain asymptomatic at 5 years). Medical therapy for anemia with symptoms includes transfusion with packed RBCs if RBC mass is low. Androgens (oxymetholone 50 mg tid or danazol) and prednisone 40 mg/day improve anemia in one-third to one-half of patients. Corticosteroids may be of benefit in one-third of patients with hemolysis or thrombocytopenia. In the evaluation of anemia, check stool for occult blood loss due to esophageal varices and microinfarcts of the gut, and treat vitamin B_{12} and folate deficiency if indicated.

Pressure symptoms occur in 23% of patients and may be managed with hydroxyurea or splenic irradiation. Hydroxyurea is indicated with symptomatic hepatosplenomegaly, leukocytosis, and thrombocytosis.

Bleeding with or without thrombocytopenia is managed with platelet transfusions.

Treat disseminated intravascular coagulopathy appropriately if present (may be present in up to 40% of patients).

Splenectomy may be of benefit in major hemolysis, pressure symptoms, life-threatening thrombocytopenia, portal hypertension, and refractory thrombocytopenia. Splenectomy is contraindicated in disseminated intravascular coagulopathy. Bone marrow transplantation may be helpful in some patients.

The prognosis is good if the patient is asymptomatic, hemoglobin concentration is greater than 10, platelet count is greater than 100,000, and the liver is less than 5 cm below the costal margin.

Essential Thrombocythemia (Primary Thrombocythemia)

Essential thrombocythemia is a clonal hematologic disorder in which patients present with asymptomatic thrombocytosis, thrombotic disorders, or hemorrhage. The median survival is more than 10 years, with about 75% of patients alive at 5 years. The overall risk of bleeding is 3% and of thrombosis, 20%. The risk factors include age, previous thrombosis, and short remission. The risk of acute leukemic transformation is less than 2%.

Diagnosis—Platelet count is greater than 600 x 10^9/L; megakaryocytic hyperplasia in the bone marrow; splenomegaly; absence of the Philadelphia chromosome, which is a translocation between chromosome 9 and 22 or M*bcr* rearrangement (100% of patients); normal RBC mass (100%); no collagen fibrosis and stainable iron in the bone marrow. Also, there is no other secondary cause of thrombocytosis, including acute or chronic inflammatory disease; acute or chronic bleeding; iron deficiency; chronic bone marrow stimulation (e.g., hemolysis); rebound after thrombocytopenia; disseminated malignancy; splenectomy, congenital asplenia, or functional hyposplenism; postoperative state; and intense exercise, parturition, trauma, and epinephrine. An increased C-reactive protein level in patients with thrombocytosis suggests a reactive process.

Treatment—Platelet apheresis should be used in the emergent management of acute bleeding or thrombosis. Treatment of patients younger than 30 years is controversial. These patients may be observed if there are no hemorrhagic or thrombotic problems, no significant trauma, and no emergency or elective surgery. Platelet apheresis is indicated in cases of elective surgery for patients of any age and in pregnant women during the course of delivery. Treatment is recommended for patients with thrombotic symptoms, a previous history of thrombotic events, cardiovascular risk factors, and those older than 60 years who have a platelet count greater than 600 x 10^9/L. Currently, hydroxyurea is the treatment of choice for most patients. Anagrelide is a therapeutic alternative. Patients who are asymptomatic and have a platelet count less than 600 x 10^9/L and asymptomatic and of childbearing age may be observed. Chronic treatments available for the management of essential thrombocythemia include hydroxyurea; anagrelide; antiaggregating agents for mild thrombotic symptoms, including aspirin and dipyridamole; radioactive phosphorus at a dose of 2.7 mCi/m^2; and interferon alfa-2a or 2b recombinant.

Erythrocytosis

An increased hematocrit due to a reduced plasma cell volume and normal RBC mass is "relative polycythemia." Absolute erythrocytosis is almost always present with a hemoglobin concentration in males of 18 g/dL and in females, 16.5 g/dL. The history, physical examination, CBC, arterial blood gases, leukocyte alkaline phosphatase score, and the marrow can determine the diagnosis of polycythemia in a high percentage of patients, as shown in Table 12-11.

The differential diagnosis of erythrocytosis with a normal oxygen saturation value and normal leukocyte alkaline phosphatase score includes the following: hypernephroma, renal adenoma, hydronephrosis, renal cyst, transplantation, Bartter syndrome, cerebellar hemangioblastoma, adrenal cortical adenoma or hyperplasia, ovarian carcinoma, hepatoma, pheochromocytoma, uterine fibroids, and hemoglobinopathies. Administration of erythropoietin to healthy persons may cause erythrocytosis. Patients with unexplained erythrocytosis should have intravenous pyelography or computed tomography (CT) of the abdomen to exclude hypernephroma.

- Polycythemia rubra vera: very low erythropoietin.
- Cerebral blood flow decreases at a hematocrit of >46.
- Smoking 1.5 packs of cigarettes per day can raise hematocrit to 60% (check carboxyhemoglobin).
- RBC mass returns to normal when smoking is stopped.

Polycythemia Rubra Vera

Clinical features include postbathing pruritus, weakness, erythromelalgia, acral dysesthesias, erythema, headache,

Table 12-11.—Differential Diagnosis of Erythrocytosis

	Polycythemia rubra vera	Apparent or stress erythrocytosis	Anoxic polycythemia	Tumor
History	Multiple symptoms	Nervousness Hypertension Obesity	High-altitude COPD Fibrosis Congenital heart disease Sleep apnea Hemoglobinopathy	
Gout	Occasionally	Occasionally		
Other history	Postbathing pruritus[*]			
Examination	Plethora skin, mucous membrane	±Plethora	Cyanosis	No cyanosis, clubbing, or COPD
	Distention of retinal vein		Clubbing[*]	Mass in left upper quadrant
	Hepatomegaly (50%) Splenomegaly (75%);[*] not others			
Laboratory				
Oxygen saturation	Normal	Normal	<88% (±88%-92%)[*]	Normal
LAP score	+++ (almost invariably)[*]	Normal	Normal	Normal
Red blood cell mass	++	Normal	+ to ++	+ to ++
Plasma volume	Normal or slightly increased	Reduced	Normal	Normal
Excretory urogram	Normal	Normal	Normal	Tumor
Erythrocyte sedimentation rate	0-1[*]	Normal	Normal, low	
Bone marrow	Pancytosis	Erythrocytosis	Erythrocytosis	Erythrocytosis
Platelets	+ to ++ (50%)	Normal	Normal	± Normal

COPD, chronic obstructive pulmonary disease; LAP, leukocyte alkaline phosphatase.
[*]Most important differentiating factors.
Modified from Dameshek W: Comments on the diagnosis of polycythemia vera. Semin Hematol 3:214-215, 1966. By permission of WB Saunders Company.

dizziness, weight loss, joint symptoms, dyspnea, and epigastric distress. Classification: category A, increased RBC mass, splenomegaly, normal arterial oxygen saturation; category B, platelet count greater than 400×10^9/L, WBC greater than 12×10^9/L (no fever or infection), leukocyte alkaline phosphatase score higher than 100, serum level of vitamin B_{12} greater than 900 ng/L. The presence of all three criteria in category A establishes the diagnosis. If the patient has increased RBC mass (category A) with either of the other two category A criteria, then two of the four category B criteria are necessary to establish the diagnosis. Unfavorable prognostic signs are previous thrombotic disease, age older than 60 years, diabetes mellitus, vascular diseases, and hypertension.

Bone marrow is normal in up to 10% of patients; 90% to 95% have absent iron stores in the bone marrow even if not phlebotomized. Cytogenetic abnormalities are present in 11%. The erythropoietin (epo) level is low or normal, and increased levels are unusual. The Philadelphia chromosome in the bone marrow is negative. Morphologically, the bone marrow may resemble chronic myelogenous leukemia in 10% to 40% of patients. The leukocyte alkaline phosphatase score is increased.

● The leukocyte alkaline phosphatase score may be increased in polycythemia rubra vera, leukemoid reactions, agnogenic myeloid metaplasia, idiopathic thrombocytopenic purpura, pregnancy, pyogenic infections, and stress erythrocytosis.

● Think of polycythemia rubra vera with microcytosis, absent iron stores, and splenomegaly. Other features include postbathing puritus, unusual thrombosis, and erythromelalgia.

- Laboratory evaluation for polycythemia rubra vera: previous results to document interval change, erythropoietin level, and bone marrow evaluation.
- Erythropoietin is increased in secondary erythrocytosis.

Treatment in patients who are asymptomatic is phlebotomy to maintain the hematocrit from below 42 to 45. Patients are phlebotomized every 2 to 4 months, because there is 250 mg of iron in 1 pint of blood. If the normal daily absorption is 4 mg, then phlebotomizing every 2 months will maintain the hematocrit in an appropriate range. A phlebotomy program starts at 500 mL every other day for 3 to 6 phlebotomies and the goal is to maintain the hematocrit at 42 to 45. In the elderly, start phlebotomies at 250 mL. There is a risk of thrombosis in older patients with vascular lesions, with the rate and volume of phlebotomy, and in patients with a history of thrombosis. In patients with asymptomatic thrombocytosis, anagrelide decreases the platelet count in 96% of those treated. Other agents available include hydroxyurea and interferon alfa-2a or 2b recombinant.

In patients who are symptomatic or who are at risk for thrombosis, hydroxyurea, anagrelide, and ^{32}P are the treatment approaches. Hydroxyurea is the treatment of choice. All patients 60 years and younger with cardiovascular risk factors or a previous history of thrombosis should be considered for treatment. With ^{32}P, the number of platelets decreases in 2 weeks and the number of RBCs decreases in 1 month. This treatment is indicated for patients older than 60, because of the 2.3-fold risk of acute nonlymphocytic leukemia in younger patients treated with ^{32}P. Chlorambucil is not indicated because of a 5.3-fold risk of developing acute nonlymphocytic leukemia when compared with phlebotomy.

- Sequence of ordering tests in erythrocytosis—If the hematocrit is greater than 58% in males or more than 52% in females, then proceed with an erythrocytosis evaluation. If the arterial oxygen saturation is greater than 92%, then check carboxyhemoglobin (smoker's polycythemia). If the arterial blood gases are normal, measure the erythropoietin level. Determining the RBC mass and plasma volume may aid in diagnosis, especially in the more difficult cases.

Oncogenesis

Environmental influences, viruses, and genetic predisposition affect proto-oncogenes and tumor suppressor genes, resulting in aberrations in proliferation, differentiation, and apoptosis. The hallmark of neoplastic disease is clonal proliferation of cells. Balanced reciprocal translocations affect specific sites on the genome. The consequences of these translocations are transcriptional deregulation. The series of events

induce DNA damage that have the potential to affect neoplastic transformation of cells. Alkylating agents and radiation involve activation of many of the same cellular oncogenes that are homologous to the oncogenes carried by retroviruses. Many oncogenes have been shown to be associated with specific chromosomal breakpoints or translocations (Table 12-12). Therefore, a silent oncogene can come to be involved at an active chromosomal site, resulting in unregulated expression (cell division) or expression of an inappropriate cell type (cell differentiation). Also, there are proteins that convert an extracellular signal into an intracellular biochemical event, leading to a neoplastic event such as epidermal growth factor. Oncogenesis is likely a multistep process. Principles of malignancy include prolongation of cellular life span, tumor promoters, and genetic instability.

In diseases with oncogene-related viral-induced transformation, viral gene sequences encode a product thought to activate transcription of many different cellular genes. Examples include HTLV-I, causative agent in adult T-cell leukemia; HTLV-II, associated with one T-cell hairy cell leukemia line; and Epstein-Barr virus infection in Burkitt lymphoma, nasopharyngeal carcinoma, Hodgkin disease, and post-transplantation lymphoproliferative disorders. Oncogene activation may occur with rearrangements of an oncogene, mutation of an oncogene, or through altered expression of an oncogene.

- Oncogenes are gene loci with the potential to affect neoplastic transformation of cells.
- Viral associations with hematologic malignancies: HTLV-I in adult T-cell leukemia; Epstein-Barr virus in Burkitt lymphoma, Hodgkin disease, and post-transplantation lymphoproliferative disorders.
- Many oncogenes are associated with chromosomal breakpoints or translocations.

COAGULATION

Prolonged Bleeding Time

The coagulation mechanism does not participate in the bleeding time. An abnormal bleeding time is a reflection of vascular defects, quantitative disorders of platelets (including thrombocytopenia and thrombocytosis), or functional disorders of platelets. Qualitative platelet defects result in an abnormal bleeding time but normal partial thromboplastin time, prothrombin time, thrombin time, and platelet count (except von Willebrand disease and disseminated intravascular coagulopathy).

- Prolonged bleeding time differential diagnosis includes Glanzmann thrombasthenia, von Willebrand disease,

Table 12-12.—Chromosome Rearrangement and Increase of Specific Oncogenes

Disease	Rearrangement	Oncogene	Gene product
Burkitt lymphoma	t(8,14)	c-*myc*	Cell cycle progression
	t(8,22)		Translocation into transcriptionally active immuno-globulin heavy or light chain loci
Chronic myelogenous leukemia	t(9,22)	c-*abl*	Tyrosine kinase
Follicular small cleaved cell lymphoma	t(14,18)	*bcl*-2	Anti-apoptosis
Diffuse large cell non-Hodgkin lymphoma	---	*bcl*-6	Transcriptional repression
Mantle cell lymphoma	t(11,14)	*bcl*-1	Overexpression of PRAD-1 Increase in cyclin D1

Bernard-Soulier syndrome, disseminated intravascular coagulopathy, thrombocytopenia, storage pool disease, drugs (aspirin, etc.), and uremia.

von Willebrand disease

von Willebrand disease is the most common inherited bleeding disorder; numerous subtypes have been described. In most subtypes of von Willebrand disease, the inheritance pattern is autosomal dominant with incomplete penetrance (parent of either sex). The bleeding is usually mild, but hemorrhage postoperatively can be severe. The most common bleeding symptoms are epistaxis, skin ecchymoses, cutaneous hematomas, prolonged bleeding from trivial wounds, oral cavity bleeding, bleeding from tooth extractions, and menorrhagia. Severe hemorrhage after surgery is less common. Bleeding may be exacerbated by aspirin. Hemarthroses are rare.

To understand von Willebrand disease, it is helpful to review platelet activity. The steps are platelet attachment, followed first by platelet adhesion and then by platelet aggregation. Collagen and factor VIII-related antigen are involved in adhesion. Factor VIII-related antigen is found in plasma, platelets, and endothelial regions and is detected functionally by its ability to cause aggregation of washed platelets when ristocetin is administered. Aggregation requires ADP and thromboxane A_2. The activation of the clotting mechanism and generation of thrombin seem to result from the activation of the platelet membrane during adhesion and aggregation. Platelets make available platelet factor III and catalyze the activation of other coagulation factors. von Willebrand factor (vWF) is a multimeric protein that circulates in blood plasma and is stored in endothelial cells and platelets. The factor VIII complex is composed of the following: 1) VIII:C, the coagulant activity which is missing in hemophiliac plasma; this is decreased in hemophilia and von Willebrand disease and circulates in the plasma with von Willebrand factor VIII (VIII vWF). 2) VIII C:Ag, antigenic determinants of VIII:C; this is decreased in von Willebrand disease and is normal in hemophilia. 3) VIII vWF antigen (vWF:Ag); vWF is a carrier protein for VIII:C, protecting it from rapid proteolytic destruction, and is the mediator of the initial platelet adhesion to the blood vessel wall. The adhesive function is contained largely within large multimers. 4) VIII vWF activity: ristocetin cofactor, the activity necessary for ristocetin-induced platelet aggregation that is not present in von Willebrand disease. The ristocetin cofactor is the closest measurement of vWF. 5) VIII R:Ag, antigenic determinant of VIII R:vWF and/or VIII R:RCo; factor VIII-related antigen is important in adherence, and it is likely that the activities of VIII R:vWF and VIII R:RCo are properties of this protein. All platelet-related activities of the VIII molecule are referred to as "vWF." vWF plays an essential role in the adhesion of platelets to the subendothelium. Factor VIII coagulant activity and vWF activity reside in two separate molecules that are noncovalently bound in the plasma. Therefore, von Willebrand disease represents a defect in hemostasis involving the interaction of the platelet membrane glycoprotein, subendothelial tissues, and vWF. There is either decreased synthesis, decreased release, or abdominal production of vWF. Defects in vWF may cause bleeding because platelets cannot adhere to sites of vascular injury.

The many distinct variants can be divided into three different subtypes. The classification is intended to reflect differences in the von Willebrand phenotype. Type 1 von Willebrand disease is characterized by a partial deficiency of vWF, type 2 is characterized by a qualitative deficiency in vWF, and type 3 by a complete deficiency in vWF. This classification is intended to reflect differences in the pathophysiology of the von Willebrand disease phenotypes. Type 1 is characterized by a quantitative abnormality in vWF, accounting for 70% of patients. It is the most common type and is autosomal dominant in inheritance pattern. The total amount of circulating vWF multimers are 50% or less. The distribution and function of vWF are normal. The definitive diagnosis of type 1 von Willebrand disease requires documentation of bleeding, low levels of qualitatively normal vWF, and inheritance. Patients who do not meet all three criteria may have a possible von Willebrand type 1 disease. The broad normal ranges for vWF levels and the variation in levels over time may complicate the diagnosis of vWF type 1. Type 2 (A, B, M, and N) is characterized by a qualitative dysfunctional abnormality in vWF. In type 3 von Willebrand disease, there is virtually no detectable von Willebrand protein. Heterozygous von Willebrand disease (1% of the population) is characterized clinically by mild to moderate bleeding. It is autosomal dominant in inheritance pattern. The laboratory diagnosis of von Willebrand disease includes abnormal activated partial thromboplastin time (APTT) and prothrombin time (PT), prolonged bleeding time, reduced VIII:C, VIII vWF antigen (vWF:Ag), vWF activity (ristocetin-cofactor activity), normal platelet aggregation except in the presence of ristocetin, and a mildly prolonged partial thromboplastin time.

- vWF has two functions in hemostasis: adhesion and aggregation of platelets and the transportation and stabilization of VIII:C in the plasma.
- The tests for the diagnosis and exclusion of von Willebrand disease are: VIII vWF antigen and ristocetin cofactor activity (vWF:RCo).
- Supplementary tests that may be needed for the type of von Willebrand disease: activated partial thromboplastin time, bleeding time, platelet count, vWF multimer analysis, and ristocetin-induced platelet aggregation response.

Treatment—The goal of treatment is to correct the coagulant defect, the result of the subnormal VIII:C levels. Restoration of VIII:C levels results in control of hemorrhage in the absence of a consistent correction of the bleeding time. Mild and moderate cases of von Willebrand disease require treatment only at the time of an operation or bleeding. For menorrhagia, birth control pills are effective. For dental extractions, local hemostasis and local fibrinolytic agents are effective. In pregnancy, there is no need to transfuse in mild to moderate cases of the disease, because the levels of vWF increase with the duration of pregnancy. The mainstays of treatment are 1-desamino-8-D-arginine vasopressin (DDAVP) and factor VIII concentrates rich in vWF. DDAVP causes the release of preformed vWF multimers from the subendothelium and is useful in type 1 von Willebrand disease. Side effects include facial flushing, headache, mild decrease in blood pressure, mild tachycardia, and hyponatremia. Repeated doses at intervals of less than 24 hours may result in a decrease or loss of response (tachyphylaxis). DDAVP may be delivered intranasally, subcutaneously, or intravenously. A trial should be conducted before it is used as primary therapy. The levels increase for 4 to 8 hours. This usually is effective only in type 1 von Willebrand disease. For patients with type 2B and 3 von Willebrand disease or for those with type 1 disease who have become transiently unresponsive to DDAVP, viral-inactivated factor VIII preparations rich in high molecular weight multimer vWF are recommended. Humate-P (antihemophilic factor [human], pasteurized) is being evaluated. Cryoprecipitate from carefully selected and repeatedly tested donors is more desirable than cryoprecipitate from random donors.

Glanzmann Thrombasthenia

Glanzmann thrombasthenia results from a defect in the first phase of platelet aggregation, secondary to marked reduction or absent platelet glycoproteins IIb and IIIa. It is autosomal recessive in inheritance pattern. Early hemorrhagic complications occur in the neonatal period, and epistaxis, purpura, petechiae, and ecchymoses persist throughout life. The laboratory findings include no clumping of platelets on the peripheral blood smear, normal platelet number and morphology, and no aggregation with ADP, epinephrine, thrombin, or collagen. There is aggregation with ristocetin/factor VIII R:vWF. Treatment consists of nasal packing, local measures, and cryoprecipitate, with or without platelets, when local measures are not successful.

Bernard-Soulier Syndrome

Bernard-Soulier syndrome is the result of the absence of glycoprotein Ib/IX complexes on the surface of human platelets that mediate ristocetin-induced vWF-dependent platelet aggregation. Glycoprotein Ib/IX is the platelet receptor for vWF. These platelets are unable to react with subendothelial vWF. It is more common in whites and blacks and is autosomal recessive in inheritance pattern. This disorder is characterized by moderate to severe bleeding with surgery and menstruation. Bleeding typically is from mucous membranes, the gums, and the gastrointestinal tract. The bleeding time is markedly prolonged. Characteristically, there is thrombocytopenia with giant platelets. The aggregation pattern is the opposite of that of Glanzmann thrombasthenia with normal platelet aggregation with ADP, collagen, epinephrine, and thrombin but no aggregation with ristocetin. There is no specific treatment for

Bernard-Soulier syndrome other than local measures and platelets.

Storage Pool Disease

Normally, ATP, ADP, serotonin, and calcium are stored by platelets and released from them. In storage pool disease, there is a marked decrease in platelet ADP and a lesser decrease in ATP. Because of the profound decrease in ADP, the amount released from the platelets is insufficient to bring uninvolved platelets into larger aggregates.

Disseminated Intravascular Coagulopathy

Disseminated intravascular coagulopathy is characterized by a dynamic process caused by many diseases with microvascular clotting secondary to thrombin deposition. The laboratory findings are variable. No single laboratory test can confirm or exclude the diagnosis, which depends on the clinical setting and laboratory findings. The manifestations vary from patient to patient and from time to time in the same patient. These may be of little clinical significance or cause life-threatening bleeding or clotting. The mortality rates of severe disseminated coagulopathy range from 50% to 85%.

The pathophysiology of disseminated intravascular coagulopathy is complex. Thrombin is formed in the vascular system and alters platelets. The platelets aggregate, agglutinate, and secrete many products, resulting in thrombocytopenia and platelets that do not function well. Plasmin circulates systematically degrading fibrin and fibrinogen, creating the D-dimer and X, Y, D, and E fragments known as "fibrinogen degradation products." Thrombin cleaves fibrinopeptides A and B from fibrinogen to form fibrin monomers. These monomers may complex with fibrinogen (polymerization) to form insoluble fibrin, which is deposited in capillaries and small blood vessels, resulting in microangiopathy. Activated factor XIII cross-links fibrin to make it more resistant to fibrinolysis. Thrombin increases the activity of factors V and VIII. Therefore, thrombin accounts for the decreased fibrinogen, platelets, and factors II, V, VIII, and XIII. Secondary fibrinolysis may occur. Bleeding occurs because the coagulation factors are depleted or fibrinolysis with vessel damage results in decreased control proteins, such as antithrombin III and protein C. Activated factor XII leads to kallikrein production, resulting in the conversion of plasminogen to plasmin, which is capable of digesting fibrinogen, clotting factors, and complement. The clinical picture depends on a balance: if thrombin activity is greater than plasmin activity, there is thrombosis; or, if plasmin activity is greater than thrombin activity, there is hemorrhage.

The following occur in acute disseminated intravascular coagulopathy: bleeding from wounds and perivenipuncture sites, ecchymoses, petechiae, hematomas, hematuria, intracranial hemorrhage, intrapleural hemorrhage, intraperitoneal hemorrhage, hemoptysis, vaginal melena, and hematemesis. Thromboembolic complications, as manifested by necrotic skin lesions, pulmonary emboli, acute arterial occlusions, ischemia, stroke, and myocardial infarction, may occur in 8% of patients. Thrombosis is more common than bleeding in chronic disseminated intravascular coagulopathy.

Causes—Malignancies are the most common cause: prostate, breast, lung, leukemia (acute progranulocytic [M3]), pancreas, and lymphoma. Infections are the second most common cause (gram-negative and gram-positive organisms, e.g., *Staphylococcus*, *Streptococcus*, pneumococcus, typhoid, *Rickettsia*, viral, fungal, histoplasmosis, *Aspergillus*). Surgery/trauma is the third leading cause. Other causes are liver disease, pregnancy, acute renal failure associated with cardiogenic shock, gun shots, endothelial injury (giant hemangiomas, aortic aneurysms, angiography), hemolytic transfusion reactions, burns, crush injuries, acidosis, and alkalosis.

Tests—The best screening study results are thrombocytopenia in 90% of patients, increased prothrombin time in 90% of patients, and hypofibrinogenemia in 70% of patients. The best available confirmatory test is the fibrin D-dimer assay, which detects fibrinogen fragments that are formed by the lysis of cross-linked fibrin. More sensitive techniques include detection of products of fibrinolysis or fibrin degradation products (D-dimer products) and coagulation activation (soluble fibrin monomers). The values obtained with these two tests may be increased in the postoperative state and in patients with recent thrombi because of fibrinolysis that may not be a reflection of a pathologic state.

- Screening tests for disseminated intravascular coagulopathy: thrombocytopenia (90%), increased prothrombin time (90%), and hypofibrinogenemia (70%).

Treatment—The first goal in treatment is to treat the underlying disease. Next, the approach depends on the clinical situation. If the patient has a low level of fibrinogen, low platelet count, or low levels of clotting factor and is not bleeding or undergoing a surgical procedure, no treatment is necessary. If the patient is bleeding or undergoing a surgical procedure, treat with cryoprecipitate, fresh frozen plasma, and platelets. Monitoring the effect of replacement therapy with platelet and fibrinogen levels 30 minutes to 1 hour after transfusion and every 4 to 6 hours thereafter provides a guide to further replacement therapy. If the patient continues to bleed and the above measures do not cause an increase in coagulation factors, it may be necessary to continue factor and platelet replacement therapy and to start a continuous infusion of heparin. Heparin is contraindicated in central nervous system lesions. If there is evidence of fibrin deposition or thrombosis (such as dermal necrosis in purpura fulminans, acral ischemia, livedo reticularis, or venous thromboembolism), heparin therapy is indicated. Both full-dose therapy (a loading dose of 5,000 units followed by 1,000 units per hour) and subcutaneous heparin have been advocated. Monitoring is a problem. The initial approach is to follow the prothrombin time, fibrinogen level, and platelet count. A heparin assay to achieve a level of 0.2 to 0.4 M/mL is an alternative approach that is not advocated as a routine practice. The thrombotic events of disseminated intravascular coagulopathy in solid tumor malignancy can be treated effectively with heparin, but warfarin anticoagulation may not be as effective. Other instances in which heparin is indicated are retained dead fetus with hypofibrinogenemia before induction of labor, excessive bleeding associated with giant hemangioma, promyelocytic leukemia, and mucinous adenocarcinoma. Heparin is not indicated in more than 95% of patients.

Chronic disseminated intravascular coagulopathy is common. Routine tests of hypercoagulability are abnormal in a significant number of patients with cancer. Increased levels of fibrinogen are common. The syndrome of coexisting cancer and thrombotic disease is called "Trousseau syndrome," which is associated with mucin-producing neoplasms.

Coagulation and Liver Disease

The most important factor is the condition of the blood vessels. There is no tendency to bleed unless and until blood vessels are damaged, such as by needle, surgical procedure, or gastric acid. The three main coagulation patterns are 1) portal hypertension, which is characterized by thrombocytopenia and normal coagulation factor synthesis; 2) cholestasis, which results in impaired absorption of fat-soluble vitamins with vitamin K deficiency and an increase in prothrombin time and activated partial thromboplastin time; and 3) acute and chronic hepatocellular disease, which is characterized by a normal fibrinogen level (until late in the course of the disease), thrombocytopenia, and an increase in prothrombin time and activated partial thromboplastin time because of multiple factor deficiencies. Liver disease is contrasted with disseminated intravascular coagulopathy in Table 12-13.

Factor-Deficiency States

Factor XIII Deficiency

Factor XIII deficiency is characterized by normal blood tests but significant bleeding. There is a history of umbilical cord bleeding, ecchymoses, and prolonged hemorrhage from cuts. It is autosomal recessive in inheritance. All routine clotting tests, including bleeding time, may give normal results. Treatment is with fresh frozen plasma.

Factor XII Deficiency

Factor XII deficiency is characterized by a prolonged APTT but no bleeding complications.

Factor XI Deficiency (Hemophilia C)

Factor XI deficiency is a rare autosomal recessive disorder that occurs predominantly in Ashkenazi Jews. This is a mild bleeding disorder that usually becomes manifest after surgery or trauma. The indications for replacement therapy depend on several variables. Treatment options included fresh frozen plasma and virally inactivated factor XI concentrate.

Factor IX Deficiency (Christmas Disease, Hemophilia B)

This X-linked disorder accounts for 15% of all cases of hemophilia. It is clinically indistinguishable from factor VIII deficiency. The laboratory abnormalities include an abnormal partial thromboplastin time. Patients undergoing a surgical procedure or who have major bleeding could receive purified factor IX complex. There may be an increased risk of thrombosis, because of the presence of activated factors VII and X. Factor IX-complex products developed from a monoclonal antibody purifying process are available. They are safe from contamination with the AIDS virus, and the risk of hepatitis is significantly reduced.

Table 12-13.—Differences in Laboratory Findings Between Liver Disease and Disseminated Intravascular Coagulopathy

Tests	Liver disease	Disseminated intravascular coagulopathy
Thrombocytopenia	Mild, decreased in 50% of patients, <50,000 uncommon	90% of patients
Increased prothrombin time	Common	90% of patients
Decreased fibrinogen	Late in disease	70% of patients
Factor V	Decreased	Regularly decreased
Factor VIII	Normal	Regularly decreased
Factors VII, X	Decreased	Normal

Factor VIII Deficiency (Hemophilia A)

This disease results from a defect in factor VIII:C, is X-linked recessive in inheritance pattern, and accounts for 85% of cases of hemophilia. If a hemophiliac male has children from a normal female, all daughters are obligatory carriers and all sons are normal. If a normal male marries a carrier, each daughter has a 50% chance of being a carrier and each son has a 50% chance of having hemophilia. At birth, there are no bleeding manifestations; however, 50% of males bleed at the time of circumcision. Bleeding occurs in 75% of severely affected infants by age 18 months. The severity of hemophilia runs true in families. Severe hemophiliacs have less than 1% factor VIII and clinically have hemarthroses, atrophied muscles, subcutaneous hematomas in the tongue and neck, and hematomas in the genitourinary and gastrointestinal tracts. Mild hemophiliacs have factor VIII levels of 5% to 25% (55%-145%) and may bleed heavily, even fatally, postoperatively or after dental extractions unless the factor is adequately replaced.

Laboratory studies reveal an abnormal partial thromboplastin time, abnormal factor VIII:C, normal prothrombin time, normal bleeding time, and normal thrombin time. One treatment consists of factor VIII concentrate, which has a half-life of 8-12 hours. Current factor VIII:C concentrates are regarded as safe from HIV transmission. However, three highly purified products, all produced by monoclonal antibodies, are available and no cases of AIDS or hepatitis B or C have been reported with the use of these products. There have been no seroconversions to HIV with any of the products in the U.S., including products that have been heated in aqueous solution, solvent-detergent treated, and/or immunoaffinity purified. Heat- and solvent-detergent-treated concentrates appear to be free from transmission of hepatitis B, hepatitis C, and HIV. Hepatitis A and parvovirus are not inactivated by these techniques. Recombinant factor VIII products (Recombinate, Kogenate) are available and appear to be free from human virus transmission and are the standard treatment of choice.

The management of patients with factor VIII inhibitors is complex. Porcine factor VIII should be considered in the initial management if the patient does not have an inhibitor to this factor. When porcine factor VIII cannot be used, prothrombin complex concentrates (I, VII, IX, and X) may be administered to bypass the need for factor VIII. These agents have a risk of thrombotic complications. Always check Bethesda unit assay before any general surgery in patients with hemophilia. From 5% to 20% of hemophiliacs develop inhibitors (IgG antibodies) that inactivate factor VIII:C (Bethesda units). If the inhibitor is less than 3 Bethesda units/mL, then treat with higher doses or replacement therapy. If the value is higher (>10 Bethesda units), one can attempt to use prothrombin complex concentrates (II, VII, IX, X) to "bypass." Hemophilia A is contrasted with von Willebrand disease in Table 12-14.

- Factor VIII and factor IX deficiencies are X-linked.
- Management of hemophilia A: a desmopressin trial should be undertaken in cases of mild-to-moderate hemophilia A.
- For other patients, factor VIII products that are heat treated, solvent-detergent treated, immunoaffinity purified, or produced by recombinant techniques.
- Recombinant techniques appear to be free from human virus transmission and are the treatment of choice.

Acquired factor VIII deficiency states may occur and are secondary to the following causes: idiopathic, post partum, collagen vascular diseases (rheumatoid arthritis, systemic lupus erythematosus, temporal arteritis), drug hypersensitivity (penicillin, sulfonamides), malignancies (lymphoproliferative, solid tumors), and old age. Clinically, bleeding is intramuscular, retropharyngeal, retroperitoneal, and cerebral. Also, hematuria occurs. The treatment is very difficult and requires the combination of steroids, cyclophosphamide, plasmapheresis, prothrombin-complex concentrate, activated prothrombin-complex concentrate, and porcine factor VIII. The combination of cyclophosphamide and prednisone may be effective in the outpatient setting in patients with an acquired factor VIII inhibitor.

Factor XII deficiency is an autosomal recessive disorder in which thromboembolic complications are more important than bleeding complications. The APTT is abnormal, and the PT is normal.

Factor VII Deficiency

Factor VII deficiency is characterized clinically by epistaxis, gingival bleeding, bleeding after trauma, menorrhagia, and hemarthroses. The APTT is normal, and the PT is abnormal.

Factor X Deficiency

Factor X deficiency is characterized by bleeding that is the same as that in factor VII deficiency. An acquired factor X deficiency state may occur in amyloidosis. The APTT and PT are abnormal.

Table 12-14.—Differences Between Hemophilia A and von Willebrand Disease

	Hemophilia A	von Willebrand disease
Inheritance	Sex-linked	Autosomal
Bleeding time	Normal	Prolonged
Factor VIII:C	Decreased	Decreased
Factor VIII rag	Normal	Decreased
Ristocetin cofactor	Normal	Decreased

Factor V Deficiency

Factor V deficiency may be acquired in myeloproliferative disorders. Bruising occurs with severe bleeding postoperatively and at the onset of menstruation. Treatment consists of administering platelets and fresh frozen plasma.

Causes of an increased thrombin time include heparin, heparin-like anticoagulants, increase in fibrin degradation products, and decreased or defective fibrinogen.

The hemorrhagic disorders are summarized in Table 12-15.

Treatment of Factor Deficiency States

Circulatory overload problems must be taken into consideration when transfusing into patients materials used to treat deficiency states. To control major bleeding or to prepare patients for a surgical procedure, it is advised that the plasma level of factor VIII be increased to 60% in patients with factor VIII deficiency. The number of factor VIII units is calculated by multiplying the patient's weight in pounds by 12 (example, 160 pounds x 12 = 1,920 units of factor VIII).

Fresh frozen plasma is a good source of all factors. It has been used in treating congenital deficiencies in factors II, V, VII, IX, X, XI, and XIII and multiple coagulation deficiencies, including oral anticoagulant overdose, liver disease, massive transfusion, disseminated intravascular coagulopathy, plasmapheresis, and vitamin K deficiency. One should suspect multiple coagulation factor deficiencies in patients with prolonged PTs and partial thromboplastin times greater than 1.5 times normal if not due to known coagulation factor deficiency or circulating lupus-like anticoagulant. In dosing fresh frozen plasma, 1 or 2 units is usually not sufficient to replace coagulation factors, as in patients with liver disease, which requires 3 to 9 units. The maximal effect declines 2 to 4 hours after transfusion. Purified antihemophilic concentrates are derived from fresh frozen plasma of paid donors and are lyophilized or freeze-dried in form. Complications include hepatitis and factor VIII inhibitors. Cryoprecipitate is a good source of factors V, VIII, and fibrinogen. The activity per gram of protein is 12 to 60 times that of fresh frozen plasma. One bag will increase the factor VIII level 2.5% or one bag per 6 kg of body weight twice a day in factor VIII deficiency. Factor IX complex contains factors II, VII, IX, and X. Activated factor IX-complex products include KONyNE and anti-inhibitor coagulant complex, heat treated (Autoplex T). This is indicated in severe factor IX deficiency and in the management of factor VIII inhibitors. Complications include hepatitis, disseminated intravascular coagulopathy, and thrombosis.

Hypercoagulable States

Thrombophilia refers to the tendency to have recurrent venous thromboembolism. Clinical indications of hypercoagulable states include a family history of thrombosis, recurrent thrombosis without other precipitating risk factors, thrombosis at unusual sites, and postpartum thrombosis. With the congenital states, the initial episode of venous thromboembolism is rare before the age of 18 years and uncommon after the age of 50 years and occurs in high-risk situations. Risk factors for thrombosis are noncongenital, congenital, and acquired. Noncongenital risk factors include age, trauma, obesity, immobilization, pregnancy, diabetes mellitus, and oral contraceptive pills. Congenital risk factors include the deficiency states of

Table 12-15.—Summary of Test Results in Hemorrhagic Disorders and Anticoagulant Therapy

	Prothrombin time	Activated partial thromboplastin time	Thrombin time	Fibrinogen	Bleeding time
Classic hemophilia A	Normal	Abnormal	Normal	Normal	Normal
von Willebrand disease	Normal	Normal or abnormal	Normal	Normal	Abnormal
Afibrinogenemia	Abnormal	Abnormal	Abnormal	Absent	Normal
Hypofibrinogenemia	Normal	Normal	Normal	Low	Normal
Dysfibrinogenemia	Normal or abnormal	Normal or abnormal	Abnormal	Normal	Normal
Factor XIII deficiency	Normal	Normal	Normal	Normal	Normal
Heparin	Slightly abnormal	Abnormal	Abnormal	Normal	Normal or abnormal
Warfarin (Coumadin)	Abnormal	Normal or abnormal	Normal	Normal	Normal

protein S, protein C, hyperhomocysteinemia, plasminogen deficiency, antithrombin III deficiency, and congenital resistance to activated protein C (80% of all cases of activated protein C [APC]-resistance are caused by heterozygosity or homozygosity for a single point mutation in the factor V gene, factor V Leiden). Acquired conditions include lupus anticoagulant, disseminated intravascular coagulopathy, paroxysmal nocturnal hemoglobinuria, pregnancy, malignancy, inflammatory bowel disease, myeloproliferative disorders, cryoglobulinemia, and aberrant blood flow.

Protein S deficiency is more common than deficiency of protein C or antithrombin III. Routine coagulation assays fail to detect these patients. A 50% decrease in either protein S or C increases thrombotic tendencies. Family studies are requisite. Assays are available for all three. Protein S is a vitamin K-dependent factor that is required for expression of APC anticoagulant activity. There is an increased incidence of thrombosis, with venous complications greater than arterial. APC destroys activated factors V and VIII and, thus, is a potent plasma anticoagulant. APC requires a second vitamin K-dependent factor, or cofactor, protein S. Antithrombin III deficiency is an uncommon cause of venous thromboembolism. The management of protein S deficiency, protein C deficiency, and antithrombin III deficiency requires heparin and oral anticoagulant agents. There is an increased incidence of warfarin (Coumadin) necrosis that is a rare complication in nonhospitalized patients and occurs 2 to 10 days after initiating treatment with warfarin.

Resistance to APC is a condition of autosomal dominant inheritance resulting from a point mutation in the gene encoding coagulation factor V, commonly known as the factor V "Leiden" mutation. This mutation renders factor V resistant to proteolytic down-regulation by APC, and so the clotting mechanism continues to generate the clotting enzyme thrombin. The heterozygous mutation has a prevalence of 2% to 5%. There is approximately a tenfold increased prevalence (20%-50%) among persons with familial or recurrent venous thromboembolism and a 20% to 25% increased prevalence among those with deep venous thrombosis. Homozygotes have an 80-fold increased risk for venous thromboembolism. The risk of venous thromboembolism is increased 30-fold among heterozygotes receiving oral contraceptive therapy. The diagnosis is established by an APTT-based APC-resistance ratio or DNA-based testing. DNA-based testing is recommended for patients with an abnormal APTT-based APC-resistance ratio, in patients with an abnormally prolonged APTT, and in patients taking anticoagulants. Asymptomatic patients with APC resistance should have prophylactic intervention when clinical thrombosis risk factors are present. APC-resistant persons with an initial deep venous thrombosis are managed in a standard fashion. Those who are homozygotes or heterozygotes with additional thrombophilic predispositions should be considered for lifelong anticoagulation prophylaxis.

The antiphospholipid antibodies include anticardiolipin antibodies, lupus anticoagulants, protein-phospholipid reactivity, and anti-reagin antibodies. The lupus anticoagulant is an immunoglobulin (IgG, IgA, or IgM) that interferes with in vitro phospholipid steps of coagulation, causing a prolonged clotting time in the APTT, dilute Russell viper venom time, or plasma clot time. Patients with the lupus anticoagulant are at a higher risk for thrombosis. This is an interfering inhibitor of the APTT that does not correct with equal volumes of normal plasma. These react with anionic phospholipids, prothrombin, and β_2 glycoprotein 1. The screening test is the prolonged APTT. Clinically, venous thrombosis of the lower extremities is more common than arterial thrombosis. The clinical approach to lupus anticoagulant and antiphospholipid antibody syndrome is as follows. If it is possible that the plasma sample is contaminated by heparin, perform a thrombin time. The diagnosis is confirmed with a failure to correct with a 1:1 mixture of normal plasma. The best confirmatory test is the dilute Russell viper venom time, which is prolonged in patients with lupus-like anticoagulants. The dilute Russell viper venom time is also abnormal in patients receiving heparin. If there is no history of thrombotic disease, check the APC-resistant factor Va, antithrombin III, protein C, and protein S. If normal, observe. Prophylactic anticoagulant therapy is indicated for times of increased risk, such as postoperative state and long bone fracture. Alternatives to oral contraceptives should be considered. If the patient develops thrombosis and is receiving heparin, follow the anti-Xa test. If the patient requires oral warfarin, regulate with an arbitrary International Normalized Ratio (INR) of 3 to 4 or with the prothrombin-proconvertin test. After thrombotic events, long-term warfarin is indicated.

The clinical syndromes of the antiphospholipid antibody syndromes include major (venous and arterial thromboses, spontaneous abortions, and thrombocytopenia) and minor (livedo reticularis, multistroke dementia, and chorea) components. The thrombotic manifestations are venous (deep venous thrombosis, cutaneous thrombosis, renal vein thrombosis, and Budd-Chiari syndrome) or arterial (central nervous system, coronary thrombosis, and renal artery or vein thrombosis). Hematologic associations include thrombocytopenia, hemolysis, and hypocomplementemia. Obstetrical associations are maternal (deep venous thrombosis, chorea, eclampsia, and pulmonary embolus) and fetal (spontaneous abortion, fetal death, and second and third trimester premature birth).

There is no indication for the treatment of asymptomatic patients without a history of associated conditions. Initial treatment with heparin followed by anticoagulation with warfarin with an INR greater than 3.0 is the treatment for thrombosis.

Low doses of aspirin and heparin are recommended for the management of pregnant patients.

Who should be tested? Patients who should be considered for further testing include persons younger than 40 years with thrombotic events and those with a strong family history of thrombosis, recurrent thromboses at different sites, skin necrosis, recurrent fetal loss, and thrombosis at unusual sites (sagittal sinus thrombosis, mesenteric thrombosis, etc.).

Warfarin

Warfarin is a vitamin K antagonist, which limits the gamma-carboxylation of the vitamin K-dependent coagulation proteins II, VII, IX, and X and anticoagulant proteins C and S, impairing their biologic function in blood coagulation. This drug is contraindicated in pregnancy. Complications include embryopathy. Other relative contraindications include patients with a hemorrhagic tendency such as thrombocytopenia or coagulation factor abnormalities, diastolic blood pressure greater than 110 mm Hg, gastrointestinal tract lesions liable to bleed, severe liver disease, severe renal disease, malabsorption, subacute bacterial endocarditis, diverticulosis, or colitis. It is also contraindicated if the patient recently had a surgical procedure performed on the central nervous system or eye.

In venous thromboembolism, warfarin treatment should be started within 24 hours after the initiation of heparin. The appropriate dose of warfarin for preventing systemic embolism and myocardial infarction, for prophylaxis for venous thrombosis, and for treating venous thrombosis and pulmonary embolism is that which maintains PT at an INR of 2 or 3, which corresponds to a PT ratio of 1.3 to 1.5. A loading dose of 5 mg avoids the development of a potential hypercoagulable state caused by a precipitous decrease in the levels of protein C. Patients should receive 3 to 6 months of warfarin treatment. Patients with metastatic cancer with venous thromboembolism are candidates for long-term therapy, as are patients with recurrent thromboembolism. Warfarin has been demonstrated to be efficacious in atrial fibrillation. The therapeutic INR in patients with artificial heart valves is controversial.

Bleeding occurs in 2% to 4% of patients. In patients with a prolonged PT with or without bleeding, use of the drug should be stopped for 24 to 72 hours. Available information suggests that patients taking warfarin with an INR greater than 8 are at a substantially increased risk for bleeding. In patients who have taken a suicidal dose or have a suspected cerebral hemorrhage and who need no further anticoagulation, vitamin K given intravenously at a dose of 20 to 30 mg may be administered with fresh frozen plasma. Fresh frozen plasma may be administered to patients taking warfarin who require continued anticoagulation but who have life-threatening bleeding. Drugs that potentiate warfarin include those that prolong the PT, such

as phenylbutazone, metronidazole, sulfinpyrazone, trimethoprim/sulfamethoxazole, and disulfiram. Drugs that inhibit platelet function, such as aspirin, may also potentiate the toxic effects of warfarin. Some drugs antagonize warfarin, for example, cholestyramine decreases the absorption of warfarin. Other drugs, such as barbiturates, carbamazepine, and rifampin, increase the clearance of warfarin. Acetaminophen may be a cause of over anticoagulation in the outpatient setting.

Unfractionated Heparin

Heparin inhibits thrombin by binding to anti-thrombin III and forming a heparin-antithrombin III complex, which interrupts the clotting cascade by deactivating thrombin (factor IIa) and factor Xa. The heparin is then reused. In the initial treatment of deep venous thrombosis or pulmonary embolus, the goal is to prolong the APTT at a level of 1.5 to 2.5 times normal within the first 24 hours of treatment. If this is not accomplished, the risk of recurrent thromboembolism is 15-fold, and the risk persists for weeks. Heparin and warfarin may be given simultaneously and be overlapped for 5 days, after which treatment should be warfarin alone. Heparin should be administered for a minimum of 4 days and not be discontinued until the INR has been in therapeutic range for 2 consecutive days because of the half-lives of the vitamin K-dependent factors. Warfarin treatment should be maintained for 3 months if there are no risk factors. Prolonged treatment may be indicated when risk factors such as prolonged immobilization, hypercoagulable state, and recurrent deep venous thrombosis exist.

Heparin is indicated for the treatment of venous thrombosis and pulmonary emboli. It is also used to prevent venous thrombosis and pulmonary emboli (prophylactic doses of 5,000 units subcutaneously every 8 to 12 hours in cases of abdominal surgery or for medical patients with a history of thrombosis, prolonged bed rest, congestive heart failure, or cancer). A dose of 12,000 units is administered subcutaneously twice a day for the prevention of mural thrombosis after myocardial infarction. Heparin is indicated in the prevention of coronary artery rethrombosis after thrombolysis, and it is the treatment of choice in venous thrombosis and pulmonary emboli in pregnancy (17,500 U subcutaneously twice a day). Impedance plethysmography, ultrasonography, or venography may document this complication of pregnancy. (Warfarin is contraindicated in pregnancy because of the risks of embryopathy, including nasal hypoplasia and central nervous system abnormalities.) Heparin is indicated after treatment with thrombolytic therapy. The normal dose is a 5,000-U bolus followed by 30,000 to 35,000 U/24 hours by continuous infusion. Side effects include hemorrhage (which occurs in 6.8% of patients treated by continuous infusion), osteoporosis, and skin necrosis. A hypersensitivity reaction may convert antithrombin III from a slow inhibitor to a very rapid inhibitor.

Resistance to heparin is defined as the need for more than 40,000 units per day. There may be a reactivation of the thrombotic process when heparin is discontinued. Heparin resistance is secondary to increased plasma concentrations of factor VIII and heparin-binding proteins. Approaches include monitoring the plasma heparin concentration or low-molecular-weight heparin (LMWH).

Low-Molecular-Weight Heparin

LMWH has advantages over unfractionated heparin, with a more predictable dose response allowing for fixed doses without laboratory monitoring. There is a lower risk of heparin-induced thrombocytopenia, because nonspecific binding of heparin to other proteins and cells causes variability. The LMWHs do not cause significant change in the measured APTT because of their propensity toward factor Xa inhibition over thrombin inhibition. In most circumstances, blood monitoring is not required. If monitoring is necessary, anti-factor Xa levels should be measured. In general, twice-daily dosage should give better coverage for prophylaxis and treatment, although single dosage for prophylaxis is adequate for dalteparin and enoxaparin. Subcutaneous dosages for prophylaxis for the available LMWHs include endoxaparin (30 mg bid or 40 mg daily), dalteparin (2,500 anti-Xa units/day to 5,200 anti-Xa units/day), ardeparin (50 anti-Xa units/day), and danaparoid (750 anti-Xa units/day).

Thrombolytic Therapy

The thrombolytic agents are streptokinase, urokinase, recombinant tissue plasminogen activator and urokinase-like activator, and anisolyated streptokinase-plasminogen activator complex. Fibrin is the major target of thrombolytic therapy. Anticoagulation does *not* dissolve or prevent the growth of thrombi (even at recommended doses), eliminate the source of subsequent emboli in the deep veins during an acute attack, alleviate hemodynamic problems, prevent valvular damage, prevent persistent venous hypertension, or prevent persistent pulmonary hypertension. The primary role of anticoagulation is prophylaxis against further propagation of the clot.

Thrombolytic therapy lyses thrombi and emboli and restores the circulation to normal, normalizes hemodynamic disturbances, reduces morbidity, decreases systemic and mean pulmonary artery pressures at 72 hours, prevents venous vascular damage and subsequent venous hypertension in the lower extremities, and prevents permanent damage to the pulmonary vascular bed, reducing the likelihood of persistent pulmonary hypertension. Residual emboli usually persist with heparin therapy alone. Tissue plasminogen activator has a relative fibrin specificity; yet, significant fibrinolysis and bleeding may occur. There is an initial fibrinolysis of the plug followed by proteolysis of fibrinogen and factors V and VIII. In general,

venous thrombi are rich in fibrin and are potentially more suitable than platelet thrombi to fibrinolytic therapy. The age of the thrombus is also important in that it is essential to start these agents within 48 hours in cases of pulmonary emboli and in less than 7 days in cases of deep venous thrombosis. In cases of pulmonary emboli, this treatment improves hemodynamics and pulmonary perfusion; it may be indicated with more lobar pulmonary arteries or an equivalent amount of emboli in other vessels with or without shock or submassive emboli accompanied by shock or impending shock or persistent hypotension. In deep venous thrombosis, these agents may minimize valvular dysfunction and decrease the risk of recurrent and postphlebitic syndrome. At this time, these agents are not recommended for routine use in pulmonary emboli and deep venous thrombosis. Currently, it should be restricted to and considered in patients with extensive iliofemoral venous thrombosis with a low risk of bleeding and patients with hemodynamic compromise due to pulmonary embolism.

If the timing is appropriate, these agents may be administered in thrombosis of the hepatic, renal, mesenteric, cerebrovenous, sinus, and central retinal veins. Of arterial disorders, acute myocardial infarction has been the most excessively studied. The SCAT 1 trial demonstrated that mortality was significantly lower in patients randomly assigned to heparin after thrombolytic therapy in acute myocardial infarction. The GUSTO trial revealed that a rapid infusion of tissue plasminogen activator with intravenously given heparin was most favorable.

Thrombolytic therapy is monitored with fibrinogen levels. The absolute contraindications to this therapy include active internal bleeding and a cerebral vascular accident within the preceding 2 weeks. Relatively major contraindications include the following if they have occurred within less than 10 days: major surgical procedure, obstetrical delivery, pregnancy, the first 10 days post partum, organ biopsy, burns, skin grafts, previous puncture of noncompressible vessels, thoracentesis, paracentesis, gastrointestinal tract bleeding, ulcerative colitis, diverticulosis, serious trauma, systolic blood pressure greater than 200 mm Hg, diastolic pressure greater than 110 mm Hg, intracranial neoplasms, or thrombocytopenia. Relatively minor contraindications include a high likelihood of left-sided heart thrombus such as mitral stenosis with atrial fibrillation, subacute bacterial endocarditis, severe hepatic or renal disease, age older than 75 years, diabetic hemorrhagic retinopathy, active and progressive cavitating lung lesions, ulcerative cutaneous and mucous membrane lesions, recent intra-arterial diagnostic procedure except arterial blood gases. Bleeding may be superficial or internal; it occurs because of the indiscriminate lysis of fibrin. Thrombolytic agents are not substitutes for heparin and warfarin and, therefore, the morbidity is additive. Approaches to hemorrhage control include volume replacement, manual techniques, and RBC transfusions. If bleeding is massive, replace with cryoprecipitate and fresh frozen plasma and discontinue use of heparin. With central nervous system bleeding, discontinue fibrinolytic therapy, administer cryoprecipitate and fresh frozen plasma, and avoid anticoagulants and antiplatelet agents.

Aplastic Anemia

Aplastic anemia may develop as a consequence of a defect in the stem cell population, defective marrow environment, or immune suppression. This group of disorders with failure of hematopoiesis is characterized by peripheral pancytopenia, bone marrow hypocellularity, and absence of malignant or myeloproliferative diseases. No primary disease of hematopoietic tissue is evident.

Before the use of allogeneic bone marrow transplantation and antithymocyte globulin, the natural history of the disease was that 80% of patients with severe aplastic anemia were not alive at 1 or 2 years, and 20% had partial recovery.

- Aplastic anemia: pancytopenia, hypocellular bone marrow, and absence of primary disease of hematopoietic tissue.
- Full recovery is uncommon without allogeneic bone marrow transplantation or antithymocyte globulin.

Clinical features include weakness, fatigue, easy bruising or bleeding, fever, and infections. Lymphadenopathy and splenomegaly are uncommon. In 40% to 70% of patients, the cause of aplastic anemia is idiopathic. This is more frequent in adults. Drugs are the second most common cause of aplastic anemia. These include chloramphenicol, phenylbutazone, methylphenylethylhydantoin, trimethadione, sulfonamides, gold, and benzene. Paroxysmal nocturnal hemoglobinuria and infections are the third and fourth most common causes, respectively. Infectious hepatitis is the most common infection to cause aplastic anemia. Non-A, non-B, non-C hepatitis followed by hepatitis A are the most common types of hepatitis to cause aplastic anemia. Hepatitis B is the least common hepatitis that causes aplastic anemia. These patients have a poor prognosis. Other infectious agents causing aplastic anemia include Epstein-Barr viral infections, influenza, and mycobacterial infections. Ionizing irradiation may also be a cause.

If transfusion is needed, select nonrelated donors and use leukocyte-poor RBC transfusions and single-donor platelet transfusions. Transfusions should be given with considerable care and concern. Family members should not be donors, because they are more likely to sensitize the patient to minor histocompatibility antigens present in the donor but absent in the patient. The survival rate is better for those not receiving transfusion.

Immunosuppressive treatments include antithymocyte globulin and steroids with or without cyclosporine. These are not curative. In a trial of moderate to severe aplastic anemia patients, 11 of the 21 treated with antithymocyte globulin alone had sustained improvement, whereas none of the 21 in the control population improved.

In patients who are not eligible for bone marrow transplantation, treatment with antithymocyte globulin, methylprednisolone, and cyclosporine has been reported to result in 70% to 80% partial recovery in the peripheral blood counts. Blood count recovery usually is not complete; however, transfusions are not required, and the absolute neutrophil count is at a level to protect against infectious complications. About 30% of patients have relapse.

The allogeneic bone marrow transplantation success rate is 66% in young patients. This is the therapy of choice in all patients with a homozygous twin and should be considered immediately for all patients younger than age 20, and this treatment should be considered in high-risk patients between the ages of 20 and 45 with an HLA match. A trial of immunosuppressive therapy is indicated in other patients, including those with moderate disease and those 45 to 55 years old. Cyclosporine or corticosteroids, at a dose of 0.2 to 1.0 mg/kg daily, and androgens are other therapeutic modalities. Androgens are not effective in severe aplastic anemia. The toxic effects include virilization and hepatic toxicity. The 17-alpha derivative is responsible for hepatic adenomas and hepatocellular carcinoma.

- With severe aplastic anemia, avoid transfusions.
- If the patient is younger and has an HLA-matched donor or identical twin, consider bone marrow transplantation with cyclophosphamide alone or cyclophosphamide plus irradiation in previously transfused patients as preconditioning. If the patient is older or has no HLA match, treat with a combination of antithymocyte globulin and methylprednisolone with or without cyclosporine.
- Long-term survival in patients with severe disease has increased from <25% in patients treated with androgens to 75% in those treated with intensive immunosuppressive therapy and to 66% in those treated with bone marrow transplantation.

Neutropenia

The differential diagnosis of nonmalignant acute neutropenia includes drugs, infections (HIV, parvovirus, and hepatitis), autoimmune neutropenia (Felty syndrome, rheumatoid arthritis, systemic lupus erythematosus, and Sjögren syndrome), ulcerative colitis, hemodilution, hypersplenism, and hematologic disorders (cyclic neutropenia and aplastic anemia). Drug-induced neutropenia is associated with sulfonamides, semisynthetic penicillins (nafcillin, ampicillin), phenothiazines, nonsteroidal anti-inflammatory agents (indomethacin), and antithyroid medications (propylthiouracil, methimazole). Drug-induced neutropenia becomes manifest 1 to 2 weeks after initial drug exposure or sooner following a recent repeat exposure. The treatment of choice is to discontinue the drug. Corticosteroids characteristically are not efficacious.

The differential diagnosis of chronic neutropenia includes cyclic neutropenia and chronic idiopathic neutropenia. Cyclic neutropenia is characterized by oscillations in the neutrophil counts every 19 to 23 days. It is a disorder of neutrophil production at a regulation phase. The typical clinical syndrome is manifested as furuncles, cellulitis, chronic gingivitis, and abscesses. Patients can predict the timing of successive episodes. Treatment involves timely antibiotics, avoidance of dental and surgical work at nadirs, oral hygiene, and dental care. Granulocyte colony-stimulating factor (filgrastim) may be effective in increasing the neutrophil count in cyclic neutropenia and chronic idiopathic neutropenia.

In the adult population, the recommended dose of granulocyte colony-stimulating factor (G-CSF, filgrastim) is 5 µg/kg per day subcutaneously. The 1996 American Society of Clinical Oncology colony-stimulating factor guidelines emphasized the following: primary prophylaxis is recommended when the incidence of febrile neutropenia is greater than 40% of the control group. Therefore, in general, for previously untreated patients receiving most chemotherapy regimens, primary administration of colony-stimulating factors should not be used routinely. Special circumstances for patients who might benefit from these agents include preexisting neutropenia due to disease, extensive previous chemotherapy, previous irradiation to the pelvis, a history of recurrent febrile neutropenia while receiving earlier chemotherapy, and conditions that potentially enhance the risk of infection (poor performance status, decreased immune function, open wounds, or active tissue infections). There is evidence that colony-stimulating factors can decrease the probability of febrile neutropenia in subsequent cycles of chemotherapy after a documented occurrence in a previous cycle. These agents are effective adjuncts in progenitor-cell transplantation. The data are inadequate to support the routine use of these agents in afebrile patients or to routinely use them in dose-intensity programs. The colony-stimulating factors should be avoided with concomitant chemotherapy or radiation therapy.

Neutropenia in the black population is common, and if patients are asymptomatic, this need not be evaluated further. Other causes of neutropenia include autoimmune neutropenia (which is secondary to an antibody), antigens, rheumatoid arthritis, and chronic active hepatitis.

Thrombocytopenia

The causes of thrombocytopenia in adults are multiple and broadly include autoimmune idiopathic thrombocytopenic purpura, drug-induced thrombocytopenia, pseudothrombocytopenia, refractoriness to platelet transfusion therapy, posttransfusion purpura, and secondary causes. Secondary causes include systemic lupus erythematosus (in which 14%-26% of patients develop thrombocytopenia), infections (HIV, rubella, infectious mononucleosis), chronic lymphocytic leukemia, non-Hodgkin lymphoma, sarcoidosis, ovarian carcinoma, and purpura of septicemia.

The diagnosis of pseudothrombocytopenia should be excluded with examination of a peripheral blood smear. Causes of pseudothrombocytopenia include EDTA-induced platelet clumping, platelet satellitosis, May-Hegglin anomaly, Bernard-Soulier syndrome, and large platelets in myeloproliferative disorders.

A spuriously low platelet count may be reported in EDTA-induced platelet agglutination. This is an antibody-mediated phenomenon caused by antibodies that bind to the patient's platelets after withdrawal of calcium. Patients have a spuriously low platelet count by automated techniques only but a normal number of platelets on the peripheral smear.

Idiopathic thrombocytopenic purpura is an autoimmune disease characterized by thrombocytopenia with a normal WBC count and hemoglobin (Table 12-16). In 1996, the American Society of Hematology guidelines for this disorder were published. This group defined idiopathic thrombocytopenic purpura as "isolated thrombocytopenia with no clinically apparent conditions." The diagnosis of idiopathic thrombocytopenic purpura is a diagnosis of exclusion. Patients with risk factors should be tested with HIV antibody tests. The clinical manifestations include purpura, mucous membrane hemorrhage, and cerebromeningeal bleeding. From 7% to 28% of children and up to 40% to 60% of adults have progression to a chronic state of idiopathic thrombocytopenic purpura. In most patients, the platelet count is less than 50,000/µL, and 30% are less than 10,000/µL. The mean platelet volume is increased. Splenomegaly is present in only 10% of patients. If it is present, one should think of other causes. Bone marrow examination reveals a normal to increased number of megakaryocytes. Antibodies to specific platelet-membrane glycoproteins, usually the IIb-IIIa complex, and platelet IgG (erroneously called antiplatelet-antibody tests) measurements are detected in most patients but are unnecessary in the diagnosis or treatment. Up to 10% of patients with chronic idiopathic thrombocytopenic purpura may have accessory spleens. The absence of Howell-Jolly bodies on a peripheral blood smear of patients who have previously undergone splenectomy suggests the diagnosis, which is confirmed by radionuclide imaging or CT scan. Surgical removal may be beneficial.

Table 12-16.—Idiopathic Thrombocytopenic Purpura

Characteristics	Acute	Chronic
Presentation	Abrupt onset of petechiae, purpura, mucosal bleeding	Insidious petechiae, menorrhagia
Usual age	Children (2-6 years old)	Adults (20-40 years old)
Sex	Male = female	Female:male = 3:1
Antecedent infection	Common 85%	Uncommon
	Typically an upper respiratory tract infection	
Platelet count, $x10^9/L$	$<20 \times 10^9/L$	$30\text{-}80 \times 10^9/L$
Duration	2-6 weeks	Months to years
Spontaneous remission	80% within 6 months	Uncommon, fluctuates

From Lee GR, Bithell TC, Foerster J, Athens JW, Lukens JN: Wintrobe's Clinical Hematology. Vol 2. Ninth edition. Philadelphia, Lea & Febiger, 1993, p 1331. By permission of publisher.

The American Society of Hematology guidelines for treatment are as follows: patients with platelet counts of 50,000 or higher do not routinely require treatment. Those with a platelet count less than 50,000 but greater than 30,000 should be treated if there is mucous membrane bleeding or when there are risk factors for bleeding, including hypertension, peptic ulcer disease, and vigorous lifestyle. Patients with platelet counts less than 30,000 should be treated. Corticosteroids are the mainstay of initial treatment; 70% of patients initially respond, with about a 40% chance of long-term remission at an initial dose of prednisone of 1 mg/kg daily for up to 1 month. Steroids decrease antibody production in the reticuloendothelial system and decrease reticuloendothelial clearance. Patients with severe life-threatening bleeding should be treated with intravenous immunoglobulin and platelets and transfusion alone or in combination with high-dose intravenous corticosteroids (methylprednisolone at a dose of 1g/day for 3 days).

The management of patients who do not respond completely to these measures is difficult and controversial. The American Society of Hematology had no formal recommendations. Splenectomy removes the predominant site of antibody production and platelet destruction and is followed by a 75% chance of long-term remission. Dexamethasone (40 mg/day for 4 sequential days every 28 days for 12 months) is an option for the treatment of resistant or relapsed idiopathic thrombocytopenic purpura. Danazol decreases the number of phagocytic cell IgG Fc receptors. A slow infusion of vincristine or vinblastine may be given to patients who do not respond to the above measures. Other agents used in refractory cases include azathioprine (Imuran), cyclophosphamide, colchicine, cyclosporine, and immunoadsorption apheresis on staphylococcal protein A columns.

- Spontaneous bleeding may occur with platelet counts less than 10,000.
- Idiopathic thrombocytopenic purpura is a diagnosis of exclusion.
- The diagnosis rests on the history, physical examination, the CBC, and examination of the peripheral blood smear.
- A bone marrow examination is appropriate to establish the diagnosis of idiopathic thrombocytopenic purpura in patients older that 60 years and in patients considered candidates for splenectomy.
- In idiopathic thrombocytopenic purpura with severe life-threatening bleeding, intravenous immunoglobulin is the treatment of choice, with platelet transfusions, and high-dose corticosteroids.

In drug-induced thrombocytopenia, the pathophysiology is secondary to haptens bound to a carrier protein. Clinically, there is acute bleeding with a hemorrhage syndrome characterized by bleeding from mucous membranes, petechiae, and oozing after brushing the teeth. These problems subside after use of the drug is discontinued. Drug-induced thrombocytopenia subsides in 4 to 14 days except for gold, which may take much longer. In contrast, viral-induced thrombocytopenia resolves in 2 weeks to 3 months. The drugs most commonly implicated include heparin, quinidine, gold, trimethoprim/sulfamethoxazole, amphotericin B, carbamazepine, chlorthiazide, chlorpropamide, procainamide, quinidine, rifampin, and vancomycin. Glycoprotein IIb/IIIa antagonists may cause thrombocytopenia (abciximab [ReoPro], epifibatide [Integrilin], tirofiban [Aggrastat]) and may cause acute (within 24 hours) or delayed (up to 14 days after initiating chronic therapy) thrombocytopenia.

Heparin-induced thrombocytopenia is a clinicopathologic syndrome that has a variable incidence of 1% to 7.8% and is patient-population dependent. Type I heparin-associated thrombocytopenia occurs early, is associated with intravenous heparin, and is a common transient nonimmunologic event of no clinical relevance due to direct heparin-induced platelet aggregation. Type II heparin-associated thrombocytopenia is an immunologic reaction caused by IgG antibodies to an antigen (platelet factor 4 bound to heparin) that activates platelets through their Fc receptors. The platelet counts usually decrease 50% or more and such a decrease should raise clinical suspicion, even if the count is greater than 150,000. The coagulation system may be activated, increasing the production of thrombin. Venous thrombosis (deep venous thrombosis and pulmonary embolus) is more common than arterial thrombosis. Other clinical events include warfarin-induced venous limb damage, acute platelet activation syndromes (fevers, chills, or transient amnesia) 5 to 30 minutes after an intravenous bolus of heparin, or skin lesions at the site of injection of heparin (necrosis or erythematous plaques). The diagnosis may be confirmed by functional assays (serotonin release assay) or antigen assays (antibody against platelet factor 4). The treatment of heparin-associated thrombocytopenia is complex. Heparin should be discontinued. The subsequent risk of thrombosis with discontinuing heparin or substituting warfarin is as high as 50%. Lepirudan, the recombinant form of hirudin, has a half-life of 1.3 hours and is metabolized by the kidney. It is monitored by the APTT (1.5 to 3.0 times normal). Thromboembolectomy may be considered. Danaproid, an LMWH, has been used in heparin associated thrombocytopenia. The risk varies with the dose of heparin, the type of heparin (unfractionated > LMWH > bovine > porcine) and clinical associations (higher risk for surgical than medical patients). This complication is usually mild, and the patients are asymptomatic. It develops 3 to 15 days after therapy, with a median time of 10 days. It is not dose-related and can occur at very low doses. There are no reliable risk factors. Patients are at higher risk if there is a history of this problem. It is essential to pay attention to any substantial decrease in platelet number while patients are taking heparin.

- 6%-8% of pregnant women at term and 25% of women with preeclampsia have mild thrombocytopenia with platelets >80,000/μL.
- Drug-induced thrombocytopenia subsides in 4-14 days with the exception of gold.
- Viral-induced thrombocytopenia resolves in 2 weeks to 3 months.
- Heparin is the drug that most commonly causes thrombocytopenia.

The management of idiopathic thrombocytopenic purpura in pregnancy is complex. The ASH consensus panel recommends intravenous immunoglobulin for pregnant women with severe and symptomatic thrombocytopenia. The recommendations for percutaneous umbilical sampling, fetal scalp vein monitoring at the time of delivery, and the route of delivery are controversial. Neonatal hemorrhagic complications are low. After delivery, infant platelet counts should be followed for 4 days. Intravenous immunoglobulin is recommended for platelet counts less than 20,000 and brain imaging of the infant is recommended for platelet counts less than 50,000.

Thrombocytopenia in Pregnancy

The most common cause of thrombocytopenia in pregnancy is incidental thrombocytopenia of pregnancy, which occurs in 5% of pregnancies and accounts for 75% of cases and is not associated with adverse maternal or fetal outcomes. The diagnosis is one of exclusion. No treatment is required.

Other common causes include preeclampsia, idiopathic autoimmune thrombocytopenia (idiopathic thrombocytopenic purpura), HIV, and thrombotic thrombocytopenic purpura. Fifty percent of patients with preeclampsia are thrombocytopenic. No specific therapy is required, and platelet recovery occurs 72 hours after delivery. Thrombocytopenia may occur in 3% of pregnant women with HIV infection. Intravenous immunoglobulin is an effective therapy.

Other causes of thrombocytopenia in pregnancy include acute fatty liver of pregnancy, drugs (quinine/quinidine, cocaine, and heparin), folate deficiency, infections (cytomegalovirus), and antiphospholipid antibody-related thrombocytopenia. HELLP syndrome is a variant of preeclampsia, consisting of hemolysis, elevated liver function tests, and low platelet counts. Disseminated intravascular coagulopathy develops in up to 38% of patients. The primary treatment of HELLP syndrome is stabilization of the patient's condition and delivery of the fetus.

Post-Transfusion Purpura

In post-transfusion purpura, thrombocytopenia occurs 5 to 8 days after blood transfusion in patients alloimmunized against the platelet antigen HPA-1a. The treatment of choice is intravenous administration of immunoglobulin and corticosteroids.

Postsplenectomy State

Postsplenectomy complications include sepsis secondary to pneumococcus, meningococcus, *Haemophilus influenzae*, *Escherichia coli*, and *Staphylococcus aureus*. Hematologic features include such RBC abnormalities as Howell-Jolly bodies present on the peripheral blood smear. Leukocytes show a postsplenectomy surge and then return to normal numbers. Platelets also show a postsplenectomy surge; the value usually returns to normal in 1 month. If there is a history of splenectomy but no Howell-Jolly bodies on a peripheral blood smear, suspect an accessory spleen and confirm it with a liver-spleen scan.

Spontaneous Splenic Ruptures

Spontaneous splenic ruptures have been reported to occur in infectious mononucleosis (Plate 12-10), cytomegalovirus infections, acute and chronic myelogenous leukemia, acute and chronic lymphocytic leukemia, myeloproliferative diseases, and non-Hodgkin lymphoma.

Transfusion Reactions

The major transfusion reactions include acute hemolytic transfusion reactions, transfusions associated with anti-IgA antibodies, transfusion-associated adult respiratory distress syndrome, delayed hemolytic transfusion reactions, febrile transfusion reactions, urticarial transfusion reactions, and circulatory overload (Table 12-17).

Acute hemolytic transfusion reactions are the most life-threatening. The most common cause is human error (51%), especially when blood is released on an emergency basis, and these are secondary to ABO mismatches. Other causes include antibodies not detected before transfusion, such as Kell, Duffy, and Kidd. ABO mismatches are less frequent than with Kell, Duffy, and Kidd and have virtually disappeared from transfusion reaction complications, but clerical error may play a role in these reactions. Intravascular hemolysis is caused by problems related to ABO, Kell, Duffy, and Kidd. Females are at greater risk than males, because sensitization through pregnancy leads to a higher frequency of preformed antibodies. Obstetrical complications with massive bleeding also predispose females. Age is a factor because older people receive more transfusions. Transfusion of large amounts of blood products given urgently also increases the risk. Clinically,

Table 12-17.—Risks of Complications From Transfusions in the U.S.

Complication	Risk per unit
Minor allergic reaction	1/100
Circulatory overload	Unknown
Febrile, nonhemolytic	1/200
Viral hepatitis	1/3,000
Hemolytic transfusion reaction	1/6,000
Transfusion-related acute lung injury (TRALI)	1/10,000
Fatal hemolytic reaction	1/100,000
HIV infection	1/225,000
HTLV I/II infection	1/200,000
Bacterial infections	1/2,500
IgA-related anaphylaxis	1/100,000
Graft-versus-host disease	Rare
Immunosuppression	Unknown
Post-transfusion purpura	Rare

there is pain at the intravenous site, apprehension, back pain, abdominal pain, fever, chills, chest pain, hypotension, nausea, flushing, and dyspnea. The Coombs test gives positive results in all but anti-A. Complications include oliguria in 33.3% of patients, acute postischemic renal failure, and disseminated intravascular coagulopathy in 4%. In one series, the mortality rate was 17%. Treatment includes immediate termination of the transfusion, intravenous access, vigorous administration of fluids, and furosemide to increase renal cortical blood flow. It is difficult to distinguish between an acute hemolytic transfusion reaction and a febrile nonhemolytic transfusion reaction at the time fever occurs. Therefore, fevers occurring during transfusion should be worked up for hemolysis.

Transfusion reactions associated with anti-IgA antibodies and anaphylactic reactions are secondary to IgA deficiency, the development of a class-specific anti-IgA antibody, normal IgA levels with anti-IgA antibodies acquired through pregnancy or previous transfusions, and ataxia telangiectasia, in which 44% of patients have class-specific anti-IgA antibodies. The pathogenesis is secondary to anti-IgA antibodies of IgG type that are capable of binding complement. Clinically, patients develop apprehension, hives, hypotension, chest pain, abdominal pain, lumbar pain, flushing of the face and neck, dyspnea, and cyanosis. Wheezing, diarrhea, vomiting, unconsciousness, and chills may occur. Fevers are uncommon. The treatment includes stopping the transfusion and giving antihistamines and conventional anti-anaphylactic drugs. Transfusion policy for patients with this problem includes washed RBCs, frozen RBCs, and IgA-deficient plasma.

Transfusion-associated adult respiratory distress syndrome or transfusion-related acute lung injury (TRALI) is a complication of transfusion, with respiratory distress in 1 to 6 hours, hypotension, bilateral pulmonary infiltrates, normal or low pulmonary capillary wedge pressure, hypotension, and fever. Recovery is rapid, occurring in 24 to 48 hours. Most blood donors implicated in this complication have had multiple pregnancies. Possible mechanisms include leukoagglutins in plasma or HLA-specific lymphocytotoxic antibodies passively transfused from the donor to the recipient, resulting in polymorphonuclear-leukocyte-complement-triggered microvascular injury and pulmonary edema. The treatment is supportive. Many patients require a ventilator with positive end-expiratory pressure and dopamine. This disorder may be misdiagnosed as circulatory overload. From 5% to 8% of patients die of complications of the pulmonary injury.

Delayed hemolytic transfusion reactions occur because of the inability to detect clinically significant recipient antibodies before transfusion. This is less dramatic and less dangerous than acute hemolytic reactions and is more common in females. The recipient's plasma already contains antibody before transfusion because of previous transfusion, or previous pregnancy. It usually involves the Rh or Kidd systems, which become rapidly undetectable and increase quickly in titer on rapid stimulation. Results of the Coombs test are positive. There is evidence of hemolysis. One-third of patients are asymptomatic, and the others present with anemia, chills, jaundice, and fever. Management consists of monitoring hemoglobin and renal output. Urticarial reactions are a complication of 1% to 3% of all transfusions. Glottal edema and asthma are rarely associated. The cause is an antibody in the recipient against foreign-donor serum proteins. Treatment consists of stopping the transfusion, which is not absolutely necessary, and giving antihistamines (premedication with antihistamines if patient had previous reaction).

Febrile reactions are characterized by chills and fever an hour after the transfusion starts, with accompanying flushing, headache, tachycardia, and discomfort lasting 8 to 10 hours. This occurs in 1% of all transfusions. The causes include previous transfusions or pregnancy with acquired antibodies against donor leukocyte antigens, antiplatelet antibodies, and antiserum protein antibodies. Treatment consists of stopping the transfusion to evaluate the problem further, because one cannot initially distinguish a febrile reaction from a hemolytic transfusion reaction because both conditions may present with fever.

Circulatory overload may cause tightness in the chest, dry cough, and acute edema in patients with an already increased intravascular volume or decreased cardiac reserve. This is a frequently overlooked diagnosis. Symptoms generally develop within several hours after transfusion. Management includes slowing the transfusion to 100 mL/h, placing the patient in the sitting position, and giving diuretics.

Post-transfusion purpura is a rare syndrome characterized by the abrupt onset of severe thrombocytopenia 5 to 10 days after blood transfusion, with an estimated mortality of 10% to 15%. Most cases involve patients whose platelets lack the P1A1 antigen and who have developed an antibody from a previous pregnancy or transfusion. Therapy is usually successful. Intravenous immunoglobulin at a dose of 400 to 500 mg/kg is the treatment of choice. Plasma exchange and corticosteroids are alternative choices.

Thrombopoietin

Thrombopoietin and interleukin-11 are approved for secondary prophylaxis against chemotherapy-induced thrombocytopenia. In clinical practice, even severe treatment-related thrombocytopenia only rarely leads to death or life-threatening illness. Transfusion of platelet concentrates ensures that very few patients with thrombocytopenia die as a result of hemorrhage.

Gaucher Disease

Adults have type I Gaucher disease, with no neurologic symptoms, splenomegaly, and no symptoms; 50% have anemia or thrombocytopenia. Bone lesions are present in 75%, with the femur being most common with an Erlenmeyer flask deformity. Avascular necrosis and pathologic fractures may occur. The pathogenesis is related to an accumulation of glucosylceramide due to deficient β-glucuronidase. The Gaucher cell is large and has an eccentric nucleus and fibrillar cytoplasm that is wrinkled like tissue paper (Plate 12-18). Treatment options include alglucerase (Ceredase) (an enzyme replacement therapy that is extraordinarily expensive), hemisplenectomy, and allogeneic bone marrow transplantation.

● Differential diagnosis of asymptomatic massive splenomegaly includes Gaucher disease, agnogenic myeloid metaplasia, portal hypertension, splenic cyst, non-Hodgkin lymphoma, and hairy cell leukemia.

Porphyria

The porphyrias are enzyme disorders, which are autosomal dominant with low disease penetrance, except for congenital erythropoietic porphyria which is autosomal recessive and porphyria cutanea tarda which may be acquired. Most persons remain biochemically and clinically normal throughout life. Clinical expression is linked to environmental and acquired factors. Disease manifestation depends on the type of the excess porphyrinogen intermediate and related porphyrin. When there is an excess of the earlier precursor molecules (δ-aminolevulinic acid and porphobilinogen), the clinical manifestations are neuropsychiatric. These symptoms include autonomic dysfunction (abdominal pain, vomiting, constipation, tachycardia, and hypertension), psychiatric symptoms, fever, leukocytosis, syndrome of inappropriate antidiuretic hormone, and neurologic symptoms (proximal paresis and paresthesias). If the excess is in the distal intermediates (uroporphyrins, coproporphyrins, and protoporphyrins), then the manifestations are cutaneous (photosensitivity, blister formation, facial hypertrichosis, and hyperpigmentation). If the excess is early and late, then there are neuropsychiatric and cutaneous manifestations. Porphobilinogen production and excretion are invariably increased during significant symptoms caused by the three neuropathic porphyrias, which include acute intermittent porphyria, hereditary coproporphyria, and porphyria variegata. In hereditary coproporphyria and porphyria variegata, there is an accumulation of coproporphyrinogen/coproporphyrin or protoporphyrinogen/protoporphyrin and a concomitant increase in δ-aminolevulinic acid and porphobilinogen. In the acute porphyrias, urinary porphobilinogen is increased during the attacks. Acute intermittent porphyria lacks skin lesions. It is important to check fecal porphyrins in protoporphyria, variegate porphyria, and coproporphyria. The porphyrias are compared in Table 12-18.

Secondary coproporphyrinuria has multiple causes, including impaired hepatobiliary transport of coprophyrin (steroids) or increased hepatic or erythroid synthesis (alcohol, liver disease, or hemolytic anemia).

- Determine the 24-hour urinary porphobilinogen during the acute episode.

Cardiac Toxicity of Chemotherapeutic Agents

Doxorubicin (Adriamycin) has the greatest potential for cardiac toxicity. It is dose-limited at a dose of 450 mg/m^2 to 500 mg/m^2. The course is characterized by cardiomyopathy to congestive heart failure to death. The pathologic features are characterized by a diffuse patchy myocardial cell degeneration that antedates any alteration in left ventricular function. Risk factors include age older than 70 years, coronary artery disease, hypertension, combination chemotherapy and previous or concomitant mediastinal radiation therapy, and the use of other cardiotoxic agents. Weekly and prolonged continuous infusion schedules may decrease the risk of toxicity. Acutely, there may be transient and reversible nonspecific ST-segment changes, decrease in ejection fraction, or arrhythmias. The dilated cardiomyopathy is dose-dependent: a 3.5% risk at a total dose of 400 mg/m^2, 7% at a dose of 500 to 550 mg/m^2, and 36% at a total dose of 600 mg/m^2 or greater. The clinical features of the cardiomyopathy vary widely. Follow-up examination requires evaluating left ventricular ejection fraction by radionuclide ventriculography or echocardiography. The former is more sensitive.

- Doxorubicin has the greatest potential for cardiac toxicity.
- The incidence of cardiomyopathy is dose-dependent.
- Age >70 years, coronary artery disease, and previous radiation may potentiate toxicity.

Table 12-18.—Comparison of Porphyrias

Porphyria cutanea tarda	Acute intermittent porphyria	Porphyria variegata
Features		
Most common	Increased urinary δ-aminolevulinic acid (ALA) and porphobilinogen (PBG)	Clinically: skin, sun-exposed, mechanical fragility; abdominal pain; neurologic problems (e.g., acute intermittent porphyria)
Iron overload		
Skin lesions on light-exposed areas	Triad: abdominal pain of 3-5 days' duration, neurologic problems of polyneuropathy and motor paresis, psychiatric problems with hallucinations, confusion, psychosis, seizures	Increased protoporphyrin and coproporphyrin in stool
Hypertrichosis		
Increased uroporphyrins in urine		
No neuropathic features	Decreased porphobilinogen deaminase	
Most common of porphyrias	Normal protoporphyrin and coproporphyrin in stool	
Associations		
Alcoholic liver disease	Drugs: sulfonamides, barbiturates, alcohol	Common in South Africa, Holland
Estrogens: females, males treated for prostatic carcinoma	Menstrual cycle	
	Infection	
Hexachlorobenzene	Inadequate nutrition	
	Stress: infections, surgery	
Treatment		
Phlebotomy, to remove iron	Avoid prolonged fasting and crash diets	
Chloroquine	Large amounts of carbohydrate (400 g/day)	
	Intravenous hematin	
	Luteinizing hormone-releasing hormone agonists	

Superior Vena Cava Syndrome

Most cases (78%) of superior vena cava syndrome are caused by malignancy. Extrinsic compression of the thin superior vena cava, which has a low intravascular pressure, in a rigid compartment is the pathophysiologic basis of this syndrome. The causes include bronchogenic carcinoma (75% of cases, with small cell and squamous cell carcinoma most common), lymphoma (15%), testicular carcinoma (consider this if biopsy shows anaplastic or undifferentiated carcinoma; check the β-subunit of human chorionic gonadotropin and alpha-fetoprotein), carcinoma, and adenocarcinoma of undetermined primary. The symptoms include suffusion of the face and conjunctiva, dyspnea, facial swelling, other swelling, cough, dysphagia, syncope, orthopnea, stridor, and lethargy. Physical examination reveals thoracic vein distention, neck vein distention, facial edema, cyanosis, edema of the upper extremities, paralyzed vocal cord, Horner syndrome, and heart murmurs. The diagnosis is established by the history and physical examination. Superior vena cava venography is not useful. A tissue diagnosis is essential to establish the diagnosis precisely. Mediastinotomy is the safest way to obtain histologic diagnosis. If the syndrome is rapid in onset, then treatment must be rapid. In patients with lymphoma, testicular carcinoma, or small cell carcinoma of the lung, treat the underlying disease initially with chemotherapy. If life-threatening problems are present, such as tracheal obstruction or increased intracranial pressure, emergency radiation therapy may be necessary in any disorder presenting with superior vena cava syndrome. Steroids may be helpful. Initial treatment with radiation therapy is indicated for solid tumors, with a total dose of 30 to 50 Gy or a single dose of 7 to 12 Gy. Anticoagulation is indicated only if a blood clot has been implicated in the pathophysiology. Diuretics and surgical decompression are not indicated.

- For superior vena cava syndrome, establish a tissue diagnosis.
- Features: edema of the face and neck and venous engorgement of the upper torso.
- Medical emergency in certain situations; may require immediate radiation.

Hypercalcemia

Virtually any malignancy may lead to hypercalcemia. Specific causes include carcinomas of the breast and lung (squamous and large cell carcinoma are common and adenocarcinoma and small cell carcinoma are uncommon causes), hypernephroma, other tumors (head and neck, cervix, prostate, neuroblastoma, hepatoma, and melanoma), lymphoma, Burkitt lymphoma, multiple myeloma, Hodgkin disease, chronic myelogenous leukemia, and Waldenström macroglobulinemia.

The signs and symptoms include lassitude, somnolence, weakness, anorexia, nausea, vomiting, constipation, abdominal pain, peptic ulcer, pancreatitis, polyuria, polydipsia, poor intake, renal failure, hyporeflexia, Babinski sign, myopathy, stupor, coma, occasional localizing signs, visual abnormalities, psychotic behavior, bradycardia, tachycardia, shortened QT interval, digitalis sensitivity, arrhythmias, hypertension, fractures, pain, skeletal deformities, loss of height, poor skin turgor, calcinosis, and band keratopathy. It is misdiagnosed as terminal disease, brain metastases, drug toxicity, renal failure, diabetes insipidus, acute abdomen, and intractable peptic ulcer disease. The diagnosis can be confirmed by measuring serum levels of parathyroid hormone (PTH). In malignancy, these levels are low, and in primary hyperparathyroidism, the level is increased.

- Misdiagnoses include terminal disease, brain metastases, drug toxicity, renal failure, diabetes insipidus, acute abdomen, and intractable peptic ulcer disease.

The mechanisms of action of hypercalcemia are multiple. Osteolytic metastases may produce accelerated skeletal resorption. Osteoclast activating factors are associated with multiple myeloma, lymphoma, and Burkitt non-Hodgkin lymphoma. Other factors include dehydration, mobilization, adrenal insufficiency secondary to tumor metastases, estrogens, androgens, progestins, and tamoxifen.

Most hypercalcemia is related to increased bone resorption. Intestinal absorption is low or low-normal in most cases. There usually is no increase in renal tubular reabsorption, but the kidney may be involved in hyperparathyroidism, breast cancer, metabolic alkalosis, and salt depletion. The course is short and rapidly progressive. There may be moderate to severe weight loss and no renal calculi; pancreatitis is rare. The serum level of calcium is greater than 14 mg/dL in 75% of patients. The serum level of alkaline phosphatase may be increased, normal, or decreased. Anemia and metabolic alkalosis may be present. The alkaline phosphatase level is increased in 50% of patients but can be increased in primary hyperparathyroidism. Hypophosphatemia can occur whether or not there is a PTH-secreting tumor. Hypoalbuminemia must be considered, and for every gram of albumin below 4, add 1 to the ionized calcium.

Treatment is multifaceted. The use of such precipitating factors as vitamins A and D, lithium, thiazides, absorbable antacids, and estrogens should be discontinued. The patient should be mobilized. Also, the patient should be hydrated with a minimum of 2.5 to 4 L of fluid in the first 24 hours. To each liter of normal saline, add 20 to 40 mEq of KCl and 10 to 20 mEq of magnesium. Experimentally, if the sodium is increased from 25 mEq to 250 mEq, calcium excretion is increased threefold and is not related to the glomerulofiltration rate. Treat the underlying disease. Glucocorticoids are efficacious in multiple myeloma and non-Hodgkin lymphomas. The typical dose is 80 mg of prednisone in divided doses daily. The mechanisms of action include antitumor effects, an antivitamin D effect, inhibition of prostaglandin synthesis or release, inhibition of osteoclast activating factor production, anti-PTH activity, and an inhibitory effect on osteoprogenitor cells. Furosemide should be administered after 2 L of fluid. The dosages are variable, ranging from 20 mg to 40 mg up to every 4 hours. Furosemide blocks the tubular reabsorption of calcium, depletes sodium, depletes potassium, and depletes magnesium. The bisphosphonates have an inhibitory effect on osteoclast function and viability. Etidronate at a dose of 7.5 mg/kg over 4 hours is given intravenously up to 7 days. This decreases calcium within 2 days. Pamidronate is given by intravenous infusion at a dose of 15 to 45 mg/day for up to 6 days. Alternatively, 90 mg may be given over 24 hours or it may be administered orally at a dose of 1,200 mg for up to 5 days. In general, the bisphosphonates are more potent than calcitonin and less toxic than plicamycin. Plicamycin inhibits RNA synthesis in osteoclasts. There may be subjective improvement within 12 hours and improvement in the serum levels of calcium in 36 hours. The dose is 25 µg/kg over 4 hours and may be repeated once if necessary. Side effects include thrombocytopenia, hemorrhage, renal complications, increased liver enzymes, sudden arterial occlusion, and toxic epidermal necrolysis. Contraindications include thrombocytopenia and coagulopathy. The use of phosphate should be restricted to extreme life-threatening hypercalcemia. Calcium phosphate complexes are deposited in vessels, lungs, and kidneys.

HEMOCHROMATOSIS

Hemochromatosis is the end result of a pathologic process that evolves over years and is secondary to the excessive absorption of dietary iron. The causes of hemochromatosis include hereditary hemochromatosis (idiopathic), secondary anemia and ineffective erythropoiesis (thalassemia major, thalassemia minor), hereditary spherocytosis, idiopathic refractory sideroblastic anemia and myelodysplasia, oral intake of iron (medicinal), liver disease (alcoholic cirrhosis, portal caval anastomosis), drugs (isoniazid, chloramphenicol), and copper deficiency. Patients with end-stage disease present with endocrine complications and hepatic fibrosis.

Hereditary hemochromatosis is a potentially fatal disorder that is among the most prevalent of deleterious genes in whites of European ancestry and is as prevalent as the sickle cell gene in African-Americans. The prevalence is 1:300. The gene for hereditary hemochromatosis has been identified. These homozygotes typically develop clinical evidence of hemochromatosis. It is inherited as an autosomal recessive trait. Males present in the fourth to fifth decade. The transferrin saturation is greater than 55% even early in life and before tissue iron loading occurs. Screening appears to be effective and should be considered at about age 30 in men.

The most advocated screening test for homozygotes is a transferrin saturation greater than 55%. Urine iron is increased in the range of 5 to 20 mg/24 hr (normal, <2 mg/24 hr). Liver biopsy defines the degree of iron overload and the status of the liver (fibrosis, cirrhosis, and hepatitis). The reference standard for diagnosis is liver biopsy, and hepatic iron by dry weight is markedly increased at 200 to 1,800 µg/100 ng dry weight (normal, 30-140). Supporting evidence is also provided by the amount of iron removed by venesection therapy (>5 g) and pedigree studies.

The goal of treatment is to improve prognosis and the clinical course in patients with established liver damage. The mainstays of treatment are phlebotomy and chelation until the ferritin level is less than 50 µg/L; 224 mg of iron are removed per phlebotomy unit. Patients initially have venesection once to twice weekly. Maintenance phlebotomies are required, typically every 3 months. Deferoxamine (10 mg/day by continuous infusion) is the chelation agent used most often. Timely diagnosis and therapy can prevent irreversible organ failure. Features not altered by chelation include arthropathy, hypogonadism, development of hepatocellular carcinoma, and hepatic cirrhosis. Patients who begin treatment before end-organ damage have a normal life span. The role of genetic testing is under investigation. Genotyping can be used as a confirmatory test in a patient of suspected iron overload.

- Endocrine dysfunction: 50% with diabetes mellitus at presentation and a minority have vascular sequelae; hypogonadism (decreased libido, impotence, and amenorrhea); hypopituitarism.
- Cardiac: congestive heart failure and arrhythmias.
- Skin: bronze, "slate gray."
- Arthropathy: chondrocalcinosis, bone cysts, and irregularity.
- Hepatomegaly, abdominal pain, cirrhosis, and hepatocellular carcinoma.
- Lethargy, weight loss.
- Transferrin saturation >55% on at least two occasions should raise clinical suspicion.
- After an index case is identified, family members must be screened.
- The gene for hereditary hemochromatosis and two mutations have been defined.
- 82% of patients of European descent are homozygous for the hemoglobin H mutation.

- The molecular genetics of non-HLA-linked African hemochromatosis has yet to be elucidated.

HEMATOLOGY OF ACQUIRED IMMUNE DEFICIENCY

In AIDS, lymphocytopenias are the hallmark of the disease. There is an absolute decrease of T4 lymphocytes, with a relative reduction of the T4-to-T8 ratio. Also, there is functional impairment of T4 lymphocytes. Whereas T8 lymphocytes may increase early in the disease in infections, they decrease in number late in the disease. Neutropenia occurs in 50% of the patients. Natural killer cells are normal in number but altered in function. Neutropenia may be due to autoimmune destruction with antigranulocyte antibodies in two-thirds of patients, decreased production, zidovudine (AZT), ganciclovir, trimethoprim/sulfamethoxazole, pentamidine, coexisting infections, non-Hodgkin lymphoma, or antineoplastic chemotherapy. Neutrophil dysfunction is also manifested by decreased chemotaxis, granulation, and phagocytosis.

Anemia occurs in 70% of HIV-infected patients. Most commonly, the anemia is normochromic normocytic. The degree of anemia is a prognostic factor in the patients. Anemia occurs in 10% of asymptomatic HIV-positive patients, 50% of patients with AIDS-related complex, and more than 75% of patients with overt AIDS. HIV-associated RBC problems include decreased RBC production; 70% of AIDS patients have decreased erythropoietin levels. Approximately 25% of patients have positive results on the Coombs test, but significant hemolysis is not common. Of patients treated with zidovudine, 30% develop significant anemia, which is characteristically macrocytic. Decreased RBC production is a principal cause. Erythropoietin has been used successfully in those with an erythropoietin level less than 500 IU/mL. Clinical studies have demonstrated that transfusions may decrease survival and increase the risk of cytomegalovirus infection. Anemia is also associated with infections from *Mycobacterium avium* complex, parvovirus, B19, *Mycobacterium tuberculosis*, and histoplasmosis. Anemia may be malignancy-related. Decreased vitamin B_{12} levels are present in 20% of HIV-infected patients and are due to altered serum transport of vitamin B_{12} and not to a deficiency in body stores unless there has been prolonged malabsorption. Microangiopathic hemolytic anemia is milder than in other causes of this disorder. Plasmapheresis with plasma exchange is the treatment of choice. Vincristine may be efficacious in refractory cases.

Thrombocytopenia occurs in 40% of HIV-infected patients and is often detected early in the disease. Platelet survival is decreased in HIV-infected patients. The serum and cell-bound antibodies are frequently positive. Circulating complexes are either the cause of or are associated with immune cytopenias. Idiopathic thrombocytopenic purpura is usually accompanied by platelet-associated antibodies and responds to zidovudine (80% of patients), prednisone (90%), danazol, dapsone (60%), immunoglobulin given intravenously, and splenectomy (80%). Other HIV associations include thrombotic thrombocytopenic purpura, decreased platelet production, and peripheral platelet sequestration. Other non-HIV associations include therapy, infection, and malignancy. Coagulation disorders may complicate HIV disorders. The lupus-like anticoagulant is present in 20% of HIV patients, usually in association with opportunistic infections, and is rarely associated with thrombosis or bleeding. Vitamin K deficiencies due to nutritional abnormalities, drugs, or hepatic dysfunction may occur. Other problems include increased level of vWF:Ag (with a poor prognosis if >200%), increased level of tissue plasminogen activator (with a poor prognosis if >20 ng/mL), and increased level of fibrinogen.

Non-Hodgkin lymphoma is the second most common HIV-associated malignancy, occurring in 2.9% of patients. Extranodal disease occurs in 66% of patients. Up to one-third of patients with lymphoma may have bone involvement. There is also an increased risk of Hodgkin disease among HIV patients, which is not one of the diagnostic criteria for AIDS.

Microangiopathic hemolytic anemia is milder than in other causes of this disorder. Plasmapheresis with plasma exchange is the treatment of choice. Vincristine may be efficacious in refractory cases.

PARVOVIRUS INFECTION

Parvovirus infection (B19), or fifth disease, is a highly contagious disease in children. Adults with this infection may develop a polyarthralgia syndrome or cytopenia. Abnormalities in the erythroid line include severe anemia, reticulocytopenia, and RBC hypoplasia in the marrow. Pancytopenia may occur. Immunoglobulin therapy administered intravenously is the treatment of choice.

REVIEW OF CHEMOTHERAPEUTIC AGENTS

Chemotherapeutic agents—alkylating agents, antibiotics, and hormones—and their effects are reviewed in Table 12-19.

Table 12-19.—Chemotherapeutic Agents

Drug	Toxic effects	Other
Alkylating agents		
Carmustine	Delayed marrow suppression, nausea, vomiting, pulmonary, hepatic toxicity, secondary leukemia	Cumulative marrow suppression, crosses blood-brain barrier
Busulfan	Pulmonary fibrosis	Hepatic metabolism, renal excretion
Carboplatin	Marrow suppression, nausea and vomiting, less nephrotoxicity and neurotoxicity than cisplatin	Renal excretion
Chlorambucil	Pulmonary, secondary leukemia	Hepatic metabolism
Cisplatin	Nephrotoxicity, peripheral neuropathy, ototoxicity, magnesium depletion, hand-foot syndrome	Renal excretion Raynaud phenomenon
Cyclophosphamide	Acute nonlymphocytic leukemia and dysmyelopoietic syndromes (monosomy 5 and 7), bladder cancer, leukopenia, cystitis, pulmonary fibrosis, syndrome of inappropriate antidiuretic hormone, alopecia, nausea, vomiting	Hepatic metabolism to active compound, renal excretion, lower dose with renal failure, late transitional cell carcinoma of bladder
Dacarbazine	Marrow suppression, flu-like syndrome, severe nausea and vomiting, fever	
Melphalan	Marrow suppression, secondary leukemia	The absence of renal clearance allows the use of high-dose melphalan in patients with renal failure, erratic oral absorption
Nitrogen mustard	Marrow suppression, nausea and vomiting, sterility, secondary leukemia	
Streptozocin	Diabetes, marrow suppression, severe nausea and vomiting, renal	Leads to pancreatic and endocrine insufficiency
Procarbazine	Secondary leukemia	
Antibiotics		
Bleomycin	Pulmonary fibrosis (threshold 400 µg/lifetime) but may recur at lower doses, fever and chills, myalgias, skin pigmentation, alopecia, adult respiratory distress syndrome with oxygen	Lower dose with renal insufficiency
Dactinomycin	Marrow suppression, radiation recall, nausea and vomiting, mucositis, alopecia	
Daunorubicin	Marrow suppression, radiation recall, cardiomyopathy, mucositis, nausea and vomiting, alopecia, acute nonlymphocytic leukemia	Decrease dose by 50% if bilirubin >1.5 mg/dL or by 75% if bilirubin >3.0 mg/dL
Doxorubicin	Dose-related cardiomyopathy, marrow suppression, alopecia, nausea and vomiting, stomatitis, radiation recall, acute nonlymphocytic leukemia	Hepatic metabolism, biliary excretion, decrease dose by 50% if bilirubin >1.5 mg/dL or by 75% if bilirubin >3.0 mg/dL

Table 12-19 (continued)

Drug	Toxic effects	Other
Mitomycin C	Delayed marrow suppression, nausea and vomiting, alopecia, hepatic toxicity, microangiopathic hemolytic anemia	Vesicant, alkylator, forms free radicals
Mitoxantrone	Marrow suppression, cardiac toxicity, nausea and vomiting, mucositis, alopecia, blue sclera and urine	

Hormones

Corticosteroids	Diabetes, hepatic toxicity, aseptic necrosis, adrenal insufficiency, myopathy, infection, osteoporosis, peptic ulcer disease, hypokalemia, psychosis, cataract	

Podophyllotoxin

Etoposide (VP-16)	Acute nonlymphocytic leukemia t(11q23)	

Adenosine deaminase inhibitors

2'-Deoxycoformycin Fludarabine 2-Chlorodeoxyadenosine	Myelosuppression and immunosuppression Opportunistic infections	

Biologic agents

G-CSF	Fever, bone pain, myalgias, arthralgias	
GM-CSF	Fever, bone pain, myalgias, arthralgias	
Interferon-α	Fever, fatigue, pain, headache, anorexia, nausea, diarrhea, allergic reactions, central and peripheral neuropathy	

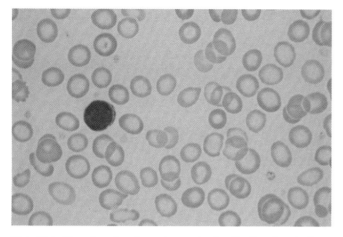

Plate 12-1. Hypochromic-microcytic anemia. Small cells, <6 μm in diameter, with increased central pallor and assorted aberrations in size (anisocytosis) and in shape (poikilocytosis). (Courtesy of Curtis A. Hanson, M.D., Mayo Clinic.)

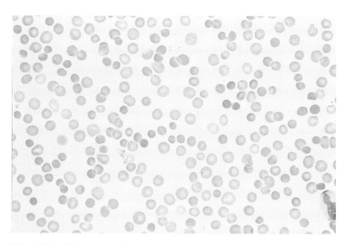

Plate 12-2. Spherocytes. Smooth, small, and spheroidal darkly stained cells with minimal or no central pallor. (Courtesy of Curtis A. Hanson, M.D., Mayo Clinic.)

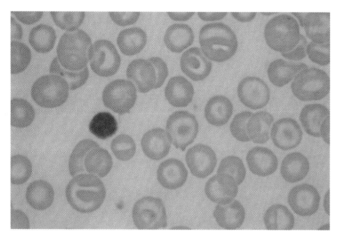

Plate 12-3. Target cells. Red blood cells with a broad diameter and a dark center. (Courtesy of Curtis A. Hanson, M.D., Mayo Clinic.)

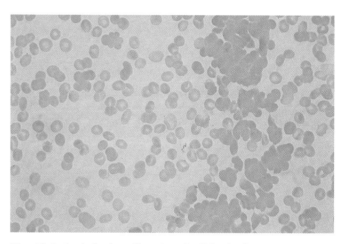

Plate 12-4. Agglutination. Clumping of red blood cells.

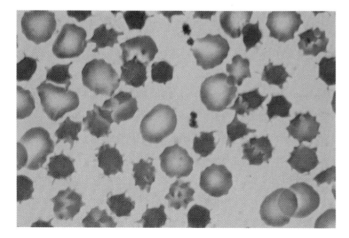

Plate 12-5. Acanthocytes. Note the thin, thorny, or finger-like projections. (Courtesy of Curtis A. Hanson, M.D., Mayo Clinic.)

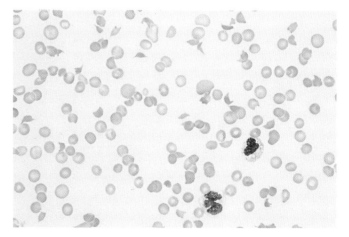

Plate 12-6. Schistocytes. Fragmented red blood cells shaped like helmets, triangles, or kites. (Courtesy of Curtis A. Hanson, M.D., Mayo Clinic.)

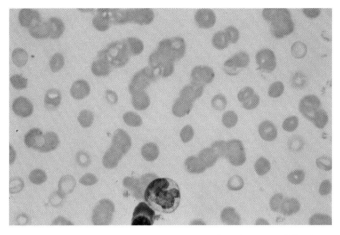

Plate 12-7. Rouleaux. Stacking of red blood cells. (Courtesy of Curtis A. Hanson, M.D., Mayo Clinic.)

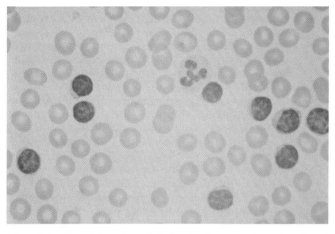

Plate 12-8. Chronic lymphocytic leukemia. Large number of small and agranular mature lymphocytes whose nuclei are approximately the same size as red blood cells.

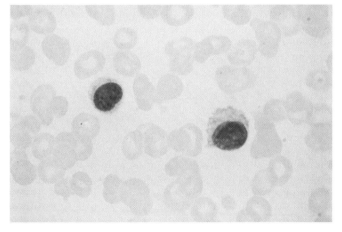

Plate 12-9. Hairy cell leukemia. Mature lymphocytes with eccentrically placed nuclei and pale cytoplasm that have characteristic projections.

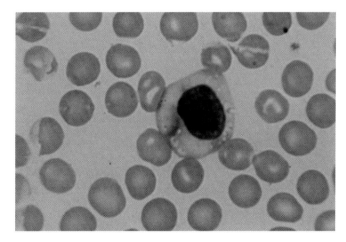

Plate 12-10. Infectious mononucleosis. Large atypical lymphocyte has a large amount of pale cytoplasm, which may be vacuolated, and a large oblong nucleus.

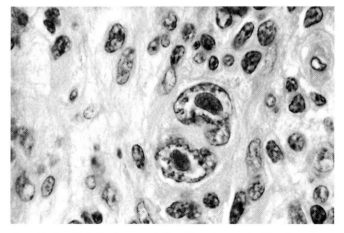

Plate 12-11. Hodgkin disease. A Reed-Sternberg cell, a binucleate large cell. (Courtesy of Curtis A. Hanson, M.D., Mayo Clinic.)

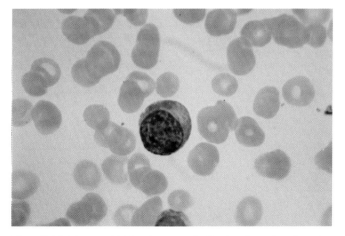

Plate 12-12. Plasma cell. Note the eccentrically placed round nucleus; the copious, dark blue cytoplasm has a characteristic pale-staining area adjacent to the nucleus.

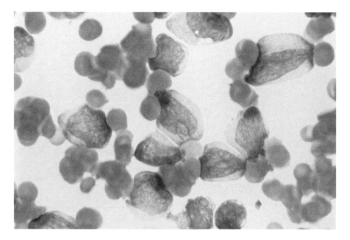

Plate 12-13. Acute nonlymphocytic leukemia. Large pleomorphic cells with large nuclei and a barely visible nuclear membrane.

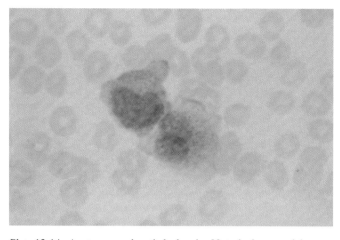

Plate 12-14. Acute promyelocytic leukemia. Note the large nuclei; more than half of the leukemic cells have large atypical granulations. (Courtesy of Curtis A. Hanson, M.D., Mayo Clinic.)

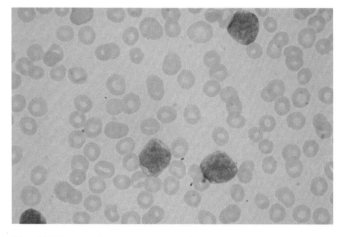

Plate 12-15. Acute lymphocytic leukemia. Large, rounded, and indented nuclei with diverse shapes and scant, darker blue cytoplasm.

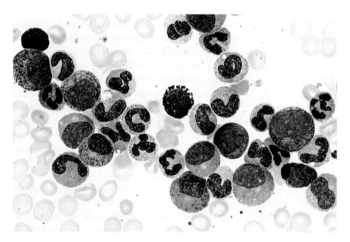

Plate 12-16. Chronic myelogenous leukemia. Normal-appearing myeloid cells representing all stages of maturation, with a decreased number of erythropoietic cells and one basophil precursor in the center. (Courtesy of Curtis A. Hanson, M.D., Mayo Clinic.)

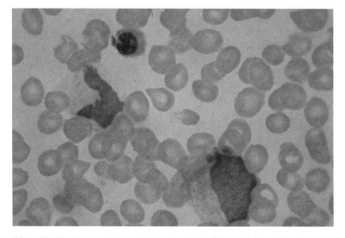

Plate 12-17. Agnogenic myeloid metaplasia. The peripheral blood smear is leukoerythroblastic with dacrocytes.

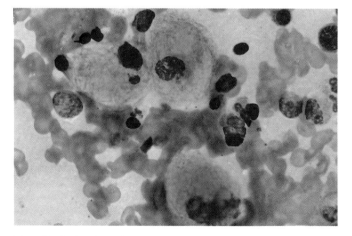

Plate 12-18. Gaucher cells. Large cell with characteristic pale, foamy, and fibrillar cytoplasm. (Courtesy of Curtis A. Hanson, M.D., Mayo Clinic.)

QUESTIONS

Multiple Choice (choose the one best answer)

1. A 55-year-old woman has had a history of anemia since childhood. Seven years ago, the folate level was 0.9 µg/L (normal, 2.0-14). The patient has had a long history of psoriasis. Physical examination revealed only psoriatic plaques. The complete blood count showed hemoglobin of 10.2 g/dL, mean corpuscular volume of 68 fL, and red blood cell count of 3.59 x 10⁶/L. The ferritin level was 1 (normal, 20-120). Fecal hemoglobin levels were within normal limits. The most likely diagnosis is:
   a. Peptic ulcer disease
   b. Arteriovenous malformation of the small bowel
   c. Glucose-6-phosphatase dehydrogenase deficiency
   d. Celiac sprue
   e. Pernicious anemia

2. A 75-year-old man was referred for medical evaluation before cataract surgery. Review of previous records indicated that the complete blood count was within normal limits. The hemoglobin was 9.5 g/dL; mean corpuscular volume, 65.1 fL; and red blood cell count, 4.59 x 10⁶/L. Ferritin was 4 µg/L (normal, 20-300). The most likely diagnosis is:
   a. Peptic ulcer disease
   b. Beta thalassemia trait
   c. Glucose-6-phosphatase dehydrogenase deficiency
   d. Celiac sprue
   e. Pernicious anemia

3. A 72-year-old man was referred with a diagnosis of hemolytic anemia. He has had severe osteoarthritis and is taking nonsteroidal anti-inflammatory agents. The diagnosis of Crohn disease was established 4 years ago. Six months ago, anemia developed. Currently, he has six bowel movements per day. Laboratory values revealed hemoglobin of 7.0 g/dL, mean corpuscular volume of 81.4 (normal, 81.6-98.3), reticulocyte count of 7.8%, a normal bilirubin, and normal lactic dehydrogenase. The fecal hemoglobin was increased. The most likely diagnosis is:
   a. Peptic ulcer disease
   b. Voltaren-induced colonic ulcers
   c. Glucose-6-phosphatase dehydrogenase deficiency
   d. Crohn disease
   e. Pernicious anemia

4. Four months earlier, a 31-year-old woman developed abdominal distention, hepatomegaly, and anemia. At this time, she presented with abdominal swelling. A complete blood count revealed hemoglobin, 10.4 g/dL and mean corpuscular volume, 96.7 fL. The white blood cell count and platelet count were normal. Indirect bilirubin was increased. Blood smear revealed regeneration with no spherocytes. The reticulocyte count was 10.4. The Coombs test was negative. Fecal hemoglobin was normal. The most likely diagnosis is:
   a. Peptic ulcer disease
   b. Arteriovenous malformation of the small bowel
   c. Paroxysmal nocturnal hemoglobinuria
   d. Celiac sprue
   e. Pernicious anemia

5. A 63-year-old man presented with a 27-lb weight loss. He had diabetes mellitus of 20 years' duration. Physical examination revealed a fissured tongue and loss of vibratory sensation. Complete blood count showed hemoglobin of 10.1 g/dL and a mean corpuscular volume of 124 fL. The most likely diagnosis is:
   a. Erosive gastritis
   b. Alcoholism
   c. Hypothyroidism
   d. Celiac sprue
   e. Pernicious anemia

6. A 73-year-old woman had a 22-year history of deforming polyarthritis. About 2.5 years ago, she developed an acute fulminating generalized erythematous exfoliative dermatitis. Now, she was admitted with postural dizziness and severe refractory edema of her legs. Hemoglobin was 5.9 g/dL; red blood cell count 1.05, and mean corpuscular volume, 158.7 fL. The most likely diagnosis is:
   a. Laboratory error
   b. Hyperglycemia
   c. Hypothyroidism
   d. Folate deficiency
   e. Pernicious anemia

7. A 28-year-old woman was well until 3 weeks ago, when she was treated with ampicillin for a sore throat. Two weeks ago, she developed intermittent headaches. One week ago, she had petechia. Yesterday, she had weakness and confusion. Hemoglobin was 9.4 g/dL and the platelet count was 10,000. A blood smear revealed schistocytes. Creatinine was 1.0. Urinalysis revealed +2 proteinuria. The next best approach to this patient would be:
   a. Heparin
   b. Estrogen/progesterone to prevent menses
   c. Plasmapheresis
   d. Plasmapheresis with replacement with fresh frozen plasma
   e. Steroids

8. A 67-year-old woman had a diagnosis of polycythemia rubra vera in January 1991. Treatment was started with hydroxyurea, 1 g daily. She now returns for follow-up. A complete blood count shows the following: hemoglobin, 12.6 g/dL; mean corpuscular volume, 112.3 fL; white blood cell count, 5,600; and platelet count, 294,000. The most likely cause of the macrocytosis is:
   a. Vitamin B_{12} deficiency
   b. Hydroxyurea
   c. Folate deficiency
   d. Liver disease
   e. Myelodysplasia

9. A 21-year-old man has well-documented sickle cell anemia. Which of the following factors is not associated with a risk of early death?
   a. Acute chest syndrome
   b. Renal failure
   c. A high level of fetal hemoglobin
   d. A baseline white blood cell count >15,000
   e. Hemorrhagic stroke

10. A critically ill 25-year-old African-American man was admitted to the hospital with fever, tachypnea, chest pain, and an increased white blood cell count. The peripheral blood smear showed sickle cells. The most common cause of death in this clinical situation is:
   a. Acute pain and chest syndrome
   b. HIV infection
   c. Stroke
   d. Pneumococcal sepsis
   e. *E. coli* sepsis

11. A 72-year-old woman has an increased white blood cell count. The complete blood count revealed the following: hemoglobin, 13.0 g/dL; white blood cell count, 20,000; and platelet count, 178,000. The differential showed 96% lymphocytes. On physical examination, there was no palpable lymphadenopathy or splenomegaly. The treatment of choice is:
   a. Observation
   b. Prednisone
   c. Chlorambucil/prednisone or fludarabine
   d. ABVD
   e. CHOP

12. A 63-year-old woman has lymphadenopathy and a white blood cell count of 63,000. The differential showed 90% lymphocytes. The platelet count was 80,000. Physical examination showed that the spleen was 1 cm below the costal margin. The treatment of choice is:
   a. Observation
   b. Prednisone
   c. Chlorambucil/prednisone or fludarabine
   d. ABVD
   e. CHOP

13. A 52-year-old man has massive splenomegaly, normochromic-normocytic anemia, severe pancytopenia, and temperatures to 40°C. The most likely diagnosis is:
   a. Follicular small cleaved cell non-Hodgkin lymphoma
   b. Gaucher
   c. Agnogenic myeloid metaplasia
   d. Hairy cell leukemia
   e. Splenic cyst

14. A 64-year-old woman has asymptomatic lymphadenopathy. The complete blood count and lactic dehydrogenase level were normal. Computed tomography showed mild lymphadenopathy, and biopsy revealed follicular small cleaved cell non-Hodgkin lymphoma. Bone marrow biopsy showed 10% involvement with non-Hodgkin lymphoma. The cells in the bone marrow were small. The treatment of choice is:
   a. Observation
   b. Oral chlorambucil
   c. CVP
   d. Anti-CD20 antibody therapy
   e. CHOP

15. A 50-year-old woman presented with a 2- by 2-cm high anterior cervical lymph node. This was resected. The biopsy showed diffuse large cell non-Hodgkin lymphoma. Lactic dehydrogenase level, computed tomography, and bilateral bone marrow examination were all normal. The treatment of choice is:
   a. Observation
   b. Chlorambucil
   c. CVP
   d. Anti-CD20 antibody therapy
   e. CHOP

16. A 28-year-old woman presented with cervical adenopathy and night sweats. Computed tomography showed a mediastinal mass, splenomegaly, and lymphadenopathy in the lower abdomen. Biopsy revealed nodular sclerosing Hodgkin disease. The treatment of choice is:
   a. CHOP
   b. MOPP
   c. ABVD
   d. Autologous bone marrow transplant
   e. Total nodal radiation therapy plus ABVD

17. A 19-year-old college student presented with temperatures to 39°C and a sore throat. Physical examination showed an exudative tonsillitis, bulky lymphadenopathy, and a rash. The complete blood count revealed lymphocytosis. The results of a lymph node biopsy are pending. The most likely treatment would be:
    a. Observation
    b. CHOP
    c. Fludarabine
    d. Prednisone
    e. Acyclovir

18. A 72-year-old woman presented with melena. She had no lymphadenopathy. Hemoglobin was 10.5 g/dL, and the lactic dehydrogenase level was normal. Gastric biopsy revealed MALTOMA. *Helicobacter pylori* was identified in the biopsy specimen. The initial treatment of choice is:
    a. Observation
    b. Oral chlorambucil
    c. CVP
    d. A double or triple oral antibiotic regimen
    e. Gastrectomy

19. A 52-year-old woman was found to have an IgG kappa monoclonal protein of 0.45 g/dL in the gamma region. The complete blood count, creatinine, and calcium were normal. The initial treatment of choice is:
    a. Observation
    b. Melphalan/prednisone
    c. Alpha recombinant interferon
    d. VBMCP
    e. VBMCP followed by autologous bone marrow transplantation

20. A 64-year-old man had fatigue, weight loss, and dizziness when standing. Physical examination revealed +2 edema of the lower extremities. Creatinine was 3 mg/dL. Urinalysis showed proteinuria. The next best test is:
    a. Computed tomography of the abdomen
    b. Bone marrow
    c. Fat aspiration of the abdominal wall
    d. Renal biopsy
    e. Autonomic studies

21. A 35-year-old man has had a 7-year history of transitional cell carcinoma of the bladder. After being lost to follow-up, he presented with gross hematuria, severe abdominal pain, and an increased white blood cell count. The spleen was not palpable. The white blood count was 129,000. The differential showed 83% neutrophils, 13%

lymphocytes, 1% monocytes, 1% basophils, 1% metamyelocytes, and 1% myelocytes. The platelet count was 518,000. The next test in his evaluation should be:
    a. Bone marrow
    b. Peripheral blood cytogenetics
    c. Erythrocyte sedimentation rate
    d. Leukocyte alkaline phosphatase score
    e. *Bcr-abl* molecular genetic studies

22. An asymptomatic 56-year-old woman was found to have splenomegaly. The spleen was 3 cm below the costal margin. The complete blood count revealed the following: hemoglobin, 12.9 g/dL; hematocrit, 39; mean corpuscular volume, 72 fL; total red blood cell count, 5.45; platelet count, 500,000; and white blood cell count, 16,000. The differential on the complete blood count was within normal limits. The erythrocyte sedimentation rate was 0. The most likely diagnosis is:
    a. Polycythemia rubra vera
    b. Stress erythrocytosis
    c. Anoxic polycythemia
    d. Hypernephroma
    e. Uterine fibroids

23. A 48-year-old woman was referred for rectal surgery. She had a 40-pack-year history of smoking. Physical examination showed +2 forced expiratory wheezing on examination of the lungs. There was no palpable lymphadenopathy or hepatosplenomegaly. Hemoglobin was 16.4 g/dL (normal, 11.6 to 14.9) and the hematocrit was 50.3% (normal, 34.5-43.9), with a normal white blood cell count and platelet count. The most likely diagnosis is:
    a. Polycythemia rubra vera
    b. Stress erythrocytosis
    c. Anoxic polycythemia
    d. Hypernephroma
    e. Uterine fibroids

24. A 56-year-old man presented with asymptomatic lymphadenopathy. The biopsy findings were morphologically consistent with follicular small cleaved cell non-Hodgkin lymphoma. The following cytogenetic results and oncogenes would be expected:
    a. t(8,14), c-*myc*
    b. t(8,22), c-*myc*
    c. t(14,18), *bcl*-6
    d. t(14,18), c-*myc*
    e. t(14,18), *bcl*-2

25. A 68-year-old woman had a life-long history of mild bleeding. Over the last 4 to 5 years, she has developed frequent

epistaxis and ecchymoses. Two years ago, she had a hysterectomy. Ten days after the operation, there was a re-exploration. At that time, she had rectal bleeding. Prothrombin time was normal. The partial thromboplastin time was 80 seconds (normal, 45-60). There was correction with 1/10 volumes. Factor VIII activity was 10% (normal, 55%-145%). Bleeding time was longer than 15 minutes. The diagnosis is:

a. Hemophila A
b. von Willebrand disease
c. Hemophila B
d. Glanzmann thrombasthenia
e. Disseminated intravascular coagulopathy

26. A 62-year-old man presented with epistaxis and extensive purpura and ecchymoses. Laboratory tests showed the following: hemoglobin, 7.0 g/dL; platelet count, 40,000; fibrinogen, 47. Aspartate aminotransferase was 29 (normal). The initial treatment approach would be:

a. Transfusion with red blood cells, platelets, and fresh frozen plasma and cryoprecipitate
b. Transfusion with red blood cells and platelets
c. Plasmapheresis, with replacement with fresh frozen plasma
d. Transfuse with red blood cells and platelets and administer heparin intravenously
e. Administer heparin intravenously

27. A 23-year-old man presented with a 2-week history of rectal bleeding. He had been treated with 9 units of red blood cells before transfer. Seven years ago, he bled excessively after repair of an abscessed tooth. Five years ago, he bled after removal of a sebaceous cyst. Activated partial thromboplastin time was 49 seconds (normal 25-40); prothrombin time was normal. Bleeding time was normal. Factor VIII coagulant activity was 27%. Factor VIII antigen was 132% (normal, 45%-184%). The treatment of choice in the long-term management of this patient is:

a. Humate P
b. Recombinant factor VIII
c. Heat-treated factor VIII concentrate
d. Solvent-detergent-treated factor VIII
e. Desmopressin (DDAVP) if an initial trial demonstrates a response

28. The following are characteristic results in a patient receiving a full dose of heparin intravenously:

a. Normal prothrombin time (PT), activated partial thromboplastin time (APTT), thrombin time (TT), fibrinogen, and bleeding time
b. Abnormal APTT only

c. Abnormal PT, APTT, TT, and fibrinogen
d. Slightly abnormal PT, abnormal APTT, abnormal TT, normal fibrinogen, and normal or abnormal bleeding time
e. Abnormal APTT and thrombin time only in all cases

29. A 56-year-old woman presented with anemia, a leuko-erythroblastic blood smear, dacrocytes on the peripheral blood smear, and splenomegaly. The most likely diagnosis is:

a. Chronic myelogenous leukemia
b. Hypernephroma
c. Agnogenic myeloid metaplasia
d. Active nonlymphocytic leukemia
e. Polycythemia rubra vera

30. A 70-year-old man presented with splenomegaly, post-bathing pruritus, and an erythrocyte sedimentation rate of 1 mm/hr. Erythrocytosis was demonstrated. The most likely diagnosis is:

a. Chronic myelogenous leukemia
b. Hypernephroma
c. Agnogenic myeloid metaplasia
d. Stress erythrocytosis
e. Polycythemia rubra vera

31. A 58-year-old man presented with the following history: 3 months ago, he was treated with phenylbutazone for a potential painful right shoulder. Two months ago, he developed fatigue, dyspnea on exertion, and exercise intolerance. Currently, he has ecchymoses. Physical examination showed hepatosplenomegaly. The laboratory evaluation showed the following: hemoglobin, 9.0 g/dL; white blood cell count, 3,700; and platelet count, 16,000. There were 24.5% neutrophils and 65.5% lymphocytes in the differential. The most likely treatment for this patient would be:

a. Steroids
b. Cyclophosphamide
c. Transfusion support with red blood cells and platelets only
d. Allogeneic bone marrow transplantation
e. Antithymocyte globulin

32. A 33-year-old woman is 36 weeks pregnant. She had a 2- to 3-month history of edema, increasing blood pressure, and decreased red blood cell count. At that time, she had significant abdominal pain. She was admitted to the hospital. On admission to the hospital, the platelet count was 75,000, with an aspartate aminotransferase of 108 (normal, 12-31). In 72 hours, the platelet count had

decreased to 12,000, with an aspartate aminotransferase of 1,024 (normal, 12-31). The treatment of choice is:
a. Observation and treatment of hypertension
b. Heparin given intravenously
c. Platelet transfusion
d. Prednisone
e. Stabilization and delivery of the fetus

33. A 23-year-old gravida 1, para 0 woman presented in the late second trimester. Blood pressure was normal. The platelet count was 100,000. The optimal management is:
a. Oral prednisone
b. Cesarean section when fetal maturation is documented
c. Observation
d. Bone marrow examination
e. Antiplatelet antibody tests

34. A 56-year-old woman had an 8-year history of non-Hodgkin lymphoma, with six different treatment regimens. Currently, she has somnolence, anorexia, weakness, nausea, vomiting, poor intake, and polyuria. Physical examination showed that the patient was in a stupor and skin turgor was poor. The most likely diagnosis is:
a. Brain lymphoma
b. Renal failure
c. Hypercalcemia
d. Drug toxicity
e. Diabetes insipidus

35. A 55-year-old man was admitted to the coronary care unit with congestive heart failure. Work-up documented cardiomyopathy, diabetes mellitus, and hypogonadism. Family members should have which screening test?
a. Serum ferritin
b. Transferrin saturation
c. Molecular studies for the hemoglobin H mutation
d. Complete blood count, glucose, and liver function tests only
e. Liver biopsy

36. A 45-year-old woman had a diagnosis of diffuse large cell non-Hodgkin lymphoma. She received CHOP chemotherapy. On the 7th day of her second cycle, she was found to have an absolute neutrophil count of 300×10^9/L. The patient has been checking her temperature, and she is afebrile. The management of this patient should be:
a. Observation

b. Oral ciprofloxacin
c. Trimethoprim/sulfamethoxazole
d. Granulocyte colony-stimulating factor (G-CSF)
e. No further chemotherapy in the future

37. A 37-year-old man presented with thrombocytopenia and an otherwise normal complete blood count. The platelet count was 67,000. The peripheral blood smear confirmed thrombocytopenia. The next best test in this clinical situation is:
a. Antiplatelet antibodies
b. HIV serology
c. Erythropoietin level
d. Ferritin
e. Bone marrow

38. In the anemia of AIDS:
a. Anemia occurs in 10% of asymptomatic HIV-positive patients
b. Decreased erythropoietin levels are uncommon
c. Significant hemolysis is common
d. Red blood cell transfusions have no effect on overall survival or cytomegalovirus infection
e. Decreased levels of vitamin B_{12} reflect a deficiency in body stores unless there has been prolonged malabsorption

39. A 35-year-old man has received chemotherapy for Hodgkin disease. After the 6th full cycle, he had dyspnea. The most likely cause of the dyspnea is:
a. Nitrogen mustard
b. Adriamycin
c. Prednisone
d. Bleomycin
e. Vincristine

40. A 32-year-old man received chemotherapy. At this time, he presented with pancytopenia. It has been 7 years since the diagnosis of Hodgkin disease. The most likely diagnosis is:
a. Relapse of Hodgkin disease
b. Aplastic anemia
c. Non-Hodgkin lymphoma
d. Acute nonlymphocytic leukemia secondary to a monosomy 5 translocation due to cyclophosphamide
e. Acute nonlymphocytic leukemia with a related monosomy 5 translocation secondary to MOPP chemotherapy.

ANSWERS

1. Answer d.

The low mean corpuscular volume and ferritin level are consistent with iron deficiency. This with the low folate suggests small-bowel disease. Small-bowel radiographs and biopsy confirmed the diagnosis of celiac sprue.

2. Answer a.

This anemia is characterized by a low mean corpuscular volume, and the red blood cell count is less than 5×10^6/L. The low ferritin level is consistent with iron deficiency. Upper gastrointestinal tract endoscopy confirmed peptic ulcer disease.

3. Answer b.

This patient has an anemia with a minimally decreased mean corpuscular volume. Fecal hemoglobin was 20.1 mg/Hg per gram of stool (2-4). A barium enema demonstrated a 3-cm colon ulcer. On colonoscopy, there were multiple right colonic ulcerations. The biopsy specimens showed inflammatory tissue and granulation. This diagnosis is consistent with diclofenic (Voltaren)-induced colonic ulceration.

4. Answer c.

This patient has a normochromic-normocytic anemia. The reticulocyte count is increased. Fecal hemoglobin is normal, and the Coombs test was negative. The patient has a Budd-Chiari syndrome and a Coombs-negative hemolytic anemia. The most likely diagnosis is paroxysmal nocturnal hemoglobinuria.

5. Answer e.

This patient has a macrocytic anemia. This, a fissured tongue, and decreased vibratory sensation are clinically consistent with pernicious anemia. The next best test is determining serum vitamin B_{12} level which was <50 pg/mL (normal, 200-1,000). The intrinsic factor-blocking antibody was positive.

6. Answer d.

This patient presented in high-output congestive heart failure. The folate value was low. The etiology of this folate deficiency was extensive skin disease and diet.

7. Answer d.

This patient has thrombotic thrombocytopenic purpura as manifested by neurologic symptoms, microangiopathic hemolytic anemia (schistocytes), thrombocytopenia, and abnormal bilirubin. The picture is most compatible with thrombotic thrombocytopenic purpura. The treatment of choice in thrombotic thrombocytopenic purpura is plasmapheresis, with replacement with fresh frozen plasma.

8. Answer b.

All the answers listed are causes of macrocytosis. Hydroxyurea is the most likely cause in this clinical situation.

9. Answer c.

The Cooperative Study of Sickle Cell Disease reported that a high level of fetal hemoglobin predicted for improved survival in young persons. The other factors listed are associated with the risk of early death in patients 20 years or older.

10. Answer a.

This clinical scenario is consistent with sickle cell anemia. The most common cause of death in sickle cell anemia is acute pain and chest syndrome.

11. Answer a.

Observation. This patient has Rai stage 0 chronic lymphocytic leukemia, or International Workshop on Chronic Lymphocytic Leukemia Classification clinical stage A disease. The treatment of choice in this situation is observation.

12. Answer c.

This patient has Rai stage IV, or International Workshop on Chronic Lymphocytic Leukemia Classification stage C disease. The treatment of choice is chlorambucil and prednisone or fludarabine. The long-term results of a randomized study of fludarabine versus chlorambucil are pending at this time.

13. Answer d.

This is a presentation of massive splenomegaly. All the listed diagnoses are in the differential diagnosis of this presentation. The presence of fevers with pancytopenia is more consistent with hairy cell leukemia.

14. Answer a.

This patient has stage IVA low-grade non-Hodgkin lymphoma, with no evidence of bulky disease or symptoms. The treatment of choice is observation. Early treatment has not been shown to improve survival.

15. Answer e.

This patient has diffuse large cell non-Hodgkin lymphoma. The treatment of choice is CHOP. The disease of this patient is potentially curable. In the International Prognostic Factor data set, this was the most favorable group.

16. Answer c.

This patient has advanced stage Hodgkin disease. Currently,

the treatment of choice is ABVD. Autologous bone marrow transplantation or peripheral stem cell transplantation is used for patients who have relapse.

17. Answer a.

This is the classic presentation of infectious mononucleosis. Lymph node interpretation may be difficult to differentiate. The mono spot test was positive. The treatment of choice is observation.

18. Answer d.

This patient has MALTOMA. *H. pylori* is associated with gastric MALTOMA. The initial treatment of choice is an antibiotic regimen. Studies are evaluating different double and triple regimens.

19. Answer a.

This patient has a monoclonal gammopathy of undetermined significance as manifested by an M-protein level <3 g/dL, normal calcium, normal hemoglobin, and normal creatinine. Twenty-three percent of patients may go on to develop a malignancy (multiple myeloma, amyloidosis, non-Hodgkin lymphoma, etc.). This patient should be observed and followed with serum protein electrophoresis studies.

20. Answer c.

The clinical presentation of postural hypotension in nephrotic syndrome is most consistent with primary systemic amyloidosis. There is an 80% yield in the diagnosis of primary systemic amyloidosis with a fat aspirate.

21. Answer d.

The differential diagnosis in this case is leukemoid reaction versus chronic myelogenous leukemia. The nonpalpable spleen suggests leukemoid reaction. The leukocyte alkaline phosphatase score differentiates these two disorders. In this case, the score was 217 (normal, 40-100). Therefore, the diagnosis is consistent with leukemoid reaction. At operation, the patient was found to have metastatic transitional cell carcinoma of the bladder.

22. Answer a.

The differential diagnosis includes all the following answers. Splenomegaly is present in up to 75% of cases of polycythemia rubra vera, and the erythrocyte sedimentation rate is 0 to 1 in uncomplicated cases.

23. Answer c.

Anoxic polycythemia was subsequently documented. The oxygen saturation was 88%. The red cell mass was 23.9 (normal, 21-29.7). The plasma volume was 33.2 (normal, 38-50.6)

24. Answer e.

Follicular small cleaved cell non-Hodgkin lymphoma is associated with the t(14,18) in 90% of patients and *bcl*-2 oncogene abnormality. An altered *bcl*-2 results in aberrations in the process of programmed cell death, apoptosis.

25. Answer b.

Prolonged activated partial thromboplastin time and normal prothrombin time with the prolonged bleeding time are all compatible with von Willebrand disease. The treatment of choice in this patient is humate P.

26. Answer a.

This patient has disseminated intravascular coagulopathy. Replacement of all the missing factors and products is the initial treatment of choice. If these measures fail, then heparin is indicated. Plasmapheresis with replacement with fresh frozen plasma is the treatment of choice in thrombotic thrombocytopenic purpura (TTP). This is not a case of TTP because the prothrombin time and fibrinogen are very abnormal.

27. Answer e.

The findings are consistent with mild hemophilia A with a factor VIII level that is the range of mild hemophila. Mild to moderate hemophiliacs should undergo a trial of desmopressin. If there is a response, this should be used in the long-term management of these patients.

28. Answer d.

Slightly abnormal prothrombin time, abnormal activated partial thromboplastin time, abnormal thrombin time, normal fibrinogen, and normal or abnormal bleeding time are the characteristic findings in patients receiving heparin intravenously.

29. Answer c.

These are the classic findings in agnogenic myeloid metaplasia.

30. Answer e.

This patient has the classic findings of polycythemia rubra vera.

31. Answer e.

This patient had bone marrow with less than 5% cellularity, consistent with aplastic anemia. The treatment of choice in this age group is antithymocyte globulin with or without cyclosporine.

32. Answer e.

This patient has HELLP syndrome. The treatment of choice

in this case is stabilization of the patient's condition, followed by delivery of the fetus.

33. Answer c.

It is most likely that this patient has the incidental thrombocytopenia of pregnancy. The patient should be followed up, but no further work-up or treatment is necessary at this time.

34. Answer c.

The most likely diagnosis in this clinical scenario is transformation of a low-grade lymphoma to diffuse large cell lymphoma with a clinical presentation secondary to hypercalcemia. The calcium was 15 mg/dL (normal, 8.9-10.1).

35. Answer b.

This patient has hemochromatosis. The most accepted screening test is transferrin saturation.

36. Answer a.

This patient should be observed and not treated with granulocyte colony-stimulating factor (G-CSF) at this time. The patient has afebrile neutropenia. The current American Society of Clinical Oncology practice guidelines and randomized studies do not support the routine use of G-CSF in this situation. To date, randomized trials with oral antibiotics have not supported this indication. Myelosuppression is an expected toxic affect of CHOP chemotherapy in this potentially curable disease. CHOP is usually given for six to eight cycles. In this situation, treatment should be continued with potential dose modifications.

37. Answer b.

Patients with HIV may initially present with thrombocytopenia with or without other cytopenias. The diagnosis may require a significant degree of clinical suspicion.

38. Answer a.

Anemia occurs in 10% of asymptomatic HIV-positive patients, 50% of patients with AIDS-related complex, and more than 75% of patients with overt AIDS. Of AIDS patients, 70% have decreased erythropoietin levels. Clinical studies have demonstrated that transfusions may decrease survival but increase the risk of cytomegalovirus infection. Decreased vitamin B_{12} levels are present in 20% of HIV-infected patients and are due to altered serum transport of vitamin B_{12} and not to a deficiency in body stores unless there has been prolonged malabsorption.

39. Answer d.

ABVD is the chemotherapeutic treatment most commonly used in Hodgkin disease. Bleomycin is the most common cause of pulmonary toxic effects in this regimen

40. Answer e.

This patient has a complication of survival of Hodgkin disease, which is acute nonlymphocytic leukemia secondary to nitrogen mustard with a monosomy 5 cytogenetic abnormality. Cyclophosphamide is an alkylator agent that can cause secondary leukemia, but this is not used in the treatment of Hodgkin disease. ABVD has replaced MOPP as the treatment of choice in Hodgkin disease.

CHAPTER 13

HYPERTENSION

Gary L. Schwartz, M.D.

HYPERTENSION

Definition

Systolic blood pressures between 130 and 139 mm Hg and diastolic blood pressures between 85 and 89 mm Hg are considered high-normal. Hypertension is defined as average blood pressure of 140/90 mm Hg or greater. It is stratified further on the basis of pressure level (Table 13-1).

- Hypertension is average blood pressure ≥140/90 mm Hg.

Isolated systolic hypertension, mainly a problem of the elderly, is defined as systolic blood pressure of 140 mm Hg or greater with diastolic blood pressure less than 90 mm Hg. Secondary causes of isolated systolic hypertension include disorders associated with either increased cardiac output (anemia, thyrotoxicosis, arteriovenous fistula, Paget disease of bone, beriberi) or increased cardiac stroke volume (aortic insufficiency, complete heart block).

- Isolated systolic hypertension affects mainly the elderly.
- Secondary causes: 1) increased cardiac output (anemia, thyrotoxicosis, arteriovenous fistula, Paget disease of bone, beriberi) and 2) increased cardiac stroke volume (aortic insufficiency, complete heart block).

Epidemiology

Blood pressure increases with age. Systolic blood pressure increases throughout the seventh decade, but diastolic blood pressure plateaus in the fifth decade. Hypertension is a major risk factor for cardiovascular morbidity and mortality (myocardial infarction, congestive heart failure, stroke, and renal disease). Risk is continuous and proportionate over both systolic and diastolic blood pressure levels. Systolic blood pressure is as good or better a predictor of risk than diastolic blood pressure. In young adulthood and early middle age, high blood pressure is more common in men than in women. In older persons, the reverse is true. High blood pressure is more common in blacks than in whites at all ages, and in both races, it is more common in less educated than in more educated persons. For any given level, men have greater morbidity and mortality than women and blacks, greater than whites. It is estimated that 50 million Americans have hypertension or are taking medication to decrease blood pressure.

- Hypertension is a major risk factor for cardiovascular morbidity and mortality.
- Risk is continuous and proportionate over both systolic and diastolic blood pressure levels.
- Men and blacks have greater morbidity and mortality.

In persons with hypertension, the most common causes of death are due to complications of coronary artery disease.

Table 13-1.—Classification of Blood Pressure for Adults 18 Years and Older*

Category	Systolic blood pressure, mm Hg		Diastolic blood pressure, mm Hg
Optimal	<120	and	<80
Normal	<130	and	<85
High normal	130-139	or	85-89
Hypertension			
Stage 1	140-159	or	90-99
Stage 2	160-179	or	100-109
Stage 3	≥180	or	≥110

*Not taking antihypertensive drugs and not acutely ill. When systolic and diastolic blood pressures fall into different categories, the higher category should be selected to classify the person's blood pressure status.
From The Sixth Report of the Joint National Committee on Prevention, Detection, Evaluation, and Treatment of High Blood Pressure. Arch Intern Med 157:2413-2446, 1997.

Factors that add to this risk are tobacco use, hyperlipidemia, diabetes mellitus, obesity, sedentary lifestyle, sex (men and postmenopausal women), age older than 60 years, and a family history of premature cardiovascular disease (women younger than 65, men younger than 55). Target organ damage (stroke, left ventricular hypertrophy, ischemic heart disease, congestive heart failure, renal disease, retinopathy, peripheral vascular disease) increases the risk of cardiovascular events even if blood pressure is controlled. This fact argues for early treatment of mild hypertension. Therefore, in addition to the level of blood pressure, the risk in an individual patient is determined by the presence of additional cardiovascular risk factors and target organ damage.

- The most common causes of death in persons with hypertension are related to complications of coronary artery disease.
- Other risk factors for coronary artery disease: tobacco use, hyperlipidemia, diabetes mellitus, obesity, sedentary lifestyle, male sex, postmenopausal state, older age, and family history of premature cardiovascular disease.
- Target organ damage increases the risk of cardiovascular events even if blood pressure is controlled.

Left ventricular hypertrophy is a powerful predictor of sudden death and myocardial infarction in persons with hypertension. Other factors associated with increased left ventricular muscle mass include increasing age, obesity, and increased physical activity. Echocardiography is more sensitive than electrocardiography in detecting left ventricular hypertrophy.

- Left ventricular hypertrophy is a powerful predictor of sudden death and myocardial infarction in persons with hypertension.
- Echocardiography is more sensitive than electrocardiography in detecting left ventricular hypertrophy.

Diagnosis

Because blood pressure varies, the diagnosis of hypertension requires several measurements made on different occasions. The person should be at rest in the sitting position for at least 5 minutes before the measurement. Recent physical activity, use of tobacco or caffeine, or a full urinary bladder can transiently increase blood pressure. Some persons have increased blood pressure when it is measured in a physician's office but have normal blood pressure at all other times. This is called "office hypertension" or "white coat hypertension." Whether these people suffer the adverse consequences of hypertension is uncertain; therefore, they usually require no treatment initially but need to be followed and periodically assessed for target organ damage. Older persons

may have pseudohypertension, a falsely increased systolic and diastolic blood pressure when measured by the cuff method; it is the result of a stiff vascular tree caused by atherosclerosis. Pseudohypertension may exist if the radial artery remains palpable after the brachial artery is occluded by inflating the blood pressure cuff until the radial pulse is obliterated (Osler maneuver).

- The diagnosis of hypertension requires several measurements made on different occasions.
- Recent physical exercise, use of tobacco or caffeine, or a full urinary bladder can increase blood pressure.
- Office (white coat) hypertension: increased blood pressure only when measured in a physician's office.
- Older patients may have pseudohypertension, the result of a stiff vascular tree.

Evaluation

After the diagnosis of hypertension has been established, 1) determine, if possible, the duration and severity of hypertension and any previous therapies and reasons for discontinuation, 2) assess for target organ damage, 3) identify associated cardiovascular risk factors, and 4) consider the possibility of secondary hypertension. Secondary hypertension accounts for fewer than 5% of all cases of increased blood pressure.

- Secondary hypertension explains <5% of all cases of increased blood pressure.

Clues to secondary hypertension are features that are not consistent with essential hypertension. Essential hypertension usually occurs in the fourth or fifth decade. There is often a family history of hypertension. Usually, blood pressure is mildly increased initially and easily controlled with one or two medications. Target organ damage is rare, and routine laboratory findings are normal. Blood pressure does not progress to higher levels over a short period of time. Factors inconsistent with essential hypertension are listed in Table 13-2.

- Recognition of secondary hypertension is important.

Drugs

Certain drugs can cause or aggravate hypertension or interfere with the action of antihypertensive medications. These drugs and their mechanism of action are listed in Table 13-3.

- Certain drugs can cause or aggravate hypertension or interfere with the action of antihypertensive medications.
- Oral contraceptives induce sodium retention, increase renin substrate, and facilitate the action of catecholamines.

Table 13-2.—Factors Inconsistent With Essential Hypertension

Age at onset—before 30 or after 50 years
Blood pressure >180/110 mm Hg at time of diagnosis
Significant target organ damage at time of diagnosis
    Hemorrhages and exudates on funduscopic examination
    Renal insufficiency
    Cardiomegaly
    Left ventricular hypertrophy
Features suggesting secondary hypertension
    Primary aldosteronism (unprovoked hypokalemia,
      Chvostek sign, Trousseau sign)
    Pheochromocytoma (labile blood pressure with sweating,
      tremor, tachycardia, pallor, neurofibromatosis, orofacial
      neuromas [MEN II])
    Renovascular disease (abdominal bruits)
    Cushing disease (truncal obesity, pigmented stria)
    Coarctation of aorta (delayed/absent femoral pulses)
    Polycystic kidney disease (abdominal or flank masses,
      family history of renal disease)
Poor response to appropriate three-drug therapy

- Nonsteroidal anti-inflammatory drugs induce sodium retention by blocking the formation of renal vasodilating, natriuretic prostaglandins.
- Tricyclic antidepressants block the uptake of guanethidine and inhibit the action of centrally acting agents (methyldopa, clonidine).

Laboratory Studies

Routine laboratory tests should include: complete blood cell count, sodium potassium, glucose, creatinine or BUN, uric acid, calcium, cholesterol (total and HDL), triglycerides, urinalysis, and electrocardiography (ECG). Additional studies should not be performed unless abnormalities are identified on initial screening tests or the history or examination suggests a secondary form of hypertension.

Treatment

The goal of therapy is to eliminate the cardiovascular morbidity and mortality attributable to hypertension by decreasing blood pressure to less than 140/90 mm Hg. A lower goal of less than 130/85 mm Hg is appropriate for patients with diabetes mellitus, renal disease, or heart failure.

Lifestyle Modifications

Lifestyle modifications may be sufficient for some patients with stage 1 hypertension. It is adjunctive therapy for those with more severe hypertension. Restriction of daily sodium intake to 100 mEq (2 g sodium, 4 g salt) decreases blood pressure in some but not all hypertensive persons. Although salt sensitivity is more common among persons who are black, obese, elderly, or who have low renin hypertension, higher blood pressure levels, or renal failure, the antihypertensive effect of many medications is enhanced by sodium restriction. Also, sodium restriction minimizes diuretic-induced potassium losses. The prevalence of hypertension is increased in the obese. An increase in blood pressure often parallels weight gain. Weight loss may decrease blood pressure. Weight reduction to within 15% of ideal body weight is the goal, although losses of as little as 10 lb may produce a decrease in blood pressure. Restriction of daily alcohol intake to less than 1 oz (30 mL) of ethanol (<1/2 oz for women or lighter weight men) is often associated with a decrease in blood pressure. Alcohol is a source of calories, and its use is often associated with poor compliance. Excessive alcohol intake may cause labile hypertension that is difficult to control in association with other symptoms (flushing, tachycardia) that suggest pheochromocytoma. Regular aerobic exercise may decrease blood pressure directly and by facilitating weight loss. Because coronary artery disease is the most common cause of mortality in hypertensive persons, all cardiovascular risks need to be addressed. The benefits of blood pressure reduction are diminished in smokers. Dyslipidemia (increased low-density lipoprotein [LDL] cholesterol, decreased high-density lipoprotein [HDL] cholesterol, increased triglycerides) and glucose intolerance coexist more often in hypertensive than in normotensive persons.

- Restriction of daily sodium intake to 100 mEq decreases blood pressure in some, not all, hypertensive persons.
- Weight reduction to within 15% of ideal body weight is the goal.
- Restriction of alcohol intake to <1 oz daily is often associated with a decrease in blood pressure.
- Regular aerobic exercise may decrease blood pressure directly.
- Address all cardiovascular risk factors.

A diet deficient in potassium may increase blood pressure; therefore, an adequate intake of potassium should be encouraged. There is little evidence to support a role for increased intake of calcium or magnesium. Studies do not support the use of biofeedback or relaxation therapies for blood pressure control.

A trial of lifestyle modifications alone for up to 12 months is appropriate for patients with stage 1 hypertension who do not have diabetes or other cardiovascular risk factors, target organ involvement, or clinical cardiovascular disease. If lifestyle modifications fail to decrease blood pressure to less than 140/90

Table 13-3.—Drugs That Can Increase Blood Pressure or Interfere With Antihypertensive Therapy

Drug	Mechanism
Oral contraceptives	Induce sodium retention Increase renin substrate Facilitate action of catecholamines
Alcohol (>1 oz daily)	Activation of sympathetic nervous system Increase cortisol secretion Increase intracellular calcium levels
Sympathomimetics and amphetamine-like substances (cold formulas, allergy medications, diet pills)	Increase peripheral vascular resistance Interfere with action of guanethidine and guanadrel
Nonsteroidal anti-inflammatory drugs	Induce sodium retention by blocking formation of renal vasodilating, natriuretic prostaglandins, thus interfering with action of diuretics, β-blockers, and angiotensin-converting enzyme inhibitors
Corticosteroids	Iatrogenic Cushing disease
Tricyclic antidepressants	Block uptake of guanethidine Inhibit action of centrally acting drugs such as methyldopa and clonidine
Ephedrine	Competitive antagonist of guanethidine
Monoamine oxidase inhibitors (in combination with tyramine—found in aged cheeses and some red wines)	Prevent degradation and metabolism of norepinephrine released by tyramine-containing foods Increase blood pressure when combined with reserpine/guanethidine
Cocaine	Vasoconstriction Interferes with action of adrenergic inhibitors
Marijuana	Increases systolic blood pressure
Cyclosporine	Renal and systemic vasoconstriction
Erythropoietin	Systemic vasoconstriction
Serotonin	Systemic vasoconstriction

mm Hg, drug treatment should be initiated. For patients at increased risk because of additional cardiovascular risk factors, drug treatment should be started if lifestyle modifications are ineffective after 3 to 6 months. Drug treatment should be considered initially in addition to lifestyle modifications for patients with stage 2 or higher hypertension or for those with stage 1 hypertension who also have target organ involvement or clinical cardiovascular disease. Drug treatment should be considered together with lifestyle modifications for blood pressure in top high-normal range or higher ($\geq$130 mm Hg systolic or $\geq$85 mm Hg diastolic) in patients with congestive heart failure, renal disease, or diabetes. Significant changes in lifestyle (weight loss, reductions in salt or alcohol intake, exercise) may allow tapering of an established drug program.

- A 3- to 12-month trial of lifestyle modifications alone is appropriate for stage 1 hypertension in the absence of diabetes or other cardiovascular risk factors, target organ involvement, or clinical cardiovascular disease.
- If this fails to decrease blood pressure to <140/90 mm Hg, drug therapy should be initiated.

Pharmacologic Therapy

More than 50% of cases of stage 1 hypertension can be controlled with one drug. Important factors in selecting a drug for initial therapy are 1) effectiveness as monotherapy, 2) side effects, and 3) cost. Proper drug selection is important in maintaining long-term compliance.

Drugs appropriate for monotherapy are diuretics, β-blockers, calcium channel antagonists, angiotensin-converting enzyme (ACE) inhibitors, α-blockers, α-β-blockers, and angiotensin receptor (AII) antagonists. Low-dose combinations may also be used for initial therapy. Because thiazide diuretics and β-blockers are the only classes of drugs that have been demonstrated in prospective clinical trials to reduce morbidity and mortality, they are preferred. Other classes of drugs should be considered if diuretics or β-blockers are ineffective, contraindicated, or in settings in which the efficacy of the drug has been established (e.g., ACE inhibitors in a hypertensive person with congestive heart failure). Centrally acting α-agonists (clonidine, methyldopa, guanfacine, guanabenz) and traditional vasodilators (hydralazine, minoxidil) may be associated with pseudotolerance—that is, reflex stimulation of the renin-angiotensin-aldosterone system and/or the sympathetic nervous system that causes fluid retention, increased vascular resistance, or increased cardiac output and loss of efficacy with prolonged use—and so ordinarily are not used as monotherapy. Centrally acting α-agonists are appropriate when used in combination with diuretics, whereas traditional vasodilators are best as a third drug in combination with diuretics and adrenergic inhibitors. Additional important factors influencing drug selection include the recognition that certain drugs work better according to a person's age and race (diuretics and calcium antagonists are more effective in blacks and the elderly; β-blockers and ACE inhibitors are more effective in whites and younger patients), the presence of concomitant diseases, and drug-drug interactions. If the first drug chosen fails to control blood pressure, increase the dose or discontinue it and substitute a drug from a different class or add a second drug. With combination therapy, make certain that the chosen drugs work in combination and that two drugs of the same class are not used simultaneously. Fatigue and impotence are potential side effects of all antihypertensive drugs.

- Drugs for monotherapy: diuretics, β-blockers, calcium channel antagonists, ACE inhibitors, α-blockers, α-β-blockers, and AII antagonists.

- Centrally acting α-agonists ordinarily are not used as monotherapy but are appropriate in combination with diuretics.
- Traditional vasodilators are best as a third drug in combination with diuretics and adrenergic inhibitors.

Thiazide Diuretics

Thiazide diuretics have been the mainstay for treatment of mild-to-moderate hypertension. Concomitant diseases for which these drugs should be considered are edema states and congestive heart failure due to systolic dysfunction. Metabolic disturbances associated with their use are hypokalemia, hyperuricemia, hypercalcemia, hypomagnesemia, hyponatremia, glucose intolerance, hypochloremic metabolic alkalosis, and increased levels of LDL cholesterol and triglycerides. Because of these potential adverse effects, relative contraindications to the use of thiazide diuretics include the coexistence of diet-controlled type 2 diabetes, gout, hyperlipidemia, cardiac arrhythmias, and ischemic heart disease. Drug interactions include potentiation of lithium toxicity (thiazides decrease the renal clearance of lithium), lessening of the anticoagulant effect of warfarin, enhancement of digitalis toxicity, and enhancement of the effects of skeletal muscle relaxants. Nonsteroidal anti-inflammatory drugs decrease the antihypertensive effect of thiazide diuretics. The use of thiazide diuretics is associated with volume depletion, pancreatitis, vasculitis, mesenteric infarction, hepatitis, intrahepatic cholestasis, interstitial nephritis, and photosensitivity. Rarely, they cause blood dyscrasias. Thiazide diuretics are usually ineffective when the serum level of creatinine is greater than 2.0 mg/dL. An exception is indapamide, a thiazide-like diuretic that is effective in states of decreased renal function and that is less likely to increase blood lipids. When the serum level of creatinine is greater than 2.0 mg/dL, a more potent loop diuretic or metolazone is more effective. Volume expansion is often important etiologically in hypertension associated with renal insufficiency.

- Metabolic disturbances associated with diuretics: hypokalemia, hyperuricemia, hypercalcemia, hypomagnesemia, hyponatremia, glucose intolerance, hypochloremic metabolic alkalosis, and increased levels of LDL cholesterol and triglycerides.
- Drug interactions: potentiation of lithium toxicity, lessening of anticoagulant effect of warfarin, enhancement of digitalis toxicity, and enhancement of effects of skeletal muscle relaxants.
- Use of diuretics is associated with pancreatitis, vasculitis, mesenteric infarction, hepatitis, and photosensitivity.

Loop Diuretics

1. Furosemide. The major indication for furosemide is hypertension associated with renal insufficiency. Because of its

short duration of action, furosemide must be given twice daily to avoid rebound sodium retention. Similar to thiazide diuretics, furosemide can cause volume depletion, hypokalemia, hyperuricemia, increased fasting blood glucose, and hypochloremic alkalosis. Unlike thiazide diuretics, furosemide causes calciuresis. Potential adverse effects include reversible deafness, postural hypotension (especially in older patients), photosensitivity, pancreatitis, blood dyscrasias, nephrocalcinosis, and interstitial nephritis. Furosemide enhances salicylate clearance and the effects of skeletal muscle relaxants. It is synergistic when used with metolazone. Avoid using with aminoglycosides or other ototoxic drugs. Nonsteroidal anti-inflammatory drugs reduce the antihypertensive response of all diuretics.

- Major indication for furosemide: hypertension associated with renal insufficiency.
- Furosemide can cause: hypokalemia, hyperuricemia, increased fasting blood glucose, enhanced salicylate clearance, and enhanced effect of skeletal muscle relaxants.
- Adverse effects: reversible deafness and postural hypotension.

2. Bumetanide. The actions (including adverse effects, electrolyte alterations, and drug interactions) of bumetanide are identical to those of furosemide; however, bumetanide is a more potent diuretic on a milligram-per-milligram basis (1 mg is equivalent to 40 mg furosemide) and has twice the bioavailability of furosemide.

3. Ethacrynic acid. The actions of ethacrynic acid are similar to those of furosemide. Although permanent hearing loss is a risk, ethacrynic acid is an alternative diuretic for patients with sulfa sensitivity because it is not a sulfonamide derivative.

4. Torsemide. Torsemide is different from the other loop diuretics in that it is eliminated mainly by liver metabolism, which gives it a duration of action as long as 12 hours, considerably longer than that of other diuretics in this class. Otherwise, its action is similar to that of other loop agents.

Potassium-Sparing Diuretics

1. Spironolactone. Spironolactone is an aldosterone antagonist used specifically in persons with primary aldosteronism or with severe secondary aldosteronism. Its diuretic effect is antagonized by the concomitant use of salicylates. Adverse effects include hyponatremia, hyperkalemia, hyperchloremic acidosis, gynecomastia (but not breast cancer), and skin rash. Spironolactone is often combined with thiazides to limit hypokalemia.

- The diuretic effect of spironolactone is antagonized by the concomitant use of salicylates.
- Adverse effects: hyperkalemia, gynecomastia, and skin rash.

2. Triamterene. Triamterene inhibits renal potassium-wasting independent of aldosterone. Side effects include hyperkalemia and skin rash.

- Triamterene inhibits renal potassium-wasting independent of aldosterone.

3. Amiloride. The actions of amiloride are similar to those of triamterene. Side effects are hyperkalemia, gastrointestinal distress, and skin rash.

Of the potassium-sparing diuretics, only spironolactone causes gynecomastia. In general, these drugs should be avoided in cases of renal failure and when ACE inhibitors or AII antagonists are used.

- Avoid potassium-sparing diuretics in renal failure and when ACE inhibitors or AII antagonists are used.

Adrenergic Inhibitors

When a diuretic alone fails to control blood pressure, an adrenergic inhibitor can be added. Adrenergic inhibitors are divided into centrally acting and peripherally acting drugs.

1. Peripherally acting inhibitors.
   a. Reserpine. Reserpine blocks the transport of norepinephrine into storage granules in peripheral neurons, causing decreased sympathetic nervous system tone. Side effects include depression, nasal congestion, and stimulation of gastric acid secretion, which can precipitate or aggravate peptic ulcer disease. A history of depression or peptic ulcer disease should contraindicate its use.

- Major side effects of reserpine: depression, nasal congestion, and stimulation of gastric acid secretion.

   b. Guanethidine. Guanethidine generally is used only as part of a combination drug program to treat resistant hypertension. It decreases blood pressure by causing degranulation of catecholamine storage granules in nerve endings. It does not enter the central nervous system. It has a long half-life. The maximal hypotensive effect of a given dose may not be manifested for 2 or 3 weeks. It should be given only once daily, and titration requires several weeks. Major side effects are postural hypotension, fluid retention, diarrhea, and retrograde ejaculation. Tricyclic antidepressants, antihistamines, and ephedrine interfere with its action. Guanadrel, a short-acting form of guanethidine, is easier to titrate to an effective dose because it has a shorter half-life.

- Major side effects of guanethidine: postural hypotension, fluid retention, diarrhea, and retrograde ejaculation.
- Tricyclic antidepressants, antihistamines, and ephedrine interfere with its action.

    c. α_1-Blockers. These drugs block α_1-adrenergic receptors on vascular smooth muscle cells to blunt catecholamine-induced vasoconstriction. The first dose can precipitate hypotension and syncope; therefore, it should be given before bedtime. Longer acting peripheral α_1-blockers (doxazocin, terazosin) allow single daily dosing. Prazosin, an older drug, must be used at least twice daily. These drugs may lessen voiding symptoms associated with benign prostatic hypertrophy. Although the use of α_1-blockers in the elderly is frequently associated with orthostatic hypotension, they do not have adverse metabolic side effects. Other side effects include gastrointestinal distress and, rarely, sedation, edema, and dry mouth.

- Because the first dose of prazosin can cause hypotension and syncope, it should be given before bedtime.
- Use in the elderly is often associated with orthostatic hypotension but no adverse metabolic side effects.

    d. β-Blockers. Many β-blockers are available, differing in cardioselectivity (affinity for cardiac β_1 receptors greater than for noncardiac β_2 receptors), lipid solubility, and whether they have partial intrinsic (agonist) sympathomimetic activity (ISA). Non-ISA β-blockers decrease blood pressure by reducing cardiac output, inhibiting sympathetically mediated renin release from the kidneys, and inhibiting central sympathetic outflow. β-Blockers with ISA activity do not decrease cardiac output and cause mild peripheral vasodilatation. As lipid solubility increases, more drug is metabolized by the liver, more of it enters the brain, and its duration of action is shorter. As lipid solubility decreases, the drug is eliminated mainly by renal excretion, less of it enters the brain, and its duration of action is longer. Very lipid-soluble drugs are propranolol, metoprolol, and timolol. Intermediate lipid-soluble drugs are pindolol, carvedilol, bisoprolol, and acebutolol. The least lipid-soluble drugs are atenolol, betaxolol and nadolol.

- As lipid solubility increases, more drug is metabolized by the liver, more of it enters the brain, and its duration of action is shorter.

- As lipid solubility decreases, the drug is eliminated mainly by renal excretion, less enters the brain, and its duration of action is longer.
- Very lipid-soluble drugs: propranolol, metoprolol, and timolol.
- Least lipid-soluble drugs: atenolol, betaxolol, and nadolol.

    Cardioselective β-blockers include acebutolol, atenolol, betaxolol, bisoprolol, and metoprolol. Cardioselectivity is relative; at high doses, all β-blockers are nonselective (block both cardiac β_1 and noncardiac β_2 receptors). β-Blockers with ISA activity are pindolol and acebutolol. Three β-blockers—propranolol, timolol, and metoprolol—prevent sudden death and myocardial infarctions in patients with a history of myocardial infarction. β-Blockers should be considered for use in hypertensive patients with concomitant angina, supraventricular arrhythmia, glaucoma, migraine headaches, or hypertrophic cardiomyopathy. Contraindications to the use of β-blockers are asthma, severe chronic obstructive pulmonary disease, congestive heart failure with decreased systolic function, conduction system disease of the heart, angina due to coronary vasospasm, Raynaud phenomenon, severe occlusive peripheral vascular disease, pheochromocytoma (in absence of α-blockade), and depression. Because β-blockers may mask the symptoms of hypoglycemia and delay recovery from it, caution is required when given to patients with diabetes who are taking hypoglycemic drugs or insulin. Side effects include cold extremities (non-ISA β-blockers), fatigue, insomnia, nasal congestion, and, possibly, depression.

- Cardioselectivity is relative; all β-blockers are nonselective at high doses.
- Propranolol, timolol, and metoprolol prevent sudden death and myocardial infarction in persons with a history of myocardial infarction.
- Contraindications: asthma, severe chronic obstructive pulmonary disease, congestive heart failure with decreased systolic function, conduction system disease of the heart, angina due to coronary vasospasm, Raynaud phenomenon, severe occlusive peripheral vascular disease, pheochromocytoma, and depression.
- β-Blockers may mask hypoglycemia and delay recovery from it, so use them carefully in diabetics taking insulin or oral hypoglycemic drugs.
- Side effects: cold extremities, fatigue, insomnia, nasal congestion, and, possibly, depression.

    e. Labetalol. Labetalol is a combination of a nonselective β-blocker and a postsynaptic α_1-blocker. The ratio of α-to-β blocking action is between 1:3 and 1:7. It induces decreased cardiac output and peripheral vascular resistance. Labetalol can be used intravenously to treat hypertensive crisis. All the precautions applying to β-blockers apply to this drug. Orthostatic hypotension and scalp itching are its most common side effects. It may interfere with metanephrine and catecholamine assays.

- Labetalol can be used intravenously.
- All precautions applying to β-blockers apply to labetalol.
- Common side effects: orthostatic hypotension and scalp itching.
- It may interfere with metanephrine and catecholamine assays.

  f. Carvedilol. Carvedilol is a weak β_1-selective blocker with α_1-blocking activity. It may be of benefit in the treatment of heart failure with systolic dysfunction.

- Carvedilol may be helpful in heart failure.

 2. Centrally acting inhibitors.
    a. Methyldopa. Methyldopa inhibits central sympathetic outflow. Its side effects include sedation, dry mouth, hepatitis, fever, positive Coombs test, hemolytic anemia, leukopenia, thrombocytopenia, and antinuclear antibody positivity. Doses should not exceed 3 g/day. Hemoglobin and liver enzymes should be checked periodically. Methyldopa potentiates lithium and haloperidol toxicity, increases prolactin levels with consequent breast stimulation, interferes with metanephrine assays, and can induce orthostatic hypotension (especially in the elderly).

- Methyldopa side effects: sedation, dry mouth, hepatitis, fever, positive Coombs test, hemolytic anemia, leukopenia, thrombocytopenia, and antinuclear antibody positivity.
- It potentiates lithium and haloperidol toxicity and increases prolactin levels.
- It can induce orthostatic hypotension, especially in the elderly.

    b. Clonidine. Clonidine also inhibits central sympathetic outflow and has the side effects of dry mouth and sedation, but it is not associated with liver toxicity or a positive Coombs test. Because sudden discontinuation of clonidine may induce rebound hypertension, accompanied by symptoms of tachycardia, flushing, and diaphoresis, it should be slowly tapered. (Rebound hypertension can occur with all centrally acting agents and with β-blockers.) Taper and discontinue use of clonidine preoperatively for anticipated surgical procedures in which the

patient will not be able to take the medication. Alternatively, patients can be converted preoperatively to the transdermal form of clonidine. Treatment of rebound hypertension usually involves reinstituting clonidine therapy (or whatever agent was discontinued suddenly).

- Sudden discontinuation of clonidine may induce rebound hypertension.
- It should be tapered slowly.
- Taper and discontinue or convert to the transdermal form preoperatively.

    c. Guanabenz. Guanabenz, a newer centrally acting α_2 agonist, is similar in action to clonidine and methyldopa. It may also have weak peripheral neuronal blocking properties. Its side effects are similar to those of clonidine and methyldopa, but, unlike methyldopa, it is not associated with liver toxicity or a positive Coombs test.

- The side effects of guanabenz are similar to those of clonidine.

    d. Guanfacine. Guanfacine, another new clonidine-like drug, can be given once daily and may have fewer central nervous system side effects. Similar to guanabenz and clonidine, it is not associated with liver toxicity or a positive Coombs test.

Vasodilators

Vasodilators are usually used as step 3 agents in combination with a diuretic and an adrenergic inhibitor.

 1. Hydralazine. Hydralazine decreases blood pressure by directly dilating arterioles. Doses should not exceed 200 mg daily. Its side effects include headache, palpitations, tachycardia, fluid retention, lupus-like syndrome, and peripheral neuropathy. Hydralazine should not be used in patients with a recent cerebral hemorrhage, acute myocardial infarction, or a dissecting aortic aneurysm because of its tendency to increase cardiac output and cerebral blood flow.

- Hydralazine: direct dilatation of arterioles.
- Dose should not be >200 mg daily.
- Side effects: headache, palpitations, tachycardia, fluid retention, lupus-like syndrome, and peripheral neuropathy.
- Do not give to patients with recent cerebral hemorrhage, acute myocardial infarction, or dissecting aortic aneurysm.

 2. Minoxidil. Minoxidil is a very potent, direct vasodilator used to treat severe hypertension with or without

renal insufficiency. Its side effects include significant volume expansion with edema, hirsutism, and pericardial effusion. It may cause atrial fibrosis and pulmonary hypertension, but this has not been proved.

- Side effects: volume expansion with edema, hirsutism, and pericardial effusion.

ACE Inhibitors

ACE inhibitors decrease blood pressure by inhibiting the enzyme that converts angiotensin I to angiotensin II, a potent vasoconstrictor. These drugs are appropriate initial therapy for hypertension and work well in combination with other antihypertensive agents, particularly diuretics. ACE inhibitors retard progression of nephropathy in type I diabetes mellitus and prevent the development of congestive heart failure and recurrent myocardial infarction in persons who have had an initial myocardial infarction associated with reduced left ventricular function. They are an important treatment for established congestive heart failure. ACE inhibitors may slow the progression of nondiabetic renal diseases and lessen proteinuria. Captopril is the only sulfhydryl-containing ACE inhibitor. Because it is eliminated by renal excretion, dose reduction is necessary in cases of renal insufficiency (this is true for most available ACE inhibitors). The side effects presumed to be due to the sulfhydryl group in captopril are skin rash, loss of taste, proteinuria with membranous glomerulonephropathy, and leukopenia. Leukopenia is more likely to occur in patients with collagen vascular disease and renal insufficiency. Side effects shared by all ACE inhibitors are orthostatic hypotension, hyperkalemia, cough, angioedema, and loss of renal function. In patients with bilateral renal artery stenosis, ACE inhibitors can precipitate acute renal failure because of disruption of autoregulation of glomerular filtration in the setting of severe renal ischemia. ACE inhibitors are contraindicated in pregnancy because they can cause fetal toxicity.

- ACE inhibitors inhibit the enzyme that converts angiotensin I to angiotensin II.
- ACE inhibitors are appropriate initial therapy for hypertension.
- Dose reduction is necessary in renal insufficiency.
- Side effects of captopril: skin rash, loss of taste, proteinuria with membranous glomerulonephropathy, and leukopenia.
- Side effects of all ACE inhibitors: orthostatic hypotension, hyperkalemia, cough, angioedema, and loss of renal function.
- ACE inhibitors retard progression of nephropathy in type I diabetes mellitus.
- ACE inhibitors reduce proteinuria and may slow the progression of nondiabetic renal diseases.

- ACE inhibitors are important in the treatment of congestive heart failure.
- ACE inhibitors prevent recurrent myocardial infarctions and the development of congestive heart failure in persons who have had an initial myocardial infarction complicated by reduced left ventricular function.
- ACE inhibitors are contraindicated in pregnancy.

Calcium Channel Antagonists

Calcium channel antagonists are direct vasodilators. They are divided into dihydropyridines (nifedipine, nicardipine, isradipine, felodipine, nisoldipine, and amlodipine) and nondihydropyridines (verapamil, diltiazem). Long-acting forms of these drugs can be used as initial therapy for hypertension in patients with concomitant ischemic heart disease and chronic, stable angina (amlodipine, nicardipine, and extended release forms of nifedipine, diltiazem, and verapamil), variant angina due to coronary vasospasm (amlodipine, extended release forms of nifedipine, and diltiazem), supraventricular arrhythmias (verapamil, diltiazem), Raynaud phenomenon (nifedipine), and migraine headaches (verapamil). Verapamil decreases the risk of a second myocardial infarction in patients whose initial myocardial infarction was not associated with pulmonary congestion. Diltiazem decreases the risk of a second myocardial infarction in patients who had a non-Q-wave infarction. The long-term use of nifedipine delays the need for surgery in patients with chronic aortic insufficiency and may be of benefit for patients with primary pulmonary hypertension. Long-acting dihydropyridine calcium channel antagonists lessen the risk of stroke in older patients with systolic hypertension. Verapamil (and to a lesser extent, diltiazem) has a negative effect on the proximal cardiac conduction system and is a negative inotrope. Verapamil should not be used in patients with conduction system disease (sick sinus syndrome, second-degree or greater heart block) and should be avoided in patients with congestive heart failure (ejection fraction <40%). Verapamil in combination with β-blockers can produce profound cardiodepression. Because it decreases the renal and nonrenal elimination of digoxin, verapamil increases the risk of digoxin toxicity. Quinidine and verapamil in combination can cause serious hypotension in patients with idiopathic hypertrophic subaortic stenosis.

- Calcium channel antagonists are direct vasodilators.
- Verapamil should not be used in sick sinus syndrome or second-degree or greater heart block.
- Avoid using verapamil with congestive heart failure (ejection fraction <40%).
- Verapamil increases the risk of digoxin toxicity.

Verapamil and other calcium channel antagonists can cause an increase in liver enzymes associated with hepatic necrosis.

The most common side effect of verapamil is constipation. Most of the side effects associated with nifedipine and other dihydropyridine calcium channel antagonists are related to their potent peripheral vasodilator properties. These side effects include headache, tachycardia, flushing, and edema. Cimetidine and other drugs that decrease blood flow to the liver may increase the biologic effects of calcium channel antagonists. All calcium channel antagonists are metabolized by the liver, and dose adjustments may be necessary in the presence of liver disease. They can be used safely in renal insufficiency.

- Calcium channel antagonists can cause an increase in liver enzymes associated with hepatic necrosis.
- The most common side effect of verapamil: constipation.
- Other side effects: headache, tachycardia, flushing, and edema.
- Calcium channel antagonists are metabolized by the liver, so dose adjustments are necessary in liver disease.

Angiotensin II Antagonists

Angiotensin II antagonists (losartan, valsartan, candesartan, irbesartan) lower blood pressure by blocking the cell surface receptors that angiotensin II interacts with to produce all of its known effects on blood pressure. Unlike ACE inhibitors, these drugs may not be associated with cough. Therefore, angiotensin II antagonists are alternatives for persons who develop cough with ACE inhibitors. The most common side effect is dizziness. Diuretics or salt and volume depletion can potentiate their hypotensive action. Angiotensin II antagonists can cause fetal toxicity and should be avoided in pregnancy. They can precipitate acute renal failure in persons with bilateral renal artery stenosis. Risks of hyperkalemia are similar to those of ACE inhibitors. Losartan is uricosuric. These drugs have no adverse effect on plasma lipids or glucose.

- Angiotensin II antagonists inhibit the actions of angiotensin II by blocking its cell surface receptors.
- Angiotensin II antagonists do not cause cough.
- Side effects of angiotensin II antagonists: dizziness, hyperkalemia, acute renal failure.
- Avoid in pregnancy because of fetal toxicity.

CAUSES OF SECONDARY HYPERTENSION

Renovascular Hypertension

Renovascular hypertension is the most common form of potentially curable secondary hypertension. It occurs in 1% to 2% of the hypertensive population. Stenosis of a renal artery increases renin production from the ischemic kidney. Renin acts on circulating renin substrate to produce angiotensin I, that is converted to angiotensin II, a potent vasoconstrictor, by ACE found in lung and other tissues. In addition to vasoconstriction, angiotensin II stimulates aldosterone production, which causes renal sodium retention and volume expansion. Angiotensin II also stimulates thirst and release of vasopressin.

- Renovascular disease: the most common form of potentially curable secondary hypertension.
- Renal artery stenosis increases renin production.
- Renin increases angiotensin II.
- Angiotensin II is a potent vasoconstrictor and stimulates aldosterone production, causing renal sodium retention and volume expansion.

Correcting renal ischemia eliminates the stimulus for excess renin release and often cures or lessens hypertension. In unilateral renal artery stenosis, prolonged hypertension eventually causes nephrosclerosis in the nonischemic kidney. If this occurs, relieving renal arterial stenosis may not cure hypertension. The longer the duration of hypertension before diagnosis, the less likely that correction of renal ischemia will be beneficial for blood pressure control.

- Correcting renal ischemia eliminates excess renin release.
- The longer the duration of hypertension, the less likely that correction of renal ischemia will be beneficial.

Fibromuscular dysplasia is the most common cause of renovascular hypertension in younger persons, especially women. Lesions usually affect the middle and distal portions of the main renal vessels, often extending into branches. Medial fibroplasia, the most common subtype in adults, has a classic string-of-beads appearance on angiography. Except for rare subtypes, fibromuscular dysplasia progresses slowly over time; however, dissection and thrombosis can occur. Renal artery occlusion is rare.

- Fibromuscular dysplasia: the common cause of renovascular hypertension in younger persons.
- Dissection and thrombosis of the renal artery can occur, but occlusion is rare.

Atheromatous disease is the most common cause of renovascular hypertension in older persons. The lesions usually are in the proximal third of the renal artery, often near the orifice. Although atheromatous renal artery disease may occur in 50%-75% of older persons with hypertension, it causes or aggravates hypertension less frequently. The disease is frequently bilateral and, in 50% of cases, progresses over time, even if blood pressure is controlled. Bilateral disease can progress and lead to end-stage renal disease.

- Atheromatous disease: the common cause of renovascular hypertension in older persons.
- The disease is frequently bilateral and, in 50% of cases, progresses over time.

Clinical clues suggesting renovascular hypertension include the onset of hypertension before age 30 (consider fibromuscular dysplasia, especially in women), onset of hypertension after age 50 (consider atherosclerotic renovascular disease), presentation of accelerated or malignant hypertension, or sudden worsening of hypertension (renovascular hypertension superimposed on essential hypertension). The most important physical finding is an abdominal bruit, especially a high-pitched systolic/diastolic bruit in the upper abdomen or flank. However, 50% of patients with renovascular hypertension do not have this finding. Other physical clues include severe retinopathy of accelerated malignant hypertension (hemorrhages, exudates) or evidence of atherosclerotic occlusive disease in other vascular beds. Laboratory abnormalities consistent with renovascular hypertension include hypokalemia (due to secondary aldosteronism) and, rarely, ischemia-induced polycythemia or nephrotic range proteinuria.

- For hypertension before age 30, consider fibromuscular dysplasia, especially in women.
- The most important physical finding: abdominal bruit.
- Laboratory abnormalities: hypokalemia, ischemia-induced polycythemia, or nephrotic range proteinuria.
- For hypertension after age 50, consider atherosclerotic renovascular disease.

An acute decline of renal function with the use of an ACE inhibitor or an AII blocker or with a sudden decrease in blood pressure may indicate bilateral renal artery stenosis. Other presentations of bilateral renal artery stenosis (ischemic nephropathy) include the sudden development of pulmonary edema associated with severe hypertension (flash pulmonary edema) and subacute decline in renal function with or without worsening hypertension. Atheroembolic renal disease may also present with a sudden onset or worsening of hypertension and a subacute decline in renal function. Historical clues (e.g., occurrence after angiography or aortic surgery), physical findings (livedo reticularis, peripheral emboli), and laboratory abnormalities (increased erythrocyte sedimentation rate, anemia, hematuria, eosinophilia, eosinophiluria) help identify these patients.

- Sudden decline in renal function with the use of an ACE inhibitor or AII blocker or flash pulmonary edema may indicate bilateral renal artery disease.
- Sudden onset or worsening of hypertension and subacute decline in renal function may be due to atheroembolic renal disease.

In young persons with hypertension (even if not severe) of short duration who have suggestive clinical features, evaluation for renovascular hypertension is indicated because identification and correction of renal artery stenosis can be performed with low risk of morbidity and mortality and correction is associated with a high probability of cure. Evaluation for renovascular hypertension in older patients must be done on a selective basis. Selection should be restricted to patients with suggestive clinical features whose blood pressure cannot be controlled medically or who have an unexplained, observed decline in renal function and who are considered reasonable risks for (and are willing to undergo) interventional therapy.

- In young patients with hypertension of short duration, evaluate for renovascular hypertension.
- Evaluation for renovascular hypertension in older patients must be done on a selective basis.

Screening Tests

Intravenous Pyelography
Intravenous pyelography has been replaced by captopril renography or duplex renal ultrasonography as the initial screening test of choice. Characteristic abnormalities are 1) unilateral reduction in renal mass, with the pole-to-pole diameter of the smaller kidney decreased by 1.5 cm or more; 2) delayed appearance of contrast agent in the collecting system of the ischemic kidney; 3) hyperconcentration of contrast agent in the ischemic kidney on delayed films; 4) ureteral scalloping by collateral vessels; and 5) cortical thinning or irregularity. Sensitivity is 70% to 75%; thus, normal findings on intravenous pyelography do not exclude the diagnosis. Specificity is 85%. It is a reasonable choice if renal obstruction, infarction, calculus disease, or parenchymal disease is of concern.

- Abnormalities on intravenous pyelography: unilateral reduction in renal mass (≥1.5-cm decrease in pole-to-pole diameter of the smaller kidney), delayed appearance of contrast agent in the collecting system of the ischemic kidney (hyperconcentration of this agent in the ischemic kidney), ureteral scalloping by collateral vessels, and cortical thinning or irregularity.

Captopril Radionuclide Renal Scan
Some consider the captopril radionuclide renal scan the screening method of choice. Sensitivity of captopril renography is 90%; specificity is 90% to 95%. Pretest treatment of patients with captopril increases the sensitivity of the scan compared with that of standard renography. The rationale is that glomerular filtration in an ischemic kidney depends on the vasoconstricting effect of angiotensin II on the efferent arteriole of the nephron. Acute treatment with an ACE

inhibitor causes efferent arteriolar dilatation, with loss of filtration pressure in the nephron. This causes a decline of glomerular filtration in the ischemic kidney, with less of an effect on renal blood flow. These changes are identified with the scanning technique. The radionuclides that are used most commonly are ^{131}I orthoiodohippuric acid (OIH), which is a marker for renal blood flow, and ^{99m}Tc diethylenetriamine pentaacetic acid (DPTA), which is a marker for glomerular filtration rate. The criteria for a positive test with DPTA are time to peak activity in the kidney of 11 minutes or more and a ratio of the glomerular filtration rate between the kidneys of 1.5 or greater. The criterion for a positive test with OIH is residual cortical activity at 20 minutes of 30% or more of peak activity. The renal scan is safe for patients with renal insufficiency or a history of contrast allergy. Its interpretive value is reduced by azotemia and bilateral or branch renal artery disease. Urinary outflow obstruction may mimic renal artery stenosis.

- Some consider captopril radionuclide scan the screening method of choice.
- It has a sensitivity of 90% and a specificity of 90%-95%.
- It is safe for patients with renal insufficiency or a history of contrast allergy.
- Urinary outflow obstruction may mimic renal artery stenosis.

Duplex Ultrasonography

Duplex ultrasonography is considered the screening method of choice by some, especially in persons with renal insufficiency. It is noninvasive and does not use contrast media. It should be considered for patients with renal insufficiency or a history of contrast allergy. This method measures flow-velocity changes in renal vessels that occur with renal artery stenosis. Criteria for a positive test are 1) a ratio of peak flow velocity in the renal artery to peak flow velocity in the aorta greater than 3.5 and 2) renal artery peak systolic flow 180 cm/s or greater. In up to 50% of cases, one or both renal arteries cannot be visualized because of technical problems. Accessory renal arteries often are not identified. Sensitivity is 80% to 90% and specificity is 90%.

- Consider duplex ultrasonography for patients with renal insufficiency or a history of contrast allergy.
- In up to 50% of patients, one or both renal arteries cannot be visualized.
- It has a sensitivity of 80%-90% and a specificity of 90%.

Digital Venous Subtraction Angiography

Digital venous subtraction angiography uses contrast media, but access to the circulation is through a peripheral vein. Thus, it can be performed safely as an outpatient procedure. It allows visualization of the proximal main renal arteries (usual location of atherosclerotic disease) in 90% of patients but is not good for assessing distal or branch renal arteries (usual location of fibromuscular dysplasia). This technique is expensive, and in 20% to 30% of cases, renal arteries are not identified because of superimposition of abdominal vessels or patient motion. The sensitivity is 85% to 90% and the specificity is 85% to 90%.

- Digital venous subtraction angiography: the proximal main renal arteries are visible in 90% of patients.
- It is not good for assessing distal or branch renal arteries.
- It is expensive.
- Renal arteries not identified in 20%-30% of cases.
- It has a sensitivity of 85%-90% (same for specificity).

Captopril Test

Acute blockade of angiotensin II formation by ACE inhibitors produces a reactive increase in plasma renin activity. The magnitude of this increase is greater in patients with renovascular hypertension than in those with essential hypertension. This is the basis for the captopril test. The use of antihypertensive agents that influence the renin-angiotensin-aldosterone axis must be discontinued several days before the test. Plasma renin activity is measured at baseline and at 60 minutes after administering captopril orally. Criteria for a positive test include 1) post-captopril plasma renin activity greater than 12 ng/mL per hour, 2) absolute increase in plasma renin activity over baseline of 10 ng/mL per hour or greater, and 3) 150% or greater increase in plasma renin activity if the baseline plasma renin activity is greater than 3 ng/mL per hour or 400% or greater if baseline renin activity is less than 3 ng/mL per hour. The results are compromised in the presence of renal insufficiency. The sensitivity is 39% to 100% and the specificity is 72% to 100%.

- Plasma renin activity is measured at baseline and at 60 minutes after administering captopril orally.
- With renal insufficiency, the results are compromised.
- It has a sensitivity of 39%-100% and a specificity of 72%-100%.

Renal Vein Renins

Lateralization of renal vein renins is the best predictor of a good interventional outcome in unilateral renal artery stenosis; however, because many factors can influence renin secretion and are difficult to control for, this is not a good screening test. It is invasive and expensive. Lateralization is present if the ratio of renin activity on the affected side compared with that on the normal side is 1.5:1.0 or greater. The sensitivity is 63% to 77% and the specificity is 60% to 95%.

- Lateralization of renal vein renins: the best predictor of good interventional outcome in unilateral renal artery stenosis.
- It is invasive and expensive.
- Lateralization is present if the ratio of renin activity of the affected side to the normal side is ≥1.5:1.0.

Magnetic Resonance Angiography

This technique visualizes the main renal arteries without the need for radiocontrast agents or radiation exposure. It should be considered in persons who are at risk from radiocontrast exposure because of renal insufficiency or radiocontrast allergy. It also is a good choice for patients with severe diffuse atherosclerosis who are at risk for atheroembolization with angiography. Field limitations may limit the ability to see lesions in the distal main renal artery or lesions in branches. Accessory renal arteries may not be identified. The degree of arterial stenosis may be overestimated by this method. Persons prone to claustrophobia may not tolerate being placed in the magnetic resonance equipment. This is an expensive screening test.

- Magnetic resonance angiography: visualizes the renal arteries without radiocontrast agents or radiation exposure.
- Good choice for persons with renal insufficiency or radiocontrast allergy.
- May cause claustrophobia and is expensive.

Spiral CT Angiography

Spiral CT angiography offers excellent three-dimensional images but requires a considerable contrast load and patient cooperation. This is an alternative for patients with normal renal function who do not have a contrast allergy.

- Spiral CT requires considerable contrast.

Renal Arteriography

Renal arteriography is the standard method for identifying renal arterial lesions. Renal artery stenosis must be demonstrated in combination with clinical features and, in some cases, lateralization of renal vein renins. If the clinical suspicion for renal vascular hypertension is high, proceeding directly to arteriography is appropriate.

- Renal arteriography: the standard method for identifying renal arterial lesions.

Therapy for Renovascular Hypertension

Options for the management of renovascular hypertension include medical and interventional therapies. Percutaneous balloon angioplasty, stent placement, and surgical procedures to relieve renal ischemia are the nonmedical treatments. Goals of interventional therapy are to cure or to improve hypertension and to preserve renal function. Interventional therapy should be reserved for good surgical candidates. Medical therapy is reserved for patients not considered candidates for interventional therapy (because of the extent or location of the vascular lesions, medical/surgical risk, or uncertainty about the causative significance of the lesion).

Percutaneous transluminal angioplasty is the treatment of choice for amenable lesions due to fibromuscular dysplasia and is an option with or without stent placement in some cases of atherosclerotic renovascular disease. Complications of angioplasty include groin hematoma, dye-induced azotemia, dissection of the renal artery, renal infarction, and, rarely, rupture of the renal artery, with loss of the kidney and the need for immediate surgery. Cholesterol embolization is a risk in older patients with diffuse atherosclerosis.

- Angioplasty is the treatment of choice for amenable lesions due to fibromuscular dysplasia and is an option for some lesions caused by atherosclerosis.
- Its complications: groin hematoma, dye-induced azotemia, dissection of the renal artery, renal infarction, and, rarely, rupture of the renal artery.

Surgical treatment is best for most cases of atheromatous renal artery disease. Stent-supported angioplasty is an option for some patients. Kidneys 8 cm or less in pole-to-pole length should be removed, not revascularized, if intervention is indicated and removal will not jeopardize overall renal function.

- Surgical treatment is best for most cases of atheromatous renal artery disease.
- Stent-supported angioplasty is an option for some patients.

The medical treatment of renovascular hypertension differs little from that of essential hypertension. Volume retention and vasoconstriction (due to activation of the sympathetic nervous system and angiotensin II) both contribute to the hypertension. ACE inhibitors can precipitate acute renal failure if unrecognized bilateral renal artery stenosis is present. Medical treatment does not correct the underlying ischemia of the affected kidney, and decreasing systemic blood pressure without correcting renal vascular stenosis may aggravate further loss of renal function.

- The medical treatment of renovascular hypertension is similar to that of essential hypertension.
- If there is bilateral renal artery stenosis, ACE inhibitors can precipitate acute renal failure.

- Medical treatment does not correct the underlying ischemia of the affected kidney.

Renal Parenchymal Disease

Renal parenchymal disease is the most common cause of secondary hypertension. At least three mechanisms are involved in the hypertension of renal disease: volume expansion, renin oversecretion, and decreased production of renal vasodilators (prostaglandins, kallikrein, kinin). Treatment should include sodium restriction and diuretics. Oversecretion of renin occurs in a small proportion of patients with chronic renal disease. In advanced renal insufficiency, avoid the use of lipid-insoluble β-blockers, which rely on the kidney for excretion. ACE inhibitors reduce proteinuria and may retard further loss of renal function. However, they should be used with caution and in a reduced dose because they can cause hyperkalemia and acute declines in renal function.

- Renal parenchymal disease: the most common cause of secondary hypertension.
- Treatment should include sodium restriction and diuretics.
- Renin oversecretion occurs in a small proportion of patients with chronic renal disease.
- Use ACE inhibitors cautiously and at a reduced dose.

Primary Aldosteronism

Hypertension, hypokalemia, suppressed plasma renin activity, and increased aldosterone excretion form the syndrome of primary aldosteronism. Its main subtypes are unilateral aldosterone-producing adenoma and bilateral idiopathic zona granulosa adrenal hyperplasia. Rarer subtypes are unilateral hyperplasia, glucocorticoid suppressible hyperplasia, and aldosterone-producing cortical carcinoma. Primary aldosteronism should be suspected in any hypertensive patient presenting with spontaneous hypokalemia or significant hypokalemia precipitated by the usual dose diuretic therapy. One should consider other hypokalemic hypertensive syndromes: diuretics, renovascular hypertension, Cushing disease, exogenous steroids, and ingestion of licorice containing glycyrrhizinic acid (renal cortisol catabolism inhibitor). Primary aldosteronism may be the cause of resistant hypertension even in the absence of hypokalemia.

- Primary aldosteronism: hypertension, hypokalemia, suppressed plasma renin, and increased aldosterone secretion.
- Main subtypes: unilateral aldosterone-producing adenoma and bilateral adrenal hyperplasia.
- Suspect primary aldosteronism in patients with spontaneous hypokalemia, significant hypokalemia precipitated by the usual dose diuretic therapy, or resistant hypertension.

Clinical Features

Clinical symptoms are uncommon. Significant hypokalemia may cause muscle weakness, cramps, headache, palpitations, polydipsia, polyuria, or nocturia. Hypertension is usually moderate but may be severe; it is often resistant to pharmacologic intervention. Retinal vascular changes of significant hypertension may be present. The sign of Trousseau or Chvostek may be present if marked alkalosis is associated with the hypokalemia. Peripheral edema is rare.

- Significant hypokalemia may cause muscle weakness, cramps, headache, palpitations, polydipsia, polyuria, or nocturia.
- Peripheral edema is rare.

Laboratory Features

Characteristic laboratory abnormalities include hypokalemia, mild metabolic alkalosis (serum bicarbonate >31 mEq/L), and relative hypernatremia (serum sodium concentration >142 mEq/L). Relative hypernatremia is related to decreased vasopressin release as the result of volume expansion, resetting of the central osmostat for vasopressin release, altered thirst, and hypokalemia-induced suppression of vasopressin release or action. A mild increase in the fasting blood glucose level is seen in about 25% of patients (hypokalemia suppresses insulin release). ECG may show changes of left ventricular hypertrophy and hypokalemia (prolongation of the ST segment, U waves, and T-wave inversions).

- Laboratory abnormalities: hypokalemia, mild metabolic alkalosis, and relative hypernatremia.
- In about 25% of patients, a mild increase in blood glucose.
- ECG shows left ventricular hypertrophy and hypokalemia (prolongation of the ST segment, U waves, T-wave inversions).

Diagnosis

Investigation for primary aldosteronism is divided into three series of studies: 1) screening for primary aldosteronism, 2) confirming the diagnosis, and 3) performing imaging studies to distinguish between the two main subtypes of primary aldosteronism. Screening studies should include measurement of serum sodium, potassium, random plasma renin activity (PRA), and plasma aldosterone concentration (PAC). In a hypokalemic, hypertensive patient, a PAC-to-PRA ratio greater than 20 (with PAC >15 ng/dL and PRA <2.0 ng/mL per hour) suggests the diagnosis of primary aldosteronism. The diagnosis of primary aldosteronism rests on demonstrating hypokalemia, renin suppression, and increased aldosterone excretion in a sodium replete state (24-hour sodium excretion >200 mg) in hypertensive persons. Before initiating a diagnostic evaluation, the use of potentially interfering drugs must be discontinued and plasma volume status assessed. Spironolactone influences the renin-angiotensin-aldosterone axis and must be discontinued for at least 6 weeks before investigation. ACE inhibitors may increase plasma renin activity levels in persons with primary aldosteronism. If hypertension must be treated in the interim, guanadrel, α-blockers, or calcium channel antagonists may be used. After a high salt diet for 3 days (and with concomitant vigorous potassium supplementation), patients should submit a 24-hour urine collection for measurement of sodium, potassium, creatinine, and aldosterone. Creatinine can be used as an approximation of the adequacy of the collection. A 24-hour urine aldosterone greater than 12 μg (when urine sodium is >200 mEq/24 hr) confirms the diagnosis of primary aldosteronism.

- In a hypokalemic, hypertensive patient, a PAC-to-PRA ratio >20 suggests primary aldosteronism.
- The diagnosis of primary aldosteronism: hypokalemia, renin suppression, and increased aldosterone secretion in a sodium replete state in a hypertensive patient.
- Before diagnostic evaluation: discontinue interfering drugs and assess plasma volume status.
- After a 3-day high salt diet, measure sodium, potassium, creatinine, and aldosterone in a 24-hour urine collection.
- 24-Hour urine aldosterone >12 μg (if urine sodium is >200 mEq/24 hr) confirms the diagnosis of primary aldosteronism.

Adenoma and bilateral hyperplasia must be distinguished. Removing an aldosterone-producing adenoma normalizes blood pressure and hypokalemia in 70% of cases. Unilateral or bilateral adrenalectomy seldom corrects hypertension when bilateral adrenal hyperplasia is present. An adrenal CT scan is the initial study for distinguishing between subtypes. CT is effective in localizing adenomas larger than 1 cm in diameter when the adrenal glands are imaged at 0.3-cm intervals. Generally, if a single adenoma larger than 1 cm in diameter is clearly identified, surgical treatment is the choice. If no mass is identified, assume the diagnosis of bilateral hyperplasia and prescribe spironolactone or other potassium-retaining diuretics. Often, additional medications are needed for blood pressure control.

- Removing an aldosterone-producing adenoma normalizes hypertension and hypokalemia in 70% of cases.
- Unilateral or bilateral adrenalectomy seldom corrects hypertension in cases of bilateral adrenal hyperplasia.
- Adrenal CT scanning is the initial study for distinguishing between subtypes.
- If a single adenoma is >1 cm in diameter, treatment is surgical.

- If no mass is seen, prescribe spironolactone or other potassium-retaining diuretics.

If the results are equivocal or the gland opposite that containing the presumed adenoma is abnormal or if CT findings are normal in a young patient with severe hypertension and hypokalemia, suggesting the presence of an adenoma, then sampling blood from the adrenal veins for aldosterone may distinguish between subtypes. In these settings, subspecialty consultation should be sought.

- If the results are equivocal, sampling blood from the adrenal veins for aldosterone may distinguish between subtypes.

Pheochromocytoma

Pheochromocytomas are tumors of chromaffin cell origin that produce paroxysmal or sustained hypertension. A "rule of 10" is often quoted for this tumor: 10% are extra-adrenal (90% are located in one or both adrenal glands), 10% occur in children (90% in adults between the third and fifth decades of life; equal occurrence in males and females), 10% are multiple or bilateral, 10% recur after the initial resection, 10% are malignant, and 10% are familial. Extra-adrenal pheochromocytomas may occur anywhere along the sympathetic chain and occasionally in aberrant sites (superior para-aortic region [46%], inferior para-aortic region [29%], bladder [10%], and thorax [10%]). Chromaffin cells synthesize catecholamines from tyrosine. Norepinephrine is the end product in all sites except in the adrenal medulla, where 75% of norepinephrine is metabolized further to epinephrine. Extra-adrenal tumors produce only norepinephrine, whereas adrenal pheochromocytomas may produce an excess of one or both chemicals. Patients with tumors that secrete predominantly epinephrine tend to have mainly systolic hypertension, tachycardia, sweating, flushing, and tremulousness and may present with hypotension. Patients with tumors that secrete mainly norepinephrine tend to have both diastolic and systolic hypertension, less tachycardia, and fewer paroxysms of anxiety and palpitations.

- Remember the "rule of 10."
- 80%-90% of pheochromocytomas are in the adrenal glands.
- They may occur anywhere along the sympathetic chain.
- They are malignant in up to 10% of cases.
- Extra-adrenal tumors produce only norepinephrine.
- Adrenal pheochromocytomas produce an excess of epinephrine or norepinephrine or both.

Familial pheochromocytomas tend to be bilateral. Familial syndromes include 1) a simple form inherited as an autosomal dominant trait unassociated with other glandular abnormalities; 2) multiple endocrine neoplasia type IIA (medullary carcinoma of the thyroid [increased plasma level of calcitonin], pheochromocytoma, hyperparathyroidism) and type IIB (pheochromocytoma, medullary carcinoma of the thyroid, mucosal neuromas, thickened corneal nerves, intestinal ganglioneuromatosis, marfanoid body habitus); 3) neurofibromatosis (café au lait spots); and 4) von Hippel-Lindau disease (pheochromocytoma, retinal hemangiomatosis, cerebellar hemangioblastomas, renal cell carcinoma).

- Familial tumors: tend to be bilateral.
- Pheochromocytoma associated with neurofibromatosis, and von Hippel-Lindau disease (retinal angiomas, cerebellar hemangioblastomas, and renal cell carcinoma), and multiple endocrine neoplasia types IIA and IIB.

Symptoms

Headache, sweating, or palpitations are common, and all may occur in paroxysms. Paroxysms of hypertension occur in fewer than 50% of persons; most persons have sustained hypertension. Exercise, bending, urination, defecation, induction of anesthesia, smoking, or infusion of intravenous contrast media can induce a paroxysm. Some patients have a history of weight loss and hypermetabolism. Others have both hypertension and orthostatic hypotension, and some have retinopathy of accelerated hypertension.

- Common symptoms of pheochromocytoma: headache, sweating, and palpitations.
- Exercise, bending, urination, defecation, induction of anesthesia, smoking, or infusion of contrast media can induce a paroxysm.
- Some patients have a history of weight loss and hypermetabolism; others have both hypertension and orthostatic hypotension.

Screening

Patients who should undergo screening for pheochromocytoma are those with a history of paroxysmal hypertension, progressive or treatment-resistant hypertension, hypertension with diabetes mellitus, hypermetabolism and weight loss, marked hypertension in response to anesthesia induction, neurocutaneous lesions and hypertension, family history of pheochromocytoma, medullary carcinoma of the thyroid or hyperparathyroidism, or hypertension with orthostatic hypotension. Patients with a history of paroxysmal symptoms and hypertension should also be screened for pheochromocytoma, as should children with hypertension. The best screening test is 24-hour urine metanephrine excretion. Because pheochromocytomas may secrete intermittently, multiple samples may be required. Urine should be collected immediately after a paroxysm. In addition to urine metanephrine concentration, urine vanillylmandelic acid and catecholamine concentrations should be measured in selected patients. Medications that can interfere with these assays are listed in Table 13-4.

- Screening for pheochromocytoma: history of paroxysmal hypertension, progressive or treatment-resistant hypertension, hypertension with diabetes mellitus, hypermetabolism and weight loss, or marked hypertension in response to anesthesia induction.
- Screen children with hypertension.
- The best screening test is 24-hour urine metanephrine excretion.
- Medications interfering with assays: sympathomimetics, methyldopa, phenothiazines, tricyclic antidepressants, labetalol, and levodopa.

Diagnosis and Treatment

Computerized abdominal imaging (CT or MRI) is the initial test used to locate a tumor. The treatment is surgical. Preoperatively, administer α-blockers followed by β-blockers if needed for blood pressure and cardiac rhythm control. Patients with hypertensive crisis can be given α-blockers or sodium nitroprusside intravenously. β-Blockers can be used if tachycardia is excessive.

- Use computerized abdominal imaging to locate the tumor.
- The treatment is surgical.
- Preoperatively, administer α-blockers, followed by β-blockers.

Table 13-4.—Medications That Interfere With Results of Catecholamine and Metabolite Measurements

Associated with increased values
Amphetamines
Phenothiazines
Labetalol
Drugs containing catecholamines (decongestants)
Levodopa
Methyldopa
Withdrawal from clonidine or related drugs
Ethanol
Tricyclic antidepressants
Benzodiazepines
Sotalol
Associated with decreased values
Metyrosine
Methylglucamine (iodinated contrast medium)

Coarctation of the Aorta

Coarctation of the aorta is commonly just beyond the takeoff of the left subclavian artery. It is detected most often in childhood but may escape detection until adulthood. The classic feature of coarctation is increased blood pressure in the upper extremities, with low or unobtainable blood pressure in the lower extremities. The mechanism of hypertension involves volume expansion and inappropriate renin secretion. Symptoms of coarctation include headache, cold feet, and exercise-induced leg pain (claudication). Clinical signs include hypertension, murmurs in the front or back of the chest, visible pulsations in the neck or chest wall, and weak femoral pulses or delay when simultaneously palpating the radial and femoral pulse. Chest radiography can be diagnostic. A characteristic "3 sign" due to dilatation above and below the constriction plus notching of the ribs by enlarged collateral vessels may be identified. The diagnosis is proved by aortography, and the treatment is surgical. Postoperative hypertension is usually transient and may be associated with mesenteric vasculitis and bowel infarction. Plasma renin activity levels are usually high. β-Blockers or ACE inhibitors are recommended treatments.

- Coarctation of the aorta is usually just beyond the takeoff of the left subclavian artery.
- Usually, it is detected in childhood but may not be detected until adulthood.
- Classic feature: increased blood pressure in the upper extremities and low/unobtainable blood pressure in the lower extremities.
- Mechanism of hypertension: volume expansion and inappropriate renin secretion.
- Symptoms: headache, cold feet, and exercise-induced leg pain.
- Signs: hypertension, murmurs in front or back of the chest, visible pulsations in the neck or chest wall, and weak femoral pulses.
- Chest radiography can be diagnostic.

Hypertension in Pregnancy

Normally, blood pressure decreases early in pregnancy and then gradually increases to prepregnant levels toward term. During pregnancy, renin substrate, renin activity, and aldosterone levels increase. Vessels during normal pregnancy are hyporesponsive to angiotensin, perhaps because of prostaglandins produced by the uteroplacental unit. Although aldosterone levels increase, renal sodium retention is not marked, probably because progesterone and prostaglandins are natriuretic. Progesterone is also a vasodilator. During normal pregnancy, plasma volume and cardiac output increase 50% to 60% of baseline. The renal blood flow and glomerular filtration rate increase by 35%. Blood pressure decreases in normal pregnancy because of reduced peripheral vascular resistance. Other substances that increase during normal pregnancy are estrogen, deoxycorticosterone, and vasodilating prostaglandins produced by the uteroplacental unit.

- Blood pressure decreases early in pregnancy, gradually increasing to prepregnant levels toward term.
- Renin substrate, renin activity, and aldosterone increase.
- During pregnancy, vessels are hyporesponsive to angiotensin.
- Renal sodium retention is not marked, probably because progesterone and prostaglandins are natriuretic.
- In normal pregnancies, blood pressure decreases because of reduced peripheral vascular resistance.

Definition

Hypertension during pregnancy is when systolic blood pressure increases 30 mm Hg or more and diastolic blood pressure increases 15 mm Hg or more compared with values before 20 weeks' gestation. When previous blood pressure levels are unknown, a pressure of 140/90 mm Hg or greater is abnormal. Four major hypertensive syndromes in pregnancy are 1) chronic hypertension—high blood pressure known to be present before pregnancy or diagnosed before the 20th week of gestation, 2) preeclampsia-eclampsia (described below), 3) chronic hypertension with superimposed preeclampsia, and 4) transient hypertension (or gestational hypertension)—increase in blood pressure without significant edema or proteinuria, with return of blood pressure to normal within 10 days after delivery. This is a predictor for the future development of essential hypertension.

- Hypertension: systolic blood pressure increases ≥30 mm Hg and diastolic blood pressure increases ≥15 mm Hg, as compared with values before 20 weeks' gestation.
- Transient hypertension is a predictor for future development of essential hypertension.

Preeclampsia is characterized by the triad of hypertension, edema, and proteinuria developing after the 20th week of gestation. Eclampsia consists of these symptoms plus convulsions. Warning symptoms of eclampsia include headache, blurring of vision, epigastric pain, hyperreflexia, or cerebral symptoms. The risk of developing eclampsia is markedly increased in women with severe proteinuria (>5 g), oliguria, or absolute blood pressures greater than 160/110 mm Hg. Preeclampsia occurs more commonly in women who are relatively young or old to be pregnant, first pregnancy, twin pregnancy, obesity, diabetes mellitus, family history of eclampsia or preeclampsia in the mother, preeclampsia with a previous pregnancy, renal disease, or pregnancy in the setting of chronic hypertension. Preeclampsia developing before the

20th week of gestation suggests the possibility of molar pregnancy, fetal hydrops, α-thalassemia, or renal disease.

- Preeclampsia: characteristic triad of hypertension, edema, and proteinuria after the 20th week of gestation.
- Eclampsia: same symptoms as preeclampsia plus convulsions.
- Preeclampsia is more common in women relatively young or old for pregnancy, first or twin pregnancy, obesity, diabetes mellitus, family history of eclampsia or preeclampsia in the mother, preeclampsia with a previous pregnancy, renal disease, pregnancy in the setting of chronic hypertension.

In preeclampsia, an immune reaction prevents trophoblastic invasion of the spiral arteries. This leads to underperfusion of the placenta. Circulating mediators produced by the hypoperfused placenta act on vascular endothelial cells, which produce several factors (procoagulants, vasoconstrictors, mitogens) that constrict and obstruct vascular beds, producing the characteristic pathologic changes (hemorrhage, necrosis) that may be seen in the brain, heart, and liver of women with preeclampsia.

Unlike normal pregnant women, those with preeclampsia are sensitive to the pressor effects of angiotensin. There is a marked increase in peripheral resistance. Renal blood flow and glomerular filtration rate are decreased. Vascular volume is decreased. There is often hemoconcentration. Placental prostaglandin levels decrease. Uric acid is most often increased and distinguishes patients with preeclampsia from those with chronic hypertension in pregnancy. Uric acid elevation and declining platelet counts are the earliest laboratory findings associated with preeclampsia. The HELLP syndrome (**H**emolysis, **E**levated **L**iver enzymes, and **L**ow **P**latelet count) occurs when intravascular coagulation and liver ischemia develop in preeclampsia.

- Unlike normal pregnant women, those with preeclampsia are sensitive to the pressor effects of angiotensin.
- Peripheral resistance markedly increases.
- Uric acid is most often increased: this distinguishes women with preeclampsia from those with chronic hypertension in pregnancy.
- Uric acid elevation and declining platelet counts are the earliest laboratory abnormalities in preeclampsia.

Treatment of Hypertension in Pregnancy

For previously untreated women, consider drug therapy if diastolic blood pressure is 100 mm Hg or greater. Methyldopa (most completely studied) is recommended as initial therapy. If this drug is ineffective or not tolerated, consider other drugs. Except for ACE inhibitors and angiotensin II inhibitors, none

of the currently available drugs are known to increase perinatal morbidity or mortality. Most of the concern about these drugs is theoretical. There is evidence that β-adrenergic blocking drugs and α-β-blocking drugs are safe and effective for treating chronic hypertension in pregnancy. There is some concern that the use of β-adrenergic blockers early in pregnancy can retard fetal growth and in late pregnancy could slow the fetal heart rate.

- For previously untreated women, use drug therapy if diastolic blood pressure is ≥100 mm Hg.
- Recommended initial therapy: methyldopa.
- ACE inhibitors and angiotensin II blockers are contraindicated during pregnancy.

Treatment of Preeclampsia-Eclampsia

Prevention strategies for preeclampsia have limited value. In recent studies, aspirin and calcium supplements have not been shown to lessen the risk for preeclampsia. It is important to identify the high-risk woman and to monitor her closely to identify preeclampsia early. Early recognition of preeclampsia is based primarily on diagnostic blood pressure increases in the late second or early third trimester of pregnancy. Proteinuria is an important sign of progression, usually warranting hospitalization. The woman should be kept at rest in bed. Monitor blood pressure, urine output, and fluid retention (estimated by daily weights) daily. Periodically determine the platelet count, creatinine level, uric acid level, and urine protein excretion. Evidence of central nervous system involvement (headache, disorientation, visual symptoms) or liver distention (abdominal pain, liver tenderness) are important findings that suggest progression of preeclampsia. Hepatic rupture is associated with a 65% mortality and can be prevented only by delivery of the fetus. Evidence of progressive preeclampsia after the 30th week of gestation is an indication for delivery. When gestational age is critical (25-30 weeks), delivery is indicated by worsening maternal symptoms, laboratory evidence of end-organ dysfunction, or deterioration of the fetal condition. If a fetus is immature and preeclampsia is nonprogressive, a period of observation is warranted. Hypertension should be treated with drugs if diastolic blood pressure is greater than 100 mm Hg. The treatment of choice is methyldopa. Calcium channel antagonists, β-adrenergic blockers, or hydralazine are reasonable alternatives.

- Proteinuria is an important sign of progression, usually warranting hospitalization.
- Keep the woman at bed rest.
- Central nervous system progression or liver distention suggests progression of preeclampsia.
- Progressive preeclampsia after the 30th week of gestation is an indication for delivery.

- Delivery is indicated by worsening maternal symptoms, laboratory evidence of end-organ dysfunction, or deterioration of the fetal condition.
- If diastolic blood pressure is >100 mm Hg, treat with drugs.
- Treatment of choice: methyldopa.

Magnesium sulfate is the treatment of choice for impending eclampsia. It can be administered intravenously as 20 mL of a 20% solution over 4 minutes. Intermittent doses of a 50% solution given intramuscularly every 4 hours can also be used. Monitor the patient's patellar reflex, urine output, and respirations while giving magnesium. Calcium gluconate is the treatment of choice for magnesium toxicity.

- Magnesium sulfate: treatment of choice for impending eclampsia.
- Calcium gluconate: treatment of choice for magnesium toxicity.

Treatment of Hypertensive Crisis

The drug of choice for the treatment of a hypertensive crisis during pregnancy is hydralazine administered intravenously. Initially administer a 5-mg bolus. This can be followed by 5 to 10 mg every 20 to 30 minutes. Side effects include tachycardia and headache. For hypertension refractory to hydralazine, diazoxide is recommended. Miniboluses (30 mg) should be used. Side effects include arrest of labor and neonatal hyperglycemia. Labetalol may replace diazoxide as the second-line drug. Calcium antagonists can be used, but the concomitant use of magnesium sulfate may cause severe hypotension. Diuretics and sodium nitroprusside (cyanide poisoning in the fetus) should be avoided. However, maternal well-being may override these concerns.

- The drug of choice for treating hypertensive crisis: hydralazine given intravenously.
- For hypertension refractory to hydralazine, use diazoxide.
- Avoid diuretics and sodium nitroprusside.

Hypertensive Emergencies and Urgencies

Acute, severe increases in blood pressure are a medical emergency; prompt therapy may be lifesaving.

Definitions

Hypertensive Emergency

The term "hypertensive emergency" is defined as severe hypertension with evidence of acute injury to target organs (brain, heart, kidneys, retina). It implies the need for hospitalization and immediate reduction of blood pressure with parenteral therapy. Examples include malignant hypertension, hypertensive encephalopathy, and severe hypertension in association with dissection of the aorta, unstable angina, acute myocardial infarction, pulmonary edema, or acute renal failure. In malignant hypertension, retinal examination reveals hemorrhages, exudates, and, often, papilledema. Hypertensive encephalopathy may be present; it is cerebral edema due to breakthrough hyperperfusion of the brain caused by severely increased blood pressure. Manifestations include papilledema, headache, confusion, gastrointestinal distress, visual loss, focal neurologic deficits, coma, and seizures. Fibrinoid necrosis of blood vessels is the characteristic pathologic finding of malignant hypertension, and microangiopathic hemolysis may occur.

- Hypertensive emergency: severe increase in blood pressure associated with acute injury to target organs.
- Hospitalization and parenteral therapy to decrease blood pressure immediately are required.
- Hypertensive encephalopathy: papilledema, headache, confusion, gastrointestinal distress, visual loss, focal neurologic deficits, coma, and seizures.

Hypertensive Urgency

The term "hypertensive urgency" is defined as severe hypertension without evidence of acute target organ injury but occurring in a setting in which it is important to decrease blood pressure to safer levels over 24 hours. Treatment is with oral or parenteral therapy, and hospitalization may not be required. Examples include accelerated hypertension and severe hypertension in association with known coronary artery disease, aortic aneurysm, history of congestive heart failure, or postoperative state. Accelerated hypertension is a sudden increase in blood pressure not associated with acute organ damage. Retinal examination reveals hemorrhages and exudates but not papilledema. If untreated, it may progress to malignant hypertension.

- Hypertensive urgency: severe hypertension without acute target organ injury.
- Treatment is with oral or parenteral therapy, and hospitalization may not be required.
- Accelerated hypertension may progress to malignant hypertension if untreated.

Causes

The causes of hypertensive urgencies and emergencies include the development of accelerated malignant hypertension on the background of neglected essential hypertension, sudden discontinuation of antihypertensive therapy (especially clonidine and β-blockers), renovascular disease, collagen diseases (especially scleroderma), monoamine oxidase inhibitors and tyramine-containing foods, intracerebral or subarachnoid hemorrhage, acute aortic dissection, pheochromocytoma crisis, acute head injury, and acute stroke.

- Causes of hypertensive urgencies and emergencies: neglected essential hypertension, discontinuation of antihypertensive therapy, renovascular disease, collagen diseases, pheochromocytoma crisis, and stroke.

Pathophysiology of Malignant Hypertension

Malignant hypertension is a rapidly progressive vasospastic disorder associated with a marked increase in peripheral vascular resistance and increased levels of renin and angiotensin. Locally generated vasoconstricting factors such as endothelin may be important. If not reversed, the necrosis of blood vessel walls occurs (fibrinoid necrosis), with severe damage to organs, particularly the brain and kidneys. With progressive increases in blood pressure, the autoregulation of cerebral blood flow breaks down. Normally, as blood pressure increases, cerebral blood vessels constrict to maintain constant blood flow. When blood pressure increases to a critical level, the cerebral blood vessels suddenly dilate, causing marked hyperperfusion of the brain and leakage of fluid. This leads to cerebral edema and the clinical presentation of hypertensive encephalopathy.

- Malignant hypertension: a rapidly progressive vasospastic disorder.
- Renin and angiotensin levels are increased.
- If not reversed, necrosis of blood vessel walls occurs.

Evaluation and Management

Patients with hypertensive emergencies and evidence of acute organ injury should be hospitalized in an intensive care unit. An arterial catheter should be established to monitor blood pressure closely. Initial studies should include chest radiography, ECG, creatinine or BUN, urinalysis, glucose, sodium, potassium, and hemoglobin. Studies to determine the underlying cause should be deferred; however, a spot urine for catecholamines is reasonable. The challenge of treating hypertensive emergencies is to decrease blood pressure promptly without compromising the function of vital organs. Blood pressure should be decreased quickly to a diastolic level of approximately 110 mm Hg (decrease mean blood pressure by 20%), after which the patient's condition should be monitored for evidence of worsening cerebral, renal, or cardiac status. Blood pressure is then gradually decreased to a diastolic level of 90 to 100 mm Hg. Ischemic pancreatitis and intestinal infarction are complications in some patients.

Generally, sodium nitroprusside is the drug of choice. It must be given in an intensive care setting, with an arterial catheter in place. This balanced arterial and venous dilator

decreases both preload and afterload. The initial dose is 0.5 to 10.0 μg/kg per minute. It is titrated to a maximal dose of 500 μg/kg per hour. The infusion must be protected from light. Toxicity is related to the development of cyanide in erythrocytes, and thiocyanate levels should be monitored every 48 hours. Therapy should be discontinued if the blood level is greater than 12 mg/dL. Sodium nitrate or hydroxycobalamin can be infused in case of toxicity. Side effects of sodium nitroprusside include nausea, vomiting, agitation, muscular twitching, coarse tremor, and flushing. Frequently, patients with malignant hypertension are volume constricted because of pressure natriuresis. However, as blood pressure decreases, fluid retention occurs and the addition of a loop diuretic is often required.

- Sodium nitroprusside: the drug of choice.
- Toxicity is related to the development of cyanide in erythrocytes.
- Monitor thiocyanate levels every 48 hours.
- In case of toxicity, infuse sodium nitrate or hydroxycobalamin.
- Sodium nitroprusside side effects: nausea, vomiting, agitation, muscular twitching, coarse tremor, and flushing.

Several alternative parenteral agents are available for the management of hypertensive emergencies and urgencies.

Labetalol is a combination α-blocker and nonselective β-blocker with an onset of action of 5 to 10 minutes. It can be given in repetitive intravenous miniboluses of 20 to 80 mg or as a constant infusion at a dose of 0.5 to 2 mg/min. Its duration of action is 3 to 6 hours. It can be used in most situations except acute heart failure. It is especially useful for postoperative hypertension and in hypertensive crises of pregnancy. β-Blocker cautions and contraindications apply. Adverse effects include scalp tingling, vomiting, heart block, and orthostatic hypotension.

Glyceryl trinitrate is a direct arteriolar and venous vasodilator with an onset in 2 to 5 minutes and duration of action of 3 to 5 minutes. It is given as a constant infusion of 5 to 100 μg/min. This drug decreases myocardial oxygen demand by decreasing preload and afterload. It dilates epicardial coronary arteries and collaterals. Tolerance can develop with prolonged infusion. It is especially useful if acute coronary ischemia is present or in acute congestive heart failure. Adverse effects include headache, flushing, nausea, and methemoglobinemia.

Hydralazine is a direct arteriolar vasodilator with onset of action of 10 to 20 minutes if given intravenously and 20 to 30 minutes if given intramuscularly. The usual dose is 10 to 20 mg intravenously or 10 to 50 mg intramuscularly. Its duration of action is 3 to 8 hours. Hydralazine is used primarily in treating hypertensive crisis of pregnancy. Adverse effects include headache, flushing, nausea, vomiting, and myocardial ischemia. Hydrozones form when hydralazine is mixed with dextrose.

Esmolol is a cardioselective β-blocker with an onset of action of 1 to 2 minutes and a duration of action of 10 to 20 minutes. It is given as a constant intravenous infusion in a dose of 50 to 300 μg/kg per minute. Esmolol is useful in postoperative hypertension, aortic dissection, and ischemic heart disease. It is often combined with vasodilators for effective blood pressure control. β-Blocker cautions and contraindications apply. Adverse effects include nausea and bradycardia.

Enalaprilat is an ACE inhibitor with an onset of action of 15 minutes and a duration of action of 6 hours. It is given intravenously in doses of 1.25 to 5 mg every 6 hours, with a maximal dose of 20 mg in 24 hours and less if renal disease is present. It is useful in postoperative hypertension and in settings of acute heart failure. Adverse effects include ACE inhibitor side effects, a precipitous decrease in blood pressure in high renin states, and an acute decline in renal function if renal artery disease is present.

Nicardipine is a dihydropyridine calcium channel antagonist with an onset of action of 5 to 10 minutes and a duration of action of 1 to 4 hours. It is given as a constant intravenous infusion of 5 to 15 mg/hr. It is useful for postoperative hypertension. Nicardipine should not be used in acute heart failure. Adverse effects include headache, nausea, flushing, and phlebitis.

Phentolamine is an α-blocker that is administered intravenously in doses of 5 to 15 mg. It is most effective in states of catecholamine excess and is the drug of choice if pheochromocytoma is suspected. Adverse effects include tachycardia and flushing.

Diazoxide is considered obsolete, with the availability of newer and safer drugs. If used, it should be given by minibolus technique (50-100-150 mg every 5 to 10 minutes). This method avoids excessive hypotension with the initial dose. The blood sugar level should be monitored in diabetic persons. Adverse effects include nausea, hypotension, flushing, tachycardia, and chest pain.

- Glyceryl trinitrate is useful in acute congestive heart failure or coronary ischemia.
- Tolerance can develop to glyceryl trinitrate.
- Hydralazine is used for the hypertensive crisis of pregnancy.
- Esmolol, enalaprilat, and nicardipine are useful for postoperative hypertension.
- Phentolamine is the drug of choice if pheochromocytoma is suspected.

Conditions Requiring Avoidance of Specific Drugs
- Acute myocardial infarction or angina—hydralazine (increases cardiac work), diazoxide (increases cardiac work).
- Dissecting aortic aneurysm—hydralazine (increases cardiac output), diazoxide (increases cardiac output).
- Stroke, head injury, hypertensive encephalopathy—methyldopa (sedation, increases cerebral blood flow), diazoxide (decreases cerebral blood flow).

As soon as possible, initiate regular oral treatment and taper intravenous treatment. After blood pressure has been controlled, search for secondary causes of hypertension.

QUESTIONS

Multiple Choice (choose the one best answer)

1. A 35-year-old woman is referred for management of hypertension. She has a history of high blood pressure but discontinued drug therapy 2 months ago when she discovered she was pregnant. Her blood pressure was initially normal but has gradually risen and is now averaging 150/105 mm Hg. All the following statements are true *except*:

   a. She is at increased risk for preeclampsia
   b. Her current blood pressure level is high enough to justify drug treatment, and methyldopa is the initial drug of choice
   c. If she is intolerant to methyldopa, diuretics, angiotensin-converting enzyme inhibitors, or β-blockers would be appropriate alternatives for treatment
   d. An increasing plasma level of uric acid and decreasing platelet count would be worrisome for preeclampsia
   e. If hypertensive crisis develops, intravenous hydralazine, diazoxide, or labetalol is the treatment option

2. An obese 54-year-old business executive is evaluated for resistant hypertension. Blood pressure control has been poor despite treatment with three drugs: hydrochlorothiazide 25 mg/day, atenolol 50 mg/day, and lisinopril 20 mg/day. He admits that he does not restrict his dietary intake of sodium. He drinks alcohol daily with lunch and dinner and does not exercise on a regular basis. He uses indomethacin daily for treatment of gout. He admits to using diet pills containing phenylpropanolamine for weight control. Routine laboratory studies reveal an increased plasma level of triglycerides. All the following are true *except*:

   a. Daily consumption of alcohol in excess of 1 oz may increase blood pressure
   b. A high sodium intake and indomethacin may interfere with the blood pressure lowering effects of diuretics and angiotensin-converting enzyme inhibitors
   c. Phenylpropanolamine does not affect blood pressure and, if it leads to weight loss, will be beneficial
   d. Diuretics, β-blockers, and alcohol may increase triglycerides
   e. Hydrochlorothiazide can cause gout

3. A 62-year-old man with a history of well-controlled hypertension has induction of anesthesia for an elective hernia repair. Sinus tachycardia suddenly develops, and his blood pressure increases to 250/140 mm Hg. Intravenous sodium nitroprusside is administered, and blood pressure decreases to 100/60 mm Hg. The patient is taken to the intensive care unit where his condition stabilizes. What is the most appropriate next step in evaluation?

   a. Contrast computed tomography of the abdomen
   b. Consider oral treatment of his hypertension with labetalol
   c. Determine the plasma level of calcitonin
   d. Obtain a 24-hour urine collection for metanephrines, catecholamines, and vanillylmandelic acid (VMA)
   e. Renal angiogram

4. A 27-year-old woman is evaluated for the recent onset of headache. Physical examination discloses a blood pressure of 180/115 mm Hg and a systolic-diastolic bruit in the right upper quadrant of the abdomen. There is no personal or family history of hypertension. She is not taking any medications. What is the most appropriate first test in evaluating a possible cause of her hypertension?

   a. 24-Hour collection for metanephrines
   b. Captopril radionuclide renal scan
   c. Renal angiography
   d. Plasma aldosterone/renin activity ratio
   e. Magnetic resonance imaging of the head

5. A 55-year-old man came to the emergency department complaining of severe substernal chest pain for the past 2 hours. He has a 3-year history of hypertension but stopped treatment 2 months ago when his prescriptions lapsed. He has smoked 2 packs of cigarettes daily for 35 years. He has been told of increased cholesterol and fasting blood glucose levels. His blood pressure measures 210/130 mm Hg and electrocardiography demonstrated changes consistent with acute anterior wall myocardial infarction. All the following are true *except*:

   a. Intravenous glyceryl trinitrate or esmolol would be appropriate antihypertensive therapy
   b. Intravenous hydralazine would be inappropriate for antihypertensive therapy
   c. Use of sodium nitroprusside can be associated with cyanide toxicity
   d. Renal vascular hypertension is a possibility
   e. Diazoxide is an appropriate alternative therapy for decreasing blood pressure

6. A 56-year-old man is evaluated for the recent onset of headache. He has no personal history of hypertension. His blood pressure is 190/120 mm Hg. Retinal examination shows hemorrhages without papilledema. Initial laboratory studies are normal except for plasma potassium, which is decreased at 3.2 mEq/L (normal, 3.6-4.8). Other than headaches, the patient is asymptomatic. All

the following statements are true *except*:

a. The patient can be managed safely as an outpatient with oral medication

b. This presentation is compatible with essential hypertension

c. Primary aldosteronism should be considered

d. Pheochromocytoma should be considered

e. Hypokalemia can occur in renal vascular hypertension as the result of secondary aldosteronism

7. A 76-year-old woman complains of fatigue, weakness, and cough. She has a history of hypertension of 20 years' duration that had been controlled with hydrochlorothiazide, 25 mg daily. Recently, because of increased blood pressure values, the dose of hydrochlorothiazide was increased to 50 mg daily and lisinopril 5 mg was started. Blood pressure is 130/70 mm Hg in the sitting position and decreases to 100/60 mm Hg on standing. Laboratory studies reveal decreased plasma sodium at 129 mEq/L, normal plasma potassium, increased fasting blood glucose at 110 mg/dL, and increased serum creatinine at 2.4 mg/dL. Before the recent change in medications, her serum creatinine was 1.0 mg/dL. All the following statements are true *except*:

a. Volume depletion from hydrochlorothiazide could account for the increased creatinine and the symptoms of fatigue and weakness

b. Her cough could be a side effect of lisinopril

c. Thiazide diuretics can cause hyponatremia and hyperglycemia

d. The increase in creatinine likely indicates bilateral renal artery stenosis

e. The combination of diuretics and angiotensin-converting enzyme inhibitors can cause orthostatic hypotension

8. A 42-year-old man has a 6-month history of spells and hypertension. The spells are abrupt in onset, last 15 to 30 minutes, and are abrupt in offset. Symptoms consist of headache, tachycardia, and diaphoresis. Blood pressure has been noted to increase markedly to as high as 240/140 mm Hg during the spells. Evaluation includes a 24-hour urine for metanephrines, which are markedly increased. All the following statements are true *except*:

a. This condition can occur in patients with von Hippel-Lindau disease or neurofibromatosis

b. Tricyclic antidepressants or labetalol can increase metanephrines

c. This is likely a familial syndrome

d. Most often this condition is due to a tumor present in one or both adrenal glands

e. This condition can be associated with medullary carcinoma of the thyroid and hyperparathyroidism

9. At a community screening, a 44-year-old woman is found to have increased blood pressure. This has been confirmed on follow-up visits. She has no family history of hypertension. Her physical examination findings are normal. Initial laboratory studies included the following blood studies: sodium, 144 mEq/L; potassium, 3.0 mEq/L; fasting blood glucose, 106 mg/dL. All the following statements regarding this case are true *except*:

a. The ingestion of licorice containing glycyrrhizinic acid could cause this presentation

b. Hypokalemia can cause glucose intolerance

c. The next step in evaluation would be to determine a random plasma renin activity and aldosterone concentration

d. If both the plasma renin activity and aldosterone concentration are increased, computed tomography of the abdomen should be performed to look for an adrenal adenoma

e. The use of spironolactone should be avoided until additional tests are performed

10. A 37-year-old woman is referred for evaluation of new-onset hypertension. She is asymptomatic. Her mother and an older sister have hypertension. She has been taking an oral contraceptive for birth control for the past 10 years. She is moderately overweight and sedentary. She does not use tobacco and has no history of dyslipidemia or diabetes mellitus. She has no history of cardiovascular disease. Physical examination and routine laboratory studies are normal except for a blood pressure of 140/94 mm Hg. The following statements are true *except*:

a. Oral contraceptives can cause hypertension by inducing sodium retention and increasing angiotensinogen levels

b. Weight loss and regular aerobic exercise may lower her blood pressure

c. If secondary to the oral contraceptive, discontinuation should lead to blood pressure improvement within a few weeks

d. A family history of hypertension increases a person's risk of developing high blood pressure with oral contraceptives

e. Discontinuation of the oral contraceptive should be discussed, and alternative methods of birth control should be offered

ANSWERS

1. Answer c.

Generally, drug therapy for hypertension during pregnancy is recommended if the diastolic blood pressure is 100 mm Hg or greater. Methyldopa is the oral drug of choice. The only two antihypertensive drug classes that are absolutely contraindicated in pregnancy are angiotensin-converting enzyme inhibitors and angiotensin II receptor blockers. These drugs can cause significant fetal anomalies.

2. Answer c.

Alcohol use in amounts that exceed 1 oz daily is associated with higher blood pressure in some persons. Alcohol activates the sympathetic nervous system, increases cortisol secretion, and may increase intracellular calcium levels, leading to an increase in vascular reactivity and peripheral vascular resistance. Nonsteroidal anti-inflammatory drugs interfere with the formation of renal vasodilating and natriuretic prostaglandins and, thus, can induce sodium retention and interfere with the action of most antihypertensive drugs, especially diuretics and angiotensin-converting enzyme inhibitors. Phenylpropanolamine can increase peripheral vascular resistance and blood pressure. Diuretics can have an adverse effect on plasma lipids by increasing total and LDL cholesterol and triglycerides. This may be a short-term effect. β-Blockers can increase triglycerides and lower HDL cholesterol levels. Alcohol use may be associated with hypertriglyceridemia. Hydrochlorothiazide increases the plasma levels of uric acid and can precipitate gout in susceptible persons.

3. Answer d.

This patient's history of severe hypertension occurring with induction of anesthesia suggests the possibility of pheochromocytoma. The next step in evaluation would be to obtain biochemical evidence for a functioning tumor. Because the patient had a recent paroxysm, a urine collection should be started immediately. Because suspicion for pheochromocytoma is high, the urine collection should be comprehensive and include measures of metanephrines, catecholamines, and VMA. Imaging studies should not be performed unless there is biochemical evidence of pheochromocytoma. Contrast computed tomography or renal angiography could stimulate another paroxysm. Also, contrast exposure may interfere with urinary metanephrine measurement. The initial treatment of choice for pheochromocytoma is α-blockers. Although labetalol may be beneficial, it is a combination of an α- and a β-blocker and may have a predominately β-blocking effect. Measuring the calcitonin level would be appropriate if multiple endocrine neoplasia is a consideration.

4. Answer c.

The clinical presentation is highly suggestive of renal vascular hypertension likely due to fibromuscular dysplasia. Because the pretest probability of this diagnosis is high, it is most appropriate to proceed directly to renal angiography.

5. Answer c.

Because hydralazine and diazoxide increase cardiac work, they are not ideal drugs to use in the setting of myocardial infarction or ischemia. Intravenous glyceryl trinitrate or esmolol would be more appropriate. Cyanide toxicity can occur with the use of sodium nitroprusside. With prolonged use, thiocyanate levels should be monitored. This patient is at risk for renal vascular disease due to atherosclerosis, and if severe hypertension or declining renal function is noted in follow-up, further evaluation would be reasonable.

6. Answer b.

Although the patient's blood pressure is increased severely, there is no evidence for acute organ damage and he can be treated safely with oral medications as an outpatient. Any patient who presents with hypertension and spontaneous hypokalemia should be considered for primary aldosteronism as well as other hypertensive hypokalemic syndromes such as Cushing disease or renal vascular disease. Hypokalemia is rare, but it can occur in renal vascular hypertension as a result of significant secondary aldosteronism. Pheochromocytoma should be considered in patients with severe hypertension and headaches, even in the absence of classic paroxysms. Only 50% of patients with pheochromocytoma have paroxysms. This presentation argues against essential hypertension. Features inconsistent with essential hypertension include age of onset (usually under age 50 years for essential hypertension), stage 3 hypertension at diagnosis (usually stage 1 or 2 in essential hypertension), the presence of retinal hemorrhages, and the presence of spontaneous hypokalemia.

7. Answer d.

Although an increase in the serum level of creatinine associated with the use of an angiotensin-converting enzyme inhibitor always raises the possibility of bilateral renal artery disease, the findings in this case strongly suggest volume contraction as the more likely explanation.

8. Answer c.

This patient has a pheochromocytoma. Only 10% of pheochromocytomas are familial; the majority are sporadic. These tumors occur with increased frequency in patients with von Hippel-Lindau disease and neurofibromatosis. Various drugs can interfere with the measurement of metanephrines. Tricyclic antidepressants and labetalol can increase metanephrines in the absence of a pheochromocytoma. Although pheochromocytomas can be found anywhere along the sympathetic chain and in aberrant sites, 90% are located in one or both adrenal glands. Pheochromocytoma can be part of the multiple endocrine neoplasia syndromes.

9. Answer d.

If both plasma renin activity and aldosterone concentration are increased, the patient has secondary aldosteronism. Further evaluation for causes of secondary aldosteronism (renovascular disease) should be considered, but primary aldosteronism is excluded. Therefore, computed tomography of the abdomen would not be indicated. Glycyrrhizinic acid is a renal cortisol catabolism inhibitor and prevents the conversion of cortisol to cortisone. Cortisol has significant mineralocorticoid activity and can cause hypertension and hypokalemia. In this setting, both plasma renin activity and plasma aldosterone concentration are low. Hypokalemia can suppress insulin secretion and lead to hyperglycemia. Approximately 25% of patients with primary aldosteronism and hypokalemia have mild glucose intolerance. The initial step in screening for primary aldosteronism is to obtain a random plasma renin activity and simultaneous plasma aldosterone concentration. If the ratio of aldosterone-to-renin concentrations is greater than 20, with a plasma aldosterone concentration greater than 15 mg/dL and plasma renin activity less than 2.0 ng/mL per hour, primary aldosteronism is likely and confirmatory testing is indicated. Spironolactone is an aldosterone receptor blocker and causes marked increases in aldosterone levels. Its use should be avoided until the work-up for primary aldosteronism is complete.

10. Answer c.

Hypertension due to an oral contraceptive may require up to 6 months to resolve after discontinuation. In a patient with mild hypertension who is at low risk, discontinuation of the oral contraceptive and lifestyle modifications for up to 6 months would be an appropriate strategy. Whenever oral contraceptives are discontinued, alternative methods of birth control should be discussed.

NOTES

CHAPTER 14

INFECTIOUS DISEASES

William F. Marshall, M.D.
Zelalem Temesgen, M.D.
Lynn Estes, Pharm. D.
Abinash Virk, M.D.
Douglas R. Osmon, M.D.

This chapter approaches the ever expanding field of infectious diseases from four perspectives. The first section reviews the characteristics of specific pathogenic organisms, the second section covers clinical syndromes associated with various infections, the third section discusses the human immunodeficiency virus, and the fourth section describes anti-infective agents.

SPECIFIC MICROORGANISMS

GRAM-POSITIVE COCCI

Group A β-Hemolytic Streptococci: *Streptococcus pyogenes*

Infections

Group A streptococci are reemerging as an important cause of human disease. They are responsible for several different clinical syndromes. *S. pyogenes* is the most common cause of bacterial pharyngitis. Although the pharyngitis is usually self-limited, antibiotic therapy (penicillin) should be given to prevent subsequent acute rheumatic fever. Penicillin will shorten the duration of infection if it is given within the first 24 hours of infection. Rapid diagnostic tests for streptococcal pharyngitis are easily administered and specific but not overly sensitive (50%-70%) for detecting *S. pyogenes*. Common complications of streptococcal pharyngitis are paratonsillar abscesses, otitis media, and sinusitis.

- Common complications of streptococcal pharyngitis are paratonsillar abscesses, otitis media, and sinusitis.

S. pyogenes is responsible for many skin and soft tissue infections. These can be differentiated by the depth of infection and resulting clinical appearance.

Impetigo is a superficial skin infection caused by group A β-hemolytic streptococci (plate 14-1). *Staphylococcus aureus* may be detected in culture but probably plays no role in the pathology or pathogenesis. Antibiotic therapy shortens the duration of infection and prevents suppurative complications but probably does not prevent poststreptococcal glomerulonephritis.

- Antibiotics probably do not prevent poststreptococcal glomerulonephritis.

Erysipelas is deeper than impetigo. It is an infection of the skin with involvement of cutaneous lymphatic vessels. It often occurs on the face. It has a sharp border, is raised, violaceous, and painful, and most often occurs in the elderly. It recently has been associated with toxic strep syndrome.

Cellulitis involves the skin and subcutaneous tissue and occurs in tissue damaged by trauma, in operative wounds, and in tissue with poor venous and lymphatic drainage (postmastectomy cellulitis of the arm and cellulitis of the leg after saphenous vein harvest for coronary artery bypass grafting may recur). Tinea pedis also may serve as a portal of entry.

Invasive Group A Streptococcal Infection

Since the mid-1980s there have been increasing reports of severe group A streptococcal infection, including necrotizing fasciitis, myonecrosis, and a toxic shock-like syndrome. Suggested causes for the increase include the spread of virulent strains (especially M1 and M3), specific virulence factors (streptococcal pyogenic exotoxin and proteases), and a lack of immunity to these strains in the affected patients. In a recent outbreak of streptococcal necrotizing fasciitis in Minnesota, schoolchildren served as a reservoir for the responsible organism. Victims were mostly older and in poor health. The overall mortality rate is 30%, even in previously healthy patients and with appropriate treatment. Many victims need amputation of extremities or have major tissue loss.

Treatment requires early intervention with admission to an intensive care unit, management of shock, prompt initiation of antibiotics, and early and aggressive surgical debridement of devitalized tissue when indicated.

Group A streptococcal pneumonia is rare but can be extremely severe. It frequently is associated with preceding viral infections, including influenza, measles, and chronic lung disease.

Penicillin is the drug of choice for treatment of group A streptococcal infection. Cephalosporins (first-generation), erythromycin, and vancomycin are alternatives. There are no reports of penicillin resistance to date. There have been reports of an increased prevalence of erythromycin-resistant strains. There is mounting evidence that clindamycin may be useful for treating streptococcal necrotizing fasciitis.

- There are no reports of penicillin resistance in group A streptococci to date.

Toxins

Group A streptococci produce many toxins. Scarlet fever may develop in patients with no previous immunity to erythrogenic toxin. Production of hyaluronidase causes the rapidly advancing margins characteristic of cellulitis due to β-hemolytic streptococci. Exotoxin A is similar to the toxin that causes toxic shock syndrome in patients with *S. aureus* infection (toxic strep syndrome).

Nonsuppurative Complications

The nonsuppurative complications of group A streptococcal infection are acute rheumatic fever and acute glomerulonephritis. In the United States, there was a resurgence of acute rheumatic fever among children and military recruits during the 1980s. *Rheumatic fever* occurs only after pharyngitis, never after skin infections. The diagnostic criteria for rheumatic fever are described in Table 14-1. Treatment is with aspirin and steroids, depending on clinical circumstances and the severity of symptoms and organ involvement.

- Resurgence of acute rheumatic fever among children and military recruits in the 1980s.

The approach to prophylaxis of rheumatic fever is controversial. One approach, if a murmur is present, is indefinite prophylaxis with benzathine penicillin G, 1.2 million units by intramuscular injection monthly (alternative, oral penicillin V potassium, 250 mg twice a day). Sulfonamides and erythromycin are alternatives for the penicillin-allergic patient. If there is no murmur, no attack within previous 5 years, and no carditis with previous attack, prophylaxis may be discontinued after the age of 25. Note that patients with significant rheumatic valvular disease require endocarditis prophylaxis for dental and other procedures.

Acute glomerulonephritis may occur after infection with nephritogenic strains of *S. pyogenes*. Both cutaneous infections and pharyngitis can cause acute glomerulonephritis (Table 14-2).

- Prophylactic antibiotics are used to prevent recurrent acute rheumatic fever.
- Acute glomerulonephritis may occur after both skin infections and pharyngitis.
- Patients with significant rheumatic valvular disease require endocarditis prophylaxis for dental or other procedures.

Group B: *Streptococcus agalactiae*

This organism is an important cause of maternal and neonatal bacteremia and neonatal meningitis. It is part of the normal flora of the female genital tract and gastrointestinal tract. It is somewhat less susceptible to penicillin than group

Table 14-1.—Jones Criteria for Diagnosis of Initial Attack of Rheumatic Fever[*] (1992 Update)

Major manifestations
Carditis
Polyarthritis
Chorea
Erythema marginatum
Subcutaneous nodules
Minor manifestations
Clinical findings
Arthralgia
Fever
Laboratory findings
Elevated acute-phase reactants (erythrocyte sedimentation rate, C-reactive protein)
Prolonged P-R interval
Supporting evidence of antecedent group A streptococcal infection
Positive throat culture or rapid diagnostic test
Elevated or rising streptococcal antibody titer

[*]If supported by evidence of recent group A streptococcal infection, two major, or one major and two minor, criteria are enough for diagnosis. Three exceptions in which Jones criteria do not need to be fulfilled: 1) recurrent rheumatic fever (single major or several minor criteria in patient with a reliable history of previous rheumatic fever if supporting evidence of recent group A streptococcal infection), 2) isolated chorea, and 3) indolent carditis.
From Special Writing Group of the Committee on Rheumatic Fever, Endocarditis, and Kawasaki Disease of the Council on Cardiovascular Disease in the Young of the American Heart Association: Guidelines for the diagnosis of rheumatic fever: Jones Criteria, 1992 update. JAMA 268:2069-2073, 1992. By permission of American Medical Association.

Table 14-2.—Differences Between Acute Glomerulonephritis and Acute Rheumatic Fever Caused by Group A Streptococcal Infection

| | After infection | | Recurrence of disease | Antibiotics prevent disease |
	Skin	Pharynx		
AGN	Yes	Yes (<skin)	Rare, if ever	?
ARF	No	Yes	Often	Yes

AGN, acute glomerulonephritis; ARF, acute rheumatic fever.

A streptococci, although penicillin is still the treatment of choice. Treatment of meningitis is with penicillin or ampicillin plus gentamicin. Prepartum vaginal culture for group B streptococcus may identify women at highest risk and allow eradication of the organism before delivery.

Group D Streptococci

Enterococci are no longer considered group D streptococci. The taxonomy differences also are reflected in the differences in susceptibility to penicillin between enterococci and group D streptococci. Remember that both can cause endocarditis. *Streptococcus bovis* endocarditis and bacteremia may be associated with carcinoma of the colon or other colonic disease. Treatment of *S. bovis* and *Streptococcus equinis* is with penicillin (alone or with an aminoglycoside). If the patient is allergic to penicillin, a cephalosporin or vancomycin is effective. This approach is as opposed to that for enterococci, which are always resistant to cephalosporins.

- *S. bovis* endocarditis and bacteremia may be associated with carcinoma of the colon or other colonic disease.
- Treatment of *S. bovis* and *S. equinis* is with penicillin (alone or with an aminoglycoside).

Enterococci

In the 1990s, enterococci are an important cause of nosocomial infections. Enterococci are intrinsically resistant to many antimicrobial agents. Recently, strains that are effectively resistant to *all* antibiotics (vancomycin-resistant enterococci) are spreading worldwide. *Enterococcus faecium* is usually more resistant than is *Enterococcus faecalis*. This resistance allows the organisms to proliferate in the hospital setting. Although endocarditis rarely complicates nosocomial enterococcal bacteremia, it should be suspected in all community-acquired bacteremias.

Enterococci are only inhibited, not killed, by penicillin or vancomycin alone. When bactericidal activity is needed (endocarditis), an aminoglycoside must be added. Increasing numbers of enterococci are resistant to aminoglycosides (aminoglycoside-modifying enzymes), produce β-lactamase, or are resistant to

glycopeptides (that is, vancomycin, particularly among *E. faecium*). There is no proven effective antimicrobial therapy for infections caused by vancomycin-resistant enterococci.

- Some strains of enterococci (vancomycin-resistant enterococci) are resistant to all available antibiotics.

Enterococcal endocarditis is best treated with a combination of penicillin (or ampicillin) plus streptomycin or gentamicin. The choice of which aminoglycoside depends on the results of susceptibility testing. Duration of therapy depends on how long the patient has been ill with endocarditis. Treatment should be continued for 4 weeks if the illness is less than 3 months in duration. If longer, then 6 weeks of therapy is better. Vancomycin can be used in place of penicillin in the allergic patient, but it is significantly less effective. Optimal regimens for isolates resistant to both gentamicin and streptomycin are unknown. A valve replacement procedure may increase the chance for successfully treating subacute bacterial endocarditis due to drug-resistant enterococci.

- Enterococcal endocarditis is best treated with a combination of penicillin (or ampicillin) plus streptomycin or gentamicin.

Enterococcal urinary tract infections or bacteremia without evidence of endocarditis usually can be treated with a penicillin or vancomycin alone as long as the strains are susceptible in vitro. Options for treatment of uncomplicated urinary tract infection in penicillin-allergic patients include ciprofloxacin, nitrofurantoin, or vancomycin.

Streptococcus pneumoniae

S. pneumoniae (pneumococcus) is a ubiquitous organism and remains a leading cause of pneumonia, meningitis, otitis media, and sinusitis. Like many organisms, it is now becoming more resistant to common antibiotics. Complications of pneumococcal pneumonia include empyema and pericarditis from direct extension of infection. Empyema should be suspected when fever persists despite appropriate antibiotic therapy of pneumococcal pneumonia.

S. pneumoniae is the most common cause of bacterial meningitis in adults (plate 14-2), including those with recurrent meningitis due to cerebrospinal fluid leaks. Meningitis due to susceptible *S. pneumoniae* can still be treated successfully with high-dose penicillin G. However, given the spread of penicillin-resistant strains, high-dose cefotaxime or ceftriaxone in combination with vancomycin should be initiated while awaiting the results of susceptibility testing.

- *S. pneumoniae* is the most common cause of bacterial meningitis in adults.
- Always consider a patient to have a cerebrospinal fluid leak if recurrent *S. pneumoniae* meningitis is present.

S. pneumoniae is one of the most common causes of otitis media, especially in children. Spontaneous peritonitis due to *S. pneumoniae* is reported in children with ascites from nephrotic syndrome.

- Spontaneous peritonitis due to *S. pneumoniae* is reported in children with ascites from nephrotic syndrome.

Asplenia predisposes individuals to severe infections with *S. pneumoniae* (and other encapsulated organisms). After splenectomy, fulminant, usually fatal, pneumococcal bacteremia with disseminated intravascular coagulation is more common. Similarly, *S. pneumoniae* infections are more frequent and unusually severe in patients with sickle cell anemia. Multiple myeloma, alcoholism, and hypogammaglobulinemia also increase the risk.

S. pneumoniae is the leading cause of invasive bacterial respiratory disease in patients with human immunodeficiency virus (HIV) infection. The diagnosis of pneumococcal bacteremia precedes the diagnosis of HIV infection in 50% to 80% of cases. Recurrent invasive disease occurs in 8% to 25% of cases. Serotypes causing the invasive disease are similar to those causing invasive disease in normal hosts. Clinical presentation and treatment are similar to those in normal hosts. Secondary prophylaxis for recurrent episodes (penicillin) may be necessary. Prophylaxis for *Pneumocystis carinii* pneumonia with trimethoprim-sulfamethoxazole may provide effective primary or secondary prophylaxis, but breakthrough infections with resistant organisms are not uncommon.

- After splenectomy, fulminant, usually fatal, pneumococcal bacteremia with disseminated intravascular coagulation may develop.
- *S. pneumoniae* infections are more frequent and unusually severe in patients with sickle cell anemia.
- Patients with multiple myeloma, alcoholism, and hypogammaglobulinemia also are at increased risk of infection.

- *S. pneumoniae* is the leading cause of invasive bacterial respiratory disease in patients with HIV.

Most infections due to *S. pneumoniae* are best treated with penicillin G. A cephalosporin, vancomycin, erythromycin, or newer fluoroquinolones such as levofloxacin or trovafloxacin may be used when there is a penicillin allergy. As mentioned above, penicillin resistance (minimal inhibitory concentration, >2 µg/mL) is increasing. Vancomycin, cefotaxime, ceftriaxone, levofloxacin, or trovafloxacin may be effective against resistant strains. The mechanism of resistance is thought to be alteration of the penicillin-binding proteins. Risk factors for development of penicillin-resistant pneumococci include previous use of β-lactam antibiotics, nosocomial acquisition, and multiple previous hospitalizations.

The pneumococcal vaccine is polyvalent, containing capsular polysaccharide from the 23 serotypes that most commonly cause pneumococcal infection. It is recommended for adults with chronic lung or heart disease and immunosuppressed patients, especially patients who have had splenectomy and patients with sickle cell disease and hereditary spherocytosis. It can be given simultaneously with influenza virus vaccine. Pneumococcal vaccine booster is recommended 5 years after the initial dose in high-risk patients.

Viridans Streptococci

Several species of non-Lancefield typable streptococci are referred to as the "viridans group streptococci." They are normal oral and enteric flora. This group of organisms is a common cause of subacute bacterial endocarditis, which should be suspected in cases of viridans streptococcal bacteremia. Like the pneumococci, these organisms are increasingly likely to display resistance to penicillin. Resistance is most common in patients with hematologic malignancies and others with a history of frequent antibiotic use.

One species of viridans streptococci, *Streptococcus milleri*, frequently is associated with pyogenic abscesses, especially of the liver. This is often a monomicrobial abscess and not necessarily associated with endocarditis.

STAPHYLOCOCCI

Staphylococcus aureus (Coagulase-Positive *Staphylococcus*)

Toxins

Preformed enterotoxins produced by *S. aureus* are a common cause of food poisoning in the United States. The toxin is heat stable and, therefore, is not destroyed by cooking food. Exfoliatins are exotoxins produced by *S. aureus* belonging to phage group II which cause "scalded skin syndrome," an erythematous rash that progresses to bullous lesions. It should be differentiated from toxic epidermal necrolysis (skin biopsy). It occurs most frequently in pediatric patients and is rare in adults. Therapy is with local skin care and antistaphylococcal antibiotics. Toxic shock syndrome is due to an exotoxin (TSST-1) usually produced by *S. aureus*.

- Preformed enterotoxins produced by *S. aureus* are not destroyed by cooking food.
- Toxic shock syndrome is due to an exotoxin (TSST-1) usually produced by *S. aureus*.

Clinical Syndromes

Superficial infections with *S. aureus* include folliculitis (infection of hair follicles without involvement of skin or subcutaneous tissues), furuncles (more extensive follicular infection, often involves subcutaneous tissues and occurs in areas of friction and poor personal hygiene), carbuncles (infection in thick inelastic tissues of the scalp or upper back), and impetigo (most commonly caused by group A β-hemolytic streptococci). Drainage of infected lesions occasionally is required.

S. aureus is the most common cause of acute hematogenous osteomyelitis in pediatric patients and is a common cause of chronic osteomyelitis in adults. It is the second most common cause of prosthetic joint infection, after coagulase-negative staphylococci.

- *S. aureus* is a common cause of chronic osteomyelitis in adults.
- *S. aureus* is the second most common cause of prosthetic joint infection.

Most cases of community-acquired *S. aureus* bacteremias should be treated for 4 to 6 weeks with parenteral antibiotics because of the potential for 1) metastatic abscesses and 2) infective endocarditis. If nosocomial *S. aureus* bacteremias have a removable focus (such as an intravenous catheter), it should be removed and treatment given for 10 to 14 days. *S. aureus* infrequently causes community-acquired pneumonia, but it may develop after a case of influenza. Along with the aerobic gram-negative rods, *S. aureus* is a common cause of nosocomial infection. These are primarily postoperative wound infections, line-associated bacteremias, and ventilator-associated pneumonia. When *S. aureus* causes urinary tract infection, consider the possibility of *S. aureus* bacteremia with seeding of the kidneys.

- Cases of community-acquired *S. aureus* bacteremia should be treated for 4-6 weeks with parenteral antibiotics.
- *S. aureus* infrequently causes community-acquired pneumonia, but it may develop after a case of influenza.

Mechanisms of Resistance

Most *S. aureus* strains produce β-lactamase, and thus they are resistant to penicillin G. Semisynthetic penicillins (nafcillin, oxacillin) and first-generation cephalosporins remain active against such strains. Since the 1970s there has been a worldwide increase of methicillin resistance. This is an intrinsic resistance caused by alteration of the penicillin-binding proteins in the cell wall. Methicillin-resistant strains of *S. aureus* are resistant to all β-lactam drugs. Methicillin resistance often is associated with resistance to multiple agents, including quinolones.

Treatment

If *S. aureus* is penicillin-susceptible (rare), penicillin G is the most active agent. In penicillin-allergic patients, alternatives are cefazolin and vancomycin. If the isolate is methicillin-susceptible, nafcillin, oxacillin, cephalosporins (first-generation), vancomycin, and imipenem are effective. Vancomycin is the only available agent reliably active for treating serious infection with methicillin-resistant *S. aureus*. Occasional strains may still be susceptible to trimethoprim-sulfamethoxazole, minocycline, or macrolides. However, these antibiotics are mostly used for nonserious infections or for chronic suppression.

Methicillin-resistant *S. aureus* nasal colonization can be a difficult problem in hospitals and long-term-care facilities. Topical mupirocin ointment or other therapies (such as cotrimoxazole with or without rifampin) may temporarily eradicate the nasal colonization, but relapse is common.

- Vancomycin is the only available agent reliably active for treating serious infection with methicillin-resistant *S. aureus*.

Coagulase-Negative Staphylococci

Although *Staphylococcus epidermidis* is the most common of the coagulase-negative staphylococci, many species of *Staphylococcus* other than *S. aureus* are included in this group of organisms. For clinical purposes they are interchangeable. Coagulase-negative staphylococci are normal skin flora that rarely cause disease in healthy persons.

Clinical Syndromes

Coagulase-negative staphylococci are a common cause of intravascular device-related bacteremia, prosthetic valve endocarditis, osteomyelitis (usually after joint arthroplasty or other prosthetic implantations), and meningitis after neurosurgical procedures and are associated with wound infection. Treatment usually requires removal of the foreign body and administration of appropriate antibiotics. They can cause peritonitis in patients undergoing chronic ambulatory peritoneal dialysis.

Staphylococcus saprophyticus is a coagulase-negative staphylococcus that is associated with urinary tract infections in young women.

Treatment

Coagulase-negative staphylococci are frequently methicillin-resistant, especially when acquired in the hospital. Unless in vitro susceptibility testing shows other active agents, they should be treated with vancomycin. Ciprofloxacin may be active against some strains, but when used alone emergence of resistance occurs rapidly. *S. saprophyticus* is an exception because it is usually susceptible to many antibiotics.

Determining the significance of blood cultures growing coagulase-negative staphylococci can be difficult. True infections generally result in multiple positive blood cultures, whereas single positive cultures usually are considered contaminants.

Prosthetic valve endocarditis often is caused by coagulase-negative staphylococci. This is best treated with a regimen of vancomycin plus rifampin for 6 weeks and gentamicin for at least the first 2 weeks.

● Unless in vitro susceptibility testing shows other active agents, coagulase-negative staphylococci should be treated with vancomycin.

GRAM-NEGATIVE BACILLI

Escherichia coli Infections

E. coli organisms are part of the normal flora of the gastrointestinal tract. Disease may result from ascending infection (such as in the urinary tract) or a break in a mucosal barrier (such as intra-abdominal infection). *E. coli* bacteremia is often due to focal infection elsewhere. *E. coli* is the most common cause of urinary tract infections and spontaneous bacterial peritonitis. Like most gram-negative bacilli, *E. coli* is variably susceptible to ampicillin, cephalosporins (including first-generation agents), trimethoprim-sulfamethoxazole, aminoglycosides, and fluoroquinolones.

E. coli O157:H7 causes hemorrhagic colitis, which may be complicated by hemolytic-uremic syndrome in approximately 10% of cases. Undercooked hamburger, unpasteurized apple cider, and other food products have been implicated in outbreaks. Treatment is supportive only. Antibiotics are of no benefit in this illness.

● *E. coli* is the most common cause of urinary tract infections and spontaneous bacterial peritonitis.

Proteus, Morganella, Providencia Infections

These organisms are part of the normal fecal flora. They cause urinary tract infections, often associated with an alkaline urine, which enhances production of ammonium-magnesium phosphate stones.

Proteus mirabilis is sensitive to ampicillin. The other types are not sensitive to ampicillin but are usually susceptible to gentamicin, ticarcillin, mezlocillin, third-generation cephalosporins, imipenem, and ciprofloxacin.

Klebsiella, Enterobacter, Serratia Infections

Klebsiella pneumoniae is an important cause of both community-acquired and nosocomial pneumonia. It often is associated with alcoholism, diabetes mellitus, and chronic obstructive pulmonary disease. Red currant jelly sputum is characteristic. Lung abscess and empyema are more frequent with *K. pneumoniae* than with other pneumonia-causing organisms. Cephalosporins are the drugs of choice for treating most types of *Klebsiella*. Strains of *Klebsiella* resistant to ceftazidime have emerged. This resistance is caused by a broad-spectrum β-lactamase. Susceptibility results for such strains may erroneously report that they are susceptible to cefotaxime. If resistant to ceftazidime, consider them resistant to all cephalosporins.

● Lung abscess and empyema are more frequent with *K. pneumoniae* than with other pneumonia-causing organisms.

Enterobacter and *Serratia* primarily are associated with nosocomial infections. Recent reports indicate increased resistance to third-generation cephalosporins in *Enterobacter*. *Enterobacter* often is resistant to third-generation cephalosporins such as cefotaxime, despite in vitro data suggesting susceptibility. *Enterobacter* species are capable of inducing β-lactamases after exposure to β-lactam antibiotics. Carbapenems such as imipenem or meropenem or combining an extended-spectrum penicillin (mezlocillin, piperacillin) with an aminoglycoside may be a more effective therapy. Trimethoprim-sulfamethoxazole, quinolones, or imipenem also may be effective.

● *Enterobacter* species often are resistant to third-generation cephalosporins such as cefotaxime, despite in vitro data suggesting susceptibility.

Pseudomonas aeruginosa

This organism predominantly causes nosocomial infection and is resistant to many common antibiotics. *Pseudomonas*, together with *Staphylococcus aureus*, is the most frequent cause of infections complicating severe burn injuries. Other infections caused by *P. aeruginosa* include folliculitis associated with hot tubs, osteomyelitis (particularly in injection drug users), malignant otitis externa in patients with diabetes mellitus, complicated urinary tract infections, ventilator-associated pneumonia, and pulmonary infections in patients with cystic fibrosis. Patients with neutropenia are also at particularly high risk for *Pseudomonas* infection, especially bacteremia. Hence, the febrile neutropenic patient should empirically be treated with antipseudomonal antibiotics while awaiting culture results. Ecthyma gangrenosum is a necrotizing skin lesion that may develop in neutropenic patients with bacteremia due to *P. aeruginosa*.

- *Pseudomonas*, together with *S. aureus*, is most frequent cause of infections complicating massive burns.
- *P. aeruginosa* is a cause of malignant otitis externa in patients with diabetes mellitus.
- Ecthyma gangrenosum is a necrotizing skin lesion that may develop in neutropenic patients with bacteremia due to *P. aeruginosa*.

Agents active against most *P. aeruginosa* include the extended-spectrum penicillins (piperacillin, ticarcillin), aminoglycoside, ceftazidime and cefepime (the only cephalosporins reliably active against this organism), aztreonam, imipenem, and quinolones. Two drugs, usually a β-lactam and an aminoglycoside, should be used when treating serious infections caused by *P. aeruginosa*. Antibiotic resistance commonly emerges during and after treatment.

Stenotrophomonas (Xanthomonas) maltophilia

This organism most commonly causes nosocomial infections. Its most notable point is intrinsic resistance to imipenem and meropenem (as well as the aminoglycosides, quinolones, and most β-lactam drugs). *Stenotrophomonas maltophilia* usually is susceptible to trimethoprim-sulfamethoxazole and ticarcillin/clavulanate.

- *S. maltophilia* is intrinsically resistant to imipenem and meropenem.

Salmonella

Salmonella infections are increasing in the United States. Well-identified outbreaks have been associated with food contamination. Undercooked chicken or eggs are often sources of infection. Gastroenteritis is the most common manifestation. However, more serious illnesses, including infections of atherosclerotic aortic aneurysms, may occur.

Salmonella typhi is rare in this country. Patients with typhoid fever have relative bradycardia and rose spots (50%). The leukocyte count may be decreased. Blood cultures usually are positive within approximately 10 days of symptom onset, whereas stool cultures are positive after 10 days of symptoms. Bone marrow biopsy and culture also may reveal the diagnosis.

Salmonella choleraesuis causes chronic bacteremia and mycotic aneurysms. *Salmonella typhimurium* and *Salmonella enteritidis* produce gastroenteritis and occasionally bacteremia. Urinary tract infections caused by *Salmonella* occur in patients

from the Middle East who are infected with *Schistosoma haematobium*.

- In typhoid fever, findings on physical examination include fever with relative bradycardia and rose spots (50%).

As with many organisms, antimicrobial resistance is increasingly common with salmonellas. Most cases of *Salmonella* gastroenteritis should not be treated with antibiotics, because treatment prolongs the carrier state. Serious infections should be treated with third-generation cephalosporins or fluoroquinolones while awaiting the results of susceptibility testing.

- Most cases of *Salmonella* gastroenteritis should not be treated with antibiotics because treatment prolongs the carrier state.

Haemophilus influenzae

Widespread use of the vaccine against *Haemophilus influenzae* B has dramatically reduced the incidence of disease in children. Nontypable strains of *H. influenzae* more commonly cause disease in adults (primarily respiratory infection). Other infections include meningitis, obstetrical infections, epiglottitis, and primary bacteremia. Chronic lung disease, pregnancy, human immunodeficiency virus (HIV) infection, splenectomy, and malignancy are risk factors for invasive disease.

- Chronic lung disease, pregnancy, HIV infection, splenectomy, and malignancy are risk factors for invasive disease.

β-Lactamase production is found in up to 40% of isolates recovered from adults with invasive disease. Ampicillin resistance is mostly related to production of β-lactamase. If a strain is β-lactamase-negative, ampicillin can be used. *Haemophilus* infections that are positive or negative for β-lactamase can be treated with cotrimoxazole, cefuroxime, third-generation cephalosporins, imipenem, ciprofloxacin, aztreonam, or a β-lactam-β-lactamase inhibitor combination.

- β-Lactamase production is found in up to 40% of isolates recovered from adults with invasive disease.
- Ampicillin resistance is mostly related to production of β-lactamase.

H. influenzae is an uncommon cause of meningitis in adults. When it occurs, consider the possibility of hypogammaglobulinemia, asplenia, or cerebrospinal fluid leak. Third-generation cephalosporins (cefotaxime or ceftriaxone) are the drugs of choice. Cefuroxime is not as effective. Prophylactic treatment with rifampin is recommended for all household contacts of patients with *H. influenzae* meningitis.

Other *Haemophilus* Species

Haemophilus parainfluenzae, *Haemophilus aphrophilus*, and *Haemophilus paraphrophilus* are normal oral flora that can cause endocarditis. They are part of the HACEK group of organisms. Large valvular vegetations with systemic emboli are common with HACEK endocarditis. Treatment is with ampicillin (if the organism is susceptible) or a third-generation cephalosporin for 3 weeks.

Most cases of pneumonia and tracheobronchitis are caused by nontypable β-lactamase-negative strains of *Haemophilus*. Most are susceptible to amoxicillin.

Bordetella pertussis

The number of reported cases of whooping cough is increasing as immunization is neglected. Twelve percent of cases occur in patients older than 15 years. *B. pertussis* can cause prolonged bronchitis in older children and adults. As many as 50 million adults are now susceptible to infection as a result of waning immunity. Whooping cough may cause severe lymphocytosis (>100,000 lymphocytes/mm^3). Diagnosis of *B. pertussis* infection depends on nasopharyngeal culture. Direct fluorescence antibody testing is relatively insensitive. Treatment is with erythromycin and supportive care. Isolates resistant to erythromycin are becoming increasingly common.

- *B. pertussis* may cause severe lymphocytosis (>100,000 lymphocytes/mm^3).
- *B. pertussis* can cause prolonged bronchitis in older children and adults.

Brucella

Although rare in the United States, brucellosis may occur in meat-handlers, persons exposed to livestock, or persons who drink unpasteurized milk. Most cases occur in four states (Texas, California, Virginia, and Florida). It may cause a chronic granulomatous disease with caseating granulomas. Brucellosis (along with tuberculosis) is a cause of "sterile" pyuria. Chronic brucellosis is one of the infectious causes of fever of undetermined origin. Calcifications in the spleen may be an indication of the presence of infection (although histoplasmosis also causes splenic calcifications). Serologic testing, blood cultures, and bone marrow cultures are helpful in making the diagnosis. Treatment is with doxycycline and streptomycin or rifampin. Cotrimoxazole is sometimes also useful.

- Brucellosis is a chronic granulomatous disease and may cause fever of unknown origin.

Legionella

Legionellae are fastidious gram-negative bacilli. *Legionella pneumophila* is a cause of both community-acquired and nosocomial pneumonia, typically occurring in the summer months. Nosocomial legionellosis may be due to contaminated water supplies. Immunocompromised patients, especially those receiving chronic steroid therapy, are especially susceptible to *Legionella* infections. Typical clinical features of legionellosis include weakness, malaise, fever, dry cough, diarrhea, pleuritic chest pain, relative bradycardia, diffuse rales bilaterally, and patchy bilateral pulmonary infiltrates.

Characteristic laboratory features include decreased sodium and phosphorus values, increased leukocyte level, and increased liver enzyme values. Legionellae cannot be cultured on standard media. Diagnosis depends on results of special culture, demonstrating organisms by direct fluorescent antibody staining, or detecting an increase in anti-*Legionella* antibody titers. Urine antigen detection promises a more sensitive (80%) and simple diagnostic test for *L. pneumophila*.

Legionellae are intracellular parasites. As such, they are resistant to all β-lactam drugs and aminoglycosides in vivo. Effective agents for treating *Legionella* include macrolides, fluoroquinolones, and, to a lesser extent, doxycycline. Some authorities recommend adding rifampin for severe infection.

- Immunocompromised patients, especially those receiving chronic steroid therapy, are especially susceptible to *Legionella* infections.
- Laboratory features of legionellosis include decreased serum sodium and phosphorus values, increased leukocyte level, and increased liver enzyme values.

Tularemia

Francisella tularensis is spread by the bite of a tick or deer fly, by aerosol droplet, or by direct contact with tissues of infected animals (rabbits, muskrat, squirrels, beaver). Typically, infection causes an eschar at the site of inoculation, regional lymphadenopathy, and high fevers. Pneumonia also can occur. Streptomycin and gentamicin are the most effective therapies. Tetracycline is active but is associated with a 10% relapse rate.

- *F. tularensis* is spread by arthropod bite, aerosol droplets, or direct contact with tissues of infected animals.

Plague: *Yersinia pestis*

From 1950 to 1991, there were 336 cases in the United States, and more than 50% of these occurred after 1980. It is enzootic in the southwestern United States. New Mexico had 56% of cases, and 29% of cases are among American Indians. Rats and fleas are the vectors. Clinical presentations include 1) lymphadenopathy with septicemia—the most common form and 2) the pneumonic form (high case-fatality rate). Treatment is with streptomycin or tetracycline.

Pasteurella multocida

A cat bite is the most common mode of acquisition. It causes rapidly progressing cellulitis, bacteremia, and, rarely, infective endocarditis. It is sensitive to penicillins and cephalosporins.

Capnocytophaga (Formerly DF-2)

These gram-negative bacilli have difficulty growing in routine media. They are normal oral flora of domestic animals (especially dogs) and humans. *Capnocytophaga* causes bacteremia and fulminant sepsis, primarily in splenectomized persons. Dog and cat bites are associated with 50% of cases. Occasionally, bacteremia with human oral *Capnocytophaga* species occurs in neutropenic patients with mucositis. Treatment with a penicillin or a cephalosporin is most effective.

- *Capnocytophaga* causes bacteremia and fulminant sepsis, primarily in splenectomized persons.
- Dog and cat bites are associated with 50% of cases.

Cat-Scratch Disease

Bartonella henselae (formerly *Rochalimaea henselae*) has been identified as the primary causative agent of cat-scratch disease. The disease is characterized by a papule or pustule at the site of inoculation, followed by tender enlargement of the regional lymph nodes draining an extremity. Low-grade fever and malaise also may be present. Exposure to domestic cats (especially kittens) is the main risk factor. About 10% of patients may have extranodal manifestations. Disseminated infection has been described in patients with acquired immunodeficiency syndrome (AIDS).

Diagnosis is based on the clinical picture and serologic evidence of antibodies to *B. henselae*. A biopsy finding of organisms positive for Warthin-Starry stain or culture also can be helpful. Treatment is indicated in patients with symptoms and bothersome adenopathy. The antibiotic of choice is ciprofloxacin, 500 mg twice daily for 10 to 14 days. Trimethoprim-sulfamethoxazole, rifampin, and gentamicin are alternative agents.

Helicobacter pylori

H. pylori infects the mucous layer of the stomach in almost all persons with duodenal ulcers or gastritis. Chronic infection increases the risk for gastric adenocarcinoma. Several methods exist for detecting this organism: culture, polymerase chain reaction assay, or histologic study of a gastric biopsy specimen, labeled urea breath test, and serologic testing. Remember that this organism produces large amounts of urease. Eradicating *H. pylori* allows healing of the associated gastritis. Effective therapeutic regimens include omeprazole with clarithromycin, and bismuth subsalicylate plus metronidazole plus tetracycline or amoxicillin.

GRAM-POSITIVE BACILLI

Listeria

Listeria monocytogenes is a small, gram-positive, motile rod. Meningitis and bacteremia are common clinical manifestations. *Listeria* may be difficult to visualize on Gram stain of spinal fluid. The elderly, neonates, pregnant women, and persons taking steroids are at highest risk for disease due to *Listeria*. Epidemics have been associated with consumption of contaminated dairy products. Diarrhea may be a feature of epidemic listeriosis.

Penicillin and ampicillin are the most effective agents against *Listeria*. Combination with an aminoglycoside is often recommended. Note that *Listeria* is always resistant to cephalosporins. Cotrimoxazole is an effective alternative for the penicillin-allergic patient. Treatment should be continued for 2 to 4 weeks.

- The elderly, neonates, pregnant women, and those taking steroids are at highest risk for disease due to *Listeria*.
- Epidemics mainly are associated with consumption of contaminated dairy products.
- Diarrhea may be a feature of epidemic listeriosis.

Corynebacterium diphtheriae

Diphtheria is a classic infectious disease that is easily prevented with vaccination. Epidemics of diphtheria are now reported from several areas of the world, particularly states of the former Soviet Union. Diphtheria causes a focal infection of the respiratory tract (pharynx in 60% to 70% of cases, larynx, nasal passages, or tracheobronchial tree). A tightly adherent, gray pseudomembrane is the hallmark of the disease, but disease can occur without pseudomembrane formation. Manifestations depend on the extent of involvement of the upper airway and the presence or absence of systemic complications due to toxin. Toxin-mediated complications include myocarditis (10%-25%), which causes congestive heart failure and dysrhythmias, and polyneuritis (bulbar dysfunction followed by peripheral neuropathy). Respiratory muscles may be paralyzed.

- In diphtheria, toxin-mediated complications include myocarditis (10%-25%), which causes congestive heart failure and dysrhythmias, and polyneuritis.
- Respiratory muscles may be paralyzed.

Diagnosis is definitively established by culture with Löffler's medium. Rapid diagnosis sometimes can be made with methylene blue stain or fluorescent antibody staining of pharyngeal swab specimens. Diphtheria is highly contagious. Equine antiserum is still the main therapy. Although there is no evidence that antimicrobial agents alter the course of disease, they may prevent transmission to susceptible hosts. Erythromycin and penicillin G are active against *Corynebacterium diphtheriae*. Non-immune persons exposed to diphtheria should be evaluated and treated with erythromycin or penicillin G if culture results are positive. The diphtheria-tetanus toxoid should be given.

● Non-immune persons exposed to diphtheria should be evaluated and treated with erythromycin or penicillin G if culture results are positive.

Cutaneous infection with *C. diphtheriae* can occur in indigent patients and alcoholics. Preexisting dermatologic disease (most often in the lower extremities) is a risk factor. Lesions may appear "punched-out" and with membrane, but they may be indistinguishable from other infected ulcers. Toxin-mediated complications (such as myocarditis and neuropathy) are uncommon. Diagnosis is established with methylene blue staining and culture in Löffler's medium.

Erythromycin or penicillin is used for therapy. Antitoxin also should be administered, and an immunization series with diphtheria-tetanus toxoid should be given.

● Cutaneous diphtheria is reported in indigent patients and alcoholics.

Erysipelothrix rhusiopathiae

This nonmotile, gram-positive rod is a saprophyte that causes the infection known as "erysipeloid of Rosenbach." Infection usually occurs by traumatic inoculation of the skin. Most human cases are related to occupational exposure (fish handlers, veterinarians, slaughterhouse workers, and butchers). Localized cellulitis around a purple-red papule occurs at the site of inoculation, often a finger or upper extremity (erysipeloid). If untreated, dissemination with subsequent bacteremia, endocarditis, and septic arthritis can occur. Most strains of the organism are susceptible to penicillins, cephalosporins, clindamycin, and ciprofloxacin. *Erysipelothrix rhusiopathiae* is resistant to vancomycin.

● *E. rhusiopathiae* infection occurs with traumatic inoculation of organism after a person comes in contact with dead animals and fish.

Bacillus Species

These are increasingly recognized as a cause of bacteremia in patients with indwelling catheters or prosthetic devices and in injection drug users. Other syndromes include ocular infections (posttraumatic endophthalmitis) and gastroenteritis. Anthrax (*Bacillus anthracis*) causes cutaneous disease in handlers of animal skins (also "woolsorters' disease"). It also

may be used as a biological warfare agent.

Although many strains of *Bacillus* are susceptible to penicillins and cephalosporins, infection should be treated with vancomycin or clindamycin while awaiting the results of susceptibility tests.

Rhodococcus equi (Corynebacterium equi)

This organism causes necrotizing pneumonia in immunocompromised hosts, such as those with acquired immunodeficiency syndrome (AIDS) or those taking corticosteroids. The associated mortality rate is 30%. Clinical features include fever, nonproductive cough, and cavity or nodular infiltrates on chest radiography (concomitant brain abscesses have been reported). Bronchoscopy or open lung biopsy usually is required for diagnosis. Optimal therapy is unknown, but in vitro data suggest that the combination of erythromycin and rifampin is the most active. Vancomycin, aminoglycosides, and chloramphenicol also may be effective.

GRAM-NEGATIVE COCCI

Moraxella

Moraxella catarrhalis (*Branhamella catarrhalis*) is a respiratory tract pathogen primarily causing bronchitis and pneumonia in persons with chronic obstructive pulmonary disease. It also may cause otitis media, sinusitis, meningitis, bacteremia, and endocarditis in immunosuppressed patients. β-Lactamase production is prevalent. Trimethoprim-sulfamethoxazole, ciprofloxacin, and ampicillin-clavulanate are useful for therapy.

Neisseria

Neisseria meningitidis and *N. gonorrheae* are discussed in the section on Clinical Syndromes, page 548.

ANAEROBIC BACTERIA

Bacteroides and *Provotella*

Bacteroides species are anaerobic gram-negative rods that are normal colonic flora (*Bacteroides fragilis* group). Related organisms also reside in the mouth (such as *Provotella melaninogenica*). Infections caused by these organisms are often polymicrobial and result from disruption or perforation of mucosal surfaces. These anaerobes often produce abscesses containing foul-smelling pus. *Bacteroides* species also are associated with pelvic infections, particularly in females (such as septic abortion, tubo-ovarian abscess, or endometritis). Bacteremia usually is associated with focal infection elsewhere (such as intra-abdominal abscess) or with gastrointestinal operation. Osteomyelitis due to *Bacteroides* usually results from a contiguous source and is often polymicrobial (such as diabetic foot ulcer or osteomyelitis of the maxilla or mandible after dental infection). Pleuropulmonary infections include aspiration pneumonia and lung abscess, most commonly with *P. melaninogenica* and other oral anaerobes.

- *Bacteroides* species are associated with intra-abdominal and pelvic abscesses.
- Bacteremia usually is associated with focal infection elsewhere (such as intra-abdominal abscess) or with gastrointestinal operation.
- Pleuropulmonary infections with *Bacteroides* species include aspiration pneumonia and lung abscess.

Many strains of *Bacteroides* and *Provotella* produce penicillinase, making them resistant to penicillin. Therefore, penicillin is no longer the drug of choice for the treatment of putrid lung abscess. In one study, clindamycin was more effective than penicillin or metronidazole for curing lung abscess.

Metronidazole, clindamycin (increasing resistance), ampicillin-sulbactam, chloramphenicol, and imipenem are active against most anaerobic gram-negative rods. Some cephalosporins (cefoxitin, cefotetan) are active in vitro against *B. fragilis*. Third-generation cephalosporins have little activity against *B. fragilis*. The new fluoroquinolone, trovafloxacin, has activity against these anaerobic bacteria.

Peptococcus

These anaerobic streptococci often are involved in polymicrobial infection. Like *Bacteroides*, they are part of the normal flora of the mouth and colon and are associated with anaerobic pleuropulmonary infection and intra-abdominal abscess. *Peptostreptococcus* can be a part of the polymicrobial flora of anaerobic cellulitis.

Peptococcus is exquisitely sensitive to penicillin G. In patients allergic to penicillin, the alternatives are clindamycin, chloramphenicol, vancomycin, and cephalosporins. The organism is often resistant to metronidazole.

- *Peptococcus* and other anaerobic gram-positive cocci are often resistant to metronidazole.

Clostridia

Clostridium tetani and Tetanus

This is a strictly anaerobic gram-positive rod that produces neurotoxin (tetanospasmin). The neurotoxin produced by organisms in infected wounds is responsible for the clinical manifestations of disease. Although rare in the United States, tetanus still occurs among the elderly who have never been immunized.

In generalized tetanus, the first muscles involved are controlled by cranial nerves (trismus, lockjaw, risus sardonicus). Eye muscles (cranial nerves III, IV) rarely are involved. Other muscles soon are involved (generalized rigidity, spasms, opisthotonos). Sympathetic overactivity is common (labile hypertension, hyperpyrexia, arrhythmias). In wound tetanus, manifestations are restricted to muscles near the wound. Diagnosis is based on clinical findings, although a characteristic electromyogram is suggestive.

- Diagnosis of tetanus is based on clinical findings.

Treatment of tetanus includes supportive care, proper wound management, and administration of antiserum (human tetanus immune globulin). Hypersensitivity reactions to tetanus immune globulin are very rare. Penicillin G should be administered to eradicate vegetative organisms in the wound. Metronidazole is an alternative agent. Active tetanus does not induce protective immunity to subsequent episodes. Therefore, a primary immunization series should be given after an episode of tetanus.

- Active tetanus does not induce protective immunity to subsequent episodes of tetanus.

Botulism

Clostridium botulinum produces a heat-labile neurotoxin that inhibits acetylcholine release from cholinergic terminals at the motor end plate. Major modes of acquisition in adults include ingestion of contaminated food (home-canned products and improperly prepared or handled commercial foods) and wound botulism (contaminated traumatic wounds, injection drug users). Neonatal botulism can result from consumption of contaminated honey.

- Neurotoxin of *C. botulinum* inhibits acetylcholine release from cholinergic terminals at the motor end plate.

Clinical manifestations can be mild or severe. The diagnosis is considered in patients with unexplained diplopia; fixed, dilated pupils; dry mouth; and descending flaccid paralysis with normal sensation. Patients are usually alert and oriented and have intact deep tendon reflexes. Fever is rare.

- Diagnosis of *C. botulinum* infection is considered in patients with unexplained diplopia; fixed, dilated pupils; dry mouth; and descending flaccid paralysis with normal sensation.

Treatment is primarily supportive. An equine antitoxin is available. In food-borne cases, purging the gut with cathartics, enemas, and emetics to remove unabsorbed toxin also may be of value. Antibiotic therapy is not effective.

Other Clostridial Infections

Clostridium perfringens may cause a food-associated illness. *Clostridium difficile* causes antibiotic-associated diarrhea. Bacteremia with *Clostridium septicum* is associated with colonic malignancies. Clostridial bacteremia may be transient and clinically not significant.

- *C. perfringens* may cause a food-associated illness.
- *C. difficile* causes antibiotic-associated diarrhea.
- In patients with *C. septicum* bacteremia, occult bowel carcinoma should be suspected.

ACTINOMYCOSIS

Actinomyces israelii, an anaerobic, gram-positive, branching, filamentous organism, is the most common cause of human actinomycosis. *A. israelii* is part of the normal flora of the mouth. Infections are associated with any condition that creates an anaerobic environment (such as trauma with tissue necrosis, pus). The pathologic characteristic is formation of "sulfur granules," which are clumps of filaments. Infection is not characterized by granuloma formation.

- Pathologic characteristic of actinomycosis is "sulfur granules" (clumps of filaments).

"Lumpy jaw" is caused by a paramandibular infection with *A. israelii*. It is characterized by a chronic draining sinus and may follow a dental extraction. Pulmonary actinomycosis develops when aspirated material reaches an area of lung with decreased oxygenation (such as in atelectasis, infection). Chronic suppurative pneumonitis may develop with cavitation, empyema, and, finally, a draining sinus through the chest wall. There may be subsequent perforation into the esophagus, pericardium, ribs, and vertebrae. Hematogenous spread to the brain is a rare but often lethal complication. Ileocecal perforation from focal actinomycosis has been reported. Appendicitis may be a predisposing factor.

- "Lumpy jaw" is caused by a paramandibular infection with *A. israelii*. It is characterized by a chronic draining sinus and may follow a dental extraction.

Vertebral actinomycosis has a characteristic sieve-like appearance on radiographs because it attacks bodies of vertebrae and not intervertebral spaces. The infection progresses slowly, allowing new bone to be formed as fast as it is destroyed. Vertebral collapse is rare. These findings help differentiate vertebral actinomycosis from spinal disease due to malignancy, tuberculosis, or other infections.

A. israelii also may be found in culture of tubo-ovarian abscesses and other pelvic infections. It is especially associated with pelvic inflammatory disease developing in a woman with an intrauterine device.

Actinomyces organisms have special growth requirements. Therefore, *Actinomyces* culture must be specifically requested because the organism may not grow on routine anaerobic cultures. Although morphologically similar to *Nocardia*, it has several distinguishing characteristics (*Nocardia* is a gram-positive, filamentous, branching organism that is *aerobic* and partially acid-fast).

Penicillin is the preferred agent for treating actinomycosis. Alternatives include tetracyclines, macrolides, and cephalosporins. Therapy is prolonged, often for a year or more.

MYCOBACTERIAL DISEASES

Mycobacterium tuberculosis

Epidemiology

There was a 13% increase in tuberculosis cases in the United States from 1985 through 1992. Increased numbers of persons infected with human immunodeficiency virus (HIV) were responsible for most of this increase. At the same time, drug resistance in *M. tuberculosis* is increasingly common. Nosocomial outbreaks of multiple drug-resistant tuberculosis (MDR-TB) occurred in several cities. In a recent national survey, 14.4% of tuberculosis isolates were resistant to one drug and 3.3% were resistant to both isoniazid and rifampin.

- In cases of *M. tuberculosis* in the United States, approximately 14.4% of strains are resistant to one drug and 3.3% are resistant to both isoniazid and rifampin.

Because of the highly infectious nature of pulmonary tuberculosis, all patients suspected of having it should be placed in respiratory isolation while hospitalized. Cutaneous tuberculosis, although rare, also may result in nosocomial transmission of disease. Transmission is by droplet inhalation. Infectious droplets are 1 to 5 μm in diameter. Droplets remain suspended in room atmosphere for 30 minutes to 2 hours.

- Tuberculosis is transmitted by droplet inhalation.

Clinical Disease

M. tuberculosis infections in adults may be due to new infection, reactivation of previously latent infection, or reinfection. Common sites of reactivation are the apices of the lungs, the vertebrae, and the kidneys. Tuberculosis should be suspected as a cause of unexplained pleural effusions. Diagnosis is made by thoracentesis with culture of pleural fluid and pleural biopsy with special stains and culture. Extrapulmonary manifestations are protean. Common sites include the spine, kidneys, large joints, meninges, and peritoneum.

The caseating (necrotizing) granuloma is the main histologic characteristic in tissues infected with *M. tuberculosis*.

- Tuberculosis should be suspected as a cause of unexplained pleural effusion.

Screening

An intermediate-strength purified protein derivative (PPD) test is a helpful adjunct for diagnosing exposure to or infection with *M. tuberculosis*. Persons at highest risk include those infected with HIV, the foreign-born, close contacts (household) of persons known to have tuberculosis, low-income populations (including high-risk minority populations, especially Native Americans), the homeless, alcoholics, injection drug users, residents of institutions (such as nursing homes, prisons), and persons with medical conditions that predispose to infection with tuberculosis (Table 14-3).

Prevention

Isoniazid prophylaxis significantly reduces the incidence of subsequent tuberculosis. Lack of compliance is the major source of failure. The treatment dosage is 300 mg/day (or 15 mg/kg twice a week under direct supervision) for 6 months to 1 year. Optimal prophylaxis for exposure to isoniazid-resistant strains or exposure to MDR-TB is unknown. An outline for preventive therapy with positive results of PPD testing is given in Table 14-4.

- Isoniazid prophylaxis significantly reduces the incidence of subsequent tuberculosis.

Treatment (Table 14-5)

General principles:

- Isoniazid and rifampin should be a part of all regimens, unless there are contraindications or the organism is resistant.
- Consider directly observed therapy in all patients.
- For extrapulmonary tuberculosis and tuberculosis in HIV-infected patients, use the same regimens as for pulmonary disease.
- Manage children similar to adults, with appropriate adjustment of drug doses.
- For compliant patients with susceptible organisms, a 6-month regimen consisting of isoniazid, rifampin, and pyrazinamide given for 2 months followed by isoniazid and rifampin for an additional 4 months is recommended. For alternative regimens, see Table 14-5.

Table 14-3.—Medical Conditions That Predispose Patients to *Mycobacterium tuberculosis* Infection

Silicosis	Immunosuppression (T-cell)
Gastrectomy	Hematologic malignancy
Jejunoileal bypass	Other malignancies
Weight 10% or more below ideal body weight	Person with chest radiograph compatible with old tuberculosis
Chronic renal failure	
Diabetes mellitus	

- Start treatment with at least three drugs until drug susceptibility results are known, and include either ethambutol or streptomycin as the fourth drug if isoniazid resistance is suspected or the prevalence of isoniazid resistance in the area is more than 4%.
- Treatment of MDR-TB should be individualized based on in vitro susceptibility testing. Therapy must be extended to 18 to 24 months or longer.

The initial cure rate in a recent study of MDR-TB in persons without acquired immunodeficiency syndrome (AIDS) was 65%. Among these initial responders, 14% later had relapse, most within 2 years. Relapse and treatment failure were associated with a 46% mortality rate. In many of the MDR-TB outbreaks (70%-80% of HIV-infected persons), the mortality rate has been 70% to 80%. Patients in whom treatment is unsuccessful but who survive pose a major public health problem and must be isolated. Earlier surgical options may need to be considered.

Mycobacterial Diseases Other Than Tuberculosis (Atypical *Mycobacteria*)

Mycobacterium marinum causes swimming pool granuloma and may occur after cleaning an aquarium. It presents with a chronic indurated nodule on the finger or hand. Treatment is excision of the nodule. Rifampin plus ethambutol, doxycycline, or trimethoprim-sulfamethoxazole may be effective.

- *M. marinum* causes swimming pool granuloma.

Mycobacterium kansasii produces pulmonary disease resembling that caused by *M. tuberculosis*. *M. kansasii* is more resistant to isoniazid than is *M. tuberculosis*. Standard treatment regimens include isoniazid, rifampin, and ethambutol and continue for 12 to 24 months.

- *M. kansasii* pulmonary disease resembles *M. tuberculosis* clinically.

Table 14-4.—Criteria for Determining Need for Preventive Therapy for Persons With Positive Tuberculin Reactions, by Category and Age Group

Category	Age	
	<35 yr	≥35 yr
With risk factor[*]	Treat at all ages if PPD ≥10 mm (if PPD >5 mm in HIV positive, recent contact, chest radiographic evidence of old not active TB)	Treat at all ages if PPD ≥10 mm (if PPD >5 mm in HIV positive, recent contact, chest radiographic evidence of old not active TB)
No risk factor (high incidence group)[†]	Treat if PPD ≥10 mm	No treatment
No risk factor (low incidence group)	Treat if PPD ≥15 mm[‡]	No treatment

[*] 1) Persons with HIV infection or with multiple HIV risk factors, 2) intravenous drug users, 3) recent contact with infected person, 4) recent PPD converters, 5) persons with abnormal chest radiographic finding likely to represent old tuberculosis, 6) persons with certain medical conditions (see Table 14-3).
[†] 1) Foreign-born persons, 2) medically underserved, low-income populations, 3) residents of long-term-care facilities.
[‡] Controversial; some investigators use cutoff of 10 mm. Depends on relative prevalence of cross-reactivity with other mycobacterial organisms in the population.
HIV, human immunodeficiency virus; PPD, purified protein derivative; TB, tuberculosis.
From Centers for Disease Control: Screening for tuberculosis and tuberculous infection in high-risk populations, and the use of preventive therapy for tuberculous infection in the United States. MMWR 39 (no. RR-8):1-12, 1990.

Table 14-5.—Treatment Options for Tuberculosis Infections*

Option 1	Option 2	Option 3
INH, RIF, and PZA daily for 8 weeks, followed by INH + RIF daily or 2-3 times/week for 16 weeks[†]	INH, RIF, PZA, and STM or EMB daily for 2 weeks, followed by twice weekly administration of same drugs for 6 weeks, then followed by twice weekly administration of INH and RIF for 16 weeks	INH, RIF, PZA, and EMB or STM three times weekly for 6 months

[*] Based on the joint statement of the American Thoracic Society and the Centers for Disease Control and Prevention (MMWR 42 [no. RR-7]:1-8, 1993).
[†] All twice and thrice weekly regimens should be monitored by directly observed therapy for the duration of treatment.
INH, isoniazid; RIF, rifampin; PZA, pyrazinamide; STM, streptomycin; EMB, ethambutol.

Mycobacterium avium-intracellulare (MAI or MAC) is an important cause of infection in patients with advanced AIDS. MAC also can cause pulmonary infections in patients with underlying lung diseases. There are four characteristic chest radiographic appearances: multiple discrete nodules (71% of patients), bronchiectasis, upper lobe infiltrates, and diffuse infiltrates. When MAC is recovered from respiratory specimens, it often merely represents colonization of the respiratory tract. Defining true infection may be difficult. Treatment of MAC is often problematic because the organism is resistant to many agents. The newer macrolides (clarithromycin and azithromycin) are the most active drugs against MAC.

- When MAC is recovered from respiratory specimens, it often merely represents colonization of the respiratory tract.

Rapid-growing mycobacteria include *Mycobacterium fortuitum* and *Mycobacterium chelonei*. Typically they cause indolent subcutaneous infections of an extremity. They also are associated with osteomyelitis and nosocomial infection (sternal osteomyelitis after cardiac operation, intramuscular injection). Treatment often requires incision and drainage. They are resistant to antituberculosis drugs. Clarithromycin, with or without other agents, is the most effective treatment.

SPIROCHETES

Leptospirosis

Leptospira interrogans infection is acquired by contact with urine from infected animals (rats, dogs), and it causes a biphasic disease. The *leptospiremic phase* is characterized by abrupt-onset headache (98%), fever, chills, conjunctivitis, severe muscle aching, gastrointestinal symptoms (50%), changes in sensorium (25%), rash (7%), and hypotension. This phase lasts 3 to 7 days. Improvement in symptoms coincides with disappearance of *Leptospira* organisms from blood and cerebrospinal fluid. The *second phase* (immune stage) occurs after a relatively asymptomatic period of 1 to 3 days, when fever and generalized symptoms recur. Meningeal symptoms often develop during this period. The second phase is characterized by the appearance of IgM antibodies. Most patients recover after 1 to 3 days. However, in serious cases, hepatic dysfunction and renal failure may develop. Death in patients with leptospirosis usually occurs in the second phase as a result of hepatic and renal failure.

- *L. interrogans* infection is acquired by contact with urine from infected animals (rats, dogs).
- Leptospirosis is a biphasic disease.

Diagnosis of leptospirosis is made with cultures of blood and, rarely, cerebrospinal fluid in the first 7 to 10 days of infection. Urine cultures become positive after the second week of illness. Serologic testing is not helpful until the second phase of disease. Treatment with penicillin G is effective *only* if given within the first 1 to 5 days from onset of symptoms.

- Treatment of leptospirosis with penicillin G is effective *only* if given within the first 1- 5 days from onset of symptoms.

Lyme Disease

Epidemiology

Lyme disease is the most common vector-borne (*Ixodes* ticks) disease reported in the United States. The incidence of disease is highest in the spring and summer, when exposure to the tick vector is most common. Experimental evidence suggests ticks must be attached for more than 24 hours to transmit infection. Although Lyme disease has been reported from most states, it is most common in coastal New England and New York, the mid-Atlantic states, Oregon, Northern California, and the Upper Midwest. The white-footed mouse and the white-tailed deer serve as zoonotic reservoirs for the etiologic agent, *Borrelia burgdorferi*.

- *B. burgdorferi* is the etiologic agent of Lyme disease.

Clinical Syndromes

Stage 1 (*early*) occurs from 3 to 32 days after the tick bite. Erythema migrans (solitary or multiple lesions) is the hallmark of Lyme disease and occurs in 80% or more of infected persons. It can be associated with fever, lymphadenopathy, and meningismus. The rash of erythema migrans usually enlarges and resolves over 3 to 4 weeks. *B. burgdorferi* disseminates hematogenously early in the course of the illness.

- Erythema migrans develops in 80% of patients with Lyme disease.

Stage 2 occurs weeks to months after stage 1. In 10% to 15% of cases, neurologic abnormalities develop (facial nerve palsy, lymphocytic meningitis, encephalitis, chorea, myelitis, radiculitis, peripheral neuropathy). Carditis (reversible atrioventricular block) occurs in 10% of patients. Dilated cardiomyopathy has been reported, and conjunctivitis and iritis also occur.

- During stage 2, 10%-15% of cases have neurologic abnormalities.
- Carditis occurs in 10% of patients.

Stage 3, although uncommon, can develop months to years after initial infection. Monarticular or oligoarticular arthritis occurs in 50% of patients who do not receive effective therapy. It becomes chronic in 10% to 20%. Chronic arthritis is more common in those with HLA-DR2 and HLA-DR4. Other manifestations are acrodermatitis chronica atrophicans (primarily with European strains), progressive, chronic encephalitis, and dementia (rare). Most patients will have detectable serum antibodies against *B. burgdorferi*. Magnetic resonance imaging may show demyelination.

Diagnosis

Anti-*B. burgdorferi* antibodies can be detected by enzyme-linked immunosorbent assay after the first 2 to 6 weeks of illness. Response may be diminished by antimicrobial therapy early in the course. Antibody testing is not standardized. False-positive results occur with infectious mononucleosis, rheumatoid arthritis, systemic lupus erythematosus, echovirus infection, and other spirochetal disease. The Western blot test is an adjunct in diagnosis when antibody response is equivocal or when a false-positive result is suspected. It is particularly useful in the first few months of illness.

Treatment

For stage 1 (early) Lyme disease, doxycycline (100 mg twice a day for 10-21 days), amoxicillin (500 mg three times a day for 10-21 days), and cefuroxime axetil (500 mg twice a day for 10-21 days) are effective therapeutic agents. Erythromycin is less effective than doxycycline or amoxicillin. Because of the risk of vertical transmission, all pregnant women with active Lyme disease should be treated.

In Lyme carditis, the outcome is usually favorable. If first-degree atrioventricular block is present or the PR interval is more than 0.30 second, ceftriaxone, 2 g a day for 14 to 21 days, or penicillin G, 20 million units a day for 14 to 21 days, is recommended.

● In Lyme carditis, the outcome is usually favorable.

The outcome in patients with facial palsy is also usually favorable. In one series, 105 of 122 affected patients completely recovered. Corticosteroids have no role. If only facial nerve palsy is present (no symptoms of meningitis, radiculoneuritis), use oral therapy with doxycycline or amoxicillin. The treatment applied if other neurologic manifestations are present is described below.

● The outcome in patients with facial palsy due to Lyme disease is usually favorable.

If Lyme meningitis is present, ceftriaxone, 2 g a day for 14 to 21 days, or penicillin G, 20 million units a day for 14 to 21 days, should be given. Radiculoneuritis and peripheral neuropathy may have a greater tendency for chronicity and often occur with meningitis. Treatment is the same as that for Lyme-associated meningitis. The regimens for encephalopathy and encephalomyelitis are identical to those for meningitis.

● Radiculoneuritis and peripheral neuropathy may have a greater tendency for chronicity and often occur with meningitis.

Optimal regimens for Lyme arthritis (oral vs. intravenous) are not established. Intra-articular corticosteroids may cause treatment failures. Joint rest and aspiration of reaccumulated joint fluid are often needed. Response to antibiotics may be delayed. If no neurologic disease is present, doxycycline is given (100 mg orally twice a day for 30 days). An alternative regimen is amoxicillin and probenecid (500 mg each, four times a day for 30 days) or ceftriaxone (2 g per day intravenously for 14-21 days).

Prevention

Prophylactic antibiotic therapy after a tick bite is not recommended. The vast majority of tick bites do not transmit disease. Appropriate use of repellents and protective clothing are recommended.

● Prophylactic antibiotic therapy after a tick bite is not recommended.

NOCARDIOSIS

Nocardia are aerobic, gram-positive, filamentous, branching organisms that are visualized with a modified acid-fast stain. *Nocardia asteroides* is the cause of most human infections in the United States (plate 14-3). *Nocardia brasiliensis* and *Nocardia madurae* cause mycetomas. Infections are most often opportunistic, occurring in immunosuppressed patients, but they can occur in normal hosts also.

● *Nocardia* infections are most often opportunistic, occurring in immunosuppressed patients.

The respiratory tract is the usual portal of entry for *Nocardia* infection. Chronic pneumonitis and lung abscess are the most common findings. Hematogenous spread to the brain is relatively common. In patients with chronic pneumonia who have neurologic symptoms or signs, *Nocardia* brain abscess should be considered.

● In patients with chronic pneumonia who have neurologic symptoms, *Nocardia* brain abscess should be considered.

Nocardiosis is not diagnosed until autopsy in up to 40% of cases. Antemortem diagnosis depends on obtaining appropriate stains and cultures (the organism will grow on fungal media). Because sputum culture is relatively insensitive, bronchoscopically obtained specimens or open lung biopsy may be needed to confirm the diagnosis. The disease must be differentiated from other causes of chronic pneumonia (such as bacterial, actinomycotic, tuberculosis, fungal infections). Therapy involves drainage of abscesses and high doses of sulfa drugs (trimethoprim-sulfamethoxazole is the current drug of choice). Some species of *Nocardia* show evidence of sulfa resistance.

● Nocardiosis is diagnosed at autopsy in up to 40% of cases.

RICKETTSIAL INFECTIONS

All rickettsial infections are transmitted by an insect vector except Q fever (respiratory spread). All are associated with a rash except Q fever and ehrlichiosis. The rash of Rocky Mountain spotted fever (RMSF) may be indistinguishable from that of meningococcemia. RMSF rash begins on the extremities and moves centrally. The rash of typhus (both murine and endemic typhus) begins centrally and moves toward the extremities. RMSF is most common in the mid-Atlantic states and Oklahoma, not the Rocky Mountain states. The pathophysiology of all rickettsial infections includes vasculitis and disseminated intravascular coagulation. Rickettsial pox is a common, although usually unrecognized, disease in urban areas of the United States. It is the only rickettsial disease characterized by vesicular rash. The mouse mite is the vector for rickettsial pox. A small eschar is present at the site of inoculation in 95% of patients.

- All rickettsial infections have an insect vector except Q fever.
- All are associated with a rash except Q fever and ehrlichiosis.
- RMSF rash begins on the extremities and moves centrally.
- RMSF is most common in the mid-Atlantic states and Oklahoma, not the Rocky Mountain states.

Coxiella burnetii, the cause of Q fever, is acquired by inhalation after exposure to animal products, especially infected placentas. Sheep are common sources, but other animals, including cats, can harbor the disease (for example, a small outbreak occurred in a group of poker players after a cat gave birth beneath their card table). Disease manifests most commonly as pneumonitis, but up to 15% of patients have hepatitis (granulomatous), and 1% have endocarditis. Q fever is one of the causes of culture-negative endocarditis. It usually is diagnosed by serologic testing. Treatment is with tetracycline or chloramphenicol.

- Among persons with Q fever, most have pneumonitis, 15% have hepatitis.
- Q fever is one of the causes of culture-negative endocarditis.

Ehrlichia species are gram-negative intracellular bacteria that resemble rickettsial organisms and preferentially infect lymphocytes, monocytes, and neutrophils. The species that cause human ehrlichiosis are *E. chaffeensis* (which infects monocytes) and *Ehrlichia equi* and *phagocytophila* (which causes human granulocytic ehrlichiosis, or HGE).

The disease is seasonal; the peak incidence is from May through July. The vectors are the common dog tick (*Dermacentor variabilis*), the lone star tick (*Amblyomma americanum*) for *E. chaffeensis*, and *Ixodes* ticks for the agent of HGE. The incubation period is approximately 7 days, followed by fever, chills, malaise, headache, and myalgia. Less than 50% of patients have a rash. Important laboratory features include leukopenia, thrombocytopenia, and increased levels of hepatic transaminases.

The severity of the disease is variable, but severe complications, including death, can occur. Coinfection with HGE and *Borrelia burgdorferi* (Lyme disease) does occur and can

be especially severe. Diagnosis depends on serologic analysis (indirect immunofluorescent assay) or detection by polymerase chain reaction amplification. Treatment is with doxycycline, 100 mg twice a day. Unlike the rickettsial diseases, chloramphenicol is often not effective against *Erhlichia*.

MYCOPLASMA PNEUMONIAE

This is one of the smallest microorganisms capable of extracellular replication. Mycoplasmas lack a cell wall. Therefore, cell-wall-active antibiotics such as penicillin are not effective treatment. *Mycoplasma* infection is spread by droplet inhalation. It primarily infects young, previously healthy persons and presents with rapid onset of headache, dry cough, and fever. Results of physical examination are often unremarkable, with the possible exception of bullous myringitis. Chest radiography usually shows bilateral, patchy pneumonitis. The chest radiographic findings are often out of proportion to the physical findings. Pleural effusion is present in 15% to 20% of cases. Neurologic complications include Guillain-Barré syndrome, cerebellar peripheral neuropathy, aseptic meningitis, and mononeuritis multiplex. Hemolytic anemia may occur late in the illness as a result of circulating cold hemagglutinins.

- *Mycoplasma pneumoniae* infection is spread by droplet inhalation.
- Chest radiography usually shows bilateral, patchy pneumonitis.
- Pleural effusion is present in 15%-20% of cases.
- Neurologic complications include Guillain-Barré syndrome, cerebellar peripheral neuropathy, aseptic meningitis, and mononeuritis multiplex.

The diagnosis is established by specific complement fixation test. Cold agglutinins are nonspecific and unreliable for diagnosing *Mycoplasma* infections. Macrolides and tetracyclines are effective therapies. Because immunity to *Mycoplasma* infection is transient, reinfection may occur. Clinical relapse of pneumonia occurs in up to 10% of cases of *Mycoplasma* pneumonia.

CHLAMYDIA PNEUMONIAE (TWAR AGENT)

This is a new agent, distinct from *Chlamydia trachomatis* and *Chlamydia psittaci*. In young adults, it causes 10% of cases of pneumonia and 5% of cases of bronchitis. It has been a cause of community outbreaks, and nosocomial transmission has occurred. Fifty percent of adults are seropositive for *Chlamydia pneumoniae*. Birds are the source of infection with *C. psittaci* (psittacosis), but there is no reservoir for *C. pneumoniae*. Clinical manifestations of infection are usually mild and may resemble those caused by *M. pneumoniae*. Pharyngitis occurs 1 to 3 weeks before the onset of pulmonary symptoms, and cough may last for weeks. The diagnosis is based on serologic testing. Treatment is with doxycycline or a macrolide.

- In young adults, *C. pneumoniae* causes 10% of cases of pneumonia and 5% of cases of bronchitis.

FUNGAL INFECTIONS

Coccidioidomycosis

Coccidioides immitis is a dimorphic fungus: in tissue it exists as spherule, and in culture at room temperature it is mycelial (filamentous). It forms arthrospores that are highly infectious. *C. immitis* is endemic in the southwestern United States, especially the San Joaquin Valley of California and central Arizona. Disseminated disease is most likely to occur in males (especially Filipino and black), pregnant females, and immunocompromised hosts regardless of sex. Nonpregnant white females seem to be more resistant than white males.

- *C. immitis* is endemic in the southwestern United States.
- Disseminated disease is most likely to occur in males (especially Filipino and black), pregnant females, and immunocompromised hosts regardless of sex.

Primary infection with *C. immitis* causes pneumonitis that is usually self-limited. Common manifestations are dry cough and fever (valley fever) that may resemble influenza. Associated findings include hilar adenopathy, pleural effusion (12%), thin-walled cavities (5%), and solid "coin" lesions. Disseminated infection predominantly affects the central nervous system, skin, bones, and joints.

- Primary infection with *C. immitis* causes pneumonitis that is usually self-limited.

Coccidioidomycosis is one of the causes of erythema nodosum. When present, it usually indicates an active immune response that will control the infection. Erythema nodosum is more common in females and is often associated with arthralgias, especially of the knees and ankles.

- Coccidioidomycosis is one of the causes of erythema nodosum.

The diagnosis of coccidioidomycosis is based on detecting the organism by culture or biopsy with silver stains. A *C. immitis* serologic (complement fixation) titer more than 1:4 is suggestive of infection. Skin testing is of epidemiologic value only. Detection of cerebrospinal fluid anticoccidioidal antibodies is the usual means for diagnosing coccidioidomycosis meningitis.

Fluconazole and amphotericin B are effective for therapy of coccidioidomycosis. The acute pulmonary form is usually self-limited. Therapy may be indicated if a patient is pregnant, has human immunodeficiency virus (HIV) infection, has received an organ transplant, or has worsening infection without therapy. Ketoconazole is effective for non-life-threatening, nonmeningeal disease in a dosage of 400 to 800 mg per day for 6 months. For meningitis, therapy with high-dose fluconazole is beneficial and has largely replaced intrathecal amphotericin B. Because of the high relapse rate of *C. immitis* meningitis, chronic suppressive therapy is necessary, usually with fluconazole. *Coccidioides* meningitis may be complicated by adhesive arachnoiditis.

Histoplasmosis

Histoplasma capsulatum is also a dimorphic fungus that grows as a small (3 mm in diameter) yeast in tissue. Culture at room temperature produces the mycelial form. Although present in many areas of the world, histoplasmosis is especially prevalent in the Ohio and Mississippi River valleys. Outbreaks have been associated with large construction projects and exposure to bird droppings. Histoplasmosis is acquired by inhalation of spores. Although healthy individuals may acquire histoplasmosis, patients with acquired immunodeficiency syndrome (AIDS) are particularly susceptible. *H. capsulatum* infection is one of the causes of caseating granulomata.

- Outbreaks of histoplasmosis have been associated with large construction projects and exposure to bird droppings.
- Although healthy individuals may acquire histoplasmosis, patients with AIDS are particularly susceptible.

Primary (acute) histoplasmosis may be clinically indistinguishable from influenza or other respiratory tract infections. After resolution, multiple small, calcified granulomas may be seen on subsequent chest radiography. The progressive (disseminated) form of histoplasmosis is uncommon but serious. It is most likely to occur in infants, elderly men, and immunosuppressed persons. Manifestations may resemble those of lymphoma, with weight loss, fever, anemia, increased erythrocyte sedimentation rate, and splenomegaly. Mucosal surface lesions, especially in the mouth, are not infrequent. As with tuberculosis, the adrenal glands may be infected, with resulting adrenal insufficiency. Chronic cavitary pulmonary disease due to *Histoplasma* may resemble tuberculosis.

- Primary (acute) histoplasmosis may be indistinguishable from influenza or other upper respiratory tract infections.
- As with tuberculosis, the adrenal glands may be infected by *H. capsulatum,* with resulting adrenal insufficiency.

Serologic testing is of limited sensitivity and specificity and plays little role in the diagnosis of active infection unless increasing or markedly increased titers are detected. Biopsy, silver staining, and cultures of infected tissues are the best means of diagnosis. Bone marrow stains and cultures and fungal blood cultures are frequently helpful. Biopsy specimens of mouth lesions can be diagnostic. Detection of *Histoplasma* antigen in urine or serum is promising as a diagnostic test but is not yet widely available.

The mild, acute forms of histoplasmosis are usually self-limited and do not require therapy. Amphotericin B in a total dose of 35 mg/kg is the drug of choice for all severe, life-threatening cases. Itraconazole is effective for most non-meningeal, non-life-threatening cases and has largely replaced ketoconazole. The dosage is 200 to 400 mg per day for 6 to 12 months. Patients with AIDS require chronic maintenance therapy.

Blastomycosis

Yet another dimorphic fungal pathogen is *Blastomyces dermatitidis*. In tissue the yeast forms are thick-walled and have broad-based buds ($\pm$10 μm in diameter) (plate 14-4). In culture at room temperature, a mycelial form is found. Blastomycosis is endemic in the southeastern and upper midwestern sections of the United States. Primary pulmonary blastomycosis may be asymptomatic and may disseminate hematogenously to bone, skin, or prostate. Granulomas occur, but calcification is less frequent than with histoplasmosis or tuberculosis.

Blastomycosis affects lung, skin, bone (especially the vertebrae), male genitalia (prostate, epididymis, testis), and the central nervous system. The pulmonary form has no characteristic findings: pleural effusion is rare, hilar adenopathy develops occasionally, and cavitation is infrequent. It often mimics carcinoma of the lung. Cutaneous involvement with blastomycosis is common. Lesions, especially on the face, are characteristically painless and nonpruritic and have a sharp, spreading border. Chronic, crusty lesions may occur.

- Blastomycosis affects lungs, skin, bone (especially the vertebrae), and male genitalia (prostate, epididymis, testis).
- The most common clinical forms of blastomycosis are pulmonary and cutaneous.

The diagnosis of blastomycosis is based on the results of biopsy, stains, and cultures. Serologic and skin testing are rarely helpful.

Amphotericin B (total dose is 20-25 mg/kg) and itraconazole (200-400 mg per day for 6 months) are effective as therapy for blastomycosis. Amphotericin B primarily is reserved for life-threatening infections.

Sporotrichosis

A fourth dimorphic fungal pathogen, *Sporothrix schenckii*, in tissue is a round, cigar-shaped yeast. In culture at room temperature it is mycelial. Sporotrichosis is transmitted by cutaneous inoculation ("rose gardener's disease") and, rarely, through inhalation. It manifests as a suppurative and granulomatous reaction.

Cutaneous infection produces characteristic crusty lesions ascending the lymphatics of the extremities from the initial site of infection. Similar lesions may be produced by infection with *Mycobacterium marinum*, *Nocardia*, or cutaneous leishmaniasis. Joint spaces rarely are involved. Sporotrichosis occasionally may cause chronic pneumonitis (with cavitation and empyema) or meningitis.

- Cutaneous sporotrichosis produces characteristic crusty lesions ascending the lymphatics of the extremities from the initial site of infection.
- Sporotrichosis occasionally may cause chronic pneumonitis (with cavitation and empyema) or meningitis.

The diagnosis of sporotrichosis may be difficult and depends on clinical recognition of the cutaneous lesions in most instances. Biopsy, culture, or serologic testing may aid in the diagnosis.

For the cutaneous form, itraconazole or supersaturated solution of potassium iodine is effective. Amphotericin B is recommended for disseminated disease (pulmonary, joint), although it may respond poorly to therapy.

Aspergillosis

Aspergillus is an opportunistic pathogen that causes infection in immunocompromised persons. Although any species of *Aspergillus* can cause disease, *Aspergillus fumigatus* is the most common pathogenic species. The organisms have large, septated hyphae (phycomycetes are nonseptated) branching at 45° angles (plate 14-5). Especially in neutropenic hosts, they may invade blood vessels, producing a striking thrombotic angiitis similar to phycomycosis. Metastatic foci may cause suppurative abscess formation.

- *Aspergillus* organisms may invade blood vessels, producing a striking thrombotic angiitis.

The form of disease produced by aspergillosis primarily is determined by the nature of the immunologic deficit in the infected individual. Neutropenia predisposes to rapidly invasive bronchopulmonary disease with early dissemination to the brain and other tissues. The longer the duration of neutropenia, the higher the risk for invasive aspergillosis. Prompt therapy with high doses of amphotericin B and resolution of the neutropenia are necessary to control the disease. Diagnosis should be suspected when *Aspergillus* is isolated from any source in a susceptible individual.

T-cell deficiencies (primarily from corticosteroids) predispose to somewhat more indolent, although no less dangerous, forms of aspergillosis. Progressive pulmonary infiltrates, necrotic skin lesions, wound infections, and brain abscesses may result. Sinus infections with *Aspergillus* may be localized or invasive in these patients.

Serologic testing is not helpful for diagnosing invasive *Aspergillus* in the compromised host.

- Neutropenia predisposes to rapidly invasive bronchopulmonary disease with early dissemination to the brain and other tissues.

Aspergillus also can cause localized disease in persons with normal immunologic function. Chronic necrotizing pulmonary aspergillosis occurs in patients with pulmonary emphysema. The chronic, progressive infiltrates of this condition often require tissue sampling for diagnosis. Treatment with surgical resection and systemic antifungal therapy is sometimes curative.

Aspergillus may produce a "fungus ball" in preexisting lung bullae (such as from ankylosing spondylitis, previous tuberculosis, or emphysema). Hemoptysis is the main symptom. Surgical excision may be necessary to prevent lethal hemorrhage.

Localized colonization with *Aspergillus* is common and usually does not produce disease. However, otitis externa (swimmer's ear) and allergic bronchopulmonary aspergillosis are exceptions. The symptoms of allergic bronchopulmonary aspergillosis resemble those of asthma. It is characterized by migratory pulmonary infiltrates, thick, brown, tenacious mucous plugs in the sputum, eosinophilia, and high titers of anti-*Aspergillus* antibodies. Endophthalmitis due to *Aspergillus* may develop after ocular operation or trauma.

Aspergillus frequently colonizes the respiratory tract. Isolating the organism from the sputum of a noncompromised host usually does not indicate disease and does not require treatment.

- Chronic necrotizing pulmonary aspergillosis occurs in patients with pulmonary emphysema.
- *Aspergillus* may produce a "fungus ball" in preexisting lung bullae (such as from ankylosing spondylitis, previous tuberculosis, or emphysema).

Aspergillus infections may respond poorly to currently available antifungal medications. Amphotericin B is the most effective, but it must be given in high doses. Itraconazole is promising as the first oral agent with significant activity against *Aspergillus*. Surgical debridement of infected tissues is often

necessary for cure. Allergic bronchopulmonary aspergillosis responds to corticosteroid therapy.

Cryptococcosis

Cryptococcus neoformans is the only species of *Cryptococcus* that is pathogenic for humans. It is a yeast in both tissue and culture, is 4 to 7 μm in diameter, and has thin-walled buds and a capsule (plate 14-6). It is an opportunistic pathogen infecting persons with T-cell deficiencies or dysfunction (patients with Hodgkin disease, hematologic malignancy, organ transplantation, exogenous corticosteroids, chronic liver disease, and AIDS). The respiratory tract is the probable portal of entry. Cryptococcosis does not incite much inflammatory reaction, and calcification is rare.

- *C. neoformans* is an opportunistic pathogen.
- *Cryptococcus* primarily infects persons with T-cell deficiencies or dysfunction (Hodgkin disease, hematologic malignancy, organ transplantation, exogenous corticosteroids, chronic liver disease, and AIDS).

C. neoformans is acquired by inhalation. From the lungs it disseminates widely and easily crosses into the central nervous system. Pneumonia and meningitis are the most common forms of cryptococcosis. Meningitis may be insidious with headache as the only symptom. Cranial nerve involvement may develop (including blindness with involvement of the optic nerve). *Cryptococcus* also may cause an indolent form of cellulitis.

- Pneumonia and meningitis are the most common forms of *C. neoformans* infection.

Cryptococcal infection can be diagnosed with fungal culture (cerebrospinal fluid, blood, sputum, urine), silver staining of biopsy tissue, or detection of *Cryptococcus* antigen in body fluids. The cryptococcal antigen test is the most helpful of all fungal serologic tests. It measures capsular *antigen*, whereas most other fungal serologic tests measure antibody response. Remember that *Cryptococcus* very commonly spreads to the central nervous system. Therefore, if *C. neoformans* is isolated from any source (such as sputum, urine, blood) in a susceptible patient, simultaneous meningitis should be suspected. India ink preparation largely has been replaced by antigen detection assay.

Cryptococcal infections respond to treatment with amphotericin B or fluconazole. Combining oral flucytosine (100-150 mg/kg per day) with amphotericin B for 6 weeks allows a lower dose of amphotericin to be used. Unfortunately, relapse rates are high regardless of the treatment regimen given. In a recent study comparing fluconazole (200 mg/day) with amphotericin B for 10 weeks, fluconazole was as effective as amphotericin B ("effective" is defined as clinical improvement or resolution of symptoms with negative results for culture of cerebrospinal fluid). However, mortality in the first 2 weeks of therapy was higher with fluconazole (15% vs. 8%).

Cryptococcosis in patients with AIDS is virtually impossible to cure. The goal of therapy is to get the infection under control and then suppress it with long-term antifungal agents. A common approach is to initiate therapy with amphotericin B (with or without flucytosine). Amphotericin therapy is continued until cerebrospinal fluid cultures are negative or there is unacceptable toxicity from the drug. Oral fluconazole (200-400 mg/day) is then given indefinitely. Disappointingly, relapse remains frequent even with maintenance therapy.

Candidiasis

Candida is a normal part of the human microflora. It grows as both yeast and hyphal forms simultaneously. Although *Candida albicans* is the most common species, numerous other species can cause human disease. *Candida* causes mucosal and cutaneous infections in both normal and compromised hosts. Invasive disease primarily occurs in neutropenic hosts and as a nosocomial bloodstream infection.

Examples of candidiasis in the normal host include diaper rash and intertrigo, where *Candida* growth on moist skin surfaces produces irritation. Vulvovaginal candidiasis is common, especially after a woman takes a course of antibiotics for an unrelated infection. Treatment with topical antifungal agents or a single dose of oral fluconazole is usually curative. Diabetes, corticosteroids, oral contraceptives, obesity, and HIV infection predispose to recurrent vulvovaginal candidiasis. Oral thrush may result from the same conditions.

Candida species cause 5% to 10% of nosocomial bloodstream infections. Candidemia most often occurs in critically ill patients receiving broad-spectrum antibiotics and parenteral nutrition. Neutropenia is another predisposing factor. Current blood culture techniques usually detect *Candida*, but culture results may be delayed. Always remove or replace all intravenous catheters when bloodstream infection with *Candida* is discovered. Metastatic abscesses can occur in any site after an episode of candidemia. *Candida* osteomyelitis or joint infections can occur as complications after an episode of line-related fungemia. Endophthalmitis may occur as long as 1 month after initial fungemia. For central venous catheter-related candidemias, catheter removal followed by amphotericin B (250-500 mg) or fluconazole is indicated.

Candida tropicalis, *Candida parapsilosis*, *Torulopsis glabrata*, and multiple other species cause nosocomial illness, especially in immunocompromised patients. Note that these non-*albicans* species of *Candida* are more often resistant to fluconazole therapy.

Injection drug use is a risk factor for *Candida* endocarditis

(and joint space infections, especially of the sternoclavicular joint). It is often caused by species other than *C. albicans*.

- Fungemia develops from infected intravenous catheters, especially in the immunosuppressed host.
- Risk factors for *Candida* bloodstream infection include previous antibacterial therapy, cytotoxic or corticosteroid therapy, and parenteral nutrition.
- *Candida* endocarditis occurs most often in injection drug users.
- Diabetes, corticosteroids, oral contraceptives, obesity, and HIV infection predispose to recurrent vulvovaginal candidiasis.

Candida urinary tract infection is common in patients with urinary catheters and those receiving antibacterial drugs. Removal of the catheter is the primary therapy. If necessary, treatment with fluconazole or bladder irrigation with dilute amphotericin B may be curative, though recurrence is common.

Hepatosplenic candidiasis occurs in patients after prolonged chemotherapy-induced neutropenia. Symptoms of fever and increasing liver enzyme values manifest as the leukocyte count recovers. Typical "bull's-eye lesions" can be seen with ultrasonography or computed tomography of the infected liver. The preferred treatment is with at least 2 g of intravenous amphotericin B, but fluconazole or lipid complex amphotericin B also may be effective.

Candida esophagitis is a common cause of odynophagia in immunosuppressed patients, especially those with AIDS. Endoscopy is necessary to prove the diagnosis. *Candida* esophagitis is clinically indistinguishable from, and may coexist with, cytomegalovirus and herpes simplex virus esophagitis. Fluconazole is effective therapy for oral or esophageal candidiasis.

- Hepatosplenic candidiasis typically develops as chemotherapy-induced neutropenia resolves.
- *Candida* esophagitis is clinically indistinguishable from, and may coexist with, cytomegalovirus and herpes simplex virus esophagitis.

Mucormycosis (*Rhizopus* species, Zygomycetes)

Mucormycosis is another disease of compromised hosts. Pulmonary, nasal, and sinus infections are the most common. Rhinocerebral mucormycosis results from direct extension into the brain. Diabetic ketoacidosis, neutropenia, renal failure, and deferoxamine therapy are all risk factors for this dreaded infection. The diagnosis of mucormycosis depends on finding the typical black necrotic lesions (usually in the nose or on the palate) and is confirmed by biopsy. Treatment involves reversing the predisposing condition as much as possible, surgical debridement of necrotic tissue, and amphotericin B.

- The diagnosis of mucormycosis depends on finding the typical black necrotic lesions (usually in the nose or on the palate) and is confirmed by biopsy.
- Diabetic ketoacidosis, neutropenia, renal failure, and deferoxamine therapy are all risk factors for mucormycosis.

VIRAL DISEASES

Herpesviruses

There are now eight known herpesviruses: *herpes simplex virus* (HSV) types 1 and 2, *Epstein-Barr virus* (EBV), *cytomegalovirus* (CMV), *varicella-zoster virus* (VZV), *human herpesvirus* 6 (HHV-6), HHV-7 (not yet known to be associated with clinical disease), and HHV-8. All herpesviruses are DNA viruses that share the characteristic of establishing latency after primary infection, whether symptomatic or not.

Serologic evidence of infection is common by adulthood: HSV 1, 87%; HSV 2, 5%; EBV, 95%; CMV, 50%; and VZV, 90%. The rate of infection increases in populations of lower socioeconomic status.

Herpes Simplex Virus

Primary infection with HSV results from exposure of skin or mucous membranes to intact viral particles. Latent infection is then established in sensory nerve ganglia. Genital HSV infection is caused by HSV type 2 in 80% of cases and by HSV type 1 in the remaining 20%. The reverse is true for oral HSV. Genital HSV is more likely to recur when caused by HSV type 2. Recurrence rates can be decreased by 80% with chronic use of antiviral drugs. In normal hosts, this does not promote emergence of acyclovir-resistant strains.

Herpes simplex encephalitis (HSE) is a nonseasonal, life-threatening illness usually caused by HSV type 1. HSE causes confusion, fever, and, frequently, seizures. Simultaneous herpes labialis is present in 10% to 15% of cases. Antemortem diagnosis may be difficult. Although a definitive diagnosis traditionally requires a brain biopsy, new techniques such as magnetic resonance imaging of the temporal lobes and amplification of HSV DNA from cerebrospinal fluid are often helpful. Detecting periodic lateralized epileptiform discharges with electroencephalography is suggestive of HSE. Poor neurologic status, age older than 30 years, and encephalitis of more than 4 days in duration before initiation of therapy are associated with a poor outcome.

Neonatal HSV infection is acquired at the time of vaginal delivery. The mortality rate is high (20%) despite antiviral therapy. In neonates who survive, neurologic sequelae and recurrent

HSV lesions are common. Cesarean section is recommended if a woman has active herpetic lesions at the time of delivery.

Replication of both HSV types 1 and 2 is inhibited by acyclovir, famciclovir, valacyclovir, ganciclovir, foscarnet, and vidarabine. Acyclovir resistance may develop in patients with acquired immunodeficiency syndrome (AIDS) who are treated with multiple courses of acyclovir. Resistance usually is conferred by a mutation in the thymidine kinase gene, preventing phosphorylation of acyclovir to its active form.

- Recurrence rates of oral HSV can be decreased 80% with chronic suppressive therapy with acyclovir.
- Herpes simplex encephalitis can be diagnosed with magnetic resonance imaging and polymerase chain reaction amplification of HSV DNA from spinal fluid.
- Delivery by cesarean section is recommended if active genital lesions are present at the end of pregnancy.

HSV pneumonia is rare and usually occurs in immunosuppressed patients. When HSV is isolated from a respiratory source, it most commonly represents shedding from the oral mucosa rather than the lungs. HSV also is associated with visceral disease (such as esophagitis). Biopsy is required to reliably distinguish HSV from CMV or *Candida* esophagitis. *Eczema herpeticum* (Kaposi varicelliform eruption) occurs in areas of eczema. Large areas of skin are involved. *Herpetic whitlow* is a painful HSV infection of a finger, often caused by inoculation with a contaminated needle. Although nosocomial transmission of HSV is rare, recent reports stress the importance of mucous membrane precautions when treating all patients with HSV, particularly those with respiratory infection who undergo invasive procedures.

- *Herpetic whitlow* is painful HSV infection of a finger, often caused by inoculation with a contaminated needle.

HSV can cause outbreaks among participants in contact sports (in wrestlers it is called *herpes gladiatorum*). The infection is transmitted by skin-to-skin contact. Lesions appear on the head (78%), trunk (28%), and extremities (42%). The rash may be atypical. Large, ulcerative, perianal lesions can develop in patients with AIDS. Some of the lesions are mistaken for decubitus ulcers.

- HSV can cause outbreaks among participants in contact sports.
- Large, ulcerative, perianal lesions can develop in patients with AIDS.

Epstein-Barr Virus

Most acute EBV infections are asymptomatic. Symptomatic

infectious mononucleosis causes the clinical triad of fever, pharyngitis (80%), and adenopathy. Splenomegaly occurs in 50% of cases. One of the most serious complications of mononucleosis is splenic rupture. Other complications include hemolytic anemia, airway obstruction, encephalitis, and transverse myelitis. Associated laboratory abnormalities include atypical lymphocytosis, thrombocytopenia, and mild increases in liver enzyme values. Corticosteroids may be beneficial for treatment of hemolytic anemia and acute airway obstruction. Ampicillin or amoxicillin given during infectious mononucleosis commonly causes a diffuse macular rash.

Table 14-6 differentiates EBV from other causes of mononucleosis. The diagnosis of infectious mononucleosis depends on detection of heterophile antibodies (monospot test) or specific EBV IgM antibodies. False-negative results of the monospot test are more likely with increasing age.

- Infectious mononucleosis has the clinical triad of fever, pharyngitis, and adenopathy.
- Splenomegaly occurs in 50% of cases.
- One of the most serious complications is splenic rupture.
- If ampicillin is given, a rash often develops.

Uncomplicated cases require symptomatic care only. The patient should not participate in contact sports for several months because of the risk for splenic rupture. Corticosteroids are not indicated for uncomplicated infection. Acyclovir and other antiviral drug therapy is not effective.

Chronic fatigue syndrome is a syndrome characterized by various nonspecific symptoms. Studies have definitively shown that EBV does not cause chronic fatigue syndrome.

- No therapy is indicated for uncomplicated cases of infectious mononucleosis.
- Chronic fatigue syndrome is not caused by EBV.

EBV infection in males with X-linked lymphoproliferative syndrome is a rare disorder of young boys in whom fulminant EBV infections develop and are associated with a 57% mortality rate. Complications include severe EBV hepatitis with liver failure and hemophagocytic syndrome with bleeding. In survivors, hypogammaglobulinemia, malignant lymphoma, aplastic anemia, and opportunistic infections develop. Death occurs by age 40 years in all cases. Acyclovir and corticosteroids do not seem to be beneficial.

In EBV-associated Burkitt lymphoma and nasopharyngeal carcinoma, patients have high titers of IgA antibodies to EBV. *Polyclonal and monoclonal B-cell lymphoproliferative syndromes* have been associated with EBV in patients who have had organ transplantation and in patients with AIDS. Oral hairy leukoplakia in patients with AIDS is associated with EBV infection and responds to acyclovir therapy. EBV recently has been associated with leiomyosarcomas in transplant recipients.

- Polyclonal and monoclonal B-cell lymphoproliferative syndromes have been associated with EBV.

Cytomegalovirus

Primary CMV infection is usually asymptomatic in immunocompetent patients, but it can cause a heterophile-negative mononucleosis syndrome. It is a significant cause of neonatal disease. Perinatal infection can occur in utero, intrapartum, or post partum and can cause congenital malformations. Primary infection of the mother during pregnancy results in a 15% chance of fetal cytomegalic inclusion disease. Young children in day care centers commonly shed CMV in their urine and saliva. Their parents are at risk of acquiring primary infection from an asymptomatic child.

CMV can be transmitted by leukocytes in blood transfusions. Use of leukocyte-poor packed red blood cells or blood from CMV-seronegative donors decreases the risk of transmission via this route. Symptomatic infection develops about 4 weeks after transfusion and manifests as fever with atypical

Table 14-6.—Infectious Mononucleosis-Like Syndromes

Disease	Pharyngitis	Adenopathy	Splenomegaly	Atypical lymphocytes	Heterophile	Other test
Infectious mononucleosis	++++	++++	+++	+++	+	Specific EBV antibody + (VCA IgM)
CMV	-	-	+++	++	-	CMV IgM
Toxoplasmosis	-	++++	+++	++		Toxoserology

-, absent; +, ++, +++, and ++++, present to varying degrees; CMV, cytomegalovirus; EBV, Epstein-Barr virus; VCA, viral capsid antigen.

lymphocytes in the peripheral blood smear. Serologic testing confirms the diagnosis. Viral cultures are rarely helpful in diagnosing CMV disease in the noncompromised patient.

- CMV can cause heterophile-negative mononucleosis syndrome.
- CMV can be transmitted by blood transfusion.
- Fever and infectious mononucleosis-like picture on peripheral smear are characteristics in postoperative patients who have received blood transfusions.

In persons with impaired cellular immunity (such as those with AIDS or organ and bone marrow transplant recipients), CMV causes serious infections (CMV syndrome, retinitis, pneumonia, gastrointestinal ulcerations, encephalitis, adrenalitis). The diagnosis most often is established by isolation of CMV from blood or from culture, by histopathologic evidence of CMV infection in involved tissue (such as liver, lung, gastrointestinal tract), or from clinical findings alone (CMV retinitis).

- CMV causes serious infections (retinitis, pneumonia, gastrointestinal ulcerations, encephalitis, adrenalitis) in patients who have AIDS or take immunosuppressive medications.

The manifestations of CMV disease in persons with advanced AIDS are protean. Disease is almost always caused by reactivation of latent infection in this setting. Finding CMV in the blood or urine from patients with AIDS is common and has a low predictive value for symptomatic CMV disease. CMV retinitis occurs in 20% to 30% of patients with advanced AIDS. Diagnosis is based on ophthalmologic examination. The relapse rate for CMV retinitis in AIDS is very high, even with chronic antiviral therapy.

Solid organ and bone marrow transplant recipients are another group of patients at risk for CMV disease. It is the most common infection encountered after solid organ transplantation (occurring primarily in the first 6 months after transplantation). Those at highest risk are seronegative before transplantation and receive an organ from a seropositive donor. Latent virus is present in almost all tissues and begins replicating shortly after transplantation. Symptomatic disease (CMV syndrome) usually develops in the first 4 to 8 weeks after a solid organ transplantation and causes fever, leukopenia, increases in liver enzyme values, and end-organ involvement. CMV found in blood culture or serum antigen testing helps confirm the diagnosis. Patients who have had bone marrow transplantation are especially at risk for CMV pneumonia. The mortality rate approaches 50% despite therapy. Prophylactic ganciclovir and, possibly, CMV immune globulin may decrease or delay posttransplantation CMV disease.

- CMV retinitis occurs in 20%-30% of patients with advanced AIDS.
- CMV is the most common infectious complication of organ transplantation.

Ganciclovir is the treatment of choice for most CMV infections in compromised hosts. A recent randomized, placebo-controlled trial found that foscarnet and ganciclovir are equally efficacious for halting the progression of CMV retinitis in patients with AIDS but that patients taking foscarnet lived longer (12 vs. 8 months). Both drugs are now approved for this indication. Full-dose "induction" therapy is given for 2 to 3 weeks, followed by chronic suppressive therapy indefinitely (usually as once-daily dosing). Transplant recipients usually do not require suppressive medication after an episode of CMV disease. In patients with CMV pneumonia after bone marrow transplantation, combining ganciclovir with intravenous immune globulin is more effective than ganciclovir alone. Non-immunocompromised patients with CMV do not require treatment.

- Ganciclovir and foscarnet are the treatments of choice for most CMV infections.

Varicella-Zoster Virus

Primary infection with VZV usually occurs in childhood and causes chickenpox. Illness with chickenpox is more likely to be severe in adults and immunocompromised hosts. Varicella pneumonia occurs in 5% to 50% of cases. Pregnant women are especially vulnerable. They should be treated with high-dose acyclovir (10 mg/kg every 8 hours). Acyclovir is not associated with toxicity to the fetus. Pneumonia develops within 1 to 6 days after the onset of illness and usually recedes as the rash does. Encephalomyelitis is another serious complication of varicella infection, occurring predominantly in children. Onset is 3 to 14 days after the appearance of rash.

- Varicella pneumonia occurs in 5% to 50% of adults with chickenpox.
- Pneumonia begins to improve with disappearance of rash.

After primary infection, VZV DNA persists in a latent state in sensory neuron ganglia. Reactivated infection causes zoster (shingles), which manifests as a painful vesicular rash in a dermatomal distribution. Involvement of the fifth cranial nerve, especially the ophthalmic branch, may be sight-threatening. In non-immune persons exposed to zoster, primary VZV infection may develop. Neurologic complications of herpes zoster include motor paralysis (localized to the dermatomal distribution of rash), encephalitis, and myelitis.

- Herpes zoster infection often involves the fifth cranial nerve, especially the ophthalmic branch.

Varicella immune globulin can prevent primary VZV infection. It is indicated for 1) VZV-seronegative immunocompromised hosts who have had close contact with a person with chickenpox and 2) newborns of mothers with varicella infection that occurs 5 days before or 2 days after delivery.

Ten percent of mothers with active varicella will transmit the infection to the fetus. Infection during the first trimester may result in limb hypoplasia, cortical atrophy, and chorioretinitis. During the third trimester, multiple visceral abnormalities can occur, including pneumonia. The fetal and neonatal mortality rate is 31%.

- 10% of mothers with active varicella will transmit the infection to the fetus.

Treatment for *varicella (primary varicella-zoster) infection* is based on whether the patient is immunocompetent. Two recent randomized clinical trials showed that oral acyclovir (800 mg 5 times a day or equivalent) reduced the duration of skin lesions and viral shedding in adults and children. Its efficacy for reducing visceral complications (pneumonia) remains unknown. Early treatment (<24 hours) is necessary. The cost of therapy may limit its usefulness, but it is advocated by some to decrease the duration of illness. Acyclovir may reduce the risk of dissemination and of complications in immunocompromised patients. Treatment of zoster ophthalmicus reduces the incidence of uveitis and keratitis. For immunocompetent patients with zoster, three antiviral drugs (acyclovir, famciclovir, and valacyclovir) speed healing and reduce pain. Preliminary data suggest that the new antiviral agent famciclovir might decrease the duration of postherpetic neuralgia. Corticosteroids do not prevent postherpetic neuralgia. For disseminated infections (encephalitis, cranial neuritis), a recent controlled trial showed that high-dose intravenous acyclovir decreases the duration of hospitalization. Acyclovir-resistant VZV infection (which can occur in patients with AIDS) can be treated with intravenous foscarnet.

An effective live virus vaccine for VZV is now available. Although recommended for children, appropriate adult populations for vaccination have yet to be defined.

Human Herpesvirus 6

HHV-6 is a recently discovered lymphotropic virus. It causes the mild childhood infectious exanthem known as roseola infantum. Like CMV, reactivation of infection occurs after organ transplantation. HHV-6 has been associated with pneumonitis after bone marrow transplantation.

Human Herpesvirus 8

HHV-8 is also known as Kaposi sarcoma-associated virus. As the name implies, it is thought to be the causative agent of Kaposi sarcoma. It is related to EBV. Most recently, HHV-8 has been linked to body cavity-based lymphomas in patients with AIDS and Castleman disease.

Influenza

Type A is the most common. Epidemics occur every 2 to 4 years; pandemics occur every 20 to 30 years. Epidemics and pandemics are a result of a major antigenic shift in the influenza virus. About 80% to 90% of deaths due to influenza occur in persons older than 65 years. Complications include 1) primary influenza pneumonia (interstitial desquamative pneumonia) and 2) secondary bacterial infection, which usually is caused by *Streptococcus pneumoniae*, *Haemophilus*, or *Staphylococcus aureus*. A typical history is as follows: an elderly patient, often with chronic obstructive lung disease, develops influenza, which may or may not improve; then, the severity of symptoms increases substantially, with high fever, marked leukocytosis, and often respiratory failure. Rare cases of toxic shock syndrome have been reported when *S. aureus* pneumonia complicated influenza.

- About 80%-90% of deaths due to influenza occur in persons older than 65 years.
- Secondary infection usually is caused by *Streptococcus pneumoniae* or *Staphylococcus aureus*.

Amantadine and rimantadine are effective against only influenza A virus, not influenza B. Therapy is most beneficial if begun within 48 hours of onset of symptoms. Vaccine, together with amantadine, can give ± 95% protection against influenza A infection.

The influenza vaccine can be given simultaneously with pneumococcal vaccine (Pneumovax). Adverse reactions to influenza vaccination include fever, myalgias, and hypersensitivity. Target groups are persons older than 65 years, residents of chronic care facilities, persons with cardiopulmonary disorders, children 6 months to 18 years old receiving long-term aspirin therapy (to prevent Reye syndrome), health care personnel, employees of chronic care facilities, providers of home health care, and those sharing the same household as high-risk persons. Amantadine also is used prophylactically at a dose of 200 mg/day (if the person is older than 65 years, give only 100 mg/day to decrease the risk of side effects). The decreased dosage also is used for patients with impaired renal function or seizure disorders. Toxicity manifests as dizziness, restlessness, and insomnia.

- Influenza vaccine can be given simultaneously with pneumococcal vaccine.

- Target groups are persons older than 65 years, residents of chronic care facilities, persons with cardiopulmonary disorders, health care personnel, employees of chronic care facilities, providers of home health care, and household members of high-risk persons.

Hantavirus Infection, *Hantavirus* Pulmonary Syndrome

In May 1993, an outbreak of an acute illness consisting of fever, rapidly progressive respiratory failure, and death was reported in the four-state area of New Mexico, Arizona, Colorado, and Utah. Most of the initial cases occurred in young Navajo Indians. The causative agent is a virus belonging to the genus *Hantavirus* (family Bunyaviridae) and is now called the Sin Nombre virus. Infection is transmitted through inhalation of aerosolized secretions from the common deer mouse (*Peromyscus maniculatus*).

Since the early reports, cases also have been identified in most other states and Canada. The disease begins with a non-specific prodrome (fever and generalized myalgia) followed in 4 to 5 days by respiratory symptoms (cough, dyspnea, and tachypnea). This progresses rapidly to an adult respiratory distress syndrome. Diagnosis is possible with serologic studies (such as enzyme-linked immunosorbent assay for anti-virus IgM and IgG antibodies). Treatment is mainly supportive. Ribavirin, a guanosine analog, has been used effectively for treating hemorrhagic fever with renal syndrome caused by other related types of *Hantavirus*, but its efficacy in *Hantavirus* pulmonary syndrome is not yet established.

Poliovirus

Although wild-type polio has been eliminated from the Western Hemisphere, it remains epidemic in parts of Asia and Africa. Disease still can be imported from these areas. There was a recent outbreak in the Netherlands among members of religious groups who were not vaccinated. Remember that polio is most often an asymptomatic infection. The virus affects the nuclei of cranial nerves and anterior motor neurons of the spinal cord, causing a flaccid paralysis. When paralysis develops, it is usually asymmetric. Vaccine-related polio, although rare, can occur with the live virus vaccine.

Rabies

Rabies is difficult to diagnose ante mortem. Manifestations are hydrophobia and copious salivation. It should be considered in any case of encephalitis or myelitis of unknown cause, especially in persons who have recently traveled outside the United States. The virus spreads along peripheral nerves to the central nervous system. The most common sources of exposure are dogs, cats, skunks, foxes, raccoons (Florida, Connecticut), wolves, and bats. Spread by other animals is *very rare*. Rodents rarely, if ever, transmit rabies. From 1980 to 1989, 9 of 13 cases in the United States were due to exposure to rabid animals outside the country. Rabies also has been reported to occur in patients after corneal transplantation. Aerosol spread is possible; it is most often due to exposure to bats during spelunking or in medical laboratories. The risk of nosocomial transmission is low. Definitive diagnosis is established by finding Negri bodies on biopsy of the hippocampus. Serum and cerebrospinal fluid can be tested for rabies antibodies when trying to diagnose the disease. Direct fluorescent antibody testing of a skin biopsy specimen from the nape of the neck is used to detect rabies antigen.

- Rabies should be considered in any case of encephalitis or myelitis of unknown cause.
- Most common sources of exposure are dogs, cats, skunks, foxes, raccoons, wolves, and bats.
- Definitive diagnosis is established by the presence of Negri bodies on biopsy of the hippocampus.

Human diploid vaccine is more effective and less toxic than the older duck embryo vaccine. Human rabies immune globulin is now widely available, mitigating the need to use horse serum immune globulin. Human rabies immune globulin and vaccine are not of benefit after onset of clinical disease.

Slow Viruses and Prion-Associated Central Nervous System Diseases

Progressive Multifocal Leukoencephalopathy (PML)

PML is associated with AIDS, leukemia, lymphoma, and immunosuppression for organ transplantation. It is caused by a papovavirus (JC virus). PML can cause either diffuse or focal central nervous system abnormalities. Despite its name, PML usually causes solitary brain lesions, as seen on computed tomography or magnetic resonance imaging. Cerebrospinal fluid is normal in most cases. The diagnosis is based on brain biopsy, although detection of JC virus DNA in the cerebrospinal fluid is suggestive of PML. There is no proven effective therapy.

- PML is associated with AIDS, leukemia, lymphoma, and immunosuppression for organ transplantation.
- PML is caused by a papovavirus (JC virus).

Subacute Sclerosing Panencephalitis (Inclusion Body Encephalitis)

This is a progressively fatal disease of children and adolescents. It is thought to be due to rubeola (measles) virus. Patients are younger than 11 years in 80% of cases. Onset is insidious with progressive mental deterioration. Later, myoclonic jerks and diffuse abnormalities occur. Measles antibody levels in sera and cerebrospinal fluid are markedly increased. Brain biopsy is necessary for diagnosis (inclusion body encephalitis). There is no treatment. The disease is uniformly fatal.

Creutzfeldt-Jakob Disease

This is a rare, fatal, degenerative disease of the central nervous system. It occurs equally in both sexes, usually at older ages. There are both familial and sporadic forms of the disease. Creutzfeldt-Jakob disease usually presents as rapidly evolving dementia with myoclonic seizures. Prions (small proteinaceous infectious particles without nucleic acid) have been proposed as the cause of this disease. Nosocomial transmission of Creutzfeldt-Jakob disease can occur via corneal transplant recipients and exposure to cerebrospinal fluid. Several recent cases in Great Britain were linked to consumption of beef from cattle that had bovine spongiform encephalopathy. There is no treatment.

● Creutzfeldt-Jakob disease presents as rapidly evolving dementia with myoclonic seizures.

Measles (Rubeola)

There was a substantial increase in measles cases in the late 1980s and early 1990s in unvaccinated preschool children and vaccinated high school and college students (1990: 27,786 cases). Prodromal upper respiratory tract symptoms are prominent. Oral lesions (Koplik spots) precede the rash. Both measles infection and measles vaccine cause temporary cutaneous anergy (false-negative purified protein derivative test). Infection may cause more significant immunologic suppression as exemplified by cases of reactivated tuberculosis in persons with measles.

● In measles, oral Koplik spots precede the rash.
● Measles vaccine may cause temporary cutaneous anergy.

Complications of measles include encephalitis and pneumonia. Encephalitis is often severe. It usually occurs after a period of apparent improvement of measles infection. In primary measles pneumonia, large, multinucleated cells (Warthin-Finkeldey cells) are found on lung biopsy. Secondary bacterial infection is more common than primary measles pneumonia. *Staphylococcus aureus* and *Haemophilus influenzae* are the most common bacterial pathogens.

● Complications of measles include encephalitis.
● Secondary bacterial infection is more common than primary measles pneumonia.

Atypical measles occurs in patients vaccinated before 1968. After exposure to measles, atypical rash, fever, arthralgias, and headache (aseptic meningitis) may develop. The presence of a high titer of measles antibody in serum helps confirm the diagnosis.

Rubella

The prodromal symptoms of rubella are mild (unlike those of rubeola). Posterior cervical lymphadenopathy, arthralgia (70% in adults), transient erythematous rash, and fever are characteristic. Infection is subclinical in many cases. Central nervous system complications and thrombocytopenia are rare.

● Characteristics of rubella: posterior cervical lymphadenopathy, arthralgia (70% in adults), transient erythematous rash, and fever.

The greatest danger from rubella is to the fetus. When a pregnant female is exposed to rubella, rubella serology testing should be done. If the titer indicates immunity, there is no danger and no further testing is indicated. If the titer indicates non-immunity, the patient should be followed for evidence of clinical rubella. The serum titer should be checked again in 2 to 3 weeks to look for evidence of asymptomatic infection. If the titer is not increased and there is no evidence of clinical rubella, then no intervention is indicated. If clinical rubella develops or seroconversion is demonstrated, there is a high risk of congenital abnormalities or spontaneous abortion. The risk varies from 40% to 60% if infection occurs during the first 2 months of gestation to 10% by the 4th month. Intravenous gamma globulin may mask symptoms of rubella, but it does not protect the fetus.

● Gamma globulin does not protect the fetus after exposure to rubella.

From 6% to 11% of young adults remain susceptible to rubella after receiving rubella vaccine. A pregnant female should not be given rubella vaccine because it causes congenital abnormalities. Females of childbearing age should be warned not to become pregnant within 2 to 3 months from the time of immunization. Transient arthralgias develop in 25% of immunized women. Fever, rash, and lymphadenopathy also may develop. Symptoms may occur as long as 2 months after vaccination. They may be confused with other forms of arthritis.

Viral Meningoencephalitis

Etiologic agents of viral meningitis include mumps, enteroviruses, herpes simplex, and, in summer months, the equine encephalitis viruses. Lymphocytic choriomeningitis is acquired by exposure to rodent urine. Lactate levels in cerebrospinal fluid are normal in viral meningitis. The lactate level usually is increased in bacterial meningitis.

Mumps

Mumps virus commonly affects glandular tissue. Parotitis, pancreatitis, and orchitis are characteristic manifestations. Orchitis occurs in 20% of males with mumps. It is unilateral in approximately 75%. Orchitis often is associated with recrudescence of malaise and the appearance of chills, fever, headache, nausea, vomiting, and testicular pain. Sterility is *uncommon*, even after bilateral infection.

Mumps meningoencephalitis is one of the most common nonseasonal viral meningitides. It can cause low glucose values in the cerebrospinal fluid, mimicking bacterial meningitis. Deafness is a rare complication of mumps.

● Mumps meningoencephalitis is one of the most common viral meningitides.

Mumps polyarthritis is most common in men between the ages of 20 and 30 years. Joint symptoms begin 1 to 2 weeks after subsidence of parotitis, and large joints are involved. The condition lasts approximately 6 weeks, and complete recovery is usual. This condition may be confused with other forms of arthritis.

● Mumps polyarthritis is most common in men between the ages of 20 and 30 years.

Parvovirus B19

Parvovirus is a single-stranded DNA virus that infects the erythrocyte precursors in bone marrow with resulting reticulocytopenia. It is the cause of erythema infectiosum (fifth disease) in children, transient arthritis in adults, and aplastic crisis in persons with hemolytic anemias. Infection during pregnancy results in a 5% chance of hydrops fetalis or fetal death. Serologic testing is the preferred diagnostic method in immunologically competent persons.

Parvovirus B19 infection may persist in immunosuppressed patients, resulting in red blood cell aplasia. Diagnosis is established by demonstration of giant pronormoblasts in bone marrow or identification of viral DNA in bone marrow or peripheral blood. Most patients respond to administration of commercial immune globulin infusions for 5 to 10 days. No treatment is recommended for parvovirus infections in the noncompromised host.

● Parvovirus B19 is the cause of erythema infectiosum (fifth disease) and transient arthritis.
● B19 virus can cause red blood cell aplasia in patients with AIDS.

Human T-Cell Lymphotropic Viruses (HTLV)

HTLV-I and II are non-HIV human retroviruses. HTLV-I is endemic in parts of Japan, the Caribbean basin, South America, and Africa. It may be transmitted by sexual contact, infected cellular blood products (not clotting factor concentrates), and injection drug use. Vertical transmission (breast-feeding, transplacental) also occurs. HTLV-I is associated with human T-cell leukemia/lymphoma and tropical spastic paraparesis (also known as HTLV-I-associated myelopathy). However, 96% of persons infected with HTLV-I never develop any clinical disease. HTLV-II causes no known clinical disease. The seroprevalence of HTLV-I or -II is as high as 18% in certain high-risk groups (injection drug users, patients attending sexually transmitted disease clinics) (HTLV-II is 2.5 times more prevalent than HTLV-I). Among voluntary blood donors, the seroprevalence in the United States is estimated at 0.016%. With current screening practices, the risk of transmission of HTLV-I or -II through blood transfusion is estimated to be 0.0014% (1/70,000 units).

● HTLV-I may be transmitted by sexual contact, infected blood products, and injection drug use.
● HTLV-I infection is usually asymptomatic but is associated with human T-cell leukemia and chronic myelopathy.

PARASITIC DISEASES

Helminths

Neurocysticercosis is an infection of the central nervous system with a larval stage of the pork tapeworm (*Taenia solium*). It is acquired by ingesting tapeworm eggs from fecally contaminated food. It is endemic in Latin America, Asia, and Africa. Recent cases have been reported among household contacts of foreign-born persons (working as domestic employees). The infected persons had not traveled to an endemic area. Most common presentation is seizures. Brain imaging reveals cystic or calcified brain lesions. Serum or cerebrospinal fluid serologic testing can aid in the diagnosis. Treatment with praziquantel or albendazole may be beneficial. The coadministration of corticosteroids often is used to decrease cerebral inflammation associated with therapy.

● Seizures are the most common symptom of neurocysticercosis.

Strongyloides stercoralis is unique among the intestinal nematode infections. Unlike the other helminths, the larvae of this organism can mature in the human host (auto-infection). In compromised hosts (neutropenia, steroids, acquired immunodeficiency syndrome [AIDS]), a superinfection can develop with larval migration throughout the body. Gram-negative bacteremia is a common coinfection, resulting from disruption of the intestinal mucosa by the invasive larvae.

Trichinosis is acquired from eating undercooked meat, especially pork or bear. Features include muscle pain (especially chest and tongue), eosinophilia, and periorbital edema.

Hookworm (Necator americanus) causes anemia. It is found mainly in tropical and subtropical regions. The larval form penetrates the skin. Walking barefoot is a risk factor.

Ascariasis infection may cause intestinal obstruction or pancreatitis (worm migrates up the pancreatic duct).

Schistosomiasis is a tropical disease that causes hepatic cirrhosis, hematuria, and carcinoma of the bladder. Transverse myelitis may develop as a result of schistosomiasis.

- Trichinosis is acquired from eating undercooked meat, especially pork or bear.
- Transverse myelitis may develop as a result of schistosomiasis.

Protozoan Parasites

Acanthamoeba, a free-living ameba, causes amebic keratitis in persons swimming in fresh water while wearing soft contact lenses. The diagnosis is based on microscopic examination of scrapings of the cornea. Treatment is with topical antifungal agents. Patients often respond poorly to therapy and have progressive corneal destruction.

Symptomatic infection with *Entamoeba histolytica* (*amebiasis*) may cause diarrhea (often bloody), abdominal pain, and fever. Metronidazole, followed by a lumenocidal agent such as iodoquinol or paromomycin, is the preferred therapy (metronidazole does not kill amebae in the intestinal lumen). Asymptomatic carriage of amebic cysts should be treated with one of the lumenocidal agents.

- Metronidazole, followed by a lumenocidal agent such as iodoquinol or paromomycin, is the preferred therapy for symptomatic amebiasis.

Invasive amebiasis may lead to distant abscesses (primarily the liver, but other organs can be involved). An amebic liver abscess usually is single and is commonly located in the posterior portion of the right lobe of the liver. The anatomical location, the fact that it is usually a single abscess, and the absence of other signs of bacterial infection help to distinguish amebic hepatic abscess from bacterial abscess. Serologic tests (complement fixation) are positive in more than 90% of patients with amebic abscess. Hepatic abscess may rupture through the diaphragm into the right pleural cavity.

- Amebic liver abscess may rupture through the diaphragm into the right pleural cavity.

Giardia lamblia is the parasite most frequently detected in state parasitology laboratories. Infection characteristically produces sudden onset of watery diarrhea with malabsorption, bloating, and flatulence. Prolonged disease that is refractory to standard therapy may occur in patients with IgA deficiency. The organism may be detected in stool specimens, but examination of duodenal aspirates is more sensitive. Treatment with metronidazole usually cures giardiasis.

- *G. lamblia* is the parasite most frequently detected in state parasitology laboratories.
- Giardiasis causes sudden onset of watery diarrhea and malabsorption, bloating, and flatulence. Prolonged disease is particularly common in patients with IgA deficiency.

Toxoplasma gondii is acquired from eating undercooked meat or exposure to cat feces. Primary toxoplasmosis is usually asymptomatic. In non-immunocompromised persons it may cause a heterophile-negative mononucleosis-like syndrome. Toxoplasmosis causes brain lesions and pneumonia in patients with AIDS. Immunocompromised patients with toxoplasmosis can be treated effectively with pyrimethamine in combination with either sulfadiazine or clindamycin.

- Toxoplasmosis is acquired from eating undercooked meat or exposure to cat feces.
- Toxoplasmosis may cause an infectious mononucleosis-like syndrome.

Malaria is endemic and spreading in many parts of the world. Spiking fever is the hallmark of malaria. With falciparum malaria, the fevers may be irregular or continuous. *Plasmodium vivax* and *Plasmodium malariae* infections cause regular episodic fevers (malarial paroxysms). Malaria is diagnosed by examination of thick and thin blood smears (plate 14-7).

- Diagnosis of malaria is based on examination of thick and thin blood smears.

Prophylaxis for malaria is increasingly difficult because of resistant *Plasmodium falciparum*. Personal protection should always be used (such as mosquito nets). For travelers to chloroquine-sensitive areas (Central America [north of Panama], Mexico, Haiti, Dominican Republic, and the Middle East), chloroquine phosphate is still effective. In chloroquine-resistant areas, mefloquine, doxycycline, or sulfadoxine-pyrimethamine (Fansidar) is suggested. Travelers to the mefloquine-resistant areas of the Thai-Myanmar and Thai-Cambodian borders should use doxycycline. Mefloquine should be avoided in patients taking β-adrenergic blockers. No regimen guarantees 100% prophylaxis. All patients should be advised to seek medical attention if fever develops within

1 year after return from an endemic area. Prophylaxis should begin 2 weeks before travel and continue through 4 to 6 weeks after leaving an endemic area.

Chloroquine is the preferred treatment of infection caused by *P. vivax, P. malariae,* and known susceptible strains of *P. falciparum.* Chloroquine-resistant strains may respond to quinine and sulfadoxine-pyrimethamine or doxycycline. For severe *P. falciparum* infections, intravenous quinidine or quinine is effective. Primaquine is used to eradicate the exoerythrocytic phase of *Plasmodium ovale* and *P. vivax* infections, preventing later relapses. Be aware that primaquine can cause hemolysis in persons with glucose-6-phosphate dehydrogenase (G-6-PD) deficiency. Exchange transfusion may be beneficial as treatment for cases with overwhelming parasitemia.

Cryptosporidium parvum is an important cause of diarrhea, especially in persons with AIDS. Cryptosporidiosis is also a cause of self-limited diarrhea in otherwise healthy patients. Waterborne outbreaks (Georgia; Milwaukee, Wisconsin) have been reported. They occur most often in late summer or fall. Thirty-five percent of patients have another pathogen simultaneously, most often *Giardia.* The diagnosis may be missed on standard stool examination for ova and parasites.

- Cryptosporidiosis is an important cause of diarrhea in AIDS.

Cyclospora cayetanensis is a recently described cause of persistent diarrhea, fever, and profound fatigue. First described in travelers to tropical areas of the world, disease due to *Cyclospora* also has been linked to consumption of contaminated food in the United States (raspberries from Guatemala). Like *Cryptosporidium,* the organism may not be detected on routine stool examinations. The illness can be effectively treated with cotrimoxazole.

- Infection with *Cyclospora cayetanensis* causes persistent diarrhea, fever, and profound fatigue.

Leishmaniasis is a protozoan disease transmitted by the sand fly bite. Visceral leishmaniasis (kala-azar; caused by *Leishmania donovani*) causes fever, hepatosplenomegaly, hypergammaglobulinemia, cachexia, and pancytopenia. It has been reported in patients with AIDS in Spain. Bone marrow examination (Giemsa stain) is often diagnostic. The cutaneous leishmaniasis (caused by *L. tropica, L. major, L. braziliensis,* and *L. mexicana*) may be self-limited. However, South and Central American forms of cutaneous leishmaniasis are often destructive and should be treated.

Babesia microti is a tick-borne (same vector as Lyme disease, *Ixodes dammini*) parasite that infects erythrocytes and causes fever, myalgias, and hemolytic anemia. Often asymptomatic in normal hosts, severe disease may develop in asplenic individuals. Babesiosis is endemic in the northeastern United States, especially around Nantucket and Cape Cod. Cases of transfusion-transmitted babesiosis have been documented. The diagnosis is established with examination of peripheral blood smear or polymerase chain reaction amplification of babesial DNA from peripheral blood. Treatment is with clindamycin and quinine. Simultaneous infection with babesiosis and Lyme disease may be especially severe.

- Babesiosis infects erythrocytes and causes fever, myalgias, and hemolytic anemia.

CLINICAL SYNDROMES

INFECTIVE ENDOCARDITIS

Native Valve Infective Endocarditis

Native valve infective endocarditis is more common in males and patients older than 65 years. The age- and sex-adjusted incidence rate of infective endocarditis is 4.9 cases per 100,000 person-years. In 60% to 80% of cases, there is a predisposing cardiac lesion. The mitral and aortic valves are most commonly involved. Congenital heart disease is present in 10% to 20% of cases, and rheumatic heart disease is present in less than 15% of cases. The risk of infective endocarditis from mitral valve prolapse is low, but the prevalence of mitral valve prolapse makes it the most common underlying cardiac condition. Infective endocarditis may present with acute or subacute manifestations, depending on the virulence of the infecting organism. The diagnosis of infective endocarditis is often difficult and is based on clinical, microbiologic, and echocardiographic findings. Diagnostic criteria have been developed to aid the clinician in the diagnosis of infective endocarditis (Tables 14-7 and 14-8).

- The risk of infective endocarditis from mitral valve prolapse is low, but the prevalence of mitral valve prolapse makes it the most common underlying cardiac condition.
- Diagnostic criteria have been developed to aid in the diagnosis of infective endocarditis.

Microorganisms causing native valve infective endocarditis include viridans group streptococci (that is, *Streptococcus sanguis, S. mutans,* and *S. mitis*), 30% to 40% of cases; enterococci (that is, *Enterococcus faecalis* and *E. faecium*), 5% to 18%; other streptococci (that is, *Streptococcus bovis* and *S. pneumoniae*), 15% to 25%; *Staphylococcus aureus,* 10% to 27%; coagulase-negative staphylococci, 1% to 3%; gram-negative bacilli, 1.5% to 13%; fungi, 2% to 4%;

Table 14-7.—Duke Criteria for the Diagnosis of Infective Endocarditis

Definite infective endocarditis
    Pathologic criteria
        Microorganisms: demonstrated by culture *or* histology in vegetation, *or* in vegetation that has embolized, *or* in an intracardiac abscess, *or*
        Pathologic lesions: vegetation or intracardiac abscess present, confirmed by histology showing active endocarditis
    Clinical criteria, using specific definitions listed in Table 14-8
        2 major criteria, *or*
        1 major and 3 minor criteria, *or*
        5 minor criteria

Possible infective endocarditis
    Findings consistent with infective endocarditis that fall short of "definite," but not "rejected"

Rejected
    Firm alternative diagnosis for manifestations of endocarditis, *or*
    Resolution of manifestations of endocarditis, with antibiotic therapy for 4 days or less, *or*
    No pathologic evidence of infective endocarditis at surgery or autopsy, after antibiotic therapy for 4 days or less

From Durack DT, Lukes AS, Bright DK, Duke Endocarditis Service: New criteria for diagnosis of infective endocarditis: utilization of specific echocardiographic findings. Am J Med 96:200-209, 1994. By permission of Excerpta Medica.

Table 14-8.——Definitions of Terminology Used in the Proposed New Criteria

Major criteria
    1. Positive blood culture for infective endocarditis
        a. Typical microorganism for infective endocarditis from two separate blood cultures
            1) Viridans group streptococci,* *Streptococcus bovis*, HACEK[†] group, *or*
            2) Community-acquired *Staphylococcus aureus* or enterococci, in the absence of a primary focus, *or*
        b. Persistently positive blood cultures, defined as recovery of a microorganism consistent with infective endocarditis from:
            1) Blood cultures drawn more than 12 hours apart, *or*
            2) All of three or a majority of four or more separate blood cultures, with first and last drawn at least 1 hour apart
    2. Evidence of endocardial involvement
        a. Positive echocardiogram for infective endocarditis
            1) Oscillating intracardiac mass, on valve or supporting structures, *or* in the path of regurgitant jets, *or* on implanted material, in the absence of an alternative anatomical explanation, *or*
            2) Abscess, *or*
            3) New partial dehiscence of prosthetic valve, *or*
        b. New valvular regurgitation (increase or change in preexisting murmur not sufficient)

Minor criteria
    1. Predisposition: predisposing heart condition *or* intravenous drug use
    2. Fever: 38.0°C (100.4°F)
    3. Vascular phenomena: major arterial emboli, septic pulmonary infarcts, mycotic aneurysm, intracranial hemorrhage, conjunctival hemorrhages, Janeway lesions
    4. Immunologic phenomena: glomerulonephritis, Osler nodes, Roth spots, rheumatoid factor
    5. Microbiologic evidence: positive blood culture but not meeting major criterion as noted previously[‡] *or* serologic evidence of active infection with organisms consistent with infective endocarditis
    6. Echocardiogram: consistent with infective endocarditis but not meeting major criterion as noted previously

*Including nutritional variant strains.
[†]HACEK, *Haemophilus* spp., *Actinobacillus actinomycetemcomitans*, *Cardiobacterium hominis*, *Eikenella* spp., and *Kingella kingae*.
[‡]Excluding single positive cultures for coagulase-negative staphylococci and organisms that do not cause endocarditis.
From Durack DT, Lukes AS, Bright DK, Duke Endocarditis Service: New criteria for diagnosis of infective endocarditis: utilization of specific echocardiographic findings. Am J Med 96:200-209, 1994. By permission of Excerpta Medica.

miscellaneous bacteria, less than 5%; mixed infections, 1% to 2%; and "culture-negative," less than 5% to 24% (data from Scheld WM, Sande MA: Endocarditis and intravascular infections. *In* Principles and Practice of Infectious Diseases. Vol I. Fourth edition. Edited by GL Mandell, JE Bennett, R Dolin. New York, Churchill Livingstone, 1995, pp 740-783).

- The organisms most commonly involved in native valve infective endocarditis are viridans group streptococci.

Treatment of native valve infective endocarditis includes an emphasis on short-course therapy in patients with uncomplicated left-sided native valve infective endocarditis caused by penicillin-susceptible viridans group streptococci. For enterococcal endocarditis, combination therapy with penicillin G or ampicillin in addition to gentamicin is recommended. Testing for high-level aminoglycoside resistance (gentamicin, >500 µg/mL; streptomycin, >2,000 µg/mL) and penicillin and vancomycin resistance is mandatory.

Table 14-9 shows the recommended treatment regimens for native valve infective endocarditis.

Prosthetic Valve Infective Endocarditis

Prosthetic valve endocarditis occurs in up to 3% to 6% of patients with a prosthetic cardiac valve. The aortic valve is affected more often than the mitral valve. Early-onset endocarditis is defined as infection occurring 60 days or less after implantation, and late-onset endocarditis is infection occurring more than 60 days postoperatively. Early infection tends to have a more acute presentation. Microorganisms that cause prosthetic valve endocarditis are outlined in Table 14-10. Treatment regimens for prosthetic valve infective endocarditis are given in Table 14-11.

Additional Information About Infective Endocarditis
- Transthoracic echocardiography (TTE) and transesophageal echocardiography (TEE) visualize vegetations in approximately 60% and 90% of patients, respectively. TEE is superior to TTE for diagnosing complications of infective endocarditis such as cardiac abscesses and fistulas.
- Infective endocarditis in injection drug users is caused by *S. aureus* (60%), streptococci (16%), gram-negative bacilli (13.5%), polymicrobial infection (8.1%), and *Corynebacterium JK* (1.4%). *Candida* spp. endocarditis also occurs in this patient population. Tricuspid valve involvement is common. Short-course (2 weeks) therapy with a penicillinase-resistant penicillin with or without an aminoglycoside may be as effective as longer courses of therapy in uncomplicated right-sided endocarditis due to methicillin-susceptible *S. aureus* in injection drug users who are not infected with human immunodeficiency virus (HIV).

- "Culture-negative" endocarditis may be the result of previous use of antibiotics (most common) and endocarditis due to the following organisms: HACEK organisms, nutritionally deficient streptococci, *Neisseria* spp., *Listeria monocytogenes*, *Brucella* spp., fungi, mycobacteria, *Legionella* spp., *Coxiella burnetii*, *Chlamydia* spp., *Mycoplasma* spp., *Nocardia* spp., *Rothia dentocariosa*, and *Bartonella* spp.

Surgical Therapy

If cardiac valve replacement is needed, it should not be delayed to allow additional days of antimicrobial therapy. Surgical treatment is often indicated in cases of congestive heart failure refractory to medical management. Other generally accepted indications for cardiac valve replacement include evidence of more than one serious systemic embolic episode, uncontrolled bacteremia despite effective antimicrobial therapy, and inadequate antimicrobial therapy. Other indications include invasive perivalvular infection as manifested by abscess or fistula on echocardiography, new or persistent electrocardiographic changes, persistent unexplained fever, fungal endocarditis, and relapse of appropriately treated prosthetic valve endocarditis due to penicillin-sensitive streptococci.

- Surgical treatment is indicated in cases of congestive heart failure refractory to medical management.
- Intractable congestive heart failure is the most common indication for cardiac valve replacement.

Prevention

Most cases of infective endocarditis are not due to invasive procedures. The incidence of endocarditis after invasive procedures is low, and the reported efficacy, in large retrospective studies, of antimicrobial prophylaxis in preventing infective endocarditis is approximately 50%. The lowest-risk group for which antibiotic prophylaxis is currently recommended is patients with mitral valve prolapse with a cardiac murmur or echocardiographic evidence of regurgitation or thickened leaflets. American Heart Association guidelines for the prevention of bacterial endocarditis after invasive dental and medical procedures have been published (JAMA 277:1794-1801, 1997). Significant changes from prior guidelines include the following for oral or dental procedures that require prophylaxis: the initial dose of amoxicillin has been reduced to 2.0 g, a follow-up antibiotic dose is not recommended, and erythromycin is not recommended for penicillin-allergic persons.

- Significant changes from prior guidelines include the following for oral or dental procedures that require prophylaxis: the initial dose of amoxicillin has been reduced to 2.0 g, a follow-up antibiotic dose is not recommended, and erythromycin is not recommended for penicillin-allergic persons.

Table 14-9.—Treatment of Native Valve Infective Endocarditis

Microorganisms	Therapy*	Alternative therapy*
Penicillin-sensitive viridans group streptococci and *Streptococcus bovis* (MIC, ≤0.1 µg/mL)	Aqueous crystalline penicillin G, 12-18 x 10^6 U/24 hr i.v. either continuously or in six equally divided doses for 4 wk *Or* Ceftriaxone sodium 2 g i.v. or i.m. for 4 wk‡ *Or* Aqueous penicillin G, 12-18 x 10^6 U/24 hr i.v. either continuously or in six equally divided doses for 2 wk *Plus* Gentamicin sulfate,§ 1 mg/kg i.v. or i.m. every 8 hr for 2 wk	Vancomycin,† 30 mg/kg i.v. in two equally divided doses, not to exceed 2 g/24 hr unless serum levels are monitored for 4 wk Vancomycin therapy is recommended for patients allergic to β-lactams (immediate-type hypersensitivity); serum concentration of vancomycin should be obtained 1 hr after completion of the infusion and should be in the range of 30-45 µg/mL for twice-daily dosing
Relatively penicillin-resistant viridans group streptococci (MIC, >0.1 µg/mL and <0.5 µg/mL)	Aqueous crystalline penicillin G, 18 x 10^6 U/24 hr i.v. either continuously or in six equally divided doses for 4 wk *Plus* Gentamicin sulfate,§ 1 mg/kg i.v. or i.m. every 8 hr for 2 wk	Vancomycin,† 30 mg/kg i.v. in two equally divided doses, not to exceed 2 g/24 hr unless serum levels are monitored for 4 wk Vancomycin therapy is recommended for patients allergic to β-lactams (immediate-type hypersensitivity); serum concentration of vancomycin should be obtained 1 hr after completion of the infusion and should be in the range of 30-45 µg/mL for twice-daily dosing
Enterococci (gentamicin- or vancomycin-susceptible) or viridans group streptococci with MIC ≥0.5 µg/mL or nutritionally variant streptococci (All enterococci causing endocarditis must be tested for antimicrobial susceptibility in order to select optimal therapy)	Aqueous crystalline penicillin G, 18-30 x 10^6 U/24 hr i.v. either continuously or in six equally divided doses for 4-6 wk *Or* Ampicillin sodium 12 g/24 hr i.v. either continuously or in six equally divided doses *Plus* Gentamicin sulfate,§ 1 mg/kg i.v. or i.m. every 8 hr for 4-6 wk (4-week therapy recommended for patients with symptoms <3 months in duration; 6-week therapy recommended for patients with symptoms >3 months in duration)	Vancomycin,† 30 mg/kg i.v. in two equally divided doses, not to exceed 2 g/24 hr unless serum levels are monitored for 4-6 wk *Plus* Gentamicin,§ 1 mg/kg i.v. or i.m. every 8 hr for 4-6 wk Vancomycin therapy is recommended for patients allergic to β-lactams (immediate-type hypersensitivity); serum concentration of vancomycin should be obtained 1 hr after completion of the infusion and should be in the range of 30-45 µg/mL for twice-daily dosing Cephalosporins are not acceptable alternatives for patients allergic to penicillin
Staphylococcus aureus// Methicillin-sensitive	Nafcillin sodium or oxacillin sodium, 2.0 g i.v. every 4 hr for 4-6 wk *Plus* Gentamicin sulfate (optional),§ 1 mg/kg every 8 hr i.v. or i.m. for first 3-5 days. Benefit of additional aminoglycoside has not been established	Cefazolin (or other first-generation cephalosporins in equivalent dosages), 2 g i.v. every 8 hr for 4-6 wk *Plus* Gentamicin (optional),§ 1 mg/kg every 8 hr i.v. or i.m. for first 3-5 days Cephalosporins should be avoided in patients with immediate-type hypersensitivity to penicillin Vancomycin,† 30 mg/kg i.v. in two equally divided doses, not to exceed 2 g/24 hr unless serum levels are monitored for 4-6 wk Vancomycin therapy is recommended for

Table 14-9.—continued

Microorganisms	Therapy*	Alternative therapy*
		patients allergic to β-lactams (immediate-type hypersensitivity); serum concentration of vancomycin should be obtained 1 hr after completion of the infusion and should be in the range of 30-45 µg/mL for twice-daily dosing
Methicillin-resistant	Vancomycin,[†] 30 mg/kg i.v. in two equally divided doses, not to exceed 2 g/24 hr unless serum levels are monitored for 4-6 wk	Consult infectious diseases specialist
HACEK group	Ceftriaxone sodium, 2 g i.v. or i.m. for 4 wk[†] *Or* Ampicillin,[¶] 12 g/24 hr i.v. either continuously or in six divided doses for 4 wk *Plus* Gentamicin sulfate,[§] 1 mg/kg i.v. or i.m. every 8 hr for 4 wk Cefotaxime sodium or other third-generation cephalosporins may be substituted	Consult infectious diseases specialist
Neisseria gonorrhoeae	Ceftriaxone, 1-2 g every 24 hr for ≥4 wk	Aqueous crystalline penicillin G, 20 x 10[6] U/24 hr i.v. either continuously or in six equally divided doses for 4 wk, for penicillin-susceptible isolates
Gram-negative bacilli	Most effective single drug or combination of drugs i.v. for 4-6 wk	
Urgent empiric treatment for culture-negative endocarditis	Vancomycin,[†] 30 mg/kg i.v. in two equally divided doses, not to exceed 2 g/24 hr unless serum levels are monitored for 6 wk *Plus* Gentamicin sulfate,[‡] 1.0 mg/kg i.v. every 8 hr for 6 wk	
Fungal endocarditis	Amphotericin B *Plus* Flucytosine (optional) *Plus* Cardiac valve replacement (flucytosine levels should be monitored)	

*Dosages recommended are for patients with normal renal function. i.v., intravenous; i.m., intramuscular.

[†]Vancomycin dosage should be reduced in patients with impaired renal function. Vancomycin given on a mg/kg basis produces higher serum concentrations in obese patients than in lean patients. Therefore, in obese patients, dosing should be based on ideal body weight. Each dose of vancomycin should be infused over at least 1 hr to reduce the risk of the histamine-release "red man" syndrome.

[‡]Patients should be notified that i.m. injection of ceftriaxone is painful.

[§]Dosing of gentamicin on a mg/kg basis produces higher serum concentrations in obese patients than in lean patients. Therefore, in obese patients, dosing should be based on ideal body weight. (Ideal body weight for men is 50 kg + 2.3 kg per inch over 5 feet, and ideal body weight for women is 45.5 kg + 2.3 kg per inch over 5 feet.) Relative contraindications to the use of gentamicin are age older than 65 years, renal impairment, or impairment of the eighth nerve. Other potentially nephrotoxic agents (such as nonsteroidal anti-inflammatory drugs) should be used cautiously in patients receiving gentamicin.

[//]For treatment of endocarditis due to penicillin-susceptible staphylococci (MIC, < 0.1 µg/mL), aqueous crystalline penicillin G, 12-18 x 10[6] U/24 hr i.v. either continuously or in six equally divided doses for 4-6 wk can be used instead of nafcillin or oxacillin. Shorter antibiotic courses have been effective in some injection drug users with right-sided endocarditis due to *S. aureus*. The routine use of rifampin is not recommended for the treatment of native valve staphylococcal endocarditis.

[¶]Ampicillin should not be used if laboratory tests show β-lactamase production.

Abbreviations: HACEK, *Haemophilus* spp., *Actinobacillus actinomycetemcomitans, Cardiobacterium hominis, Eikenella* spp., and *Kingella kingae*; MIC, minimal inhibitory concentration.

Data from Wilson WR, Karchmer AW, Dajani AS, Taubert KA, Bayer A, Kaye D, Bisno AL, Ferrieri P, Shulman ST, Durack DT: Antibiotic treatment of adults with infective endocarditis due to streptococci, enterococci, staphylococci and HACEK microorganisms. JAMA 274:1706-1713, 1995; and Modified from Steckelberg JM, Giuliani ER, Wilson WR: Infective endocarditis. *In* Cardiology: Fundamentals and Practice. Vol. 2. Second edition. Edited by ER Giuliani, V Fuster, BJ Gersh, MD McGoon, DC McGoon. St. Louis, Mosby Year Book, 1991, pp 1739-1772. By permission of Mayo Foundation.

Table 14-10.—Organisms That Cause Prosthetic Valve Endocarditis

Organism	Onset, %		All, %
	Early	Late	
Coagulase-negative staphylococci	35	26	29
Staphylococcus aureus	17	12	14
Enterococci and group D streptococci	3	9	7
Streptococcus pneumoniae	1	<1	1
Other (i.e., viridans group streptococci)	4	25	17
Gram-negative bacilli	16	12	13
Diphtheroids	10	4	7
Other bacteria	1	2	2
Candida	8	4	5
Other fungi	1	<1	1
"Culture negative"	1	4	3

From Threlkeld MG, Cobbs CG: Infectious disorders of prosthetic valves and intravascular devices. *In* Principles and Practice of Infectious Diseases. Fourth edition. Edited by GL Mandell, JE Bennett, R Dolin. New York, Churchill Livingstone, 1995, pp 783-793. By permission of publisher.

Table 14-11.—Treatment of Prosthetic Valve Infective Endocarditis

Organism	Therapy*	Alternative therapy/comments
Staphylococcus aureus or coagulase-negative staphylococci Methicillin-resistant	Vancomycin,[†] 30 mg/kg i.v. in two equally divided doses, not to exceed 2 g/24 hr unless serum levels are monitored for ≥6 wk *Plus* Rifampin,[‡] 300 mg orally every 8 hr for ≥6 wk *Plus* Gentamicin sulfate,[§] 1 mg/kg i.v. or i.m. every 8 hr for first 2 wk of therapy. (If organism is not susceptible to gentamicin, ciprofloxacin may be substituted if the organism is susceptible in vitro)	Rifampin increases the amount of warfarin sodium required for anti-thrombotic therapy
Staphylococcus aureus or coagulase-negative staphylococci Methicillin-susceptible	Nafcillin sodium or oxacillin sodium, 2 g i.v. every 4 hr for ≥6 wk *Plus* Rifampin,[‡] 300 mg orally every 8 hr for ≥6 wk *Plus* Gentamicin sulfate,[§] 1 mg/kg i.v. or i.m. every 8 hr for first 2 wk of therapy. (If organism is not susceptible to gentamicin, ciprofloxacin may be substituted if the organism is susceptible in vitro)	Rifampin increases the amount of warfarin sodium required for anti-thrombotic therapy First-generation cephalosporins or vancomycin should be used in patients allergic to β-lactams Cephalosporins should be avoided in patients with immediate-type hypersensitivity to penicillin or to methicillin-resistant staphylococci

Table 14-11.—continued

Organism	Therapy*	Alternative therapy/comments
Enterococci (gentamicin- or vancomycin-susceptible) or viridans group streptococci or nutritionally variant streptococci or *Streptococcus bovis* (All streptococci causing endocarditis must be tested for antimicrobial susceptibility in order to select optimal therapy)	Aqueous crystalline penicillin G, 18-30 x 10^6 U/24 hr i.v. either continuously or in six equally divided doses for 4-6 wk *Or* Ampicillin sodium, 12 g/24 hr i.v. either continuously or in six equally divided doses *Plus* Gentamicin sulfate,§ 1 mg/kg i.v. or i.m. every 8 hr for 4-6 wk (4-week therapy recommended for patients with symptoms <3 months in duration; 6-week therapy recommended for patients with symptoms >3 months in duration)	Vancomycin,[†] 30 mg/kg i.v. in two equally divided doses, not to exceed 2 g/24 hr unless serum levels are monitored for 4-6 wk *Plus* Gentamicin sulfate,§ 1 mg/kg i.v. or i.m. every 8 hr for 4-6 wk Vancomycin therapy is recommended for patients allergic to β-lactams (immediate-type hypersensitivity); serum concentration of vancomycin should be obtained 1 hr after completion of the infusion and should be in the range of 30-45 µg/mL for twice-daily dosing Cephalosporins are not acceptable alternatives for patients allergic to penicillin

*Dosages recommended are for patients with normal renal function. i.v., intravenous; i.m., intramuscular.

[†]Vancomycin dosage should be reduced in patients with impaired renal function. Vancomycin given on a mg/kg basis produces higher serum concentrations in obese patients than in lean patients. Therefore, in obese patients, dosing should be based on ideal body weight. Each dose of vancomycin should be infused over at least 1 hr to reduce the risk of the histamine-release "red man" syndrome.

[‡]Rifampin plays a unique role in the eradication of staphylococcal infection involving prosthetic material; combination therapy is essential to prevent emergence of rifampin resistance.

§Dosing of gentamicin on a mg/kg basis will produce higher serum concentrations in obese patients than in lean patients. Therefore, in obese patients, dosing should be based on ideal body weight. (Ideal body weight for men is 50 kg + 2.3 kg per inch over 5 feet, and ideal body weight for women is 45.5 kg + 2.3 kg per inch over 5 feet.) Relative contraindications to the use of gentamicin are age older than 65 years, renal impairment, or impairment of the eighth nerve. Other potentially nephrotoxic agents (such as nonsteroidal anti-inflammatory drugs) should be used cautiously in patients receiving gentamicin.

Data from Wilson MR, Karchmer AW, Dajani AS, Taubert KA, Bayer A, Kaye D, Bisno AL, Ferrieri P, Shulman ST, Durack DT: Antibiotic treatment of adults with infective endocarditis due to streptococci, enterococci, staphylococci, and HACEK microorganisms. JAMA 274:1706-1713, 1995.

MENINGITIS

Bacterial Meningitis

The incidence of bacterial meningitis is estimated to be 3.0 cases/100,000 person-years. The overall case fatality rate was 25% in a recent report of 443 cases of bacterial meningitis in adults between 1962 and 1988. Forty percent of cases were nosocomial. Common predisposing conditions for community-acquired meningitis include acute otitis media, altered immune states, alcoholism, pneumonia, diabetes mellitus, sinusitis, and a cerebrospinal fluid leak. Risk factors for death among adults with community-acquired meningitis include age 60 years or older, obtundation on admission, and occurrence of seizures within 24 hours of symptom onset. In 66% of patients, fever, nuchal rigidity, and altered mental status are present (N Engl J Med 328:21-28, 1993).

Typical initial cerebrospinal fluid characteristics include a cell count of 1,000 to 5,000/µL (range, <100-10,000) and a glucose value less than 40 mg/dL or a cerebrospinal fluid-serum glucose ratio less than 0.31. The leukocyte differential is more likely to show a predominance of polymorphonuclear neutrophils. The Gram stain is positive in 60% to 90% of cases. Countercurrent immunoelectrophoresis or latex agglutination tests are useful for the detection of *Haemophilus influenzae* type B, *Streptococcus pneumoniae*, and *Neisseria meningitidis* types A, B, C, and Y, *Escherichia coli* K1, and group B streptococci. Cerebrospinal fluid cultures are positive in 85% to 90% of cases. Blood cultures often are positive. Polymerase chain reaction has been used to diagnose meningitis due to *Listeria monocytogenes* and *N. meningitidis*.

Organisms most commonly causing community-acquired meningitis in adults are *S. pneumoniae* (38%), *N. meningitidis* (14%), *L. monocytogenes* (11%), streptococci (7%),

Staphylococcus aureus (5%), *H. influenzae* (4%), and gram-negative bacilli (4%).

In some studies, dexamethasone has decreased the incidence of neurologic sequelae or sensorineural hearing loss in children with bacterial meningitis due to *H. influenzae*. Treatment with dexamethasone for bacterial meningitis in adults remains controversial. If administered, dexamethasone should be given before or with the first dose of antibacterial therapy.

- Risk factors for death in bacterial meningitis: age 60 years or older, decreased mental status at admission, seizures within 24 hours of symptom onset.
- Gram stains of cerebrospinal fluid are positive in 60%-90% of cases.
- Organisms most commonly causing community-acquired infection in adults: *S. pneumoniae, N. meningitidis, H. influenzae, L. monocytogenes*.

The causative organisms, affected age groups, and predisposing factors in bacterial meningitis are shown in Table 14-12, and empiric treatment in various age and patient groups is outlined in Table 14-13.

Meningococcal Meningitis

Meningitis often occurs in patients who are carriers of meningococci in the nasopharynx. Terminal component complement deficiencies predispose to repeated episodes of infection. Serotypes A, B, C, and Y cause most disease. Many patients have a petechial rash. The pathogenesis of Waterhouse-Friderichsen syndrome is related to disseminated intravascular coagulation. Treatment is with penicillin G. If a patient is allergic to penicillin, ceftriaxone or cefotaxime can be used. If the risk of the carrier state is high (close contacts of the index case, hospital workers with significant respiratory exposure), chemoprophylaxis should be given. Rifampin, minocycline, ciprofloxacin (use only in patients 18 years or older), and ceftriaxone have been used. The carrier state is not eliminated by penicillin. Immunization for certain populations (such as military recruits, epidemics) is also of benefit.

- In meningococcal meningitis, terminal component complement deficiencies predispose to repeated episodes of infection.
- If the risk of the carrier state is high (household contacts), rifampin or minocycline should be used for prophylaxis.

Aseptic Meningitis

This is a syndrome characterized by an acute onset of meningeal symptoms, fever, cerebrospinal fluid pleocytosis (usually lymphocytes), and negative bacterial cultures from the cerebrospinal fluid. There are many infectious and noninfectious causes, but most often the cause is viral. Viral menin-gitis is usually a self-limited illness. Common causes include enteroviruses (most common in summer; cause 80%-85% of cases in which a pathogen is identified), mumps virus (most common in winter and spring; decreased incidence with use of vaccine), and others, including arboviruses, lymphocytic chori-omeningitis virus (contact with rodents), herpes simplex virus types 1 and 2, human herpes viruses 6 and 7, cytomegalovirus, human immunodeficiency virus, varicella-zoster virus, Epstein-Barr virus, and Colorado tick fever virus.

- Characteristics of aseptic meningitis: meningeal symptoms, fever, cerebrospinal fluid pleocytosis, negative bacterial cultures.
- Cause is most often viral, but there are many infectious and noninfectious causes.
- Viral meningitis is usually self-limited.

SEXUALLY TRANSMITTED DISEASES

Neisseria gonorrhoeae

Common uncomplicated infections include urethritis and cervicitis. Symptoms are indistinguishable from those of nongonococcal disease. Gram stain and culture or detection by molecular detection formats is required for diagnosis. The asymptomatic carrier state occurs in both males and females, but it is more common in females. Asymptomatic carriers are primarily responsible for continued transmission of the infection. In females, concomitant proctitis is common (rectal cultures should be done in all women). Gonococcal pharyngitis is often asymptomatic. Coexistence of chlamydial infection is common (both conditions should be treated). For diagnosis, in males, a Gram stain of urethral exudate showing intracellular gram-negative diplococci has high sensitivity and specificity. Gram staining of cervical exudate has a sensitivity of only 50%, but the specificity is high. Definitive diagnosis requires culture on modified Thayer-Martin medium.

- *N. gonorrhoeae* commonly causes urethritis, cervicitis, pharyngitis, and proctitis.
- Asymptomatic carrier rate occurs in both males and females, but it is more common in females.

The prevalence of multiply resistant gonococcal strains is increasing. Resistance to penicillin and tetracycline is frequent, and quinolone resistance is rare but is increasing. Primary treatment is ceftriaxone (125 mg intramuscularly) or appropriate doses of cefixime, ciprofloxacin, or ofloxacin plus doxycycline (100 mg orally twice a day for 7 days) or azithromycin (a single 1-g dose). Alternative drugs include spectinomycin and other oral and injectable cephalosporins and fluoroquinolones. Pharyngeal infection is best treated

Table 14-12.—Organisms Involved, Affected Age Groups, and Predisposing Factors in Bacterial Meningitis

Organism	Age group	Comment	Predisposing factors
Streptococcus pneumoniae	Any age, but often elderly	Most common cause of recurrent meningitis in adults	Cerebrospinal fluid leak, alcoholism, splenectomy, functional asplenia, multiple myeloma, hypogammaglobulinemia, Hodgkin disease, HIV*
Neisseria meningitidis	Infants to 40 yr	Petechial rash is common. Epidemics occur in closed populations	Terminal component complement deficiency
Haemophilus influenzae type B	>Neonate to 6 yr	Significant decrease in incidence since licensure of *H. influenzae* B vaccine	Hypogammaglobulinemia in adults, HIV,* splenectomy, functional asplenia
Escherichia coli, group B streptococci	Neonates		Maternal colonization
Gram-negative bacilli	Any age	*Staphylococcus aureus* and coagulase-negative staphylococci also common after neuro-surgical procedure	Neurosurgical procedures, bacteremia due to urinary tract infection, pneumonia, etc., *Strongyloides* hyperinfection syndrome
Listeria monocytogenes	Neonates; immuno-suppressed		

*HIV, human immunodeficiency virus.

Table 14-13.—Empiric Therapy for Bacterial Meningitis

Age group/patient group	Common pathogens	Antimicrobial therapy
0-4 weeks	Group B streptococci, *Escherichia coli*, *Listeria monocytogenes*, *Klebsiella pneumoniae*, *Enterococcus* spp., *Salmonella* spp.	Ampicillin plus cefotaxime or ampicillin plus an aminoglycoside
4-12 weeks	Group B streptococci, *E. coli*, *L. monocytogenes*, *Haemophilus influenzae*, *Streptococcus pneumoniae*, *Neisseria meningitidis*	Ampicillin plus cefotaxime or ceftriaxone
3 months-18 yr	*H. influenzae*, *N. meningitidis*, *S. pneumoniae*	Cefotaxime or ceftriaxone or ampicillin plus chloramphenicol
18-50 yr*	*H. influenzae*, *S. pneumoniae*	Cefotaxime or ceftriaxone ± ampicillin
Immunocompromised host	*S. pneumoniae*, *N. meningitidis*, *L. monocytogenes*, aerobic gram-negative bacilli (including *Pseudomonas aeruginosa*)	Vancomycin plus ampicillin plus ceftazidime
Basilar skull fracture	*S. pneumoniae*, *H. influenzae*, group A β-hemolytic streptococci	Cefotaxime or ceftriaxone
Post-neurosurgery	Coagulase-negative staphylococci, *Staphylococcus aureus*, aerobic gram-negative bacilli (including *P. aeruginosa*)	Vancomycin plus ceftazidime

*Vancomycin should be added to empiric therapeutic regimens when highly penicillin-resistant or cephalosporin-resistant strains of *S. pneumoniae* are suspected.
Modified from Tunkel AR, Schield WM: Central nervous system infections. *In* A Practical Approach to Infectious Diseases. Fourth edition. Edited by RE Reese, RF Betts. New York, Little Brown, 1996, pp 133-183. By permission of publisher.

with ceftriaxone, ciprofloxacin, or ofloxacin. Spectinomycin, ciprofloxacin, and ofloxacin may not be active against incubating syphilis. Therapy in pregnant patients involves ceftriaxone (125 mg intramuscularly) plus erythromycin (500 mg orally four times a day for 7 days). Follow-up gonococcal cultures need to be performed only if nonstandard regimens are used. All patients with sexually transmitted diseases should be considered at risk for human immunodeficiency virus (HIV) infection and testing should be offered. Sexual partners should be offered evaluation and treatment.

- Primary treatment of *N. gonorrhoeae*: ceftriaxone (125 mg intramuscularly) plus doxycycline (100 mg orally twice a day for 7 days) or azithromycin as a single 1-g dose.

Disseminated gonococcemia occurs in 1% to 3% of infected patients and is most likely to occur in females during menstruation (sloughing of endometrium allows access to blood supply, enhanced growth of gonococci due to necrotic tissue, and change in pH). There are two distinct phases. The bacteremic phase may manifest as tenosynovitis (often around the wrists or ankles), skin lesions (usually less than 30 in number), and polyarthralgias. Results of synovial fluid are usually negative. The nonbacteremic phase follows in approximately 1 week and may present as monarticular arthritis of the knee, wrist, and ankle; results of joint culture are positive in ± 50%. Culture specimens should be obtained from the urethra, cervix, rectum, and pharynx.

- Disseminated gonococcemia is most likely to occur in females during menstruation.
- Bacteremic phase may manifest as tenosynovitis, skin lesions, and arthralgias; joint cultures usually negative.
- Nonbacteremic phase may present as monarticular arthritis of knee, wrist, ankle; positive results of joint cultures in ± 50%.

Treatment is with ceftriaxone (1 g intravenously daily for 7-10 days); alternatives include ceftriaxone (for 3 or 4 days or until improvement is noted) followed by cefixime or ciprofloxacin to complete a course of 7 to 10 days. If the strain is tested and found to be penicillin-susceptible, treatment includes penicillin G (10 million units intravenously daily) for 7 to 10 days, or it is given for 3 or 4 days and then oral amoxicillin is used to finish a 7- to 10-day course. If the patient is allergic to cephalosporins, spectinomycin, ciprofloxacin, or ofloxacin can be given. Chlamydial infection can coexist with gonococcal infection and should be treated. For meningitis, treatment includes ceftriaxone (1 to 2 g intravenously every 12 hours for at least 10 to 14 days). Alternative drugs are penicillin, if the strain is susceptible,

or chloramphenicol. For endocarditis, ceftriaxone or penicillin is used for at least 28 days.

- Treatment of disseminated gonococcal infection: ceftriaxone (1 g intravenously daily for 7-10 days).
- Chlamydial infections can coexist with gonococcal infection and should be treated.

Nongonococcal Urethritis and Cervicitis

The most common etiologic agent is *Chlamydia trachomatis*. Infection is often asymptomatic. Diagnosis can be made with culture, antigen detection, or molecular detection formats. Doxycycline (100 mg twice a day for 7 days) or azithromycin as a single 1-g dose is standard treatment. *Trichomonas vaginalis, Mycoplasma genitalium,* and herpes simplex virus are less common causes of nongonococcal urethritis. If urethritis does not resolve and reinfection or relapse of a chlamydial infection has been excluded, consider *Trichomonas* or *Ureaplasma* infection, among others.

- Nongonococcal urethritis and cervicitis are most commonly caused by *C. trachomatis*.

Herpes Genitalis

Seventy percent to 90% of cases are caused by herpes simplex virus type 2. For the first episode, therapy with acyclovir (400 mg orally three times a day or 200 mg orally five times a day for 7-10 days) or famciclovir (250 mg orally three times a day or valacyclovir 1 g orally twice a day) shortens the duration of pain, viral shedding, and systemic symptoms. If symptoms are severe, acyclovir at a dosage of 5 mg/kg intravenously every 8 hours for 5 to 7 days is used. Topical acyclovir has marginal benefit for decreasing viral shedding and has no effect on symptoms or healing time. For recurrent episodes with severe symptoms, therapy can be started at prodrome or within 1 day of the onset of symptoms (acyclovir, 400 mg orally three times a day, 200 mg orally five times a day, or 800 mg orally twice a day, or famciclovir, 125 mg orally twice a day, or valacyclovir, 500 mg orally twice a day, all for 5 days). Recurrence after therapy is usually not related to the development of in vitro resistance of herpes simplex to acyclovir. For suppression, in selected patients with more than six recurrences a year, acyclovir (400 mg twice a day), famciclovir (250 mg orally twice a day), or valacyclovir (250 mg, 500 mg, or 1 g orally twice a day) is used for up to 1 year.

Syphilis

The etiologic agent of syphilis is *Treponema pallidum*. The incidence of syphilis increased between 1985 and 1990 but has decreased since that time. It is estimated that half of the cases are not reported. The incidence of syphilis is increased in large cities among sexually active persons, particularly among inner city minority populations.

The fluorescent treponemal antibody absorption (FTA-ABS) test is the most helpful serologic test for the diagnosis of syphilis (Table 14-14). Results of this test are positive before those on VDRL testing, and thus they may be positive without a positive VDRL result in primary syphilis.

- FTA-ABS is the most helpful serologic test for the diagnosis of syphilis.
- VDRL results may be negative in 30% of patients with primary syphilis.

A chancre (clean, indurated ulcer) is the main manifestation of *primary syphilis*. It occurs at the site of inoculation and is usually painless. The incubation period is 3 to 90 days. It should be distinguished from herpes simplex virus and chancroid (painful exudative ulcer, *Haemophilus ducreyi*). Diagnosis is made by dark field examination.

The manifestations of *secondary syphilis* result from hematogenous dissemination and usually occur 2 to 8 weeks after appearance of the chancre. Constitutional symptoms occur, in addition to rash, mucocutaneous lesions, alopecia, condylomata lata, lymphadenopathy, and various other symptoms and signs. The diagnosis is based on the clinical picture and serologic testing. The condition resolves spontaneously without treatment.

Latent syphilis is the asymptomatic stage after symptoms of secondary syphilis subside. Those that occur after 1 year are classified as late. The diagnosis is based on serologic testing. A cerebrospinal fluid examination before treatment in patients with latent syphilis is indicated in those with neurologic or ophthalmologic abnormalities, in patients with other evidence of active syphilis, before re-treatment of relapses, and in patients with HIV infection.

Tertiary syphilis can involve all body systems (cardiovascular—aortitis involving the ascending aorta, which can cause aneurysms and aortic regurgitation; gummatous osteomyelitis; hepatitis). However, neurosyphilis is the most common manifestation in the United States.

Neurosyphilis is often asymptomatic. Symptomatic disease is divided into several clinical syndromes that may overlap and occur at any time after primary infection. The diagnosis is made from cerebrospinal fluid examination; abnormalities include mononuclear pleocytosis and an increased protein value. VDRL testing of cerebrospinal fluid is only 30% to 70% sensitive. The FTA-ABS test on cerebrospinal fluid is highly sensitive but not specific. Any cerebrospinal fluid abnormality in a patient who is seropositive for syphilis must be investigated. Syndromes include 1) meningovascular syphilis (occurs 4-7 years after infection and presents with focal central nervous system deficits such as stroke or cranial nerve abnormalities) and 2) parenchymatous syphilis (general paresis or tabes dorsalis). Parenchymatous syphilis occurs decades after infection and may present as general paresis (chronic progressive dementia) or as tabes dorsalis (sensory ataxia, lightning pains, autonomic dysfunction, optic atrophy).

- Neurosyphilis is the most common manifestation (in tertiary disease) in the United States.
- Diagnosis is made from cerebrospinal fluid examination.
- VDRL testing of cerebrospinal fluid is only 30%-70% sensitive.

Treatment of syphilis is based on whether the disease is early or late. For early syphilis (primary, secondary, or early latent [<1 year]), benzathine penicillin is used—2.4 million units intramuscularly; follow-up serologic testing is done. (Some experts recommend a second dose in 7 days in patients with HIV infection.) Alternatives are doxycycline (100 mg twice a day for 14 days) or tetracycline (500 mg orally four times a day for 14 days). Erythromycin (500 mg orally four times a day) is less effective.

Treatment for late disease (>1 year in duration, cardiovascular disease, gumma, late latent syphilis) is with benzathine penicillin, 2.4 million units intramuscularly weekly for 3 weeks. Alternatives are doxycycline (100 mg orally twice a day) or tetracycline (500 mg orally four times a day) for 4 weeks.

Treatment for neurosyphilis is with aqueous penicillin G (12-24 million units intravenously per day for 10-14 days), or procaine penicillin (2.4 million units intramuscularly per day) plus probenecid (500 mg four times a day) for 10 to 14 days.

For early and secondary syphilis, follow-up clinical and serologic testing should be performed at 6 and 12 months. Retreatment with three weekly injections of 2.4 million units of benzathine penicillin G should be given to patients with

Table 14-14.—Laboratory Diagnosis of Syphilis

| Syphilis | Test, % positive | | |
	VDRL*	FTA-ABS[†]	MHA-TP[‡]
Primary	70	85	50-60
Secondary	99	100	100
Tertiary	70	98	98

*VDRL, Venereal Disease Research Laboratories.
[†]FTA-ABS, fluorescent treponemal antibody absorption.
[‡]MHA-TP, Microhemagglutination assay for *Treponema pallidum*.
From Hook EW III: Syphilis. *In* Cecil Textbook of Internal Medicine. Twentieth edition. Edited by JE Bennett, F Plum. Philadelphia, WB Saunders, 1996, pp 1705-1714. By permission of publisher.

signs or symptoms that persist or whose VDRL result has a sustained fourfold increase in titer. HIV testing should be performed if not done previously. If the VDRL titer does not decrease fourfold by 6 months, consideration also should be given to re-treatment.

Patients with latent syphilis should have a follow-up examination at 6, 12, and 24 months. If the VDRL result increases fourfold, if a high titer (>1:32) fails to decrease fourfold within 12 to 24 months, or if signs or symptoms attributable to syphilis occur, the patient should be examined for neurosyphilis and re-treated.

Follow-up in cases of neurosyphilis should include testing of cerebrospinal fluid every 6 months if cerebrospinal fluid pleocytosis was present initially; this testing is done until results are normal. If the cell count is not decreased at 6 months or if the cerebrospinal fluid is not entirely normal at 2 years, retreatment should be considered.

Pelvic Inflammatory Disease

In this condition, proximal spread of infection from the endocervix causes endometritis, salpingitis, tubo-ovarian abscess, or pelvic peritonitis in various combinations. Organisms responsible are *N. gonorrhoeae, C. trachomatis, Mycoplasma hominis,* and various aerobic gram-negative rods and anaerobes. *Actinomyces israelii* can be a pathogen in patients with an intrauterine device. Tuberculosis in older women, including postmenopausal women, should be considered. Clinical signs and symptoms include lower abdominal tenderness, adnexal tenderness, cervical motion tenderness, oral temperature more than 38.3°C, abnormal cervical discharge, increased erythrocyte sedimentation rate, and evidence of *N. gonorrhoeae* or *C. trachomatis* infection. Laboratory evidence includes laparoscopic or ultrasound documentation.

- In pelvic inflammatory disease, responsible organisms are *N. gonorrhoeae, C. trachomatis,* and anaerobes.
- The emphasis on early diagnosis is meant to decrease the incidence of infertility as a complication of pelvic inflammatory disease.

Treatment for inpatients includes cefoxitin (2 g intravenously every 6 hours) or cefotetan (2 g intravenously every 12 hours) or clindamycin and gentamicin plus doxycycline (100 mg intravenously every 12 hours) followed by doxycycline (100 mg orally twice a day) for 14 days. For outpatients, treatment is with ofloxacin (400 mg orally twice a day) plus metronidazole (500 mg orally twice a day) or ceftriaxone (250 mg intramuscularly once) or cefoxitin (2 g intramuscularly plus probenecid, 1 g orally as a single dose daily once, or another third-generation cephalosporin) plus doxycycline (100 mg orally twice a day) for 14 days.

Hospitalization is indicated when the outpatient therapy is precluded by severe nausea and vomiting, the diagnosis is uncertain, pelvic abscess or peritonitis is present, the patient is pregnant, the patient is an adolescent, HIV infection is present, or noncompliance is suspected.

Tubo-ovarian abscess may be characterized by an adnexal mass on physical examination or radiographic examination or by failure of antimicrobial therapy. Medical treatment is successful in 50% of cases. Careful follow-up is required.

- Tubo-ovarian abscess is characterized by an adnexal mass on physical examination or radiographic examination or by failure of antimicrobial therapy.

Trichomonas vaginalis

Infection with this organism produces a yellow, purulent discharge in 5% to 40% of cases. Dysuria and dyspareunia occur in 30% to 50% of cases. Petechial lesions on the cervix are noted with colposcopy (strawberry cervix) in 50% of cases. The vaginal pH is usually more than 4.5. The diagnosis is established with wet mount preparation of vaginal secretion (80% sensitive). Culture is done in difficult cases. Treatment is with metronidazole (2 g as a single dose or 500 mg twice a day for 7 days). All partners should be examined and treated if necessary.

- *T. vaginalis* infection often is characterized by yellow, purulent discharge.
- Diagnosis is established with wet mount of vaginal secretion.
- Treatment: metronidazole orally.

Gardnerella vaginalis (Bacterial Vaginosis)

This condition is characterized by a malodorous "fishy" smell and a grayish white discharge that is homogeneous and coats the vaginal walls. Dysuria and pain are relatively uncommon. Organisms associated with the syndrome are *Mobiluncus* spp., *M. hominis, G. vaginalis,* and *Prevotella* spp. The diagnosis is determined by excluding *Candida* and *Trichomonas* infections and other sexually transmitted diseases. The following are characteristics of the vaginal secretion: demonstration of "clue" cells on wet mount examination, pH more than 4.5 and often more than 6.0, and a "fishy" smell when secretion is mixed with KOH. Recommended treatment regimens include metronidazole (500 mg orally twice a day for 2 days) or topical clindamycin cream or metronidazole gel. A single 2-g dose of metronidazole or clindamycin, 300 mg orally twice a day for 7 days, is an alternative. Treatment of asymptomatic carriers is not recommended.

- Diagnosis of *G. vaginalis* is established by excluding *Candida, Trichomonas,* and other sexually transmitted diseases.

- Vaginal discharge has "clue" cells and a "fishy" smell when mixed with 10% KOH and has a pH more than 4.5.

Vulvovaginal Candidiasis

The predominant symptom of this condition is pruritus. It is typically caused by *C. albicans*. Seventy-five percent of women will have one episode and 40% to 45%, two or more episodes. Usually there is no odor, and discharge is scant, watery, and white. "Cottage cheese curds" may adhere to the vaginal wall. The diagnosis is made by the addition of 10% KOH to the discharge to demonstrate pseudohyphae. Culture may detect an asymptomatic carrier. Treatment is with various topical agents from 1 to 7 days, depending on the dose and agent. Single-dose fluconazole therapy also is available, although the cost and potential toxicities of the oral azoles must be considered. Multiple-dose oral azole therapy also is used for severe, refractory cases. In severe or recurrent cases, consider HIV infection or drug-resistant candidal species.

- In vulvovaginal candidiasis, "cottage cheese curds" may adhere to the vaginal wall.
- In severe or recurrent cases, consider HIV infection.

Epididymitis

This condition usually is unilateral. It should be distinguished from testicular torsion. In young, sexually active men, *C. trachomatis* and *N. gonorrhoeae* are the common pathogens. In older men, aerobic gram-negative rods and enterococci predominate. Urologic abnormality is more common in this population than in younger men. Doxycycline, 100 mg orally twice a day for 7 days, plus ceftriaxone, 250 mg intramuscularly, is the treatment of choice in young males. In older men, treatment is individualized on the basis of results of urine Gram stain, results of culture, local susceptibility patterns, and presence of recent instrumentation.

- Epididymitis is usually unilateral; should be distinguished from testicular torsion.
- In young, sexually active men, *C. trachomatis* and *N. gonorrhoeae* are the common pathogens.

GASTROINTESTINAL INFECTION

Bacterial Diarrhea

The principal causes of toxigenic diarrhea are listed in Table 14-15, and those of invasive diarrhea are listed in Table 14-16. Fecal leukocytes usually are absent in toxigenic diarrhea. In invasive diarrhea, fecal leukocytes usually are present. The travel history is often important.

Campylobacter jejuni is being recognized with increasing frequency as a common cause of bacterial diarrhea. Outbreaks are associated with consumption of unpasteurized dairy products and undercooked poultry. The incidence of disease peaks in summer and early fall. Diarrhea may be bloody. Fever usually is present. The diagnosis is established by isolation of the organism from stool; a special medium is required. Treatment is with erythromycin. Alternatives are ciprofloxacin and norfloxacin (emergence of resistance to fluoroquinolones has been reported). Supportive care also is needed.

- Outbreaks of bacterial diarrhea caused by *C. jejuni* are associated with consumption of unpasteurized milk and undercooked poultry.

In bacterial diarrhea caused by *Staphylococcus aureus*, preformed toxin is ingested in contaminated food. Onset is abrupt, with severe vomiting (often predominates), diarrhea, and abdominal cramps. The duration of infection is 8 to 24 hours. Diagnosis is based on *rapid onset*, absence of fever, and history. Treatment is supportive.

- Bacterial diarrhea due to *S. aureus* is caused by ingestion of preformed toxin in contaminated food.

Bacterial diarrhea caused by *Clostridium perfringens* is associated with ingestion of bacteria that produce toxin in vivo, often in improperly prepared or stored precooked foods (meat and poultry products). Food is precooked and toxin is destroyed but spores survive; when food is rewarmed, spores germinate. When food is ingested, toxin is produced. Diarrhea is worse than vomiting, and abdominal cramping is prominent. Onset of symptoms is later than with *S. aureus* infection. Duration of illness is 24 hours. The diagnosis is based on the later onset of symptoms, a typical history, and Gram staining or culture of incriminated foods. Treatment is supportive.

- In diarrhea caused by *C. perfringens*, ingested bacteria produce toxin in vivo in precooked food.
- Diarrhea is worse than vomiting; abdominal cramping is prominent.

Two types of food poisoning are associated with *Bacillus cereus* infection. A short incubation period (1 to 6 hours) is followed by profuse vomiting; this is associated with the ingestion of a preformed toxin (usually in fried rice). A disease with a longer incubation occurs 8 to 16 hours after consumption; profound diarrhea develops and usually is associated with eating meat or vegetables. The diagnosis is confirmed by isolation of the organism from contaminated food. The illness is self-limited and treatment is supportive.

Diarrhea caused by *Escherichia coli* can be either enterotox-

Table 14-15.—Bacterial Diarrhea: Toxigenic

Organism	Onset after ingestion, hr	Preformed toxin	Fever present	Vomiting predominates
Staphylococcus aureus	2-6	Yes	No	Yes
Clostridium perfringens	8-16	No	No	No
Escherichia coli	12	No	No	No
Vibrio cholerae	12	No	Due to dehydration	No
Bacillus cereus				
a.	1-6	Yes	No	Yes
b.	8-16	No	No	No

Table 14-16.—Bacterial Diarrhea: Invasive

Organism	Fever present	Bloody diarrhea present	Antibiotics effective
Shigella species	Yes	Yes	Yes
Salmonella (non-*typhi*)	Yes	No	No
Vibrio parahaemolyticus	Yes	Yes (occasional)	No
Escherichia coli O157:H7	Yes	Yes	No
Campylobacter	Yes	Yes	Yes
Yersinia	Yes	Yes (occasional)	±

igenic or enterohemorrhagic. Enterotoxigenic *E. coli* is the most common etiologic agent in traveler's diarrhea. Treatment consists of fluid and electrolyte replacement along with loperamide plus trimethoprim-sulfamethoxazole, ciprofloxacin, or norfloxacin. Medical evaluation should be sought if fever and bloody diarrhea occur. For prophylaxis, water, fruits, and vegetables need to be chosen carefully. Routine use of trimethoprim-sulfamethoxazole, ciprofloxacin, and doxycycline is not recommended because the risks outweigh the benefits in most travelers. Bismuth subsalicylate reduces the incidence of enterotoxigen *E. coli*-associated diarrhea by up to 60%. Patients who are allergic to salicylates or who are taking therapeutic doses of salicylates or anticoagulants should not use bismuth subsalicylate.

- Enterotoxigenic *E. coli* is the most common etiologic agent in traveler's diarrhea.

A relatively uncommon form of bloody diarrhea is caused by *E. coli* O157:H7. This agent has been identified as the cause of waterborne illness, outbreaks in nursing homes and child care centers, and sporadic cases. It also has been transmitted by eating undercooked beef. This enterohemorrhagic illness is characterized by bloody diarrhea, severe abdominal

cramps, fever, and profound toxicity. It may resemble ischemic colitis. At extremes of age (old and young), the infection may produce hemolytic-uremic syndrome, thrombocytopenic purpura, and death. This organism should be considered in all patients with hemolytic-uremic syndrome. Antibiotics are not known to be effective.

- *E. coli* O157:H7 has been identified as the cause of waterborne illness, outbreaks in nursing homes and child care centers, and sporadic cases.
- *E. coli* is also transmitted by eating undercooked beef.
- Characterized by bloody diarrhea, severe abdominal cramps, profound toxicity; may resemble ischemic colitis.
- Infection should be considered in all patients with hemolytic-uremic syndrome.

Vibrio cholerae causes the only toxigenic bacterial diarrheal disease in which antibiotics (tetracycline) clearly shorten the duration of disease. However, fluid replacement therapy is the mainstay of management. It is associated with consumption of undercooked shellfish. Recently, there was an epidemic in Peru and other parts of South America, and cases in the United States have occurred because of this epidemic.

Diarrhea caused by *Shigella* species is often acquired outside the United States. It often is spread by person-to-person transmission but also has been associated with eating contaminated food or water. Bloody diarrhea is characteristic, bacteremia may occur, and fever is present. The diagnosis is based on results of stool culture and blood culture (occasionally positive). Treatment is with ampicillin (ampicillin-resistant strains are common), trimethoprim-sulfamethoxazole (in some countries, increasing resistance is being reported), norfloxacin, or ciprofloxacin. The illness may precede the onset of Reiter syndrome. Neurotoxin may cause seizures in pediatric patients.

- Diarrhea caused by *Shigella* species is associated with person-to-person transmission and the consumption of contaminated food or water.
- Bloody diarrhea is characteristic, bacteremia may occur, and fever is present.
- Illness may precede onset of Reiter syndrome.

Salmonella (non-*typhi*)-associated illness most commonly is caused by *Salmonella enteritidis* and *Salmonella typhimurium* in the United States. It is associated with consumption of contaminated foods or with exposure to pet turtles, ducklings, and iguanas. *Salmonella* infection is a common cause of severe diarrhea and may cause septicemia in patients with acquired immunodeficiency syndrome (AIDS). Fever is usually present, and bloody diarrhea is often absent (a characteristic distinguishing it from *Shigella* infection). The diagnosis is based on stool culture. Treatment is supportive. Antibiotics only prolong the carrier state and do not affect the course of the disease. Antibiotics are used if results of blood culture are positive. Reactive arthritis may be a complication of this illness.

- *Salmonella* infection is common cause of severe diarrhea.
- May cause septicemia in patients with AIDS.
- Bloody diarrhea is often absent (feature distinguishing it from *Shigella* infection).

Vibrio parahaemolyticus infection is acquired by eating undercooked shellfish. It is a common bacterial cause of acute food-borne illness in Japan and is appearing with increasing frequency in the United States (Atlantic Gulf Coast and on cruise ships). Acute onset of explosive, watery diarrhea and fever are characteristic. The diagnosis is determined with stool culture. Antibiotic therapy is not required.

- *V. parahaemolyticus* infection is acquired by eating undercooked shellfish.
- Acute onset of watery diarrhea and fever are characteristic.
- Antibiotic therapy is not required.

Clinical syndromes associated with *Vibrio vulnificus* include bacteremia, gastroenteritis, and cellulitis. Most patients with bacteremia have distinctive bullous skin lesions and underlying hepatic disease (cirrhosis). The condition is associated with consumption of raw oysters. The mortality rate is high. Wound infections occur in patients who have had contact with seawater, such as with fishing injuries or contamination of wound with seawater. Affected patients have intense pain and cellulitis in the extremities. Gastrointestinal illness is associated with consumption of raw oysters. The incubation period is approximately 18 hours. Vomiting, diarrhea, and severe abdominal cramps are features. Treatment is with tetracycline or chloramphenicol.

- *V. vulnificus* bacteremia can cause distinctive bullous skin lesions and occurs in patients who are immunocompromised or have cirrhosis.
- Associated with consumption of raw oysters.

Yersinia enterocolitica is the etiologic agent of four major clinical syndromes. Acquisition of infection is thought to be associated with eating contaminated food products. The organism has been cultured from chocolate milk, meat, mussels, poultry, oysters, and cheese. Recently, the illness was associated with transfusion-related bacteremia.

The four syndromes that result from *Y. enterocolitica* infection are as follows:

1. Enterocolitis is the most common, especially in young children. Diarrhea is bloody in 25% of cases. Infection itself is limited. Antibiotic therapy is not necessary.
2. Mesenteric adenitis (pseudoappendicitis syndrome) develops in older children and young adults. Antibiotic therapy is not helpful.
3. Postinfectious syndromes usually occur in adults; these include erythema nodosum, polyarthritis, and Reiter syndrome. Postinfectious syndromes usually begin 1 to 2 weeks after gastrointestinal symptoms. The polyarthritis often includes weight-bearing joints (knees and ankles). Symptoms may last 1 to 4 months or longer. HLA-B27 antigen may be positive in patients with polyarthritis or Reiter syndrome but is not associated with erythema nodosum. Cultures of synovial fluid are negative. Diagnosis is by stool culture or serologic testing.
4. Bacteremia is associated with contaminated blood products and alcoholism. Many patients have underlying disease such as cirrhosis. Treatment with trimethoprim-sulfamethoxazole, tetracycline, gentamicin, ciprofloxacin, and third-generation cephalosporins has been effective.

- In adults with *Y. enterocolitica* infection, erythema nodosum, polyarthritis, and Reiter syndrome can develop.

Colitis caused by *Clostridium difficile* should be distinguished from other forms of antibiotic-associated diarrhea (watery stools, no systemic symptoms, negative tests for *C. difficile* toxin). Symptoms often occur 2 to 4 weeks after stopping use of antibiotics. The illness is associated with antibiotic exposure in 99% of cases (any antibiotic can cause it). Nosocomial spread has been documented. Typical features are profuse, watery stools; crampy abdominal pain; constitutional illness; the presence of fecal leukocytes; and a positive *C. difficile* toxin. In toxin-negative disease, proctoscopy or flexible sigmoidoscopy can be used to look for pseudomembranes. Disease can be localized to the cecum (postoperative patient with ileus) and can present as fever of unknown origin. Treatment consists of vancomycin (125 mg orally four times a day for 7-10 days) or metronidazole (250-500 mg orally three or four times a day for 7-10 days). The emergence of vancomycin-resistant enterococci and cost differences favor the use of metronidazole as a first-line agent in most circumstances. Antiperistalsis drugs should not be used. If a patient is unable to take drugs orally, intravenous metronidazole (not vancomycin) or vancomycin enemas can be used. Relapse is frequent and requires re-treatment. Treatment of asymptomatic carriers to decrease the nosocomial spread of infection or to reduce the risk of pseudomembranous colitis is not recommended.

- Colitis caused by *C. difficile* often occurs 2-4 weeks after stopping use of antibiotics.
- Illness is associated with antibiotic exposure in 99% of cases (any antibiotic can cause it).
- Features: profuse, watery stools; crampy abdominal pain; constitutional illness; fecal leukocytes; and a positive *C. difficile* toxin.
- Treatment: vancomycin (125 mg orally four times a day for 7-10 days) or metronidazole (250-500 mg orally three or four times a day for 7-10 days).
- Relapse is frequent (about 15% of cases).

Viral Diarrhea

Rotavirus infection is the most common cause of sporadic mild diarrhea illness in children. It may be spread from children to adults. It usually occurs during the winter. Vomiting is a more common early manifestation than watery diarrhea. Hospitalization for dehydration is common in young children. Diagnosis is made by detection of antigen in stool. Treatment is symptomatic.

Norwalk virus is a common cause of epidemic diarrhea and "winter vomiting disease" in older children and adults. It occurs in families, communities, and institutions. Outbreaks have been associated with eating shellfish, undercooked fish, cake frosting, and salads and with drinking contaminated water. It is the cause of up to 10% of gastroenteritis outbreaks. Illness is characterized by nausea, vomiting, and watery diarrhea. It is a mild, self-limited (<36 hours) illness.

Currently, no diagnostic test is available. Treatment is symptomatic.

- Outbreaks of Norwalk virus are associated with eating shellfish, undercooked fish, cake frosting, and salads and with drinking contaminated water.
- Illness is mild and self-limited (<36 hours).

BACTEREMIA, SEPSIS, AND SEPTIC SHOCK

Bacteremia, or bloodstream infection in general, is defined as the presence of living bacteria or other organisms in the blood and is established by a positive blood culture or other microbiologic techniques. The systemic inflammatory response syndrome (SIRS) is characterized by a group of physiologic responses due to several infectious and noninfectious causes. If SIRS is caused by an infection, then sepsis is said to be present. Some of the common manifestations of SIRS or sepsis include tachypnea, tachycardia, irritability, lethargy, fever or hypothermia, hypoxemia, and leukocytosis. Septic shock is sepsis with hypotension (blood pressure <90 mm Hg or a reduction of 40 mm Hg from baseline) despite adequate fluid replacement.

Severe sepsis and septic shock are characterized by impaired tissue perfusion, hypotension, and multiorgan dysfunction in the setting of infection (blood cultures positive in 50% to 60% of cases). Endotoxin activates endogenous mediators of inflammation with catastrophic consequences. The result can be increased vascular permeability, a decrease in peripheral vascular resistance, profound hypotension with progressive lactic acidosis, and death.

Common causative organisms of community-acquired bloodstream infections include *Escherichia coli, Staphylococcus aureus*, and *Streptococcus pneumoniae*. Nosocomial infections most often are due to gram-negative aerobic bacilli, coagulase-negative staphylococci, *S. aureus*, enterococci, and *Candida* spp. The frequency of any one organism depends on the host (that is, neutropenia is associated with *P. aeruginosa*, central lines are associated with coagulase-negative staphylococci, *S. aureus*, and *Candida* spp.). The overall mortality rate is 20% to 30%. Management involves maintaining intravascular volume, administering appropriate bactericidal antimicrobials, and correcting any problems that lead to infection (such as draining abscesses). Corticosteroids are of no benefit and may be harmful.

- In septic shock, blood cultures are positive in 50% to 60% of cases.
- Most frequent blood isolates: *E. coli, Klebsiella-Enterobacter, Proteus, Pseudomonas, S. aureus, S. pneumoniae.*

- Endotoxin activates endogenous mediators of inflammation with catastrophic consequences.

GRANULOCYTOPENIA

This condition is characterized by an absolute polymorphonuclear neutrophil value less than 500/mm^3, most often in the setting of chemotherapy for malignancy. Bacteremia is documented in approximately 20% of neutropenic fever episodes. If ecthyma gangrenosum is present, *Pseudomonas* infection should be considered. Other gram-negative aerobic rods (such as *Escherichia coli*) also cause bacteremia. The frequency of bacteremia due to aerobic gram-positive organisms is increasing. Bloodstream infection with these organisms (*Staphylococcus aureus*, coagulase-negative staphylococci, enterococci, viridans streptococci, *Corynebacterium jeikeium*) often is associated with central venous catheters or quinolone antibacterial prophylaxis. *Candida* species should be considered in cases associated with nodular skin lesions, fluffy white chorioretinal exudates, and fever unresponsive to empiric antibacterial agents. Anaerobic organisms are uncommon, except in cases of perirectal abscess and gingivitis. Empiric antimicrobial therapy after an attempt to identify the source of the infection is required for fever of 38.3°C or higher. Monotherapy with ceftazidime, cefepine, or imipenem alone is the preferred initial empiric antibacterial regimen. Alternative therapy with antipseudomonal penicillin plus an aminoglycoside is also acceptable. Vancomycin can be added to the initial regimen if there is severe mucositis, quinolone prophylaxis has been utilized, the patient is known to be colonized with methicillin-resistant *S. aureus* or penicillin-resistant *S. pneumoniae*, an obvious catheter-related infection is present, or the patient is hypotensive. If subsequent cultures show the presence of aerobic gram-positive organisms, vancomycin can be added to the regimen. If there is no response after 5 to 7 days of treatment and the patient remains neutropenic, empiric therapy with amphotericin B should be considered.

URINARY TRACT INFECTION

Females

Because urethritis or cystitis can occur with low colony counts of bacteria, routine urine cultures in young women with dysuria are not recommended. Urinalysis should be done with or without a Gram stain. If pyuria and uncomplicated urinary tract infection (UTI) are present, short-course treatment should be initiated. Only if occult upper urinary tract disease, a complicated UTI, or sexually transmitted disease is suspected should appropriate culture and sensitivity testing be performed.

Risk factors for occult infection and complications include emergency room presentation, low socioeconomic status, hospital-acquired infection, pregnancy, use of Foley catheter, recent instrumentation, known urologic abnormality, previous relapse, UTI at age less than 12 years, acute pyelonephritis or three or more UTIs in 1 year, symptoms for more than 7 days, recent antibiotic use, diabetes mellitus, and immunosuppression. Causative organisms include *Escherichia coli* and *Staphylococcus saprophyticus* (susceptible to ampicillin and trimethoprim-sulfamethoxazole), *P. mirabilis,* or *K. pneumoniae.*

- Routine urine cultures are not recommended in young women with dysuria.
- Associated organisms: *E. coli, S. saprophyticus* (susceptible to trimethoprim-sulfamethoxazole), *P. mirabilis,* or *K. pneumoniae.*

For the first episode of cystitis or urethritis, treatment is given but no investigation is needed. Trimethoprim-sulfamethoxazole or an oral fluoroquinolone is more effective than ampicillin. Short-course treatment (single-dose) has fewer side effects than standard (7 to 10 days) therapy, but the risk of relapse (due to retention of viable organisms in the vaginal or perivaginal area) is higher. Three-day therapy may be associated with relapse rates equal to those with treatment for 7 to 10 days with less toxicity. If recurrence develops after 3-day therapy, subclinical pyelonephritis is likely and treatment is then given for 14 days. Urologic evaluation is usually not necessary. It should be performed in patients with multiple relapses, painless hematuria, a history of childhood UTI, renal lithiasis, and recurrent pyelonephritis.

- For first episode of cystitis or urethritis, trimethoprim-sulfamethoxazole or an oral fluoroquinolone is more effective than ampicillin.
- Short-course treatment (3 days) has fewer side effects than standard (7-10 days) therapy, and risk of relapse of infection may be the same.
- Urologic evaluation should be done in patients with multiple relapses, painless hematuria, history of childhood UTI, renal lithiasis, and recurrent pyelonephritis.

For acute pyelonephritis, 2 weeks of therapy is equal in efficacy to 6 weeks of therapy. Most patients are sufficiently ill to require hospitalization. Many are bacteremic. Unless gram-positive cocci are seen on Gram stain (?enterococci), a third-generation cephalosporin, cotrimoxazole, or a fluoroquinolone can be used as empiric therapy. If enterococci are suspected, use ampicillin or mezlocillin with or without gentamicin. Oral regimens can be substituted quickly as the patient improves. A urine culture is recommended 1 to 2 weeks after the completion of therapy. If relapse occurs, treatment is given for 6 weeks and a urologic evaluation is done. For recurrent lower UTI (more than two episodes per year), single-dose therapy, 3-day therapy, or 6-week therapy is used. For treatment failure, chronic suppressive therapy may be used; however, the risk of resistant organisms must be weighed. Asymptomatic bacteriuria ($>10^5$ cfu/mL) in a midstream urine specimen should be treated only in pregnant women, diabetic patients, and immunocompromised adults.

- For acute pyelonephritis, 2 weeks of therapy is equal in efficacy to 6 weeks of therapy.
- A follow-up urine culture is recommended.

Males

UTI is less common in males than females. Urologic abnormalities (such as benign prostatic hyperplasia) are common. Symptoms are unreliable for localization. Physical examination should include prostate examination, retraction of the foreskin to look for discharge, and palpation of the testicles and epididymides. When a UTI is suspected, urine culture and sensitivity testing should always be done. Causative organisms include *E. coli* in 50% of cases, other gram-negative organisms in 25%, enterococci in 20%, and others in 5%. If signs and symptoms of epididymitis, acute prostatitis, and pyelonephritis are present, treat accordingly. If uncomplicated lower UTI is present, treat for 10 to 14 days. If symptoms persist or relapse, repeat the urine culture. If results are positive, treat for a minimum of 6 weeks. If culture results are negative, consider chronic prostatitis or nonbacterial or noninfectious diseases and treat accordingly.

- Causes of UTI in males: *E. coli* in 50%, other gram-negative organisms in 25%, enterococci in 20%, others in 5%.

BONE AND JOINT INFECTIONS

Acute Bacterial Arthritis (Nongonococcal)

This is most commonly due to hematogenous spread of bacteria. The hip and knee joints are commonly involved. Bacteria involved are gram-positive aerobic cocci (about 75% of cases): *Staphylococcus aureus* (most common) and β-hemolytic streptococci. Gram-negative aerobic bacilli also can cause infection (about 20% of cases); *Pseudomonas aeruginosa* is a common cause in injection drug users. Anaerobes, fungi, and mycobacteria are unusual. Clinical features include involvement usually of monarticular, large joints. Fever, pain, swelling, and restriction of motion are the most frequent signs and symptoms. The synovial fluid is usually turbid, and the leukocyte count generally exceeds 40,000 cells/mm^3 ($\geq$75% polymorphonuclear neutrophils).

The condition may overlap and be confused with other inflammatory arthropathies. Gram stain is 50% to 95% sensitive. Culture results are positive unless antibiotics have been used previously or the pathogen is unusual. Blood culture results are often positive. Radiographs are not helpful in routine cases because destructive changes have not had time to occur. Specific antimicrobial therapy is based on results of Gram stain, culture, and sensitivity testing. The duration of therapy is dependent on individual circumstances, such as the presence of complicating osteomyelitis. Usually, treatment is given for 2 to 4 weeks. Empiric therapy should include agents directed against *S. aureus* and gram-negative bacilli. Drainage is essential. Percutaneous, arthroscopic, or open procedures are used. Hip, shoulder, and sternoclavicular joint involvement, development of loculations, and persistently positive culture results (not due to resistant organisms) are the usual indications for arthroscopy or open debridement.

- Acute bacterial arthritis (nongonococcal) is most commonly due to hematogenous spread of bacteria.
- Bacteria involved are gram-positive aerobic cocci (about 75% of cases): *S. aureus* is most common.
- Monarticular, large joints usually are involved.
- Fever, pain, swelling, and restriction of motion are frequent.
- Synovial fluid is turbid; leukocyte count is 10,000-300,000/mm^3.
- Blood culture results are positive in 50% of cases.
- Drainage is essential.

Viral Arthritis

This is usually transient, self-limited polyarthritis. It may be caused by rubella (also may occur after vaccination), hepatitis B, mumps, coxsackievirus, adenovirus, parvovirus B19, and human immunodeficiency virus, among others.

Chronic Monarticular Arthritis

Organisms involved include *Mycobacteria* (*Mycobacterium tuberculosis* is more common than *Mycobacterium aviumintercellulare, Mycobacterium kansasii, Mycobacterium marinum*), fungi (*Coccidioides immitis* and *Sporothrix schenckii* are more common than *Histoplasma capsulatum, Blastomyces dermatitidis*—acute, and *Candida* spp.—acute), and others (*Brucella, Nocardia*).

- *M. tuberculosis, C. immitis*, and *S. schenckii* often are involved in chronic monarticular arthritis.

Osteomyelitis

Acute hematogenous osteomyelitis is more common in infants and children than adults. The metaphysis of long bones (femur, tibia) most commonly is affected. *S. aureus* is the most common organism. Acute onset of pain and fever are typical features. The illness can present with pain only. Compatible radiographic changes and bone biopsy for culture and pathologic examination are used to establish the diagnosis. Results of blood culture may be positive. Specific parenteral antibiotic therapy is used for 3 to 6 weeks on the basis of culture and sensitivity test results. Debridement is usually not necessary unless sequestrum is present.

- *S. aureus* is the most common organism in acute hematogenous osteomyelitis.
- Acute onset of pain and fever are typical features.

Chronic osteomyelitis is more common in adults. It results from direct inoculation caused by trauma or adjacent soft tissue infection, for example. Open fractures and diabetic foot ulcers are common predisposing factors. *S. aureus* is the most common organism. Coagulase-negative staphylococci are often pathogens if a foreign body (such as plate, screws) is present. Often, osteomyelitis complicating a foot ulcer is polymicrobial, including aerobic gram-positive and gram-negative organisms and anaerobes. Local pain, tenderness, erythema, and draining sinuses are common. Fever is atypical unless there is concurrent cellulitis. The condition can present with pain only. Compatible radiographic changes (often vague) and bone biopsy for culture and pathologic examination are used to establish the diagnosis. Results of blood culture are rarely positive. Adequate debridement, removal of dead space, soft tissue coverage, and fixation of infected fractures are essential. Specific parenteral antibiotic therapy is given for 4 to 6 weeks on the basis of culture and sensitivity test results.

- *S. aureus* is the most common organism in chronic osteomyelitis.
- Coagulase-negative staphylococci are common pathogens if foreign body is present.
- Local pain, tenderness, erythema, and draining sinuses are common.
- Specific parenteral antibiotic therapy is given for 4-6 weeks.

Vertebral Osteomyelitis

This condition often results from hematogenous dissemination from a focal source of infection (such as urinary tract, pneumonia). *S. aureus* and gram-negative bacilli are the major pathogens. Only 10% of cases have positive results of blood culture. Symptoms include pain and local tenderness. Fever may be present. The leukocyte count may be normal or increased. The sedimentation rate often is increased. Plain radiographs do not show destruction early in the course of disease. Gallium scan is approximately 80% sensitive.

Magnetic resonance imaging is the diagnostic test of choice because it is sensitive and specific and shows anatomical detail (coexistent epidural abscess). Percutaneous needle biopsy (computed tomography-guided) or open biopsy of bone or disc tissue is usually needed to define the microbiology of the infection. Treatment includes appropriate parenteral antimicrobial therapy for 4 to 6 weeks. Drainage may be necessary if a concomitant epidural abscess is present.

- In vertebral osteomyelitis, *S. aureus* and gram-negative bacilli are major pathogens.
- Gallium scan is about 80% sensitive; magnetic resonance imaging is diagnostic test of choice.

SINUSITIS IN ADULTS

The physician's overall impression as to the presence or absence of sinusitis is the best clinical predictor of disease. Independent clinical predictors of disease are maxillary toothache, poor transillumination, poor response to decongestants, and a history or examination finding of purulent discharge. Pertinent sinus radiographic findings include membrane thickening of more than 6 mm (maxillary sinus), opaque sinuses, or air-fluid level. Organisms that are usually involved are *Haemophilus influenzae*, *Streptococcus pneumoniae*, and oral anaerobes. Treatment is with oral trimethoprim-sulfamethoxazole, amoxicillin, amoxicillin-clavulanate, and levofloxacin, among many others.

- Organisms involved in sinusitis in adults are *H. influenzae*, *S. pneumoniae*, oral anaerobes.

HEPATIC (BACTERIAL) ABSCESS

Mechanisms of bacterial abscess include portal vein bacteremia resulting from, for example, appendicitis and diverticulitis, bacteremia caused by a primary focus elsewhere in the body, ascending cholangitis, direct extension (subphrenic abscess), or trauma. Fever is common. Right upper quadrant pain, tenderness on percussion, and increased values on liver function tests may or may not be present. Computed tomography and ultrasonography are very helpful in diagnosis. Bacteriology depends on the mechanism of abscess formation. Infection is often polymicrobial and is due to aerobic gram-negative rods, anaerobic streptococci, and *Bacteroides* species. Treatment is individualized and depends on suspected and isolated organisms. Empiric therapy with clindamycin or metronidazole plus a third-generation cephalosporin or aminoglycoside, a β-lactam/β-lactamase inhibitor combination, or a carbapenem is appropriate. If the hematogenous route is suspected, an agent should be used in the regimen that is active against staphylococci. Drainage (surgical or percutaneous) is of primary importance.

TOXIC SHOCK SYNDROME

This syndrome is caused by the establishment or growth of a toxin-producing strain of *Staphylococcus aureus* in a non-immune person. Clinical scenarios associated with this syndrome include young menstruating women with prolonged, continuous use of tampons, postoperative and nonoperative wound infections, localized abscesses, and *S. aureus* pneumonia developing after influenza. It is a multisystem disease. Clinical criteria include fever, hypotension, erythroderma (often leads to desquamation, particularly on palms and soles), and involvement in three or more organ systems. Onset is acute; blood culture results are usually negative. Condition is caused by production of staphylococcal toxin (TSST-1). Treatment is supportive; subsequent episodes are treated with a β-lactam antibiotic, which decreases the frequency and severity of subsequent attacks. The relapse rate may be as high as 30% to 40% (menstruation-related disease). The mortality rate is 5% to 10%.

- Toxic shock syndrome is caused by toxin-producing strain of *S. aureus* in non-immune person.
- Multisystem disease: fever, hypotension, erythroderma (often leads to desquamation, particularly on palms and soles).
- Onset is acute; results of blood culture are usually negative.
- Toxic shock syndrome is caused by production of staphylococcal toxin (TSST-1).

STREPTOCOCCAL TOXIC SHOCK SYNDROME

This syndrome is similar to staphylococcal toxic shock syndrome. Patients have invasive group A streptococcal infections with associated hypotension and two of the following: renal impairment, coagulopathy, liver impairment, adult respiratory distress syndrome, rash (may desquamate), or soft tissue necrosis. It is caused by group A streptococci. Symptoms are caused by production of streptococcal toxin (pyrogenic exotoxin A). Most patients have skin or soft tissue infection, are younger than 50 years, and are otherwise healthy compared with patients with invasive group A streptococcal infections without the toxic streptococcal syndrome. Most patients are bacteremic (different from toxic shock syndrome due to *Staphylococcus aureus*). Treatment is with appropriate antibiotics, supportive care, and surgical debridement in some cases. The case-fatality rate is 30%.

- Toxic streptococcal syndrome is caused by group A streptococci.

- Symptoms are caused by production of streptococcal toxin.
- Most patients are bacteremic (different from toxic shock syndrome due to *S. aureus*).

INFECTIONS IN SOLID ORGAN TRANSPLANTATION

The spectrum of potential pathogens in patients after solid organ transplantation is diverse. The individual risk of specific infection can be classified according to the following: symptoms and signs of illness at presentation (i.e., meningitis vs. pneumonia), posttransplantation time course, serostatus of recipient and donor for certain infections (such as cytomegalovirus, toxoplasmosis), type of organ transplantation, type and duration of immunosuppression, type of antimicrobial prophylaxis patient has received, and travel history and previous exposure to pathogens (such as tuberculosis, cocci). The time of occurrence of opportunistic infections after solid organ transplantation is given in Table 14-17. Pathogens associated with various immunodeficiency states are shown in Table 14-18.

HUMAN IMMUNODEFICIENCY VIRUS (HIV)

Human immunodeficiency virus (HIV) belongs to the family of Retroviridae, subfamily Lentiviridae.

The viruses share a distinct biologic characteristic: an initial stage of primary infection followed by a relatively asymptomatic period of months to years, culminating in a final and generally fatal stage of overt disease.

There are two types of HIV: HIV-1 and HIV-2. Most reported cases of HIV disease around the world are caused by HIV-1. HIV-2 is found predominantly in western Africa. Although HIV-1 and HIV-2 are clinically indistinguishable and have identical modes of transmission, HIV-2 appears to be less easily transmitted than HIV-1, and the progression to acquired immunodeficiency syndrome (AIDS) may be slower in HIV-2 infection.

Epidemiology

HIV infection is a global epidemic affecting more than 22.6 million people in more than 190 countries. According to estimates by the joint United Nations Program on HIV/AIDS (UNAIDS), more than 3.1 million new HIV infections occurred during 1996 (8,500 daily). Most newly infected adults are younger than 25 years, and approximately 42% of the adults who currently have HIV or AIDS are women. Around 70% of all cases of AIDS are thought to occur in sub-Saharan Africa. The epidemic is now spreading most rapidly in Asia, affecting countries such as India, Thailand, Cambodia, Vietnam, and Myanmar. Approximately 1 million Americans are now infected with HIV. Through January 1, 1997, 581,429 cases of AIDS in the United States have been reported to the

Table 14-17.—Opportunistic Infections in Solid Organ Transplantation

Month	Type of infection after transplantation
1	Bacterial infections (related to wound, intravenous lines, urinary tract), herpes simplex virus, hepatitis B
1-4	Cytomegalovirus, *Pneumocystis carinii, Listeria monocytogenes, Mycobacterium tuberculosis, Aspergillus, Nocardia, Toxoplasma*, hepatitis B, *Legionella*
2-6	Epstein-Barr virus, varicella-zoster virus, hepatitis C, *Legionella*
>6	*Cryptococcus neoformans, Legionella*

Centers for Disease Control and Prevention (CDC), and 362,004 AIDS deaths have been reported.

In recent years, heterosexual transmission has become the most rapidly increasing transmission category in the United States. This increase in heterosexual transmission explains the dramatic increase in HIV infection in women. In 1994, 62% of reported cases of heterosexual transmission of AIDS were among women. The proportion of women with AIDS attributable to heterosexual contact increased from 15% in 1983 to 43% in 1994. Among men who have sex with men, new infections occur predominantly in young men and in minorities. In the United States, HIV/AIDS is the leading cause of death for Americans between the ages of 25 and 44 years and is the fourth leading cause of years of potential life lost among all Americans before age 65 years. The prevalence of HIV infection continues to be disproportionately high in racial and ethnic minorities.

Transmission

HIV is transmitted sexually, perinatally, by parenteral inoculation (intravenous drug injection, occupational exposure), through blood products, and, less commonly, through donated organs or semen. Sexual transmission is the most common means of infection. Female-to-male sexual transmission of HIV is less efficient than male-to-female, as is true for other sexually transmitted diseases. Some of the conditions that may increase the risk of sexually acquiring HIV infection are traumatic intercourse (such as receptive anal), ulcerative genital infections such as syphilis, herpes simplex, and chancroid, and lack of circumcision. The use of latex condoms, especially if used properly, reduces the risk of HIV transmission.

HIV infection develops in 16% to 30% of infants born to HIV-infected mothers. Infection also can be transmitted through breast milk. Recently, zidovudine treatment of HIV-infected pregnant women in the second and third trimesters and zidovudine treatment of their infants in the first 6 weeks of life resulted in a significant reduction of maternal-infant transmission of HIV (zidovudine group 8.3% and placebo group 25.5%, $P < 0.00006$).

In the United States, all blood donations have been tested routinely for HIV-1 antibody since early 1985. Since June 1, 1992, all U.S. blood centers have tested for antibodies to both HIV-1 and HIV-2. Today, the estimated risk of acquiring HIV through blood transfusion is 1 in 225,000. No cases of transfusion-associated HIV-2 infection have been reported in the United States.

Occupational exposure occurs through needle sticks. The average risk associated with needle injury is approximately 0.32%. Factors that influence transmission include stage of HIV infection in the source case (this relates to virus titer in the specimen), size and type of needle (hollow needle or suture needle), and depth of injury. The risk associated with mucous membrane and non-intact skin contact is low but is not zero.

Laboratory Diagnosis

Routine Tests

The enzyme-linked immunosorbent assay (ELISA) is the standard screening test for HIV-1 infection. It detects specific HIV antibodies (primarily antibodies against gp160, gp41, and p24). It is 99% sensitive and specific, but its positive predictive value is low in low-prevalence populations. False-positive results occur because of the presence of cross-reacting antibodies in certain patients (such as multiparous women, patients with multiple transfusions). False-negative results are caused by testing patients before seroconversion, patients who have undergone replacement transfusions or bone marrow transplantation, or by poorly manufactured testing equipment.

Individuals with positive or indeterminate results of ELISA should have the test repeated. If the results are still positive, they should undergo additional confirmatory testing, usually Western blot testing. The Western blot test detects antibodies directed against specific viral proteins, such as gag (p18, p24, p55), pol (p31, p51, p66), and env (gp41, gp120/gp160) gene products. The CDC guidelines for interpretation of the Western blot (adopted in 1989) are as follows: the presence of antibody against any two of the three major viral gene products (p24, gp41, or gp120/gp160) is classified as positive. A Western blot result is classified as negative if no bands are present. Results that cannot be classified as positive or negative based on these criteria are categorized as indeterminate. If results are indeterminate, the clinician should assess the risk of HIV infection in the individual patient and retest at 3 to 6 months. HIV-RNA assays may be of additional help in these cases. The risk of HIV infection is extremely low in patients with repeatedly indeterminate results of Western blot testing.

Table 14-18.—Pathogens Associated With Immunodeficiency

Condition	Usual conditions	Pathogens
Neutropenia (<500/mL)	Cancer chemotherapy, adverse drug reaction, leukemia	**Bacteria:** Aerobic gram-negative bacilli (coliforms and pseudomonads, *S. aureus*, *S. viridans*, *S. epidermidis*) **Fungi:** *Aspergillus*, *Candida* spp.
Cell-mediated immunity	Organ transplantation, human immunodeficiency virus infection, lymphoma (especially Hodgkin disease), corticosteroid therapy	**Bacteria:** *Listeria, Salmonella, Nocardia*, Mycobacteria (*M. tuberculosis* and *M. avium*), *Legionella* **Viruses:** CMV, *H. simplex*, varicella-zoster, JC virus **Parasites:** *Pneumocystis carinii, Toxoplasma, Strongyloides stercoralis, Cryptosporidium* **Fungi:** *Candida, Cryptococcus, Histoplasma, Coccidioides*
Hypogammaglobulinemia or dysgammaglobulinemia	Multiple myeloma, congenital or acquired deficiency, chronic lymphocytic leukemia	**Bacteria:** *S. pneumoniae, H. influenzae* (type B) **Parasites:** *Giardia* **Viruses:** Enteroviruses
Complement deficiencies C2, 3 C5 C6-8 Alternative pathway	Congenital	**Bacteria:** *S. pneumoniae, H. influenzae*, *S. pneumoniae, S. aureus*, Enterobacteriaceae *Neisseria meningitidis* *S. pneumoniae, H. influenzae*, *Salmonella*
Hyposplenism	Splenectomy, hemolytic anemia	*S. pneumoniae, H. influenzae*, DF-2
Defective chemotaxis	Diabetes, alcoholism, renal failure, lazy leukocyte syndrome, trauma; SLE	*S. aureus*, streptococci, *Candida*
Defective neutrophilic killing	Chronic granulomatous disease, myeloperoxidase deficiency	Catalase-positive bacteria: *S. aureus, E. coli*, *Candida* spp.

CMV, cytomegalovirus; SLE, systemic lupus erythematosus.
From Bartlett JG: Pocket Book of Infectious Disease Therapy. Baltimore, Williams & Wilkins, 1998, p 236. By permission of the publisher.

Clinical Syndromes

Primary HIV Infection

Synonyms for this syndrome are acute HIV infection and acute retroviral syndrome. Within 4 to 8 weeks after exposure to HIV, 40% to 60% of infected individuals present with a brief illness that may last for a few days to a few weeks. This period of illness is associated with a huge amount of circulating virus, a rapid decline in CD4 cell count, and a vigorous immune response. Patients usually present with a mononucleosis-like illness, but the clinical manifestations may be protean (Table 14-19). An atypical lymphocytosis is present in approximately 50% of patients. Results of ELISA may be negative (usually positive at 6 to 12 weeks); p24 antigen, HIV culture, or polymerase chain reaction results may be positive. The differential diagnosis includes infection due to Ebstein-Barr virus, cytomegalovirus, primary herpes simplex virus, toxoplasmosis, rubella, viral hepatitis, secondary syphilis, and drug reactions. Currently, treatment with the most potent antiretroviral combination regimen available is recommended with the hope of intervening before the HIV infection is fully established, when the viral population is relatively homogeneous, and the host immune system is relatively intact.

Infections Associated With HIV Infection

Pneumocystis carinii Pneumonia

Pneumocystis carinii pneumonia (PCP) is one of the most common opportunistic infections in patients with AIDS (plate 14-8). It occurs in approximately 80% of patients who do not receive primary prophylaxis. Onset is insidious with several weeks of fever, weight loss, malaise, and night sweats. Chest radiography typically shows bilateral interstitial pulmonary infiltrates, but a lobar distribution and spontaneous pneumothoraces may occur. Arterial blood gas analysis usually reveals hypoxia and respiratory alkalosis. A wide A-a gradient (>35 mm Hg) and low Po_2 (<70 mm Hg) are associated with increased mortality. Several methods are used for the diagnosis of PCP. Staining for PCP in hypertonic saline-induced expectorated sputum is 30% to 85% sensitive. The sensitivity improves with liquefaction and the use of monoclonal antibody staining, and it decreases with use of PCP prophylaxis. Bronchoalveolar lavage is 85% to 90% sensitive. If the patient is receiving PCP prophylaxis, transbronchial lung biopsy may be needed to make the diagnosis. Open lung biopsy rarely is needed.

The treatment of choice for both severe and mild to moderate disease is trimethoprim-sulfamethoxazole, 15 mg/kg per day (trimethoprim component) in 3 or 4 equally divided doses for 21 days. Other treatment options for PCP include oral trimethoprim-dapsone, oral primaquine plus clindamycin, intravenous pentamidine, trimetrexate plus folinic acid, and atovaquone. If there is no improvement 5 to 7 days after beginning treatment, switching to or adding an alternative agent should be considered. Adverse reactions to trimethoprim-sulfamethoxazole include fever, rash, neutropenia, thrombocytopenia, increased results of liver function tests, and renal dysfunction. Intravenous pentamidine is an alternative to cotrimoxazole (3-4 mg/kg per day for 21 days). The adverse reactions noted with intravenous pentamidine include hypotension, nephrotoxicity, hypoglycemia, and pancreatitis.

Controlled studies have shown that adjunctive corticosteroid therapy increases survival in patients with moderate to severe disease. Benefit was shown when the Pao_2 in room air was less than 70 mm Hg or the alveolar-arterial Po_2 difference (A-a gradient) was more than 35 mm Hg. When indicated, adjunctive corticosteroid therapy should be started immediately; a delay may compromise its effectiveness. The recommended dosage of oral prednisone is 40 mg twice a day on days 1 to 5, 20 mg twice a day on days 6 to 10, and 20 mg each day on days 11 to 21.

Primary prophylaxis of PCP is indicated in all HIV-infected patients with a CD4 count less than 200 cells/mm^3 and in HIV-infected persons with higher CD4 cell counts but with symptoms of fever, weight loss, night sweats, or oral candidiasis. Treatment options are as follows: 1) trimethoprim-sulfamethoxazole is the drug of choice (1 double-strength tablet each day, 1 double-strength tablet 3 times per week, or 1 single-strength tablet daily); 2) dapsone, 100 mg daily; 3) aerosolized pentamidine, 300 mg inhaled monthly via Respirgard II nebulizer; 4) dapsone, 100 mg orally each day plus pyrimethamine 25 mg orally three times a week.

Recent trials of trimethoprim-sulfamethoxazole compared with inhaled pentamidine for primary and secondary prophylaxis showed conclusively that trimethoprim-sulfamethoxazole was more effective than inhaled pentamidine. Trimethoprim-sulfamethoxazole has the additional benefit of potential protection against other infectious agents (*Nocardia, Toxoplasma gondii, Staphylococcus aureus, Streptococcus*

Table 14-19.—Clinical Manifestations of Primary Human Immunodeficiency Virus Infection

General	Neuropathic	Dermatologic	Gastrointestinal
Fever	Headache, retro-orbital pain	Maculopapular rash	Oral candidiasis
Pharyngitis	Meningoencephalitis	Roseola-like rash	Nausea, vomiting
Lymphadenopathy	Peripheral neuropathy	Diffuse urticaria	Diarrhea
Myalgia	Radiculopathy	Desquamation	
Lethargy	Guillain-Barré syndrome	Alopecia	
Anorexia, weight loss	Cognitive impairment	Mucocutaneous ulceration	

From Tindall B, Imrie A, Donovan B, Penny R, Cooper DA: Primary HIV infection. *In* The Medical Management of AIDS. Third edition. Edited by MA Sande, PA Volberding. Philadelphia, WB Saunders Company, 1992, pp 67-86. By permission of publisher.

pneumoniae, Haemophilus influenzae, Listeria monocytogenes, Isospora belli) and prevention of extrapulmonary pneumocytosis.

Mycobacterial Infections

The resurgence of tuberculosis in the United States is not entirely explained by the HIV epidemic. Factors such as socioeconomic conditions, immigration, breakdown of the public health infrastructure, and lack of interest of the medical and scientific community in tuberculosis all play a role. In addition to the impact of HIV on the incidence of tuberculosis, there are other important interactions between HIV infection and *Mycobacterium tuberculosis*: tuberculosis may accelerate the course of HIV infection; unlike many of the opportunistic infections in patients with HIV infection, tuberculosis can be cured if diagnosed promptly and treated appropriately; tuberculosis can be successfully prevented. Tuberculosis may occur relatively early in HIV infection. When it occurs later, it tends to have atypical features, such as extrapulmonary disease, disseminated disease, and unusual chest radiographic appearance (lower lung zone lesions, intrathoracic adenopathy, diffuse infiltrations, lower frequency of cavitation).

Outbreaks of multiple drug-resistant tuberculosis have been reported. Patients may have a fulminant course with high mortality (>70%) and a rapid course to death in 2 to 3 months.

Treatment of tuberculosis in patients with AIDS is the same as that in normal hosts, unless drug resistance is suspected. In initial regimens, isoniazid, rifampin, pyrazinamide, and ethambutol are used until drug sensitivity results are available. For drug-susceptible organisms, isoniazid and rifampin are continued for an additional 4 months, for a total of at least 6 months. For isoniazid-resistant organisms, rifampin and ethambutol with or without pyrazinamide are used for 18 months, or for 12 months after cultures are negative, whichever is longer. If there is a potential for noncompliance, directly observed therapy should be strongly considered. Optimal regimens for multiple drug-resistant tuberculosis are unknown. Prophylaxis with isoniazid for 12 months is recommended for all patients who are HIV-positive and have skin reactions of more than 5 mm to 5 tuberculin units of purified protein derivative.

Mycobacterium avium complex causes infection when immunosuppression is severe (CD4 cell count <50/mm^3). Disseminated *M. avium* complex infection is the most common systemic bacterial infection in HIV-infected patients. Common presentations include low-grade fever, night sweats, weight loss, and diarrhea. Blood cultures are usually positive; however, organisms also can be isolated from stool, respiratory tract secretions, bone marrow, liver, and other biopsy specimens. The organism is resistant to conventional antimycobacterial agents. Treatment involves multiple drugs with many side effects. Some studies have shown an increase in survival with treatment, but symptoms often can be ameliorated. The current recommended treatment regimen includes one of the newer macrolides (clarithromycin, azithromycin) plus ethambutol, and one or two additional drugs with activity against *M. avium* complex. These include rifabutin, ciprofloxacin, amikacin, rifampin, and clofazimine. Rifabutin is thought to be the best option for a third agent. Treatment with full therapeutic doses is continued for life. For patients with AIDS whose CD4 cell count is less than 100 (some would prefer <50) cells/mm^3, prophylaxis with clarithromycin 500 mg twice daily, azithromycin 1,200 mg weekly, or rifabutin 300 mg daily is recommended. The combination of clarithromycin and rifabutin is not more effective than clarithromycin alone for prophylaxis in *M. avium* complex.

Treponema pallidum

Sexually transmitted diseases, including syphilis, that cause genital ulceration may be co-factors for acquiring HIV infection. There are reports of false-negative and false-positive serologic tests for syphilis in patients with HIV. Neurosyphilis has been reported to occur earlier and more frequently in patients with AIDS than in HIV-negative patients. Patients with AIDS also have been reported to have unusually severe manifestations of all stages of syphilis. Recent studies, however, suggest that these phenomena are rare. Serologic response to standard treatment regimens was the same in HIV-positive and HIV-negative persons in a recent study of 50 injection drug users. However, because of these concerns, some physicians advocate cerebrospinal fluid examination in all patients before initiating treatment and using regimens with better cerebrospinal fluid penetration, at higher doses, and for a longer duration. Penicillin-based regimens, whenever possible, are recommended by the CDC for all stages of syphilis in HIV-infected individuals.

Fungal Infections
Cryptococcus neoformans

Cryptococcus neoformans is a round or oval yeast that is acquired from the environment. It is inhaled into the lungs, where it usually causes asymptomatic infection, but it has a strong propensity for dissemination to the central nervous system. Other sites for potential dissemination include skin, bone, and the genitourinary tract. Disease caused by *C. neoformans* occurs in approximately 10% of patients with AIDS. The most common presentation is cryptococcal meningitis. The onset is insidious, symptoms are nonspecific (fever, headache, malaise), and symptoms may have a waxing and waning course. Meningismus may not be present. Brain imaging studies are also nonspecific; cerebral atrophy and ventricular enlargements are the most common findings. Cerebrospinal fluid findings may be minimal or include an increased opening pressure, mild mononuclear pleocytosis, and increased protein value. The India ink preparation is positive in more than 70% of cases. The serum and cerebrospinal fluid cryptococcal antigen test has a sensitivity of 93% to 99%. Cultures of cerebrospinal fluid are usually positive. In up to 80% of patients, results of blood cultures are positive for *C. neoformans*. Adverse prognostic factors include altered mental status on presentation and high fungal burden (positive result of India ink test, high antigen titers, extraneural disease). Initial therapy includes amphotericin B with or without flucytosine for at least 2 weeks, followed by fluconazole 400 mg daily for a total of 8 to 10 weeks. Fluconazole (200 mg daily) is more effective than amphotericin B (1 mg/kg weekly) for chronic suppression. Itraconazole 200 mg by mouth daily is another alternative. Persistence of infection in the prostate may be a cause of relapse of infection.

Dimorphic Fungi (Histoplasma capsulatum, Coccidioides immitis, Blastomyces dermatitidis)

Coccidioidomycosis and histoplasmosis are reported more often than blastomycosis. Disease with all three pathogens usually presents as disseminated infection and can even present as septic shock (histoplasmosis). Localized pulmonary involvement occurs but is much less common, except with blastomycosis (50% of cases). Disseminated disease often involves the central nervous system (blastomycosis, coccidioidomycosis). Organisms may be seen in the buffy coat of blood (histoplasmosis) in some cases. Travel history and geographic location are important clues to the diagnosis. A test for the detection of *Histoplasma capsulatum* polysaccharide antigen is currently available. This test can be applied to serum, urine, and other body fluids. It is used not only for diagnosis but also for following the response to therapy. Initial therapy with intravenous amphotericin B is recommended for all three pathogens. For nonmeningitic and nonseptic histoplasmosis, itraconazole (200 mg twice daily) can be used as initial treatment. For chronic suppression, itraconazole or amphotericin B is effective for histoplasmosis. Treatment of blastomycosis is the same as that of histoplasmosis. For coccidioidomycosis, fluconazole or itraconazole can be used for maintenance therapy after initial control with intravenous amphotericin B. An acid environment is required for optimal absorption of itraconazole, and clinicians should be aware of potential interactions with H_2-receptor antagonists, antacids, phenobarbital, rifampin, and other drugs. The routine use of fluconazole or itraconazole for the prevention of systemic mycosis is not currently recommended.

Candida albicans

Mucocutaneous disease (such as oral thrush or recurrent vaginitis) is common. Esophagitis is also frequent and is a common cause of dysphagia. Systemic candidal infection, including candidemia, is rare unless additional risk factors for disseminated fungal infection such as severe neutropenia and indwelling catheters are involved. Candidal esophagitis is an AIDS-defining condition. Treatment is with clotrimoxazole troches or nystatin initially for mucocutaneous disease. Fluconazole or itraconazole is used for treatment of candidal esophagitis and topical treatment failures. Amphotericin B can be used for azole failures.

Cytomegalovirus

Cytomegalovirus disease usually affects persons with advanced HIV disease (CD4 cell count <100/mm³). Chorioretinitis is the most common clinical manifestation of cytomegalovirus disease, occurring in as many as 40% of patients with AIDS. The usual symptoms are floaters, visual field deficits, and painless loss of vision. Funduscopic examination reveals yellowish white granules with perivascular exudates and hemorrhages. Cytomegalovirus gastrointestinal disease most commonly involves the esophagus and colon and manifests with abdominal pain, dysphagia, and bloody diarrhea. Cytomegalovirus also can cause hepatitis, pneumonitis, sclerosing cholangitis, encephalitis, adrenalitis, polyradiculopathy, and myelopathy. Current agents available for the treatment of cytomegalovirus disease include ganciclovir, foscarnet, and cidofovir. The limiting side effect of ganciclovir is bone marrow suppression, and the major adverse effect of foscarnet is renal toxicity. Ganciclovir can be administered intravenously, through intravitreal injection, or in a sustained-release form through a surgically implantable device. Cidofovir is a recently approved agent and has a longer half-life than either ganciclovir or foscarnet; administration once weekly to once every 2 weeks is thus possible. Renal toxicity is a significant problem with cidofovir, and for this reason vigorous hydration and coadministration of probenecid is required. In a recently published report, combination therapy with ganciclovir and foscarnet was significantly better than either agent alone for delaying progression of relapsed cytomegalovirus retinitis.

Enteric Infections

Differential diagnoses for various clinical syndromes are outlined in Table 14-20.

Initial evaluation of patients with AIDS who have abdominal pain, large-volume diarrhea, and weight loss should include stool cultures for bacteria, three separate stool specimens for ova and parasites, specific examination for cryptosporidiosis, and *Clostridium difficile* toxin. In cases of persistent diarrhea despite routine studies, cytomegalovirus or *M. avium-intracellulare* should be considered. If no diagnosis is made, upper and lower gastrointestinal endoscopy and biopsy may yield pathogens that are treatable.

Salmonellosis presents with fever, severe diarrhea, abdominal pain, or typhoidal illness without diarrhea. Bacteremia is common. Ciprofloxacin is used for treatment for 10 to 14 days; however, recurrence is common and maintenance therapy may be needed.

Cryptosporidiosis and *Isospora belli* infections often cause massive, watery diarrhea, crampy abdominal pain, anorexia, flatulence, and malaise. Fever and bloody diarrhea are uncommon, but malabsorption and dehydration are common. Cryptosporidiosis is diagnosed by identification of *Cryptosporidium parvum* oocysts in fecal samples or biopsy specimens. The specimens are stained with either a modified acid-fast procedure or a fluorescent assay utilizing monoclonal antibodies to *Cryptosporidium* antigens. Biliary tract involvement may occur with cryptosporidiosis. If the CD4 cell count is more than $180/mm^3$, cryptosporidium infection is usually self-limited (<4 weeks); if it is less than $140/mm^3$, persistent disease develops in 80% to 90%. There are no proven regimens for the treatment of cryptosporidiosis, but paromomycin, a nonabsorbable aminoglycoside used for the treatment of *Entamoeba histolytica*, has been effective in some patients. Trimethoprim-sulfamethoxazole is effective for the treatment of *I. belli* infections.

Two species of *Microsporidia*, *enterocytozoon bieneusi* and *septata intestinalis*, cause enteric disease in patients with AIDS. Infection with these *Microsporidia* resembles infection with *Cryptosporidium parvum*. Microscopy of biopsy specimens and special stains are required for diagnosis. There is no effective therapy for microsporidiosis, but albendazole is being studied for this purpose.

Table 14-20.—Differential Diagnoses of Enteric Infections in Association With Human Immunodeficiency Virus

Proctitis	Proctocolitis	Enteritis
Neisseria gonorrhoeae	*Campylobacter*	*Giardia*
Herpes simplex	*Shigella*	Cryptosporidiosis
Chlamydia	*Chlamydia*	*Isospora*
Treponema pallidum	*Entamoeba histolytica*	Microsporidia
Cytomegalovirus	*Clostridium difficile*	
	Salmonella typhimurium	
	Cytomegalovirus	

Central Nervous System Infections

AIDS dementia complex consists of a triad of cognitive, motor, and behavioral dysfunction. In its mildest form, it may begin early in the course of HIV disease, but it is otherwise a late manifestation of HIV disease. It can progress from subtle cognitive impairment to severe dementia with marked motor dysfunction. Computed tomography and magnetic resonance imaging of the brain show diffuse atrophy. No specific therapy has proved to be effective. Its prevalence may have been reduced by antiretroviral therapy.

Progressive multifocal leukoencephalopathy is a demyelinating disease caused by papovavirus (JC virus). Symptoms and signs are variable and consist of focal neurologic deficits without altered sensorium or a systemic toxic state. Fever is absent. Symptoms evolve over weeks to months. Magnetic resonance imaging shows characteristic white matter changes without contrast enhancement or mass effect. Prognosis is poor; there is no proven effective treatment.

Toxoplasma gondii, a protozoan, is the most common cause of focal central nervous system lesions in patients with AIDS. The most common symptoms of *Toxoplasma* encephalitis include headache and confusion, and fever may be absent. Focal neurologic deficits occur in 69% of cases. The median CD4 cell count at diagnosis is $50/mm^3$. Multiple ring-enhancing lesions usually are noted on brain imaging studies. Magnetic resonance imaging is more sensitive than computed tomography for identifying lesions. Empiric anti-toxoplasmosis therapy is indicated in patients with AIDS and positive *Toxoplasma* serologic testing who present with multiple intracranial lesions. Effective treatment should result not only in amelioration of symptoms but also in a reduction of the number, size, and contrast enhancement of the brain lesions. If the patient is seronegative for *Toxoplasma*, or has a single mass lesion on both computed tomography and magnetic resonance imaging, or did not achieve the desired response after an empiric course of anti-*Toxoplasma* therapy for 10 to 14 days, the presumptive diagnosis of *Toxoplasma* encephalitis becomes doubtful and a diagnostic brain biopsy is indicated. The treatment of choice for *Toxoplasma* encephalitis is the combination of pyrimethamine (with folinic acid) plus sulfadiazine or clindamycin. Alternatives include either trimethoprim-sulfamethoxazole or the combination of pyrimethamine with various other agents, including the macrolides, atovaquone, and dapsone. Lifelong suppressive therapy (secondary prophylaxis), with the same agents used for primary therapy but at a reduced dose, is necessary to prevent relapse. All *Toxoplasma* seropositive HIV-infected individuals with a CD4+ lymphocyte count of less than $100/mm^3$ should receive primary prophylaxis against *Toxoplasma* encephalitis. The agent of choice for this is trimethoprim-sulfamethoxazole in the doses recommended for PCP prophylaxis and dapsone plus pyrimethamine as an alternative regimen. HIV-infected patients should be tested for IgG antibody to *Toxoplasma* as part of their initial workup; if the result is negative, they should be counseled about the various potential sources of *Toxoplasma* infection.

The differential diagnosis of *central nervous system mass lesions* in patients with AIDS includes toxoplasmosis, lymphoma, and bacterial brain abscesses and infections caused by *C. neoformans*, *Coccidioides immitis*, *M. tuberculosis*, and *Nocardia asteroides*, among others.

AIDS-Associated Malignancies

Kaposi sarcoma is a tumor of uncertain origin; vascular proliferation is its most prominent feature. It is the most common neoplasm affecting HIV-infected persons. It is most common in the homosexual population with AIDS. Clinical manifestations include nodules, plaques, lymph node enlargement, and signs and symptoms of visceral involvement. Skin, lung, and the gastrointestinal tract are the commonly affected organs. Lung involvement may mimic infection. Treatment options include local therapy (radiotherapy, intralesional chemotherapy, cryotherapy) and systemic therapy (chemotherapy, interferon-α). Liposome-encapsulated anthracycline chemotherapeutic agents recently have become available, potentially enabling delivery of higher doses of effective drug with fewer toxic side effects. Herpes-like DNA sequences have been identified in AIDS-associated Kaposi sarcoma. These are thought to represent a new human herpesvirus, now designated human herpesvirus 8 (HHV-8).

The vast majority of *non-Hodgkin lymphomas* in patients with HIV are of B-cell origin. Intermediate- or high-grade B-cell non-Hodgkin lymphoma is a CDC-defined AIDS diagnosis. As patients with AIDS live longer, this complication will become more frequent. It commonly presents with constitutional symptoms (fever, night sweats, weight loss) and involvement of extranodal sites, the most commonly involved sites being the central nervous system, bone marrow, gastrointestinal tract, and liver. The optimal treatment of HIV-associated non-Hodgkin lymphoma has not been well defined. It has become clear, however, that high-intensity chemotherapeutic regimens do not necessarily translate into better outcome when compared with lower-dose regimens, especially in patients with profound immunosuppression. The most important predictor of outcome is the underlying immune status of the HIV-infected patient.

Primary central nervous system lymphoma, associated with Epstein-Barr virus in almost 100% of cases, is a complication of advanced AIDS (CD4 count <50/mm^3) and occurs in 1% to 3% of all patients with AIDS. Clinical presentation includes headache, focal neurologic deficits, and seizure. Brain imaging studies show single or multiple contrast-enhancing lesions. Biopsy is required for diagnosis. Whole-brain radiation is the primary treatment of primary central nervous system lymphoma. Even with treatment, the mean duration of survival is usually less than 6 months.

Miscellaneous Infections and Clinical Syndromes

Bacillary angiomatosis was first described in 1983, and the causative organisms, *Bartonella quintana* and *Bartonella henselae*, were isolated for the first time in 1992. Bacillary angiomatosis is characterized by vascular proliferative lesions that can involve any organ in the body. The most commonly involved site is the skin, where it may present as nodules or plaques that are sometimes difficult to differentiate from Kaposi sarcoma. Other sites include bone, lymph nodes, brain, respiratory tract, and gastrointestinal tract. Characteristic, fluid-filled spaces occasionally are noted in the liver and spleen and are called peliosis hepatis or peliosis splenis. Diagnosis is established by biopsy, demonstration of the organism on Warthin-Starry stain, and cultivation of the causative organisms. Results of blood culture (lysis centrifugation technique) also may be positive if incubation is prolonged. Treatment is with erythromycin or doxycycline.

Oral disease is common and can occur at any stage of HIV disease. Oral lesions in HIV-infected persons can be caused by fungi, bacteria, virus, or neoplasms. Recurrent aphthous ulcers and salivary gland disease also occur in this population. The clinical manifestations of oral candidiasis are varied and include pseudomembranous candidiasis, erythematous candidiasis, and angular cheilitis. Treatment is either local (clotrimazole, nystatin) or systemic (fluconazole). Periodontal disease also is common, causing linear gingival erythema and necrotizing periodontitis. The causative oral flora are similar to those in non-HIV-infected persons. Treatment includes local debridement, daily chlorhexidine mouth rinses, and, in cases of necrotizing periodontitis, the addition of metronidazole, amoxicillin-clavulanate, or clindamycin. The etiologic agent of *oral hairy leukoplakia* is Ebstein-Barr virus. It usually responds to acyclovir therapy.

Gynecologic complications in women with HIV infection include recurrent or chronic genital infections (vulvovaginal candidiasis, trichomoniasis, herpes simplex virus type 2), anogenital infections with human papilloma virus, and invasive cervical cancer. Note that, as of January 1993, invasive cervical cancer is an AIDS-defining condition.

Recent Advances

Advances in the management of HIV during the past 2 years have led to a new perception of the disease and the establishment of new treatment paradigms. These advances include 1) an improved understanding of the pathogenesis of HIV infection, 2) the development of reliable assays to detect and quantify HIV-1 RNA (viral load), 3) the availability of new and potent drugs to treat HIV infection, and 4) results from recently completed trials of antiretroviral therapy demonstrating that treatment of HIV does translate into clinical benefit as defined by reductions in the risk of progression to AIDS and death.

Pathogenesis

Contrary to previously held beliefs, HIV is not dormant during the so-called clinical latency period. Studies (with use of nucleic acid hybridization techniques) of lymph node biopsy specimens from HIV-infected persons have demonstrated active virus application at all stages of disease. As many as 10 billion viral particles are produced and cleared daily in an HIV-infected person throughout all stages of disease. Concurrent with this rapid turnover of the HIV virus, more than 2 billion CD4 lymphocytes are produced every day.

Quantitative Plasma HIV RNA (Viral Load)

The ability to reliably quantify plasma HIV RNA is a significant advance that permits individualized management of HIV-infected persons. Currently, three assays are available for measurement of the viral load: reverse transcriptase polymerase chain reaction (RT-PCR), branched DNA (bDNA) assay, and nucleic acid sequence-based amplification (NASBA). The methods differ, but all three are thought to be reliable and reproducible. Of the three assays, RT-PCR is the only one that has, as of yet, been approved by the Food and Drug Administration for use in clinical practice, but the others are available through commercial laboratories.

New Antiretroviral Drugs

Before November 1995, the antiretroviral drugs available and approved for clinical use in the United States consisted of only four nucleoside analogue reverse transcriptase inhibitors: zidovudine (Retrovir, ZDV, AZT), zalcitabine (Hivid, ddC), didanosine (Videx, ddI), and stavudine (Zerit, d4T). Since then, two new classes of agents and 11 new agents have been approved (Table 14-21).

Antiretroviral Treatment Trials

In the early years of antiretroviral therapy, the use of single drugs was the standard, and sequential single-drug substitutions were used for clinical failure or adverse reactions. This monotherapy approach resulted in weak suppression of HIV replication, rapid development of drug resistance, and a short-lived clinical benefit. Since then, several clinical trials using combination antiretroviral drug regimens have clearly demonstrated that these regimens are associated with greater declines in viral replication and sustained clinical benefits as measured by a delay in progression to AIDS and a reduction in the risk of death.

Guidelines for Use of Antiretroviral Therapy for HIV Infection

Recent advances in the management of HIV infection have made earlier state-of-the-art guidelines and recommendations obsolete. In recent months, guidelines addressing the issue of antiretroviral therapy in different populations and situations have become available.

Guidelines for Use of Antiretroviral Agents in HIV-Infected Adults

A panel of leading AIDS specialists, convened by the Department of Health and Human Services in collaboration with the Henry J. Kaiser Family Foundation, has developed recommendations for use of antiretroviral agents in HIV-infected adults and adolescents. There is general consensus for treating patients with the acute HIV syndrome, those within 6 months of seroconversion, and those with symptoms ascribed to HIV infection. Although the HIV RNA level that should trigger initiation of treatment in an asymptomatic HIV-infected individual with a high CD4 cell count is still being debated, it is generally recommended that treatment should be offered to those HIV-infected individuals with a CD4 count less than 500 cells/mm^3 or a plasma HIV RNA value more than 10,000 copies/mL (bDNA assay) or 20,000 copies/mL (RT-PCR assay). Additionally, patients must actively participate in all therapeutic decisions, understand the benefits and risks of treatment, and make an informed commitment to a complex, long-term treatment.

The goal of treatment is maximal viral suppression for as long as possible. On the basis of currently available clinical trial data, the regimen of choice for initiation of antiretroviral therapy is the combination of a protease inhibitor or efavirenz in combination with two nucleoside analogue reverse transcriptase inhibitors. The combination of ritonovir plus saquinavir with one or two nucleoside analogue reverse transcriptase

Table 14-21.—Currently Approved Antiretroviral Drugs

Nucleoside analogue reverse transcriptase inhibitors	Non-nucleoside analogue reverse transcriptase inhibitors	Protease inhibitors
Zidovudine	Nevirapine	Saquinavir
Didanosine	Delavirdine	Fortovase*
Zalcitabine	Efavirenz	Indinavir
Stavudine		Ritonovir
Lamivudine		Nelfinavir
Abacavir		Amprenavir

*Fortovase is the brand name of a soft gel formulation of saquinavir.

inhibitors provides another option. The role of other alternative combinations is yet to be fully defined. Response to treatment is evaluated with plasma HIV RNA (viral load) levels. HIV RNA testing should be performed at baseline and repeated every 3 to 4 months during therapy and at more frequent intervals if the situation warrants. In general, successful regimens are expected to decrease the plasma HIV RNA level by at least 1 log (10-fold) at 8 weeks and to less than 500 copies/mL at 4 to 6 months. In cases of therapy failures, a new regimen consisting of at least two new agents, without cross-resistance to the drugs in the failed regimen, should be substituted.

Recommendations for the Use of Antiretroviral Drugs in Pregnant Women

In the past few years, perinatal transmission of HIV has dramatically decreased in the United States. This decrease is a result of recommendations from the U.S. Public Health Service for universal prenatal HIV counseling, testing with consent for all pregnant women, and the use of ZDV for reduction of perinatal HIV transmission. These recommendations were based on the results of the Pediatric AIDS Clinical Trial Group (PACTG) protocol 076. This trial demonstrated that the administration of ZDV to the mother during the antepartum and intrapartum periods and to the newborn for the first 6 weeks of life reduced the perinatal transmission of HIV by two-thirds. The advances in understanding the pathogenesis of HIV and the changes in antiretroviral therapy and monitoring of disease have made the establishment of new guidelines necessary.

Consequently, the U.S. Public Health Service has updated its recommendations for the use of antiretroviral drugs in pregnant women (MMWR 47:No. RR-2; 1998). The recommendations note that health care providers of pregnant HIV-infected women must address two separate but related issues: treatment of the mother's HIV infection and reduction of the risk for HIV transmission to the fetus. The benefits of therapy must therefore be weighed against the potential risk for adverse events to the fetus or newborn. In its guidelines, the U.S. Public Health Service presents various clinical scenarios and recommendations and discussions relevant to these scenarios.

Recommendations for Postexposure Prophylaxis

Numerous studies have estimated that the average risk for HIV transmission is approximately 0.3% after a percutaneous exposure to HIV-infected blood and 0.09% after a mucous membrane exposure. A retrospective case-control study of health care workers documented that the use of ZDV was associated with a 79% decrease in the risk for HIV transmission. Results of that study and studies in animals and data from PACTG on the efficacy of ZDV in preventing perinatal transmission of HIV prompted the U.S. Public Health Service to issue recommendations for postexposure prophylaxis for health care workers after occupational exposure to HIV. With the availability of new drugs and the accumulation of more knowledge, these 1996 guidelines were recently updated (MMWR 47:No. RR-7; 1998). The risk of infection is a function of the type of exposure and the infectivity of the exposure source. The guidelines provide an algorithm to guide clinicians in assessing risk and deciding when to offer postexposure prophylaxis. Systems, including written protocols, should be in place to prompt reporting and facilitate management of exposed health care workers. For most HIV exposures, a 4-week regimen of two antiretroviral drugs (ZDV and 3TC) is recommended. The addition of a protease inhibitor (indinavir or nelfinavir) is recommended for exposures with an increased risk of transmission or when resistance to one of the recommended drugs is known or suspected. Individual clinicians may, of course, prefer other antiretroviral drugs or combinations according to local knowledge and experience.

These recommendations are based on information available at the time they were developed. A mechanism has been put in place, through the HIV/AIDS Treatment Information Service Web site (http://www.hivatis.org), to refine and update the recommendations regularly in tandem with the evolution of knowledge about HIV infection.

ANTIMICROBIALS

The mechanisms of action, spectrum of activity, route of excretion, and toxicities of various antimicrobial agents are emphasized. Some of this information is given in Tables 14-22 through 14-25.

SPECIFIC ANTIBACTERIAL AGENTS

Penicillins

Natural Penicillins

These **agents** include penicillin G (intravenous, IV), penicillin V (oral), procaine penicillin (intramuscular, IM), and benzathine penicillin (IM, repository formulation).

Their **spectrum of activity** includes non-penicillinase-producing staphylococci (rare); β-hemolytic streptococci (group A, B, C, G); viridans streptococci; group D streptococci; penicillin-susceptible *Streptococcus pneumoniae* (incidence of penicillin resistance is increasing); most *Neisseria meningitidis*; non-penicillinase-producing *Neisseria gonorrhoeae*; and susceptible anaerobes (*Clostridium* species, most oral *Bacteroides* and *Fusobacterium* species, and *Peptostreptococcus*).

Enterococci are inhibited but not killed by the natural penicillins. Less common microbes that these agents are active against include *Erysipelothrix, Listeria monocytogenes, Pasteurella multocida, Streptobacillus, Spirillum, Treponema pallidum, Borrelia burgdorferi,* and *Actinomyces israelii.*

Hypersensitivity reactions are the most common **adverse reactions** (3%-10% of cases). These reactions include maculopapular rash, urticaria, angioedema, serum sickness, and

anaphylaxis. True anaphylaxis occurs in 0.004% to 0.015% of patients receiving penicillin. Intravenous preparations cause more frequent allergic reactions than oral agents. Skin testing in difficult cases can be used to predict subsequent severe (type I) penicillin allergy but will not predict maculopapular drug eruptions. Patients allergic to one penicillin should be considered allergic to all penicillins. Furthermore, there is a cross-allergenicity rate of 3% to 7% with cephalosporin compounds and also with the carbapenems. Cephalosporins should be avoided when possible in patients who have had a severe, immediate penicillin allergy (type I anaphylaxis or urticarial eruption). Gastrointestinal side effects include nausea, vomiting, and diarrhea—including *Clostridium difficile* colitis. Rare hematologic side effects include neutropenia, platelet dysfunction, and hemolytic anemia. Drug fever also can occur with penicillin therapy. Electrolyte disturbances, especially hyperkalemia, can occur when high doses of penicillin potassium are used in patients with renal dysfunction. Central nervous system side effects with penicillin G, when given in high doses, may involve tremors, lowered seizure threshold, and neuromuscular irritability.

- With natural penicillins, intravenous preparations cause more frequent allergic reactions than oral agents.
- There is a cross-allergenicity rate of 3%-7% with cephalosporin compounds.

Aminopenicillins

The **agents** are ampicillin and amoxicillin. The advantages of amoxicillin over oral ampicillin are increased gastrointestinal

Table 14-22.—Routes of Excretion of Antimicrobial Agents

Antimicrobial	Major route of excretion
Acyclovir, valacyclovir, famciclovir	Renal
Aminoglycosides	Renal
Aztreonam	Renal
Carbapenems (imipenem, meropenem)	Renal
Cephalosporins*	Renal
Chloramphenicol	Liver
Clarithromycin	Liver/renal
Clindamycin	Liver
Cotrimoxazole (trimethoprim-sulfamethoxazole)	Renal
Cytomegalovirus agents: foscarnet, ganciclovir, cidofovir	Renal
Didanosine	Liver/renal
Doxycycline	Liver, intestine
Erythromycin, azithromycin, dirithromycin	Liver
Fluconazole	Renal
Flucytosine	Renal
Fluoroquinolones†	Renal
Itraconazole, ketoconazole	Liver
Metronidazole	Liver
Non-nucleoside reverse transcriptase inhibitors (nevirapine, delaviridine, efavirenz)	Liver
Penicillins‡	Renal
Protease inhibitors	Liver
Rifamycins (rifampin, rifabutin)	Liver
Tetracycline	Renal
Vancomycin	Renal
Zalcitabine, stavudine, lamivudine	Renal
Zidovudine	Liver/renal

*Ceftriaxone has renal and biliary excretion, and cefoperazone is excreted primarily in the bile.
†Sparfloxacin and grepafloxacin are eliminated primarily by the liver and in the feces; ciprofloxacin and enoxacin have a heptic and renal elimination.
‡Nafcillin and oxacillin are excreted by the liver.

Table 14-23.—Antimicrobials That Do Not Require Dose Adjustment in Renal Failure

Cefoperazone, ceftriaxone
Choramphenicol
Clindamycin
Dapsone
Doxycycline
Erythromycin, dirithromycin, azithromycin
Grepafloxacin
Itraconazole
Ketoconazole
Metronidazole
Minocycline
Nafcillin, oxacillin, dicloxacillin
Non-nucleoside reverse transcriptase inhibitors
Protease inhibitors
Rifampin, rifabutin
Trovafloxacin

Table 14-24.—Mechanisms of Action of Antimicrobials

Cell wall	Protein synthesis	Cell membrane	Cell synthesis	RNA synthesis
Penicillins	Macrolides	Amphotericin B	Naladixic acid	Rifampin
Cephalosporins	Aminoglycosides	Azole antifungals	Quinolones	
Carbapenems	Tetracyclines		Flucytosine	
Vancomycin	Chloramphenicol			
Aztreonam	Metronidazole			

Table 14-25.—Selected Pharmacologic Properties of Azole Antifungals

| Factor | Antifungal | | |
	Ketoconazole	Fluconazole	Itraconazole
Route of administration	Oral	Oral, intravenous	Oral
Requires gastric acidity for absorption	Yes	No	Yes (capsules only)
Protein binding	99%	12%	99%
Cerebrospinal fluid concentrations	Nil	About 80%	Nil
Half-life, hr	9	25-30	15-42
Clearance route	Hepatic	Renal	Hepatic
Urinary levels of active drug	Low	High	Low
Dose reduction in renal dysfunction	No	Yes	No

absorption, decreased incidence of diarrhea, and dosing three versus four times a day.

Their **spectrum of activity** extends the antibacterial spectrum of the natural penicillins to include certain strains of *Escherichia coli, Proteus mirabilis, Salmonella, Shigella* (amoxicillin is less active than ampicillin), and β-lactamase-negative *Haemophilus influenzae* and *Moraxella catarrhalis*. Production of β-lactamase by the organism or alterations in binding to the penicillin-binding proteins have resulted in increasing resistance by some of these organisms.

Toxicities are the same as outlined under Natural Penicillins (page 576). Rash is common when these agents are given to patients with infectious mononucleosis—this is not a true allergy.

Penicillinase-Resistant Penicillins

Agents include methicillin (IV), oxacillin (IV), nafcillin (IV), dicloxacillin (oral), and cloxacillin (oral).

The **spectrum of activity** includes methicillin-susceptible *Staphylococcus aureus* and most nonenterococcal streptococci. Treatment of serious infections caused by methicillin-susceptible coagulase-negative staphylococci with these agents is controversial because of the difficulty of detecting resistance

in the laboratory. Penicillinase-resistant penicillins have no gram-negative or anaerobic activity.

Their **toxicities** are the same as outlined under Natural Penicillins (page 576). In addition, nephritis (methicillin), phlebitis (nafcillin), hepatitis (oxacillin), and transient neutropenia can occur.

● Penicillinase-resistant penicillins primarily are used for treatment of methicillin-susceptible *S. aureus*. They are also active against most nonenterococcal streptococci.

Carboxypenicillins

Agents include carbenicillin and ticarcillin.

The carboxypenicillins have a broader gram-negative **spectrum of activity** than ampicillin. When used as antipseudomonal agents, they should be used in combination with an aminoglycoside to provide synergism and to prevent the emergence of resistant organisms. They have little or no activity against staphylococci, streptococci, enterococci, or *Klebsiella* species. Because ticarcillin has more (2 to 4 times) antipseudomonal activity in vitro, it is more effective in smaller quantities than carbenicillin against *Pseudomonas aeruginosa*; thus, the adverse effects of large quantities of carbenicillin can be avoided.

Toxicities are similar to those described under Natural Penicillins (page 576). Additional side effects for the carboxypenicillins include sodium overload, hypokalemia, and platelet dysfunction.

- Carboxypenicillins have little or no activity against staphylococci, streptococci, enterococci, or *Klebsiella* species.

Ureidopenicillins

Agents include mezlocillin, piperacillin, and azlocillin.

These agents have a wide **spectrum of activity** against gram-negative bacteria. Compared with carbenicillin and ticarcillin, they have a lower sodium content per gram, less associated hypokalemia, less platelet inhibition, and greater hepatic excretion. Compared with penicillin G and ampicillin, they are slightly less active against streptococci and enterococci (except mezlocillin), but they are more active against *H. influenzae*. Mezlocillin and piperacillin are more active than carbenicillin and ticarcillin against Enterobacteriaceae, including most strains of *Klebsiella*. In addition, they are more active than ticarcillin against *Bacteroides fragilis*. Against *Pseudomonas*, piperacillin is the most active of this group, followed by mezlocillin and then azlocillin. Similar to the carboxypenicillins, combination therapy with the ureidopenicillins and an aminoglycoside is suggested because of the frequent emergence of resistance by *Pseudomonas* and *Enterobacter* species. Because of the cost of ureidopenicillins, the need for frequent dosing, and the frequency of primary resistance (20% to 40%) among certain Enterobacteriaceae, their use is becoming less common.

Toxicities are the same as detailed under Natural Penicillins (page 576). Other effects are hypokalemia (less common than with carbenicillin and ticarcillin), bleeding (less than with carbenicillin and ticarcillin), and hepatitis (similar to that with carbenicillin and ticarcillin).

β-Lactam/β-Lactamase Inhibitors

Agents in this group are amoxicillin-clavulanate, ampicillin-sulbactam, ticarcillin-clavulanate, and piperacillin-tazobactam.

The **spectrum of activity** of the parent drug is increased by the addition of β-lactamase inhibitors; this results in activity against β-lactamase-producing organisms such as *S. aureus* (nonmethicillin-resistant), *B. fragilis*, most *Klebsiella pneumoniae*, *H. influenzae*, and *M. catarrhalis*. These agents are not active against methicillin-resistant *S. aureus* and do not change the activity of the parent compound against most strains of *Pseudomonas* or *Enterobacter*.

Toxicities are similar to those of the parent compounds. Clavulanate may cause diarrhea and rarely hepatitis.

- β-Lactamase inhibitors are not active against methicillin-resistant *S. aureus*.

- These agents have good activity against β-lactamase-producing strains of *S. aureus*, *B. fragilis*, *K. pneumoniae*, *H. influenzae*, and *M. catarrhalis*.
- The addition of the β-lactamase inhibitor does not change the activity of the parent compound against most strains of *Pseudomonas* or *Enterobacter*.

Cephalosporins

First-Generation Cephalosporins

Representative agents include the injectable agents cefazolin (long serum half-life allows dosing every 8 hours) and cephalothin and the oral agents cephalexin and cefadroxil.

The **spectrum of activity** of the first-generation agents includes activity against methicillin-susceptible staphylococci, β-hemolytic streptococci, penicillin-susceptible pneumococci, and many strains of *P. mirabilis*, *E. coli*, and *Klebsiella* species. Similar to all cephalosporins, the first-generation agents are not active against methicillin-resistant staphylococci, enterococci, *L. monocytogenes*, *Legionella* species, *Chlamydia pneumoniae*, *Mycoplasma pneumoniae*, and *C. difficile*. The first-generation agents do not penetrate the blood-brain barrier and should not be used to treat meningitis.

Cephalosporins are usually well tolerated. The most common **toxicities** include adverse reactions related to the gastrointestinal tract (such as nausea, vomiting, diarrhea). Hypersensitivity reactions, primarily rashes, occur in 1% to 3% of patients taking cephalosporins. Anaphylaxis is rare. Cross-allergenicity may occur with penicillins. Other adverse reactions associated with cephalosporins include drug fever and *C. difficile* colitis.

- First-generation cephalosporins are active against methicillin-susceptible staphylococci and most streptococci.
- First-generation cephalosporins are not active against methicillin-resistant staphylococci or enterococci.

Second-Generation Cephalosporins

Representative IV agents include cefamandole, cefoxitin, cefuroxime, and cefotetan. Oral second-generation agents include cefuroxime axetil, cefprozil, cefaclor, and loracarbef. **Toxicities** with these agents are similar to those with the first-generation cephalosporins, unless specified.

In general, the second-generation agents have improved gram-negative activity but slightly less gram-positive activity than the first-generation agents. Of the second-generation agents, cefuroxime has the best activity against *S. aureus* and β-lactamase-producing *H. influenzae* and *M. catarrhalis*.

Cefamandole has limited advantage over cefazolin and is more expensive. It has some increase in activity against *E. coli*, *Klebsiella*, indole-positive *Proteus*, *Enterobacter*, and non-β-lactamase-producing *H. influenzae*. The methylthi-otetrazole (MTT) side chain causes bleeding problems and a disulfiram-like reaction.

Cefoxitin has some increase in activity over first-generation agents against *E. coli, Klebsiella*, indole-positive *Proteus*, and *Serratia*. It is less active against *S. aureus* and streptococci than first-generation cephalosporins. It is active against most strains of *B. fragilis*. It is used for treatment of intra-abdominal infections and pelvic inflammatory disease (in combination with doxycycline).

Cefotetan is similar to cefoxitin in activity against gram-positive cocci and *B. fragilis*, but it has better activity than cefoxitin against aerobic gram-negative rods. It has the MTT side chain with the associated toxicities described for cefamandole.

The oral second-generation agents have improved gram-negative activity over first-generation agents. Their activity generally includes β-lactamase-producing *H. influenzae* and *M. catarrhalis*, penicillin-sensitive streptococci, and many community-acquired strains of *E. coli, Klebsiella*, and *P. mirabilis*. Of these agents, cefaclor probably is the least stable against the β-lactamases of *H. influenzae* and *M. catarrhalis*, and treatment failures have been reported. Cefprozil and cefuroxime axetil have the greatest gram-positive activity of the oral second-generation agents.

Third-Generation Cephalosporins

Representative agents are the IV agents cefotaxime, ceftizoxime, ceftriaxone, cefoperazone, and ceftazidime and the oral agents cefixime, cefpodoxime proxetil, ceftibuten, and cefdinir. Their **toxicities** are similar to those of the first-generation cephalosporins, unless specified. The third-generation cephalosporins have improved gram-negative activity versus the second-generation agents. Of note is that some organisms, most notably *Enterobacter*, have developed an inducible resistance to these agents. Extended-spectrum β-lactamases have been seen in some strains of *Klebsiella* and *E. coli*, and they can cause resistance to ceftazidime. Their gram-positive activity varies as described below.

Cefotaxime, ceftizoxime, and ceftriaxone have very similar coverage. The primary difference among these agents is their pharmacokinetics. These agents are less active against *Pseudomonas* than ceftazidime or cefoperazone. However, they have better activity against methicillin-susceptible staphylococci and streptococci (including *S. pneumoniae*, which are intermediately resistant to penicillin) than ceftazidime and cefoperazone. Cefotaxime, ceftizoxime, and ceftriaxone have good cerebrospinal fluid penetration. Cefotaxime or ceftriaxone (± vancomycin) is the drug of choice for community-acquired meningitis (except *Listeria*). These third-generation agents are more effective than cefuroxime in *H.*

influenzae meningitis. The active desacetyl metabolite of cefotaxime allows dosing every 8 hours except in life-threatening infections. Ceftizoxime also is dosed every 8 hours, whereas the long half-life of ceftriaxone allows for dosing every 24 hours in most circumstances. Cefotaxime and ceftizoxime are primarily eliminated renally. Ceftriaxone has combined renal and hepatobiliary excretion and dosage reduction is generally unnecessary unless hepatic and renal dysfunction coexist. Ceftriaxone has been reported to cause pseudocholelithiasis, cholelithiasis, biliary colic, and chole-cystitis as a result of biliary precipitation of ceftriaxone as the calcium salt in up to 2% of cases, especially in children. This effect usually resolves with discontinuation of therapy.

Cefoperazone has some activity against *Pseudomonas*. Penetration into cerebrospinal fluid is less than that of other available third-generation cephalosporins. This agent is excreted primarily in the bile; therefore, no change in dose is needed with abnormal renal function. Cefoperazone has the MTT side chain with the associated toxicities described for cefamandole.

In regard to its spectrum of activity, ceftazidime is much more active than any other third-generation cephalosporin against *Pseudomonas*. It is less active against *S. aureus* and streptococci than most other third-generation cephalosporins. Pseudomonads may acquire resistance if the drug is used alone (less often than with the antipseudomonal penicillins). It often is used empirically in patients with neutropenic fever. It penetrates into cerebrospinal fluid as well as cefotaxime and ceftriaxone.

Oral agents in this class include cefpodoxime proxetil, cefdinir, cefixime, and ceftibuten. They have improved gram-negative activity over the second-generation oral cephalosporins, but they are not as active as the injectable third-generation agents. None of these are effective against *Pseudomonas*. Cefixime and ceftibuten have the best gram-negative activity of any oral cephalosporins. However, neither is very active against staphylococci, and ceftibuten has poor streptococcal activity. Cefpodoxime proxetil and cefdinir have better gram-positive activity than the other oral third-generation cephalosporins, particularly against staphylococci and streptococci. Although they have somewhat less gram-negative activity, they are active against *H. influenzae, M. catarrhalis, N. gonorrhoeae*, and many other gram-negative organisms.

- Ceftazidime is more active than any other third-generation cephalosporin against *Pseudomonas*.

Fourth-Generation Cephalosporins

Cefepime is the first of the fourth-generation cephalosporins. Its **spectrum of activity** includes gram-positive activity (*S.*

aureus and *Streptococcus*) similar to cefotaxime and gram-negative activity (including *P. aeruginosa*) similar to or better than ceftazidime. In addition, cefepime has a lower potential for inducible resistance and may be active against some gram-negative organisms, such as *Enterobacter*, which are resistant to third-generation agents. **Toxicities** associated with cefepime are similar to those with other cephalosporins. The agent does penetrate into the cerebrospinal fluid.

● Cefepime has gram-positive activity similar to cefotaxime and gram-negative activity similar to ceftazidime.

Carbapenems

Imipenem and Meropenem

Imipenem and meropenem are very broad-spectrum β-lactams. Their mechanism of action is similar to that of other β-lactam antibiotics (that is, inhibition of cell wall synthesis). Bacterial resistance, particularly among *P. aeruginosa*, is increasing and is mediated by various mechanisms. Imipenem is administered intravenously and is hydrolyzed in the kidney by a peptidase located in the brush border of renal tubular cells. Administration with cilastatin, a dihydropeptidase inhibitor, solves this problem and allows imipenem to have activity in the urine. Meropenem does not require the addition of cilastatin.

The carbapenems have the broadest antibacterial activity of any antibiotic currently available. Their **spectrum of activity** includes excellent activity against anaerobes, including *B. fragilis*, β-hemolytic streptococci, pneumococci, methicillin-susceptible *S. aureus*, *Enterococcus faecalis* (inhibited only), Enterobacteriaceae, *H. influenzae*, *Nocardia*, and most *P. aeruginosa*. They are not active against methicillin-resistant *S. aureus*, *Enterococcus faecium*, *Legionella*, *Chlamydia* species, *Mycoplasma* species, *Pseudomonas cepacia*, or *Stenotrophomonas maltophilia*. Differences in spectra between these agents include slightly better gram-positive activity for imipenem (probably only clinically significant for *Enterococcus faecalis*) and slightly better gram-negative activity for meropenem (including *P. aeruginosa*).

Toxicities of imipenem include nausea and vomiting (1% of cases), diarrhea (3%), rash or drug fever (2.7%), and dysgeusia. Seizures occur in 1.5% of patients, particularly in those with a history of previous seizures, renal insufficiency, or structural central nervous system defects. Nausea and vomiting may occur with less frequency with meropenem. In addition, meropenem is associated with a lower incidence of seizures than imipenem and has been used for pediatric meningitis.

● The carbapenems are the broadest spectrum agents to date—including gram-positive, gram-negative, and anaerobic organisms.

● Meropenem has a lower risk of seizures than imipenem.

Aztreonam

The monobactam antibacterial agents, of which aztreonam is the only one commercially available, are derivatives of naturally occurring monocyclic β-lactam compounds. The mechanism of action of aztreonam, like that of β-lactam antimicrobial agents, is the inhibition of cell wall synthesis. Aztreonam is administered intravenously and is excreted by the kidneys.

Its **spectrum of activity** involves only aerobic gram-negative bacteria, including *P. aeruginosa*. It has minimal activity against *Acinetobacter, Alcaligenes, Flavobacterium, Pseudomonas fluorescens*, and *S. maltophilia*. Furthermore, it has no activity against gram-positive aerobic or anaerobic bacteria, and it is not synergistic with penicillins against the enterococci, as are gentamicin and streptomycin.

The **toxicities** of aztreonam are similar to those of other β-lactams. Patients with a penicillin allergy may tolerate aztreonam because cross-reactivity is uncommon.

● Aztreonam is active only against gram-negative aerobes.
● Aztreonam may be useful in cases of penicillin or cephalosporin allergy because cross-reactivity is uncommon.

Aminoglycosides

Agents in this group are gentamicin, tobramycin, amikacin, netilmicin, streptomycin, kanamycin, and neomycin.

The **spectrum of activity** of these agents includes aerobic gram-negative bacilli, mycobacteria (*Mycobacterium tuberculosis*, streptomycin; *Mycobacterium avium-intracellulare*, amikacin; *Mycobacterium chelonei*, amikacin), *Brucella* (streptomycin), *Nocardia* (amikacin), *Francisella tularensis* (streptomycin), and *Yersinia pestis* (streptomycin). They are synergistic with certain β-lactams and vancomycin in the treatment of serious infections due to susceptible enterococci (gentamicin, streptomycin), staphylococci, and several aerobic gram-negative species.

The major **adverse reactions** to aminoglycosides include nephrotoxicity and auditory or vestibular toxicity. Neuromuscular blockade, drug fever, and hypersensitivity reactions are much less common. The risk of nephrotoxicity varies among the different aminoglycosides; neomycin is the most nephrotoxic, and streptomycin is the least nephrotoxic. Gentamicin, tobramycin, and amikacin have intermediate nephrotoxicity. Risk factors include increased serum trough levels, total cumulative dose, old age, hypotension, concomitant use of other nephrotoxic drugs, and liver disease. Aminoglycoside nephrotoxicity is almost always reversible with discontinuation of use of the drug, and it can be minimized if dosages are adjusted to achieve desired serum concentrations and if renal function is carefully monitored. Nephrotoxicity may be delayed or decreased when the entire daily dose is administered at once (single daily dosing of aminoglycosides). Nephrotoxicity is potentiated by other nephrotoxic drugs such as cisplatin, amphotericin B, vancomycin, and cyclosporine. Ototoxicity is almost always irreversible. Streptomycin, gentamicin, and tobramycin are preferentially toxic to the vestibular system, whereas amikacin and neomycin are primarily toxic to the auditory nerve. Advanced age and concomitant use of ethacrynic acid or furosemide seem to be risk factors for ototoxicity. Because of the imprecision of bedside testing for auditory and vestibular toxicity, routine audiographic and vestibular function evaluation should be considered when prolonged administration is anticipated and in patients predisposed to ototoxicity.

- Aminoglycosides are active against aerobic gram-negative bacilli and are synergistic with β-lactams or vancomycin against susceptible enterococci and staphylococci.
- Major adverse reactions to aminoglycosides are nephrotoxicity and auditory or vestibular toxicity.
- Aminoglycoside nephrotoxicity is almost always reversible with discontinuation of drug.
- Ototoxicity is almost always irreversible.

Tetracyclines

Agents are short-acting (tetracycline, chlorotetracycline, oxytetracycline), intermediate-acting (demeclocycline, methacycline), and long-acting (doxycycline, minocycline).

Spectrum of activity: These agents are drugs of choice for *Rickettsia, Chlamydia* species (including pelvic inflammatory disease), spore *M. pneumoniae, Vibrio cholerae, Vibrio vulnificus, Brucella* species (with streptomycin or rifampin), *Borrelia burgdorferi* (early stages), and *Borrelia recurrentis*. These agents are also *effective therapy* or *alternatives* for *Actinomyces*, anthrax, *Campylobacter, P. multocida, Spirillum minus, Streptobacillus moniliformis, Treponema pallidum, F. tularensis*, Whipple disease, *Y. pestis, Nocardia* (minocycline), and *Mycobacterium marinum*. Minocycline also may be active against methicillin-resistant staphylococci (in patients who cannot tolerate vancomycin). The tetracyclines sometimes are used as *prophylaxis* for traveler's diarrhea and meningococcal disease (minocycline only; rifampin is drug of choice). Although the tetracyclines are active in vitro against many aerobic gram-positive and gram-negative organisms as well as some anaerobes, they are usually not the drugs of choice to treat the infections caused by these organisms because of the presence or emergence of resistant strains.

Toxicities include gastrointestinal upset, rash, and photosensitivity. Uremia is increased in patients with renal failure.

Other, more rare side effects include acute fatty liver of pregnancy, Fanconi syndrome (old tetracycline), or pseudotumor cerebri. The tetracyclines are not used in pregnant females or in children because they impair bone growth of the fetus and stain the teeth of children. Minocycline is associated with vestibular toxicity, and recently cell-mediated hypersensitivity pneumonitis was reported.

Chloramphenicol

The **spectrum of activity** of this agent includes inhibition of most strains of clinically important aerobic and anaerobic bacteria. Exceptions include methicillin-resistant *S. aureus*, many *Klebsiella* isolates, *Enterobacter, Serratia*, indole-positive *Proteus*, and *P. aeruginosa*. It is active against *Rickettsia* organisms and has bactericidal activity against *S. pneumoniae, H. influenzae*, and *N. meningitidis*. Major indications are few (severe *Salmonella typhi* infection, bacterial meningitis or abscess due to susceptible organisms in patients who cannot tolerate penicillin or cephalosporins, and rickettsial infections in patients who cannot take tetracyclines) because of the availability of less toxic alternative therapies. Use has increased recently because of potential activity against vancomycin-resistant enterococcal infections.

Toxicities include two types of hematologic manifestations: idiosyncratic aplastic anemia (not dose-related; severe, often fatal; incidence approximately 1/24,000 to 1/40,000) and dose-related, reversible bone marrow suppression (much more common with a dose >4 g/day or increased serum levels). Gray syndrome (abdominal distention, cyanosis, vasomotor collapse) occurs in premature infants and possibly in patients with profound liver failure who cannot conjugate chloramphenicol and who have high serum levels. Rare toxic effects are hemolytic anemia, retrobulbar neuritis, peripheral neuritis, and potentiation of oral hypoglycemic agents.

- Toxicities with chloramphenicol include two main types of hematologic manifestations: idiosyncratic aplastic anemia (very rare and usually fatal) and dose-related bone marrow suppression.

Clindamycin

Clindamycin has good anaerobic **activity**. However, 10% to 20% of *B. fragilis* organisms, 10% to 20% of non-*Clostridium perfringens* organisms, and 10% of peptostreptococci organisms are resistant to clindamycin. Clindamycin also is active against many strains of staphylococci and streptococci. However, emergence of resistance by staphylococci is common during treatment. Gram-negative aerobic bacteria and enterococci are resistant to clindamycin.

Toxicities most commonly include rash and gastrointestinal side effects. Antibiotic-associated diarrhea can occur in up to

20% of patients, and *C. difficile* colitis occurs in 1% to 10%. Minor increases of transaminase levels, reversible neutropenia, thrombocytopenia, and neuromuscular blockade when the agent is given concurrently with neuromuscular blocking agents are much less common.

- Emergence of resistance to clindamycin by staphylococci is common during treatment.
- About 10% to 20% of *B. fragilis* organisms are resistant to clindamycin.
- Antibiotic-associated diarrhea can occur in up to 20% of patients, including *C. difficile* colitis in 1% to 10% of patients.

Metronidazole

Metronidazole has very good antimicrobial **activity** against most anaerobic microorganisms, including *B. fragilis*. The exceptions include some anaerobic gram-positive non-spore-forming bacilli and peptostreptococci, *Actinomyces*, and *Propionibacterium acnes*. The agent is also effective in infections due to *Entamoeba histolytica*, *Giardia lamblia*, and *Gardnerella vaginalis*.

Toxicities include nausea, vomiting, reversible neutropenia, metallic taste, a disulfiram reaction when coadministered with alcohol, and potentiation of the effects of oral anticoagulants. Major adverse reactions are rare and usually include central nervous system effects (seizures, cerebellar ataxia, peripheral neuropathy).

Macrolides

Erythromycin

Indications for this agent include infections caused by *Legionella* species, *M. pneumoniae*, and *Campylobacter jejuni*. It is an effective or alternative agent for *Chlamydia* species, group A hemolytic streptococci, many *S. pneumoniae* (resistance is increasing), methicillin-sensitive *S. aureus* (mild skin and soft tissue infections), *N. gonorrhoeae*, and *T. pallidum*. It may eradicate the carrier state of *Corynebacterium diphtheriae* and shorten the duration of *Bordetella pertussis* disease (whooping cough). It does not have good coverage for *H. influenzae*.

Toxicities may include gastrointestinal upset (dose-related), cholestatic jaundice (especially the erythromycin estolate compound), and transitory deafness (especially with large doses, such as 4 g/day). It can increase the serum levels of several drugs that are metabolized through the P450 system, including theophylline, carbamazepine, and cyclosporine, and the potentially fatal interaction (may cause ventricular arrhythmias) with cisapride and astemizole.

Dirithromycin

The **spectrum of activity** for dirithromycin appears to be very similar to that of erythromycin. **Toxicities** are also similar to those of erythromycin, although gastrointestinal toxicity may be slightly less frequent with dirithromycin. Possible advantages of dirithromycin over erythromycin are the once-daily dosing regimen and lack of reported drug interactions. However, there is considerably less clinical experience with dirithromycin.

Clarithromycin

This agent provides good **activity** against most *S. pneumoniae* (resistance is increasing), β-hemolytic streptococci, viridans streptococci, *S. aureus* (methicillin-sensitive), *M. catarrhalis*, *Legionella pneumophila*, *M. pneumoniae*, *C. pneumoniae*, *Chlamydia trachomatis*, *B. burgdorferi*, *M. avium-intracellulare*, and *M. chelonei*. It is superior to erythromycin for *S. pneumoniae* and β-hemolytic streptococci. It is moderately effective against *H. influenzae* and *N. gonorrhoeae*. It provides poor activity against *S. aureus* (methicillin-resistant).

In regard to **bioavailability**, excellent concentrations are achieved in many body fluids. The drug penetrates macrophages and polymorphonuclear neutrophils. Food has no effect on absorption. The half-life is 4 to 6 hours, which allows twice-daily dosing. Excretion is through the liver and kidney.

Adverse effects include nausea (3%) and other gastrointestinal complaints (less often than with erythromycin). As with erythromycin, reversible hearing loss may occur at high dosages. Drug interactions (less severe than with erythromycin), including with theophylline and carbamazepine, may occur with concomitant use of clarithromycin, and serious toxicity can result from the combination of clarithromycin with cisapride or astemizole (arrhythmias).

Clinical uses include mild to moderate upper and lower respiratory tract infection (may not be appropriate initial therapy if *H. influenzae* is the expected pathogen). Others are pharyngitis, skin and soft tissue infection, *M. avium-intracellulare*, and other atypical mycobacterial infections.

Azithromycin

The **spectrum of activity** is similar to that of clarithromycin. It is twofold to fourfold less active against streptococci, including pneumococci, than erythromycin. It is more active against *H. influenzae* than clarithromycin.

In regard to **bioavailability**, excellent concentrations are achieved in many body fluids. The agent penetrates macrophages and polymorphonuclear neutrophils. Food decreases absorption. Its half-life is 68 hours, which allows once-daily dosing. In addition, for many mild to moderate infections, a 5-day course of oral azithromycin is as effective as a 10-day course with an alternative drug. Excretion is hepatic. **Adverse effects** are similar to those for clarithromycin. Intravenous azithromycin can cause pain at the injection site.

Clinical uses include treatment of mild to moderate upper and lower respiratory tract infection (may not be appropriate initial therapy if *H. influenzae* is the expected pathogen), pharyngitis, skin and soft tissue infection, nongonococcal urethritis and cervicitis (single 1-g dose), treatment or prophylaxis of *M. avium-intracellulare*, other atypical mycobacteria, and *Toxoplasma gondii*.

Vancomycin

Vancomycin, a glycopeptide antibiotic, has a **spectrum of activity** against most aerobic and anaerobic gram-positive organisms, with the exception of certain strains of *Lactobacillus, Leukonostoc, Actinomyces*, and enterococci (vancomycin-resistant strains). Vancomycin is the drug of choice for infections caused by methicillin-resistant *S. aureus*, methicillin-resistant coagulase-negative staphylococci, highly penicillin-resistant *S. pneumoniae, Bacillus* species, *Rhodococcus equi*, and other multiply resistant gram-positive organisms such as *Corynebacterium jeikium*. It is also an alternative agent for infections caused by methicillin-sensitive staphylococci, enterococci (synergistic with aminoglycosides), or streptococci in patients intolerant of β-lactam antimicrobials. Recent data suggest that vancomycin may be less effective than antistaphylococcal β-lactams for methicillin-susceptible *S. aureus* infections. Vancomycin-resistant strains of *Enterococcus* are becoming a major issue. Of great concern is the fact that vancomycin-resistant staphylococci have now also been reported. Because use of vancomycin is a risk factor for the development of vancomycin-resistant organisms, the Centers for Disease Control has developed guidelines designed to minimize unnecessary use of this agent. Oral vancomycin is not absorbed and is used to treat only *C. difficile* colitis.

Although rare, ototoxicity is the major **toxicity** with vancomycin. This side effect is more common in the elderly and when vancomycin and aminoglycosides are administered concurrently. Infusion-related pruritus and the production of an erythematous rash or flushing involving the face, neck, and upper body ("red man" syndrome) are due to non-immunologic-related release of histamine. Its frequency can be reduced by slowing the rate of infusion and by the administration of antihistamines before vancomycin infusion. Nephrotoxicity is rare, except when vancomycin and aminoglycosides (or other nephrotoxic agents) are administered concurrently. Chemical thrombophlebitis (13%) and reversible neutropenia (2%) are also known side effects.

- Vancomycin is bactericidal against most aerobic and anaerobic gram-positive organisms.
- Vancomycin is the drug of choice for infections caused by methicillin-resistant *S. aureus*, methicillin-resistant coagulase-negative staphylococci, ampicillin-resistant enterococci, highly penicillin-resistant *S. pneumoniae*, and *Bacillus* species.

- Major toxic effect is ototoxicity. Nephrotoxicity can occur when vancomycin is coadministered with other nephrotoxic agents.
- "Red man" syndrome is due to non-immunologic-related release of histamine. This is not an allergy.

Cotrimoxazole (Trimethoprim-Sulfamethoxazole)

Cotrimoxazole consists of two separate antimicrobials, trimethoprim and sulfamethoxazole, combined in a fixed (1:5) ratio. Both trimethoprim and sulfamethoxazole inhibit microbial folic acid synthesis, and when combined they have a synergistic effect.

The **spectrum of activity** of cotrimoxazole includes a wide variety of aerobic gram-positive cocci and gram-negative bacilli, including *S. aureus* (moderate activity), many coagulase-negative staphylococci, most *S. pneumoniae, H. influenzae, M. catarrhalis, L. monocytogenes*, and many Enterobacteriaceae. It is not active against anaerobic bacteria and many strains of *Citrobacter freundii, Proteus vulgaris*, and *Providencia*. It is inactive against *P. aeruginosa* and enterococci. It is active against *Pneumocystis carinii, Isospora belli, S. maltophilia*, and *Nocardia asteroides*.

Toxicities with the agent include the common adverse reactions of nausea and vomiting (3.2%) and rash (3.4%). Hypersensitivity reactions are common in patients with acquired immunodeficiency syndrome (AIDS). Diarrhea, nephrotoxicity, neutropenia, drug fever, and cholestatic hepatitis are less common. Its use is contraindicated during the last month of pregnancy and in patients with known glucose-6-phosphatase dehydrogenase deficiency. In some patients treated for *P. carinii* pneumonia, hyperkalemia due to the trimethoprim component may occur. Cotrimoxazole has several known drug interactions, including increasing the activity of oral anticoagulants, increasing plasma phenytoin concentrations, enhancing hypoglycemia in patients taking oral hypoglycemics, and contributing to pancytopenia when coadministered with chemotherapeutic agents.

- The spectrum of activity of cotrimoxazole includes a wide variety of gram-positive and gram-negative aerobic organisms.
- With cotrimoxazole, hypersensitivity reactions are common in patients with AIDS.

Fluoroquinolones

Agents include norfloxacin, ciprofloxacin, ofloxacin, lomefloxacin, enoxacin, sparfloxacin, grepafloxacin, levofloxacin, and trovafloxacin.

Fluoroquinolones are derivatives of nalidixic acid, the first quinolone. They are bactericidal against a wide variety of microorganisms because of their ability to inhibit DNA gyrase and topoisomerase IV.

The **spectrum of activity** of fluoroquinolones varies from drug to drug. In general, they are active against most Enterobacteriaceae (including most strains that cause bacterial gastroenteritis), *H. influenzae, S. aureus* (including many methicillin-resistant), many coagulase-negative staphylococci, and enterococci (urinary tract isolates only, because of high drug levels achieved in the urine). Of concern is that bacterial resistance to fluoroquinolones is increasing, particularly among *P. aeruginosa* and staphylococci.

The first-generation agent norfloxacin achieves good concentrations in the urine, kidney tissue, bile, and feces. However, levels are poor in other sites. Thus, it is used only for treatment of complicated and uncomplicated urinary tract infection, prostatitis, bacterial diarrhea, and bowel decontamination (in immunocompromised patients).

The second-generation agents include ofloxacin, enoxacin, lomefloxacin, and ciprofloxacin. These agents achieve good tissue and fluid concentrations and can be used for infections at numerous sites. Ciprofloxacin has the best gram-negative activity (including *Pseudomonas*) of the currently available fluoroquinolones. Neither ciprofloxacin nor enoxacin has good activity against *S. pneumoniae*, but ofloxacin and lomefloxacin have somewhat improved streptococcal coverage. These agents do offer some atypical pneumonia coverage.

Available third-generation agents include levofloxacin, sparfloxacin, and grepafloxacin. These agents have improved gram-positive activity, providing improved streptococcal coverage, and better activity also against staphylococci and enterococci. They also retain good gram-negative coverage, but somewhat less than that of ciprofloxacin. These agents have good activity against atypical pneumonia pathogens such as *C. pneumoniae, Mycoplasma,* and *Legionella*. They have variable activity against anaerobes, but generally less than fourth-generation agents.

To date, the available fourth-generation agent is trovafloxacin. This agent has an enhanced spectrum that includes good gram-positive, gram-negative, and anaerobic activity, as well as activity against atypical pneumonia organisms. Its coverage includes many strains of *P. aeruginosa*; it may be slightly less active than ciprofloxacin against this pathogen. Unfortunately, use of this agent has been limited by reports of liver damage, including transplants and death.

Intravenous formulations of ciprofloxacin, ofloxacin, levofloxacin, and trovafloxacin (alatrofloxacin) are currently available. In general, oral formulations should be used whenever possible because they attain plasma levels similar to the IV formulations and are much less costly.

Fluoroquinolones are generally safe. The most common adverse effects are nausea, vomiting, abdominal pain, and diarrhea (1%-5%). Central nervous system effects are also fairly common and can include headache, dizziness, light-headedness, confusion, restlessness, tremors, and seizures. Patients who experience seizures usually have a previous history of a seizure disorder, have a central nervous system structural defect, or are taking another drug that lowers the seizure threshold. *C. difficile* colitis is uncommon. Hypersensitivity reactions, nephrotoxicity, and serum sickness can occur but are uncommon. Phototoxicity can occur with the fluoroquinolones, and its frequency varies among the various agents. QTc prolongation and subsequent dysrhythmias have been reported with grepafloxacin and sparfloxacin; concomitant medications that can increase the QT interval (such as cisapride, astemizole, and erythromycin) should be avoided. Quinolones can cause erosions in cartilage in animals and thus are not recommended in pregnant women or in patients younger than 18 years. Tendinitis and tendon rupture are rare complications of fluoroquinolones.

There are several important **drug interaction**s with fluoroquinolones. Gastrointestinal absorption of the quinolones may be decreased by coadministration of divalent or trivalent cations, which are found in aluminum- and magnesium-containing antacids, multivitamin preparations that include zinc, oral iron preparations, and calcium supplements. Concurrent administration of sucralfate also inhibits quinolone absorption. Spacing administration of the quinolone and interacting drug by several hours can minimize these absorption interactions. Some quinolones, particularly ciprofloxacin, enoxacin, grepafloxacin, and, to a lesser extent, ofloxacin, increase serum theophylline and caffeine concentrations. Morphine, and possibly other narcotic agents, can decrease oral absorption and area under the curve of trovafloxacin. This is likely a class effect that may apply to all quinolones. Whether this interaction affects other quinolones is unknown. Studies are ongoing to further delineate these interactions.

- Bacterial resistance to fluoroquinolones is increasing, particularly among *P. aeruginosa* and staphylococci.
- Gastrointestinal absorption of quinolones may be decreased by coadministration of aluminum-, calcium-, and magnesium-containing antacids, oral iron preparations, sucralfate, and multivitamin preparations with minerals.

ANTIFUNGAL THERAPY

Amphotericin B

Amphotericin B is a fungicidal antifungal agent whose **mode of action** is binding of ergosterol in cell walls and increasing cell wall permeability. It is used for most serious or life-threatening fungal infections. Exceptions include *Pseudallescheria boydii*, chromoblastomycosis, *Candida lusitaniae*, and *Candida guillermondii*, which have inherent resistance to amphotericin.

Toxicities include infusion-related toxicities such as fever, chills, nausea, and vomiting. Pretreatment options (such as diphenhydramine and acetaminophen) are available which may lessen these adverse reactions if a patient experiences problems. Nephrotoxicity is the other major side effect of amphotericin B. This can be lessened by sodium loading, every other day dosing, or using a lipid formulation of amphotericin B. Nephrotoxicity is increased with concomitant use of cyclosporine or other nephrotoxic agents. Other adverse effects include hypokalemia (may exacerbate digitalis toxicity), hypomagnesemia, phlebitis, and pulmonary infiltrates when given to patients who have had a leukocyte transfusion.

Three lipid formulations of amphotericin B are currently available: amphotericin B lipid complex (Abelcet), amphotericin B cholesteryl sulfate (Amphotec), and liposomal amphotericin (Ambisome). These agents are considerably less renal toxic than amphotericin B, but they have variable effects on infusion-related toxicities. Unfortunately, these newer agents are very expensive and should be used judiciously.

Flucytosine

The **mode of action** of this agent involves conversion to 5-fluorouracil intracellularly. Resistance develops rapidly when it is used alone. It has **activity** against cryptococci, *Candida* species, and chromoblastomycosis. **Indications** include cryptococcal meningitis (used in combination with amphotericin B), *Candida* meningitis (good cerebrospinal fluid penetration, in combination with amphotericin B), *Candida* cystitis (urinary levels are high), and chromoblastomycosis.

Toxicity is associated with high serum levels (>100 μg/mL). Neutropenia, thrombocytopenia, diarrhea, nausea, gastrointestinal upset, colitis, and hepatotoxicity (idiosyncratic, uncommon) are possible side effects. Serum levels should be monitored to minimize toxicity.

Azole Antifungals

The azole antifungal agents produce their fungistatic effect by interfering with the synthesis and permeability of fungal cell membranes. They do this through inhibition of the fungal cytochrome P450 enzyme responsible for conversion of lanosterol to ergosterol, which is a major constituent of fungal cell membranes. This results in leakage of intracellular contents. The azole antifungal agents are less toxic alternatives to amphotericin for many types of fungal infections.

Ketoconazole

Ketoconazole was the first of the azole antifungals. It has a broad spectrum of action; however, because of its toxicities and the improved pharmacologic characteristics of newer agents, ketoconazole is typically not a drug of choice. It is currently second-line therapy (itraconazole is drug of choice)

for nonmeningeal and non–life-threatening *Histoplasmosis* and *Blastomycosis* in immunocompetent patients. The drug is also used as an alternative for chronic mucocutaneous candidiasis, paracoccidioidomycosis, and *Pseudallescheria boydii*. It has poor cerebrospinal fluid penetration and should not be used to treat central nervous system fungal infections.

Ketoconazole requires gastric acid for absorption. Antacids, H_2 receptor antagonists, proton pump inhibitors, and didanosine (contains buffers) increase gastric pH and inhibit absorption of this agent. Coadministration of isoniazid, phenytoin, or rifampin can decrease drug levels. In addition, ketoconazole can increase the levels of several drugs metabolized through the P450 system (CYP3A4 isoenzyme). Drugs whose metabolism may be inhibited include cyclosporine, tacrolimus, calcium channel blockers, hydroxymethylglutaryl-coenzyme A (HMG-CoA) reductase inhibitors, and others. It is contraindicated in patients receiving astemizole or cisapride because concomitant therapy can lead to potentially fatal dysrhythmias. Warfarin levels also can be significantly increased.

The most common **toxic effect** of ketoconazole is dose-related gastrointestinal upset. Decreased synthesis of adrenal corticosteroids, most notably androgenic steroids, may occur with ketoconazole. This may lead to gynecomastia, menstrual irregularities, and loss of libido with impotence, especially with higher dosages of ketoconazole. Arterial hypertension, edema, and hypokalemia also have been reported. Acute hepatitis, which can be fatal, occurs rarely.

- Ketoconazole requires gastric acid for absorption.
- Ketoconazole potentiates the effect of warfarin and has serious interactions with astemizole and cisapride.
- Gynecomastia is a fairly common side effect.

Fluconazole

Fluconazole is a newer azole antifungal with fewer side effects and drug interactions. It has activity against *Candida*, *C. neoformans*, *C. immitis*, *H. capsulatum*, *B. dermatitidis*, and paracoccidioidomycosis.

Clinical uses include treatment of many types of susceptible candidal infections. The drug is also used for prophylaxis of candidal infection in neutropenic patients, patients undergoing bone marrow transplantation, and patients with AIDS. A concern is emergence of resistant fungi (such as *C. krusei*, resistant *C. glabrata*). In serious infections, speciation and susceptibility testing of *Candida* organisms should be considered.

Fluconazole is also used for treatment of cryptococcal meningitis. For this infection, most experts recommend initial therapy with amphotericin B, followed by maintenance therapy with fluconazole. In addition, this agent has been used successfully for treatment of *Coccidioides* meningitis. It is second-line therapy for non–life-threatening cases of histoplasmosis and blastomycosis (itraconazole is preferred).

Because of the long half-life of fluconazole, it can be administered in a once-per-day dose. It is available in oral tablet, oral suspension, and IV formulations. Because of its excellent oral absorption and the considerably higher expense of IV therapy, fluconazole should be given via the oral route whenever possible.

This agent is generally well tolerated. **Adverse effects** can occur in up to 16% of patients. However, discontinuation of therapy is necessary in only 1% to 2% of patients. Most common effects are gastrointestinal (1.5% to 3.5%), rash (1.8%), and headache (1.9%). Fatal hepatic necrosis and exfoliative rash also have been reported. There is no interference with adrenocortical function or synthesis of testosterone, which can occur with ketoconazole.

Fluconazole inhibits metabolism of several other drugs. It increases serum levels of phenytoin, oral hypoglycemic agents, carbamazepine, cyclosporine, tacrolimus, calcium channel blockers, and warfarin. It also can increase concentrations of rifabutin, leading to potential uveitis (dose should be decreased). Coadministration with rifampin and isoniazid decreases serum concentrations of fluconazole.

Itraconazole

A major advantage of itraconazole over fluconazole is its greater activity against *Aspergillus, S. schenckii, H. capsulatum*, and *B. dermatitidis*. **Clinical uses** include histoplasmosis, in which it is used for chronic cavitary pulmonary disease and disseminated, non–life-threatening nonmeningeal disease. Itraconazole also is effective maintenance therapy in patients with AIDS. Itraconazole is now the drug of choice for pulmonary and nonpulmonary (bone, joint, skin) blastomycosis. For coccidioidomycosis (pulmonary, bone, and joint), the efficacy rate is 57% to 72%. A small number of patients with coccidioidal meningitis also have been effectively treated. When used for sporotrichosis, itraconazole is effective in lymphocutaneous and bone and joint disease, although relapse may occur in disseminated disease. As therapy for *Aspergillus*, success rates of 44% to 77% have been reported for invasive pulmonary and sinus disease. Amphotericin B remains the drug of choice, at least for initial use, for most cases of aspergillosis.

Itraconazole is now available in capsule and oral solution formulations. These two formulations are not bioequivalent; the oral solution produces considerably higher serum concentrations and area under the curve. To optimize absorption, the capsule should be taken with food, and the liquid on an empty stomach.

Minor **side effects** occur in 2% to 20% of patients if doses less than 400 mg/day are used. The most common side effects involve the gastrointestinal tract: nausea, 10.6%; vomiting,

5.1%; and abdominal pain, 1.5%. Rash occurs in 8.6% of patients. Hepatitis can occur but is rare. If the dose is less than 400 mg/day, there is no effect on glucocorticoid or testosterone synthesis. At doses more than 400 mg/day, edema, hypokalemia, nausea, and vomiting can occur.

Itraconazole inhibits metabolism and increases serum levels of cyclosporine, digoxin, astemizole, and cisapride. Cyclosporine and digoxin levels should be monitored, and astemizole and cisapride should not be administered concurrently because of potentially fatal ventricular arrhythmias. Coadministration with rifampin, isoniazid, phenytoin, and carbamazepine can decrease itraconazole levels. Like ketoconazole, itraconazole capsules require gastric acid for absorption; thus, absorption is decreased with concomitant use of H_2 blockers, antacids, proton pump inhibitors, and didanosine (contains an antacid buffer). This interaction is less significant with the oral liquid formulation.

ANTIVIRAL AGENTS

Current agents are virustatic and have no activity against nonreplicating or latent viruses.

Acyclovir

This is a nucleoside analog of guanosine. After phosphorylation by virus-specific thymidine kinase to monophosphate and further phosphorylation to triphosphate by cellular enzymes, it inhibits DNA polymerase. In vitro activity and clinical efficacy correlate with the amount of viral-specific thymidine kinase produced (herpes simplex virus type 1 > herpes simplex virus type 2 > varicella-zoster virus > Epstein-Barr virus). Cytomegalovirus does not produce thymidine kinase and is therefore resistant. Other viruses can develop resistance through mutations of either viral thymidine kinase or DNA polymerase. Oral acyclovir is poorly absorbed (with a bioavailability of 15%-30%). Thus, patients with severe disease or who are immunocompromised should generally receive intravenous therapy. Acyclovir generally is well tolerated. **Toxicities** include gastrointestinal distress and headaches (oral form), phlebitis (intravenous form), and crystalline nephropathy (increased risk with high dose, bolus infusion, dehydration, and preexisting renal impairment). Confusion, delirium, lethargy, and seizures can occur in patients with a serum concentration more than 25 µg/mL.

Indications for the drug include herpes simplex virus infections. It is effective for treatment of primary and recurrent episodes of herpes genitalis and suppression of frequent recurrences. Topical acyclovir is less effective than oral in genital herpes simplex virus infection. Intravenous therapy should be considered in serious disease. If chronic suppression is used, reassess after 1 year. In immunocompromised patients, oral or intravenous acyclovir is highly effective in the prophylaxis and treatment of oral-labial disease. Intravenous acyclovir is the drug of choice for herpes simplex virus encephalitis; a high dose is used (10 mg/kg every 8 hours). Acyclovir also is used for varicella-zoster virus. Intravenous acyclovir in immunocompromised patients can halt progression and prevent dissemination of herpes zoster. In immunocompetent patients with primary varicella, it can shorten the healing time (about 1 day) and decrease the number of lesions if given early (within 24 hours). Oral therapy is effective against herpes zoster ophthalmicus (most effective within 72 hours; 600 to 800 mg five times a day). Herpes zoster in an immunocompetent host responds to acyclovir, 800 mg five times a day (decreased viral shedding, time to healing). It should be used only if given within 72 hours after onset of symptoms. There is a questionable effect on postherpetic neuralgia.

- With acyclovir, crystalline nephropathy is increased with high dose, bolus infusion, dehydration, and preexisting renal impairment.
- Intravenous acyclovir is the drug of choice for herpes simplex encephalitis.

Valacyclovir

Valacyclovir is an oral pro-drug of acyclovir which is converted extensively and almost completely to acyclovir and L-valine. Acyclovir is the active drug that inhibits viral DNA synthesis. Approximately 54% to 60% of the valacyclovir dose is available as active acyclovir, representing a twofold to fivefold increase in bioavailability over that achieved after administration of oral acyclovir. The higher bioavailability of valacyclovir also allows for less frequent administration than with oral acyclovir (3 times per day with valacyclovir versus 5 times per day with acyclovir). Like acyclovir, valacyclovir generally is well tolerated.

Toxicities with valacyclovir are very similar to those with acyclovir (see above). However, when valacyclovir was studied in high doses in immunosuppressed patients (patients who had transplantation and patients with human immunodeficiency virus [HIV]), thrombotic thrombocytopenic purpura and hemolytic-uremic syndrome were reported. Thus, valacyclovir currently is not approved for immunocompromised hosts.

Indications: Valacyclovir currently is approved by the Food and Drug Administration (FDA) for the treatment of herpes zoster infections and for the treatment and suppression of recurrent genital herpes. Some studies have suggested that valacyclovir may be more effective than acyclovir for herpes zoster.

- Valacyclovir is an oral pro-drug of acyclovir which increases bioavailability twofold to fivefold.

- Valacyclovir currently is contraindicated in immunocompromised patients because thrombotic thrombocytopenic purpura and hemolytic-uremic syndrome have been reported in this population.

Famciclovir

Famciclovir is a relatively new antiviral agent. Available only as an oral drug, famciclovir is a pro-drug that is converted to its active form, penciclovir, through tissue and hepatic enzymatic processes. A prolonged intracellular half-life allows for dosing three times daily. It has good bioavailability and is well tolerated. It may reduce the duration of postherpetic neuralgia when given early in herpes zoster. It is also useful for treatment and suppression of genital herpes.

Ganciclovir

This agent inhibits DNA polymerase and is dependent on phosphorylation by viral thymidine kinase. It is active against herpes viruses, particularly cytomegalovirus. It is available as oral and intravenous preparations.

Indications for ganciclovir include treatment of cytomegalovirus retinitis in patients with AIDS. Studies have shown beneficial results in other cytomegalovirus infections (colitis, esophagitis, gastritis, and pneumonia) in patients with AIDS and in other immunocompromised hosts. In patients with AIDS, maintenance therapy may be necessary to prevent relapse. Used in combination with hyperimmune globulin, ganciclovir reduces mortality from cytomegalovirus pneumonitis in patients who have had allogeneic bone marrow transplantation. Ganciclovir therapy given before the development of cytomegalovirus disease in patients who have had heart or bone marrow transplantation may decrease the incidence of cytomegalovirus infection.

Toxicities include neutropenia and thrombocytopenia. The incidence of neutropenia may be increased when ganciclovir is used in combination with other immunosuppressive drugs. Cytopenias are reversible after use of the drug is stopped. It is teratogenic, carcinogenic, and mutagenic in animals. Less common are fever, rash, anemia, and increased values on liver function tests.

Ganciclovir **resistance** is associated with persistent viremia and progressive disease. The mechanism of resistance is postulated to be decreased cellular phosphorylation.

Oral ganciclovir is an alternative to intravenous maintenance therapy for cytomegalovirus retinitis in patients who have only peripheral cytomegalovirus lesions. Unfortunately, the oral formulation has poor bioavailability. An oral prodrug of ganciclovir that will achieve higher systemic levels is currently under study.

Ganciclovir ocular implants are also available which provide the drug directly to the site of the infection. Vitrasert implants are surgically implanted into the pars plana and deliver a slow release of drug over 7 to 8 months. Possible disadvantages include the spread of infection to the contralateral eye, a low incidence of endophthalmitis, and the need to replace the inserts about every 8 months. Research is under way on implants that may last up to 2 years.

- Ganciclovir is used for cytomegalovirus in immunocompromised patients.
- The incidence of neutropenia is increased when ganciclovir is used in combination with other immunosuppressive drugs.

Foscarnet

This is a noncompetitive inhibitor of viral DNA polymerase and reverse transcriptase. It does not require phosphorylation and may be active against acyclovir-resistant and ganciclovir-resistant strains. It has in vitro activity against HIV, all human herpes viruses, and hepatitis B.

Indications include cytomegalovirus retinitis, including disease that is due to ganciclovir-resistant strains. It also may be effective in gastrointestinal disease in patients with AIDS. Foscarnet may be active against acyclovir-resistant strains of herpes simplex virus or varicella-zoster virus and against ganciclovir-resistant strains of cytomegalovirus. However, it is more expensive and less well tolerated than ganciclovir. It requires controlled rates of infusions and large volumes of fluid. Controlled trials in patients with AIDS and cytomegalovirus retinitis showed no difference in the progression of the retinitis between foscarnet-treated and ganciclovir-treated patients. However, there was an unexplained decrease in mortality in the foscarnet group (which may be related to antiretroviral activity).

Toxicities include nephrotoxicity, which usually develops during the second week and is reversible. The risk of nephrotoxicity is increased with concurrent use of nephrotoxic drugs (such as amphotericin B, aminoglycosides). Hydration may decrease the risk of nephrotoxicity. Electrolyte disturbances, such as hypocalcemia, hyperphosphatemia, hypophosphatemia, hypokalemia, and hypomagnesemia, also may occur. The risk of hypocalcemia is increased with concomitant use of pentamidine intravenously. Fever, nausea, vomiting, anemia, fatigue, headache, leukopenia, pancreatitis, and genital ulceration also have been reported.

- Foscarnet is effective for cytomegalovirus retinitis, including disease due to ganciclovir-resistant strains.
- With foscarnet, nephrotoxicity may occur; it usually develops during the second week and is reversible.

Cidofovir

Cidofovir is a nucleotide analogue with activity against herpes viruses, including cytomegalovirus, herpes simplex virus, varicella-zoster virus, and Epstein-Barr virus. Its FDA indication is for the treatment of cytomegalovirus retinitis in patients with AIDS. Unlike ganciclovir and acyclovir, which require activation by viral-encoded enzymes, conversion of cidofovir to its active intracellular metabolite is performed by host (rather than viral) cellular enzymes. Thus, cidofovir may retain activity against many ganciclovir-resistant strains of cytomegalovirus. The long intracellular half-life of cidofovir-active metabolites allows for weekly intravenous dosing during induction therapy and every other week intravenous administration during maintenance therapy. The dose-limiting toxicity of cidofovir is nephrotoxicity. Administration with probenecid and saline hydration can decrease the incidence and severity of nephrotoxicity. It is contraindicated in patients with preexisting renal dysfunction (serum creatinine >1.5 mg/dL, estimated creatinine clearance <55 mL/min, or urine protein ≥100 mg/dL), and renal function must be monitored closely during therapy. It also should not be given with other nephrotoxic drugs. Neutropenia also has been reported in up to 20% of patients. More rare adverse reactions include ocular hypotony and metabolic acidosis. Adverse effects to probenicid are also fairly common.

Ribavirin

Ribavirin is a purine analog. Aerosolized ribavirin is indicated for respiratory syncytial virus bronchiolitis in children, in whom treatment decreases morbidity. Adverse teratogenic and embryotoxic effects have been noted in animals. The drug is contraindicated in pregnancy, and precautions must be taken when aerosolized ribavirin is used in the hospital. A new combination product containing injectable interferon alfa-2b and oral ribavirin has been recently released for the treatment of chronic hepatitis C infection.

ANTIRETROVIRAL THERAPY

(See the section on Human Immunodeficiency Virus, page 567, for a discussion of clinical issues and guidelines for the use of these agents.)

Reverse Transcriptase Inhibitors

The **mechanism of action** of these agents is to inhibit reverse transcriptase and terminate human immunodeficiency virus (HIV) nucleic acid chain elongation.

Nucleoside Reverse Transcriptase Inhibitors

Zidovudine (AZT)

This is a dideoxynucleoside (thymidine analog) that must be phosphorylated to active triphosphate form by cellular enzymes. Central nervous system concentrations are 0.1 to 1.35 (average, about 0.5) times the serum concentrations. It is effective for treating HIV neurologic disease. It is eliminated primarily through hepatic metabolism with subsequent renal excretion. Elimination is reduced in patients with uremia and cirrhosis (dosing every 8 hours may be appropriate). **Drug interactions** include an increased half-life of AZT when used with probenecid and additive myelosuppressive effects when given with ganciclovir or other immunosuppressive agents.

Adverse effects include anemia (usually megaloblastic) and neutropenia. They are less common with the lower doses commonly used today (500-600 mg/day). With more severe bone marrow suppression, discontinuation of therapy or use of granulocyte-macrophage colony-stimulating factor and granulocyte colony-stimulating factor may be necessary. Recombinant erythropoietin in patients with low erythropoietin levels (<500 IU/L) may decrease transfusion requirements. Asthenia, headache, dizziness, insomnia, anorexia, nausea, vomiting, malaise, and myalgia are common initial events after initiation of therapy, but they usually diminish with continued therapy and seldom require stopping use of the drug. Esophageal ulceration and hyperpigmentation of the skin also have been reported. Myopathy occurs in 6% to 18% of patients who receive therapy for more than 6 months. It is difficult to distinguish from HIV-associated myopathy.

- With AZT, adverse effects are anemia and neutropenia.
- Concomitant use of ganciclovir and AZT may increase the risk of neutropenia.
- Myopathy occurs in 6%-18% of patients who receive AZT for more than 6 months.

Stavudine (d4T)

Stavudine is a thymidine analogue similar to zidovudine.

Pharmacokinetics: The bioavailability of stavudine is about 86%, and it can be taken without regard to meals. About 40% of stavudine is eliminated renally, and thus the dose requires adjustment in patients with renal dysfunction. The terminal half-life in patients with normal renal function is about 1 to 1.6 hours, whereas the intracellular half-life is about 3.5 hours. Concentrations in the central nervous system are about 10% to 70% of plasma concentrations. The dosage of stavudine is based on the patient's weight (if >60 kg, dose is 40 mg twice a day; if <60 kg, dose is 30 mg twice a day).

Drug interactions: Stavudine should be used with caution in combination with other drugs that can cause peripheral neuropathy.

Toxicities: The dose-limiting toxicity is peripheral neuropathy, which occurs in 15% to 20% of patients (usually reversible). Patients with preexisting peripheral neuropathy are at increased risk for development of this adverse reaction. Hepatotoxicity also has been noted in some patients.

- The dose-limiting toxicity with stavudine is peripheral neuropathy.

Didanosine (ddI)

Didanosine is a nonthymidine analogue that must be phosphorylated to be active.

Pharmacokinetics: The bioavailability of didanosine is about 40%, and absorption is decreased with food. Didanosine is acid labile and thus is administered in a buffered form. It penetrates poorly into the central nervous system. Serum half-life is 1.4 hours, and intracellular half-life is 8 to 24 hours. It is eliminated through hepatic metabolism and renal excretion.

Drug interactions: Because ddI tablets contain antacid to enhance absorption, drugs that require gastric acidity (such as itraconazole, ketoconazole, dapsone) should be administered at least 2 hours apart from ddI. Quinolones and tetracycline absorption also may be hindered by the didanosine buffer and should be given at intervals separate from didanosine. Drugs that can cause pancreatitis (pentamidine) may increase the risk of this adverse effect.

Toxicity: Pancreatitis (about 7% of patients) is the most severe adverse effect of didanosine, and its incidence is increased with concomitant use of intravenous pentamidine, a previous history of pancreatitis, alcohol use, or advanced HIV infection. Painful peripheral neuropathy also can occur and is characterized by distal numbness, tingling, or pain in the feet or hands which generally improves 2 to 12 weeks after discontinuation. This is less common in patients in whom didanosine is introduced early in the course of HIV. Other less common potential side effects include hypersensitivity, increased liver enzyme values, fulminant hepatitis, gastrointestinal toxicity, electrolyte abnormalities, and myalgias. Anemia and neutropenia are significantly less common than in patients administered AZT.

- Pancreatitis and peripheral neuropathy are the major adverse effects of didanosine.

Zalcitabine (ddC)

Zalcitabine is a nonthymidine analogue that must be phosphorylated to be active.

Pharmacokinetics: The bioavailability is about 90%. Central nervous system concentrations are about 14% to 20% of plasma concentrations and are lower than with zidovudine. The serum half-life is 1 to 3 hours, and the intracellular half-life is 8 to 24 hours. Elimination is through renal excretion, and the dose should be decreased with renal dysfunction.

Drug interactions occur with concomitant use of drugs that have the potential to cause peripheral neuropathy either through additive direct neurotoxicity or by decreasing the renal clearance of zalcitabine. The drug should not be used concomitantly with intravenous pentamidine because of the risk of pancreatitis.

Toxicities include painful distal peripheral neuropathy (17%-31% of cases in monotherapy studies). This is usually reversible with discontinuation of use of the drug. Pancreatitis also has been reported (1% of cases), and oral and esophageal ulcers, gastrointestinal toxicity, increased liver enzyme values, and rashes also can occur. Anemia and neutropenia are significantly less common than in patients administered AZT.

- The major toxicity associated with zalcitabine is peripheral neuropathy. Pancreatitis also has been reported, but it is less frequent than with didanosine.

Lamivudine (3TC)

This is a synthetic nucleoside analogue that is phosphorylated intracellularly to its active form.

Pharmacokinetics: Bioavailability of lamivudine is about 86%. There is no significant effect on absorption when this agent is administered with food. The major route of elimination is through renal excretion, and doses must be adjusted for renal function. The half-life of lamivudine is approximately 5 to 7 hours in patients with normal renal function.

Toxicities: Lamivudine is generally well tolerated. Adverse effects noted with lamivudine include headache, rashes, nasal signs and symptoms, cough, and gastrointestinal irritation. Pancreatitis is rare (<0.5%) in adults but occurs in about 15% of pediatric patients receiving lamivudine. Paresthesias and peripheral neuropathy have been reported rarely.

Abacavir

Abacavir is a recently released nucleoside reverse transcriptase inhibitor and is believed to be the most potent agent to date of this class.

Pharmacokinetics: The bioavailability of abacavir is about 85% and is not significantly affected by the presence or absence of food. Plasma binding of abacavir is about 50%, and data from a small number of patients indicated cerebrospinal fluid levels of 27% to 33%. This drug is metabolized primarily by alcohol dehydrogenase and glucuronyl transferase, and the inactive metabolites are subsequently eliminated in the urine.

Drug interactions: Abacavir does not inhibit or induce the P450 enzymes. As a result of inhibition of alcohol dehydrogenase, alcohol significantly increases the maximal plasma concentration and area under the curve of abacavir. In addition, there is a possible increase in the area under the curve of both agents when abacavir is administered with disulfiram, chlorpromazine, isoniazid, or chloral hydrate because of common metabolic pathways.

Toxicities: The most serious toxicity is a potentially fatal hypersensitivity reaction characterized by flu-like symptoms, fever, gastrointestinal symptoms, and myalgias with or without rash. This has been reported in about 5% of patients. Patients should be warned to discontinue use of abacavir immediately and call their physician if this reaction is suspected. Patients should not be rechallenged with abacavir because more severe symptoms (including the possibility of death) will occur.

- A severe hypersensitivity reaction has been reported with abacavir. Patients should never be rechallenged with abacavir because this can lead to more severe symptoms, including death.

Non-nucleoside Reverse Transcriptase Inhibitors

These agents are chemically distinct from the nucleoside analogue reverse transcriptase inhibitors, and their actions are specific for HIV-1 (not active against HIV-2).

Nevirapine

Nevirapine was the first of the non-nucleoside reverse transcriptase inhibitors. Because resistance occurs rapidly when used as monotherapy, nevirapine should always be used in combination with at least one other antiretroviral agent. Cross-resistance with other currently available non-nucleoside reverse transcriptase inhibitors also occurs.

Pharmacokinetics: Bioavailability of nevirapine is about 93% and is not affected by administration of food. This agent distributes widely and achieves central nervous system concentrations of about half of those in plasma. It has a long half-life of about 45 hours initially and about 23 hours after 2 weeks of therapy. This agent is extensively metabolized by the P450 system and subsequently eliminated in the urine.

Drug interactions: Nevirapine may cause induction of CYP3A and may result in lower concentrations of other drugs metabolized through this route (including the protease inhibitors). Maximal induction occurs within 2 to 4 weeks.

Toxicities: The principal adverse reaction associated with nevirapine is rash (29%—with about 8% of patients requiring discontinuation of therapy). Rash was labeled as serious in only 3% to 8% of patients. Stevens-Johnson reaction has occurred in about 0.4% of patients. Beginning therapy with a dosage of 200 mg daily for 14 days and then increasing up to 400 mg per day reduces the rate of rash. If rash develops during the lead-in period, the dosage should not be increased to 400 mg per day until the rash resolves. In many cases the rash resolves despite continued treatment. Other risk factors for rash include coadministration of trimethoprim-sulfamethoxazole (Bactrim) or amoxicillin-clavulanate (Augmentin).

Headache, fever, somnolence, and asymptomatic increases in γ-glutamyltransferase also have been noted with nevirapine.

● Nevirapine was the first non-nucleoside reverse transcriptase inhibitor. Because resistance develops rapidly with monotherapy, it should be used in combination with other agents.

Delavirdine

Delavirdine is a non-nucleoside reverse transcriptase inhibitor similar to nevirapine.

Pharmacokinetics: Absorption does not appear to be significantly affected by food or didanosine. However, delavirdine should be administered at least 1 hour apart from an antacid. Delavirdine displays nonlinear pharmacokinetics if the daily dose is more than 60 mg. It is metabolized in the liver through the P450 system (primarily CYP3A4).

Drug interactions: Rifampin and rifabutin, which are strong inducers of P450-CYP3A4, can significantly decrease delavirdine concentrations. Delavirdine can inhibit the metabolism of other drugs that are substrates for CYP3A.

Toxicities: The most frequent side effects are rash, fatigue, gastrointestinal complaints, and mild headache. Rash has developed in about one-third of patients in clinical trials. This is usually a maculopapular rash occurring between days 7 and 15. The incidence of rash is higher in patients with a CD4 count less than 300/mm^3. In most cases, treatment can continue during the rash.

Efavirenz (DMP-266)

Efavirenz is the newest addition to the non-nucleoside reverse transcriptase class of medications. This agent may be more potent than the other currently available agents of this class, and it also has the advantage of once-daily dosing.

Pharmacokinetics: The bioavailability is about 40%. Meals of normal composition do not significantly affect the absorption of efavirenz. However, concomitant administration with a very high-fat meal should be avoided because this can increase absorption up to 50%. Protein binding is more than 99%, and it achieves cerebrospinal fluid concentrations of 0.26% to 1.2% of the corresponding serum concentration. It is metabolized by P450 isoenzymes 3A4 and 2B6 and induces its own metabolism.

Drug interactions: Efavirenz can induce or inhibit metabolism of other drugs that are metabolized by P450, and the package insert should be consulted regarding drug interactions before this agent is prescribed. Drugs that are contraindicated include astemizole, cisapride, midazolam, triazolam, and ergot derivatives.

Toxicities: The most frequent side effects include rash and central nervous system symptoms. The incidence of rash may be less common than with other non-nucleoside reverse tran-

scriptase inhibitors, and treatment can often be continued despite the rash. Rash is more common and may be of a higher grade in children. Nervous system adverse reactions include dizziness, sleep disturbances, vivid dreams or nightmares, a feeling of "disconnectedness," and impaired concentration. These side effects generally subside within 1 to 2 weeks. Serious central nervous system effects (such as delusions and hallucinations) may be more frequent in patients with underlying psychiatric illness or substance abuse problems. Efavirenz is usually given in the evening to minimize side effects during the day.

Protease Inhibitors

The **mechanism of action** of these agents is to inhibit viral protease. Viral protease is necessary for the terminal maturation of infectious virions. Inhibiting protease results in production of immature, defective viral products. These agents require no intracellular processing for activation. Protease inhibitors are very potent antiretroviral agents but need to be used in combination with other agents because resistance occurs rapidly with monotherapy.

Saquinavir

Saquinavir was the first available protease inhibitor and shows synergy with reverse transcriptase inhibitors.

Pharmacokinetics: The original formulation of saquinavir (Invirase) has poor bioavailability (only about 4%). Because of this, a new formulation (Fortouase) has been developed. Administering saquinavir with a high-fat meal enhances its absorption. After administration, saquinavir undergoes extensive first-pass metabolism. It is primarily metabolized by the P450 isoenzyme CYP3A4. Only about 1% of the dose is eliminated renally. Saquinavir appears to partition extensively into tissues, but penetration into the central nervous system is minimal. This agent is highly protein-bound (about 98%).

Drug interactions: Saquinavir is an inhibitor of the P450 isoenzyme CYP3A4 and thus can increase concentrations of other drugs metabolized through this route (it is a less potent inhibitor than indinavir or ritonavir). It should not be used concomitantly with terfenadine, astemizole, or cisapride because potentially fatal arrhythmias may occur. In addition, saquinavir used in combination with enzyme inducers, such as rifampin, rifabutin, and phenobarbital, significantly reduces concentrations of saquinavir. Consult the package insert for more information on drug interactions.

Toxicities: Saquinavir is generally well tolerated. The most common adverse effects are headache, diarrhea, nausea, and gastrointestinal discomfort. These are typically mild. Lipid disturbances, body shape alterations, and rare cases of diabetes have also been reported in patients on protease inhibitors.

• Saquinavir is generally well tolerated; gastrointestinal side effects and headache are the most common adverse effects.

Ritonavir

Ritonavir appears to be the most potent of the currently available protease inhibitors.

Pharmacokinetics: The bioavailability of ritonavir is 60% and is significantly better than with saquinavir. Absorption is increased when administered with food. Ritonavir is extensively metabolized by the P450 system isoenzyme CYP3A4, and it is a very potent inhibitor of this isoenzyme. It is about 98% protein-bound and has a half-life of about 3 hours.

Drug interactions: Ritonavir is an extremely potent inhibitor of the isoenzyme CYP3A4 and can significantly increase the concentrations of other drugs metabolized through this route. It is sometimes purposefully used to boost the levels of other protease inhibitors. Ritonavir also may inhibit other isoenzymes to a lesser degree. A long list of potential drug interactions is provided on the package insert, and this should be checked carefully when any drugs are given concomitantly with ritonavir. Agents that induce liver enzymes (such as rifampin, rifabutin, phenobarbital) can decrease ritonavir levels.

Toxicities: Adverse reactions with ritonavir include circumoral and peripheral paresthesias, altered taste, gastrointestinal disturbances, and increased liver function tests. Gastrointestinal toxicities typically subside over time. Lipid disturbances, body shape alterations, and rare cases of diabetes have also been reported in patients on protease inhibitors.

• Ritonavir is a very potent inhibitor of the P450 system and has numerous potential drug interactions.

Indinavir

Pharmacokinetics: Indinavir is rapidly absorbed. Administration with a meal high in fat, protein, or calories reduces the area under the curve by about 84%. It should be taken on an empty stomach if possible. Alternatively, it can be taken with other low-fat liquids such as skim milk, coffee, tea, or juice or with a light meal. The half-life of indinavir is about 2 hours. It is primarily metabolized in the liver through the P450 system (isoenzyme CYP3A4).

Drug interactions: Like ritonavir, indinavir is an inhibitor of isoenzyme CYP3A4 and can significantly increase the concentrations of other drugs metabolized through this route. Indinavir has the potential to cause many drug interactions, and the package insert should be checked carefully for drug interactions before indinavir is prescribed. It inhibits the metabolism of drugs metabolized through the P450 isoenzyme 3A4. In addition, it should be given at least 1 hour from didanosine administration because optimal absorption of indinavir may

require gastric acidity. Because rifampin can significantly reduce indinavir concentrations, these two drugs should not be used concomitantly.

Toxicities: Indinavir is generally fairly well tolerated. Nephrolithiasis is reported in about 4% of patients treated with indinavir. It usually resolves with hydration and temporary interruption of therapy. The incidence of kidney stones can be reduced by having patients drink at least 48 ounces of water per day. Other potential side effects include asthenia, gastrointestinal disturbances, headache, insomnia or somnolence, dizziness, asymptomatic hyperbilirubinemia, and taste perversion. Lipid disturbances, body shape alterations, and rare cases of diabetes have also been reported in patients on protease inhibitors.

Nelfinavir

Nelfinavir is indicated for adults and children age 2 years or older. Like other protease inhibitors, nelfinavir should be given in combination with other antiretrovirals to maximize the antiviral effects and delay the onset of resistance.

Pharmacokinetics: Nelfinavir should be taken with food to enhance absorption. Nelfinavir is extensively protein bound (>98%). Like the other protease inhibitors, it is primarily metabolized by the P450 system. The half-life of nelfinavir is 3.5 to 5 hours.

Drug interactions: Nelfinavir is an inhibitor of the P450 isoenzyme CYP3A4. It should not be coadministered with astemizole, terfenadine, rifampin, midazolam, triazolam, or cisapride. Coadministration of nelfinavir and oral contraceptives also results in a significant decrease in estrogen and progesterone levels; alternative forms of contraception should be used. The dose of rifabutin should be decreased by 50%. Other potential drug interactions are listed on the package insert. Drug interactions should be checked carefully when changes are made to the patient's drug regimen.

Toxicities: Nelfinavir is fairly well tolerated. The most frequently reported side effect is diarrhea, which is usually of mild to moderate intensity. Nausea and rash also can occur. Lipid disturbances, body shape alterations, and rare cases of diabetes have also been reported in patients on protease inhibitors.

Amprenavir

Amprenavir is the protease inhibitor most recently approved by the FDA.

Pharmacokinetics: Amprenavir can be taken with or without food; however, it should not be taken with a high-fat meal because absorption may be reduced. It is about 90% protein-bound and has an elimination half-life of 6 to 10 hours. Amprenavir is primarily metabolized in the liver through the P450 isoenzyme CYP3A4. Dosage adjustment may be necessary in patients with impaired hepatic function.

Drug interactions: Like the other currently available protease inhibitors, amprenavir inhibits the P450 isoenzyme CYP3A4. Thus, it can inhibit the metabolism of other drugs metabolized via this pathway. In addition, other drugs that induce or inhibit CYP3A4 may affect the metabolism of amprenavir. The package insert and other information regarding drug interactions should be carefully consulted when beginning therapy with amprenavir or when starting or stopping the use of other drugs that may interact with it.

Toxicities: Patients should be instructed not to take supplemental vitamin E because the current amprenavir formulations contain vitamin E in concentrations considerably higher than the reference daily intake. Long-term consequences of high doses of vitamin E are unknown. Adverse effects of amprenavir include nausea, vomiting, diarrhea, headache, and rash. Lipid disturbances, body shape alterations (lipodystrophy), and rare cases of diabetes also have been reported in patients taking protease inhibitors. Preliminary information suggests that lipodystrophy may be less common with amprenavir than with other protease inhibitors, but studies are needed to document and confirm this.

ANTITUBERCULOSIS DRUGS: TOXICITIES

Isoniazid

Peripheral neuritis can be prevented with simultaneous use of pyridoxine. Hepatotoxicity is the most serious adverse effect and occurs in 1% to 2% of patients. In patients taking isoniazid, the approach for following them for possible hepatotoxicity is controversial. It is more likely to occur in older patients. Slow acetylators are more likely to have hepatotoxicity. Most patients have a transient increase in the aspartate aminotransferase value.

- With isoniazid, peripheral neuritis can be prevented with simultaneous use of pyridoxine.
- Hepatotoxicity occurs in 1%-2% of patients.
- Slow acetylators and older patients are more likely to have hepatotoxicity.

Risk of hepatotoxicity is 0.3% in patients 20 to 34 years old, 1.2% in those 35 to 49 years, 2.3% in those 50 to 64 years, and 4% in those older than 64 years.

Ethambutol

Toxicity is rare with this agent. If optic neuritis develops, red-green color vision may be lost first. This agent should probably not be used in young children in whom it may be difficult to assess vision.

Rifampin

Toxic effects include neutropenia, thrombocytopenia, and hepatotoxicity. Hepatotoxicity may be identical to that caused by isoniazid. Rifampin is also a hepatic enzyme inducer and thus has interactions with many medications, including warfarin, protease inhibitors, azole antifungals, and birth control pills. Fever with a flu-like syndrome is also a common toxic manifestation of rifampin, especially with intermittent administration. Body fluids are turned orange with administration of rifampin.

Pyrazinamide

Hepatotoxicity is similar to that with isoniazid. Hyperuricemia also may occur.

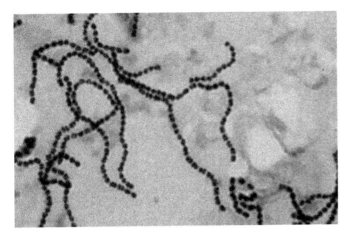

Plate 14-1. Chaining of β-hemolytic *Streptococcus* in a blood culture. (Gram stain.)

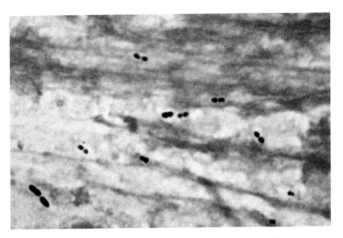

Plate 14-2. *Streptococcus pneumoniae* in sputum. (Gram stain.)

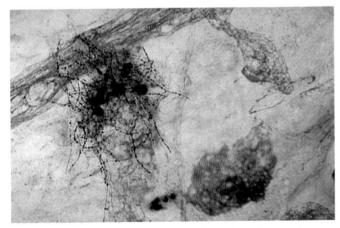

Plate 14-3. *Nocardia asteroides*. (Modified acid-fast stain; x450.)

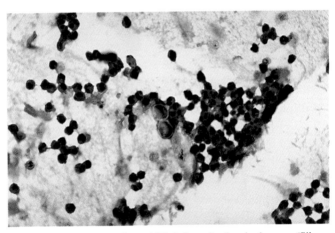

Plate 14-4. *Blastomyces dermatitidis* in bronchoalveolar lavage. (Silver stain; x450.)

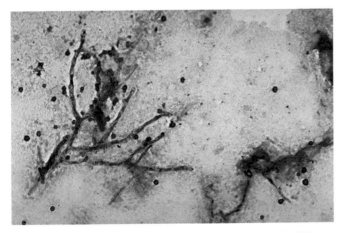

Plate 14-5. *Aspergillus fumigatus* in bronchoalveolar lavage. (x450.)

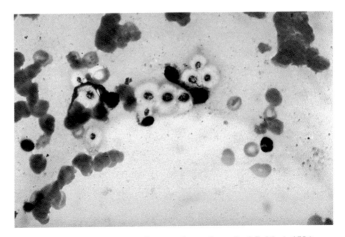

Plate 14-6. *Cryptococcus neoformans* in cerebrospinal fluid. (x450.)

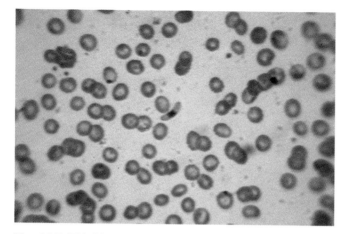

Plate 14-7. Thin blood smear showing banana-shaped gametocyte of *Plasmodium falciparum.*

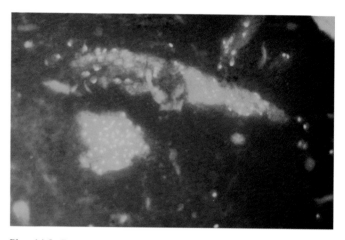

Plate 14-8. *Pneumocystis carinii* in induced sputum from a patient infected with human immunodeficiency virus. (Calcofluor white stain.)

QUESTIONS

Multiple Choice (choose the one best answer)

1. Each of the following statements regarding recurrent lower-extremity cellulitis after saphenous vein harvest for coronary artery bypass grafting is true *except*:
   a. The most common causative organisms are β-hemolytic streptococci
   b. Patients with this condition are at risk for development of rheumatic fever
   c. The cellulitis usually responds to therapy with penicillin G
   d. Coexisting tinea pedis may be a predisposing factor
   e. There is no effective vaccine to prevent this condition

2. Which of the following antibiotics or combination of antibiotics will most likely cure endocarditis caused by *Enterococcus faecalis*?
   a. Vancomycin
   b. Ciprofloxacin plus amikacin
   c. Penicillin plus tobramycin
   d. Ampicillin plus gentamicin
   e. Ceftazidime plus tobramycin

3. Risk factors for severe invasive disease due to *Streptococcus pneumoniae* include all of the following *except*:
   a. Cystic fibrosis
   b. Sickle cell disease
   c. Asplenia
   d. Multiple myeloma
   e. Human immunodeficiency virus (HIV) infection

4. Which of the following scenarios most likely depicts a true infection due to coagulase-negative staphylococci rather than colonization or contamination of cultures?
   a. A 67-year-old man with community-acquired pneumonia and one of four blood cultures growing coagulase-negative staphylococci
   b. An 18-year-old woman with symptoms of cystitis and urine cultures growing more than 10^5 cfu/mL coagulase-negative staphylococci
   c. A 46-year-old woman 3 days after mastectomy. Culture of serous drainage from the incision grows coagulase-negative staphylococci
   d. A 28-year-old man 5 days after liver transplantation for primary sclerosing cholangitis. Cultures of bile drawn through the biliary drainage tube reveal coagulase-negative staphylococci
   e. A 39-year-old woman with fever and headache. Spinal fluid examination is normal *except* for bacterial cultures, which grow coagulase-negative staphylococci

5. A 75-year-old woman receiving long-term treatment with prednisone for asthma develops acute meningitis. Empiric therapy with high-dose ceftriaxone is started. You astutely recommend that she also receive ampicillin because of your concern that she may be infected with which of the

following?

a. *Streptococcus pneumoniae*
b. *Haemophilus influenzae*
c. *Cryptococcus neoformans*
d. *Neisseria meningitidis*
e. *Listeria monocytogenes*

6. Infection with *Escherichia coli* serotype O157:H7 is associated with which of the following?

a. Gastritis and duodenal ulcers
b. Chronic, profuse, watery diarrhea
c. Hemorrhagic colitis and the hemolytic uremic syndrome
d. Recurrent cystitis and pyelonephritis
e. Broad-spectrum β-lactamase production and cephalosporin resistance

7. Which of the following illnesses is *not* caused by infection with *Bartonella henselae* (formerly *Rochalimaea henselae*)?

a. Cat-scratch disease
b. Ecthyma gangrenosum
c. Bacillary angiomatosis
d. Bacillary peliosis hepatis
e. Relapsing febrile bacteremia

8. A 19-year-old man is bit by his pet cat. The cat has received appropriate immunizations for rabies. Several hours after the injury, the wound becomes inflamed and painful. Gram stain of fluid expressed from the wound reveals gram-negative rods. All of the following antibiotics are effective for treatment of this infection *except*?

a. Cephalexin
b. Penicillin
c. Amoxicillin-clavulanic acid
d. Trimethoprim-sulfamethoxazole
e. Ciprofloxacin

9. Which of the following statements concerning tuberculosis is *true*?

a. Isoniazid prophylaxis after purified protein derivative (PPD) conversion does not significantly reduce the risk of subsequent tuberculosis
b. Corticosteroids are contraindicated as adjunctive therapy for tuberculous meningitis
c. 50% of *Mycobacterium tuberculosis* isolates in the United States are now resistant to isoniazid
d. Multidrug-resistant tuberculosis (MDR-TB) should be treated with four drugs for 6 to 9 months
e. Predisposing conditions for tuberculosis include silicosis, chronic renal failure, diabetes, and hematologic malignancies

10. All of the following statements regarding the rapid-growing mycobacteria (*Mycobacterium chelonei* and *Mycobacterium fortuitum*) are true *except*:

a. They cause indolent subcutaneous infections on the extremities
b. They are associated with bronchiectasis in HIV-infected patients
c. They are resistant to antituberculosis drugs such as isoniazid and rifampin
d. They are most often susceptible to clarithromycin
e. They may cause nosocomial infections such as sternal osteomyelitis after cardiac operation

11. Fever develops in a 53-year-old man with chronic lymphocytic leukemia, treated with fludarabine. Examination and imaging studies demonstrate multiple abscesses, including one in the left parietal lobe of the brain. Modified acid-fast stain of pus drained from an abscess reveals filamentous, branching bacilli. Which of the following antimicrobial therapies is most appropriate for this condition?

a. High-dose penicillin G
b. Trimethoprim-sulfamethoxazole
c. Amphotericin B
d. Isoniazid, rifampin, and pyrazinamide
e. Clarithromycin, rifabutin, and ethambutol

12. During the early summer, a native of northern Wisconsin presents to your office concerned about his risk for Lyme disease. Three days previously, he found a small tick crawling on his leg after an outing in the woods. He is currently asymptomatic and physical examination is normal. Which of the following courses of action do you recommend for this concerned individual?

a. Obtain a Lyme serologic test, begin empiric doxycycline therapy, and repeat the serologic testing in 6 weeks
b. Begin empiric doxycycline therapy and obtain a Lyme serologic test in 6 weeks
c. No antibiotic therapy or testing is needed unless clinical signs of early Lyme disease develop over the ensuing weeks
d. Obtain a Lyme serologic test. If positive, begin therapy with doxycycline. If negative, give no therapy
e. Explain to the patient that Lyme disease has never been reported in Wisconsin and he has nothing to worry about

13. All of the following statements match a specific fungal infection with a particular risk factor. Which match is *not* correct?

a. Coccidioidomycosis and travel to Arizona

b. Aspergillosis and neutropenia

c. Sporotrichosis and rose gardening

d. Blastomycosis and travel to northern Mexico

e. Cryptococcosis and meningitis in patients with acquired immunodeficiency syndrome (AIDS)

14. A 65-year-old woman is hospitalized with renal failure and severe metabolic acidosis. On the second hospital day, you notice a black, necrotic-appearing lesion on her soft palate. Biopsy of this lesion will most likely reveal which of the following?

a. Yeast and hyphal elements consistent with invasive candidiasis

b. Viral inclusion bodies consistent with herpes simplex virus infection

c. Large, nonseptated, branching hyphae consistent with mucormycosis

d. An acute inflammatory infiltrate with a mixture of gram-positive and gram-negative organisms

e. Necrotizing granulomas and acid-fast organisms

15. Infectious mononucleosis-like syndromes can be produced by infection with several different organisms, including Epstein-Barr virus, cytomegalovirus, and *Toxoplasma gondii*. All of the following are findings common to all three of these infections *except* one. Which of the following is found only in cases of Epstein-Barr virus infection?

a. Exudative pharyngitis

b. Splenomegaly

c. Atypical lymphocytosis

d. Fever

e. Diagnosis by specific serologic test

16. A 32-year-old man with advanced HIV infection has recurrent genital ulcers. For the past 6 months the ulcers have been quiescent while the patient was taking acyclovir (400 mg twice daily). Now the painful ulcers have returned and have not responded to an increased dose of acyclovir. Which of the following medications is most likely to help this patient?

a. Foscarnet

b. Ganciclovir

c. Famciclovir

d. Valacyclovir

e. Fluconazole

17. An 18-year-old man from Guatemala has acute lymphocytic leukemia. He is neutropenic because of the chemotherapy, and fever and pulmonary infiltrates develop. *Escherichia coli* is isolated from his blood, sputum, and spinal fluid. Despite treatment with appropriate antibiotics, his condition worsens and blood cultures remain positive. Which of these parasitic infections is most likely responsible for his condition?

a. *Entamoeba histolytica*

b. *Plasmodium falciparum*

c. *Toxoplasma gondii*

d. *Necator americanus*

e. *Strongyloides stercoralis*

18. Which of the following is a shared characteristic of Creutzfeldt-Jakob disease and progressive multifocal leukoencephalopathy (caused by JC virus)?

a. Both are caused by reactivation of a latent DNA virus

b. Both are caused by the same infectious agent

c. They have both familial and acquired forms of disease

d. Both involve significant central nervous system defects

e. Both have been linked to consumption of beef from cattle with bovine spongiform encephalopathy

19. A 54-year-old woman with non-Hodgkin lymphoma develops leukopenia and fever after a course of chemotherapy. She initially responds to empiric therapy with ceftazidime. However, as her neutrophil count recovers she has worsening fever, right upper quadrant abdominal pain, and increasing liver enzyme values. Computed tomography imaging of her abdomen reveals multiple, small, enhancing lesions throughout the liver and spleen. This complication is best treated with which of the following therapeutic agents?

a. Tobramycin and ticarcillin

b. Clarithromycin

c. Metronidazole

d. Acyclovir

e. Amphotericin B

20. A 58-year-old man with Wegener granulomatosis has received 3 months of therapy with prednisone and cyclophosphamide. He is admitted to the hospital with a new pulmonary infiltrate and neurologic changes. Biopsy of a brain lesion detected by computed tomography reveals acute inflammatory changes and filamentous branching organisms that are visualized with a weak acid-fast stain. The same organism grows from culture of respiratory secretions. Which of the following therapies is most likely to be effective?

a. Fluconazole

b. Trimethoprim-sulfamethoxazole

c. Isoniazid, rifampin, and pyrazinamide

d. Amphotericin B

e. High-dose penicillin G

21. A 20-year-old student with a history of rheumatic fever and a loud mitral regurgitation murmur presents to you for advice regarding prophylactic antibiotics to prevent bacterial endocarditis. She has no drug allergies. You suggest:
    a. Clindamycin 600 mg 1 hour before the procedure and 6 hours later
    b. Amoxicillin 3 g 1 hour before the procedure
    c. Clindamycin 600 mg 1 hour before the procedure
    d. Amoxicillin 2 g 1 hour before the procedure
    e. None of the above

22. A 40-year-old man with a history of aortic regurgitation and no drug allergies presents with fever and chills of 3 weeks' duration. Multiple blood cultures are positive for viridans group streptococci; the minimal inhibitory concentration is 0.06 μg/mL for penicillin and less than 0.25 μg/mL for ceftriaxone. Which of the following antimicrobial regimens for his infective endocarditis would not be appropriate?
    a. Penicillin G 12 to 18 x 10^6 units/24 hours for 4 weeks
    b. Ceftriaxone 2 g intravenously for 4 weeks
    c. Penicillin G 12 to 18 x 10^6 units/24 hours plus gentamicin for 2 weeks
    d. Vancomycin 30 mg/kg intravenously for 2 weeks
    e. Penicillin G 12 to 18 x 10^6 units/24 hours plus gentamicin for 4 weeks

23. A 40-year-old woman presents with fever, chills, and meningismus of 24 hours' duration. Cerebrospinal fluid examination shows a leukocyte count of 5,000/mm^3, 90% polymorphonuclear neutrophils, and glucose value of 20 mg/dL. Gram stain reveals gram-positive diplococci. The incidence of penicillin-resistant pneumococci in your community is 10%. The initial empiric antimicrobial regimen should include:
    a. Cefotaxime
    b. Ceftriaxone
    c. Cefazolin
    d. Penicillin G
    e. Vancomycin and ceftriaxone

24. All of the following are associated with the aseptic meningitis syndrome except:
    a. Enterovirus
    b. Mumps virus
    c. Nonsteroidal anti-inflammatory drugs (NSAIDs)
    d. *Neisseria meningitidis*
    e. Herpes simplex virus 2

25. All of the following are true regarding nongonococcal

urethritis and cervicitis except:
    a. *Chlamydia trachomatis* is the most common pathogen
    b. Doxycycline 100 mg orally twice a day for 7 days is effective therapy
    c. Azithromycin 1 g orally for 1 dose is effective therapy
    d. Ceftriaxone 125 mg intramuscularly for 1 dose is effective therapy
    e. Cefixime 400 mg orally x 1

26. All of the following are true about herpes genitalis except:
    a. 70% to 90% of cases are caused by herpes simplex virus 2
    b. For first-time therapy, acyclovir, famciclovir, or valacyclovir is appropriate
    c. Recurrence of disease while receiving chronic suppression therapy with acyclovir is not related to in vitro resistance to acyclovir
    d. Topical penciclovir has substantial benefit for this disease
    e. For prophylaxis of recurrence, acyclovir, famciclovir, or valacyclovir is appropriate

27. A 30-year-old white man who has just finished a 10-day course of amoxicillin therapy for sinusitis presents with abdominal cramps and watery diarrhea of 24 hours' duration. He has just returned from Mexico. All of the following are potential causes of his diarrhea except:
    a. Enterotoxigenic *Escherichia coli*
    b. *Clostridium difficile*
    c. *Clostridium perfringens*
    d. *Staphylococcus aureus*
    e. Cytomegalovirus

28. A 30-year-old woman with short bowel syndrome on receiving total parenteral nutrition through a permanent venous catheter presents with fever, chills, and purulent drainage from the exit site of the catheter. All of the following are usual causes of her infection except:
    a. *Staphylococcus aureus*
    b. Coagulase-negative staphylococci
    c. *Pseudomonas aeruginosa*
    d. *Candida albicans*
    e. *Mycobacterium avium-intracellulare* (MAI)

29. All of the following are usual causes of chronic monarticular arthritis except:
    a. *Mycobacterium tuberculosis*
    b. *Sporothrix schenckii*
    c. *Nocardia* spp.
    d. *Blastomyces dermatitidis*
    e. Parvovirus B19

30. All of the following are true about toxic shock syndrome (TSS) *except*:
    a. Bacteremia is common in patients with TSS due to group A streptococci
    b. The case fatality rate is as high as 30%
    c. Group A streptococci is a common cause of TSS after influenza
    d. The relapse rate may be as high as 30% to 40% for TSS due to *Staphylococcus aureus*
    e. All of the above

31. Which of the following statements is *not* true about transmission of HIV infection?
    a. Sexual transmission is the most common mode of acquiring HIV
    b. It is possible to acquire HIV through donated organs
    c. HIV-1 and HIV-2 differ in their modes of transmission
    d. Sexually transmitted diseases increase the risk of HIV transmission
    e. It is possible to decrease the rate of transmission of HIV from a pregnant woman to her infant through the use of antiretroviral therapy

32. Which of the following statements is *not* true about occupational exposure to HIV infection?
    a. In general, the risk of transmission of HIV from an HIV-infected person through a needle stick exposure is high
    b. The stage of infection (CD4 count, viral load) of the index patient is an important factor in assessing the risk of transmission
    c. The size and type of needle are important factors in assessing the risk of transmission
    d. The depth of injury is an important factor in assessing the risk of transmission
    e. It is possible to reduce the risk of transmission using prophylactic antiretroviral therapy.

33. Primary HIV infection:
    a. Has symptoms that usually appear within days of acquiring the infection
    b. Occurs in only a minority of patients
    c. Treatment with antiretroviral drugs is not indicated
    d. Is associated with a very large amount of circulating virus
    e. HIV antibody test is usually positive

34. Which of the following statements is true about *Pneumocystis carinii* pneumonia (PCP)?
    a. PCP is a relatively uncommon opportunistic infection in HIV-infected persons
    b. Typical presentation includes an acute illness with high fevers and cough productive of purulent sputum
    c. PCP grows within a few days of inoculation when special culture media are used
    d. An A-a gradient >35 mm is an indication for the use of adjunctive corticosteroids
    e. Inhaled pentamidine once monthly is the drug of choice for primary prophylaxis of PCP

35. Which of the following statements is true about tuberculosis?
    a. Treatment duration of tuberculosis in an HIV-infected person should be longer than in a non–HIV-infected person
    b. Prophylaxis with isoniazid is given for the same length of time in both HIV-infected and uninfected persons
    c. Tuberculosis accelerates the course of HIV disease
    d. As is the case with other opportunistic diseases, tuberculosis cannot be cured completely in HIV-infected persons and, therefore, necessitates chronic suppression to prevent recurrence
    e. In HIV-infected persons, tuberculosis occurs in those with CD4 cell counts less than 200

36. Which of the following statements is *not* true about *Cryptococcus neoformans* infections in HIV-infected persons?
    a. *C. neoformans* is a yeast that is acquired from the environment
    b. *C. neoformans* enters the body through the lungs by inhalation
    c. The most common clinical presentation is pneumonia.
    d. Serum cryptococcal antigen test is very sensitive and diagnostically useful
    e. After initial treatment, chronic suppression to prevent recurrence is necessary

37. Which of the following statements is *not* true about cytomegalovirus (CMV) infections in HIV-infected persons?
    a. CMV disease usually occurs in advanced HIV infection
    b. The most common clinical presentation is chorioretinitis
    c. Lifelong treatment with acyclovir is necessary to prevent recurrence
    d. Foscarnet and cidofovir are drugs that can be used for treating CMV
    e. Renal toxicity is the major side effect of foscarnet

38. Which of the following statements is true about central nervous system infections in HIV-infected persons?

a. Cerebrospinal fluid studies are useful for the diagnosis of AIDS dementia complex

b. High-dose AZT is indicated for the treatment of progressive multifocal leukoencephalopathy

c. *Cryptococcus neoformans* is the most common cause of focal mass lesions of the central nervous system

d. *Toxoplasma* encephalitis occurs mainly in patients with CD4 cell counts less than 100

e. Trimethoprim-sulfamethoxazole is the drug of choice for the treatment of *Toxoplasma* encephalitis

39. Which of the following is *not* a protease inhibitor?
    a. Saquinavir
    b. Nelfinavir
    c. Ritonovir
    d. Adefovir
    e. Indinavir

40. Which of the following statements is *not* true about recent advances in the management of HIV infection?
    a. There is active viral replication at all stages of HIV infection
    b. Quantitative HIV RNA assays are useful for assessing prognosis and monitoring patients' response to treatment
    c. Clinical trials have shown that combination antiretroviral regimens are superior to single-drug therapy in delaying progression to AIDS
    d. Clinical trials have shown that combination antiretroviral regimens are superior to single-drug therapy in delaying progression to AIDS but not in improving survival
    e. Since 1995, there have been new classes of antiretroviral drugs licensed for treating HIV

41. A patient who received a bone marrow transplant 6 weeks previously develops fever and progressive pulmonary infiltrates unresponsive to antibiotics. *Aspergillus* infection is diagnosed. Which of the following would be the most appropriate therapy?
    a. Ketoconazole
    b. Amphotericin
    c. Fluconazole
    d. Itraconazole
    e. Miconazole

42. Which of the following antibiotics has no activity against aerobic gram-positive organisms?
    a. Vancomycin
    b. Levofloxacin
    c. Ceftriaxone

d. Ticarcillin clavulanate

e. Aztreonam

43. Which of the following cephalosporins does not penetrate the cerebrospinal fluid?
    a. Cefazolin
    b. Ceftriaxone
    c. Cefotaxime
    d. Cefepime
    e. Ceftazidime

44. Which of the following are active against *Pseudomonas aeruginosa*?
    a. Cefotaxime
    b. Cefepime
    c. Cefuroxime
    d. Ceftazidime
    e. Cefepime and ceftazidime

45. A patient with late-stage HIV and CD4 cell count of 10 presents with cytomegalovirus retinitis. Appropriate therapy might include all of the following *except*:
    a. Ganciclovir
    b. Foscarnet
    c. Acyclovir
    d. Cidofovir
    e. Fluconazole

46. All of the following drugs are active against herpes simplex virus *except*:
    a. Acyclovir
    b. Famciclovir
    c. Valacyclovir
    d. Foscarnet
    e. Ribavirin

47. All of the following statements are true regarding itraconazole *except*:
    a. Is active against *Histoplasma capsulatum*
    b. Does not require dose adjustment in patients with renal insufficiency
    c. Is active against *Sporothrix schenckii*
    d. Requires gastric acidity for absorption
    e. The capsules have better bioavailability compared with the solution

48. Metronidazole is usually active against all the following organisms *except*:
    a. *Clostridium* spp.
    b. *Bacteroides fragilis*
    c. *Giardia lamblia*

d. *Entamoeba histolytica*
e. *Treponema pallidum*

49. All of the following statements concerning meropenem are false *except*:
    a. Seizures are less frequent with meropenem than imipenem
    b. Meropenem is active against *Stenotrophomonas maltophilia*
    c. Requires administration with cilastin

d. Is active against methicillin-resistant staphylococci
e. Is active against *Legionella* spp.

50. All of the following antibiotics require dose adjustment in renal failure *except*:
    a. Clindamycin
    b. Cefazolin
    c. Cefotaxime
    d. Cefepime
    e. Meropenem

ANSWERS

1. Answer b.

Saphenous vein removal and other conditions that impede venous and lymphatic drainage of the legs increase the risk of cellulitis, most often due to β-hemolytic streptococci. These organisms are universally susceptible to penicillin. Rheumatic fever occurs only after streptococcal pharyngitis.

2. Answer d.

Enterococcal endocarditis must be treated with a bactericidal combination of drugs. Of the agents listed, only the combination of ampicillin and gentamicin is reliably bactericidal against this organism.

3. Answer a.

Cystic fibrosis is associated with sinus and pulmonary infections predominantly due to *Staphylococcus aureus*, *Haemophilus*, and *Pseudomonas aeruginosa*. Disorders of immunoglobulins (myeloma) and splenic function (sickle cell and asplenia) cause increased susceptibility to invasive disease with pneumococci. HIV infection, even in the early stages, is similarly associated.

4. Answer b.

As normal skin flora, coagulase-negative staphylococci are the most common organisms to contaminate blood and other cultures (choices d and e). These relatively nonvirulent organisms colonize wounds (c) and drainage tubes (d). *Staphylococcus saprophyticus*, one of the many species of

coagulase-negative staphylococci, is a relatively common cause of bacterial cystitis in young women.

5. Answer e.

Listeria monocytogenes causes meningitis in the elderly, the very young, and immunocompromised hosts. It is intrinsically resistant to all cephalosporins. Choices a, b, and d are all common causes of bacterial meningitis but are usually susceptible to ceftriaxone and cefotaxime. *Cryptococcus*, a fungus, is not susceptible to β-lactam drugs.

6. Answer c.

O157:H7 is the main serotype of *E. coli* responsible for acute hemorrhagic colitis. It is not associated with chronic diarrhea. Hemolytic-uremic syndrome follows in up to 10% of cases. This strain of *E. coli* is usually susceptible to most antibiotics. Although *E. coli* is a common cause of urinary tract infection, this serotype is infrequently implicated. *Helicobacter pylori* is the agent implicated as a cause of gastritis and ulcers.

7. Answer b.

Ecthyma gangrenosum is a necrotic skin lesion found in neutropenia and is most often caused by systemic infection with *Pseudomonas aeruginosa*. All of the other conditions are associated with *Bartonella* organisms.

8. Answer a.

The infecting organism, *Pasteurella multocida*, is susceptible to many antibiotics. Those to which it is resistant include cephalexin, cefadroxil, cefaclor, dicloxacillin, erythromycin, and clindamycin.

9. Answer e.

Isoniazid prophylaxis is very effective at preventing subsequent tuberculosis if given after PPD conversion. Corticosteroids decrease mortality from tuberculous meningitis. Isoniazid resistance occurs in less than 10% of current isolates in the United States. MDR-TB is rarely cured with less than 18 months of therapy. See the table.

Medical Conditions That Predispose Patients to *Mycobacterium tuberculosis* Infection

Silicosis	Diabetes mellitus
Gastrectomy	Immunosuppression (T-cell)
Jejunoileal bypass	Hematologic malignancy
Weight 10% or more below ideal body weight	Other malignancies
	Person with chest radiograph compatible with old tuberculosis
Chronic renal failure	

10. Answer b.

The rapid-growing mycobacteria predominantly cause subcutaneous infections. HIV is not associated with these infections, nor is bronchiectasis. *M. chelonei* is often resistant to all available agents *except* clarithromycin.

11. Answer b.

The patient has a disseminated infection with *Nocardia asteroides*. Plate 14-3 demonstrates the appearance of the organism with a modified acid-fast stain. *Nocardia* organisms are bacterial despite an appearance suggestive of fungi. They are resistant to the antimicrobial effects of all described agents except trimethoprim-sulfamethoxazole. Alternative effective agents sometimes include imipenem, minocycline, and amikacin.

12. Answer c.

Lyme disease is endemic in Wisconsin. To cause infection, a tick must be attached for approximately 24 hours. Lyme serologic testing will not reveal infection in the early stages. About 1 of every 100 persons bitten by an infected tick will develop *Borrelia burgdorferi* infection. Beginning therapy in this situation would needlessly expose 99 of 100 persons to possible adverse drug effects. Waiting until symptoms develop does not affect the efficacy of therapy.

13. Answer d.

Blastomycosis is predominantly found in the southeastern and upper midwestern areas of the United States.

14. Answer c.

The appearance of the lesion in the setting of a metabolic acidosis is highly suggestive of mucormycosis (also known as zygomycosis). Although herpes simplex virus and *Candida* frequently cause oral lesions in patients with other illnesses, neither would produce the necrotic lesion described.

15. Answer a.

See Table 14-6. Pharyngitis is not characteristic of infection with either cytomegalovirus or *Toxoplasma*.

16. Answer a.

The case described is an example of acyclovir-resistant herpes simplex infection in a patients with AIDS. Acyclovir resistance also implies resistance to the other antiviral agents, which require phosphorylation to their active forms. Foscarnet retains activity against these resistant strains.

17. Answer e.

Chronic subclinical *S. stercoralis* autoinfection can progress to hyperinfection in a compromised host. In this setting, large numbers of larval organisms migrate through the gut wall causing systemic disease. Intestinal bacteria accompany the migrating larvae, resulting in disseminated bacterial infections. See page 546 of the text.

18. Answer d.

These are two distinct illnesses affecting the central nervous system. JC virus acquired its name from the initials of the first patient from whom it was isolated: it does not stand for "Creutzfeldt-Jakob." JC is a polyoma virus (DNA virus), whereas Creutzfeldt-Jakob disease is thought to be caused by a prion, an abnormal transmissible protein. Creutzfeldt-Jakob disease occurs in familial and acquired forms. Atypical cases in Britain may be related to consumption of beef from cattle with bovine spongiform encephalopathy ("mad-cow" disease).

19. Answer e.

This presentation is highly suggestive of hepatosplenic candidiasis (also called disseminated candidiasis). Antifungal therapy with amphotericin B or fluconazole is indicated.

20. Answer b.

The infection described is nocardiosis (*Nocardia asteroides*). This opportunistic infection most commonly involves the respiratory tract and the brain. Although weak acid-fast stain is used to visualize the organisms, they are not *Mycobacteria* and do not respond to antituberculous therapy.

21. Answer d.

The American Heart Association guidelines for prevention

of bacterial endocarditis were changed in 1997. This patient requires antibiotic prophylaxis for dental procedures because of her valvular heart disease caused by rheumatic fever. The initial dose recommended is amoxicillin 2 g before procedure. No follow-up antibiotic dose is recommended. (Reference: JAMA 277:1794-1801, 1997.)

22. Answer d.

Current suggested treatment of penicillin-sensitive viridans group streptococci includes answers a, b, and c. Vancomycin is recommended as alternative therapy for penicillin-allergic patients, and the duration of treatment is 4 weeks. (Reference: JAMA 274:1706-1713, 1995.)

23. Answer e.

This patient, presenting with bacterial meningitis, requires treatment for *Streptococcus pneumoniae*. In an area with a high incidence of penicillin resistance, initial empiric treatment pending antibiotic susceptibility studies should include vancomycin.

24. Answer d.

Aseptic meningitis is caused most often by viruses, but there are many infectious and noninfectious causes. *N. meningitidis* is a frequent cause of bacterial meningitis in young adults. NSAIDs can cause a chemical meningitis.

25. Answer d.

In nongonococcal urethritis and cervicitis, the most common etiologic agent is *C. trachomatis*. Treatment is with either doxycycline (100 mg orally twice a day for 7 days) as standard treatment or azithromycin as a single 1-g dose.

26. Answer d.

Herpes genitalis is caused in 70% to 90% of cases by herpes simplex virus 2. For the first episode, therapy with acyclovir, famciclovir, or valacyclovir is appropriate. Recurrence after therapy is not related to in vitro resistance of herpes simplex virus to acyclovir. Topical therapy is not appropriate.

27. Answer e.

Enterotoxigenic *E. coli* is the most common etiologic agent in traveler's diarrhea. Onset after infection may occur at 12 hours. *C. difficile* colitis may occur 2 to 4 weeks after stopping use of antibiotics. Any antibiotic may cause this illness. *C. perfringens* has an onset of diarrhea 8 to 16 hours after ingestion, and duration of illness is 24 hours. *S. aureus* has an abrupt onset (2-6 hours) with severe vomiting, diarrhea, and abdominal cramps. Duration of infection is 8 to 24 hours. CMV infection is a cause of bloody diarrhea in immunocompromised patients.

28. Answer e.

Central venous catheters may be a portal of infection for several organisms. Common associations include *S. aureus*, coagulase-negative staphylococci, *Candida* spp., and *P. aeruginosa*. MAI is a common cause of disseminated infection in patients with AIDS.

29. Answer e.

Chronic monarticular arthritis may be caused by mycobacteria (*M. tuberculosis, M. avium-intercellulare, M. kansasii, M. marinum*); fungi (*S. schenckii, Nocardia* spp., and *B. dermatitidis*). Parvovirus B19 is usually polyarticular and self-limited.

30. Answer c.

S. aureus is a common cause of toxic shock syndrome after influenza infection.

31. Answer c.

HIV-1 and HIV-2 have identical modes of transmission and clinical manifestations. HIV-2 appears to be less efficient in its transmission and progresses less rapidly to AIDS.

32. Answer a.

In general, the risk of transmission of HIV from an HIV-infected person through a needle stick is low, approximately 0.3%.

33. Answer d.

Primary HIV infection is seen in 40% to 60% of patients 4 to 6 weeks after acquiring infection. Although the results of HIV antibody tests are usually negative, HIV is associated with a very large amount of circulating virus. Antiretroviral therapy is indicated with the goal of controlling the infection before it is fully established, when the viral population is relatively monogeneous, and when the immune system is relatively intact.

34. Answer d.

PCP is the most common opportunistic infection in HIV-infected persons in the United States. Typical presentation includes low-grade fever, fatigue, malaise, and nonproductive cough. There is no reliable way of growing PCP in the laboratory. Stains are used for diagnosis. Trimethoprim-sulfamethoxazole is the drug of choice for primary and secondary prophylaxis of PCP.

35. Answer c.

Tuberculosis may accelerate the course of HIV infection; unlike many of the opportunistic infections in HIV-infected persons, tuberculosis can be cured if diagnosed promptly and treated appropriately; tuberculosis can be successfully prevented. Tuberculosis may occur relatively early in HIV infection. When it occurs later, it tends to have atypical features, such as extrapulmonary disease, disseminated disease, and unusual chest radiographic appearance (lower lung zone lesions, intrathoracic adenopathy, diffuse infiltrations, lower frequency of cavitation). Treatment of tuberculosis in patients with AIDS is the same as in normal hosts. Prophylaxis with isoniazid for 12 months is recommended (as opposed to 6 months in normal hosts) for all patients who are HIV-positive and have skin reactions of more than 5 mm to 5 tuberculin units of purified protein derivative.

36. Answer c.

Although the lungs are the port of entry, the most common clinical presentation of cryptococcosis is meningitis.

37. Answer c.

Ganciclovir, rather than acyclovir, is the drug used to treat CMV disease.

38. Answer d.

Although *C. neoformans* is the most common cause of central nervous system infection in AIDS patients, it is *Toxoplasma gondii* that is the most common cause of focal mass lesions in these patients.

39. Answer d.

Adefovir is a nucleotide analogue that has not yet been licensed for use in HIV infection. The rest are protease inhibitors.

40. Answer d.

Recent clinical trials have clearly demonstrated that combination regimens are associated with declines in viral replication and sustained clinical benefits, as measured by a delay in progression to AIDS and a reduction in the risk of death.

41. Answer b.

Amphotericin B is the drug of choice for *Aspergillus* infections in neutropenic hosts. Itraconazole has been used for mild to moderate *Aspergillus* infections.

42. Answer e.

Aztreonam has a spectrum of activity involving only aerobic gram-negative bacteria. The remainder have activity against aerobic gram-positive organisms.

43. Answer a.

Cefotaxime, ceftazidime and ceftriaxone have good cerebrospinal fluid penetration. Cefepime, a fourth-generation cephalosporin, also has cerebrospinal fluid activity. First-generation cephalosporins, including cefazolin, do not penetrate even into inflamed meninges.

44. Answer e.

Both cefepime (fourth-generation cephalosporin) and ceftazidime have activity against *P. aeruginosa*. Cefotaxime is less active against *Pseudomonas* than ceftazidime. Cefuroxime does not have activity against *Pseudomonas*.

45. Answer c.

Antiviral agents active against cytomegalovirus include ganciclovir, foscarnet, and cidofovir. Cytomegalovirus is resistant to acyclovir because it does not produce thymidine kinase. Fluconazole is an antifungal, not an antiviral agent.

46. Answer e.

Acyclovir, famciclovir, valacyclovir, and foscarnet all have activity against herpes simplex virus. Ribavirin is indicated for respiratory syncytial virus.

47. Answer e.

Itraconazole has greater activity against *H. capsulatum*, *S. schenckii*, *Aspergillus*, and *B. dermatitidis*. Similar to ketoconazole, itraconazole requires gastric acidity for absorption. A new oral solution has improved bioavailability. Itraconazole does not require renal dose adjustment.

48. Answer e.

Metronidazole has very good antimicrobial activity against most anaerobic microorganisms, including *B. fragilis*, *E. histolytica*, *G. lamblia*, and *Clostridium* spp.

49. Answer a.

Meropenem does not require administration with cilastin. Neither imipenem nor meropenem is active against *Legionella* spp., methicillin-resistant *Staphylococcus aureus*, or *S. maltophilia*. Meropenem is associated with a lower incidence of seizures and has been used for pediatric meningitis.

50. Answer a.

Clindamycin does not require dose adjustment in renal failure.

NOTES

CHAPTER 15

MEDICAL ETHICS

C. Christopher Hook, M.D.
Udaya B. S. Prakash, M.D.
William F. Dunn, M.D.

Medicine is first and foremost a relationship. It is the coming together of one individual, the patient, who is ill or has specific needs and a second individual, the physician, whose goal is to help the patient. Physicians have a long history of creating codes or oaths to provide the ethical norms and framework to support and protect the underlying relationship. Because medicine is fundamentally a relationship, it is at heart an ethical endeavor. Medical ethics is a set of principles that attempts to guide physicians in their relationships with patients and others. These principles are based on moral values shared by both the lay society (may vary from culture to culture) and the medical profession.

- Medical ethics is a set of principles that guide physicians in their relationships with patients and others.

Historically, the Hippocratic Oath has served as the foundation on which much of Western medical ethics has been built. Its principles form the framework for many of our current ethical standards, including beneficence, nonmaleficence, confidentiality, and the prohibition of active euthanasia. In recent times, there have been many other articulations of these core principles, including the Declaration of Geneva (1983), World Medical Association International Code of Medical Ethics (1983), The American College of Physicians Ethics Manual (1989), and The American Medical Association Code of Medical Ethics (1997).

ETHICAL DILEMMAS

Ethical issues in medicine are as dynamic as the scientific and technical progresses in medicine. In fact, the relentless advances in medical science are greatly responsible for the dynamism in medical ethics. These factors are partly responsible for ethical dilemmas. Furthermore, changes in societal mores and laws also have an impact on the ethical issues in medicine. An ethical dilemma can be defined as a predica-

ment in which there is no clear course to resolve the problem of conflicting moral principles because of credible evidence both for and against a certain action. Increasing emphasis is being placed on medical ethics in the certifying and licensing examinations for physicians.

- Ethical dilemma: predicament in which there is no clear course to resolve the problem of conflicting moral principles because of credible evidence both for and against a certain action.
- Ethical issues in medicine are dynamic and will continue to change.

PRINCIPLES OF MEDICAL ETHICS

Today, many schools are competing to provide a philosophical framework for deriving the rules or particulars of medical ethics. One of the major approaches has been labeled principalism. Proposed by Beauchamp and Childress, principalism, although not necessarily providing bedside guidance for each ethical dilemma, provides a useful delineation of overall principles in which to consider many or most of the ethical concerns in the physician-patient relationship. The four major principles that they list are: 1) autonomy, 2) beneficence, 3) nonmaleficence, and 4) justice.

- Four tenets of medical ethics: autonomy, beneficence, nonmaleficence, and justice.

Autonomy

Autonomy derives from two Greek words: *autos* ("self") and *nomes* ("rule"). The principle of autonomy is the articulation that all individuals have the right to determine their individual values and goals and have the right to self-determination. For autonomy to have expression, however, two requirements need to be present. First, the patient must have "agency," that is, the patient must be able to establish his or her own values and goals and be able to make appropriate decisions based on those values. From the requirement of agency, we have the clinically important concept of decision-making capacity. Decision-making capacity often is confused with the legal term "competence." Capacity is the physician's clinical determination of the patient's ability to understand his or her situation and make appropriate decisions for treatment, and competence is the legal determination that an individual has the right to make life-affecting decisions. The judges' or courts' assessment of competence is based in significant part on the clinical assessment of decision-making capacity.

- Autonomy: respecting the patient's right to self-determination and pursuit of one's own life plan.
- Autonomy implies "decision-making" capacity (the right to refuse medical therapy, even at the risk of death).
- Competence is the legal determination that an individual has the right to make life-affecting decisions.

In clinical practice, the lack of decisional capability should be proved and not presumed. Clinical evidence of confusion, disorientation, and psychosis resulting from organic diseases, metabolic disturbances, and iatrogenic interference can adversely affect decision-making ability. Decisionally capable patients have the right to refuse medical therapy, even at the risk of death. If a previously decisionally capable patient had indicated, clearly and convincingly, whether life-sustaining therapy should be administered or withheld in the event of permanent unconsciousness, that wish should be respected (see Living Will, below), unless it was subsequently clearly rescinded.

- Lack of decisional capability should be proved and not presumed.

Several clinical standards are used to assess decision-making capacity: 1) the patient can make and communicate a choice; 2) the patient understands the medical situation and prognosis, the nature of the recommended care, available alternative options, and the risks, benefits, and consequences of each; 3) the patient's decisions are stable over time; 4) the decision is consistent with the patient's values and goals; and 5) the decision is not due to delusions.

The second major element required in autonomy is liberty; that is, the patient must be free to influence the course of her or his life and medical treatment. Many recent court decisions, from the *Quinlan* case in 1976 to the *Cruzan* decision in 1990, along with strong support from the bioethical community, have established the right of patients to refuse any form of medical treatment, even if such refusal will lead to the patient's death.

- Liberty: the patient is free to influence the course of her or his life and medical treatment.

The principle of autonomy, particularly as it affects the right of an individual to die, has been reaffirmed in the recent writings of ethicists and legal judgments. Nevertheless, a survey of physicians published in 1995 reported that 34% of physicians had, at least once in the preceding 12 months, declined to withdraw life-sustaining mechanical ventilation despite being requested to do so by a capable patient or by the family of a patient lacking decision-making capacity. Nearly 20% of physicians engaged in this practice because of the fear of malpractice litigation. Unfortunately, a significant number of physicians in the United States have either a poor or no understanding of the laws of states regarding the principle of autonomy. The 1995 survey revealed that 46% of the respondents from New York incorrectly believed that withdrawal of mechanical ventilation was illegal.

- A significant number of physicians have poor understanding of the principle of autonomy.

Preservation of the Patient's Autonomy

Can a patient who now is unconscious or lacks decision-making capacity prevent unwanted treatment? Another way of asking this question is, who speaks for the patient when he or she is no longer able to articulate? Because autonomy is based on a respect for persons, caregivers should endeavor to continue treatment in accordance with what the patient would have desired if he or she were still able to interact capably with the caregivers. To preserve the patient's autonomy, patients may communicate through two means to express their wishes: advance directives and surrogate decision makers.

- The patient's autonomy is preserved by 1) advance directives and 2) surrogate decision makers.

Advance Directives

An advance directive is a document in which a person either states choices for medical treatment or designates an individual who should make treatment choices if the person should lose decision-making capacity. The term also can apply to oral statements from the patient to the caregivers, given at a time when the patient was decisionally capable. Advance directives can take several forms: 1) the living will, 2) the durable power of attorney for health care, 3) a document appointing a health care surrogate (in jurisdictions that do not formally recognize a durable power of attorney for health care), and the advance medical care directive.

- Advance directive: a document in which a person either

states choices for medical treatment or designates an individual for this purpose.

Living Will

A living will requires that two conditions be present before it takes effect: 1) the patient must be terminally ill, and 2) the patient must lack decision-making capacity. The determination of terminal varies from jurisdiction to jurisdiction, as do the laws concerning advance directives. It is therefore advised that each physician be familiar with the local statutes concerning advance directives. Because of the requirement that the patient must be terminally ill, the living will is restricted in its use and may not be useful in many circumstances in which the patient lacks decision-making capacity but cannot necessarily be described as terminally ill. When activated, the living will provides guidance to the caregivers about what treatments the patient does or does not desire. It is, however, ineffective if vaguely written or applied to patients with uncertain prognoses.

- The living will reflects a patient's autonomy.
- Legal reliability of the living will may vary from state to state.

Surrogates

1. Definition—The surrogate represents the patient's interests and previously expressed wishes in the context of the medical issues. The surrogate is optimally designated by the patient before critical illness. One type of surrogate is the durable power of attorney for health care, in which a legally binding proxy directive authorizes a designated individual to speak on behalf of the patient. The second type of surrogate is the patient's family or the court. The third type is a moral surrogate (usually a family member) who best knows the patient and has the patient's interest at heart. Difficulties may arise when the moral surrogate is not the legal surrogate. Dialogue between the physician and surrogate is important.

- Surrogate represents the patient's interests and previously expressed wishes in the context of the medical issues.
- Optimally, a surrogate is designated by patient before critical illness.

2. Standards of surrogate decision-making—How should the surrogate make decisions for the patient's health care decisions? If the patient has issued explicit directives, the surrogate should follow those instructions, unless it can clearly be demonstrated that the patient did not understand the nature of the information or choices made in that explicit directive. This situation unfortunately occurs when advance directives are completed without discussing the nature of the questions addressed with a health care provider. In the absence of such directives, the surrogate should use "substituted judgment," that is, the surrogate should decide to the best of his or her ability, based on the beliefs and values of the patient, what the choices would be if the patient were able to speak for himself or herself. In some circumstances the surrogate has not had enough communication about health care and life issues to be able to project how the patient would decide. There simply is not enough information to be able to specifically "substitute" for the patient. In these circumstances the surrogate's obligation is to try to decide what are the best interests of the patient given the clinical situation.

- Surrogate decision maker represents the patient's interest.
- In the absence of specific advance directives, the surrogate should use "substituted judgment."

Several studies have shown that surrogate decision makers often choose courses that are not what the patient would have chosen for themselves in specific circumstances. Because of this, physicians should strongly stress the importance of having patients discuss their values and health care goals with their family members or surrogates. It is also the duty of each physician to discuss these issues with her or his patients personally; this practice allows physicians to understand their patients' values to ensure that their choices are not made on misinformation.

- Each physician should discuss specific advance directives with her or his patients.

Durable Power of Attorney for Health Care

The durable power of attorney for health care (DPAHC) is a document that designates a surrogate decision maker should the patient lose decision-making capacity. It does not require that the patient be terminally ill, and therefore it is an advance directive that is more generally useful. Within the DPAHC, the patient can make specific directives concerning different types of treatments such as cardiopulmonary resuscitation (CPR), artificial nutrition, and hydration. The major value, however, is in providing an individual who can dynamically interact with the health care team regarding the great breadth of medical decisions.

- DPAHC designates a surrogate decision maker should the patient lose decision-making capacity.

Advance Medical Care Directive

In some instances, patients have specific desires never to receive certain forms of therapy. For instance, a member of the Jehovah's Witness faith wishes to refuse the administration of blood or blood products in any and all circumstances. Other individuals may want to refuse dialysis or some other intervention regardless of the circumstance. The advance medical care directive is a document that states this categorical refusal for a specific treatment. It may take the form of a no-transfusion card or a medic-alert statement, for example.

- Adults who refuse life-saving measures (such as a blood transfusion) should be allowed to maintain their religious practices.

It is always very helpful when the patient has a specific advance directive appointing a surrogate decision maker. What if there is no advance directive? Who speaks for the patient? The underlying principle is to find a person, or persons, who most likely can share with the caregivers the patient's values and how the patient would most likely choose if he or she could speak for himself or herself. Different jurisdictions may create a specific list of ranking, but a practical approach would be the following list, in descending order of authority: 1) the spouse, 2) an adult child or the majority of adult children, 3) a parent or parents, 4) an adult sibling or the majority of adult siblings, 5) an adult relative who has exhibited special care and concern, and 6) if no relative can be located, a close friend.

- A surrogate decision maker is helpful for directing or enforcing a specific advance directive.

Conflicts

Inescapably, situations arise in which a surrogate's instructions conflict with the patient's previously expressed directive or with those of other family members. Because the primary responsibility of the physician is to the patient, the physician should determine as best as possible what the patient would choose for himself or herself. In these circumstances, it may be helpful to involve an independent third-party arbitrator, such as an ethics consultant or committee or legal counsel to help work through the issues. This option is useful only if the physician is unable, for whatever reason, to resolve the conflict. In reality, every physician must learn to be a medical ethicist in dealing with her or his own patients.

- The primary responsibility of the physician is to serve the patient's interest.

The Patient Self-Determination Act of 1990

In response to the *Cruzan* decision, the U.S. Congress passed the Patient Self-Determination Act (PSDA) to ensure that patients were informed of their rights to accept or refuse medical care and to create and execute an advance directive. The PSDA requires that hospitals, nursing homes, hospices, managed care organizations, and home health care agencies provide this information to patients at the time of admission or enrollment. The organizations are required to 1) document whether patients have advance directives, 2) establish policies to implement the advance directives, and 3) educate their staffs and community about advance directives and these policies.

- The PSDA requires that all health care providers, at the time of admission, dispense information to patients about their rights to accept or refuse care and to create an advance directive.

Informed Consent

A derivative of the principle of autonomy, informed consent is the voluntary acceptance of physician recommendations for treatment or research investigations by decisionally capable patients or surrogates who have been furnished with ample truthful information regarding the risks, benefits, and alternatives of the proposed intervention. Informed consent has two preconditions on the part of the patient: 1) decision-making capacity, and 2) voluntariness (essentially the same as the agency and liberty associated with the principle of autonomy). Beyond these preconditions are the informational requirements of informed consent. Patients should receive accurate, truthful information sufficient to make a reasoned decision. The amount of information shared with the patient should not be guided by only what the physician believes is adequate (Professional Practice Standard) but that which the average prudent person would need to have in order to make an appropriate decision (Reasonable Person Standard). Included within this information is a discussion of available alternatives to the proposed treatment. For example, a patient with a cancer amenable to surgical resection, chemotherapy, or radiation therapy, all associated with a similar long-term outcome, should receive a thorough discussion of each of the options and their potential complications and side effects, even if the physician may be biased toward one of the three treatments. It is the duty of the physician to set aside personal bias and provide detailed information on each treatment to allow the patient to make a well-informed personal decision. The patient can then take the information and assess it within the context of her or his own life's goals and quality of life considerations.

- Informed consent requires decision-making capacity and voluntariness.
- Reasonable Person Standard: amount of information needed by a patient is that which the average prudent person would need to make a decision.
- Many informed-consent forms do not meet the Reasonable

Person Standard and are therefore of no value morally or legally

After a discussion of the available alternatives, the physician should present the patient with a single recommendation that the patient can accept or reject. Patients come to their physicians expecting the caregivers to use their knowledge and experience in providing them with a recommendation. Simply laying out a series of choices before the patient may lead to confusion or the perception by the patient that the physician is unconcerned with his or her welfare. If the patient refuses the recommended treatment, and chooses one of the alternatives, the physician should respect the patient's choice. The final plan should reflect an agreement between a well-informed patient and a well-informed, sympathetic, and unbiased physician. In certain circumstances, a patient may require more information than what the average reasonable person might desire. For instance, some religious belief systems may specifically preclude certain forms of medical intervention that might not trouble another individual in the least. It is important to ensure that patients receive sufficient information within the context of their beliefs to help them make an appropriate choice.

- The physician should provide all alternatives followed by a single recommendation.
- If the patient refuses the recommended treatment, the physician should respect the patient's choice.

Informed consent from surrogates is necessary to perform autopsy (except in certain instances such as coroner's cases, in which the decision is made by outside authorities) or to practice intubation, placement of intravascular lines, or other procedures on the newly dead. Informed consent is essential when performing new, innovative, nonstandard surgical procedures and research procedures. In rare exceptions, the physician can treat a patient without truly informed consent (e.g., in an emotionally unstable patient who requires urgent treatment, informing the patient of the details may produce further problems).

- Informed consent from surrogates is necessary to perform autopsy.
- Informed consent from surrogates is necessary to perform new, innovative, and nonstandard surgical procedures.

Implied Consent

The principle of implied consent is invoked when true informed consent is not possible because the patient (or surrogate) is unable to express a decision regarding treatment, specifically, in emergency situations in which physicians are compelled to provide medically necessary therapy, without which harm would result. This clarifies that there is a duty to assist a person in urgent need of care. This principle has been legally accepted, and it provides the physician a legal defense against battery (although not negligence).

- Implied consent is invoked when true informed consent is not possible.

Disclosure

Truth-telling on the part of the physician is an integral aspect of autonomy. To make the principle of autonomy function, the physician must provide decisionally capable patients with adequate and truthful information on which to base medical decisions. Without the receipt of sufficient truthful information, patients cannot make truly autonomous decisions about their life plans. Occasionally, however, the physician may withhold part or all of the truth if it is believed that telling the truth is likely to cause significant injury. This is the principle of *therapeutic privilege*. For example, if it can be well ascertained that a patient will attempt harm of himself or herself or others if certain information is received, such as the diagnosis of cancer, then the information may be withheld. However, there is a high burden of proof on the withholding physician to establish the likelihood of injury, and this decision for intentional nondisclosure must be fully and carefully recorded in the medical record.

- Truth-telling on the part of the physician is an integral aspect of patient's autonomy.

Justifiable Paternalism

Rarely, it may be necessary for the physician to withhold part or all of the truth if telling the whole truth is likely to cause more harm than good. Making such decisions that would bypass or override the patient's autonomous decision making has been described as paternalistic or parentalistic. Parentalistic behavior may be justified in certain circumstances. The following criteria should be met in these circumstances: 1) the patient is at risk of significant, preventable harm; 2) the parentalistic action probably will prevent the harm; 3) the projected benefits outweigh the risks to the patient; and 4) the least autonomy-restrictive alternative that will secure the benefits and reduce the risks is to be used.

- Paternalistic or parentalistic action: withholding information from a patient to prevent potential harm to the patient which may result if the patient knows the information.

Confidentiality

Privacy is an integral part to the protection of an individual's autonomy. Confidentiality respects that right to privacy and provides the patient the right to keep medical information solely within the realm of the physician-patient relationship. The physician is ethically and legally obliged to maintain a patient's medical information in strict confidence, a tradition dating back to the Hippocratic Oath. However, the obligation to safeguard patient confidences is subject to certain exceptions that are justified because of overriding ethical and social concerns. When a patient threatens to inflict serious bodily harm on another individual, and there is reasonable probability that the patient will carry out the threat, the physician is obligated to take reasonable precautions for the protection of the intended victim, including notification of law enforcement authorities if necessary (American Medical Association Council on Ethical and Judicial Affairs, June 1994). Also, in some exceptions, a patient's data must be shared with public health care agencies, such as in the case of the human immunodeficiency virus (HIV), *Mycobacterium tuberculosis*, and other infectious diseases. A growing area of concern regards heritable genetic traits. This concern is undergoing significant ethical and legal scrutiny at the present time. A common example that challenges the principle of confidentiality is a patient with HIV who refuses to inform third parties who may not yet be infected but certainly will have future contact with the individual. A functional solution is the following: 1) attempt to persuade the infected patient to cease endangering the third party or to notify the third party of the risk; 2) if persuasion fails, notify an authority who can intervene; 3) if the authority takes no action or is not available, notify the endangered party of the risk (American Medical Association Council on Ethical and Judicial Affairs, 1988). It must be clearly stated that this approach still may be open to legal liabilities and is based on the medical profession's obligation to prevent harm.

- Physician is obliged to maintain medical information in strict confidence.
- Exceptions include instances when data, if not released to appropriate agencies, may cause greater societal harm (e.g., positive results of HIV test, sputum culture for *Mycobacterium tuberculosis*).

Futility

It has been clearly established, both ethically and legally, that patients have the right to refuse any and all medical therapies. But does the principle of autonomy give patients, or their surrogates, the right to demand treatments? This question particularly arises when patients or families request that cardiopulmonary resuscitation, mechanical ventilation, and other aggressive treatment be performed on patients with little chance of recovery or survival to dismissal. Can physicians unilaterally withhold or withdraw medical interventions if, in the opinion of the physicians, the intervention is futile? The conflict seemingly is between the autonomy of the patients and the moral autonomy and integrity of the caregivers. Physicians are moral agents, just as much as patients, and should not be forced to violate their ethical beliefs and principles.

- Patients have the right to refuse any and all medical therapies.
- Futility: unilateral decision by the physician to withhold or withdraw medical interventions, based on predictable futile outcome.

The definition of futility states that something is futile if it is "leaky, hence untrustworthy, vain, failing of the desired end through intrinsic defect" (*Oxford English Dictionary*). Therefore, a futile intervention is one that cannot achieve the goals of intervention no matter how many times it is repeated. From this definition, it can clearly be stated that physicians are not required to provide treatments that have no pathophysiologic rationale, have already failed in a given patient in the past, or will not achieve the goals of care already agreed on by the physician and patient or surrogate. *Physiologic futility* is determined by the physician, who needs to decide whether a treatment can achieve its physiologic goal. However, most futility conflicts arise in clinical situations in which an intervention is "unlikely" to benefit the patient or there is a conflict about the goals of treatment (such as, maintaining physiologic life versus restoration of independent functioning or survival to dismissal). Many have tried to create functional definitions of futility that would cover these circumstances, but all have the flaw of establishing arbitrary thresholds that are value-laden in themselves.

- Physiologic futility is determined by the physician.

When cases of futility conflicts arise in clinical situations in which an intervention is "unlikely" to benefit the patient or there is a conflict about the goals of treatment (such as maintaining physiologic life versus restoration of independent functioning or survival to dismissal), the solution should be one of "due process." The American Medical Association Council on Ethical and Judicial Affairs endorsed such a program ("Houston Policy," JAMA 276:571-574, 1996), which requires the following:

1. Earnest attempts to deliberate over and negotiate prior understanding between patient, surrogate, and physician about what constitutes "futile" care for the patient and what falls within acceptable limits for those involved. Many times the disagreement is based on inappropriate expectations of the patient or surrogate. When appropriate data about outcomes are shared, many requests for treatments such as cardiopulmonary resuscitation decrease.

2. Joint decision making should occur to the maximal extent possible.

3. Attempts should be made to negotiate and resolve disagreements (such as through ethics consultation).

4. If disagreements are irresolvable, a consultant or end-of-life decisions committee should become involved.

5. If the committee agrees with the patient and the physician remains unpersuaded, intra- or inter-institutional transfer may be arranged.

6. If the committee agrees with the physician and the patient or surrogate remains unpersuaded, intra- or inter-institutional transfer may be arranged.

7. If transfer is not possible, the intervention need not be offered.

● Cases of futility conflicts should be resolved by due process (see above).

Beneficence

Beneficence is acting to benefit patients by preserving life, restoring health, relieving suffering, and restoring or maintaining function. The physician (acting in good faith) is obligated to help patients attain their own interests and goals as determined by the patient, *not* the physician.

● Beneficence: preservation of life, restoration of health, relief of suffering, and restoration or maintenance of function.

Nonabandonment

Abandonment connotes leaving the patient (for whom the physician has provided health care in the past) without providing for immediate or future medical care. This action has been "universally condemned as a serious and punishable infraction of both the legal and ethical obligations that physicians owe patients" (Ann Intern Med 122:377-378, 1995). In contrast, nonabandonment denotes a requisite ethical obligation of physicians to provide ongoing medical care once the patient and physician mutually concur to enter into an alliance. Nonabandonment is closely related to the principle of beneficence and is fundamental to the long-term physician-patient relationship. This tenet has several drawbacks and limitations. The degree of physician's involvement in the relationship cannot be measured as to its quantity or quality. Furthermore, the extent of the relationship is dictated by the underlying medical condition. For instance, an annual examination may require a single visit to the physician, whereas a complicated disease process may bring the physician and patient closer to each other over a long period. It would be improper for the physician to force a patient to maintain a long-term physician-patient relationship if the latter is unwilling, for whatever reason. Noncompliance, in terms of taking medications or following a physician's instructions, by the patient is not grounds for abandonment. Physicians should strive to respond to the needs of their patients over time, but they should not trespass their own values in the process.

● Nonabandonment: a requisite ethical obligation of physician to provide ongoing care once the patient and physician mutually concur to enter into an alliance.

Conflict of Interest

The principle of beneficence requires that the physician not engage in activities that are not in the patient's best interest. This is considered to be a significant problem in the United States and other countries. Some studies have suggested that physicians' prescribing practices are influenced by financial and other significant rewards from drug companies. If the physician does not ardently avoid areas of potential conflict of interest (because of the principle of beneficence), the result may be maleficence. Authorship of scientific papers and editorials to promote drugs and appliances solely for immediate or future personal financial gains also constitutes conflict of interest (Ann Intern Med 126:986-988,1997).

● Conflict of interest is contrary to the tenet of beneficence.

Nonmaleficence

Nonmaleficence requires that one should not do evil or harm. This principle is based on "do no harm, prevent harm, and remove harm." This tenet also addresses unprofessional behavior: verbal, physical, and sexual abuse of patients, and uninformed and undisclosed experimentation on patients with drugs and procedures that have the potential to cause harmful side effects. Breach of physician-patient confidentiality which results in harm to the patient is another example of maleficence.

● Nonmaleficence: "do no harm, prevent harm, and remove harm."

The Impaired Physician

According to the American Medical Association, the impaired physician is one who is "unable to practice medicine with reasonable skill and safety to patients because of physical or mental illness, including deteriorations through the aging process, or loss of motor skill, or excessive use or abuse of drugs including alcohol." Impairment is distinct from competence, which specifically concerns the physician's knowledge and skills to adequately perform his or her duties as a physician. Impairment and incompetence both may seriously compromise patient care and safety. Under the obligation to protect patients from harm, physicians must protect patients from impaired and incompetent colleagues. Physicians have a moral and legal obligation to report impaired and incompetent colleagues to the appropriate authority. Different states vary in the specifics of reporting, but all have a reporting requirement. Typical authorities to contact include the institutional chief of staff or impairment program, local or state medical society impairment programs, or the state licensing body. It is important that reporting the behavior of a colleague be based on objective evidence rather than supposition.

- Physicians have an obligation to report impaired behavior in colleagues.

The Principle of Double Effect (Beneficence Versus Nonmaleficence)

In the medical management of patients, sometimes the pursuit of a beneficent outcome risks the potential for serious injury or death. Consequently, the moral obligations for beneficence and nonmaleficence conflict. The classic example of such a situation is the terminally ill patient who may require high doses of narcotics for adequate analgesia, but such doses also have the potential for respiratory depression and an earlier death. The rule or principle of double effect is a means of trying to resolve the conflict. This principle states that 1) the act itself must be good or morally neutral, 2) the actor or agent intends only the good effect, 3) the bad effect must not be a means to the good effect (e.g., death is the only way to achieve the desired outcome), and 4) the good effect must outweigh the bad effect. By the reasoning of double effect, and the high requirement of beneficence to address the suffering of patients, adequate analgesia for the relief of suffering should always be given even if death is hastened. The analgesics are to be given, however, in such a way as to relieve the pain and not specifically to hasten the death of the patient, even in terminally ill patients.

- Adequate analgesia, particularly in patients with incurable disease, is the responsibility of the physician.
- Physician has not performed immorally if death in a terminally ill patient is result of respiratory depression from analgesic therapy; euthanasia is not the goal.

Incurable Disease and Death

Probably the most distressing aspect of medical practice is the encounter with a patient who has an incurable disease and in whom premature death is inevitable. The physician and patient (or surrogate) must formulate appropriate goals of therapy, choose what measures should be taken to maintain life, and decide how aggressive these measures ought to be. It is important to remind oneself that the patient is under enormous mental anguish and physical stress and that the ability to make solid decisions may be clouded. Furthermore, the decision(s) made by the patient may be guided by his or her understanding (whether adequate or not) of the medical condition and prognosis, religious beliefs, financial status, and other personal wishes. The patient may seek counsel from family, friends, and clergy as well as the attending physician.

- In incurable disease, recognize that the patient is under enormous mental anguish and physical stress.
- Ability of the patient to make solid decisions may be clouded.

The following guidelines are suggested in dealing with incurable disease and death. The patient and family (if the patient so desires) must be provided ample opportunity to talk with the physician and ask questions. An unhurried openness and willing-to-listen attitude on the part of the physician are critical for a positive outcome. Patients often find it easier to share their feelings about death with their physician, who is likely to be more objective and less emotional, than with family and friends. Nevertheless, the physician should not remain or "appear" completely detached from the patient's feelings and emotions. Even an attempt on the part of the physician to enter the "inner" feelings of the patient will have a soothing, if not therapeutic, effect.

- The patient and family must be provided every opportunity to talk with the physician and ask questions.
- An unhurried openness and willing-to-listen attitude on the part of the physician are critical for a positive outcome.

The physician should assume the responsibility to furnish or arrange for physical, emotional, and spiritual support. Adequate control of pain, maintenance of human dignity, and close contact with the family are crucial. The emotional and spiritual support available through local clergy (as appropriate, given the patient's personal beliefs) should not be underestimated. At no other time in life is the reality of human mortality so real as in the terminal phases of disease. It is always preferable to allay the anxiety of the dying patient through adequate emotional and spiritual support rather than by sedation. The physician should constantly remind herself or himself that despite all the medical technology that surrounds the patient, the patient must not be dehumanized.

- Adequate pain control, maintenance of human dignity, and close contact with family are crucial.
- It is better to allay anxiety by adequate emotional and spiritual support rather than by sedation.

Justice

Every patient deserves and must be provided optimal care as warranted by the underlying medical condition. Allocation of medical resources fairly and according to medical need is the basis for this principle. The decision to provide optimal medical care should be based on the medical need of each patient and the perceived medical benefit to the patient. The patient's social status, ability to pay, or perceived social worth should not dictate the quality or quantity of medical care. The physician's clear-cut responsibility is to the patient's well-being (beneficence). Physicians should not make decisions about individual care of their patients based on larger societal needs. The bedside is not the place to make general policy decisions.

- Justice: allocation of medical resources fairly and according to medical need.
- Physician should not make decisions about individual care of patients based on larger societal needs.

PHYSICIAN-ASSISTED SUICIDE AND EUTHANASIA

All four tenets of medical ethics have an impact on the issue of physician-assisted death, that is, physician-assisted suicide and euthanasia. Historically, the medical profession has taken a strong stand against physicians directly killing patients, but this prohibition has been challenged on the basis of patient autonomy, beneficence or compassion, and other grounds. Numerous opinion polls have shown that significant portions of the general population and the medical community now favor some legalization of physician-assisted suicide, if not euthanasia. The American Medical Association and other large professional medical groups have maintained their stance against these practices.

In 1997, the Supreme Court of the United States ruled that states may maintain laws prohibiting euthanasia and assisted suicide but may also pass laws allowing these practices. The Court, however, emphasized the patient's right to adequate, aggressive pain control even if it might shorten the patient's life. In the election of 1997, the people of the state of Oregon reiterated their support for physician-assisted suicide by re-approving a referendum first passed in 1994 legalizing assisted suicide but still prohibiting euthanasia. The Oregon law requires that the patient 1) be terminal, 2) be decisionally capable, 3) have initiated two verbal and one written request for a prescription for a lethal overdose, 4) undergo a second-opinion consultation, 5) receive appropriate psychiatric intervention if perceived to be depressed, and 6) undergo a 15-day waiting period after the request has been made to allow the patient to change his or her mind. At this time, assisted suicide and euthanasia remain illegal in the other 49 states.

- Euthanasia and physician-assisted suicide are legally prohibited in the United States with the exception of the state of Oregon, which permits physician-assisted suicide.

Regardless of one's final position on this difficult issue, physicians are obligated to address the underlying concerns that lead patients and physicians to believe that assisted suicide and euthanasia are necessary (the New York State Task Force on Life and the Law, 1994). Physicians should be acquainted with appropriate means of pain management and palliative care and be willing to be aggressive in the relief of a patient's symptoms. Physicians also are obligated to recognize and appropriately treat depression. Furthermore, physicians should strive to address the other issues that may lead patients to desire assisted death, such as fear of abandonment and loss of control.

"DO NOT RESUSCITATE" (DNR)

DNR orders affect administration of cardiopulmonary resuscitation (CPR) only; other therapeutic options should not be influenced by the DNR order. Every person whose medical history is unclear or unavailable should receive CPR in the event of cardiopulmonary arrest. CPR is not recommended when it merely prolongs life in a patient with terminal illness or when the fatal outcome is clinically evident (Table 15-1).

Of paramount importance are the patient's knowledge of the extent of disease and the prognosis, the physician's estimate of the potential efficacy of CPR, and the wishes of the patient (or surrogate) regarding CPR as a therapeutic tool. The DNR order should be reviewed frequently because clinical circumstances may dictate other measures (e.g., a patient with terminal cardiomyopathy who had initially turned down heart transplantation and wanted to be considered a "DNR candidate" may change her or his mind and now opt for the transplantation). Physicians should discuss the appropriateness of CPR or DNR with patients at high risk for cardiopulmonary arrest and with the terminally ill. The discussion should optimally take place in the outpatient setting, during the initial period of hospitalization, and periodically during hospitalization, if appropriate. DNR orders (and rationale) should be entered in the patient's medical records.

- DNR orders affect CPR only.
- Other therapeutic options should not be influenced by the DNR order.
- Every patient should be considered a candidate for CPR unless clear indications exist otherwise.
- CPR is not recommended when it merely prolongs life in a patient with a terminal illness.

Table 15-1.--Clinical Situations in Which Cardiopulmonary Resuscitation Is Unlikely to Prolong Life

---

Advanced, progressive, ultimately lethal illness
        Bedfast with metastatic cancer
        Child's class C cirrhosis
        Infection by human immunodeficiency virus (with ≥2 episodes of *pneumonia caused by Pneumocystis carinii*)
        Dementia requiring long-term care
Acute, near-fatal illness without evidence of improvement after admission to the intensive-care unit
        Coma (traumatic or nontraumatic) lasting ≥48 hours
        Multiple organ system failure with no improvement after 3 consecutive days in the intensive-care unit
Unsuccessful out-of-hospital cardiopulmonary resuscitation

From Murphy DJ, Finucane TE: New do-not-resuscitate policies: a first step in cost control. Arch Intern Med 153:1641-1648, 1993. By permission of the American Medical Association.

- DNR orders should be reviewed frequently.
- DNR orders (and rationale) should be entered in the patient's medical records.

WITHHOLDING AND WITHDRAWING LIFE SUPPORT

This decision may be compatible with beneficence, nonmaleficence, and autonomy. The right of a decisionally capable person to refuse lifesaving hydration and nutrition was upheld by the U.S. Supreme Court (Table 15-2), but a surrogate decision maker's right to refuse treatment for decisionally incapable persons can be restricted by states. As of mid-1997, the states of New York, Missouri, and Florida required "clear and convincing evidence" that withdrawing and withholding of the life-supporting treatment would be the patient's desire. Other states had lesser evidentiary standards for surrogates to withhold or withdraw life support. Brain death is not a necessary requirement for withdrawing or withholding life support. The value of each medical therapy (risk:benefit ratio) should be assessed for each patient. When appropriate, the withholding or withdrawal of life support is best accomplished with input from more than one experienced clinician.

- Withholding or withdrawing life support does not conflict with the principles of beneficence, nonmaleficence, and autonomy.
- Brain death is not a necessary requirement for withdrawing or withholding life support.

PERSISTENT VEGETATIVE STATE

This is a chronic state of unconsciousness (loss of self-awareness) lasting for more than a few weeks, characterized by the presence of wake/sleep cycles, but without behavioral or cerebral metabolic evidence of possessing cognitive function or of being able to respond in a learned manner to external events or stimuli. The body retains functions necessary to sustain vegetative survival, if provided nutritional and other supportive measures—note that the U.S. Supreme Court has ruled that there is no distinction between artificial feeding and hydration versus mechanical ventilation (Table 15-2).

- Persistent vegetative state: unconsciousness (loss of self-awareness) lasting for more than a few weeks.
- U.S. Supreme Court ruling states that there is no distinction between artificial feeding and hydration versus mechanical ventilation.

DEFINITION OF DEATH

Death is irreversible cessation of circulatory and respiratory function *or* irreversible cessation of all functions of the entire brain, including the brain stem. Clinical criteria (at times substantiated by electroencephalographic testing or assessment of cerebral perfusion) permit the reliable diagnosis of "cerebral death."

The family should be informed of the brain death but should not be asked to decide whether further medical therapy should be continued. One exception is when the patient's surrogate (or the patient, via an advanced directive) permits certain decisions, such as organ donation, in the case of brain death.

Once it is ascertained that the patient is "brain dead" and that no further therapy can be offered, the primary physician, preferably after consultation with another physician involved in the care of the patient, may withdraw supportive measures. This is true in general throughout the United States, with the exception of the states of New Jersey and New York, which have modified their definition of death statutes to allow a religious exemption for groups (such as Orthodox Jews) that do

Table 15-2.--Pertinent Legal Rulings

Case, yr	Legal issue	Court	Decision
Salgo, 1957	Informed consent	California Court of Appeals	First used term "informed consent"
Brooks, 1965	Jehovah's Witness refusal of blood	Illinois District Court	Patients have right to personal treatment on religious grounds
Canterbury, 1972	Degree of disclosure required for adequate informed consent	U.S. District Court	Established "prudent patient test"
Quinlan, 1976	PVS—discontinuation of mechanical ventilation, previously articulated directive	New Jersey Supreme Court	Discontinuation (based on right to privacy)
Brophy, 1986	PVS—discontinuation of gastrostomy feedings, previously articulated directive	Massachusetts Supreme Court	Discontinue feedings (based on autonomy)
Bouvia, 1986	Severely impaired, refusal of nasogastric tube feedings by a decisionally capable patient	California Court of Appeals	Removal of nasogastric tube (based on autonomy)
Corbett, 1986	PVS—discontinuation of nasogastric tube feedings, no predefined directive(s)	Florida Court of Appeals	Discontinue feedings (based on right to privacy)
Cruzan, 1990	PVS—state of Missouri required "clear and convincing" evidence of individual's wishes before allowing withdrawal of life support	U.S. Supreme Court	States have right to restrict exercise of right to refuse treatment by surrogates; decisionally capable patients may refuse life-sustaining therapy, including hydration, nutrition, and mechanical ventilation
Wanglie, 1991	PVS—family wished continued support despite objections to continued life-sustaining therapy by the physicians and institution	Minnesota District Court	Continuation (based on autonomy, substituted judgment)
Lee, 1997	Assisted suicide	U.S. Supreme Court	States have the right to make laws prohibiting physician-assisted suicide and euthanasia

PVS, persistent vegetative state.

not accept brain death as a valid criterion for death. In these states, continued care may be requested of the caregivers until circulatory and respiratory function collapse.

The imminent possibility of harvesting organs for transplantation should in no way affect any of the above-outlined decisions. When organ donation is possible after the determination of brain death, the family should be approached, preferably before cessation of cardiac function, regarding organ donation.

- Death: irreversible cessation of circulatory and respiratory function *or* irreversible cessation of all functions of entire brain, including brain stem.

- Electroencephalography is not necessary to establish death.

AUTHORS' NOTE

Laws concerning ethical issues in medicine continue to evolve, reflecting changing attitudes of society. Certainly, legal decisions will continue to influence the practice of medicine. Many states have no directly applicable statutes or court cases relating to difficult ethical issues in medical practice. This review is meant as a guide; the individual practitioner is referred to the appropriate state medical society for further information regarding state-specific mandates.

QUESTIONS

Multiple Choice (choose the one best answer)
1. A previously healthy 69-year-old white man with the new diagnosis of metastatic prostate carcinoma is admitted to the hospital for pain control. During the initial history and physical examination, the patient indicates he wants full resuscitation efforts applied should he experience a cardiopulmonary arrest. He is fully oriented and cognitively capable. Which of the following do you do?
   a. Tell the patient that you will not make him full code status because resuscitation would be futile
   b. Comply with the patient's request and write that he be full code status
   c. Say nothing further but order "do-not-resuscitate" (DNR) status in the orders and the medical record
   d. Do nothing at this time, but hope that subsequent discussions will change the patient's mind
   e. Be willing to leave the patient full code, but engage him in a discussion about his values and goals and inform him of the probable outcomes from resuscitation attempts should he have cardiopulmonary arrest

2. A 68-year-old man with end-stage, irreversible, chronic obstructive pulmonary disease is in the intensive care unit. He is severely obtunded. During a course of several weeks in the unit, repeated efforts to wean him from the ventilator have failed. Among the team of physicians caring for the patient, there is agreement that he will remain ventilator-dependent and probably not improve any further clinically. The issue of cardiopulmonary resuscitation in the event of a cardiopulmonary arrest is raised. The patient gave no prior indication of his wishes and did not execute an advance directive. The physicians should do which of the following?

   a. Tell the family that they are indicating the patient's status as DNR because a resuscitation attempt would be cruel
   b. Explain the dismal situation and prognosis to the family and advise DNR status but leave the final decision to the family
   c. Order DNR status without consultation with the family
   d. Leave the patient full code status because the family has been difficult to get along with
   e. Ask the medical student to discuss code status with the family

3. A 29-year-old married man frequently travels in the course of his business. He presents to his physician for evaluation of a lesion on his penis. The physician diagnoses primary syphilis. His physician informs him that this diagnosis will need to be reported to the State Department of Health in accordance with state law and that the Health Department may perform some contact tracing to ensure that individuals the patient has had contact with receive appropriate testing, and treatment if indicated. The patient is quite uncomfortable on learning about the reporting law. He indicates he knows from whom he must have contracted the illness, a contact on one of his business trips, and also indicates that he has not had any sexual contact with his wife since that one affair took place. He therefore does not see why reporting must occur. He suggests to his physician that he will not have any contact with his wife or anyone else until after he has undergone his treatment, and he requests that this issue be kept strictly confidential between the physician and patient. The physician should:
   a. Report the patient to the State Department of Health in accordance with the law

b. Agree with the patient's proposed plan and maintain strict confidentiality

c. Contact the patient's wife and advise her to be tested for syphilis

d. Threaten the patient that you (the physician) will tell his wife of his activities if he should ever contract a sexually transmitted disease again

e. Write a prescription for the appropriate antibiotics and indicate that you will discuss the issue further at the time of the return appointment

4. Which of the following is *not* true about a living will?

a. A patient must be terminally ill for a living will to take effect

b. A patient must lack decision-making capacity for a living will to take effect

c. A living will usually indicates that a patient does not want some form(s) of life-sustaining therapy

d. A living will may not be verbally rescinded

e. A living will does not require preparation by an attorney

5. A 61-year-old white man is admitted to the hematology service with advanced diffuse large-cell non-Hodgkin's lymphoma. There is a huge abdominal mass in addition to diffuse adenopathy. The patient is obtunded, has a high serum lactic acid level, and has rapidly progressing hepatic and renal failure. Before his transfer from another hospital, he had filled out an advance directive while still oriented. The advance directive indicated that until two independent physicians had declared the patient brain dead, all forms of life-sustaining therapy should be used. The one family member who currently accompanies the patient, a daughter, was present when the advance directive was filled out. On questioning her, it becomes clear that the patient and the other family members who were present at the time, which included the patient's wife and his other children, did not know what brain death was. When it was explained that the patient will probably soon need to be placed on a ventilator and undergo dialysis, the daughter expresses concerns that these "machines" were not what they had in mind when they talked about "life-sustaining therapies." They were thinking about things such as an intravenous or feeding tube. She is concerned that a ventilator and dialysis would be far more invasive than what her father actually desired. The physician should do which of the following?

a. Contact legal counsel to request a court-ordered surrogate be appointed

b. State that the advance directive is legally binding and that the caregivers have no choice but to do all interventions to maintain the patient's life

c. Speak with the wife and the other children to corroborate the daughter's story. If all concur, override the advance directive with a careful and detailed explanation in the medical record

d. Tear up the advance directive as invalid

e. Transfer the case to a colleague

6. A 38-year-old white woman with end-stage, refractory metastatic breast cancer is admitted to the hospital for pain management. Despite receiving a combination of multiple classes of drugs including corticosteroids, nonsteroidal anti-inflammatory agents, and narcotics, she is still in severe pain. Her physician has been increasing her morphine dosage steadily during the past 24 hours. The patient's respiratory rate is 8 per minute, and although drowsy, the patient still is able to communicate that her pain is 8 or 9 on a scale of 1 to 10. The physician should do which of the following?

a. Hold the narcotics at the current dosages because to increase them further may risk putting the patient into respiratory failure

b. Give the patient a bolus of 100 mg of morphine to end the patient's suffering and shorten the inevitable, agonizing dying process

c. Back down on the dose of morphine until her respiratory rate improves

d. Give the patient naloxone hydrochloride (Narcan) to reverse the respiratory depression and sedation

e. Continue to upwardly titrate the morphine dosage until the pain has been relieved

7. A widowed 71-year-old white woman has been your patient for several years. She has been a particularly frustrating patient because she does not take the medications you have prescribed to treat her hypertension, congestive heart failure, and adult-onset diabetes mellitus. Usually she presents after an absence of several months with significant congestive heart failure and requires hospitalization, despite numerous educational efforts and other initiatives to improve her compliance. She now presents with 2+ ankle edema, shortness of breath, and a fasting glucose value of 200 mg/dL. You should do which of the following?

a. Treat her, but tell her she has 30 days to find a new physician

b. Refuse to treat her and tell her to go to the emergency room and to find another physician

c. Provide appropriate medical care and follow-up

d. Begin legal proceedings to have the patient declared incompetent and admitted to a nursing home

e. Tell the patient she is an idiot and had better get with the program

8. A 78-year-old, right-handed, widowed woman has a history of adult-onset diabetes mellitus and coronary artery disease, having previously had two myocardial infarctions. She now has had a stroke that has rendered her paralyzed on the right side of her body and comatose. Cerebral arteriography reveals that the left hemisphere of her brain was destroyed in the stroke. Her three daughters request that use of the feeding tube be discontinued. There is no formal written advance directive, but the daughters indicate that their mother would not want to be maintained this way. The patient had taken care of her mother after a severe stroke and had stated she would never want to live like her mother had. The physician should do which of the following:

   a. Discontinue use of the tube feedings according to the children's request
   b. Refuse to discontinue the tube feedings because there is no advance directive
   c. Tell the children that a court order must be obtained before the feedings can be withheld
   d. Insist that the tube feeding be continued until the patient can regain capacity and speak for herself
   e. Refuse to comply because dehydration is a painful way to die

9. A 28-year-old woman comes to your office and complains that she has been sexually harassed by one of your partners. You should *not*:

   a. Confront your partner with this information
   b. Discuss the issue with your risk-management administrator
   c. Tell her to obtain an attorney
   d. Ask the woman to discuss why she is bringing the allegations of harassment

   e. Refer the woman to the local medical board or Department of Professional Regulation

10. Mrs. A. C. is a 64-year-old white woman with a history of diabetes mellitus and poorly controlled hypertension. She presents with a severe generalized headache. She does not have a past history of headache. Her blood pressure is 170/95 mm Hg. Her creatinine level is 2.1 mg/dL. Concerned that she may have had an aneurysmal bleed, you obtain a computed tomography (CT) scan of the head. No major abnormality is noted, but the radiologist comments that a small aneurysm with a tiny leak may escape the resolution of a plain CT scan. Magnetic resonance (MR) angiography is recommended, particularly because the contrast necessary for a cerebral angiogram may be particularly hazardous in light of her renal insufficiency. On ordering the test, you are informed that her insurance company still considers MR angiography an experimental procedure and refuses to pay for it. When you attempt to contact her insurance company to appeal, you are informed that the medical director will not be able to get back to you for another 24 hours. The patient indicates that she is widowed, has little financial reserves, and cannot pay for this test on her own. You should:

    a. Refer the patient to the business office to work out some form of financial arrangement
    b. Proceed with the MR angiography
    c. Wait the 24 hours to speak with the medical director
    d. Call the president of the insurance company and tell her you're going to tell all of your patients what a lousy company she runs
    e. Proceed with routine cerebral arteriography, which is a procedure covered by the patient's insurance.

ANSWERS

1. Answer e.

A DNR order must be consented to by the patient or the patient's surrogate. It is not appropriate to unilaterally override a patient's request concerning resuscitation. Although one could simply write that the patient be full code status, it is best to ensure that the patient understands what he or she is requesting and the probable outcome of that course. Sometimes after such a discussion, patients change their mind and want a DNR order.

2. Answer b.

Even if the prognosis is quite dismal, physicians cannot unilaterally order DNR status without the consent of the patient or a surrogate. In the situation in which coding the patient is highly unlikely to benefit the patient, it would be inappropriate to not address the issue.

3. Answer a.

Physicians have a responsibility to protect the health of the public and other specific individuals known to be at risk. The physician does not know that the patient indeed has not had contact with his wife or another individual. Therefore, failing to report not only would be illegal but also may put other individuals at unnecessary risk. Deferring the issue would not be appropriate because the patient may not return. The obligation to break confidence is limited. Because state authorities will intervene and contact the appropriate individuals at risk, the physician should not independently make those contacts.

4. Answer d.

A living will may be rescinded at any time, verbally or on paper.

5. Answer c.

This is a difficult situation in which an advance directive is ethically invalid because it does not reflect the patient's actual understanding or desires. Unfortunately, there is no check on these directives to ensure that patients do indeed understand what they are requesting, unless a physician has the opportunity to discuss these concerns with the patient during or after the document's preparation. Advance directives are legally binding, but extenuating circumstances may arise that change their interpretation. In this case, it would be very important to corroborate what the daughter is saying. If all of the family members who were present when the document was created agree that measures such as dialysis and ongoing ventilatory support were not what the patient had in mind, and would not be what he would desire, then the caregivers are obligated not to initiate those treat-

ments. The advance directive cannot be torn up, however, because once accepted it is entered into the patient's medical record. Rather, it would be important to carefully document the evidence proving that the advance directive is ethically invalid and indicating that the directive that the surrogates are stating is more in keeping with what the patient really desired.

6. Answer e.

This is a clear example of a case in which the principle of double effect comes into play. It is true that continuing to titrate the patient's narcotic dosages to achieve pain control may risk putting the patient in respiratory failure. It is not, however, the intent to simply end the patient's life, as the approach in answer b does. Decreasing her analgesic dosages or using Narcan would be inappropriate because either choice would only exacerbate the patient's suffering during her dying process. Because the intent is to enable the patient to die in comfort, the morally preferable option is to carefully push on to achieve adequate analgesia, even if that may potentially lead to the patient's earlier death. It is important to document the need for increasing analgesia in the medical record.

7. Answer c.

Even when confronted with extremely frustrating patients, physicians should never abandon them.

8. Answer a.

The daughters have provided some evidence of how their mother would respond if she could speak for herself. They also are making a request that does not seem to be inappropriate, given the clinical circumstances. Because the patient's husband is dead, her children become the appropriate proxies and they can provide guidance regarding medical interventions, including life-supporting measures. Even if the patient were more conscious, dehydration is generally not an uncomfortable way of death, particularly if the patient is debilitated and receives appropriate oral hygiene and care. (It is important to maintain a clear understanding of current state law regarding issues of withholding or withdrawing life-sustaining treatments.)

9. Answer c.

It is our obligation as physicians to pursue the best interests of our patients. This includes protecting them from inappropriate behavior of colleagues. The complaint must not be discounted, and the woman should be assisted in bringing her complaint to an independent group that can investigate the situation and intervene objectively and appropriately. It is also important to obtain the facts of the situation to help guard against subsequent complaints or incidents.

10. Answer b.

Our primary responsibility is to the best interests of our patients. Our primary fidelity must be to the patient and not to other institutions. This woman needs a study soon, and MR angiography is the most appropriate test with the least risk to the patient. Although it would be nice to work out some form of financial coverage, the insurance company is not responding appropriately. This should not deter the physician from doing what is necessary, even if it means the hospital may have to absorb the cost.

CHAPTER 16

NEPHROLOGY

Thomas R. Schwab, M.D.
Stephen B. Erickson, M.D.

ACUTE RENAL FAILURE–DEFINITIONS

Three important principles in the clinical evaluation of acute renal failure are the following: 1) It must be determined whether an increase in serum levels of creatinine or urea reflects a *genuine* and *recent* decrease in glomerular filtration rate. Many medications and substances interfere with the measurement of creatinine and urea and its renal handling. 2) If substantial irreversible renal dysfunction is to be avoided, acute renal failure must be recognized early. Remember, an increase in serum creatinine of 0.8 to 1.8 mg/dL reflects as much as a 50% loss of renal function. 3) Appropriate treatment of patients with acute renal failure demands that the cause be pinpointed promptly from the more than 100 potential causes. Currently, acute renal failure is broadly classified into prerenal, renal, and postrenal types.

- Increase in creatinine levels independently of glomerular filtration rate: ketoacidosis (acetoacetate), cefoxitin, cimetidine, trimethoprim, flucytosine, massive rhabdomyolysis, and high intake of meat.
- Increase in urea (BUN) independently of glomerular filtration rate: gastrointestinal tract bleeding, tissue trauma, glucocorticoids, and tetracyclines.
- Anuria <50 mL/day (limited differential diagnosis!): complete obstruction, rapidly progressive glomerulonephritis, cortical necrosis, and bilateral renal artery occlusion (e.g., dissection), but not acute tubular necrosis.
- Oliguria is <400 mL/day or <20 mL/hr: patients with an inability to concentrate urine may be "oliguric" with 1,000+ mL/day.
- Nonoliguric renal failure is >800 mL/day (most cases are nonoliguric).
- Polyuria is >3,000 mL/day (a clue to partial obstruction).

POSTRENAL FAILURE (OBSTRUCTION)

The pathogenesis of an obstructive uropathy is characterized by early vasoconstriction followed by vasodilatation. Obstruction may be anatomical (e.g., methysergide causing retroperitoneal fibrosis) or functional (neurogenic bladder). Wide fluctuations in urine volume may be present with partial obstruction.

- Pathogenesis of obstructive uropathy: early vasoconstriction followed by vasodilatation.
- Obstruction: anatomical or functional.

The most useful clinical test is renal ultrasonography. However, 2% of these studies are false negative (usually because of early obstruction or possible retroperitoneal fibrosis). Up to 26% of ultrasonograms are false positive. A combination of renal ultrasonography and abdominal computed tomography (CT) without contrast media is 100% diagnostic for obstruction and can pinpoint the cause of obstruction in 84% of cases. Urinalysis results are usually normal in obstructive uropathy. Hyperchloremic (normal anion gap) hyperkalemic metabolic acidosis is often a clue to obstruction.

- Renal ultrasonography: 2% of studies are false negative and as many as 26% are false positive.
- Ultrasonography plus CT (no contrast agent): 100% diagnostic, can pinpoint the cause in 84% of cases.
- Hyperkalemic metabolic acidosis: often a clue to obstruction.

Treatment

Always irrigate and change urinary catheters in evaluating obstructive uropathy. If the obstruction is relieved, replace two-thirds of the postobstructive diuresis volume. According to animal studies, treatment instituted within 1 week produces

50% recovery of the glomerular filtration rate; treatment in 2 weeks results in 30% recovery, and treatment after 8 weeks produces little, if any, recovery.

PRERENAL FAILURE

Prerenal failure is defined as a rapidly reversible cause of renal insufficiency due to renal hypoperfusion. It accounts for at least 50% of cases of acute renal failure in hospitalized patients. The urine sediment is benign (hyaline and granular casts). Urinary indices of oliguria are helpful in distinguishing prerenal from renal failure. These diagnostic indices are listed in Table 16-1. It is important in treatment to correct the underlying disorder if known and to replace fluids if hypovolemic.

- Prerenal failure: rapidly reversible renal insufficiency due to renal hypoperfusion.
- Urinary indices of oliguria help to distinguish between prerenal and renal failure.

The fractional excretion of sodium is the most helpful urinary index to distinguish prerenal oliguria from oliguria due to acute intrinsic renal failure. It is an index of the quantity of sodium excreted divided by the quantity of sodium filtered times 100. Normally, this value is less than 1%; it is also less than 1% in prerenal insufficiency. Patients with tubular dysfunction have more than 3% of the sodium filtered eventually excreted. There are some causes of acute *intrinsic* renal failure associated with a low fractional excretion of sodium. All these causes have a decrease in renal blood flow. They include renal failure due to nonsteroidal anti-inflammatory drugs (NSAIDs), angiotensin-converting enzyme (ACE) inhibitors, radiocontrast media, hemoglobinuria or myoglobinuria, early obstruction, acute glomerulonephritis, and hepatorenal failure.

HEPATORENAL SYNDROME

Hepatorenal syndrome is a severe state of prerenal hypoperfusion that occurs in 40% to 50% of patients with terminal cirrhosis. It usually occurs in the presence of jaundice, ascites, and stigmata of portal hypertension. This syndrome usually develops in the hospital, triggered by diuretics, gastrointestinal tract bleeding, or paracentesis. Hyponatremia, hypokalemia, and hypoalbuminemia commonly accompany the syndrome. The pathogenesis of this disorder is accompanied by severe vasoconstriction. Endothelin levels are ten times higher than normal. Laboratory findings include urinary sodium less than 10 mOsm/L, urinary osmolality greater than 500 mOsm/L, and only a transient response to fluids. A transition to acute tubular necrosis is possible, and recovery is only about 10%. Treatment includes liver transplantation, LaVeen shunt, dopamine, and high doses of spironolactone (Aldactone). Other causes of renal failure associated with liver disease include amyloidosis, leptospirosis, methoxyflurane, vasculitis, and acute Wilson disease.

- Hepatorenal syndrome: severe state of prerenal hypoperfusion.
- Occurs in 40%-50% of patients with terminal cirrhosis.
- Hyponatremia, hypokalemia, and hypoalbuminemia are common.
- Urinary sodium is <10 mOsm/L and urinary osmolality is >500 mOsm/L.
- 10% of patients recover.
- Pathogenesis: accompanied by severe vasoconstriction.
- Endothelin levels are 10x normal.

ACUTE INTRINSIC RENAL FAILURE

Acute Tubular Necrosis

Most patients (60%) with acute tubular necrosis are not oliguric and have a better prognosis than oliguric patients (40%). The mean incidence of acute tubular necrosis in hospitals is about 5%. It occurs in 50% of patients undergoing emergency abdominal aortic aneurysm repairs, in 10% of those undergoing elective abdominal aortic aneurysm repairs, and in 20% of patients undergoing heart operations or operations related to trauma. The pathogenesis of acute tubular necrosis is usually due to ischemia, which may occur without hypotension, as in 50% of postoperative cases. Acute tubular necrosis has more than one cause in 70% of patients. Important toxins that can cause tubular damage include endogenous toxins (calcium, uric acid, hemoglobinuria, and myoglobinuria) and exogenous toxins (antibiotics, contrast dye, chemotherapeutic agents, cyclosporin A, and acyclovir).

- Acute tubular necrosis: 60% of patients are not oliguric and 40% are.
- It occurs in 50% of emergency abdominal aortic aneurysm repairs.
- Pathogenesis: usually is ischemia.

Table 16-1.—Diagnostic Indices of Oliguria

	Prerenal	Acute tubular necrosis
Urine osmolality, mOsm/L	≥500	≤350
Urine/plasma creatinine ratio	≥40	≤20
BUN/plasma creatinine ratio	>20	<15
Fractional excretion of sodium	<1%	>3%

Ischemia affects the kidney similar to the way it affects the myocardium. We often think of ischemia being a continuum in the myocardium, going from angina to subendocardial infarction to true transmural infarction. Ischemia can affect the kidney by initially inducing prerenal insufficiency, followed by acute tubular necrosis, and then cortical necrosis. Studies have demonstrated that the redistribution of blood flow, medullary ischemia, backleak of filtrate through damaged tubules, intrarenal obstruction by necrotized tubule casts, and glomerular filter damage all have a role in acute tubular necrosis. Sublethal ischemia leads to a loss of tubular cell polarity and, therefore, lack of transport. Free radicals of oxygen and high intracellular concentrations of calcium also promote tubule cell injury.

Urinalysis often demonstrates cellular debris, tubular epithelial cell casts, granular casts, and a "muddy brown" appearance. Erythrocyte casts are associated with acute glomerular nephritis and not with acute tubular necrosis. Also, leukocyte casts, leukocytes, and eosinophils accompany acute interstitial nephritis and not acute tubular necrosis.

A stepwise approach to immediate treatment of acute renal failure is outlined in Table 16-2.

Urine alkalinization is helpful in acute tubular necrosis induced by uric acid, myoglobin, or methotrexate.

The typical course of acute renal failure includes an oliguric phase, which lasts 1 to 2 weeks but not usually longer than 4 weeks. If the oliguric phase lasts longer than 4 weeks, biopsy should be considered to look for causes of acute renal failure other than acute tubular necrosis. The diuretic phase is characterized by increases in urine flow that are not necessarily associated with improvement in creatinine levels early in the disease. Late in the disease, improvement in the creatinine level occurs as the glomerular filtration rate begins to increase. It is during this phase that severe hypercalcemia can occur in rhabdomyolysis-induced renal failure. The third and final phase is the recovery phase of intrinsic renal failure. During this phase, glomerular filtration rate improves over a period of 3 to 12 months. In general, the condition of 60% of patients stabilizes, with reduced glomerular filtration rate, especially if the patients have been oliguric for longer than 16 days. Complications of acute renal failure include infection, which is the most common cause of death and occurs in 50% to 90% of patients. It is important to note that fever may be absent and that a careful search for pulmonary and urinary tract infections, abscesses, and other sources of infection must be completed. Other complications include gastrointestinal tract bleeding, hypervolemia with congestive heart failure, hyperkalemia, hyponatremia, metabolic acidosis, and uremia.

Management of acute renal failure includes allowing 0.5 lb loss/day for catabolism. Restricting fluid and sodium, in addition to a 100-g carbohydrate diet with limitations of potassium, magnesium, phosphate, and protein, is also recommended. Treatment with thiazide diuretics, magnesium-containing antacids, and NSAIDs must stop, and contrast agents must be avoided if possible. It is also important to adjust drug doses, especially of digoxin, antibiotics, antihypertensive agents, and benzodiazepines. Phosphate binders are also helpful in patients taking oral nutrition. Although patients have low serum levels of calcium, this is rarely treated.

Dialysis can be performed with hemodialysis, continuous hemofiltration, or peritoneal dialysis. It is best to anticipate the patient's course and to maintain the predialysis BUN less than 100. Other indications include extracellular fluid volume excess, hyperkalemia, severe acidosis, pericarditis, and the need to make space for parenteral nutrition. Dialysis is often necessary daily in hypercatabolic patients.

Patients with aminoglycoside-induced renal failure are often nonoliguric. The renal failure occurs only after 5 to 7 days of therapy and correlates with the cumulative dose received. Aminoglycosides are freely filtered and absorbed partially in the proximal tubule: the more amino groups on the aminoglycoside, the more toxic the agent (streptomycin is more toxic than gentamicin, which is as toxic as tobramycin). Magnesium and potassium wasting from tubular dysfunction are common accompaniments. Regular measurement of serum creatinine concentrations is the best way to detect nephrotoxicity. Animal studies have suggested that single daily dosing reduces aminoglycoside nephrotoxicity.

Table 16-2.—Stepwise Approach to Immediate Treatment of Acute Renal Failure

1. Exclude postrenal and prerenal causes. Try a volume challenge if indicated.
2. Discontinue use of all nephrotoxic agents.
3. Treat with mannitol (12.5-25 g i.v.) and/or furosemide (20 mg i.v.); 25 g of mannitol increases plasma volume 250 mL. Do not exceed total dose of 50 g in renal failure (mannitol intoxication with hyponatremia, extracellular fluid overload).
4. No response (<60 mL/hr), treat with furosemide (400-500 mg i.v.).
5. Response (>60 mL/hr), 20% mannitol (i.v. infusion; no more than 100 g/24 hr) and furosemide (200 mg) to keep urine output >60 mL/hr. Replace urine 1:1.
6. Other—avoid high doses of furosemide, ethacrynic acid (ototoxicity); use dopamine (2-5 μg).

- Aminoglycoside-induced renal failure: often nonoliguric.
- Occurs after 5-7 days of therapy.

Acute renal dysfunction due to amphotericin B occurs after a 2- to 3-g dose of treatment and is rare if the dose is less than 600 mg. It is also associated with distal tubular dysfunction. Patients also develop nephrogenic diabetes insipidus and a type IV renal tubular acidosis. Some evidence suggests that alkalinizing the urine may be beneficial in these patients. Administering amphotericin B in liposomes may decrease its nephrotoxicity.

- Volume depletion is a principal risk factor.
- Amphotericin B-induced renal failure: occurs with a 2-3-g dose but rarely if the dose is <600 mg.

Up to 30% of the patients receiving cisplatin develop renal failure if the cumulative dose is 50 to 75 mg/m^2. Renal failure can be avoided with adequate hydration and forced diuresis; it is associated with hypomagnesemia and hypokalemia.

- Cisplatin-induced renal failure: occurs in 30% of patients receiving 50-75 mg/m^2.

Methotrexate is a dose-related (>50 mg/kg) cause of renal failure. It precipitates in the renal tubules, as do acyclovir and some sulfa compounds (treatment with an alkaline diuresis has been helpful).

- Methotrexate-induced renal failure: dose related.
- Methotrexate precipitates in the renal tubules.

Contrast dye-induced nephropathy is likely due to vasoconstriction, obstruction, and direct tubular toxicity of contrast agents. Its incidence is probably less than previously believed, but patients who are at risk can be identified, including those with severe renal insufficiency alone or diabetic patients with mild renal insufficiency. Patients who receive multiple exposures to contrast agent are at increased risk, as are those who receive high doses of contrast agent. The acute renal failure that accompanies radiocontrast dye toxicity is often associated with a low fractional excretion of sodium. The patients usually become oliguric 24 to 48 hours after exposure, with dense nephrotomograms on radiography; this reverses within 7 days. Low osmolar, low ionic contrast agents cause less allergic reactions and may be helpful in selected patients. Other measures include prevention by normal saline-induced

diuresis and decreasing the dose of contrast agent. There is some investigational evidence that calcium channel blockers and atrial natriuretic factor may be helpful in preventing acute contrast-induced nephropathy. Spacing contrast studies for several days is also an important preventive measure. Contrast agents can be removed by dialysis, but this generally is not clinically beneficial.

- Contrast dye-induced renal failure: due to vasoconstriction, obstruction, and direct tubular toxicity.
- Patients at risk: patients with severe renal insufficiency and patients with diabetes and mild renal insufficiency.
- Prevention: hydration, forced diuresis, low dose of contrast agent.

Heme pigments (Table 16-3) induce renal failure by intrarenal vasoconstriction and obstruction. Rhabdomyolysis can be due to traumatic causes (crush, seizures, alcoholic coma, and ischemia) and to nontraumatic causes (cocaine, clofibrate, lovastatin, heat stroke, sickle cell trait, carbon monoxide poisoning, spider bite, and polydermatomyositis). Hypocalcemia, frequently severe, can often accompany the acute syndrome, followed by severe hypercalcemia in the diuretic phase of recovering renal failure. Treatment includes forced diuresis and urine alkalinization, with careful attention to the patient's serum levels of calcium and potassium.

- Heme pigment-induced renal failure: due to intrarenal vasoconstriction and obstruction.
- Hypocalcemia can occur in acute phase and hypercalcemia in diuretic phase.

NSAIDs may cause reversible acute renal failure due to intense intrarenal vasoconstriction. Renal blood flow depends on prostaglandins in the setting of extracellular fluid volume contraction (especially with heart failure, cirrhosis, nephrotic syndrome, and chronic renal failure). Inhibition of prostaglandin synthesis results in acute renal failure. NSAIDs also may be associated with hyperkalemia, hyponatremia, aggravation of hypertension, acute interstitial nephritis, and acute nephrotic syndrome.

ACE inhibitors cause acute renal failure in the setting of preexisting decreased renal blood flow due to large or small vessel renal disease. The renal failure is reversed after discontinuation

Table 16-3.—Heme Pigments

	Serum color	Haptoglobin	CPK	Heme dipstick	Urine benzidine
Hemoglobin	Red	Decreased	Normal	+	-
Myoglobin	Clear	Normal	Increased	+	+

of treatment with the ACE inhibitor. Hyperkalemia may also occur.

Cyclosporine induces reversible intrarenal vasoconstriction and aggravates hypertension. This is best treated with a calcium channel blocker. Chronic cyclosporine nephrotoxicity has been associated with hyperkalemia, hyperuricemia, and hyperchloremic metabolic acidosis. Chronic interstitial fibrosis develops in some patients.

Acute renal failure may occur in 25% to 35% of patients infected with the human immunodeficiency virus (HIV). Opportunistic infections of the kidney may occur. Hypovolemia due to diarrhea may cause prerenal insufficiency. High doses of acyclovir and sulfa antibiotics may cause intrarenal obstructive renal failure. Rifampin and sulfa compound may cause acute interstitial nephritis. Pentamidine and amphotericin B have been associated with hyperkalemic metabolic acidosis and acute tubular necrosis. Foscarnet may cause acute renal failure and nephrogenic diabetes insipidus. Aggressive hydration minimizes renal injury.

Acute Renovascular Disease

Atheroembolic-induced renal failure is an increasingly recognized cause of renal failure. It generally occurs in older patients, either spontaneously or after an invasive procedure. The patients often have livedo reticularis of the extremities and emboli seen on funduscopic examination. Laboratory studies can demonstrate a high erythrocyte sedimentation rate, low level of complement, eosinophilia, eosinophiluria, and thrombocytopenia. Although contrast nephropathy is usually reversible, patients with atheroembolic-induced renal failure often have minimal reversibility. Renal biopsy specimens demonstrate cholesterol emboli in medium-sized arteries, with intense tubulointerstitial nephritis. The only treatment is to correct the source of the embolization, looking for atrial fibrillation, cardiac valve disease, endocarditis, etc. Anticoagulation may actually aggravate the tendency for embolization.

- Atheroembolic-induced renal failure: generally in older patients.
- Findings: high erythrocyte sedimentation rate, low levels of complement, eosinophilia, eosinophiluria.

DISORDERS OF WATER BALANCE

The most important principle in understanding disorders of water balance is that the serum level of sodium is the clinical index of total body water. The serum sodium level is not an index of total body sodium. Total body sodium can be determined only by physical examination. The serum sodium level is a useful clinical index to evaluate water balance, not sodium balance, disorders. Water balance is regulated by thirst, antidiuretic hormone, and renal medullary concentration of water.

- Total body sodium can be determined only by physical examination.
- Water balance is regulated by thirst, antidiuretic hormone, and renal medullary concentration of water.

Hyponatremia

Hyponatremia is the most common electrolyte abnormality in hospitalized patients. Its symptoms are protean, including lethargy, cramps, decreased deep tendon reflexes, and seizures. The diagnosis and management of hyponatremia are shown in Figure 16-1.

- Hyponatremia: the most common electrolyte abnormality in hospitalized patients.

Diagnosis

The first step in evaluating patients with hyponatremia is to measure serum osmolality. Isosmotic hyponatremia may be due to severe hypertriglyceridemia (>1,500, lipemia retinalis is always present), severe hyperproteinemia (>8.0, Waldenström macroglobulinemia, myeloma), or isotonic infusions of glucose, mannitol, or glycine. Hyperosmotic hyponatremia may be due to severe hyperglycemia (sodium decreases 1.6 for each 100 mg/dL increase in glucose) and to hypertonic infusions of glucose, mannitol, or glycine.

The second step is to assess the extracellular fluid volume of the hyposmotic hyponatremic patient and to determine whether he or she is hypovolemic, euvolemic, or hypervolemic. 1) Hyposmotic *hypovolemic* hyponatremia: check urine osmolality and sodium concentration; common causes are thiazides and adrenal insufficiency. 2) Hyposmotic *hypervolemic* hyponatremia: check urine osmolality and sodium concentration; edematous states and renal failure are common. 3) Hypotonic *euvolemic* hyponatremia: check cortisol level, thyroid, urine osmolality, hypothyroidism, Addison disease, reset osmostat, and psychogenic polydipsia.

The syndrome of inappropriate secretion of antidiuretic hormone is a diagnosis of exclusion. Patients must meet the following criteria: 1) hypotonic plasma, 2) urine less than maximally dilute (<100 mOsm/kg), 3) urine sodium matches intake, 4) absence of hypoadrenocorticism and hypothyroidism, and 5) improvement with water restriction. An important clinical hint is the presence of a low serum level of uric acid. BUN also tends to be low.

Acute hyponatremia has been described in several special clinical settings. Hyponatremia may occur in up to 5% of patients after surgery and anesthesia. Plasma vasopressin concentrations are increased because of nonosmolar stimuli. Rarely, profound hyponatremia may occur. During transurethral prostatic resection, isotonic or hypotonic fluids containing glycine, mannitol, or sorbitol can be absorbed and depress the serum level of sodium. Schizophrenic patients with severe compulsive water drinking occasionally have acute hyponatremia. Also, infusions of oxytocin during infusions of cyclophosphamide may induce acute hyponatremia.

Chronic hyponatremia may be induced by the use of thiazides, chlorpropamide, carbamazepine, and NSAIDs.

- The physical examination, osmolality of plasma and urine, and urine sodium concentration provide important information for diagnosis.
- Syndrome of inappropriate secretion of antidiuretic hormone: serum level of uric acid and BUN are low.

Patients with acute hyponatremia in the presence of neurologic symptoms generally respond to infusion of isotonic saline and a loop diuretic. Water intake should be restricted. The use of hypertonic saline and loop diuretics may be necessary in patients with severe clinical hyponatremia and should

be monitored in an intensive care unit. In symptomatic patients with acute hyponatremia, the serum level of sodium should be increased no faster than 1 to 1.5 mEq/L per hour to 100 or 125 mEq/dL. Generally, hyponatremia should be reversed cautiously at a rate similar to that at which it developed to avoid central pontine myelinolysis. In patients with chronic syndrome of inappropriate secretion of antidiuretic hormone, demeclocycline may be of benefit. Increasing protein intake also facilitates water excretion.

Hypernatremia

As in hyponatremia, the symptoms of hypernatremia are often protean, with irritability, hyperreflexia, ataxia, and seizures. All forms of hypernatremia are associated with hypertonicity, so there is no pseudohypernatremia. Cases are categorized as hypovolemic, hypervolemic, and euvolemic hypernatremia. The diagnosis and management of hypernatremia are shown in Figure 16-2.

- Hypovolemic hypernatremia: check urine sodium; may be caused by osmotic diuresis, excessive sweating, and diarrhea.

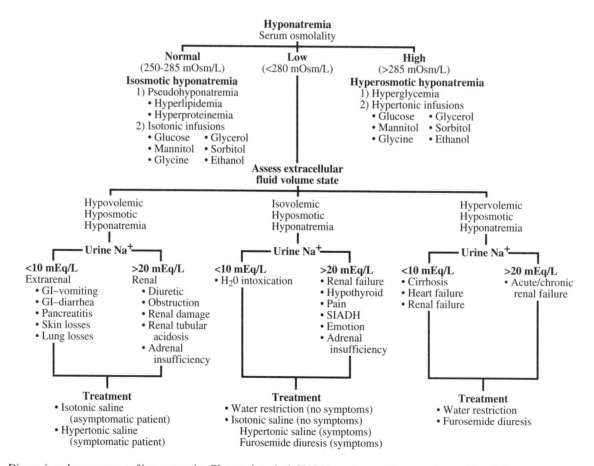

Fig. 16-1. Diagnosis and management of hyponatremia. GI, gastrointestinal; SIADH, syndrome of inappropriate antidiuretic hormone.

- Hypervolemic hypernatremia: may be caused by sodium poisoning.
- Euvolemic hypernatremia: loss of water; extrarenal (skin, lung) versus renal; diabetes insipidus, central versus nephrogenic water deprivation test.

Patients with hypovolemic hypernatremia often respond to saline followed by hypotonic solution. Patients with hypervolemic hypernatremia respond to diuretics and may or may not need dialysis. Euvolemic patients should receive free water, either orally or intravenously, to correct the serum level of sodium, generally no faster than 0.5 mEq/hr.

DISORDERS OF SODIUM BALANCE

Disorders of sodium balance can be determined only by clinical examination. Orthostatism implies volume depletion and sodium deficiency. Edema implies volume excess and sodium excess.

DISORDERS OF POTASSIUM BALANCE

Potassium is predominantly an intracellular cation. Total body potassium is approximately equal to 4,200 mEq, with only 60 mEq in the total extracellular fluid volume. Gastric fluid contains 5 to 10 mEq of potassium/L, and diarrheal fluid contains 10 to 100 mEq/L. The internal balance of potassium is regulated by endogenous factors such as acidemia, sodium, potassium, ATPase, insulin, catecholamines, and aldosterone. The external balance is regulated primarily by potassium excretion, which in large part is regulated by urinary flow rate, aldosterone, antidiuretic hormone, and sodium delivery to the distal tubule.

Hypokalemia

Symptoms of hypokalemia include weakness, ileus, polyuria, and, sometimes, rhabdomyolysis. Hypokalemia also aggravates digoxin toxicity. A stepwise approach to the diagnosis of hypokalemia is given in Table 16-4 and outlined in Figure 16-3.

- Hypokalemia symptoms: weakness, ileus, and polyuria.

Therapy—If the serum level of potassium is less than 2 mEq/L, the total potassium deficit is equal to 1,000 mEq; if the serum level of potassium is between 2 and 4 mEq/L, then a decrease of 0.3 is equivalent to a 100 to 500 mEq deficit, usually potassium chloride (diabetic ketoacidosis, potassium phosphate; potassium citrate, severe acidosis). Do not exceed 10 mEq/hr i.v. unless using a central catheter and ECG monitoring. Dietary sodium restriction decreases potassium-losing effects of diuretics.

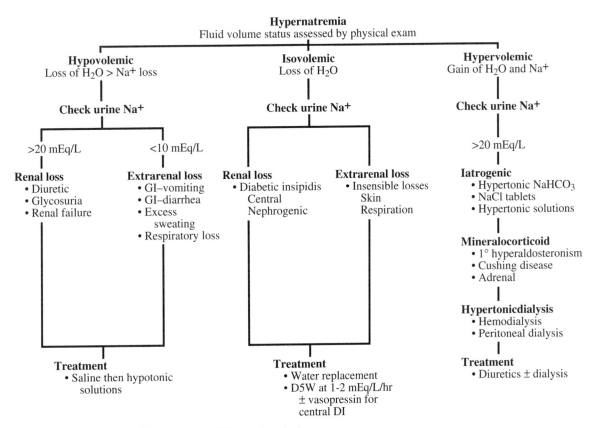

Fig. 16-2. Diagnosis and management of hypernatremia. GI, gastrointestinal.

Table 16-4.—Stepwise Approach to Diagnosis of Hypokalemia

1. Exclude redistribution—β-agonists (albuterol and terbutaline for asthma and ritodrine for labor), acute alkalosis, vitamin B_{12} therapy for pernicious anemia (especially if thrombocytopenic), barium carbonate
2. Determine whether potassium losses are renal or extrarenal—check urine potassium level on high sodium diet, is potassium > or < 20 mEq/day
3. If loss is extrarenal, determine cause (laxative screen)—usually diarrhea, enemas, laxative abuse, villous adenomas, ureterocolostomy
4. If loss is renal, determine if hypertensive or normotensive (diuretic screen)
5. If hypertensive, check plasma renin and aldosterone levels, includes primary aldosteronism or hyperplasia (glycyrrhizic acid in licorice, chewing tobacco), adrenal abnormalities
6. If normotensive, check plasma HCO_3 levels and urine chloride, includes renal tubular acidosis, vomiting, diuretic abuse, Bartter syndrome, magnesium deficiency

Hyperkalemia

A stepwise approach to the diagnosis of hyperkalemia is given in Table 16-5 and outlined in Figure 16-4.

Therapy—Antagonize the membrane effects and redistribute (treat with calcium, then sodium bicarbonate, then insulin, then resins, and finally dialysis). For chronic therapy, use loop diuretics, sodium bicarbonate, resins, fludrocortisone, or dialysis.

ACID-BASE DISORDERS

Clinically, it is absolutely critical that a stepwise approach to acid-base disorders be followed. The six steps listed in Table 16-6 should always be followed before interpreting an acid-base disorder.

Metabolic Acidosis

Metabolic acidosis is defined as a primary disturbance in which retention of acid consumes endogenous alkali stores. This is reflected by a decrease in HCO_3. The secondary response is increased ventilation with a decrease in Pco_2. Metabolic acidosis can be caused by overproduction of endogenous acid (e.g., diabetic ketoacidosis), loss of alkali stores (diarrhea, renal tubular acidosis), or failure of renal acid secretion or base resynthesis (renal failure).

- Metabolic acidosis: primary disturbance is retention of acid.
- Secondary response: increased ventilation with Pco_2.

Some of the signs and symptoms of metabolic acidosis include fatigue, dyspnea, abdominal pain, vomiting, Kussmaul respiration, myocardial depression, hyperkalemia, leukemoid

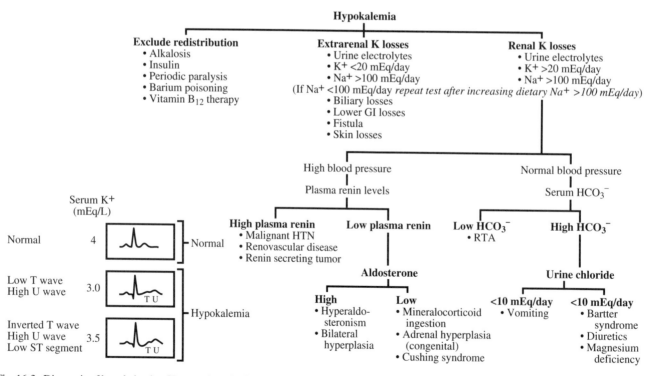

Fig. 16-3. Diagnosis of hypokalemia. GI, gastrointestinal; HTN, hypertension; RTA, renal tubular acidosis.

Table 16-5.—Stepwise Approach to Diagnosis of Hyperkalemia

1. Exclude pseudohyperkalemia—ECG is normal,
   heparinized plasma potassium is normal
   Hemolysis of clotted blood (0.3 increase), tourniquet
   ischemia, severe leukocytosis or thrombocytosis
2. Determine cause based on redistribution or excess total
   body potassium (see Fig. 16-4)

reaction, insulin resistance, and, when pH is less than 7.2, arteriolar dilatation and hypotension.

Some formulas for the predicted compensation for pure metabolic acidosis (which will take up to 24 hours) are 1) Pco_2 = last two digits of the pH, 2) Pco_2 decreases by 1 to 1.3 mm Hg for each mEq/L decrease in HCO_3, and 3) $Pco_2 \pm 2 = 1.5$ (HCO_3) + 8 (this is the best formula).

The metabolic acidoses are classified as either normal anion gap or high anion gap. Normal anion gap metabolic acidosis is defined in terms of serum levels of potassium.

Hypokalemic normal anion gap metabolic acidosis can be associated with diarrhea, ureteral diversion, or the use of carbonic anhydrase inhibitors such as acetazolamide. Renal tubular acidosis type I, or classic renal tubular acidosis, is also a cause. This is associated with nephrocalcinosis and osteomalacia. The causes of type I renal tubular acidosis include toluene sniffing, amphotericin B, lithium, Sjögren syndrome, hypergammaglobulinemia, and sickle cell disease. Type II renal tubular acidosis is also a hypokalemic anion gap metabolic acidosis. In adults, it is often associated with other proximal tubule defects, including glycosuria, uricosuria, phosphaturia, and aminoaciduria (Fanconi syndrome). Causes of type II renal tubular acidosis include myeloma, cystinosis (not cystinuria), lead, tetracycline, and acetazolamide.

The causes of hyperkalemic normal anion gap metabolic acidosis include acid loads such as NH_4Cl, arginine chloride, lysine chloride, cholestyramine, total parenteral nutrition, HCl, oral $CaCl_2$, obstructive uropathy, hypoaldosteronism (Addison disease), 21-hydroxylase deficiency, sulfur toxicity, and type IV renal tubular acidosis. Type IV renal tubular acidosis is associated with hyporenin and hypoaldosteronism, and it may be caused by diabetes mellitus, interstitial nephritis, spironolactone, amiloride, triamterene, or cyclosporin A.

High anion gap metabolic acidosis is due to several causes. In chronic renal failure, the anion gap is usually less than 25. If anion gaps are greater than 25, one should immediately think of an ingestion of a poison. Isopropyl alcohol increases the osmolar gap but not the anion gap (acetone is not an anion).

- In chronic renal failure, the anion gap usually is <25.
- A gap >25 should suggest ingestion of a poison.

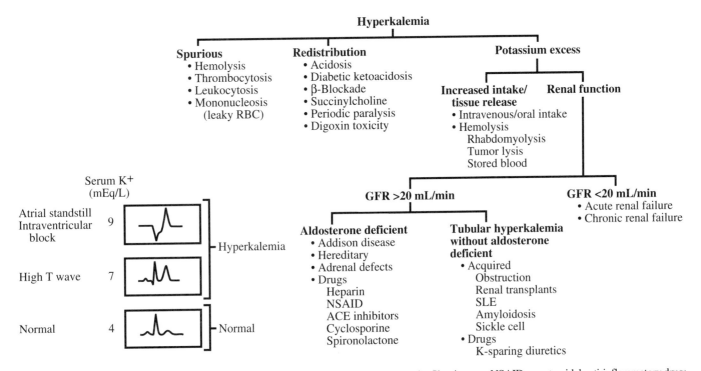

Fig. 16-4. Diagnosis of hyperkalemia. ACE, angiotensin-converting enzyme; GFR, glomerular filtration rate; NSAID, nonsteroidal anti-inflammatory drug; RBC, red blood cell; SLE, systemic lupus erythematosus.

Table 16-6.—Six Steps for Interpreting Acid-Base Disorder

1. Note the clinical presentation
2. Always check the anion (hidden acidosis) and osmolar gaps if possible
    Normal anion gap Na - (HCO$_3$ + Cl) = 8 to 12
        Cations = Na, gammaglobulins, Ca, Mg, K
        Anions = Cl, HCO$_3$, albumin, PO$_4$, SO$_4$, organic
    High anion gap >12—K-U-S-S-M-A-U-L
    Low anion gap <8—bromism, paraproteinemia, hypercalcemia/magnesemia, lithium toxicity, severe hypernatremia, severe hypoalbuminemia
    Osmolar gap >10-OLS—methanol, ethanol, ethylene glycol, isopropyl alcohol, mannitol
3. Use the Henderson equation to check the validity of the arterial blood gases values:

$$H^+ \ (nEq/L) = \frac{24 \times Lungs \ (P_{CO_2})}{Kidneys \ (HCO_3)}$$

pH	7.00	7.10	7.20	7.30	7.40	7.50	7.60	7.70
H$^+$	100	79	63	50	40	32	25	20

4. Is the pH high or low?
5. Is the primary disturbance metabolic (HCO$_3$) or respiratory (P$_{CO_2}$)?
6. Is it simple or mixed?

Metabolic acidosis is generally corrected by treating the underlying disorder, but the bicarbonate deficit can be determined by the following formula:
    Bicarbonate deficit = 0.2 x body weight (kg) x (normal HCO$_3$ [i.e., 24] - measured HCO$_3$)

Metabolic Alkalosis

Metabolic alkalosis is defined as a primary disturbance in which plasma bicarbonate is increased. This can be caused by 1) endogenous alkali, 2) acid loss through the gastrointestinal tract or kidney, or 3) loss of nonbicarbonate fluid causing contraction of the remaining fluid around unchanged total body bicarbonate. The kidney must also be stimulated to sustain the high level of plasma bicarbonate. This can occur by 1) extracellular fluid volume contraction, 2) hypercapnia, 3) potassium depletion, 4) steroid excess, 5) hypercalcemia, or 6) hypoparathyroidism. The secondary response is decreased ventilation with an increase in P$_{CO_2}$. The signs and symptoms of metabolic alkalosis include weakness, muscle cramps, hyperreflexia, alveolar hypoventilation, and dysrhythmias.

- Metabolic alkalosis: primary disturbance is increased plasma bicarbonate.
- The kidney must be stimulated to sustain the high level of plasma bicarbonate.
- Secondary response: decreased ventilation with increased P$_{CO_2}$.

The predicted compensation for pure renal metabolic alkalosis (which will take up to 24 hours) can be calculated by using the following formulas:
1. P$_{CO_2}$ ± 5 = 0.9(HCO$_3$) + 15
2. P$_{CO_2}$ increases 6 mm Hg for each 10 mEq/L increase in HCO$_3$

Metabolic alkalosis can be classified in terms of the spot urine chloride.

Mixed Acid-Base Disorders

- HCO$_3$ <15 usually is caused partly by a metabolic acidosis.
- HCO$_3$ >45 usually is caused partly by a metabolic alkalosis.
- Arterial blood gas values may be normal, but a high anion gap indicates a mixed metabolic alkalosis/acidosis.
- In metabolic acidosis and respiratory alkalosis, the P$_{CO_2}$ is lower than predicted for the acidosis.
- In metabolic alkalosis and respiratory acidosis, the HCO$_3$ is higher than predicted for acidosis.
- In mixed metabolic and respiratory alkalosis, HCO$_3$ is higher and P$_{CO_2}$ is lower than expected.
- Triple disorders: diabetic/alcoholic (vomiting) + (keto/lactic acidosis) + (sepsis or liver disease).

CLINICAL MANIFESTATIONS OF GLOMERULAR INJURY

The glomerular basement membrane is an important size barrier (MW, 70,000) and negative charge barrier, repulsing albumin and immune globulins. There is also tubular reabsorption of protein in the range of 500 to 1,500 mg/24 hr by the proximal tubule.

Orthostatic proteinuria is usually benign and remits spontaneously. The diagnosis can be made by obtaining two 12-hour urine collections for protein: one supine and one upright. Significant proteinuria is defined as more than 75 mg/12 hr. Tubulointerstitial disease is sometimes associated with proteinuria, but it is usually less than 1,500 mg/day. Overflow low molecular weight proteinuria is due to increased light chain or lysozyme excretion without nephrosis.

Renal biopsy is indicated to determine the prognosis and diagnosis of patients with greater than 2 g/day non-nephrotic-range proteinuria if it is associated with an abnormal sediment or renal insufficiency. Other indications for biopsy include nephrotic-range proteinuria, microscopic hematuria with abnormal urine sediment or renal function, progressive renal insufficiency, and acute renal failure lasting for longer than 3 to 4 weeks. Patients with an atypical course of diabetes mellitus and undiagnosed systemic diseases, which include the differential diagnosis of amyloidosis, systemic lupus erythematosus, and polyarteritis nodosa, should undergo biopsy. Renal biopsy is contraindicated in bleeding disorders, uncontrolled hypertension, urinary tract infections, solitary kidneys other than allografts, and uncooperative patients. Complications include microscopic hematuria, gross hematuria (10%-20%), need for nephrectomy, biopsy of other tissue, and death (0.001%).

- Renal biopsy: to determine the prognosis and diagnosis of patients with >2 g/day non-nephrotic-range proteinuria.
- Other indications: nephrotic-range proteinuria, microscopic hematuria, progressive renal insufficiency, acute renal failure lasting >3-4 weeks, atypical course of diabetes mellitus, and undiagnosed systemic disease.
- Contraindications: bleeding disorders, uncontrolled hypertension, urinary tract infections, solitary kidneys other than allografts, and uncooperative patients.

Nephrotic Syndrome

Nephrotic syndrome is defined by the presence of urinary protein greater than 3.5 g/1.73 m^2 per day, hypoalbuminemia (<3.0 g/dL), peripheral edema, and hypercholesterolemia (total >200 mg/dL). Urinalysis demonstrates waxy casts, free fat, oval fat bodies, and lipiduria. Other associations include hypogammaglobulinemia (increases infection risk), vitamin D deficiency due to loss of vitamin D-binding protein, and iron deficiency anemia due to hypotransferrinemia. Renal vein thrombosis may occur because of an increased thromboembolic tendency (increased factor V, VIII, fibrinogen, platelets and decreased antithrombin III and antiplasmin). Management includes controlling blood pressure and limiting sodium and lipid intake.

- Nephrotic syndrome: urinary protein >3.5 g/1.73 m^2 daily.
- Hypoalbuminemia, <3 g/dL.
- Peripheral edema.
- Hypercholesterolemia, total >200 mg/dL.

Nephritic Syndrome

Nephritic syndrome is characterized by the presence of erythrocyte casts with variable amounts of proteinuria. Because of methemoglobin formation in acid urine, it has a "Coca-Cola" or smokey appearance.

- Nephritic syndrome: erythrocyte casts with variable amounts

of proteinuria.
- Urine: "Coca-Cola" or smokey appearance.

GLOMERULAR DISEASE WITH ACUTE REVERSIBLE RENAL FAILURE

Poststreptococcal Glomerulonephritis

Poststreptococcal glomerulonephritis is usually caused by group A β-hemolytic streptococcal infections. The latent period is 6 to 21 days (type 12 pharyngeal infection) or 14 to 28 days (type 49 skin infection). The urine sediment is active, with usually less than 3 g proteinuria/24 hr and a fractional excretion of sodium less than 1%. Because of activation of the alternative complement pathway, total and C3 complements are low but only up to 8 weeks. Antistreptolysin-O is present in pharyngeal infections and anti-DNase B in skin infections. In renal biopsy specimens, light microscopy demonstrates many polymorphonuclear neutrophils, with proliferation and subepithelial deposits or humps. Immunofluorescence demonstrates a granular "lumpy-bumpy" pattern with IgG and C3. Treatment is supportive alone, with control of blood pressure and edema. Penicillin therapy for the patient and contacts may prevent new cases. The course and prognosis are excellent in children and adults unless crescents or persistent proteinuria is present.

- Poststreptococcal glomerulonephritis: usually due to group A β-hemolytic streptococcal infections.
- Urine sediment: active, <3 g proteinuria/24 hr and fractional excretion of sodium is <1%.
- Total and C3 complements are low.
- Immunofluorescence: granular "lumpy-bumpy" pattern with IgG and C3.

Other forms of postinfectious glomerulonephritis include bacterial endocarditis and infected ventriculoatrial shunts.

CRESCENTIC GLOMERULAR DISEASE WITH PROGRESSIVE RENAL FAILURE

Rapidly progressive glomerulonephritis is defined as an acute (days to weeks to months) deterioration of renal function associated with active urinary sediment and crescentic glomerulonephritis (Fig. 16-5). Usually, adults (mean age, 55 years) are affected. The pulmonary-renal syndrome is frequent, and oliguria is not uncommon. On light microscopy, there is fibrinoid necrosis and more than 50% crescents. Immunofluorescence demonstrates three patterns: type I, linear IgG (Goodpasture syndrome or anti-GBM mediated); type II, granular immune complexes (D-penicillamine); and type III, negative immunofluorescence. Treatment of rapidly progressive glomerulonephritis: pulse methylprednisolone sodium succinate (SoluMedrol), 1 g for 3 days, with or without cytotoxic agents. Plasmapheresis is helpful in Goodpasture syndrome by removing the anti-GBM antibody. The antibody is directed against the α-3 chain of type IV collagen. Prognosis—35% of patients develop end-stage renal disease, with 25% mortality, and 40% progress to chronic renal insufficiency. Oliguria, a high creatinine level (>7), and old age are poor prognostic signs.

- Rapidly progressive glomerulonephritis: subacute deterioration of renal function.
- Crescentic glomerulonephritis.
- Pulmonary-renal syndrome is common; oliguria is not uncommon.
- 25% mortality.
- 40% progress to chronic renal insufficiency.

GLOMERULAR DISEASE WITH HEMATURIA AND VARIABLE PROTEINURIA AND FUNCTION

IgA Nephropathy

IgA nephropathy is the most common glomerulopathy worldwide. Patients present with synpharyngitic hematuria (microscopic with or without macroscopic hematuria), often with erythrocyte casts. Urine sediment activity may be exacerbated by an upper respiratory tract infection. Pathogenesis may be due partly to exaggerated IgA mucosal production. Secondary causes include advanced chronic liver disease, sprue, dermatitis herpetiformis, and ankylosing spondylitis. Poor prognostic signs are heavy proteinuria, hypertension, and renal insufficiency. Plasma IgA is increased in only 50% of the patients. Skin biopsy for IgA is not helpful. Renal biopsy in IgA demonstrates mesangial proliferation on light microscopy. The immunofluorescence studies are diagnostic and demonstrate IgA within the mesangium. The prognosis is generally good for IgA nephropathy; however, 20% of patients may reach end-stage renal disease in 20 years. Progression to end-stage renal disease in those patients at high risk has been shown to be slowed by administration of fish oil capsules containing omega-3 fatty acids. This disorder often recurs in renal transplant recipients but often is not clinically significant. Poor prognostic signs are diminished renal function, heavy proteinuria, and hypertension.

- IgA nephropathy: most common glomerulopathy worldwide.

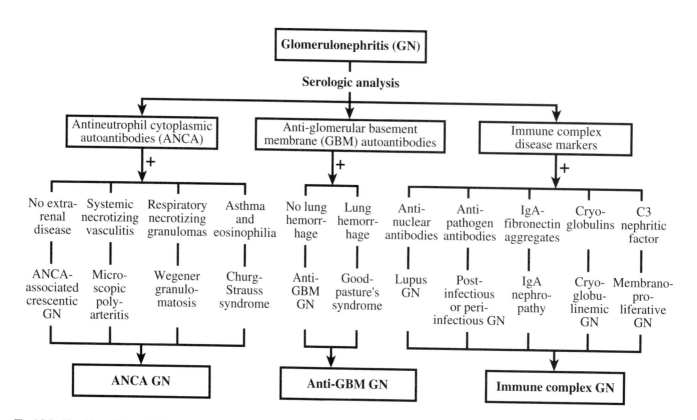

Fig. 16-5. Algorithm of the serologic and pathologic categorization of rapidly progressive (crescentic) glomerulonephritis. (From MKSAP in the Subspecialty of Nephrology and Hypertension. Book 1 Syllabus and Questions, 1994. American College of Physicians. By permission.)

- Presents with synpharyngitic hematuria, often with erythrocyte casts.
- Pathogenesis: exaggerated IgA mucosal production or regulation.
- Secondary causes: advanced chronic liver disease, sprue, dermatitis herpetiformis, ankylosing spondylitis.
- Plasma IgA increased in only 50% of patients.
- Prognosis: generally good.

Schönlein-Henoch Purpura

Patients with Schönlein-Henoch purpura present with microscopic and/or macrohematuria along with erythrocyte casts, purpura, and abdominal pain. Renal biopsy findings are similar to those of IgA nephropathy with or without vasculitis. The prognosis generally is good for children and variable for adults. Treatment is supportive only.

Membranoproliferative Glomerulonephritis

Patients with membranoproliferative glomerulonephritis present with nephrotic syndrome (50% of patients), non-nephrotic-range proteinuria (30%), or nephritic sediment (20%). Complement values are persistently low (>8 weeks). Anti-streptolysin-O may be present, and a C3 nephritic factor is present in many cases. It is an autoantibody to alternative pathway C3 convertase, resulting in persistent C3 breakdown. Secondary causes include chronic infections, "shunt nephritis," malaria, hepatitis B, systemic lupus erythematosus, congenital complement deficiency (C2, C3), mixed cryoglobulinemia, sickle cell disease, partial lipodystrophy (only type II), and α_1-antitrypsin deficiency. The two idiopathic forms are type I and type II (dense-deposit disease).

- Membranoproliferative glomerulonephritis: presents with nephrotic syndrome in 50% of patients, non-nephrotic range proteinuria in 30%, and nephritic sediment in 20%.
- Complements are persistently low.
- C3 nephritic factor is often present.
- Secondary causes: chronic infections, "shunt nephritis," hepatitis B, systemic lupus erythematosus, and sickle cell disease.

In biopsy samples of membranoproliferative glomerulonephritis, light microscopy demonstrates duplication or splitting, tramtracking, or double contouring of the glomerular basement membrane. This proliferation within the glomerulus and capillary loop thickening result in a lobular appearance of the glomeruli. Immunofluorescence demonstrates complex deposition in the mesangium and capillary walls. Electron microscopy demonstrates a distinctive ribboning or sausaging of dense material in type II membranoproliferative glomerulonephritis. Generally, adults receive supportive care; steroids have been helpful in some children. Dipyridamole (225 mg/day) and aspirin (975 mg/day) have been used to slow the progression of adult membranoproliferative glomerulonephritis. The prognosis is worse with hypertension, poor renal function, and heavy proteinuria. This disorder tends to recur in transplants (type I, 30%; type II, 90%).

- Prognosis: worse with hypertension, poor renal function, heavy proteinuria.

GLOMERULAR DISEASE WITH HEAVY PROTEINURIA AND VARIABLE RENAL FAILURE

Minimal Change Nephropathy

Patients with minimal change nephropathy present with abrupt nephrotic syndrome with normal renal function (exceptions, hypovolemia and NSAIDs). This is the number one cause of nephrotic syndrome in children and the cause of 20% of adult cases of idiopathic nephrotic syndrome. Pathogenesis may be due to an attack on the glomerular epithelial cells by T-cell lymphokines, resulting in fusion of the foot processes. The heparan sulfate basement membrane negative charge barrier is lost. Secondary causes include Hodgkin disease and NSAIDs (with interstitial nephritis). Light microscopic and immunofluorescence findings on renal biopsy specimens in minimal change nephropathy are normal. Electron microscopy shows fusion of the foot processes. A relapsing course is common (60% of patients). Patients are generally responsive, and 90% have complete remission within 4 weeks. Generally, therapy is continued for 4 weeks after remission. Although 80% of adults respond to steroid therapy, 60% have repeated relapses. Cyclophosphamide can prolong remission and may decrease steroid dependence after 8 weeks of therapy; 50% of these patients have prolonged remissions. If patients are unresponsive, another biopsy is indicated to exclude focal segmental glomerulosclerosis.

- Minimal change nephropathy: abrupt nephrotic syndrome with normal renal function.
- Number one cause of nephrotic syndrome in children and cause of 20% of adult cases of idiopathic nephrotic syndrome.
- Secondary causes: Hodgkin disease and NSAIDs (with interstitial nephritis).
- 80% of adults respond to steroid therapy; 60% have repeated relapses.

Focal Glomerular Sclerosis

Focal glomerular sclerosis accounts for 10% of cases of adult nephrotic syndrome. Mean age at disease onset is 21 years. Patients present with hypertension, renal insufficiency, proteinuria, and gross or microscopic hematuria. Secondary causes include HIV infection (more frequent in drug abusers than in homosexuals), heroin abuse, reflux nephropathy, and massive obesity. Light microscopic results of renal biopsy samples demonstrate focal and segmental sclerosis without proliferation. Foam cells are often seen. Immunofluorescence shows IgM and C3 and deposits within the mesangium. Electron microscopy demonstrates fusion of foot processes in all glomeruli. Generally, therapy is supportive, although some patients may respond to a 4- to 6-month course of corticosteroid treatment. Cyclosporine may also have a role in treating these patients. ACE inhibitors decrease heavy proteinuria independent of their effect on lowering blood pressure. In selected patients with heavy proteinuria, meclofenamate has also decreased complications due to proteinuria. This disorder can recur in renal transplant recipients, and its prognosis is poor if proteinuria is greater than 10 g/day.

HIV nephropathy is characterized by progressive renal insufficiency in patients with heavy proteinuria but often little edema. Large echogenic kidneys are seen on ultrasonography, and renal biopsy demonstrates focal and segmental glomerulosclerosis and glomerular collapse. Visceral epithelial cell swelling in the glomeruli is also present.

This predominates in intravenous drug-using HIV-infected patients. Some patients have had considerable improvement after the administration of corticosteroids.

Four other types of glomerulonephritis are seen frequently in HIV-infected patients. These include post-infectious glomerulonephritis, HIV-associated IgA nephropathy, membranoproliferative glomerulonephritis, and membranous nephropathy. Also, some patients with HIV develop a hemolytic-uremic/thrombotic thrombocytopenic purpura syndrome. Antiretroviral therapy, treatment of underlying infection, and plasmapheresis in hemolytic-uremic/thrombotic thrombocytopenic purpura may be of benefit therapeutically. It is also important to recognize the renal toxic effects of antimicrobial and antiviral therapy in HIV-infected patients.

- Focal glomerular sclerosis: 10% of cases of adult nephrotic syndrome.
- Mean age is 21 years.
- Presents with hypertension, renal insufficiency, proteinuria, and gross or microscopic hematuria.
- Secondary causes: HIV infection, heroin abuse, reflux nephropathy, massive obesity.
- Steroid therapy: <10% of patients respond.
- Prognosis is poor if proteinuria is >10 g/day.

Membranous Glomerulopathy

Membranous glomerulopathy is the primary cause of idiopathic nephrotic syndrome in adults (50% of patients).

Mean age at disease onset is 35 years. However, 25% of the patients do not have nephrotic-range proteinuria. Patients are often hypertensive (40%), with some renal insufficiency. Pathogenesis is due to in situ deposition of cationic antigens in the subepithelial space. Renal vein thrombosis (25%-50%) in some cases may cause sudden loss of renal function. Secondary causes include infections (hepatitis B, quartan malaria, syphilis), multisystem disease (systemic lupus erythematosus, Sjögren syndrome, sarcoidosis), and neoplasms (1.5% of cases, including carcinoma [lung, colon, stomach, breast] and lymphoma). Malignancies occur at five times the expected rate in adults with membranous nephropathy. Medications that cause membranous glomerulopathy are gold, D-penicillamine, captopril, probenecid, and some NSAIDs. Hereditary and metabolic causes include sickle cell disease. Renal biopsy demonstrates "spike and dome" epithelial deposits, with thickened capillary loops seen on light microscopy. Granular IgG and C3 are seen on immunofluorescence. Therapy for membranous nephropathy is generally supportive, although 8 weeks of alternate-day steroids are often recommended. ACE inhibitors are often efficacious in decreasing the degree of proteinuria. Other measures include the necessity to control hypertension and to treat any underlying disorders. Corticosteroids with or without cyclophosphamide (Cytoxan) may have a role in treatment of heavy proteinuria and worsening renal insufficiency. Without treatment, nearly 25% of the patients have spontaneous complete remission and 50% have partial remission. Approximately 20% of these patients progress to end-stage renal disease; the prognosis is related to the degree of proteinuria.

- Membranous glomerulopathy: primary cause of idiopathic nephrotic syndrome in adults.
- Mean age is 35 years.
- Pathogenesis: in situ deposition of cationic antigens in the subepithelial space.
- Renal vein thrombosis causes sudden loss of renal function in 25%-50% of patients.
- Secondary causes: infections, multisystem disease, neoplasms, and medications.
- Complete remission in 25% of patients and partial remission in 50%.

OTHER GLOMERULAR DISORDERS

Diabetes Mellitus

From 2% to 4% of U.S. citizens have diabetes mellitus. Diabetic nephropathy occurs in both insulin-dependent (30%-40%) and noninsulin-dependent (20%-30%) diabetics. More than 30% of patients hospitalized with end-stage renal disease have diabetic nephropathy, the single most common cause of end-stage renal disease in the U.S. Pathogenesis is secondary to glycosylation, renal hemodynamic changes, and hypertension. Microalbuminuria is the primary predictor of renal disease. The stages of diabetic nephropathy are listed in Table 16-7.

- Diabetic nephropathy occurs in insulin-dependent (30%-40%) and noninsulin-dependent (20%-30%) diabetics.
- Diabetes mellitus is the single most common cause of end-stage renal disease in the U.S.
- Microalbuminuria is the primary predictor of renal disease.

Renal biopsy of diabetic involvement of the kidney demonstrates a nodular and diffuse glomerular scarring or sclerosis. Capsular drop lesions and fibrin cap lesions are also pathognomonic. There is thickening of all basement membranes, with arteriolar hyalinosis and arteriosclerosis. Interstitial fibrosis and tubular atrophy may also be present. Other manifestations of diabetic urinary tract disease include papillary necrosis, perinephric abscess, acute pyelonephritis, neurogenic bladder and hydronephrosis with functional obstruction, bacteriuria, cystitis, and hypertension. Although tight glucose control by all current means available does not reverse diabetic nephropathy, it does tend to slow development of the disease. It is clear that aggressive control of blood pressure and glycemia definitely slows the progression of diabetic nephropathy. Patients with end-stage renal disease due to diabetes mellitus are kidney transplant candidates. Hemodialysis and continuous ambulatory peritoneal dialysis are also alternatives.

- Other manifestations of diabetic urinary tract disease: papillary necrosis, perinephric abscess, acute pyelonephritis, neurogenic bladder and hydronephrosis with functional obstruction, bacteriuria, cystitis, hypertension.

Table 16-7.—Stages of Diabetic Nephropathy

Stage I	Hyperfiltration, glomerular filtration rate is 20%-50% above normal, microalbuminuria (>300 mg/24 hr)
Stage II	Normalization of glomerular filtration rate with early structural damage
Stage III	Early hypertension
Stage IV	Progression to proteinuria >0.5 g/day, hypertension, declining glomerular filtration rate (lasts 10-15 years)
Stage V	Progression to end-stage renal disease (5-7 years), heavy proteinuria persists even to end-stage disease

Although tight glycemic control by all means available does not reverse diabetic nephropathy, it has been shown to delay the onset and progression of microalbuminuria. Tight glycemic control has not been shown to be effective in diabetic renal disease when overt nephropathy is present.

ACE inhibitors slow the progression from microalbuminuria to overt proteinuria in both insulin-dependent and noninsulin-dependent diabetic patients. They also have been shown to decrease the degree of microalbuminuria or proteinuria when present and to decrease the increasing level of creatinine, therefore slowing the progression from overt nephropathy to end-stage renal disease. Non-dihydropyridine calcium channel blockers (e.g., diltiazem) may have a similar effect. Dietary protein restriction (0.8 g/kg per day) may be beneficial in slowing progressive symptoms from renal disease in patients with moderate renal insufficiency.

In early insulin-dependent and noninsulin-dependent diabetics, maintenance of optimal glycemic control is recommended in addition to annual screening for microalbuminuria. Blood pressure should be treated aggressively with ACE inhibitors and non-dihydropyridine calcium channel blockers. Insulin-dependent diabetics who develop microalbuminuria should start ACE inhibitor therapy even if they are normotensive. In insulin- and noninsulin-dependent diabetics with overt proteinuria (>500 mg/day), blood pressure control and dietary protein restriction may be of benefit, but glycemic control does not limit the progression of diabetic renal disease. In patients whose condition is advancing to end-stage renal disease, kidney or kidney-pancreas transplantation should be considered when the creatinine level reaches 4 mg/dL.

Aldose reductase inhibitors and nonenzymatic glycosylation inhibitors may also be beneficial in slowing progressive renal insufficiency.

- Aggressive control of blood pressure and glycemia slows progression.
- Diabetes mellitus is the most common cause of type IV renal tubular acidosis.
- Patients with noninsulin-dependent diabetes mellitus also benefit from aggressive blood sugar and blood pressure control.

Lupus Erythematosus

Of patients with lupus erythematosus, 50% have renal disease at presentation and 90% have renal disease at some time. If renal involvement occurs with lupus, it usually presents early in the course of the disease. The presenting histologic renal lesion is fairly stable except that a focal proliferative lesion progresses to diffuse proliferative lesion in 20% of patients. An active diffuse proliferative lesion is treatable with steroids with or without cytotoxic agents. Membranous systemic lupus erythematosus usually is not treatable with immunosuppressive agents. Kidney biopsy is indicated for active urinary sediment with or without decreased glomerular function to define the renal lesion in lupus erythematosus. The five classes of renal disease that may be present are listed in Table 16-8.

- Lupus erythematosus: 50% of patients present with renal disease and 90% have renal disease some time during the course of lupus erythematosus.
- Active diffuse proliferative lesion is treatable with steroids with or without cytotoxic agents.
- Membranous systemic lupus erythematosus usually is not treatable with immunosuppressive agents.

Other manifestations of lupus include acute and chronic tubulointerstitial nephritis and vasculitis. Chronic changes include glomerular scarring, tubular atrophy, and interstitial fibrosis, all of which are untreatable. Therapy for lupus nephritis is often limited to treatment of proliferative nephritis. Patients with acute proliferative nephritis and acute renal failure should receive high doses of steroids with or without cytotoxic agents. Diffuse proliferative glomerulonephritis without azotemia is also treated with high doses of steroids for 6 to 8 weeks. Cyclophosphamide can be added to the therapy if necessary. Aside from proteinuria, membranous lupus involvement often is characterized by weakly positive or negative antinuclear antibody without red cell casts. Generally, therapy is supportive only. It is important to remember that drug-induced lupus rarely involves the kidney. Pregnancy should be delayed until after lupus is inactive for 6 months; 25% to 45% of lupus patients have exacerbations usually 8 weeks after delivery. Lupus "burns out" with end-stage renal disease and generally does not recur in transplant recipients.

- Drug-induced lupus rarely involves the kidney.
- Pregnancy should be delayed until after lupus is inactive for 6 months.

- Lupus "burns out" with end-stage renal disease and generally does not occur in transplant recipients.

Vasculitis

The types of vasculitis are listed in Table 16-9.

Microscopic polyarteritis nodosa presents with hypertension, weight loss, arthralgias, myalgias, mononeuritis multiplex, epididymitis, subcutaneous nodules, gastrointestinal tract bleeding, active urine sediment, and proteinuria. Anemia, azotemia, normal levels of complement, perinuclear ANCA (antimyeloperoxidase antibodies), and erythrocyte sedimentation rate greater than 100 mm/hr are common. Renal biopsy and not angiography is best to determine diagnosis in patients with abnormal urinalysis. Light microscopy of biopsy sample demonstrates a segmental necrotizing glomerulonephritis with or without crescents. Renal granulomas are rarely seen in Wegener granulomatosis. Prednisone with a slow taper over 6 to 12 months is often prescribed for therapy. Dialysis-dependent patients have regained renal function after treatment. Remissions are common but vasculitis may recur. Patients with Wegener granulomatosis often have positive cytoplasmic ANCA (antiproteinase 3 antibodies) and respond to steroids and cyclophosphamide (Cytoxan) given orally.

- Microscopic polyarteritis nodosa: presentation includes hypertension, weight loss, arthralgias, myalgias, mononeuritis multiplex, epididymitis, subcutaneous nodules, gastrointestinal tract bleeding, active urine sediment, proteinuria.
- Common features: anemia, azotemia, normal levels of complement, perinuclear ANCA, erythrocyte sedimentation rate >100 mm/hr.
- Renal biopsy and not angiography is best for determining diagnosis.

Table 16-8.—Five Classes of Renal Diseases Present With Lupus

Class I	Normal
Class II	Mild mesangial change (no clinical findings of renal disease in 50% of patients)
Class III	Focal and segmental proliferative glomerulonephritis (20% nephritic with or without nephrotic syndrome)
Class IV	Diffuse proliferative glomerulonephritis (70% nephritic with or without nephrotic syndrome), "wire loop"
Class V	Membranous glomerulonephritis (nephrotic but not active sediment)

Table 16-9.—Types of Vasculitis

Microscopic polyarteritis nodosa—overlap (most common form of vasculitis) (p-ANCA)
Wegener granulomatosis (c-ANCA)
Classic polyarteritis nodosa
Allergic granulomatosis (Churg-Strauss syndrome)
Hypersensitivity vasculitis
Essential mixed cryoglobulinemia
Rheumatoid arthritis, systemic lupus erythematosus-associated vasculitis
Giant cell arteritis (no renal involvement?)

MONOCLONAL GAMMOPATHIES

Amyloidosis (primary, AL; secondary, AA), multiple myeloma, light chain nephropathy, and fibrillary and immunotactoid nephropathy are renal manifestations of monoclonal gammopathies. Renal manifestations include proteinuria (λ light chains: amyloid; κ light chains: light chain nephropathy; λ and κ light chains: myeloma), nephrotic syndrome, hematuria, nephritic syndrome, acute renal failure, and tubulointerstitial disease. Patients may also have renal manifestations of myeloma, including normal- or large-sized kidneys, pseudohyponatremia, low anion gap, hypercalcemia, Fanconi syndrome (low phosphorus, urate, potassium; glycosuria; aminoaciduria; type II and renal tubular acidosis), and Bence Jones proteinuria.

Renal biopsy—The diagnostic stains for amyloid are Congo red, thioflavin T, and methyl violet. Light chain nephropathy demonstrates κ light chain deposition, and the nodular glomerulosclerosis often mimics diabetes mellitus. Immunofluorescence generally demonstrates λ light chains in amyloid and κ light chains in light chain nephropathy. Electron microscopy is helpful in further differentiating the type of light chain fibrils. Renal biopsy findings correlate poorly with the clinical course and renal function in patients with monoclonal gammopathies. Treatment is often supportive, but melphalan and prednisone have had some beneficial effect in selected patients. In secondary causes of this disorder, it is necessary to treat the underlying disorder. Colchicine is helpful in the treatment of familial Mediterranean fever.

CRYOGLOBULINEMIAS

Patients with cryoglobulinemia often present with palpable purpura and are either nephritic or nephrotic (Table 16-10). Acute renal failure can occur if the cryocrit is greater than 1 g/dL. Renal biopsy demonstrates characteristic fibrin thrombi within glomeruli. Prednisone, cytotoxic agents, and plasmapheresis are used with variable results in cryoglobulinemia.

HEMOLYTIC UREMIC SYNDROME AND THROMBOCYTOPENIC PURPURA

Patients present with severe hypertension, proteinuria, active sediment, and renal failure. Both hemolytic uremic syndrome and thrombocytopenic purpura are associated with a microhemangiopathic hemolytic anemia and thrombocytopenia. Endothelial cell injury and subendothelial deposits are present on biopsy, "endotheliosis." The glomerular lesion is also seen in malignant hypertension, scleroderma, and postpartum acute renal failure. Secondary causes include mitomycin C, bleomycin, cyclosporin A, quinine, *E. coli* O157, and radiation. Children with hemolytic uremia syndrome have a good prognosis (90% recover renal function), but adults have a poor prognosis. Thrombocytopenic purpura includes fever, neurologic signs, and purpura in addition to the above. Therapy is plasma infusion and plasmapheresis with or without antiplatelet therapy and corticosteroids. For scleroderma, therapy is limited to treating hypertension with ACE inhibitors.

- Presentation: severe hypertension, proteinuria, active sediment, renal failure.
- Associated with: microhemangiopathic hemolytic anemia and thrombocytopenia.
- Glomerular lesion also seen in malignant hypertension, scleroderma, postpartum acute renal failure.
- Therapy: plasma infusion plus plasmapheresis with or without antiplatelet therapy/corticosteroids.

ALPORT SYNDROME AND THIN GLOMERULAR BASEMENT MEMBRANE DISEASE—DISEASES WITH GLOMERULAR BASEMENT MEMBRANE ABNORMALITIES

Patients present with hematuria, proteinuria, and nephrosis (end-stage renal disease by age 16 to 30 years). High-frequency hearing loss and ocular abnormalities (anterior lenticonus and cataracts) are present. Inheritance is X-linked

Table 16-10.—Cryoglobulins and Associated Diseases

Cryoglobulin type		Ig class	Associated disease
I	monoclonal immunoglobulins	M>G>A>BJP	Myeloma, Waldenström macroglobulinemia
II	mixed cryoglobulins with monoclonal immunoglobulins	M/G>>G/G	Sjögren syndrome, Waldenström macroglobulinemia, lymphoma
			Essential cryoglobulinemia
III	mixed polyclonal immunoglobulins	M/G	Infection, systemic lupus erythematosus, vasculitis, neoplasia
			Essential cryoglobulinemia

dominant (males have a worse prognosis). Transplant recipients may develop anti-GBM-mediated renal disease. In Alport syndrome, the lack of the domain of noncollagenous type IV collagen and the absence of Goodpasture antigen mean that anti-GBM antibodies cannot be bound.

In thin glomerular basement membrane disease, the glomerular basement membrane is 200 nm thick. Patients present with hematuria.

CLINICAL MANIFESTATIONS OF TUBULOINTERSTITIAL RENAL DISEASE

Acute and chronic interstitial disease preferentially involves renal tubules. Some of the patterns of renal tubular injury are 1) tubular proteinuria, less than 1.5-2 g/day; 2) proximal tubule dysfunction (hypokalemia, hypouricemia, hypophosphatemia, acidosis, glycosuria, aminoaciduria); 3) distal tubule dysfunction (hyperchloremic acidosis, hyperkalemia or hypokalemia, salt wasting); 4) medullary concentration dysfunction, nephrogenic diabetes insipidus with decreased urine-concentrating ability; 5) urine sediment (pyuria, leukocyte casts, eosinophiluria, hematuria); and 6) azotemia, renal insufficiency.

- Tubular proteinuria, <1.5-2 g/day.
- Proximal tubule dysfunction and distal tubule dysfunction.
- Medullary concentration dysfunction.

ACUTE INTERSTITIAL NEPHRITIS

Patients with acute interstitial nephritis present with fever of mean onset of 15 days (90% of patients), pyuria (100%), hematuria (95%), proteinuria (75%), renal insufficiency (60%), eosinophilia (50%), arthralgias (25%), and rash (25%). Diagnosis sometimes requires renal biopsy. Gallium or indium scans can also be helpful.

- Acute interstitial nephritis: 100% have pyuria; 90%, fever; 60%, renal insufficiency; 50%, eosinophilia; and 25%, arthralgias.

Drug-induced acute interstitial nephritis can be due to several agents:

1. Antibiotics—penicillin, methicillin (anti-tubular basement membrane antibodies), ampicillin, rifampin, sulfa drugs, ciprofloxacin, pentamidine
2. NSAIDs—interstitial nephritis with nephrotic syndrome and renal insufficiency may have a latent period, not dose-dependent, recurs, possibly T-cell mediated, allergic signs and symptoms are absent
3. Diuretics—thiazides, furosemide, bumetanide (sulfa derivatives)
4. Cimetidine
5. Allopurinol, phenytoin, phenindione—exfoliative dermatitis, hepatitis, and acute interstitial nephritis
6. Cyclosporin A—acute renal vasoconstriction

Treatment is to discontinue use of the drug and possibly to prescribe a short course of prednisone (60 mg every other day) for 2 to 4 weeks.

- Methicillin (anti-tubular basement membrane antibodies).
- NSAIDs: interstitial nephritis with nephrotic syndrome and renal insufficiency.
- Sulfa derivatives.
- Cimetidine.

Acute interstitial nephritis can be caused by infection (streptococcosis, leptospirosis, Rocky Mountain spotted fever, legionnaire disease, Epstein-Barr virus, cytomegalovirus), lymphoma, leukemic infiltration, lupus, renal transplant rejection, toxic radiation, and acute pyelonephritis.

ANALGESIC CHRONIC INTERSTITIAL NEPHRITIS

Analgesic nephropathy is a good example of chronic interstitial nephritis and is responsible for 20% of the cases of tubulointerstitial nephritis, with 3% to 10% of patients entering end-stage renal disease. Patients have a chronic pain problem. Other features include arthritis and muscular aches, female (85% of patients), anemia (85%), headache (80%), history of peptic ulcer (40%), hypertension (40%), urinary tract infection with history of dysuria (25%), history of obstruction (10%), and premature aging. Patients generally do not admit to analgesic abuse. Findings include sterile pyuria, small kidneys (50%), papillary necrosis (30%), and normal excretory urogram (10%).

- Analgesic nephropathy: responsible for 20% of cases of chronic tubulointerstitial nephritis (3%-10% have end-stage renal disease).
- Chronic pain problem, headache (80%), arthritis and muscular aches, female (80%), history of peptic ulcer (40%).
- Patients generally do not admit to analgesic abuse.
- Findings: sterile pyuria, small kidneys (50%), papillary necrosis (30%), and normal excretory urogram (10%).

Phenacetin and its metabolites are concentrated in the renal papillae. Renal hydroperoxidases react with these metabolites and produce reactive intermediates that damage the papilla by lipid peroxidation. Aspirin diminishes local renal blood flow and decreases the concentration of glutathione, which normally inactivates phenacetin metabolites. The result is papillary ischemia and eventually necrosis. The amount necessary to cause analgesic nephropathy: total intake of 3 kg of phenacetin or 1 g/day for 3 years. Aspirin or acetaminophen alone *does not* cause this disorder but NSAIDs may. Patients with a history of analgesic ingestion may even continue ingestion after kidney transplantation. Multicentric transitional cell carcinomas of the collecting system, although rare, are more common in patients with analgesic nephropathy. Evidence suggests that these patients have accelerated arteriosclerosis.

- Phenacetin and its metabolites are concentrated in the renal papillae.
- Amount necessary to cause analgesic nephropathy: total intake of 3 kg of phenacetin or 1 g/day for 3 years.

Papillary necrosis is a common accompaniment of analgesic nephropathy. Other causes of papillary necrosis can be remembered by the mnemonic P-O-S-T C-A-R-D (pyelonephritis, obstruction, sickle cell disease or trait, tuberculosis, chronic alcoholism with cirrhosis, analgesics, renal vein thrombosis, and diabetes mellitus).

OTHER RENAL DISEASES PRESENTING WITH INTERSTITIAL NEPHRITIS

Other renal diseases presenting with interstitial nephritis are glomerular injury (lupus, mixed cryoglobulinemia, hypertension, diabetes mellitus, Sjögren syndrome, Alport syndrome, myeloma), Balkan nephropathy (as with analgesic nephropathy, increased incidence of uroepithelial cancers), granulomatous nephropathy (tuberculosis, sarcoidosis), and sickle cell trait/disease.

ELECTROLYTE- AND TOXIN-INDUCED INTERSTITIAL NEPHRITIS

Acute uric acid nephropathy is associated with the tumor lysis syndrome after chemotherapy, myeloproliferative disorders, heat stroke, status epilepticus, and Lesch-Nyhan syndrome. In this disorder, intraluminal crystals cause intrarenal obstruction, and serum uric acid is often greater than 15 mg and 24-hour urinary uric acid is greater than 1,000 mg. The spot urinary uric acid divided by spot urinary creatinine is often greater than 1.0. Prevention requires alkaline diuresis, allopurinol, and, sometimes, hemodialysis. Generally, this disorder is completely reversible. Chronic uric acid nephropathy due to saturnine gout (lead from "moonshine" or paint) or chronic tophaceous gout is due to interstitial crystal formation, microtophi present in the renal parenchyma. It has only limited reversibility. Remember that de novo gout in renal failure is rare; in this setting, it should be assumed that the patient has lead nephropathy until proved otherwise.

- Acute uric acid nephropathy associated with tumor lysis syndrome and myeloproliferative disorders.
- Serum uric acid is >15 mg and 24-hour urinary uric acid is >1,000 mg.
- The urine uric acid-to-urine creatinine ratio is >1.
- Prevention: alkaline diuresis and allopurinol.

Early on, hypercalcemia results in mitochondrial deposits of calcium in the proximal and distal tubules as well as in the collecting duct. Later, tubular degeneration with calcium deposition and obstruction occurs. Calcium inhibits sodium transport, induces nephrogenic diabetes insipidus, and causes intrarenal vasoconstriction. It also stimulates the release of renin and catecholamines, producing increased blood pressure.

Hypokalemia has been associated with vascularization of the proximal and distal tubules and possibly chronic interstitial fibrosis. Nephrogenic diabetes insipidus is also associated with chronic hypokalemia.

Oxalate deposition from primary hyperoxaluria causes renal and extrarenal oxalate deposition. Extrarenal sites include the eye, heart, bone, joint, and vascular system. Oxalate deposition from secondary causes can be due to ethylene glycol, methoxyflurane, high doses of ascorbic acid, vitamin B_6 deficiency, and enteric hyperoxaluria.

Lithium induces a nephrogenic diabetes insipidus and microcystic changes in the renal tubules. Interstitial fibrosis may be present.

Heavy metals such as cadmium, pigments, glass, plastic, metal alloys, electrical equipment manufacturing, and some cigarettes induce a proximal renal tubular acidosis and tubulointerstitial nephritis. Lead intoxication can cause lead nephropathy, as mentioned above. The organic salt of mercury can induce chronic tubulointerstitial nephritis and membranous nephritis or acute tubulonecrosis.

CYSTIC RENAL DISEASE

Autosomal-dominant polycystic kidney disease is the cause of renal failure in 10% of all patients who reach end-stage renal failure. It is the most common hereditary renal disease. Chromosome abnormalities found thus far include mutations of the short arm of chromosome 16 and mutations of chromosome 4. Patients with polycystic kidney disease have cysts that grow from birth and are present in all nephron segments. By age 25 years, the cysts are usually seen on ultrasonography or CT. Other cysts can form in the liver (more prevalent in females), spleen, and pancreas. Urinary tract infections are common in polycystic kidney disease and can be localized with CT, gallium or indium scans, or MRI. Lipid-soluble antibiotics tend to penetrate the cysts well. Hematuria may also be seen with hemorrhage into a cyst, a stone, or, sometimes, a malignancy. Uric acid and calcium oxalate stones are common. Other associations with adult autosomal-dominant polycystic kidney include diverticulosis, cardiac valve myxomatous degeneration, and intracranial aneurysms. Also, the hematocrit may be higher than expected because of production of renal erythropoietin.

- Autosomal-dominant polycystic kidney disease: cause of 10% of cases of end-stage renal failure.
- By age 25, cysts usually seen with ultrasonography or CT.
- Other cysts in liver, spleen, and pancreas.
- Other associations: diverticulosis, cardiac valve myxomatous degeneration, intracranial aneurysms, and hypertension.

Medullary sponge kidney is due to dilated collecting ducts, seen on excretory urography, and may be unilateral, bilateral, or involve a single papilla. There is no known pattern of inheritance of this disorder, which is associated with nephrolithiasis and some renotubular abnormalities.

Acquired renal cystic disease can affect up to 50% of long-term dialysis patients and may present with hematuria and an increasing hematocrit. Although these cysts sometimes have neoplastic potential, they rarely metastasize.

UROLITHIASIS

Epidemiology

The prevalence of urolithiasis is about 5% in the U.S. The annual incidence is about 0.1%. Of patients with urolithiasis who are untreated, 30% to 75% have recurrence within 10 years. Urolithiasis is strongly familial and related to diet and urine volume. Many patients have a metabolic disorder that can be demonstrated with further testing, but conservative treatment with diet and increased fluid intake eliminates the stone-forming tendency in 70% of patients. For those in whom conservative therapy fails, medications are curative in another 25% (Fig. 16-6 and 16-7).

- Prevalence of urolithiasis in the U.S.: about 5%.
- It is strongly familial and related to diet and urine volume.

Risk Factors

Urine pH is important in the pathogenesis of some renal stones. Struvite and calcium phosphate stones tend to form in alkaline urine; uric acid and cystine stones form in acid urine. Some anatomical factors predisposing to urolithiasis include medullary sponge kidney, polycystic kidney disease, and chronic obstruction.

- Struvite and calcium phosphate stones form in alkaline urine.
- Uric acid and cystine stones form in acid urine.

An evaluation of patients who have urolithiasis is important to classify the patient's activity. Surgical activity: indicated by hydronephrosis, unrelieved pain, or infection (stones <5 mm should pass). Metabolic activity: formation of new stone or growth of an existing stone within 1 year. *Stones that are not "active" do not justify treatment.* Historic factors include fluid intake, dietary intake, urinary tract infection history, drugs, family history, and other illnesses. Laboratory studies should include reviewing earlier radiographic findings; excretory urography; stone analysis; serum calcium and phosphorus; urinalysis; urine culture; 24-hour urinary volume; calcium, phosphorus, citrate, creatinine, oxalate, potassium sodium, magnesium, uric acid, and cystine analysis with usual diet.

Calcium Stones

About 70% of all renal stones contain calcium. Patients may develop calcium oxalate and calcium phosphate stones or, rarely, pure calcium phosphate stones. Causes include idiopathic hypercalciuria, other hypercalciuric states, hypouricosuria, hyperoxaluria, and reduced inhibitor excretion (see below). Conservative treatment includes correcting dietary stresses and increasing urine volume greater than 2.5 L/day. Medications include neutral sodium phosphate for idiopathic calcium urolithiasis (2 g/day, but not in cases of urinary tract infection or renal insufficiency), thiazides for patients with hypercalciuria (sodium must be restricted for urine calcium to decrease 50%), and allopurinol for patients with hyperuricosuria. Patients with primary hyperparathyroidism and urolithiasis generally should have their parathyroid adenomas resected.

Pure Uric Acid Stones

Patients with uric acid urolithiasis often have normal plasma and urinary uric acid. They often have very acidic urine. Of patients with primary gout, 25% form renal stones. Dietary protein excess also can predispose to uric acid stones, as can any cause of chronic diarrhea because of decreased urine volume and hyperacidity. Uric acid urolithiasis is treated with preventive measures such as increased intake of fluid and decreased protein intake. Alkalinizing the urine to pH 6.5 not only helps prevent uric acid urolithiasis but dissolves renal stones. Although allopurinol is not as effective as alkalinizing very acid urine, it can be helpful in patients with hyperuricosuria.

- Renal stones form in 25% of patients with primary gout.
- Colectomy and ileostomy predispose to stones because of decreased intestinal ureolysis.

Struvite Stones

All patients with magnesium ammonium phosphate stones are infected with urease-producing bacteria, which can include *Proteus*, *Staphylococcus*, *Klebsiella*, and *Pseudomonas* but only rarely *E. coli*. The urine pH of these patients is alkaline, sometimes greater than 7.8. Also, many of the patients have an underlying stone-forming tendency. Staghorn stones are not uncommon, and 50% are bilateral. Treatment includes antibiotics given preoperatively and then surgical removal of all stone material, followed by an attempt to identify the underlying stone-forming tendency, and treatment of this followed by bactericidal antibiotics for 6 to 12 months for suppression.

- All patients with magnesium ammonium phosphate stones are infected with urease-producing bacteria.
- Urine pH is very alkaline.
- 50% of staghorn stones are bilateral.

- Treatment: surgical removal, followed by bactericidal antibiotics for 6-12 months for suppression.

Urolithiasis and Bowel Disease

Hyperoxaluria: patients must have an intact colon to absorb free oxalate. Free oxalate is over-absorbed when free fatty acids complex calcium and magnesium (the usual oxalate complexers). Fatty acids and bile acids also increase the colonic permeability to oxalate. Other factors that increase hyperoxaluria and malabsorption include decreased water absorption, decreased bicarbonate absorption, and decreased absorption of magnesium, phosphate, and pyrophosphate (inhibitors). Treatment of this disorder includes correcting the underlying problem, increasing dietary calcium, decreasing dietary oxalate and fat, considering cholestyramine to bind bile acids, and increasing urine pH and inhibitors.

- Absorption of free oxalate requires an intact colon.

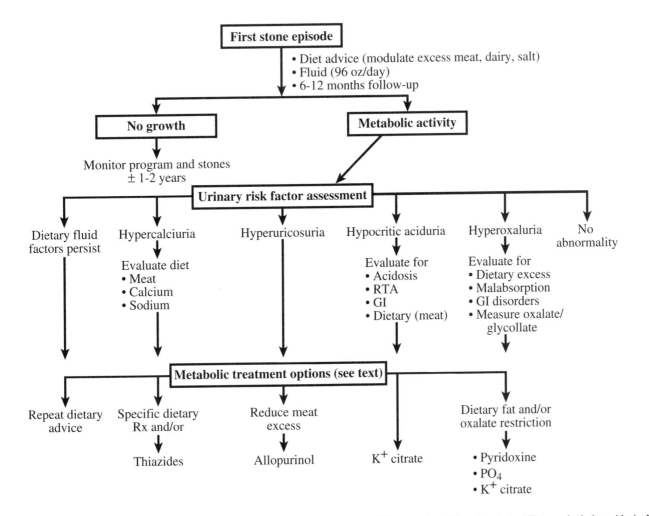

Fig. 16-6. Approach to therapy for idiopathic renal lithiasis. GI, gastrointestinal; K+, potassium; PO4, phosphate; RTA, renal tubular acidosis; Rx, therapy. (From MKSAP in the Subspecialty of Nephrology and Hypertension. Book 1 Syllabus and Questions, 1994. American College of Physicians. By permission.)

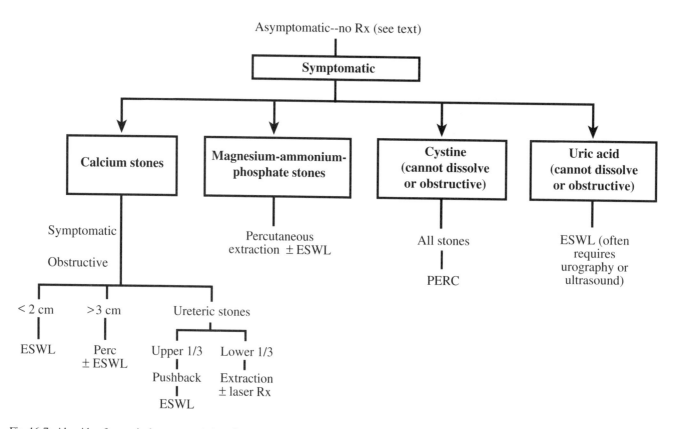

Fig. 16-7. Algorithm for surgical treatment choices for renal stones based on size, location, and type. ESWL, extracorporeal shock-wave lithotripsy; PERC, percutaneous lithotripsy; Rx, therapy. (From MKSAP in the Subspecialty of Nephrology and Hypertension. Book 1 Syllabus and Questions, 1994. American College of Physicians. By permission.)

Patients with bowel disease may also develop uric acid urolithiasis. Ileostomy patients are frequently susceptible to these stones because of the loss of alkali and water. Treatment includes alkali, fluids, and allopurinol.

Renal Tubular Disorders

Renal tubular disorders associated with urolithiasis include distal renal tubular acidosis (type I). These patients can often make pure calcium phosphate stones. They may also have nephrocalcinosis, a urine pH that is always greater than 5.3, and a hyperchloremic hypokalemic normal anion gap acidosis with decreased urinary citrate (a stone inhibitor) and high level of urinary calcium. Treatment is to correct the acidosis with alkali and to monitor urinary citrate excretion.

Cystinuria is an autosomal recessive disorder in which homozygotes develop urolithiasis. Cystine crystalluria in routine urine is diagnostic, as are positive findings on the nitroprusside test. These patients have a defect in the renal and intestinal absorption of cystine, ornithine, lysine, and arginine ("COLA"). The stones can be dissolved with urinary alkalinization, cysteine chelators such as D-penicillamine, and high intake of fluid; however, urinary alkalinization must be very intense, with urine pH maintained above 7.0. Remember

that D-penicillamine can be associated with blood dyscrasias, gastrointestinal tract upset, membranous glomerulopathy, and a Goodpasture-like syndrome. Patients with cystinuria often receive pyridoxine (25 mg/day) when taking D-penicillamine.

Some medications that increase the tendency for stone formation are listed in Table 16-11.

Enzyme Disorders

Several enzyme disorders can be associated with increased stone formation.

Primary hyperoxaluria is the most aggressive stone disease. Type I, glycolic and oxalic aciduria (glyoxylate carboxylase deficiency); type II, L-glyceric and oxalic aciduria (D-glyceric dehydrogenase deficiency). Treatment includes fluids, pyridoxine (alters glycine metabolism, an oxalate precursor), orthophosphates, and liver transplantation.

Xanthinuria, caused by xanthine oxidase deficiency, is characterized by low serum and urinary levels of uric acid. Xanthine stones are radiolucent. Treatment: fluids, alkalinization of urine, and allopurinol.

2,8-Dihydroxyadenuria is caused by deficient adenine phosphoribosyl transferase. The stones resemble urate stones. Treatment is with allopurinol.

Table 16-11.—Medications Increasing the Tendency for Stone Formation

Acetazolamide for glaucoma (calcium phosphate stones)
Calcium carbonate (milk alkali)
Allopurinol (xanthine or oxypurinol stones)
Triamterene
Methoxyflurane (oxalate)
Vitamin D, nonthiazide diuretics, steroids (hypercalciuria)
Chemotherapy (increased urate load)

CHRONIC RENAL FAILURE

Chronic renal failure is defined as a decrease in glomerular filtration rate to less than 25 to 33 mL/min. End-stage renal failure is generally defined as glomerular filtration rate less than 8 to 10 mL/min. Often, patients with chronic renal failure have small kidneys (<10 cm), as seen on KUB with tomograms. The renal size is often preserved in end-stage renal disease in diabetes mellitus, amyloidosis, myeloma, and polycystic kidney disease. Chronic renal insufficiency tends to be progressive because of the persistence of the underlying disorder and possible hyperfiltration by the remaining nephrons. The causes of end-stage renal disease include chronic glomerulonephritis (33% of patients), chronic tubulointerstitial disease (21%), polycystic kidney disease (10%), diabetes mellitus (20%), hypertension (33% blacks, 10% whites), analgesics (5%), familial (5%), and unknown (5%). One should approach chronic renal failure by first excluding any reversible cause such as heart failure, hypertension, infection, hypothyroidism, hypoadrenalism, obstruction, hypercalcemia, medications, and volume loss in salt wasters. After excluding reversible causes, management includes control of blood pressure and early treatment of metabolic acidosis and use of phosphate binders. Late treatment and management include the use of erythropoietin, fluid, sodium, potassium, and protein restrictions; treatment of acidosis; calcium and vitamin D supplements; and use of loop diuretics.

- Chronic renal failure: glomerular filtration rate <25-33 mL/min.
- End-stage renal failure: glomerular filtration rate <8-10 mL/min.
- Small kidneys, <10 cm.
- Kidney size is preserved in diabetes mellitus, amyloidosis, myeloma, and polycystic kidney disease.

UREMIC SIGNS AND SYMPTOMS

Anemia of chronic renal failure is normochromic, normocytic, and multifactorial, that is, decreased erythropoietin production, hemolysis, and blood loss.

The metabolic acidosis of chronic renal failure is first a normal then a high anion gap due to decreased ammonium secretion, followed by retention of phosphates and sulfates. Always check the anion gap in chronic renal failure; it is rarely greater than 25.

Hypertension is common and is associated with extracellular fluid excess and, in some cases, with excess renin production. Multiple agents are often necessary to control hypertension.

Heart failure is common in chronic renal failure. Thus, use caution with digoxin, long-acting calcium channel blockers, and ACE inhibitors.

Pericarditis frequently occurs in two patterns. Pattern I is a hemorrhagic pericarditis that often occurs predialysis and for which dialysis is helpful. Pattern II is sometimes hemorrhagic, occasionally with tamponade, and can occur in well-dialyzed patients. Intrapericardial steroids are often necessary. Pattern II may be due to viral pericarditis.

Hyperkalemia occurs in two patterns. Pattern I is associated with a glomerular filtration rate of less than 20 mL/min and oliguria. Pattern II occurs when the glomerular filtration rate is greater than 20 mL/min and is often associated with type IV renal tubular acidosis due to aldosterone deficiency, particularly in patients with diabetes. Other causes of hyperkalemia include NSAIDs, β-blockers, ACE inhibitors, and potassium-sparing diuretics. Emergent treatment of hyperkalemia includes the use of calcium infusion to protect the myocardium, followed by bicarbonate and then insulin to redistribute the potassium; next, resins and dialysis are used to eliminate potassium.

Bleeding tendency is common in chronic renal failure due to a platelet defect. Thus, use of antiplatelet drugs should be avoided. Treatment with desamino-D-arginine vasopressin is helpful in reversing the bleeding tendency acutely.

Renal osteodystrophy has four components: 1) osteitis fibrosa cystica—hyperparathyroidism, osteoclastic overactivity; 2) osteomalacia due to 1,25-vitamin D deficiency, in which case there is increased osteoid formation within bone; 3) osteoporosis; and 4) growth retardation. Renal disease leads to phosphate retention, which decreases urinary calcium and stimulates parathyroid hormone excretion. Bone is often poorly responsive to parathyroid hormone in chronic renal failure. Also, the 1,25-vitamin D deficiency leads to a vicious cycle of steadily increasing phosphorus and parathyroid hormone. Treatment is to bind phosphorus enterically by giving calcium-containing antacids such as calcium carbonate and calcium acetate to decrease the serum level of phosphorus and to increase calcium. Vitamin D supplements are often necessary. Selected patients who have received aluminum-containing salts for many years become hypercalcemic with low serum levels of parathyroid hormone and 1,25-vitamin D. These patients often have microcytic anemia and frequent fractures and need to have an iliac crest bone biopsy for diagnosis. Aluminum osteodystrophy is treated with deferoxamine chelation.

Endocrine abnormalities in chronic renal failure include low levels of total thyroxine and high levels of growth hormone, luteinizing hormone, and prolactin despite thyroid, adrenal, and pituitary function usually being normal. Hypergastrinemia is present, but peptic ulcer disease is not more common in these patients. Impaired fertility and sexual function and amenorrhea are common. Pregnancy is rare if the creatinine level is greater than 2.0 µg/dL. There is increased resistance to insulin but also decreased insulin degradation associated with an impaired carbohydrate tolerance.

Hyperlipidemia and accelerated atherosclerosis are common. Gastritis, not peptic ulcer disease, is common and usually drug-induced. Constipation is common and aggravated by phosphate binders that contain aluminum. Pseudogout and periarthritis are due to hydroxyapatite deposited in joint spaces.

In peripheral neuropathy of chronic renal failure, sensory fibers are affected more than motor fibers and the lower extremities are involved more than the upper extremities. It is often associated with asterixis and seizures.

DIALYSIS

Indications for dialysis include uremia, pericarditis, neuropathy, hyperkalemia, and intractable metabolic acidosis.

Complications

Hepatitis B—Patients may have mild or no symptoms and may go on to carrier state (also cytomegalovirus, Epstein-Barr virus, hepatitis C, methyldopa, anabolic steroids, azathioprine). Treatment is with vaccine and hepatitis B immune globulin. Hepatitis C is the type of hepatitis that is most common in dialysis patients. Neurologic complications include dialysis disequilibrium (brain edema and osmolar shifts), subdural hematomas, and dialysis dementia (dyspraxia, myoclonus, and gait disturbance due to aluminum overload). Infections: vascular access, peritonitis, tuberculosis (10x the frequency of that in the normal population). Carpal tunnel syndrome and diffuse arthropathy due to β_2 microglobulin amyloid deposition may occur in longer-term dialysis.

Continuous Ambulatory Peritoneal Dialysis

Indications for continuous ambulatory peritoneal dialysis are cardiovascular instability, poor hemodialysis access, and patient preference. Recent abdominal surgery, colostomy, nephrostomy, and adhesions are contraindications. Complications include peritonitis, catheter leak, hyperlipidemia, obesity, hyperglycemia, and protein malnutrition.

Continuous Arteriovenous Hemofiltration or Slow Continuous Ultrafiltration

The indications for these techniques are cardiogenic shock and pulmonary edema, diuretic unresponsive congestive heart failure, and acute renal failure with hemodynamic instability.

Dialysis and Overdoses

Dialysis can be used to treat overdoses of methanol, aspirin, ethylene glycol, lithium, sodium, mannitol, and theophylline. Dialysis is not used for overdoses of tricyclics, benzodiazepines, digoxin, dilantin, and phenothiazines.

Medications in Dialysis

Of the antibiotics, ampicillin and cephalosporins are helpful. **AVOID** using tetracyclines, nitrofurantoin, probenecid, neomycin, bacitracin, methenamine, nalidixic acid, clofibrate, lovastatin, magnesium, oral hypoglycemic agents, and antiplatelet drugs. Be careful when using ACE inhibitors, other potassium-sparing agents, metoclopramide, NSAIDs, acyclovir, long-acting calcium channel blockers, and renal-excreted β-blockers.

TRANSPLANTATION

Transplantation is the treatment of choice for eligible patients with end-stage renal disease. Since the time of the first kidney transplantation (performed in 1954), more than 100,000 of these procedures have been performed; 11,000 are performed annually (8,000 cadaveric and 3,000 living related). More than 35,000 potential recipients are awaiting kidney transplant, and this number increases annually. The main limitation is the limited number of donor kidneys. Lifetime immunosuppression is required. Recipients are from less than 1 year to more than 50 years old. The recipients must not have cancer; infections (e.g., teeth, sinuses, bladder) have to be eradicated, and cholecystectomy for gallstones has to be performed. Living donors must be older than 18 years and without systemic or renal disease. Cadaveric donors must be more than 6 months old and be without infection or malignancy (except for non-metastasizing brain cancer).

- Transplantation is the treatment of choice for eligible patients with end-stage renal disease.
- Lifetime immunosuppression is required.

Recurrent Allograft Renal Disease

Causes of recurrent allograft renal disease include membranoproliferative glomerulonephritis, membranous nephropathy, focal segmental glomerulosclerosis, diabetes mellitus, primary hyperoxaluria, hemolytic-uremic syndrome, and IgA (usually not clinically significant).

Immunosuppression

Agents for immunosuppression include the following (Fig. 16-8): 1) prednisone, which blocks interleukin-1 production by macrophages and cytokine production (complications include cataracts, psychoses, peptic ulcer disease, infection, diverticulitis, aseptic necrosis); 2) azathioprine, which inhibits proliferation of activated T cells (marrow suppression, cholestasis, infection; never treat with allopurinol); 3) cyclosporin A, which inhibits helper T cell activation and interleukin-2, -3, -4, and -5 production; it is hydrophobic and lipophilic, requiring bile acids for absorption.

Cyclosporine levels are increased or decreased by the following agents: increased levels with ketoconazole, cimetidine, ranitidine, verapamil, diltiazem, and erythromycin and decreased levels with phenytoin, phenobarbital, ethambutol, sulfamethoxazole, ethanol, and cholestyramine.

Adverse effects of cyclosporine include gum hyperplasia, hyperkalemia, hypertension, hemolytic-uremic syndrome, and thrombotic thrombocytopenic purpura.

Graft Failure (Chronic Rejection Most Commonly)

Graft failure commonly is due to chronic rejection. Acute tubular necrosis occurs after transplantation in 20% to 50% of patients. The stages of rejection are hyperacute (hours), acute (days to years), and chronic (months-years). Treat only acute stages of rejection. Recurrent disease occurs in 1% of cases. Surgical complications include renal artery stenosis, ureteral obstruction-leak, and lymphocele.

Medical complications—Opportunistic infections are the most common cause of death. *Anything is possible.* Cardiovascular problems are the number two cause. Other complications are hyperlipidemia; cancer (1%, including skin, sarcomas, lymphomas [Epstein-Barr virus-associated], solid tumors); polycythemia; proximal/distal renal tubular acidosis; and kidney stones (1%).

PREGNANCY AND THE KIDNEY

Anatomical changes associated with pregnancy are renal enlargement (1 cm) and dilatation of the calyces, renal pelvis, and ureters. Physiologic changes include 1) a 30% to 50% increase in glomerular filtration rate and renal blood flow; 2) mean creatinine level of 0.5 µg/dL and mean urea of 18 (limits: creatinine, 0.8 and urea, 26); 3) intermittent glycosuria independent of plasma glucose (<1 g/day); 4) proteinuria but less than 300 mg/day (sometimes postural); 5) aminoaciduria less than 2 g/day (most but not all amino acids); 6) increased uric acid excretion; 7) increased total body water (6-8 L) with osmostat resetting; 8) 50% increases in plasma volume and cardiac output; and 9) increased ureteral peristalsis. Bacterial growth in urine is promoted by the intermittent glycosuria and

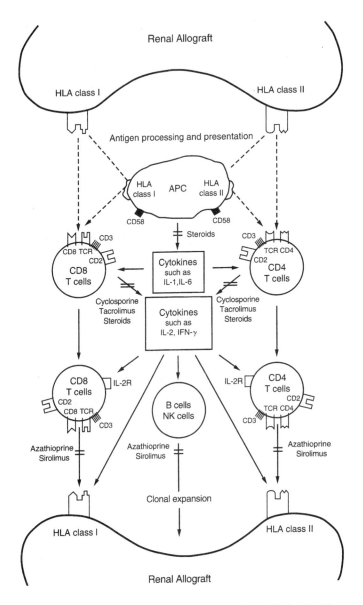

Fig. 16-8. The anti-allograft response. IFN, interferon; IL, interleukin. (From Suthanthiran M, Strom T: Renal transplantation. N Engl J Med 331:365-376, 1994. By permission of Massachusetts Medical Society.)

aminoaciduria. Hormonal effects are 1) increased levels of renin, angiotensin II, aldosterone, cortisol, estrogens, prostaglandins (E_2, I_2), and progesterone; 2) insensitivity to pressor effects of norepinephrine and angiotensin II; and 3) progesterone counteracting the kaliuretic effects of aldosterone.

Urinary Tract Infections

The prevalence of asymptomatic bacteriuria among pregnant women is similar to that among nonpregnant women, except it is higher in those with diabetes mellitus and sickle cell trait. Asymptomatic urinary tract infections progress to pyelonephritis or cystitis in 40% of pregnant women. Screen for asymptomatic bacteriuria monthly, and treat asymptomatic bacteriuria (10-14 days). Symptomatic urinary tract infections relapse and reinfect frequently. Pyelonephritis occurs in 1% to 2% of patients. Treat symptomatic urinary tract infection aggressively with antibiotics (ampicillin, cephalosporins) for 6 weeks. Perform follow-up cultures every 2 weeks. Avoid use of sulfa drugs near term and tetracyclines (because of fetal bone and teeth development and maternal liver failure).

Acute Renal Failure in Pregnancy

Conditions predisposing to acute renal failure in pregnancy are sepsis, severe preeclampsia (HELLP syndrome), abruptio placenta, intrauterine fetal death, uterine hemorrhage, and nephrotoxins. Cortical necrosis: 10% to 30% of cases of gestational acute renal failure. Patients become anuric. Although they may have partial recovery, they can have progression to end-stage renal disease years later. Postpartum hemolytic-uremic syndrome (retained placenta?) presents at 3 to 6 weeks post partum. It is characterized by acute oliguria, uremia, severe hypertension, and microhemangiopathic hemolytic anemia. There is disseminated intravascular coagulation and Schwartzman reaction, as in thrombotic thrombocytopenic purpura. Therapy includes dilatation and curettage, support, antiplatelet therapy(?), and plasma infusion. Acute renal failure and acute fatty liver of pregnancy (similar to hepatorenal syndrome) are caused by tetracyclines and possibly disseminated intravascular coagulation. Progressive hepatic failure has a mortality rate of 75%.

Parenchymal Renal Disease in Pregnancy

Lupus erythematosus—Outcome depends on clinical status prepartum. If the disease is quiescent 6 months before birth, 90% of the women have live births. If the disease is active prepartum, 50% have exacerbation and 35% have fetal loss. If the disease is stable prepartum, 30% of the women have reversible exacerbations. Congenital heart block may occur in the newborn. Glucocorticoids and cytotoxic agents have been used without teratogenicity.

Diabetes mellitus—It is associated with increased asymptomatic and symptomatic bacteriuria and increased preeclampsia. Proteinuria and hypertension may worsen, but renal function usually is stable.

Renal transplant recipients—These women should postpone pregnancy for 2 years after transplantation. Increased preeclampsia, infection, and adrenal insufficiency occur. It is usually uncomplicated if the creatinine level is less than 1.5, blood pressure is normal, and the patient is taking a low dose of immunosuppressive agent. Preeclampsia occurs in 25% of women, prematurity in 7%, and loss of renal function in 7%. Nonobstetrical abdominal pain indicates allograft stone or infection.

EVALUATION OF KIDNEY FUNCTION

Urinalysis

Causes of urine discoloration are listed in Table 16-12.

Urinary sediment: dysmorphic erythrocytes (>80%) indicate upper urinary tract bleeding. Hansel stain: urine eosinophils.

Osmolality and pH—Urine osmolality is 40-1,200 mOsm/kg and pH is 4-7.5. pH <5.5 excludes renal tubular acidosis type I. pH >7: ? infection. Acid urine is indicative of high protein diet, acidosis, and potassium depletion. Alkaline urine is associated with a vegetarian diet, alkalosis (unless potassium depleted), and urease-producing bacteria.

Glucose—Glycosuria in the absence of hyperglycemia suggests proximal tubule dysfunction.

Renal blood flow—Clearance of p-aminohippurate is a measure of renal blood flow. Ortho-iodohippurate is used in renal scans.

Glomerular filtration rate—Clearance of inulin, iothalamate, DTPA, and creatinine are measures of glomerular filtration rate. The Cockgroft-Gault Estimate formula for males is

$$GFR = \frac{(140 - \text{age in years}) \times (\text{lean body weight in kg})}{S_{Cr} \times 72}$$

Table 16-12.—Causes of Urine Discoloration

Color	Cause
Dark yellow, brown	Bilirubin
Brown-black	Homogentisic acid (ochronosis)
	Melanin (melanoma)
	Metronidazole
	Methyldopa/levodopa
	Phenothiazine
Red	Beets
	Rifampin
	Porphyria
	Hemoglobinuria/myoglobinuria
	Phenazopyridine hydrochloride (Pyridium)
	Urates
Blue-green	Indomethacin
	Amitriptyline
Turbid white	Pyuria
	Chylous fistula
	Crystalluria

in which GFR is glomerular filtration rate and S_{Cr} is serum level of creatinine. For females, the formula is males x 0.85. Creatinine levels are increased independently of the glomerular filtration rate with ketoacidosis (acetoacetate), cefoxitin, cimetidine, trimethoprim, flucytosine, massive rhabdomyolysis, high meat intake, and probenecid. Urea (BUN) levels are increased independently of glomerular filtration rate with gastrointestinal tract bleeding, tissue trauma, glucocorticoids, and tetracyclines.

Renal Imaging

KUB-plain films magnify the kidneys 30%. Normal renal size is 3.5 x height of vertebra L-2 (>11 cm). The left kidney is up to 1.5 cm longer than the right one. An enlarged kidney indicates obstruction, infiltration (amyloidosis, leukemia, diabetes mellitus), acute glomerulonephritis, acute tubulointerstitial nephropathy, renal vein thrombosis, and polycystic kidney disease. Calcifications are associated with stone, tuberculosis, aneurysms, and papillary tip necrosis.

Excretory urography provides a detailed definition of the collecting system and can be used to assess renal size and contour and to detect and locate calculi. It is also used to assess qualitative renal function. Poor screen for renovascular hypertension: rapid sequence excretory urography. Complications: large osmotic load (congestive heart failure), reactions (5%).

Premedicate with antihistamines/glucocorticoids, iodine load (hyperthyroidism).

Ultrasonography is used to measure renal size (>9 cm) and to screen for obstruction, but the results may be negative early. Ultrasonography can be used to characterize mass lesions (angiomyolipoma, solid versus cystic) and to screen for polycystic kidney disease. Use it to assess for renal vein thrombosis, that is, the presence or absence of blood flow. It is not a screen for renal artery stenosis.

CT shows calcification patterns. It is used to stage neoplasms and as an adjunct to determining the cause of obstruction (no contrast). CT assesses cysts, abscesses, and hematomas.

Magnetic resonance imaging (MRI) can be used to identify adrenal hemorrhage and to assess a mass in patients sensitive to contrast dyes. MRI angiography is a promising screen for renal artery stenosis.

Arteriography and venography are used in cases of arterial stenosis, aneurysm, fistulae, vasculitis, and mass lesions and to assess living-related donor transplants.

Gallium/indium scans are used in cases of acute interstitial nephritis, abscess, pyelonephritis, lymphoma, and leukemia.

DTPA/hippuran renal scan is used to assess post-transplant kidney, obstruction (pre- and postfurosemide), and infarct (presence or absence of blood flow).

QUESTIONS

Multiple Choice (choose the one best answer)

1. For the following patients with nephritis and renal insufficiency, select the most likely associated serologic finding: a 27-year-old woman has symmetrical arthritis, rash, and alopecia:
   a. Mixed cryoglobulins
   b. Myeloperoxidase-specific antineutrophil cytoplasm antibody (ANCA)
   c. Proteinase-3-specific ANCA
   d. Antiglomerular basement membrane antibody
   e. Anti-DS-deoxyribonucleic acid antibody

2. For the following patient with nephritis and renal insufficiency, select the most likely associated serologic finding: a 52-year-old woman has palpable purpura, arthralgias, and Raynaud phenomenon:

   a. Mixed cryoglobulins
   b. Myeloperoxidase-specific antineutrophil cytoplasm antibody (ANCA)
   c. Proteinase-3-specific ANCA
   d. Antiglomerular basement membrane antibody
   e. Anti-DS-deoxyribonucleic acid antibody

3. An 18-year-old man who has been in good general health underwent a routine physical examination and was found to have 2+ protein on a dipstick urinalysis. The urine sediment was normal and urine pH 5.0. The patient had no other abnormal physical or laboratory findings. The 24-hour urine collection demonstrated 1.3 g of protein and the creatinine clearance was normal. Which of the following procedures is most appropriate?
   a. Urine protein electrophoresis
   b. Renal biopsy
   c. Measurement of protein excretion (supine and upright)

d. Examination again in 1 year

e. Intravenous pyelography

4. A 54-year-old woman in previously good health developed a flu-like illness and diarrhea along with increasing fatigue, irritability, and tea-colored urine. Because of progressive symptoms over 7 days, including disorientation and mild dehydration, she was admitted to the hospital and found to have a blood pressure of 150/90 mm Hg, 1-2+ peripheral edema, and no evidence of pulmonary, joint, or skin disease. Laboratory studies demonstrated a new anemia and thrombocytopenia along with numerous schistocytes on the peripheral blood smear. The creatinine was 7 and there were many red cells and red cell casts on urinalysis. Indicated therapy at this time is?

a. Supportive care

b. Corticosteroids

c. Corticosteroids and plasma exchange

d. Warfarin

e. Conservative management

5. Which of the following statements is true regarding diabetic nephropathy?

a. There are no renal protective benefits of specific antihypertensive agents in human diabetes

b. Low protein diets have been shown to slow the rate of decline of renal function in patients with overt diabetic nephropathy

c. Strict control of blood glucose levels slows the rate of decline of renal function in patients with overt proteinuria and declining renal function

d. Blood pressure control is minimally beneficial in slowing the rate of decline of renal function in patients with overt diabetic nephropathy

e. Blood pressure control is not beneficial in patients with microalbuminuria

6. IgA nephropathy is characterized by mesangial cell proliferation and excess mesangial matrix production associated with positive glomerular IgA immunofluorescence. Which of the following systemic disorders is associated with a renal glomerular lesion similar to that of idiopathic IgA nephropathy?

a. Membranous nephropathy

b. Diabetes mellitus

c. HUS-TTP

d. Schönlein-Henoch purpura

e. Goodpasture syndrome

7. Each of the following renal lesions may be associated with hypocomplementemia *except*:

a. Lupus nephritis

b. Polyarteritis nodosa

c. Post-streptococcal glomerulonephritis

d. Cryoglobulinemia

e. MPGN type II

8. Monoclonal gammopathies have been associated with all the following *except*:

a. κ Light chain nephropathy

b. Myeloma kidney

c. Fibrillary nephritis

d. Amyloid kidney

e. Polycystic kidney disease

9. Patients who develop focal segmental glomerulosclerosis with nephrotic syndrome may have which of the following characteristics?

a. This histologic lesion may characteristically follow a streptococcal pharyngeal infection

b. This morphologic lesion is most common in elderly patients who present with nephrosis

c. The majority of patients with this morphologic lesion respond to corticosteroid treatment

d. Heavy proteinuria of more than 10 g daily is associated with a poor prognosis

e. This is the morphologic lesion most likely to be seen with HUS-TTP

10. Membranous nephropathy has a characteristic pattern of immune deposit deposition. Which of the following best describe this pattern?

a. "Spike-and-dome" immunofluorescence

b. Tramtracking

c. Linear staining

d. "Hair-on-end" deposits

e. Mesangial deposits and fluorescence

11. An 82-year-old man has bladder outlet obstruction due to benign prostatic hypertrophy. An indwelling urinary catheter is placed, and the patient becomes polyuric. What IV fluid rate (if any) would you choose?

a. Replace urine output mL per mL

b. Keep IV rate at 40 mL/hr

c. Push oral fluid intake and give no IV fluids

d. Replace urine two-thirds mL IV per 1 mL urine output

e. Keep IV rate at 150 mL/hr

12. Which of the following diagnostic indices can be found in acute renal failure due to both dye toxicity and pre-renal azotemia?

a. Fractional excretion of sodium <1%
b. Red blood cell casts
c. Urine/plasma creatinine ratio ≤20
d. Urinary sodium >20
e. Metabolic acidosis

13. A 40-year-old patient receiving hemodialysis has an increased parathyroid hormonal level. His serum level of phosphorus is 4.0 mg/dL (normal, 2.5-4.5 mg/dL) and calcium is 8.9 mg/dL (normal, 8.9-10.1 mg/dL). He states he follows his low phosphorus diet. What is the next step in the treatment of his secondary hyperparathyroidism?
a. Parathyroidectomy
b. Prescribe phosphate binders
c. Increase dietary phosphorus and calcium intake
d. Follow closely
e. Prescribe 1,25-dihydroxyvitamin D

14. A 70-year-old man comes for a general physical examination. He has no specific complaint. He has more than a 30-year history of hypertension. His serum level of creatinine is 3.8 mg/dL (normal, 0.8-1.2 mg/dL). Which diagnostic test would best help determine whether this is chronic or there is an acute reversible cause to his decreased renal function.
a. A dynamic nuclear renal scan
b. Renal ultrasonography
c. Fractional excretion of sodium
d. Creatinine clearance
e. Serum BUN

15. A patient you have been following with known progressive renal insufficiency complains of increased bruising, decreased appetite, increased fatigue, and lower extremity edema. Which laboratory finding is not explained by uremia?
a. Creatinine 10.0 mg/dL (normal, 0.8-1.2 mg/dL)
b. Urea 202 mg/dL (normal, 17-51 mg/dL)
c. Hemoglobin 9.0 g/dL (normal, 13.5-17.5 g/dL)
d. sTSH 14 mIU/L (normal, 0.3-5.0 mIU/L)
e. Phosphorus 6.9 mg/dL (normal, 2.5-4.5 mg/dL)

16. Nonsteroidal anti-inflammatory drugs can be associated with all of the following *except*:
a. Acute nephrotic syndrome
b. Aggravation of hypertension
c. Hypernatremia
d. Hyperkalemia
e. Acute interstitial nephritis

17. Eosinophilia, eosinophiluria, and low levels of complements

are associated with which cause of acute renal failure?
a. Atheroemboli
b. Bilateral ureteral obstruction
c. Acute tubular necrosis due to analgesic abuse
d. Dye nephrotoxicity
e. Rhabdomyolysis

18. The following information is reference for questions 18, 19, and 20: A 64-year-old patient is status-post emergency splenectomy due to traumatic splenic rupture. Preoperatively and intraoperatively, she was hypotensive. Postoperatively, her creatinine progressively increases and urine output decreases. Which urine findings test would best represent the cause to the patient's acute renal failure?
a. Red blood cell casts, >100 red blood cells, 10-20 white blood cells
b. Leukocyte casts, >100 white blood cells
c. 10-20 white blood cells, eosinophils
d. 10-20 red blood cells, fatty casts, oval fat bodies, free fat
e. Granular casts, tubular epithelial cells

19. Despite your efforts to induce urine output, the patient is now anuric. Further care of the patient includes all of the following *except*:
a. Prescribe a high fiber diet
b. Adjust all medication doses as appropriate for the patient's renal function
c. Prescribe phosphate binders
d. Avoid nonsteroidal anti-inflammatory agents for pain management
e. Avoid angiotensin-converting enzyme inhibitors to treat hypertension

20. Indications to begin hemodialysis include all of the following *except*:
a. Pericarditis
b. Serum level of creatinine >4.0 mg/dL
c. Serum level of potassium >7.0 mEq/L
d. Aspirin overdose
e. Asterixis

21. During routine follow-up, a 25-year-old woman is noted to have an increased creatinine level of 2.0 mg/dL (normal, 0.6-0.8 mg/dL). Previous creatinine levels have been normal. A review of systems is negative, and she has no history of hypertension. She usually takes no medications but is on day 6 of a course of trimethoprim sulfa for urinary tract infection. Physical examination findings are normal. Urinalysis: mosm 362, pH 5.7, red blood cells 0,

white blood cells 1-3. Her glomerular filtration rate is most likely:

a. 50 mL/min
b. 20 mL/min
c. 100 mL/min
d. 10 mL/min
e. 60 mL/min

22. A 45-year-old man is discovered in an alley beside an unlabeled plastic jug. He is brought to the emergency department comatose, with stable vital signs, without obvious signs of trauma, and with the following laboratory values: arterial blood gas, 7.20; PaO_2, 90; PCO_2, 20; electrolytes—Na, 145, K 3.8, Cl 98; HCO_3, 10; BUN, 30 mg/dL; Cr, 2.1 mg/dL; glucose, 89 mg/dL; serum osmolality, 345 mOsm/L. Which of the following characterizes his acid/base disorder?

a. Simple metabolic acidemia
b. Mixed metabolic acidosis and respiratory acidosis with acidemia
c. Mixed respiratory alkalosis and metabolic acidosis
d. "Triple disorder," with metabolic acidemia, metabolic alkalosis, and respiratory alkalosis

23. You examine the above patient's urine. It reveals many needle- and envelope-shaped crystals. The urine fluoresces under a Wood lamp (which you just happen to have available). Which of the following compounds is the cause of the toxicity induced by this patient's ingestion?

a. Formic acid
b. Oxalic acid
c. Glycyrrhizic acid
d. Lactic acid

24. A 32-year-old woman with a history of dry mouth and eyes presents to you after a screening examination revealed hypokalemia. Review of systems also reveals recent episodes of "loose stools." Laboratory studies revealed the following: Na, 140 mEq/L; K, 2.9 mEq/L; Cl, 118 mEq/L; HCO_3, 19 mEq/L; BUN, 28 mg/dL; Cr, 1.8 mg/dL. Urinalysis shows a pH of 5.7. Urine electrolytes are Na, 40 mEq/L; K, 10 mEq/L; Cl, 30 mEq/L. What is the cause of her acid/base electrolyte disorder?

a. Laxative abuse
b. Surreptitious diuretic abuse
c. Distal renal tubular acidosis (type I)
d. Proximal renal tubular acidosis (type II)

25. A 74-year-old man with congestive heart failure develops the following metabolic disorder while undergoing aggressive diuresis in the intensive care unit: pH, 7.53; PaO_2, 75; PCO_2, 46; electrolytes Na, 145 mEq/L; K, 2.5 mEq/L; Cl, 89 mEq/L; HCO_3, 34 mEq/L; BUN, 48 mg/dL; Cr, 1.9 mg/dL. Which of the following is the best option to reverse the metabolic derangement?

a. Acetazolamide
b. Dopamine drip at "renal dose"
c. Load and treat with digoxin (Lanoxin)
d. Reduction of diuretic dose as appropriate and potassium chloride repletion

26. A 35-year-old man with a history of psychosis and mania presents with polyuria and polydipsia. His serum level of Na is 137 mEq/L. He relates that "the overlords" have been warning him of "the coming plague and drought." His partner relates he drinks cold water "by the gallon." He has been treated with lithium carbonate for several months. You restrict his access to water for 3 hours and observe the changes in his electrolytes and urine chemistry values. You note his urine osmolality goes from 202 mOsm/L to 310 mOsm/L. On the basis of these results would you confidently discontinue his lithium?

a. Yes
b. No

27. An 88-year-old woman comes from a nursing home with "mental status changes." She is somnolent on examination and mumbles unintelligibly when stimulated. Your work-up reveals that she has a history of unresectable lung cancer, hypertension, and a recent history of anorexia and vomiting. She is taking a thiazide diuretic and prochlorperazine (Compazine) for her nausea. Her serum level of sodium is reported at 112 mEq/L. Which of the following is/are potential causes of her hyponatremia?

a. Nausea and vomiting
b. Thiazide diuretic
c. Paraneoplastic syndrome
d. Marked hypovolemia
e. All the above

28. Further evaluation of the above patient's hyponatremia should include which of the following?

a. Urine osmolality and sodium concentration
b. Serum osmolality
c. Physical assessment of volume status
d. Serum glucose measurement
e. All the above

29. A 64-year-old woman with diabetic nephropathy recently started treatment with an angiotensin-converting enzyme inhibitor for management of hypertension and proteinuria. She is brought to the emergency department

in cardiovascular collapse. The monitor shows a bizarre wide complex rhythm. Which of the following is the first medication you ask for?
a. Lidocaine
b. Bretylium
c. Epinephrine
d. Calcium gluconate

30. An 38-year-old diabetic with a history of asthma presents with DKA secondary to acute bronchitis with gastroenteritis. She is given IV fluids, and insulin bolus and infusion, antibiotics, subcutaneous heparin, and inhaled β-agonists. One-half hour later, her serum potassium level is reported to you as 2.3 mEq/L. Which of the following is *not* a cause of her hypokalemia.
a. Insulin therapy
b. Trancellular shifts
c. β-Agonist therapy
d. Heparin

31. A hospitalized 45-year-old man develops weakness. He has a history of leukemia and has had bone marrow transplantation. He has been taking spironolactone (Aldactone) for hypertension, amphotericin and imipenem-cilastin for neutropenic fever, cyclosporine for graft-versus-host disease prophylaxis, heparin for deep venous thrombosis prophylaxis, and trimethoprim-sulfamethoxazole for *Pneumocystis carinii* pneumonia prophylaxis, and his wife has surreptitiously been giving him ibuprofen to help ease his discomfort. His serum potassium level is 5.6 mEq/L with preserved renal function. Which of this patient's medications *likely is not* associated with the hyperkalemia?
a. Heparin
b. Ibuprofen
c. Amphotericin
d. Trimethoprim-sulfamethoxazole

Match the following patients with urolithiasis to the most appropriate drug treatment. Each answer may be used once, more than once, or not at all.

32. A 23-year-old woman with homozygous cystinuria forms recurrent cystine stones despite treatment with fluid, diet, and urinary alkalinization.
a. Thiazides
b. Allopurinol
c. Potassium citrate
d. D-penicillamine
e. Antibiotics

33. A hypercalciuric 35-year-old man forms recurrent calcium

oxalate stones despite treatment with fluid and diet.
a. Thiazides
b. Allopurinol
c. Potassium citrate
d. D-penicillamine
e. Antibiotics

34. A hyperuricosuric obese 55-year-old man with a history of gout forms stones of unknown type despite good fluid intake.
a. Thiazides
b. Allopurinol
c. Potassium citrate
d. D-penicillamine
e. Antibiotics

35. A debilitated paraplegic woman with a neurogenic bladder and chronic urinary infections has non-obstructive radiopaque staghorn calculus on intravenous pyelography. She is considered a high-risk surgical candidate.
a. Thiazides
b. Allopurinol
c. Potassium citrate
d. D-penicillamine
e. Antibiotics

36. A 43-year-old woman with ulcerative colitis after total proctocolectomy has recurrent uric acid stones. Efforts to increase fluid intake result primarily in increased ileostomy output without affecting stone formation.
a. Thiazides
b. Allopurinol
c. Potassium citrate
d. D-penicillamine
e. Antibiotics

37. Which of the following is *not* an inhibitor of calcium stone formation?
a. Citrate
b. Cystine
c. Tamm-Horsfall protein
d. Osteopontin
e. Nephrocalcin

38. Which of the following stone analyses must indicate an artifact?
a. Cystine
b. Calcium oxalate monohydrate
c. Silicate
d. Uric acid
e. Calcium phosphate

39. A risk factor for the formation of calcium nephrolithiasis is:
    a. High urine volume
    b. Hypocalciuria
    c. Hypercitraturia
    d. Hypouricosuria
    e. Hyperoxaluria

40. Which of the following stones is caused by urinary infection?
    a. Struvite
    b. Calcium oxalate monohydrate

c. Uric acid
d. Cystine
e. Calcium oxalate dihydrate

41. Which of the following is a dietary risk factor for the formation of calcium nephrolithiasis?
    a. High water consumption
    b. Moderate dairy consumption
    c. Low protein consumption
    d. Low sugar consumption
    e. High salt consumption

ANSWERS

1. Answer e.

The patient's clinical findings are consistent with a systemic disease, most likely systemic lupus erythematosus. Of the serologic findings listed, anti-DS-deoxyribonucleic antibody is most likely to be positive.

2. Answer a.

Palpable purpura is an important clinical finding that should raise the clinical suspicion of mixed cryoglobulinemia. This clinical finding helps to distinguish between systemic lupus erythematosus and other types of cutaneous vasculitis.

3. Answer c.

Orthostatic proteinuria is a benign condition that can be diagnosed easily by comparing the measurement of protein excretion when the patient is supine and upright. When this is identified, the patient can be reassured, and observation alone is necessary. There has been no evidence that it is associated with progressive renal insufficiency.

4. Answer c.

This patient clearly has findings suggestive of hemolytic uremic syndrome-thrombocytopenic purpura and will benefit from corticosteroids and plasma exchange. Dialysis may also be necessary given the patient's severe renal insufficiency. It

is also important to search for potential underlying causes of this disorder, which include medications such as quinine and, of course, enteric pathogens.

5. Answer b.

Angiotensin-converting enzyme inhibitors have been shown to be renal protective; however, their use is most beneficial in patients with microalbuminuria. Strict control of plasma glucose after development of overt nephropathy is of little benefit; however, low protein diets tend to slow the progression of renal function decline in diabetic nephropathy.

6. Answer d.

Schönlein-Henoch purpura is characterized by both renal and skin involvement. Renal biopsy specimens typically have mesangial proliferative changes associated with IgA immune complex deposition similar to those of IgA nephropathy.

7. Answer b.

Polyarteritis nodosa is associated with a p-ANCA; yet, patients do not have evidence for activation of the complement cascade. Measurement of complement is extremely useful clinically to narrow the differential of active nephritis.

8. Answer e.

Paraproteinemias may have various renal manifestations. It is important to be able to distinguish each, and renal biopsy generally is necessary to do so. There is not an increased incidence of monoclonal gammopathies in patients with autosomal dominant polycystic kidney disease.

9. Answer d.

Patients with focal segmental glomerulosclerosis are most often steroid resistant and carry a worse prognosis if proteinuria is heavy.

10. Answer a.

Membranous nephropathy is characterized by immune deposits on the epithelial side of the glomerular capillary. These deposits have a characteristic "spike-and-dome" fluorescent pattern. Linear fluorescence is characteristic of Goodpasture disease, tramtracking is seen in membranoproliferative forms of glomerulonephritis such as lupus, hair-on-end appearance often refers to the appearance of seeing an amyloidosis, and IgA nephropathy is characterized by mesangial cell immune deposits of IgA.

11. Answer d.

The patient now has post-obstructive diuresis. To avoid hypovolemia and pre-renal azotemia, urine output should initially be replaced by 2/3 mL per mL with IV fluids. This should keep the patient in fluid balance while the renal tubules recover.

12. Answer a.

During renal hypoperfusion, fractional excretion of sodium is low because of tubular reabsorption of more than 99% of filtered sodium. Radiocontrast agents have powerful vasoconstrictive effects. This may be the pathogenesis leading to a low fractional excretion of sodium with these agents.

13. Answer e.

Secondary hyperparathyroidism in patients with chronic renal failure can be caused by hyperphosphatemia or hypocalcemia. A decrease in 1,25-dihydroxyvitamin D production in patients with chronic renal failure leads to decreased intestinal absorption of calcium and hypocalcemia. Increasing dietary calcium and phosphorus would increase the serum phosphorus level and further stimulate the parathyroid gland. The patient's serum phosphorus level is normal; therefore, adding phosphate binders would not be indicated. The addition of 1,25-dihydroxyvitamin D will increase calcium absorption from the gut, leading to an increased serum level of calcium that will suppress the parathyroids. Also, 1,25-dihydroxyvitamin D is a direct inhibitor of parathyroid hormone.

14. Answer b.

A renal size of less than 10 cm as determined by ultrasonography indicates a chronic process such as nephrosclerosis (hypertension).

15. Answer d.

Endocrine abnormalities in chronic renal failure include infertility and amenorrhea. Thyroid function is usually normal.

16. Answer c.

Nonsteroidal anti-inflammatory drugs are associated with hyponatremia, hyperkalemia, aggravation of hypertension, acute interstitial nephritis, and acute nephrotic syndrome.

17. Answer a.

Atheroembolic-induced renal failure is characterized by cholesterol emboli in medium-sized arteries with an intense tubulointerstitial nephritis. Eosinophils are seen in the urine and peripheral blood. Low levels of serum complement and an increased erythrocyte sedimentation rate are also seen with renal atheroemboli.

18. Answer e.

This patient's acute renal failure is due to acute tubular necrosis secondary to hypotension leading to renal ischemia. Urinalysis reflects cellular debris. Red blood cell casts are associated with glomerular nephritis. Leukocyte casts and eosinophils can be associated with tubulointerstitial nephritis. Fatty casts, oval fat bodies, and free fat are associated with nephrotic syndromes. The management of a patient with anuric renal failure includes a diet designed to give appropriate calories but to avoid sodium, potassium, magnesium, phosphorus, protein, and fluid excesses.

19. Answer a.

Explanation same as for Question 18.

20. Answer b.

Serum creatinine level alone is a poor indicator of renal function. Patient's symptoms and signs suggestive of uremia and their acid-base and fluid balance and electrolytes all contribute to deciding when to begin hemodialysis. Salicylate is removed with dialysis, and a salicylate overdose is an indication for hemodialysis. Severe hyperkalemia, pericarditis, and asterixis are all indications to begin hemodialysis.

21. Answer c.

Trimethoprim increases the serum level of creatinine independently of the glomerular filtration rate. The patient's urinalysis is normal, excluding tubulointerstitial nephritis or acute glomerulonephritis. After the trimethoprim has been discontinued, the patient's creatinine level will normalize, reflecting her true glomerular filtration rate.

22. Answer a.

This patient has a pure metabolic acidosis with acidemia. The CO_2 level is exactly the value one would expect from application of the compensation formula. Winter formula: $P_{CO_2} = 1.5 \times HCO_3 + 8 \pm 2$ or the last 2 digits of the pH equal to the P_{CO_2}. Note the osmolar gap as well (>10), recall that the calculated osmolality = $2(Na) + (glucose/18) + (BUN/2.3)$. (Calculated Osm 305 mOsm/L versus measured = 345 mOsm/L). This "uncalculated" osmole is usually one of the "-ols"—ethanol, methanol, ethylene glycol, mannitol, sorbitol. Hence, the osmolar gap is a quick "drug screen."

23. Answer b.

The anion that accumulates in ethylene glycol intoxication/poisoning as the product of alcohol dehydrogenase is oxalic acid (also, glycolic acid). Therapy is directed at competitive inhibition of alcohol dehydrogenase (i.e., ethanol) as well as enhancing removal of ethylene glycol. The byproduct of methanol intoxication is a formate, whereas isopropyl alcohol ingestion leads to acetone formation (which is not an anion). Lactic acidosis may occur in such settings when cardiovascular collapse has begun or if a limb has become ischemic because of trauma. Glycyrrhizic acid is found in some licorice products, and although it may cause hyperkalemia (rare), it is not the culprit of this syndrome.

24. Answer c.

This patient has a "classic" type I distal renal tubular acidosis likely in conjunction with Sjögren syndrome. Calculation of the urine anion gap (UAG), $[(Na + K) - (HCO_3 + Cl)]$ allows determination of whether appropriate renal acid titration is occurring. H+ is titrated in the urine by NH_3 becoming NH_4+ which binds Cl^- to form NH_4Cl in the distal tubule. Hence, in the setting of acidosis, the urinary anion gap should be negative, as would be the case were this enteric bicarbonate loss. Note that $[HCO_3]$ plays little role in the UAG calculation in urine, which is acidic. This patient's UAG is +20, so appropriate acid titration is not occurring. Note also the urine pH is not less than 5.5 in this setting.

25. Answer d.

Metabolic alkalosis has been initiated and now is in the maintenance phase. The renin-angiotensin-aldosterone system has been activated, facilitating the distal tubular exchange of sodium for hydrogen and potassium, causing a kaluresis and a (in this case, paradoxic) acid urine. The patient's relative intravascular volume depletion also leads to nearly all of the filtered NaCl being resorbed in the proximal tubule, thus not allowing any Cl-HCO3 exchange in the distal tubule. The kaluretic effect of the loop diuretics aggravate this situation. Supplementation of potassium and chloride as well as (if possible) gentle intravascular expansion is the best option in this case.

26. Answer b.

Although lithium has the effect of causing a "nephrogenic" diabetes insipidus, prolonged water ingestion may "wash out" the counter-current gradient in the loop of Henle. Under normal circumstances, ADH acts to form the aquaporin channels in the distal collecting ducts, allowing water to pass into the hypertonic medullary interstitium by means of osmotic pull; if, however, this gradient is not present, little urinary concentration will occur. The differentiation of partial nephrogenic diabetes insipidus from chronic water intoxication may be difficult. However, the serum sodium level often tends to increase above normal in diabetes insipidus, whereas a low-normal serum sodium is often found in water intoxication. Gradual restriction of water intake over 24 to 48 hours under supervised conditions will often resolve this question.

27. Answer e.

All the answers may be possible causes of the patient's hyponatremia. Recall that thiazides may cause hyponatremia by inhibiting the kidneys' ability to dilute the urine. Severe volume depletion will cause the release of ADH, which will take precedence over tonicity. Stress, phenothiazine, emesis, and paraneoplastic syndromes are common causes of ADH secretion.

28. Answer e.

All the above need to be performed to work-up this patient's hyponatremia. Recall that hyperglycemia decreases the serum level of sodium.

29. Answer d.

This patient has a life-threatening manifestation of hyperkalemia and requires calcium parenterally as soon as possible! After this, β-agonists, sodium polystyrene sulfonate (Kayexalate), insulin, dextrose, and, possibly, dialysis will be required.

30. Answer d.

Heparin causes hyperkalemia through its inhibitory effect on angiotensin II. β-Agonists, acidosis, and insulin act to shift potassium into cells.

31. Answer c.

Amphotericin usually causes magnesium and potassium wasting. However, if amphotericin is given too rapidly, potassium may transiently shift out of cells. Trimethoprim-sulfamethoxazole causes hyperkalemia via distal tubular sodium channel blockage. Cyclosporine exerts its effects by blocking distal nephron Na-K ATPase. Aldosterone is blocked by angiotensin-converting enzyme inhibitors, heparin, and nonsteroidal anti-inflammatory drugs via angiotensin II antagonism.

32. Answer d.

D-Penicillamine. A second-generation chelator, tiopronin (Thiola), has a better safety profile. Captopril has also been used for this purpose.

33. Answer a.

Thiazides reduce hypercalciuria. (Loop diuretics increase hypercalciuria!)

34. Answer b.

Allopurinol decreases both calcium and uric acid stone formation in hyperuricosuric patients.

35. Answer e.

Struvite stones form because of the formation of ammonia from urea by certain bacteria that have the enzyme urease. (Humans do not have this enzyme, neither do *E. coli.*) If the struvite stone cannot be removed, which is the treatment of choice, the next step is to prevent the production of urease by antibiotics (as selected sensitivity studies) or acetohydroxamic acid (Lithostat), a specific enzyme inhibitor. However, acetohydroxamic acid increases the risk of deep venous thrombosis and is rarely used in paraplegics.

36. Answer c.

Most chronic diarrheal states result in the production of small volumes of highly acid urine because of copious losses of alkaline stool. This urinary environment favors the formation of uric acid stones. Decreasing urine acidity with alkali such as potassium citrate is the treatment of choice.

37. Answer b.

Cystine is a type of kidney stone. All of the other answers are inhibitors of stone formation.

38. Answer c.

Silicate, or sand, is not a stone humans can form. This finding suggests that the patient is faking stone passages for secondary gain.

39. Answer e.

Hyperoxaluria.

40. Answer a.

Struvite. It cannot form any other way. It is sometimes called an "infection stone." All the other choices are "metabolic stones."

41. Answer e.

Salt. It increases hypercalciuria through a coupling with calcium transport in the proximal tubule. All the other answers have been shown by epidemiologic studies to decrease stone formation.

NOTES

CHAPTER 17

NEUROLOGY

Eduardo E. Benarroch, M.D.
Robert D. Brown, Jr., M.D.
Frank A. Rubino, M.D.

PART I

GENERAL PRINCIPLES OF THE NEUROLOGIC EXAMINATION

INTRODUCTION

Neurologic disorders are commonly seen in general clinical practice. Because of the increasing number of older people throughout the world, cerebrovascular disorders, dementias, and Parkinson disease are assuming increasing importance. Understanding a patient with neurologic disease depends on localizing the problem on the basis of the medical history and examination findings, considering a differential diagnosis, and correlating the clinical findings with abnormalities found on diagnostic testing.

- About 10% of patients of primary care physicians in the U.S. have nervous system disorders.
- About 25% of inpatients have a nervous system disorder as a primary or secondary problem.
- Primary care physicians should have a good working knowledge of common and emergency neurologic problems.

NEUROLOGIC HISTORY

A health care provider who evaluates a patient with possible neurologic disease must use all aspects of the medical history to answer four questions. 1) Does the patient have neurologic disease? 2) If so, what is the localization of the lesion(s)? 3) What is the pathophysiology of the process? 4) What is the preliminary differential diagnosis?

The history of the present illness allows definition of the localization and pathophysiology of the problem. Clarification of the symptoms should lead to answers about the: 1) date of onset, 2) character and severity, 3) location and extension, 4) time relationships, 5) associated complaints, 6) aggravating or alleviating factors, 7) effects of previous treatment, and 8) progress, noting remissions and exacerbations.

In addition to the history of the present illness, other important factors include past medical history with specific regard to whether there is any previous history of neurologic disease. Review of neurologic symptoms that could be related to the main symptoms is also important. Review of medical systems may also lead to clarification of the cause of a specific problem. The family history is becoming increasingly important as the genetic bases of numerous diseases are defined. The social history should define a history of any use of tobacco, alcohol, caffeine, or illicit drugs. Any risk factors for sexually transmitted disorders and human immunodeficiency virus (HIV) infection should also be noted.

- The complete neurologic history allows the examiner to initially localize the lesion, which then may be confirmed by the results of the neurologic examination.

GENERAL PRINCIPLES FOR INTERPRETING NEUROLOGIC SYMPTOMS

Neurologic symptoms can be subdivided into four general categories.
1. Ill-defined, nonspecific, nonanatomical, and nonphysiologic regional or generalized symptoms.
2. Diffuse cerebral symptoms.
3. Positive focal symptoms (hyperactivity).
4. Negative focal symptoms (loss of function).

Ill-Defined Symptoms

These include such things as ill-defined dizziness, diffuse or unusual regional pain, diffuse and unusual numbness, vague memory problems, and unusual gait. Generally, no

659

serious underlying problem is found, especially if the symptoms are long-standing. Many cases have serious underlying psychopathology, but the patient often either does not recognize this fact or denies it. However, be careful in making a psychiatric diagnosis, which should be made on the basis of positive psychologic factors and not only because the physical examination findings and laboratory studies are normal.

- With ill-defined symptoms, no serious underlying problem is found in most patients.
- Many of the patients have underlying psychopathology.
- Make a psychiatric diagnosis based on positive psychologic factors, not because of normal physical examination or laboratory findings.

Diffuse Cerebral Symptoms

Diffuse cognitive problems occur in dementia and acute confusional states. However, a common diffuse symptom is syncope or presyncope, which usually implies diffuse and *not* focal cerebral ischemia. Vasovagal syncope is the major culprit, especially in the young. Syncope is *not* a transient ischemic attack (TIA). Most causes of syncope are systemic—*not* neurologic—problems. In primary autonomic dysfunction, other neurologic signs and symptoms usually help make the diagnosis (e.g., multiple system atrophy, diabetic and amyloid autonomic neuropathy).

- Diffuse cerebral symptoms imply diffuse, not focal, cerebral ischemia.
- Syncope is not a TIA.
- Systemic, not neurologic, problems usually cause syncope.

Positive Phenomena

An example of a positive sensory phenomenon is marching paresthesia, and an example of a positive motor phenomenon is tonic or clonic movement. Lights, flashes, sparkles, and formed images are examples of positive visual phenomena. An example of a positive language phenomenon is unusual vocalization. Positive central phenomena usually indicate seizures or migraine accompaniments. Positive peripheral phenomena occur with nerve damage and repair.

Negative Phenomena

They usually indicate damage to a specific central or peripheral area. TIAs and strokes usually produce negative phenomena; if there is more than one symptom, all the symptoms tend to appear at the same time. Migraine syndromes may have positive and negative phenomena; if there is more than one symptom, the symptoms tend to come on one after another and "build up."

- TIAs and strokes produce negative phenomena.
- Migraine syndromes have positive and negative phenomena.

Acute Muscular Weakness

Physicians may overlook serious underlying diseases in patients whose chief or only complaint is weakness, especially if there are few or no obvious clinical signs. Delayed or missed diagnosis can lead to life-threatening complications such as respiratory failure, irreversible spinal cord dysfunction, and acute renal failure. Respiratory muscles may be affected, although strength in the extremities is relatively normal. Patients with early Guillain-Barré syndrome may have distal paresthesias and increased respiratory effort and be given the diagnosis of hysterical hyperventilation.

- Missed diagnosis can lead to life-threatening complications: respiratory failure, irreversible spinal cord function, and acute renal failure.
- Early Guillain-Barré syndrome may be misdiagnosed as hysterical hyperventilation.

Acute muscle weakness can be classified into four groups: disease of the spinal cord, peripheral nerve, myoneural junction, or muscle.

NEUROLOGIC EXAMINATION

A complete neurologic examination includes a description of all the items noted in Table 17-1. It is useful to describe the results of the neurologic examination in usual terms that can be understood easily by others. The examination findings may then be combined with the neurologic history to clarify the localization of the disorder to the following four levels: 1) supratentorial (cerebral cortex and subcortical regions, including the basal ganglia, hypothalamus, and thalamus); 2) posterior fossa (cerebellum, brain stem, and cranial nerves); 3) spinal cord (including extramedullary, intramedullary, cauda equina, and conus medullaris lesions); and 4) peripheral (peripheral lesions may be localized further from proximal to distal—radiculopathy, plexopathy, peripheral neuropathy, myoneural junction, and muscle). One must realize that many disorders are multifocal. After the level has been determined, it should be considered whether the lesion is on the right side or the left side or on both sides based on the signs and symptoms; also, whether the lesion is bilateral or unilateral should be clarified. It then is possible to consider a differential diagnosis for the lesion and to outline the diagnostic procedures, therapeutic options, and patient education.

Neurologic abnormalities occur frequently in healthy, cognitively intact elderly persons. The following signs alone cannot be considered pathologic:

Table 17-1.—Neurologic Examination

Mental status and state of consciousness evaluation
Gait and station evaluation
Cranial nerve evaluation
Sensory evaluation
    Primary sensations
    Cortical sensations
Motor evaluation
    Strength
    Muscle bulk
    Muscle tone
Evaluation of reflexes
    Muscle stretch reflexes (deep tendon reflexes)
    Abnormal reflexes (Babinski sign, grasping of hand and
        feet)*
    Superficial reflexes (abdominal and cremasteric reflexes)
Evaluation of coordination
    Finger-to-nose and heel-to-knee tests
    Observation of abnormal movements or tremor

*Note that unusual reflexes such as snouting, sucking, and palmomental reflexes are common in elderly patients and are usually *not* pathologic. However, grasping reflexes and paratonic rigidity (gegenhalten) in *awake* patients are pathologic.

1. Decreased acuity of the special senses—olfaction, audition, and vision.
2. Decrease in upward gaze, visual pursuit, and saccadic function.
3. Abnormal gait with reduced arm swinging, shorter steps, and slow walking speed.
4. Difficulty with balance, with wider base and unsteady turns.
5. Decreased vibratory sensation in the legs.
6. Decreased pupillary response to light.
7. Atrophy of small muscles of the hand.
8. Decreased ankle reflexes.

In addition, some neurodiagnostic studies may appear abnormal in most healthy elderly people, including spondylitic abnormalities on plain cervical and lumbar radiographs and on magnetic resonance imaging (MRI) and computed tomography (CT) of the same areas, white matter changes on MRI, mild focal slowing on electroencephalography (EEG), and slowing of nerve conduction velocities on electrophysiologic testing.

● Most healthy elderly people have spondylitic abnormalities on plain cervical and lumbar radiographs.

GENERAL PRINCIPLES FROM THE LEVEL OF THE CEREBRAL CORTEX THROUGH THE NEURAXIS TO MUSCLE

Supratentorial Level: Symptoms and Clinical Correlations

The supratentorial region is large and includes all levels of the nervous system inside the skull and above the tentorium cerebelli. Symptoms and signs may be related to disorders of the cerebral cortex, leading to alterations in cognition and consciousness. Also, focal neurologic symptoms involving a single limb and a single neurologic symptom (such as numbness [sensory system] or weakness [motor system]) commonly localize to the cerebral cortex. In addition, abnormalities of speech and language are localized to the dominant cerebral hemisphere, whereas abnormalities of the nondominant hemisphere may lead to visuospatial deficits, confusion, or neglect of the contralateral side of the body. Abnormalities in the subcortical region also may lead to weakness or numbness and typically involve more than one limb. Abnormalities in the basal ganglia may lead to movement disorders, including tremor, bradykinesia (as in Parkinson disease), and chorea (as in Huntington disease). Disorders of the thalamus, another subcortical structure, typically cause unilateral sensory abnormalities. The hypothalamus is important in many functions that affect one's everyday steady-state condition: temperature, food, and water regulation; sleep; endocrine and cardiovascular functions, and regulation of the autonomic nervous system. Cortical and subcortical abnormalities may also lead to visual system deficits, usually homonymous visual deficits.

Consciousness and Cognition

Consciousness has two dimensions: arousal and cognitive content. Arousal is a vegetative function maintained by brain stem/medial diencephalic structures. Cognitive content—learning, memory, self-awareness, and adaptive behavior—depends on the functional integrity of the cerebral cortex and associated subcortical nuclei.

Coma or unconsciousness results from either bilateral dysfunction of the cerebral cortex or dysfunction of the reticular activating system in the upper brain stem (above midpons). Unconsciousness implies global or total unawareness; coma implies the lack of both wakefulness and awareness.

● Brain death is the absence of cerebral cortex and brain stem function.
● Persistent vegetative state is the absence of cerebral cortex function with normal brain stem function (deafferentated state). This is a state of wakefulness without detectable awareness, even though patients have sleep-wave cycles.

- "Locked-in" syndrome is normal cerebral cortex function with absence of brain stem function (the lesion is usually in the pons, causing quadriplegia and the inability to speak, swallow, and move the eyes horizontally—de-efferentated state).
- Acute confusional state is malfunction of the cerebral cortex and reticular activating system.
- Dementia is malfunction of the cerebral cortex but normal function of the brain stem.

Stupor and Coma

For one to stay awake, the cerebral hemispheres and reticular activating system must be intact. Patients with dysfunction of only one cerebral hemisphere have a focal neurologic deficit but are awake. The most common, important, potentially reversible causes of stupor and coma are toxic, metabolic, and infectious problems affecting both cerebral hemispheres diffusely. Thus, most patients in stupor and coma have an underlying systemic problem. In adults and children with traumatic brain injury, recovery from unconsciousness is unlikely after 12 months. Recovery is rare after 3 months in adults and children with nontraumatic brain injury.

- The most common reversible causes of stupor and coma are toxic, metabolic, and infectious causes.

Patients with systemic encephalopathies have changes in mental status and awareness before going into stupor and coma, but they have no focal signs. Their corneal reflexes are lost early, but pupillary reflexes remain. Also, ocular motility tested by the doll's eye maneuver (oculocephalic reflexes) and the cold caloric response (oculovestibular reflex) are fully intact, at least early in the disease.

- Patients with systemic encephalopathies have no focal signs.
- Their corneal reflexes are lost early, but pupillary reflexes remain.

Patients with a large unilateral cerebral lesion may go into stupor and coma if the lesion causes shifting and pressure changes in other parts of the brain, such as the opposite hemisphere or brain stem. These patients have focal neurologic signs. Patients with brain stem lesions directly affecting the ascending reticular activating system are in coma but have focal signs. Finally, people who feign coma have no focal signs, no abnormal reflexes, normal caloric responses, and a normal EEG. They are a small percentage of patients seen in stupor and coma.

- Large unilateral cerebral lesions causing a shift and pressure changes in the other hemisphere or brain stem produce focal neurologic signs together with coma.

- Brain stem lesions causing coma also produce focal signs.
- People feigning coma have no focal signs, no abnormal reflexes, normal caloric response, and normal EEG.

Dementia

Dementia is a clinical state characterized by a significant loss of function in multiple cognitive domains not due to an impaired level of arousal. The presence of dementia does not necessarily imply irreversibility, a progressive course, or any specific disease. Dementia is not a disease but an entity with various causes, which can be categorized as follows:

1. Hereditary/Degenerative: Alzheimer disease, diffuse Lewy body disease, Pick disease and other frontotemporal dementias, Huntington disease, progressive supranuclear palsy, and Wilson disease.
2. Infectious/Inflammatory: meningitis and encephalitis, HIV, brain abscess, Creutzfeld-Jakob disease, and Whipple disease.
3. Toxic/Metabolic: vitamin deficiencies (B_{12}, folate), hyponatremia, hypothyroidism, uremia, liver failure, and toxins (heavy metals).
4. Neoplastic: bilateral tumors, meningeal neoplasm, and paraneoplastic syndromes (limbic encephalitis).
5. Vascular: multiple infarcts, Binswanger disease, and vasculitis.
6. Other causes: subdural hematoma and hydrocephalus.

Reversible causes of dementia are found in a small percentage of patients and include medication-induced encephalopathy, depression, thyroid disease, infections of the central nervous system (CNS), vitamin deficiencies, and structural brain lesions (neoplasms, subdural hematomas, and symptomatic hydrocephalus).

- Dementia is not a disease.

Alzheimer disease is the most common cause of dementia. It occurs in both young and old persons and is no longer subcategorized into "presenile" and "senile" types. In general, the patients present with difficulties in several cognitive areas; they also exhibit aphasia and apraxia and may have movement disorders such as myoclonus and akinesia. Some subtypes of a genotype for apolipoprotein E may predict a higher likelihood of Alzheimer disease. Additional study is needed to clarify the association of the subtypes and the power of prediction of a specific finding.

Some symptoms of Alzheimer disease are thought to be due to partial depletion of acetylcholine in the brain. Tacrine hydrochloride and donepezil, centrally active noncompetitive reversible cholinesterase inhibitors, have been studied in persons with mild-to-moderate cognitive impairment and in patients with Alzheimer disease. These agents may improve the symptoms slightly and slow the decline of cognitive function in a small proportion of patients. Common adverse side effects of tacrine include hepatotoxicity, which requires frequent (weekly) monitoring of liver function tests. The liver toxicity is reversible if detected early. Donepezil can be given once daily and does not cause hepatotoxicity.

A typical diagnostic work-up for dementia might include a complete blood count, electrolyte survey (including calcium, glucose, BUN/creatinine), liver function tests, thyroid function tests, serum level of vitamin B_{12}, and serologic testing for syphilis. In selected patients, erythrocyte sedimentation rate, HIV testing, paraneoplastic antibody screening, chest radiography, urine collection for heavy metals, and toxicology screens should be performed. Neuroimaging should be considered in virtually all persons with dementia, depending on the medical history and examination findings. Neuropsychometric testing may also be considered. Lumbar puncture is performed in persons with a recent onset of symptoms, persons younger than 55 years who have dementia, and in those with immunosuppression, possible CNS infection, reactive serum syphilis serologic findings, and metastatic cancer without findings on an imaging study. EEG may be useful in evaluating for Creutzfeldt-Jakob disease.

Acute Confusional States

Acute confusional states are abrupt, of recent onset, and often associated with fluctuations in the state of awareness and cognition. They are manifested by confusion, inattention, disorientation, and delirium. Thus, patients may be inattentive, dazed, stuporous, restless, agitated, or excited and may have marked autonomic dysfunction and visual and tactile hallucinations. Abnormal motor manifestations are common, including paratonia, asterixis, tremor, and myoclonus. The usual etiologic factors of acute confusional states are toxic, metabolic, traumatic, infectious, organ failure of any sort, or ictal or postictal encephalopathies. Three large categories of general causes are systemic causes, neurologic causes, and psychophysiologic causes. Withdrawal states from alcohol, benzodiazepines, and barbiturates are also important causes of acute confusion or delirium.

- Three large categories of causes of acute confusional states are systemic, neurologic, and psychophysiologic causes.

Headache and Facial Pain

Headache may indicate intracranial or systemic disease, a personality or situational problem, or a combination of these. Some headaches have a readily identified organic cause. Classic migraine and cluster headaches form distinctive, easily recognized clinical entities, but their pathophysiology is not understood. The major challenge is that often neither the location nor the intensity of the pain is a reliable clue to the nature of the problem. Episodic tension headache and migraine can be difficult to distinguish.

- Neither location nor intensity of headache pain is a reliable clue to the nature of the problem.

Headache pain may be generated centrally and involve serotonergic and dopaminergic pain-modulating systems. Neurogenically mediated inflammation at the trigeminovascular junction may account for some migraine pain (sterile inflammation).

Conditions that alert physicians that a headache may have a serious cause are listed in Table 17-2. Chronic recurrent headaches are rarely, if ever, caused by eye strain, chronic sinusitis, dental problems, food allergies, high blood pressure, or temporal mandibular joint syndrome. Headache without other neurologic signs or symptoms is rarely caused by brain tumor. Serious causes of headache in which neuroimaging findings may be negative and lead to a false sense of security are listed in Table 17-3.

- "Worst or first headache of my life" is serious.
- Headache with abnormal neurologic findings, papilledema, obscuration of vision, or diplopia is serious.
- Most of the signs and symptoms in Table 17-2 can occur with chronic benign headache (tension-migraine headache).
- Headache without other neurologic signs/symptoms is rarely caused by brain tumor.

Table 17-2.—Conditions Indicating That a Headache May Have a Serious Cause

"Worst or first headache of my life"

Headache in person not prone to headache, especially middle-aged and elderly patients

Headache associated with abnormal neurologic findings, papilledema, obscurations of vision, or diplopia

Headaches that change with different positions or increase with exertion, coughing, or sneezing

Changes in headache patterns—character, frequency, severity—in someone who has had chronic recurring headaches previously

Headaches that awaken one from sound sleep

Headaches associated with trauma

Headaches associated with systemic symptoms, e.g., fever, malaise, weight loss

Most of the above signs and symptoms may occur in chronic benign headache (e.g., tension migraine)

Table 17-3.—Serious Causes of Headache in Which Neuroimaging Findings May Be Negative

Cranial arteritis

Glaucoma

Trigeminal and glossopharyngeal neuralgia

Lesions around sella turcica

Warning leak of aneurysm

Inflammation, infection, or neoplastic invasion of leptomeninges

Cervical spondylosis

Pseudotumor cerebri

Low intracranial pressure syndromes (cerebrospinal fluid leaks)

Cluster Headache

Cluster headache, unlike migraine, predominantly affects men. Onset usually is in the late 20s but may occur at any age. The main feature of cluster headache is its periodicity. On average, the cluster period lasts 2 to 3 months and typically occurs every 1 or 2 years. Attacks occur at a frequency of 1 to 3 times daily and tend to be nocturnal in more than 50% of patients. The average period of remission is about 2 years. Cluster is not associated with an aura. The pain reaches a peak in about 10 to 15 minutes and lasts 45 to 60 minutes. It is excruciating, penetrating, usually nonthrobbing, and maximal behind the eye and in the region of the supraorbital nerve and temples. Attacks of pain are typically unilateral. The autonomic features are both sympathetic paresis and parasympathetic overreaction. They may include 1) ipsilateral lacrimation, injection of the conjunctiva, and nasal stuffiness or rhinorrhea, and 2) ptosis and miosis (ptosis may become permanent), periorbital swelling, and bradycardia. The scalp, face, and carotid artery may be tender.

- Cluster headache affects men, with onset in the 20s.
- Periodicity is the main feature.
- The cluster period lasts 2-3 months.
- Cluster is not associated with an aura.
- Pain peaks in 10-15 minutes and lasts 45-60 minutes.
- Pain is typically unilateral, excruciating, penetrating, nonthrobbing, and maximal behind the eye.
- In >50% of patients, the pain is nocturnal.
- Autonomic features are present.

1. Abortive therapy includes a) oxygen inhalation, 5 to 8 L/min for 10 minutes; b) sumatriptan, a 5-HT$_{1B/1D}$ agonist; c) dihydroergotamine (DHE); d) ergotamine, especially inhalation or suppositories; e) corticosteroids (e.g., 8 mg dexamethasone); f) local anesthesia (intranasal 4% lidocaine); and

g) capsaicin in the ipsilateral nostril. Surgical intervention may be indicated under certain circumstances for *chronic* cluster headache but never for episodic headache.

2. Prophylactic treatment is the mainstay of cluster headache treatment. Calcium channel blockers (verapamil) are widely used. The usual dose of lithium is 600 to 900 mg in divided doses. Its effectiveness is known within 1 week. Methysergide (Sansert) is most effective in the early course of the disease and least effective in later years. Ergotamine at bedtime is particularly beneficial for nocturnal attacks. Corticosteroids are helpful for short-term use, especially in patients resistant to the above drugs or to a combination of the above. The usual dose is 40 mg prednisone tapered over 3 weeks. The most effective treatment for chronic cluster headache is the combination of verapamil and lithium. Valproate may also be useful.

- Prophylactic treatment is the mainstay of treatment.
- Calcium channel blockers are widely used.
- Methysergide is effective early in the disease.
- Ergotamine is effective for nocturnal attacks.
- Corticosteroids are helpful short-term.
- The combination of verapamil and lithium is best for chronic cluster headache.

Migraine and Tension Headache

Psychologic and physical therapy and pharmacotherapy are components of a systemic approach to treating headache.

1. Abortive therapy—Abortive headache medications may range from simple analgesics to anxiolytics, nonsteroidal anti-inflammatory drugs, ergots, and steroids to major tranquilizers and narcotics. Dihydroergotamine (DHE-45) as well as sumatriptan and related 5-HT$_{1B/1D}$ receptor agonists (zolmitriptan, naratriptan, rizatriptan) are effective in aborting acute migraine attacks. DHE-45 and sumatriptan can be administered parenterally or intranasally in patients with severe nausea or vomiting. Sumatriptan is the drug of choice for management of an acute attack of cluster headache. Sumatriptan and other vasoconstrictor drugs are contraindicated in patients with migraine associated with a focal neurologic deficit and in patients with coronary artery disease.

2. Prophylactic therapy—Prophylactic medication should not be used when the attacks occur no more than 2 or 3 times per month unless they are incapacitating, associated with focal neurologic signs, or of prolonged duration. When prophylactic medication is indicated, the following should be observed:

1. Begin with a low dose and increase it slowly.
2. Perform an adequate trial of medication (1-2 months).
3. Be sure that the patient is not taking drugs that might interact with the headache agent (vasodilator, estrogens, oral contraceptives).

4. Determine that a female patient is not pregnant and that she is using effective contraception.

5. Attempt to taper and discontinue prophylactic medication after the headaches are well-controlled.

6. Avoid polypharmacy.

7. Establish a strong doctor-patient relationship; emphasize that management of headache is often a team effort, with the patient playing an equal role.

8. The best medication is *no* medication.

Drugs used for prophylaxis include antiserotonergic agents, β-blockers, calcium channel blockers, antiprostaglandins, and anticonvulsant agents. The antiserotonergic agents are methysergide, cyproheptadine (Periactin), and amitriptyline (Elavil). The most widely used β-blocker is propranolol (Inderal); others are atenolol, metoprolol, and timolol. The most useful calcium channel blocker is verapamil. Naproxen (Naprosyn and Anaprox) is the most useful antiprostaglandin medication, and valproate is the most useful anticonvulsant agent.

Nonsteroidal anti-inflammatory drugs produce analgesia through alternate pathways that do not appear to induce dependence. They may be useful in 1) migraine, both for acute attacks and prophylaxis; 2) menstrual migraine (especially naproxen); 3) benign exertional migraine and sex-induced headache (especially indomethacin [Indocin]); 4) cluster variants (chronic paroxysmal hemicrania, episodic paroxysmal hemicrania, and hemicrania continua); 5) idiopathic stabbing headache, jabs and jolts, needle-in-the-eye, and ice-pick headaches (indomethacin is often useful); 6) muscle contraction headaches; 7) mixed headaches; and 8) ergotamine-induced headache.

- Begin with a low dose.
- Give an adequate trial, 1-2 months.
- Avoid polypharmacy.
- The best medication is no medication.
- Use nonsteroidal anti-inflammatory drugs for acute attacks and prophylaxis.

Transformation/Withdrawal Syndrome

Chronic daily headache (intractable headache) may occur de novo, probably as a form of tension headache or, more important, it may be part of an evolution from periodic migraine and/or tension headache. Chronic daily headache is often accompanied by sleep disturbances, depression, anxiety, and overuse of analgesics; 90% of the patients with this disorder have a family history of headache. Episodic migraine and other episodic benign headaches can evolve into a daily refractory intense headache. This syndrome is usually due to the overuse (>2 days/week) of ergotamine tartrate, analgesics (especially analgesics combined with barbiturates), and narcotics, and perhaps even benzodiazepines. Discontinuation

of the use of these medications is necessary to control the headache. Two points have to be stressed: 1) the overuse of these medications causes daily headache, and 2) the daily use of these medications prevents other useful medications from working effectively.

The treatment of daily refractory headaches usually requires hospitalization and withdrawal of the overused medication, with repetitive intravenous administration of dihydroergotamine, together with an antiemetic drug such as metoclopramide or prochlorperazine.

Nonsteroidal anti-inflammatory drugs, β-blocker drugs, calcium channel blocker drugs, and tricyclic antidepressants do *not* cause transformation/withdrawal syndrome. Also, nonheadache patients who take large amounts of analgesics for other conditions, for example, arthritis, do *not* develop analgesic/rebound headache. Simple withdrawal from analgesics produces significant improvement in patients with chronic daily headache. A nonprescription medication can be withdrawn abruptly. However, prescription medications (ergotamine tartrate, narcotics, barbiturates) have to be withdrawn gradually. When narcotics or compounds containing codeine and ergotamine tartrate are withdrawn, clonidine may be helpful in repressing withdrawal symptoms. Some think even simple analgesics (aspirin, acetaminophen [Tylenol]) taken more than 2 days/week can cause daily headache syndrome.

- Associated with daily headache are sleep disturbances, depression, anxiety, and analgesic overuse.
- 90% of patients with chronic headache have a family history of headache.
- Migraine and other headaches can become a refractory intense headache.
- Overuse of medications causes daily headache and prevents the effective action of other drugs.
- Hospitalization and withdrawal of overused drugs are usually required.
- Nonsteroidal anti-inflammatory drugs, β-blockers, calcium channel blockers, and tricyclic antidepressants do *not* cause transformation/withdrawal syndrome.
- Significant improvement after withdrawal of analgesics.

Temporal Arteritis

In an elderly person, temporal headache of new onset and mild to moderate in severity should be considered temporal arteritis. About only 50% of these persons have headache or tender temporal arteries. Common symptoms include low-grade fever, jaw claudication, weight loss, anorexia, and other systemic symptoms. The erythrocyte sedimentation rate is consistently increased. If vision loss has already occurred, emergent therapy with corticosteroids is needed. In those who do not have vision loss, prednisone therapy should be initiated immediately after the diagnosis has been made. Temporal biopsy is used to confirm the diagnosis before prescribing prednisone long-term. However, if the biopsy cannot be performed immediately, prednisone therapy may be initiated until biopsy results are available. The erythrocyte sedimentation rate may be followed, and the prednisone dose can be tapered after several months of therapy, although longer term treatment with prednisone may be needed.

Trigeminal Neuralgia

Characteristically, trigeminal neuralgia is always on the same side and is usually in the second or third division of the trigeminal nerve. The idiopathic variety occurs in middle-aged and elderly patients and is heralded by a sharp, lancinating pain that usually has a trigger point. Chewing often precipitates trigeminal neuralgia pain, whereas swallowing often precipitates glossopharyngeal neuralgia pain.

In the elderly, trigeminal neuralgia may be due to an enlarged artery (rarely a vein) compressing the trigeminal nerve. Importantly, in idiopathic trigeminal neuralgia, the results of examining the sensory and motor functions of the trigeminal nerve should be normal when the patient is examined during an asymptomatic period. If there are signs or symptoms except pain, look for other compressive lesions, for example, neoplasm. Consider the possibility of multiple sclerosis if trigeminal neuralgia is in a young person and the pain is unilateral, bilateral, or switches from side to side. Treatment options include carbamazepine, phenytoin, baclofen, gabapentin, clonazepam, and surgical management.

- Chewing often precipitates pain in trigeminal neuralgia, as does swallowing in glossopharyngeal neuralgia.
- In idiopathic trigeminal neuralgia, there should be no other signs or symptoms when the patient is examined in an asymptomatic period.
- Consider multiple sclerosis if trigeminal neuralgia is in a young person and the pain is unilateral or bilateral or switches sides.

Glossopharyngeal Neuralgia

The pain in glossopharyngeal neuralgia is similar to that in trigeminal neuralgia, but it is in the throat and neck and often radiates to the ear. Glossopharyngeal neuralgia may cause hypotension and syncope. It is usually idiopathic but has been reported with leptomeningeal metastasis or jugular foramen syndrome (head and neck malignancies). The treatment is the same as for trigeminal neuralgia, that is, carbamazepine and, occasionally, surgical treatment.

- Glossopharyngeal pain is in the throat and neck and radiates to the ear.

Intracranial Lesions

Leptomeningeal Lesions

Inflammation, infection, or neoplastic invasion of the leptomeninges may present with similar signs and symptoms, as follows:
1. Cerebral—headache, seizures, focal neurologic signs.
2. Cranial nerve—any cranial nerve (CN) can be affected, especially CN III, IV, VI, and VII (the latter is often affected in Lyme disease).
3. Radicular (radiculoneuropathy or radiculomyelopathy)—neck and back pain as well as radicular pain and spinal cord signs.

- CN VII is often affected in Lyme disease.

Parasagittal Lesions

Because the cortical leg area and cortical control for the urinary bladder are located in the interhemispheric area, parasagittal lesions can cause spastic paraparesis with urinary problems. Meningioma is a common lesion in this area and may also be manifested by seizures and headache.

- Parasagittal lesions may cause paraparesis with urinary problems.
- Meningioma may also be manifested by seizures and headache.

Cortical Lesions

Cortical lesions lead to focal signs. If the lesions are in the dominant hemisphere, they cause language dysfunction, including reading, writing, and speaking. Cortical lesions can also impair higher cortical function, producing apraxias, agnosias, and denial of illness or body parts, and impair cortical sensation. A dense loss of primary sensation (e.g., pinprick and touch) occurs with thalamic lesions.

- Cortical lesions may produce apraxia and agnosia.
- Thalamic lesions cause loss of primary sensation (e.g., touch).

Ventricular System

Hydrocephalus

A combination of signs and symptoms—impaired mental status, gait disturbance, urinary problems—suggest hydrocephalus. If it is the obstructive type, signs of increased intracranial pressure may be present, including lethargy, nausea, vomiting, and headache; obscurations of vision are often associated with changes in position.

The following are types of hydrocephalus:

1. Communicating hydrocephalus
   a. Hydrocephalus ex vacuo—due to the loss of parenchyma, either gray or white matter, and not associated with the signs listed above (if the hydrocephalus is due to aging, the findings on neurologic examination are normal; if it is due to Alzheimer disease, clinical examination reveals signs of dementia).
   b. Normal-pressure hydrocephalus—due to decreased reabsorption of cerebrospinal fluid (CSF).
   c. Hydrocephalus due to overproduction of CSF—rare and controversial; supposedly occurs with choroid plexus lesions.
2. Obstructive (noncommunicating) hydrocephalus—due to an obstructive lesion anywhere in the ventricular system.

- Hydrocephalus ex vacuo is due to the loss of parenchyma and is not necessarily associated with impaired mental status, gait disturbance, and urinary problems.

Posterior Fossa Level

Brain Stem Lesions

Brain stem lesions can produce crossed syndromes; impairment of ocular motility; medial longitudinal fasciculus syndrome (internuclear ophthalmoplegia); rotary, horizontal, and vertical nystagmus (downbeat nystagmus is highly suggestive of a lesion at the cervicomedullary junction); ataxia; dysarthria; diplopia; vertigo; and dysphagia. Cranial nerve signs are ipsilateral to the lesion, but long-tract signs are usually contralateral (crossed syndrome).

- Downbeat nystagmus is highly suggestive of a lesion at the cervicomedullary junction.
- Cranial nerve signs are ipsilateral to the lesion.
- Long-tract signs are usually contralateral to the lesion.

Cerebellar Lesions

Problems with equilibrium and coordination suggest a cerebellar lesion. Cerebellar hemisphere lesions usually produce ipsilateral ataxia of the arm and leg. Lesions restricted to the anterior superior vermis, as in alcoholism, usually cause ataxia of gait, that is, a wide-based gait and heel-to-shin ataxia, with relative sparing of the arms, speech, and ocular motility. Lesions of the flocculonodular lobe cause marked difficulty with equilibrium and walking but not much difficulty with finger-to-nose and heel-to-shin tests if the patient is lying down.

Spinal Cord Level

Sensory levels, signs of anterior horn cell involvement (atrophy and fasciculations), and long-tract signs in the posterior columns, corticospinal tract, and spinothalamic tract suggest a spinal cord lesion. Extramedullary cord lesions are usually heralded by radicular pain. Intramedullary cord lesions are usually painless but may have an ill-described nonlocalizable pain and sensory dissociation and sacral sparing. Conus medullaris lesions are often indicated by "saddle anesthesia" and early involvement of the urinary bladder.

- Extramedullary lesions heralded by radicular pain.
- Intramedullary lesions are usually painless.
- Conus medullaris lesions are indicated by saddle anesthesia and early bladder involvement.

Spinal Cord Disease-Related Weakness

A compressive or noncompressive spinal cord lesion may cause muscle weakness. Muscle weakness associated with a spinal cord disorder typically occurs in the arm and leg if the lesion is in the cervical level or in only the leg if the lesion is below the lower cervical level. The weakness is often bilateral. Bowel and bladder difficulties and numbness are frequently noted. The findings on examination include limb weakness, spasticity, and increased reflexes below the level of the lesion. Extensor plantar reflexes may also be seen. Sensory findings are often noted.

The most common noncompressive lesion is transverse myelitis, usually of unknown cause. Some patients have a history of vaccination or symptoms suggestive of viral disease, usually preceding the neurologic symptoms by a few days to 1 or 2 weeks.

Compressive myelopathy is commonly due to metastatic epidural neoplasm. Most patients present with local vertebral column pain at the level of the spinal cord lesion. This symptom is present for weeks to months before the gross neurologic deficits, although bony pain occasionally may antedate other symptoms by only a few hours.

- Weakness is due to a compressive or noncompressive lesion.
- Transverse myelitis is the most common noncompressive lesion.

Anterior Horn Cell Disease

Degenerative disorders that affect the motor neurons in the cerebral cortex and the anterior horn cells are called "motor neuron diseases." The most common one is amyotrophic lateral sclerosis (ALS). This disorder is one of the causes of weakness. It typically presents with bilateral weakness that usually begins distally, with cramps and fasciculations. Bowel and bladder difficulties are very uncommon, and sensory abnormalities are not noted. Findings on examination include weakness, severe atrophy, fasciculations, and decreased or increased reflexes and extensor plantar responses.

A mutation in the oxygen radical detoxifying enzyme, superoxide dismutase, can cause a familial form of ALS. However, no drug has been found to be effective in altering the progressive course of this disease. Recently, some beneficial effect has been noted with riluzole, especially in patients with bulbar onset of the disease. However, treating ALS with immunosuppression such as irradiation, corticosteroids, cyclophosphamide, or intravenous immunoglobulin (IVIG) is at best futile and at worst, costly and harmful. However, treatment for multifocal motor neuropathy with cyclophosphamide or perhaps IVIG can be effective. This is a syndrome of purely lower motor neuron disease. It is often distal and asymmetrical, accompanied by motor conduction block on electromyography (EMG), and is associated with high titers of serum antibodies to GM_1 gangliosides. However, antibody determinations are costly and have no therapeutic implication. Therefore, patients with purely lower motor neuron disease accompanied by the presence of conduction block on EMG should receive treatment with cyclophosphamide or IVIG.

Peripheral Level

Radiculopathy

Nerve root lesions are usually indicated by root pain that is often sharp and lancinating, follows a dermatomal pattern, and is increased by increasing intraspinal pressure (e.g., sneezing and coughing) or by stretching of the nerve root. Pain often follows a myotomal (e.g., C5 and 6 root pain in the deltoid and biceps muscles) rather than a dermatomal pattern, with paresthesias in the dermatomal pattern. Findings are in the root distribution and include weakness, sensory impairment, and decreased muscle stretch reflexes. Radiculopathies have many causes, including compressive lesions (osteophytes, ruptured disks, and neoplasms) and noncompressive ones (postinfectious and inflammatory radiculopathies and metabolic radiculopathies, as in diabetes).

- Nerve root lesions are indicated by sharp, lancinating root pain with a dermatomal pattern.
- Pain is increased by sneezing and coughing.
- Pain often has a myotomal rather than a dermatomal pattern.
- Findings are weakness, sensory impairment, and decreased muscle stretch reflexes.
- Radiculopathies have many causes.

Neuropathy

Peripheral neuropathies are usually indicated by distal weakness and distal sensory changes, usually symmetrical, more often in the legs than in the arms, and often accompanied by loss of or impaired distal muscle stretch reflexes. Neuropathy has many causes (Table 17-4), and an extensive search usually uncovers the cause in 70% to 80% of cases. A high percentage of the cases of "idiopathic neuropathy" referred to specialty centers are in fact hereditary neuropathies.

- Peripheral neuropathy: distal weakness and sensory changes more in the legs than in the arms, usually symmetrical, and absent or impaired distal muscle stretch reflexes.
- Cause of peripheral neuropathy is usually found in 70%-80% of cases.

The pattern of the neuropathy might suggest its cause.

Mononeuropathy

Mononeuropathy (impairment of a single nerve) is usually due to compression, as in compressive ulnar neuropathy at the elbow, compressive median neuropathy in the carpal tunnel, and compression of the peroneal nerve as it winds around the fibula. Mononeuropathy multiplex (asymmetrical involvement of several nerves) suggests such causes as trauma or compression, diabetes mellitus, vasculitis with or without connective tissue disease, leprosy, Lyme disease, sarcoidosis, tumor infiltration, or hereditary liability to pressure palsies.

- The pattern of neuropathy suggests its cause.
- Mononeuropathy multiplex: diabetes, vasculitis, leprosy, sarcoidosis, Lyme disease.
- Neuropathy with autonomic dysfunction: amyloidosis, diabetes, Guillain-Barré syndrome, porphyria, familial neuropathy.

Motor Neuropathy

Predominantly motor polyneuropathy suggests acute or chronic inflammatory demyelinating polyneuropathy (AIDP

Table 17-4.—Diseases Most Commonly Affecting Peripheral Nerves

Diabetes mellitus
Alcohol
Nutritional
Guillain-Barré syndrome
Trauma
Hereditary
Environmental toxins and drugs
Rheumatic (collagen vascular)
Amyloidosis
Paraneoplastic syndrome
Infectious disease
Systemic diseases
Tumors

or CIDP), hereditary neuropathy, osteosclerotic myeloma, porphyria, lead or organophosphate poisoning, or hypoglycemia. Most neuropathies are distal, but occasionally there is predominant proximal weakness, which suggests AIDP, CIDP, porphyria, diabetic proximal motor neuropathy, or idiopathic acute brachial plexopathy. Plasma exchange is the treatment preferred for acute inflammatory demyelinating polyradiculopathy (Guillain-Barré syndrome), although IVIG may become the preferred treatment. In sharp contrast to AIDP, the case for steroids in CIDP is strong; plasma exchange is also effective, and corticosteroids alone or in combination with plasma exchange remain the treatment of choice. IVIG might be beneficial to some patients.

Sensory Neuropathy

Predominantly sensory polyneuropathy suggests diabetes, cancer, Sjögren syndrome, dysproteinemias, acquired immunodeficiency syndrome (AIDS), vitamin B_{12} deficiency, cisplatin toxicity, vitamin B_6 excess, or hereditary neuropathy. More than 60% of neuropathies associated with monoclonal gammopathy of undetermined significance (MGUS) are idiopathic, but some are associated with multiple myeloma, amyloidosis, lymphoma, and leukemia. The patients are usually older than 50 years and present early with symmetrical sensory radiculoneuropathy. Later, a motor polyradiculoneuropathy develops, involving mostly the legs. CSF protein is usually increased; IgM is more common than IgG or IgA. Plasma exchange can be effective therapy in patients with IgG or IgA neuropathy. They have a better response than those with IgM neuropathy. Other immunosuppressive therapy such as IVIG may also be effective.

- Motor polyneuropathy: inflammatory demyelinating polyneuropathy, hereditary neuropathy, osteosclerotic myeloma, porphyria, lead poisoning, organophosphate toxicity, hypoglycemia.
- Sensory polyneuropathy: diabetes, cancer, Sjögren syndrome, dysproteinemias, HIV infection, vitamin B_{12} deficiency, cisplatin toxicity, vitamin B_6 excess, hereditary neuropathy.

Diabetic Neuropathy

Diabetes mellitus causes CN III neuropathy, usually including sudden diplopia, eye pain, impairment of the muscles supplied by CN III, and relative sparing of the pupil. With compressive CN III lesions, the pupil usually is involved early. Painful diabetic neuropathies include CN III neuropathy, acute thoracoabdominal neuropathy (truncal), acute distal sensory neuropathy, acute lumbar radiculoplexopathy, and chronic distal small fiber neuropathy.

- Diabetes causes CN III neuropathy.
- Pupil is involved early in compression of CN III.

Autonomic Neuropathy

Neuropathy with autonomic dysfunction (e.g., orthostatic hypertension, urinary bladder and bowel dysfunction, and impotency) suggests amyloidosis, diabetes, Guillain-Barré syndrome, porphyria, or familial neuropathy.

Acute pandysautonomia is a heterogenous, monophasic, usually self-limiting disease involving both the sympathetic and parasympathetic nervous systems. It may produce orthostatic hypotension, anhydrosis, diarrhea, constipation, urinary bladder atony, and impotence. The syndrome usually evolves over a few days to a few months, with recovery usually being prolonged and partial. This may be an immunologic disorder, but it is indistinguishable from paraneoplastic autonomic neuropathy. Some of these patients may have antibodies against the ganglion-type nicotinic acetylcholine receptor. IVIG treatment limits the duration and reduces the long-term disability for patients with acute pandysautonomia.

Peripheral Nerve Disease-Related Weakness

Weakness related to peripheral nerve disorders typically is worse distally, with foot drop and clumsy gait often associated with distal numbness and paresthesias. Examination findings include distal weakness, sensory loss, atrophy, and, sometimes, fasciculations. Reflexes usually are decreased. If a single plexus (lumbosacral or brachial) is involved, the weakness may be isolated to a single limb. However, the findings still are consistent with a "lower motor neuron" lesion, with decreased reflexes, weakness, atrophy, and sensory loss.

Guillain-Barré Syndrome

About 50% of patients typically have a mild respiratory or gastrointestinal tract infection 1 to 3 weeks before neurologic symptoms. In the other patients, the syndrome may be preceded by surgery, viral exanthems, or vaccinations. Also, the syndrome may develop in patients with autoimmune disease or lymphoreticular malignancies. This syndrome has no particular seasonal, age, or sex predilection.

Acute Intermittent Porphyria

Patients are prone to have severe, rapidly progressive, symmetrical polyneuropathy with or without psychosis, delirium, confusion, and convulsions. In most patients, weakness is most pronounced in the proximal muscles.

Tick Paralysis

This is a rapid, progressive ascending motor weakness caused by neurotoxin injected by the female wood tick. It occurs endemically in the southeastern and northwestern U.S.

After an asymptomatic period (about 1 week), symptoms develop, usually with leg weakness.

Diabetic Neuropathy

Acute or subacute muscle weakness can occur in various forms of diabetic neuropathy. Weakness, atrophy, and pain affect the pelvic girdle and thigh muscles (asymmetrical or unilateral—diabetic amyotrophy). In the second form, elderly diabetic patients have bilateral proximal and pelvic girdle weakness, wasting, weight loss, and autonomic dysfunction.

- In Guillain-Barré syndrome, 50% of patients have mild respiratory or gastrointestinal tract infection 1-3 weeks before neurologic symptoms.
- Surgery, viral exanthems, or vaccinations may precede Guillain-Barré syndrome.

Neuromuscular Junction Lesions

Lesions of the neuromuscular junction are often missed clinically. Drugs may cause problems at myoneural junctions, for example, penicillamine can cause a syndrome that looks like myasthenia gravis. Three major clinical syndromes of the myoneural junction are myasthenia gravis, botulism, and myasthenic syndrome, described below.

Myasthenia Gravis

This is usually seen in young women and older men and is often heralded by such cranial nerve findings as diplopia, dysarthria, dysphagia, and dyspnea. The deficits are usually fatigable, worsening with repetition or late in the day. However, muscle stretch reflexes, sensation, mentation, and sphincter function are normal. Because of remissions and exacerbations in this disease, patients often are considered "hysterical." Treatment strategies for myasthenia gravis include anticholinesterase, corticosteroids, azathioprine, cyclosporine, cyclophosphamide, plasma exchange, thymectomy, and IVIG. Older patients particularly derive the most benefit from azathioprine, especially when used as a steroid-sparing drug.

Botulism

This should be suspected when more than one person has a syndrome that looks like myasthenia gravis or when one person has abdominal and gastrointestinal symptoms preceding a syndrome that looks like myasthenia gravis. Botulism occurs after the ingestion of improperly canned vegetables, fruit, meat, or fish contaminated by exotoxin of *C. botulinum*. Paralysis is caused by toxin-mediated inhibition of acetylcholine release from axon terminals at the neuromuscular junction. Although an antitoxin is available, treatment is mainly supportive, especially respiratory but also psychological, because the signs and symptoms are reversible.

Myasthenic Syndrome, or the Lambert-Eaton Syndrome

There is often proximal weakness in the legs and decreased or absent muscle stretch reflexes (sometimes, reflexes are elicited after brief exercise). This syndrome is usually seen in middle-aged men, who often have such vague complaints as diplopia, impotency, urinary dysfunction, paresthesias, mouth dryness, and other autonomic dysfunctions (orthostatic hypotension). Lambert-Eaton syndrome is often associated with small cell lung carcinoma.

- Neuromuscular junction lesions are often missed clinically.
- Botulism: suspect it if more than one person has a syndrome that looks like myasthenia gravis.
- Onset of myasthenia gravis: diplopia, dysarthria, dysphagia, dyspnea, fatigability, often in young women and older men.
- In myasthenic syndrome, there is proximal weakness of the legs and decreased/absent muscle stretch reflexes.
- Myasthenic syndrome occurs in middle-aged men, who have vague complaints of diplopia, impotency, urinary dysfunction, and dry mouth.
- Myasthenic syndrome is often associated with small cell carcinoma.

Neuromuscular Junction Disease-Related Weakness

Weakness related to neuromuscular junction disorders presents as fluctuating weakness, with fatigable weakness in the limbs, eyelids (ptosis), tongue and palate (dysarthria and dysphagia), and extraocular muscles (diplopia). Sensation, muscle tone, and reflexes are typically normal except in myasthenic syndrome, in which the weakness is more constant and reflexes are diminished.

Organophosphate Toxicity

This causes the characteristic combination of miosis, excessive bodily secretions, and fasciculations. A key pathophysiologic factor is decreased acetylcholinesterase activity that causes excessive acetylcholine at the myoneural junction. The onset of symptoms varies from 5 minutes to 12 hours after exposure. The treatment is atropine.

- Ingestion of the exotoxin of *C. botulinum* causes botulism.
- Acetylcholine release is inhibited at the neuromuscular junction.
- In organophosphate toxicity, decreased acetylcholinesterase activity causes excessive acetylcholine at the neuromuscular junction.
- Atropine is the treatment for organophosphate toxicity.

Muscle Disease

Muscle disease is usually indicated by symmetrical proximal weakness (legs more than arms) and weakness of neck flexors and, occasionally, of smooth muscle and cardiac muscle. Other neurologic findings are normal. Muscle stretch reflexes are usually normal early in muscle disease.

Muscle disease may be acquired disease or progressive hereditary disease. "Myopathy" is a general term for muscle disease. If the disease is progressive and familial, it is called "dystrophy."

Two exceptions to proximal weakness in myopathy are the following:

1. Unusual distal myopathy, called "distal myopathy," occurs mainly in Scandinavian countries.
2. Myotonic dystrophy is more common and occurs everywhere. Atrophy and weakness begin distally and in the face and especially in the sternocleidomastoid muscles. An interesting feature of this dystrophy is myotonia, which is normal contraction of muscle with slow relaxation. Test for myotonia by striking the thenar eminence with a reflex hammer. Test the myotonia by shaking the patient's hand and noting that the patient cannot let go quickly.

In evaluating acquired myopathy such as inflammatory myopathy, look for the underlying cause, which often is not found in adults. There probably is an increased incidence of occult carcinomas in patients with dermatomyositis. Other important underlying causes of myopathies include collagen vascular disease, endocrinopathies (especially thyroid disease), sarcoidosis, or remote nonmetastatic effects of cancer.

Prednisone, azathioprine, and methotrexate are the standard treatments for polymyositis, dermatomyositis, and inclusion-body myositis, although the latter rarely responds to treatment. Inclusion-body myositis is seen mainly in men older than 60 years, with symmetrical weakness of proximal and distal muscles. At times, there is asymmetrical weakness, and at other times, there is a greater predominance of distal muscle involvement. Inclusion-body myositis is not associated with collagen vascular disease or neoplasms, and the creatine kinase level may be normal or slightly increased.

- In early muscle disease, stretch reflexes are normal.
- Muscle disease is "myopathy."
- If the disease is progressive and familial, it is called "dystrophy."
- Distal myopathy is unusual and occurs mainly in Scandinavia.
- Myotonic dystrophy—atrophy and weakness in the face and sternocleidomastoid muscles.
- Myotonia (normal contraction, slow relaxation) is a feature of myotonic dystrophy.
- With myotonia, the patient cannot let go quickly after a handshake.
- Acquired myopathy: no underlying cause is found in most adults.

- Increased incidence of occult carcinomas in patients with dermatomyositis.
- Causes of myopathies: collagen vascular disease, endocrinopathy, sarcoidosis, and remote nonmetastatic effects of cancer.

A classification of myopathies is given in Table 17-5.

Muscle Disease-Related Weakness

Muscle disease-related weakness typically presents as proximal greater than distal weakness, with difficulty arising from a chair or raising the arms over the head. On examination, sensation and muscle tone are normal and reflexes are affected only late. In most disorders, weakness is most prominent proximally.

Polymyalgia Rheumatica

It affects elderly patients, with aching or pain and stiffness in the neck, upper back, shoulders, upper arms, and hip girdle. Systemic symptoms include various degrees of fever, anorexia, weight loss, apathy, and depression. True muscle weakness is not present except when attributed to pain. This syndrome is sometimes associated with cranial arteritis.

Acute Alcoholic Myopathy

There is acute pain, swelling, tenderness, and weakness of mainly proximal muscles. Gross myoglobinuria may cause renal failure.

Table 17-5.—Classification of Myopathies

Dystrophies
Nonprogressive or relatively nonprogressive congenital myopathies
Inflammatory myopathies
    Infectious and viral—toxoplasmosis, trichinosis
    Granulomatous—sarcoidosis
    Idiopathic—polymyositis, dermatomyositis
    With collagen vascular disease
Metabolic myopathies
    Glycogenoses
    Mitochondrial disorders
    Endocrine
    Periodic paralyses
    Toxic—emetine, chloroquine, vincristine, lovastatin, and other HMG-CoA reductase inhibitors
    Paroxysmal rhabdomyolysis
Miscellaneous

HMG-CoA, hydroxymethylglutaryl-CoA.

Toxic Myopathies

Lovastatin and other hydroxymethylglutaryl CoA (HMG-CoA) inhibitors may produce an acute necrotizing myopathy characterized by myalgia, weakness, myoglobinuria, and a marked increase in creatine kinase. This toxic effect is potentiated by other cholesterol-lowering agents, such as fibric acid derivatives, and cyclosporine.

Electrolyte Imbalance

Severe hypokalemia (<2.5 mEq/L) or hyperkalemia (>7 mEq/L) produces muscle weakness, as do hyper- and hypocalcemia and hypophosphatemia. Familial periodic paralysis of hypo-, hyper-, or normokalemic-type episodes of acute paralysis last 2 to 24 hours and can be precipitated by a large carbohydrate meal or strenuous exercise; cranial or respiratory muscle paralysis is rare.

Endocrine Diseases

Hyper- and hypothyroidism, hyper- and hypoadrenalism, acromegaly, and primary and secondary hyperparathyroidism cause muscle weakness.

Causes of acute muscle weakness are summarized in Table 17-6.

● Polymyalgia rheumatica: an elderly patient with aching/pain and stiffness of the neck, upper back, shoulders, upper arms, and hip girdle.
● No true muscle weakness, but fever, anorexia, and weight loss.
● Gross myoglobinuria often occurs in acute alcoholic myopathy.

GENERAL PRINCIPLES OF NEUROLOGIC DIAGNOSTIC TESTING

CT and MRI

Vascular Diseases

CT is a good initial test in evaluating suspected TIA or stroke and is superior to MRI in identifying acute hemorrhage in brain parenchyma or the subarachnoid space. Subacute and chronic intracerebral hemorrhages are better defined by MRI, which is usually the first neuroimaging test to reveal abnormalities during the evolution of an ischemic cerebral infarct. CT (even with contrast enhancement) often gives equivocal or negative results in the first 24 to 48 hours after an ischemic cerebral infarct. In subacute and chronic stages of an ischemic cerebral infarct, MRI and CT give equivalent information. Vasculitic lesions or microinfarcts, as in such diseases as systemic lupus erythematosus, are often seen on MRI but missed on CT.

Table 17-6.—Important Causes of Acute Muscle Weakness

Spinal cord disease
    Transverse myelitis
    Epidural abscess
    Extradural tumor
    Epidural hematoma
    Herniated intervertebral disk
    Spinal cord tumor
Peripheral nerve disease
    Guillain-Barré syndrome
    Acute intermittent porphyria
    Arsenic poisoning
    Toxic neuropathies
    Tick paralysis
Neuromuscular junction disease
    Myasthenia gravis
    Botulism
    Organophosphate poisoning
Muscle disease
    Polymyositis
    Rhabdomyolysis-myoglobinuria
    Acute alcoholic myopathy
    Electrolyte imbalances
    Endocrine disease

From Karkal SS: Rapid accurate appraisal of acute muscular weakness. Updates Neurology 1991; pp 31-39. By permission of American Health Consultants.

Magnetic resonance angiography (MRA) is not invasive but not yet ready to replace regular angiography. Cerebral angiography is still the reference standard for evaluating the cerebral vasculature for ischemic cerebrovascular disease and hemorrhagic cerebrovascular disease (aneurysm, vascular malformation).

● For acute hemorrhage in the brain and subarachnoid space, CT is better than MRI.
● During an evolving ischemic cerebral infarct, MRI is best.
● CT scan with contrast is not useful in the first 24-48 hours after ischemic cerebral infarct.
● For subacute and chronic stages of ischemic cerebral infarct, CT and MRI are equivalent.

Trauma

MRI is competitive with but not comparable to CT for assessing the brain after craniocerebral trauma. During the first 1 to 3 days after injury, CT is preferable because the examination time is shorter and hemorrhage at this time is more reliably demonstrated by CT. Standard radiographic examination or CT is necessary to evaluate skull fractures because bone cortex is not visualized with MRI.

CT is highly dependable for subdural hematomas, which are also visualized with MRI. Coronal MRI sections are usually best for the size, shape, location, and extent of subdural hematomas.

- For the first 1-3 days after trauma, CT is best because it is more reliable for demonstrating hemorrhage.
- Radiography and CT are needed to evaluate skull fractures.
- CT is very dependable for showing subdural hematomas.

Intracranial Tumors

A wide spectrum of intracranial tumors is visualized with MRI and CT. MRI often shows more extensive involvement than CT, especially in low-grade gliomas or metastasis. CT is superior to MRI in detecting meningiomas. MRI is far superior to CT for identifying all types of posterior fossa tumors. It is the study of choice for identifying brain stem gliomas.

- MRI is superior to CT for posterior fossa tumors and brain stem gliomas.

White Matter Lesions

MRI is superior to CT in detecting abnormalities in the white matter. MRI is far superior to CT for identifying multiple sclerosis lesions and for assessing patients with isolated optic neuritis. MRI shows that Binswanger disease may be a common cause of adult-onset dementia (along with multi-infarct dementia). White matter changes in the elderly must be interpreted carefully because most of them have white matter changes on MRI.

- Most normal elderly people have white matter changes on MRI.

Cervical Cord

A wide spectrum of lesions at the cervicomedullary junction and in the cervical spinal cord can be seen clearly with MRI because of the ability to make direct sagittal and coronal sections. MRI is the study of choice for assessing cervicomedullary and cervical spinal cord regions. Generally, MRI is best for identifying intramedullary and extramedullary lesions of the spinal cord.

- MRI is best for assessing cervicomedullary and cervical spinal cord regions and intra- and extramedullary cord tumors.

Dementia

In assessing dementia, either CT or MRI can be used to demonstrate remedial lesions. MRI shows more lesions than CT in multi-infarct dementia. MRI has *not* exceeded CT in assessing dementia.

- For dementia, CT and MRI are equivalent.
- In multi-infarct dementia, MRI shows more lesions.

Disk Disease

Protruding disks are seen well on MRI sagittal sections, showing the relationship to the spine and nerve roots. MRI is equal to CT myelography in evaluating herniated disks at cervical and thoracic levels, but at the lumbar level, MRI is better than or equal to CT. In spinal stenosis, MRI and CT are roughly equal and less invasive than myelography.

CT myelography has greatest diagnostic accuracy for cervical radiculopathy due to hypertrophic degenerative changes. Bony spicules impinging on nerve roots are not directly shown by MRI, which may replace myelography for cervical and lumbar disease. Often, CT myelography is needed in defining surgical problems.

- MRI sagittal sections show protruding disks.
- For cervical and thoracic herniated disks, MRI is the same as CT myelography.
- CT myelography is best for cervical radiculopathy due to hypertrophic degenerative changes.
- CT myelography is often needed for defining surgical problems.

Electromyographic Nerve Conduction Velocity Studies

EMG studies should be performed by experts familiar with the intricacies of the procedure and who know its value and limitations. EMG tests are excellent for eliciting motor unit problems and, thus, are valuable in diseases of the anterior horn cell, nerve root, peripheral nerve, neuromuscular junction, and muscle. These tests are an extension of the neurologic examination, helping to localize and better define further diagnostic studies.

- EMG should be performed by experts.
- EMG is valuable for motor unit problems—anterior horn cell, nerve root, neuromuscular junction, and muscle.

Electroencephalography

The main use of EEG is the study of seizure disorders, but EEG is specific in only a few forms of epilepsy, such as petit mal epilepsy. Seizure disorder is a clinical diagnosis and *not* an EEG diagnosis, and a normal EEG does *not* rule out a seizure disorder. EEG has many nonspecific patterns that should not be over-interpreted.

Ambulatory EEG is available for detecting frequent unusual spells. EEG telemetry with videomonitoring is good for defining epileptic surgical candidates, nonepileptic spells (pseudoseizures), and unusual seizures. EEG is imperative in diagnosing nonconvulsive status epilepticus.

- EEG is specific in only a few forms of epilepsy.
- Seizure disorder is a clinical, not an EEG, diagnosis.
- Normal EEG does not rule out seizure disorder.
- EEG telemetry is good for defining epileptic surgical candidates, nonepileptic spells, and unusual seizures.

EEG is valuable for evaluating various encephalopathies. Many drugs cause an unusual fast pattern, and most metabolic encephalopathies cause a diffuse slow or triphasic pattern. Diffuse slow patterns also are seen in diffuse cerebral disease (Alzheimer disease). Unusual high-amplitude slow-and-spike activity helps define Creutzfeldt-Jakob disease and subacute sclerosing panencephalitis. EEG is often valuable in infectious encephalopathies (herpes simplex encephalitis).

EEG is essential for diagnosing various sleep disorders and is an *adjuvant* tool in diagnosing brain death. Remember, brain death is a clinical diagnosis. EEG is a monitoring device in surgery (during carotid endarterectomy).

At 6 hours or more after a hypoxic insult, the EEG indicates the likelihood of neurologic recovery. Poor outcome is seen with "alpha" coma, burst suppression, periodic patterns, and electrocerebral silence.

- EEG is valuable in infectious encephalopathies (herpes simplex encephalitis).
- EEG is an adjuvant tool in diagnosing brain death.
- Brain death is a clinical diagnosis.

Evoked Potentials

Evoked potentials indicate the intactness of various pathways: visual evoked potentials, somatosensory evoked potentials, brain stem auditory evoked potentials, and motor evoked potentials. Generally, these tests are not a practical clinical tool. They are excellent monitoring devices for spinal surgery and posterior fossa surgery (monitoring cranial nerve function intraoperatively). Also, they may help substantiate nonorganic disease, for example, hysterical paraplegia or hysterical blindness.

- Evoked potentials help substantiate nonorganic disease (hysterical paraplegia, hysterical blindness).

Lumbar Puncture and CSF Analysis

Perform lumbar puncture only after a thorough clinical evaluation and serious consideration of the potential value versus the hazards of the procedure.

Indicaindions for Lumbar Puncture

Urgent lumbar puncture is performed for suspected acute meningitis, encephalitis, or subarachnoid hemorrhage (unless preceding CT indicates otherwise) and for fever (even without meningeal signs) in infancy, acute confusional states, and immunocompromised patients. Another indication for lumbar puncture is unexplained dementia.

Multiple sclerosis is also an indication for lumbar puncture. If the cell count is greater than 100, look for another disease (e.g., sarcoidosis). Although IgG synthesis is increased, this is nonspecific. The demonstration of oligoclonal bands is useful, but they occur in other inflammatory diseases of the CNS. Myelin basic protein is not clinically useful.

Lumbar puncture is used to record CSF pressure. High pressure is seen in pseudotumor cerebri. Low pressure is seen in positional headache and CSF leak.

Lumbar puncture is indicated in infectious disease: AIDS, Lyme disease, and any suspected acute, subacute, or chronic infection (viral, bacterial, fungal). It is also indicated in paraneoplastic syndromes: 1) Hu and Yo antibodies to cerebellar Purkinje cells in paraneoplastic cerebellar degeneration, 2) neuronal antinuclear antibodies in subacute sensory neuronopathy and sensory neuropathy, and 3) retinal antibodies in paraneoplastic retinopathy.

Other indications for lumbar puncture are meningeal carcinomatosis, certain neuropathies (Guillain-Barré syndrome, AIDP, and CIDP), and gliomatosis cerebri.

There is *no* difference in headache frequency after immediate mobilization compared with 4 hours of bed rest after lumbar puncture; post-spinal headache is dependent on the size of the needle used and the leakage of CSF through a dural rent.

Contraindications for Lumbar Puncture

Suppuration in the skin and deeper tissues overlying the spinal canal and anticoagulation therapy or bleeding diathesis are contraindications. A minimum of 1 or 2 hours should elapse after lumbar puncture before beginning heparin therapy. If the platelet count is less than 20,000, transfuse platelets before the procedure.

Increased intracranial pressure is a contraindication. Lumbar puncture is dangerous when papilledema is due to an intracranial mass, but it is safe (and has been used therapeutically) in pseudotumor cerebri. In complete spinal block, lumbar puncture may aggravate the signs of spinal cord disease.

- Perform lumbar puncture only after a thorough clinical evaluation.
- Increased IgG synthesis is nonspecific.
- High CSF pressure in pseudotumor cerebri.
- Low CSF pressure in positional headache and CSF leak.

- Lumbar puncture is dangerous when an intracranial mass is present with or without papilledema.
- Lumbar puncture is safe in pseudotumor cerebri.
- Lumbar puncture aggravates the signs of spinal cord disease in complete spinal block.

PART II

SPECIFIC ENTITIES

SEIZURE DISORDERS

- "Seizures" refer to electroclinical events, and "epilepsy" indicates a tendency for recurrent seizures.

A classification of seizures is given in Table 17-7.

The proper treatment of epilepsy includes accurate diagnosis of the seizure type, identification of the cause (if possible), and management of psychosocial problems. The EEG can be important in deciding whether to treat a first unprovoked seizure. There is a high risk of recurrent seizures if the initial EEG shows epileptiform activity, and there is a low risk of recurrent seizures if two EEGs (one of them sleep-deprived) are normal.

Causes

Seizures occur at any age, but 70% to 90% of all epileptic patients have their first seizure before age 20. Both the cause and the type of epilepsy are related to age at onset. However, the cause may not be found in many patients. Neonatal seizures are often due to congenital defects or prenatal injury, and head trauma is often the cause of focal seizures in young adults. Brain tumors and vascular disease are major known causes of seizures in later life. Seizures often occur during withdrawal from alcohol, barbiturates, and benzodiazepines in young and old adults. Also, seizures occur during the acute use of such drugs as cocaine, usually in young adults. Metabolic derangements (e.g., hypoglycemia, hypocalcemia, hypo- and hypernatremia) can occur at any age, as can infections (e.g., meningitis, encephalitis). Metabolic abnormalities usually cause primary generalized tonic-clonic seizures and rarely focal or multifocal seizures. CNS infections usually cause partial and secondary generalized tonic-clonic seizures.

Pseudoseizures (psychogenic, nonepileptic) are sudden changes in behavior or mentation not associated with any physiologic cause or abnormal paroxysmal discharge of electrical activity from the brain. They are often the cause in so-called intractable seizures. Effective treatment remains elusive. A favorable outcome may be associated with an independent lifestyle, the absence of coexisting epilepsy, and a formal psychologic approach to therapy.

Anticonvulsant Blood Levels

Anticonvulsant blood levels are readily available and help attain best seizure control. It is extremely important to remember that therapeutic levels represent an average bell-shaped curve and that patients with well-controlled seizures are included under the bell-shaped curve. Many patients with levels below or above the therapeutic levels do well. The anticonvulsant dose should *never* be changed on the basis of blood levels alone. Remember, toxicity is a clinical, *not* a laboratory, phenomenon.

- Therapeutic levels represent an average bell-shaped curve.
- Anticonvulsant dose should never be changed on the basis of blood levels alone.
- Toxicity is a clinical, not a laboratory, phenomenon.
- 70%-90% of epileptic patients have their first seizure before age 20.
- The cause and type of epilepsy are related to age at onset.
- Head trauma is the cause of focal seizures in young adults.
- Brain tumors and vascular disease are major causes of seizures in older persons.

Table 17-7.—Classification of Seizures

Partial (focal) seizures
    Simple partial seizures
        Partial simple sensory
        Partial simple motor
        Partial simple special sensory (unusual smells or tastes)
        Speech arrest or unusual vocalizations
    Complex partial seizures
        Consciousness impaired at onset
        Simple partial onset followed by impaired consciousness
    Evolving to generalized tonic-clonic convulsions (secondary generalized tonic-clonic seizures)
        Simple evolving to generalized tonic-clonic
        Complex evolving to generalized tonic-clonic (including those with simple partial onset)
    True auras—are actually simple partial seizures
Generalized seizures—convulsive or nonconvulsive (primary generalized seizures—generalized from onset)
    Absence and atypical absence
    Myoclonic
    Clonic
    Tonic
    Tonic-clonic
    Atonic
Unclassified epileptic seizures (includes some neonatal seizures)

- Seizures occur with withdrawal from alcohol, barbiturates, and benzodiazepines.
- Seizures occur during acute use of cocaine (young adults).
- Pseudoseizures are often the basis for so-called intractable seizures.

Status Epilepticus

This is a medical emergency and a life-threatening condition. The seizure is prolonged, lasting more than 15 to 30 minutes, or there are repetitive seizures, without recovery in between. Follow the ABCs of cardiopulmonary resuscitation or trauma: **A**irway, **B**reathing, and **C**irculation. Draw a blood sample for glucose, electrolytes, BUN, and so forth. Give 50 mL of 50% dextrose with 100 mg thiamine intravenously. Slow intravenous administration of diazepam or lorazepam can be initiated. (Midazolam can also be useful, and it can be effective given intramuscularly.) You can begin with a loading dose of phenytoin or phenobarbital. If starting with benzodiazepine, then you have to go to a long-acting anticonvulsant, for example, fosphenytoin, phenytoin, or phenobarbital. Agents available include fosphenytoin, a phenytoin pro-drug. Fosphenytoin may be used either intravenously or intramuscularly. The dosage is expressed in phenytoin equivalents (if the dose of phenytoin for a particular patient would be 1,000 mg, the dose of fosphenytoin is the same but expressed as phenytoin equivalents). The recommended rate for status epilepticus is 100 to 150 mg of phenytoin equivalent per minute, which is faster than used with intravenous phenytoin. If the patient is not in status epilepticus, slower rates may be used. The dosage may also be given intramuscularly. Cardiorespiratory monitoring is required if rapid infusion with fosphenytoin is used, just as it would be with intravenous phenytoin. Other agents include phenytoin, 18 to 20 mg/kg (50 mg/minute), and phenobarbital, 10 to 20 mg/kg (100 mg/minute). Consider general anesthesia or barbiturate coma if these fail.

The most common causes of status epilepticus include withdrawal of anticonvulsant agent, alcohol and "recreational" drug toxicity, and CNS infection.

Medications for status epilepticus are outlined in Table 17-8.

Nonconvulsive status epilepticus may cause an acute confusional state or stupor and coma, especially in the elderly. EEG is a valuable diagnostic tool in these cases because nonconvulsive status epilepticus must be treated as quickly and vigorously as convulsive status epilepticus.

- Status epilepticus is life-threatening and a medical emergency.
- The seizure lasts >15-30 minutes or there are repetitive seizures without recovery.

- Give 50 mL of 50% dextrose with 100 mg thiamine intravenously.
- Slow intravenous administration of diazepam or lorazepam.
- You can begin with a loading dose of fosphenytoin, phenytoin, or phenobarbital.
- Cardiorespiratory monitoring is required if rapid infusion with fosphenytoin, as with phenytoin.

Anticonvulsant Therapy

Monotherapy is the treatment of choice, increasing the dose of the drug as high as necessary and as much as can be tolerated. The coadministration of antiepileptic drugs has *not* been proved to have more antiseizure efficacy than one drug without concurrently increasing toxicity. For a large population, one drug may be shown more efficacious and less toxic, but for a given patient, an alternate drug may be more effective or have fewer side effects.

Neurologic side effects of anticonvulsants include sedation (phenobarbital, benzodiazepines), cerebellar ataxia (phenytoin), diplopia (carbamazepine), tremor (valproate), and chorea or myoclonus (phenytoin, carbamazepine). Idiosyncratic side effects include rash (phenytoin, phenobarbital, carbamazepine, lamotrigine), bone marrow suppression (carbamazepine, valproate, felbamate), and liver toxicity (phenytoin, carbamazepine, valproate). Some anticonvulsants produce specific side effects. Phenytoin produces gum hypertrophy, hirsutism, folate deficiency, and predisposition to osteoporosis. Carbamazepine may produce hyponatremia due to inappropriate secretion of antidiuretic hormone (particularly in the elderly), and it poses the risk of cardiac blockade. Valproate produces alopecia and weight gain. Topiramate increases the risk of the development of kidney stones.

With enzyme-inducing antiepileptic drugs (e.g., carbamazepine, phenobarbital, phenytoin, primidone), oral contraceptives may be less effective in preventing pregnancy. Valproate does not cause enzyme induction and may be optimal for women using oral contraceptives.

There are special issues when dealing with epilepsy in pregnancy. Seizure control is best done with monotherapy, using the lowest possible dose of anticonvulsant and monitoring levels. There is a risk of fetal hemorrhage if the mother is taking phenytoin, phenobarbital, or carbamazepine. This risk can be minimized by the administration of vitamin K to the mother before delivery and to the fetus at delivery. Phenytoin, carbamazepine, primidone, and phenobarbital can all cause teratogenic abnormalities. In general, multiple drugs at high doses are associated with a greater frequency of anomalies. Valproate (and probably carbamazepine) can cause failure of midline structures to close (neural tube defects). Folic acid should also be given to the mother prenatally to prevent neural tube defects.

Table 17-8.—Medications for Status Epilepticus

Name	Common dose (route of administration)	Effectiveness	Advantages	Disadvantages
Benzodiazepines				
Diazepam (Valium)	5-20 mg (iv)	5-15 minutes	Rapid acting	Short effective half-life
Lorazepam (Ativan)	2-8 mg (iv)	2-8 hours	Rapid acting Longer duration of action than diazepam	May depress CNS function for hours
Midazolam (Versed)	1-10 mg (iv, im)	Minutes	Rapid acting May be given im	Short effective half-life Not FDA-approved for status epilepticus
Phenytoin (Dilantin)	500-1,000 mg (18 mg/kg) (iv)	24 hours	No CNS or respiratory depression	May be ineffective in status epilepticus from nonidiopathic causes Hypotension and arrhythmias at high infusion rates Takes 20-40 minutes to administer
Fosphenytoin (Cerebyx)	500-1,000 PE (18 PE/kg) (iv, im)	24 hours	No CNS or respiratory depression Lower risk of purple-glove syndrome than with phenytoin	Hypotension and arrhythmias at high rates of infusion
Barbiturates				
Phenobarbital (Luminal)	500-1,000 mg (iv, im)	48-120 hours	Long-lasting	Long-lasting depression of CNS function
Thiopental (Pentothal)	250-500 mg (iv)	Minutes		Short effective half-life Respiratory depression Respiratory arrest Hypotension Myocardial depression
Pentobarbital (Nembutal)	250-500 mg (iv)	Minutes		

CNS, central nervous system; im, intramuscularly; iv, intravenously; PE, phenytoin equivalents.

From Slovis CM: ED management of unstable patients with status epilepticus. Updates Neurology 1991; pp 23-30. By permission of America Health Consultants.

Anticonvulsants are outlined in Table 17-9.

- The treatment of choice is monotherapy.
- Enzyme-inducing drugs may render oral contraceptives ineffective.
- Valproate may be best for women taking oral contraceptives.
- Phenytoin, carbamazepine, primidone, and phenobarbital can cause developmental abnormalities.
- Valproate may cause neural tube defects.

New Anticonvulsant Drugs

New anticonvulsant drugs include gabapentin, vigabatrine, tiagabine, lamotrigine, topiramate, and felbamate. In general, these agents have less potential for drug interactions and fewer side effects than older drugs and are used mostly as adjuvant treatment for both partial and generalized seizures. Gabapentin increases γ-aminobutyric acid (GABA) release. Because this drug is not protein bound or metabolized in the liver, it does not affect the concentration of other anticonvulsants and may be safer than other anticonvulsants in the management of seizure of patients with porphyria. Vigabatrine inhibits GABA metabolism by GABA transaminase and may be the drug of choice for treatment of infantile spasms. Tiagabine inhibits the reuptake of GABA; it is highly protein bound and undergoes extensive liver metabolism and, thus, has higher potential for drug interactions than other new anticonvulsants. Lamotrigine

blocks voltage-gated sodium channels and the release of glutamate; it is well tolerated but is associated with a high incidence of rash. Topiramate is a partial inhibitor of carbonic anhydrase and may increase the risk of kidney stones. Felbamate is highly effective, but it has been implicated in the development of aplastic anemia. Currently it is indicated only for the treatment of Lennox-Gastaut syndrome, a refractory seizure disorder in childhood. Intravenous valproate and rectal diazepam gel are also available.

If an epileptic patient under treatment has breakthrough seizures, consider the following: 1) compliance; 2) excessive use of alcohol and other "recreational drugs"; 3) psychologic and physiologic stress (lack of sleep, anxiety, etc.); 4) combination of 1 to 3; 5) systemic disease of any type, organ failure of any type, or systemic infection; 6) a new cause of seizures (neoplasm); 7) newly prescribed medication, including other anticonvulsants (polypharmacy) and over-the-counter drugs; 8) toxic levels of anticonvulsants (with definite clinical toxicity); 9) pseudoseizures; 10) progressive CNS lesion not identified previously with neuroimaging or lumbar puncture; 11) no cause found—at this point, you must readjust anticonvulsants or replace one with another.

Surgery for Epilepsy

With improved technology, the site of seizure origin is identified more accurately, and surgical advances have made surgical management safer. Of the 150,000 patients in whom

Table 17-9.—Classic and New Anticonvulsant Medications

Drug	Indication	Maintenance dose range, mg/kg daily	Adult daily dose, mg	M/E	Half-life, hr	Therapeutic serum level range, µg/mL
Classic						
Phenytoin	GTC, P	3-5		Liver	18-24	10-20
Phenobarbital	GTC, P	2-3		Liver	48-120	10-40
Primidone	GTC, P	10-25			6-12	5-15
Carbamazepine	GTC, P	10-20		Liver	12-18	4-12
Valproic acid	GTC, A, M	20-60		Liver	6-18	40-100
Ethosuximide	A	24-36			24-36	20-40
Clonazepam	M	0.05-0.2			20-40	20-80 (mg/mL)
New						
Felbamate*	GTC, P, M, A		2,000-4,000	Kidney	14-23	20-60
Gabapentin	GTC, P		900-1,800	Kidney	5-7	>2.0
Lamotrigine†	GTC, P, M, A		300-500‡	Liver	25	1-5
Tiagabine	GTC, P		36-56	Liver	5-8	50-100
Topiramate	GTC, P		200-400	Kidney	20-24	5.0
Vigabatrine*	GTC, P		2,000	Kidney	6-8	30-80

A, absence; GTC, generalized tonic-clonic; M, myoclonic; M/E, metabolized/excreted; P, simple or partial.
*May be effective in children for infantile spasms and Lennox-Gastaut syndrome.
†Useful in Lennox-Gastaut syndrome.
‡150-300 mg if used in combination with valproate.

epilepsy develops each year, 10% to 20% have "medically intractable epilepsy." Brain surgery is an alternative therapy if antiepileptic drugs fail. However, before seizures are deemed intractable, ascertain that the correct drugs have been used in the correct amounts. Anterior temporal lobe operations and other cortical resections involve removal of the epileptic region and are performed for complex partial seizures. Corpus callosotomy (the severing of connections between the right and left sides of the brain) is used for some types of generalized epilepsy.

- If antiepileptic drugs fail, brain surgery is an alternative treatment.
- Anterior temporal lobe operations and other cortical resections remove the epileptic region.
- Resection operations are for complex partial seizures.
- Corpus callosotomy severs the connections between the left and right sides of the brain and is used for generalized epilepsy.

Vertigo and Dizziness

Accurate visual, vestibular, proprioceptive, tactile, and auditory perceptions are necessary for normal spatial orientation. These inputs are integrated in the brain stem and cerebral hemispheres. The outputs are the motor systems, extrapyramidal system, and cerebellar system. The impairment of any of these functions or their input, integration, or output causes a complaint of "dizziness" (a sensation of altered orientation or space). Dizziness, vertigo, and dysequilibrium are common complaints. The results of diagnostic tests are often normal. Diagnosis depends mainly on the medical history, with physical examination findings in some cases. Vestibular tests rarely provide an exact diagnosis. The types of dizziness are listed in Table 17-10.

Vertigo

Vertigo is an illusion of movement (usually that of rotation) and the feeling of vertical or horizontal rotation of either the person or the environment. Most patients report this as "spinning" or "rotational" feelings. Others mainly experience a sensation of staggering. In contrast to vertigo, dysequilibrium is a feeling of unsteadiness or insecurity about the environment, without a rotatory sensation. Vertigo occurs when there is imbalance, especially acute, between the left and right vestibular systems. The sudden unilateral loss of vestibular function is dramatic; the patient complains of severe vertigo and nausea and vomiting and is pale and diaphoretic. With acute vertigo, the patient also has problems with equilibrium and vision, often described as "blurred vision," or diplopia. Autonomic symptoms are common—sweating, pallor, nausea, vomiting—and can cause vasovagal syncope.

Fluctuating hearing loss and tinnitus are characteristic of Meniere syndrome. Abrupt complete unilateral deafness and vertigo occur with viral involvement of the labyrinth and/or CN VIII and with vascular occlusion of the inner ear. Patients who slowly lose vestibular function bilaterally, as with ototoxic drugs, often do not complain of vertigo but have oscillopsia with head movements and instability with walking. Even with unilateral vestibular loss, if it is slow (acoustic neuroma) patients usually do not complain of vertigo; they typically present with unilateral hearing loss and tinnitus. Vertigo invariably occurs in episodes. Common vestibular disorders with a genetic predisposition include migraine, Meniere syndrome, otosclerosis, neurofibromatosis, and spinocerebellar degeneration.

Benign positional vertigo is the most common cause of vertigo. No cause is found in about half of the patients. For the other half, the most common causes are post-traumatic and postviral neurolabyrinthitis. Brief episodes of vertigo usually last less than 30 seconds with positional change, for example, turning over in bed, getting in or out of bed, bending over and straightening up, and extending the neck to look up.

Table 17-10.—Types of Dizziness

Vertigo
Peripheral
Central
Presyncopal light-headedness
Orthostatic hypotension
Vasovagal attacks
Impaired cardiac output
Hyperventilation
Psychophysiologic dizziness
Acute anxiety
Agoraphobia (fear and avoidance of being in public places)
Chronic anxiety
Disequilibrium
Lesions of basal ganglia, frontal lobes, and white matter
Hydrocephalus
Cerebellar dysfunction
Ocular dizziness
High magnification and lens implant
Imbalance in extraocular muscles
Oscillopsia
Multisensory dizziness
Physiologic dizziness
Motion sickness
Space sickness
Height vertigo

Typically, bouts of benign positional vertigo are intermixed with variable periods of remission. Periods of vertigo rarely last longer than 1 minute, although after a flurry of episodes, patients may complain of more prolonged nonspecific dizziness lasting hours to days (light-headedness, swimming sensation associated with nausea). Management includes reassurance, positional exercises (vestibular exercises), and the canalith repositioning maneuver. Drugs are not very useful, but meclizine and phenergan may help with the nausea and nonspecific dizziness. Rarely, surgical treatment (section of the ampullary nerve) may be undertaken in intractable cases.

Vertigo of CNS origin is caused by acute cerebellar lesions (hemorrhages or infarcts) or acute brain stem lesions (especially, lateral medullary [Wallenberg] syndrome). Basilar-vertebral artery disease is also a cause, but vertigo by itself is never a TIA. Other symptoms are necessary to make the diagnosis of basilar-vertebral insufficiency—dysarthria, dysphagia, diplopia, facial numbness, crossed syndromes, hemiparesis or alternating hemiparesis, ataxia, visual field defects, and others.

Presyncopal Light-Headedness

This is best described as the "sensation of impending faint." It results from pancerebral ischemia. Presyncopal light-headedness is not a symptom of focal occlusive cerebrovascular disease, but it may indicate orthostatic hypotension, usually due to decreased blood volume, chronic use of hypotensive drugs, or autonomic dysfunction. Symptoms of vasovagal attacks are induced when such emotions as fear and anxiety activate medullary vasodepressor centers. Vasodepressor episodes can also be precipitated by acute visceral pain or sudden severe attacks of vertigo. Impaired cardiac output causes presyncopal light-headedness, as does hyperventilation. Chronic anxiety with associated hyperventilation is the common cause of persistent presyncopal light-headedness in young patients. In most subjects, only a moderate increase in respiratory rate can decrease the $Paco_2$ level to 25 mm Hg or less in a few minutes.

Five types of syncopal attacks especially common in the elderly are

1. Orthostatic—multiple causes.
2. Autonomic dysfunction due to peripheral (postganglionic) or central (preganglionic) involvement.
3. Reflex—such as carotid sinus syncope or cough or micturition syncope.
4. Vasovagal syncope—occurs less frequently in the elderly than in the young; however, the prognosis is worse in the elderly, with about 16% of them having major morbidity and mortality in the following 6 months compared with less than 1% of patients younger than 30 years;

common precipitating events in the elderly include emotional stress, prolonged bed rest, prolonged standing, and painful stimuli.
5. Cardiac syncope.

- Presyncopal light-headedness is the sensation of impending faint.
- It is not a common symptom of occlusive cerebrovascular disease.
- Vasovagal attacks occur less frequently in the elderly.
- In the young, a common cause of persistent presyncopal light-headedness is chronic anxiety with hyperventilation.
- The prognosis of vasovagal syncope is worse for the elderly; 16% have major morbidity/mortality within 6 months.
- In the elderly, vasovagal syncope is precipitated by emotional stress, bed rest, prolonged standing, and pain.

Psychophysiologic Dizziness

Patients usually describe this as "floating," "swimming," or "giddiness." They also may report a feeling of imbalance, a rocking or falling sensation, or a spinning inside the head. The symptoms are not associated with an illusion of movement or movement of the environment or with nystagmus. Commonly associated symptoms include tension headache, heart palpitations, gastric distress, urinary frequency, backache, and generalized feeling of weakness and fatigue. Psychophysiologic dizziness can also be associated with panic attacks.

Disequilibrium

Patients who slowly lose vestibular function on one side, as with an acoustic neuroma, usually do not have vertigo but often describe a vague feeling of imbalance and unsteadiness on their feet. Disequilibrium may be a presenting symptom of lesions involving motor centers of the basal ganglia and frontal lobe, for example, Parkinson disease, hydrocephalus, and multiple lacunar infarction syndrome. The broad-based ataxic gait of cerebellar disorders is readily distinguished from milder gait disorders seen with vestibular or sensory loss or with senile gait.

- Disequilibrium may be a presenting symptom of basal ganglia or frontal lobe lesions.

Multisensory Dizziness

This is commonly seen in the elderly and especially in patients with such systemic disorders as diabetes mellitus. A typical combination includes such things as mild peripheral neuropathy causing diminished touch and proprioceptive input, decreased visual acuity, impaired hearing, and decreased baroreceptor function. In such patients, an added vestibular impairment, as from an ototoxic drug, can be devastating.

The resulting sensation of dizziness is usually present only when the patient walks or moves and not present when the patient is supine or seated. There is a feeling of insecurity of gait and motion. The patient is usually helped by walking close to a wall, using a cane, or by holding on to another person. Drugs should *not* be used for this disorder. Instead, the use of a cane or walker is important to improve support and increase somatosensory signals.

- Multisensory dizziness is common in elderly diabetic patients.
- Added vestibular impairment can be devastating.
- Do not use drugs for this disorder.

PART III

DISORDERS BY MECHANISM

NEOPLASTIC DISEASE

The most common neurologic symptoms in patients with systemic cancer are back pain, altered mental status, and headache. However, the most common neurologic complication of systemic cancer is metastatic disease, of which cerebral metastasis is the most common. In patients with back pain, epidural metastasis and direct vertebral metastasis are common, but in about 15% to 20% of patients, no malignant cause is found. Nonstructural causes are the most common reasons for headache. Some identified causes include fever, side effects of therapy, postlumbar puncture headache, metastasis (cerebral, leptomeningeal, base of skull), and intracranial hemorrhage (thrombocytopenia, hemorrhage due to intracranial metastasis). The most common cause of altered mental status is metabolic encephalopathy, which is also the most common nonmetastatic manifestation of systemic cancer. Less common causes include intracranial metastatic disease (parenchymal and meningeal), intracranial hemorrhage, primary dementia, cerebral infarction, psychiatric disorder, known primary brain tumor, bacterial meningitis, and transient global amnesia.

Cancers that commonly cause neurologic problems are those of the lung and breast, leukemia, lymphoma, and colorectal cancer. Breast, lung, and prostate cancer are commonly associated with bony metastasis and epidural metastasis. The most common brain metastasis is from the lung. Meningeal metastases are common in lung and breast cancers, melanoma, leukemia, and lymphoma. Colorectal cancer causes local pelvic metastasis and is the most frequent cause of tumor plexopathy. Head and neck cancer are the most frequent cause of metastasis to the base of the skull. Proportionally, melanoma causes the most nervous system involvement. Gastrointestinal tract tumors (stomach, esophagus, pancreas) have the least number of neurologic complications.

Many neurologic problems in patients with cancer can be diagnosed on the basis of the medical history and findings on neurologic examination and require knowledge of both nonmetastatic- and noncancer-related neurologic illness. In general, neurologic complications of systemic cancer can be divided into the following categories:

1. Metastatic—parenchymal, leptomeningeal, epidural, subdural, brachial and lumbosacral plexuses, and nerve infiltration. This is *common.*
2. Infectious—unusual CNS infections because of immunosuppression.
3. Complications of systemic metastases—hepatic encephalopathy.
4. Vascular complications—cerebral infarction from hypercoagulable states, nonbacterial thrombotic endocarditis, and radiation damage to carotid arteries; cerebral hemorrhage from such entities as thrombocytopenia and hemorrhagic metastases.
5. Systemic encephalopathies—usually from multiple causes, hypercalcemia, syndrome of inappropriate secretion of antidiuretic hormone, medications, and systemic infections.
6. Complications of treatment—radiation, chemotherapy, surgery: radiation necrosis of the brain, radiation myelopathy, radiation plexopathy, fibrosis of the carotid arteries, neuropathies, encephalopathies, and cerebellar ataxia.
7. Nonmetastatic "remote" effect—syndromes have been described from the cerebral cortex through the central and peripheral neuraxes to muscle; they are rare.
8. Miscellaneous—various systemic and neurologic illnesses having nothing to do with the cancer.

- Cerebral metastasis is the most common neurologic complication of systemic cancer.
- Metabolic encephalopathy is the most common nonmetastatic manifestation of cancer.
- Cancers commonly causing neurologic problems are lung, breast, and colorectal cancers, leukemia, and lymphoma.
- The most common brain metastasis is from lung and breast cancers, melanoma, leukemia, and lymphoma.
- The most frequent cause of tumor plexopathy is colorectal cancer.
- Proportionally, melanoma causes the most nervous system involvement.
- Common metastatic sites are parenchyma of the cerebral hemispheres and cerebellum, leptomeninges, epidural and subdural spaces, brachial and lumbosacral plexuses, and nerve.
- Syndromes of nonmetastatic remote effects are rare.

Radiosurgery (gamma-knife and the LINAC-based systems) has been used to treat vascular malformations, acoustic neuromas, pituitary adenomas, and meningeal and (recently) metastatic tumors.

Primary CNS lymphoma is becoming common in both AIDS and immune competent patients. Median survival has been increased with the combination therapy of radiation and chemotherapy, including hydroxyurea, procarbazine, CCNU, vincristine, cytosine arabinoside, and intrathecal methotrexate.

PARANEOPLASTIC DISORDERS

Abnormal Antibodies

1. Anti-islet cell antibodies. They are found in high titer in stiff-person syndrome (anti-GAD antibodies).
2. Anti-calcium channel antibodies. They are positive in 80% of patients with Lambert-Eaton myasthenic syndrome who have primary lung cancer (small cell, squamous cell, adenocarcinoma) and in 36% who are *without* evidence of cancer. They are usually negative in patients with Lambert-Eaton myasthenic syndrome who have cancer other than lung cancer.
3. Purkinje cell antibodies (sometimes called "anti-Yo" antibodies). They are found in women with paraneoplastic cerebellar degeneration and are associated with ovarian, fallopian tube, endometrial, surface papillary and breast carcinoma, and occasionally with lymphoma. They are not found in men with paraneoplastic cerebellar degeneration or in women with gynecologic cancer without a neurologic syndrome. If these antibodies are positive in a woman who is without clinically known or laboratory proven cancer, exploratory laparotomy is probably warranted.
4. Antineuronal nuclear antibodies (ANNA). Type I ("anti-Hu") is a marker of various neurologic disorders occurring with small cell lung cancer, including sensory and autonomic neuropathies, mixed sensory-motor neuropathies, limbic encephalopathy, cerebellar degeneration, myelopathy, radiculopathy, and motor neuropathy. Type II ("anti-Ri") is seen with a spectrum of neurologic disorders associated with breast cancer, including cerebellar ataxia, myelopathy, opsoclonus, and other brain stem disorders.
5. Acetylcholine receptor antibodies. They are rare in conditions other than myasthenia gravis (they do not occur in patients with congenital myasthenia gravis and in only about 50% of those with purely ocular myasthenia gravis). They sometimes are found in patients with ALS, Lambert-Eaton myasthenic syndrome, and pernicious anemia. Striational antibodies are highly associated with thymoma and sometimes occur in Lambert-Eaton myasthenic syndrome or small cell lung carcinomas. They can occur in

D-penicillamine recipients, bone marrow allografts, and autoimmune liver disorders.

- If Purkinje cell antibodies are positive in a woman who is without clinically known or laboratory proven cancer, exploratory laparotomy is probably warranted.
- Acetylcholine receptor antibodies are highly associated with thymoma.
- In paraneoplastic cerebellar degeneration, Hu and Yo antibodies to cerebellar Purkinje cells.
- In paraneoplastic retinopathy, retinal antibodies.

MOVEMENT DISORDERS

Tremor

Tremor is an oscillatory rhythmical movement disorder. A simple classification of tremor is as follows:

1. Rest tremor
2. Postural tremor
3. Kinetic tremor

A rest tremor is noted with the arms lying in the patient's lap while sitting or with the arms at the patient's side while walking. Rest tremor is seen in Parkinson disease. Postural tremor is noted mainly with the arms outstretched, although there is often a kinetic component as well. Postural tremor is seen in physiologic tremor, but it is also noted pathologically in essential tremor. Drugs such as methylxanthines, β-adrenergic agonists, lithium, and amiodarone may produce postural tremor. Kinetic tremor is seen mainly in action, as in finger-to-nose testing. This type of tremor is seen in cerebellar disease and in diseases of the cerebellar connections in the brain stem.

Essential Tremor

Essential tremor is the most common movement disorder. It is often misdiagnosed and inappropriately treated. It is a monosymptomatic condition that is manifested as rhythmic oscillations of various body parts. Middle-aged and older persons are most commonly affected, and there is often a genetic component. The hands are most affected, with the tremor present in postural position and often having a kinetic component. The head and voice are often affected. Head tremor can be either horizontal (no-no) or vertical (yes-yes). It almost never occurs in Parkinson disease, but parkinsonian patients may have tremor of the mouth, lips, tongue, and jaw. The legs and trunk (orthostatic tremor) are affected less frequently in essential tremor.

Essential tremor is a slowly progressive condition with unknown pathophysiologic mechanism. It may be due to a "central pacemaker" located in the cerebellum, motor nuclei of the thalamus, or the inferior olivary nucleus.

The agent most effective in decreasing essential tremor is alcohol. Alcoholic drinks substantially reduce the tremor for 45 to 60 minutes. The rate of alcoholism in patients with essential tremor is no different from that in the general population. Propranolol (80-320 mg daily) and other β-blockers and primidone (25-250 mg at bedtime) are effective. Other drugs that have been used are the benzodiazepines, especially clonazepam and lorazepam; methazolamide has also been effective in some patients, especially in head tremor. Botulinum toxin has been used recently. Stereotactic thalamotomy can be effective in patients with severe functional disability who are unresponsive to drug therapy; surgery is probably underused. Thalamic stimulation (deep brain stimulation) is an effective surgical procedure for all types of tremor.

- Movement disorders occur mostly in middle-aged and older persons.
- There often is a genetic component.
- Hands are affected most.
- Head tremor is almost never seen in Parkinson disease.

Rest Tremor and Parkinson Disease

Patients with Parkinson disease present with tremor (the initial symptom in 50%-70% but 15% never have tremor), rigidity, and bradykinesia. Also, gait is unsteady—a slow, shuffling gait. Decreased blinking rate, lack of change in facial expression, small handwriting, and asymptomatic orthostatic hypotension are also common. Dementia is more frequent in patients with Parkinson disease, but it is noted in about only 25% of those in whom the disease develops after age 60. The detection of cerebellar findings (ataxia), corticospinal signs (increased reflexes, spasticity, extensor plantar response), lower motor neuron findings (decreased reflexes, flaccidity, or fasciculations) should all suggest a disorder other than Parkinson disease as a cause for parkinsonism. Initial treatment options for Parkinson disease include a combination of levodopa and carbidopa (Sinemet), anticholinergic agents (which are particularly useful if tremor is the most significant symptom), amantadine, and dopamine agonists. Initial doses of a combination of levodopa and carbidopa include a 25/100 tablet three times a day. Common side effects include hallucinations, confusion, dyskinesias, and orthostatic hypotension. Common side effects of the anticholinergic agents (trihexyphenidyl hydrochloride and benztropine) include memory loss, delirium, urinary hesitancy, and blurred vision. Dopamine agonists include bromocriptine, pergolide, pramipexole, and ropinirole with side effects that include confusion, hallucinations, and orthostatic hypotension.

- Tremor does not occur in 15% of those with Parkinson disease.

- If ataxia, increased reflexes, spasticity, extensor plantar responses, or lower motor neuron findings are present, consider other diagnoses.

Long-term high-dose levodopa monotherapy leads to dyskinesias and motor fluctuations. Motor fluctuations are due to variations in the plasma levels of L-dopa in the setting of severe dopaminergic cell loss and to changes in dopamine receptor sensitivity. They can be eliminated by continuous intravenous or intestinal infusions of levodopa. Management strategies include the use of 1) smaller and more frequent doses of levodopa, 2) long-acting levodopa preparations, 3) dopaminergic agonists, such as pergolide, bromocriptine, and the new nonergot derivatives pramipexole or ropinirole, and 4) inhibitors of catechol *O*-methyltransferase (COMT, an enzyme that converts peripheral levodopa in *O*-methyldopa) such as tolcapone or entacapone.

When given to a patient with newly diagnosed Parkinson disease, selegiline (a monoamine oxidase type B inhibitor) may delay the initiation of levodopa therapy as well as give mild symptomatic relief. Unpredictable off periods may also be helped with the use of a protein redistribution diet. Monotherapy with dopamine agonists (bromocriptine and pergolide) does not cause the motor side effects associated with levodopa, but the long-term use of a dopamine agonist is limited by its declining efficacy. There is also a tendency for these drugs to cause hallucinations, postural hypotension, and edema; bromocriptine has been associated with pulmonary and retroperitoneal fibrosis. Clozapine might be helpful in eliminating nocturnal akathesia and drug-induced psychosis.

Fetal dopamine cells transplanted into the caudate or putamen may be helpful, but this is still an experimental therapy. Stereotactic pallidotomy or thalamotomy can be helpful for tremor and drug-induced dyskinesia. Pallidotomy may also be useful for rigidity and bradykinesia. Recently, subthalamic stimulation has been reported to eliminate the symptoms of Parkinson disease.

Many patients with parkinsonism develop orthostatic hypotension, bladder dysfunction, and other autonomic manifestations. In these patients, Parkinson disease should be distinguished from multiple system atrophy. Findings suggestive of multiple system atrophy include lack of a predictable response to levodopa, the presence of cerebellar or pyramidal signs, severe orthostatic hypotension and urinary incontinence, sleep apnea and laryngeal stridor. The management of orthostatic hypotension includes eliminating potentially offending drugs (vasodilators, diuretics, dopaminergic agonists, clozapine), increasing sodium and water intake, performing postural maneuvers, elevating the head of the bed, and wearing support stockings. Drug treatment includes fludrocortisone (0.1-1.0 mg/day) and vasoconstrictors such as midodrine (10-40 mg/day).

Other Movement Disorders: Botulinum Toxin Therapy

Botulinum toxin is effective therapy for cervical dystonia, blepharospasm, hemifacial spasm, spasmodic dysphonia, jaw-closing oromandibular dystonia, and limb dystonia, including occupational dystonias.

NEUROLOGY OF SEPSIS

The nervous system is commonly affected in sepsis syndrome. The neurologic conditions seen are septic encephalopathy, critical-illness polyneuropathy, septic myopathy, cachexia, and panfascicular muscle necrosis. Neurologic complications also occur in an intensive care unit for critical medical illness. These complications include metabolic encephalopathy, seizures, hypoxic-ischemic encephalopathy, and stroke.

Septic Encephalopathy

Septic encephalopathy is brain dysfunction in association with systemic infection *without* overt infection of the brain or meninges. Early encephalopathy often begins before failure of other organs and is not secondary to single or multiple organ failure. Endotoxin does not cross the blood-brain barrier and so probably does not directly affect adult brains. Cytokines, important components of sepsis syndrome, may contribute to encephalopathy. Gegenhalten or paratonic rigidity occurs in more than 50% of patients and tremor, asterixis, and multifocal myoclonus occur in about 25%. Seizures and focal neurologic signs are rare.

EEG is a sensitive indicator of encephalopathy. The mildest abnormality is diffuse excessive theta low-voltage activity (4-7 Hz). The next level of severity is intermittent rhythmic delta activity (<4 Hz). As the condition worsens, delta activity becomes arrhythmic and continuous. Typical triphasic waves occur in severe cases.

Adult respiratory distress syndrome is common in severe but not in mild cases of encephalopathy.

- Brain dysfunction is associated with systemic infection.
- Encephalopathy precedes failure of other organs.
- Cytokines are an important part of sepsis syndrome.
- More than 50% of patients have paratonic rigidity.
- 25% of patients have tremor, asterixis, and multifocal myoclonus.
- EEG is a sensitive indicator of encephalopathy.

Critical Illness Polyneuropathy

This occurs in 70% of the patients with sepsis and multiple organ failure. There is often unexplained difficulty in weaning from mechanical ventilation. Nerve biopsy shows primary axonal degeneration of motor and sensory fibers without inflammation. Recovery from polyneuropathy is satisfactory if the patient survives sepsis and multiple organ failure.

- Nerve biopsy shows primary axonal degeneration of motor and sensory fibers without inflammation.
- Satisfactory recovery from polyneuropathy.

DEGENERATIVE DISEASE OF THE SPINE

Cervical Spondylosis

MRI combined with plain radiographs is the preferred approach for evaluating patients with cervical spondylosis. Surgical results for relief of the symptoms of cervical radiculopathy are better when the cause is a soft disk herniation than when spondylitic radiculopathy and myelopathy are present. In fact, surgical treatment of cervical radiculopathy due to the herniation of a soft disk is so successful that most patients and doctors prefer surgical therapy to prolonged conservative treatment. However, surgical treatment for cervical spondylitic myelopathy is much less successful, with fewer than two-thirds of patients having improvement. Cervical spondylitic myelopathy is a condition in which the spinal cord is damaged either directly by traumatic compression or indirectly by arterial deprivation or venous stasis as a consequence of proliferative bony changes in the cervical spine.

Lumbar Spine Disease

Bulging disks after the age of 30 years should be considered normal and are unlikely to cause nerve root compression. Bulging disks appear round and symmetrical compared with herniated disks, which appear angular and asymmetrical and extend outside the disk space. The criteria for surgical treatment of lumbar disk herniations include the following: 1) presence of disk herniation on anatomical imaging; 2) dermatome-specific reflex, sensory, or motor deficits; and 3) failure of 6 to 8 weeks of conservative treatment.

The lateral recess syndrome (facet syndrome) is characterized by the following: 1) it produces radicular pain; 2) it is usually caused by an osteophyte on the superior articular facet; 3) the symptoms are unilateral or bilateral pain or paresthesias in the distribution of L5 or S1; 4) the pain is brought on by standing and walking and is relieved by sitting; and 5) the results on the straight leg raising test are usually negative.

Lumbar stenosis is characterized by the following: 1) most patients are older than 50 years; 2) the occurrence of neurogenic intermittent claudication (pseudoclaudication); 3) the symptoms are usually bilateral but can be asymmetrical or unilateral; 4) the pain usually has a dull, aching quality; 5) the whole lower extremity is generally involved; 6) the pain is provoked while walking or standing; 7) sitting or leaning forward provide relief; and 8) there is often a feeling of deadness in the legs. Decompressive operations for lumbar stenosis can be performed with low morbidity despite the advanced age of most patients. A very high initial success rate can be expected, although about 25% of patients become symptomatic in a 5-year follow-up period. On reoperation, three-fourths of the patients ultimately have a successful outcome; failures result from progression of stenosis at levels not previously decompressed or restenosis at levels previously operated on.

Musculoskeletal low back pain is treated best with a formal program of physical therapy and exercise, weight reduction, and education on postural principles.

DEMYELINATING DISEASES

Idiopathic inflammatory demyelinating diseases of the CNS are as follows:

1. Multiple sclerosis
2. Isolated demyelinating syndromes—optic neuritis and transverse myelitis
3. Primary progressive demyelinating diseases—chronic progressive myelopathy and progressive cerebellar syndrome
4. Asymptomatic demyelinating diseases (revealed by MRI or autopsy)

Predictors associated with a more favorable long-term course of multiple sclerosis include age younger than 40 years at onset, female sex, optic neuritis or isolated sensory symptoms as the first clinical manifestation, and relatively infrequent attacks. Prognostic factors associated with a poor outcome include age older than 40 years at onset, male sex, cerebellar or pyramidal tract findings at initial presentation, relatively frequent attacks during the first 2 years, incomplete remissions, and a chronically progressive course. However, no single clinical variable is sufficient to predict the course or outcome of this disease. Acute transverse myelopathy is rarely the first sign of multiple sclerosis. Acute transverse myelopathy is usually a monophasic disorder. Abnormal MRI findings at the time of presentation of a clinically isolated syndrome suggestive of multiple sclerosis (isolated involvement of the optic nerve, brain stem, or spinal cord) is a strong predictor of the eventual clinical diagnosis of multiple sclerosis in the next 5 years. Interferon beta-1b, interferon beta-1a, and glatiramer acetate decrease the relapse rate and intensity of relapses in patients with remitting-relapsing type of multiple sclerosis.

A study on steroid therapy for optic neuritis found that oral prednisone therapy was *ineffective*. The recommendation is for either a 3-day course of a high dose of intravenous methylprednisolone followed by an 11-day course of oral prednisone taper or no treatment at all.

CEREBROVASCULAR DISEASE

Ischemic Cerebrovascular Disease

Pathophysiologic Mechanisms

The etiology of ischemic cerebrovascular disorders, including transient ischemic attack and cerebral infarction, can be classified on the basis of the site of the source for the arterial blockage (embolus from a proximal site or thrombosis in situ from distal causes) within the vascular system starting from most proximal to distal. First, a *cardiac* source as the most proximal site includes both arrhythmias and structural disorders such as valve disease, dilated cardiomyopathy, recent myocardial infarction, and other cardiac structural disorders. Also, paradoxical emboli with a right-to-left shunt must be considered. The second site includes *large vessel* disorders, with the most common cause being atherosclerosis or dissection in the carotid or vertebrobasilar systems. The third site involves *small vessel* occlusive disease caused by either inflammatory or noninflammatory arteriopathies (hypertension-induced disease, isolated CNS angiitis, systemic lupus erythematosus), and *hematologic* disorders, including polycythemia, sickle cell anemia, thrombocytosis, severe leukocytosis, and other disorders, including protein C and protein S deficiency, anticardiolipin antibody positivity, lupus anticoagulant positivity, and hypercoagulable states caused by carcinoma. Illicit drug use is a common cause of stroke in young persons and causes arrhythmia, inflammatory arteriopathies, and a relative hypercoagulable state.

Pathophysiologic mechanisms of ischemic cerebrovascular disease include artery-to-artery emboli (e.g., extracranial carotid bifurcation to a branch of the middle cerebral artery), cardiac embolic stroke, and lacunar infarction (small vessel disease). Other causes are hematologic disorders and states of altered coagulability (polycythemia, sickle cell anemia, thrombocytosis, severe leukocytosis, abnormalities of the cellular constituents of blood such as serologic factors like homocystinuria; deficiencies of antithrombin III, protein C, and protein S; anticardiolipin antibodies; lupus anticoagulant; and mucin produced by adenocarcinomas that can cause a hypercoagulable state). Still other causes are nonarteriosclerotic vasculopathies (fibromuscular hyperplasia, granulomatous angiitis, congophilic angiopathy, systemic lupus erythematosus, etc.), dissection of the carotid or vertebral arteries, hemodynamic crisis with impairment of distal flow, mechanical compression of arteries, steal syndromes, and AIDS. "Recreational drugs" are a major risk factor for stroke in young adults.

- Pathophysiologic mechanisms of ischemic cardiovascular disease include cardiac source, large vessel disorders, small vessel disorders, and hematologic causes.

- In young adults, "recreational drugs" are a major risk factor for stroke.

Risk Factors

Risk factors for atherosclerotic occlusive disease are similar to those predisposing to coronary artery disease: hypertension, male sex, advanced age, cigarette smoking, diabetes mellitus, hypercholesterolemia, and oral contraceptives. Emboli from intracardiac mural thrombi are also an important cause of TIA and cerebral infarct. Major cardiac risk factors include left-sided chamber enlargement or aneurysm, congestive heart failure, atrial fibrillation, transmural myocardial infarction, mitral valve disease, septic emboli, paradoxical emboli, and atrial myxoma.

Hypertension is the most powerful modifiable risk factor for stroke, but other modifiable risk factors include cigarette smoking, alcohol consumption, physical activity, and cholesterol level. Although mild-to-moderate alcohol consumption appears to have a protective effect for ischemic stroke, heavy alcohol consumption increases the risk of all types of stroke, particularly intracerebral and subarachnoid hemorrhage.

TIAs

TIAs place patients at high risk for subsequent cerebral infarctions; estimates are from 4% to 10% within 1 year to 33% within the patient's lifetime. Most TIAs are fleeting, usually lasting less than 10 to 15 minutes; 88% resolve within 1 hour. Infarcts, hemorrhages, and mass lesions can present like TIAs.

Amaurosis fugax is temporary, partial, or complete monocular blindness and is a classic symptom of a carotid artery TIA. It can be mimicked by glaucoma, vitreous hemorrhage, retinal detachment, papilledema, migrainous aura, temporal arteritis, and even ectopic floaters.

The long-term prognosis for patients with TIA generally follows the rules of 3s: 1/3 go on to have cerebral infarctions, 1/3 have at least one more TIA, and 1/3 have no more TIAs.

- With TIAs, the risk for subsequent cerebral infarction is high.
- 1/3 will have cerebral infarction, 1/3 will have one more TIA, 1/3 will have no more TIAs.
- Most TIAs last <10-15 minutes.
- Infarcts, hemorrhages, and mass lesions can present like a TIA.
- Amaurosis fugax is a classic symptom of a carotid artery TIA.

Carotid Endarterectomy

Carotid endarterectomy significantly decreases the risk of stroke and death in *symptomatic* patients who have a 70% to 99% carotid artery stenosis on angiography. For symptomatic patients with a 50% to 60% stenosis, carotid endarterectomy is moderately efficacious in selected patients. Medical treatment alone is better than carotid endarterectomy in patients with a 0% to 49% carotid artery stenosis. Symptoms must be those of a carotid territory TIA or minor stroke and must be of recent onset (<4 months). The benefits of carotid endarterectomy require a low perioperative compliction rate (4%-6%).

According to the report of a recent study (Asymptomatic Carotid Atherosclerosis Study [ACAS]), selected patients with asymptomatic carotid stenosis of at least 60% profit from carotid endarterectomy in terms of future risk for an ipsilateral stroke or death. Medical patients are treated with aspirin and risk-factor reduction. The risk for stroke was low in patients treated surgically and those treated medically (5-year risk of ipsilateral stroke or death was 11% for those treated medically and 6% for those treated surgically). This differential amounted to approximately a 1% difference per year. No trend was noted dependent on the degree of stenosis, but the number of events was small in each stenosis subdivision. Important is the fact that surgeons and hospitals were particularly chosen for having past perioperative complication rates in asymptomatic patients of less than 3%. However, most conservative neurologists advise caution in accepting the premise that patients with asymptomatic carotid stenosis less than 79% will benefit from surgical endarterectomy.

Patients with asymptomatic carotid occlusive disease who require an operation for some other reason (e.g., coronary artery bypass graft or abdominal aortic aneurysm repair) usually can have that procedure performed without a prophylactic carotid endarterectomy, because the risk of stroke in asymptomatic persons is quite low in this circumstance. If a patient has recently had symptoms in the distribution of the carotid stenosis, the decision is more complicated. Generally, if a patient with an asymptomatic carotid stenosis is experiencing cardiac symptoms such as angina, coronary artery bypass graft is performed first and carotid endarterectomy may be considered later if the patient is otherwise an excellent surgical candidate.

Antiplatelet Agents

Aspirin, ticlopidine, and clopidogrel are all effective in secondary prevention of stroke. The optimum dose of aspirin is still uncertain, with ranges recommended from 30 to 1,300 mg/day. Clopidogrel is given as a single dose, 75 mg/day. The dose of ticlopidine is 250 mg twice daily. Ticlopidine has been associated with neutropenia; thus, the complete blood count must be monitored every 2 weeks for the first 3 months of treatment. It has also been associated with thrombotic thrombocytopenic purpura. Neutropenia and thrombotic thrombocytopenic purpura have not been reported with clopidogrel.

Acute Cerebral Infarction Management

If a patient has a significant neurologic deficit caused by an acute cerebral infarction, the immediate decision in the emergency room is whether the patient is a candidate for *thrombolytic therapy* (tissue plasminogen activator [tPA]). The initial therapeutic approach to ischemic infarction depends greatly on the time from the onset of symptoms to presentation for emergency medical care. If the onset of symptoms was less than 3 hours before the evaluation, emergent thrombolytic therapy should be considered. If a patient awakens from sleep with the deficit, thrombolytic therapy should not be considered unless the duration of the deficit is clearly less than 3 hours.

The result of a CT head scan is very important in selecting patients for tPA. The scan should not reveal any evidence of intracranial hemorrhage, mass effect, or midline shift. Clinical criteria that may exclude patients are those with 1) rapidly improving deficit, 2) obtunded or comatose status or presentation with seizure, 3) history of intracranial hemorrhage or bleeding diathesis, 4) blood pressure elevation persistently greater than 185/110 mm Hg, 5) gastrointestinal tract hemorrhage or urinary tract hemorrhage within the previous 21 days, 6) a large ischemic stroke within the previous 14 days or a small ischemic stroke within the previous 4 days, and 7) mild deficit. The eligible patient should have marked weakness in at least one limb or severe aphasia. Laboratory abnormalities that may preclude treatment are 1) heparin use within the previous 48 hours with an increased activated partial thromboplastin time, 2) prothrombin time greater than 15 seconds, and 3) glucose less than 50 or greater than 400 mg/dL.

In a treatment trial of intravenous tPA, the efficacy in improving neurologic status at 3 months was defined for tPA compared with placebo, with the agent administered within 3 hours after the onset of symptoms. Although there was a greater proportion (12% greater) of people with minimal or no deficit in the tPA group at 3 months after the event, there was no increase in the proportion of persons with severe deficits or disability. This is particularly important because there was an increased occurrence of symptomatic hemorrhage in the tPA group.

Intravenous tPA should be given in a 0.9-mg/kg dose (maximum, 90 mg), with 10% given as a bolus and the rest over 60 minutes.

- Intravenous tPA should be considered in patients seen within 3 hours of onset of severe cerebral infarction symptoms.
- Do not treat with tPA if CT shows hemorrhage, mass effect, or midline shift.

Stroke Risks With Nonvalvular Atrial Fibrillation

Atrial fibrillation is associated with up to 24% of ischemic strokes and 50% of embolic strokes. The stroke rate for the entire cohort of patients with chronic atrial fibrillation is generally about 5% per year. However, patients younger than 60 years with "lone atrial fibrillation" have a lower risk of stroke than other patients with atrial fibrillation. Stroke risk factors with atrial fibrillation include a history of hypertension, recent congestive heart failure, previous thromboembolism including TIAs, left ventricular dysfunction identified on two-dimensional echocardiography, and the size of the left atrium identified on M-mode echocardiography. Patients with atrial fibrillation who have one or more risk factors should receive anticoagulation therapy (low-intensity anticoagulation is recommended) and those at low risk should receive aspirin.

In patients receiving anticoagulant therapy, the dominant risk factor for intracranial hemorrhage is the International Normalized Ratio (INR). Age is another risk factor for subdural hemorrhage. An INR of 2.0 to 3.0 is probably an adequate level of anticoagulation for all indications except for preventing embolization from mechanical heart valves. In general, the lowest effective intensity of anticoagulation should be used.

- Atrial fibrillation is associated with 24% of ischemic strokes and 50% of embolic strokes.
- Stroke rate is about 5% per year.
- Patients with "lone atrial fibrillation" have a lower risk of stroke.

HEMORRHAGIC CEREBROVASCULAR DISEASE

Intracerebral Hemorrhage

Hypertension commonly affects deep penetrating cerebral vessels, especially ones supplying the basal ganglia, cerebral white matter, thalamus, pons, and cerebellum. Common old *misconcepts* of intracerebral hemorrhage are 1) the onset is generally sudden and catastrophic, 2) hypertension is invariably severe, 3) headache is always present, 4) reduced consciousness or frank coma is usually present, 5) the CSF is always bloody, and 6) the prognosis is poor and mortality is high. None of these may be present, and the prognosis depends on the size and location of the hemorrhage.

- Prognosis depends on the size and site of the hemorrhage.

Surgical evacuation of intracerebral hematomas may be necessary in patients with signs of increased intracranial pressure or in those whose condition is worsening.

Cerebellar Hemorrhage

It is important to recognize this because drainage may be lifesaving. The important clinical findings are vomiting and inability to walk. Long-tract signs are usually *not* present. Patients may have ipsilateral gaze palsy, ipsilateral CN VI palsy, or ipsilateral nuclear type CN VII palsy and may or may not have headache, vertigo, and lethargy. Cerebellar hemorrhage may cause obstructive hydrocephalus.

- Vomiting and the inability to walk are important findings in cerebellar hemorrhage.
- Long tract signs are not present.
- Cerebellar hemorrhage may cause obstructive hydrocephalus.

Subarachnoid Hemorrhage

Subarachnoid hemorrhage accounts for about 5% of strokes, including about half of those in patients younger than 45 years, with a peak age range between 35 and 65 years. In up to 50% of cases, an alert patient with an aneurysm may have a small sentinel bleed with a warning headache, or aneurysmal expansion may cause focal neurologic signs or symptoms, for example, an incomplete CN III palsy. The prognosis is related directly to the state of consciousness at the time of intervention. The headache is characteristically sudden in onset, and although 1/3 occur during exertion, 1/3 also occur during rest and 1/3 during sleep. The peak incidence of vasospasm associated with subarachnoid hemorrhage occurs between days 4 and 12 after the initial hemorrhage. Other complications include 1) hemorrhagic infiltration into the brain, ventricles, and even subdural space, which requires evacuation; 2) hyponatremia associated with diabetes insipidus or syndrome of inappropriate secretion of antidiuretic hormone; and 3) communicating hydrocephalus.

In addition to the initial hemorrhage, vasospasm and rehemorrhaging are the leading causes of morbidity and mortality in patients who have subarachnoid hemorrhage.

The outpouring of catecholamines may cause myocardial damage with accompanying electrocardiographic abnormalities, pulmonary edema, and arrhythmias. Arrhythmias can be both supraventricular and ventricular and are most likely during the initial hours or days after a moderate-to-severe subarachnoid hemorrhage.

- About 5% of strokes are subarachnoid hemorrhage.
- In 50% of cases, an alert patient with an aneurysm may have a small sentinel bleed.
- The prognosis is related directly to the state of consciousness at the time of intervention.
- Characteristically, headache has a sudden onset.

The differential diagnosis of subtypes of hemorrhagic cerebrovascular disease is outlined in Table 17-11.

NEUROLOGIC INFECTIOUS DISEASE

Lyme Disease—Multisystem Disorder

Stage I Lyme disease begins with the bite of an infected tick. Any body area may be bitten, but the thigh, groin, and axilla are common sites. Patients often cannot recall the tick bite.

Stage II disease begins weeks to months after the initial infection and is characterized by neurologic, cardiac, and ophthalmic involvement. About 15% of the patients in the U.S.

Table 17-11.—Hemorrhagic Cerebrovascular Disease

Hemorrhage into parenchyma
    Hypertension
    Amyloid angiopathy
    Aneurysm
    Vascular malformation
        Arteriovenous malformation
        Cavernous malformation
        Venous malformation (rare cause of hemorrhage)
    Trauma—primarily frontal and temporal
    Hemorrhagic infarction
    Secondary to brain tumors (primary and secondary
      neoplasms)
    Inflammatory diseases of vasculature
    Disorders of blood-forming organs (blood dyscrasia,
      especially leukemia and thrombocytopenic purpura)
    Anticoagulant or thrombolytic therapy
    Increased intracranial pressure (brain stem) (Duret
      hemorrhages)
    Illicit drug use
    Postsurgical
    Fat embolism (petechial)
    Hemorrhagic encephalitis (petechial)
    Undetermined cause (normal blood pressure, no other
      recognizable disorder)

Hemorrhage into subarachnoid space (subarachnoid
  hemorrhage)
    Trauma
    Aneurysm
        Saccular ("berry," "congenital")
        Fusiform (arteriosclerotic)—rarely causes hemorrhage
        Mycotic
    Arteriovenous malformation
    Many of same causes as for parenchyma above

Subdural and epidural hemorrhage (hematoma)
    Mainly traumatic
    Many of same causes as for parenchyma above

Hemorrhage into pituitary (pituitary apoplexy)

---

have neurologic involvement, usually meningoencephalitis, cranial neuritis, or radiculoneuropathy. Cranial neuropathies are common, most frequently CN VII (bilaterally in 1/3 of patients). Thus, bilateral CN VII palsies in a patient from an endemic area are almost diagnostic of Lyme disease. Peripheral nervous system involvement can include the spinal roots, plexuses, and peripheral nerves.

Stage III disease marks the chronic phase and begins months to years after the initial infection. This stage is heralded by arthritic and neurologic symptoms. Any CNS symptom is possible, and there may be psychiatric symptoms and cognitive impairment. Severe fatigue is a particularly prominent feature. Rarely, a multiple sclerosis-like demyelinating illness featuring gait disturbance, urinary bladder dysfunction, spastic paraparesis, and dysarthria may develop. These symptoms may undergo exacerbations and remissions; MRI and CT reveal multifocal white matter lesions.

- Lyme disease is a multisystem disorder.
- Patients often do not recall the tick bite.
- In the U.S., 15% of patients have neurologic involvement.
- Cranial neuropathies, especially CN VII, are common.
- Bilateral CN VII palsies in an endemic area are diagnostic of Lyme disease.
- In stage III disease, severe fatigue is prominent.

The longer the duration of symptoms before diagnosis and effective antibiotic treatment, the greater the risk that serious symptoms will outlast the period of acute infection. Laboratory diagnosis can be difficult; ELISA can be undependable both in identifying new cases and in distinguishing acute from remote healed infection. Asymptomatic tick bites carry a less than 1% chance of Lyme infection, and treating such for Lyme disease is not cost-effective. However, typical erythema migrans accompanying either a tick bite or other typical symptoms is sufficiently diagnostic to warrant treatment following exposure in an endemic area, even without abnormal serologic findings.

Neurologic Complications of AIDS

The nervous system is affected clinically in up to 40% of HIV patients, and pathologic changes in the nervous system are found at autopsy in up to 90%. Neurologic features may be the presenting manifestation of the illness in 5% to 10% of the patients. HIV infection is associated with various central and peripheral nervous system disorders, and multiple levels of the nervous system can be affected simultaneously. Therapy is available for many of these syndromes. HIV dementia is treated with a high dose of zidovudine (AZT). Cytomegalovirus encephalitis is treated with ganciclovir. A

syndrome of lumbosacral polyradiculomyelopathy presenting as or manifested by progressive lumbosacral radicular symptoms (with weakness, areflexia, and sensory loss in the legs) is often due to cytomegalovirus and, thus, treated with ganciclovir. Cryptococcal meningitis is treated with amphotericin B (also flucytosine or fluconazole). CNS lymphoma in AIDS patients is treated the same as CNS lymphoma in immunocompetent patients, that is, with radiotherapy and chemotherapy. The acute inflammatory demyelinating polyradiculoneuropathy responds well to plasma exchange or prednisone. Zidovudine-induced myopathy responds to dose reduction or withdrawal of the medication. Polymyositis is treated the same as it is in other patients, that is, with steroid therapy.

The major HIV-related neurologic conditions are the following: 1) HIV dementia, 2) toxoplasma encephalitis, 3) CNS lymphoma, 4) progressive multifocal leukoencephalopathy, 5) cytomegalovirus encephalitis, 6) cryptococcal meningitis, 7) neurosyphilis, 8) vacuolar myelopathy, 9) distal symmetrical polyneuropathy, 10) inflammatory demyelinating polyradiculoneuropathy, 11) mononeuropathy multiplex, 12) progressive polyradiculopathy, and 13) myopathy. Toxoplasma encephalitis remains a common opportunistic infection in AIDS patients. Treatment for this infection is either pyrimethamine plus sulfadiazine or pyrimethamine plus clindamycin. However, CNS lymphoma and toxoplasma encephalitis can be difficult to differentiate because they are similar both in their clinical manifestations and their CT and MRI characteristics. Therefore, patients with AIDS who present with a contrast-enhancing CNS mass lesion are treated empirically for toxoplasma encephalitis and patients undergo follow-up CT or MRI scans to see if the lesion decreases in size. Patients whose lesions do not respond to medical treatment are subjected to stereotactic biopsy to exclude other causes, including lymphoma.

Patients with AIDS dementia complex have an increased concentration of CSF β_2-microglobulin. Thus, CSF β_2-microglobulin may be a valuable marker of the severity of AIDS dementia and response to treatment. Treatment with zidovudine significantly decreases the concentration of β_2-microglobulin.

NEUROLOGIC COMPLICATIONS OF ORGAN TRANSPLANTATION

Because almost all organ transplant recipients require some degree of chronic, life-long immunosuppressive therapy, the major neurologic complications of organ transplantation are due to immunosuppression. These include the direct neurotoxic side effects of immunosuppressive drugs, infections, and the development of de novo malignancies. Direct neurologic side effects include the following:

1. Cyclosporine. Tremor is the most common side effect of cyclosporine, which also may produce various motor syndromes such as hemiparesis, paraparesis, and quadriparesis. Cyclosporine may also produce encephalopathy and, less commonly, neuralgia and neuropathy; it is epileptogenic.
2. Corticosteroids. The side effects of corticosteroids include myopathy, steroid psychosis, withdrawal (myalgias, arthralgias, headache, lethargy, nausea), and spinal cord or cauda equina compression due to epidural lipomatosis.
3. Azathioprine. It has no direct neurotoxic side effects.

CNS Infections

Infection of the CNS is relatively frequent and life-threatening. The three organisms that cause more than 80% of CNS infections are *Listeria monocytogenes, Cryptococcus neoformans,* and *Aspergillus fumigatus.* The greatest risk factor for CNS infection is the magnitude and duration of immunosuppression. Severe and advanced CNS infections may present with little or no clinical evidence of infection. The period of infection risk is mainly from 1 to 6 months after transplantation. Specific infections include 1) acute meningitis, most often due to *Listeria*; 2) subacute or chronic meningitis, generally due to *Cryptococcus*; 3) slowly progressive dementia, frequently due to progressive multifocal leukoencephalopathy;

and 4) focal brain disease due to infection usually caused by *Aspergillus, Toxoplasma, Listeria,* or *Nocardia.*

CNS Involvement by de Novo Lymphoproliferative Diseases

There is an increase in non-Hodgkin lymphoma, especially primary CNS lymphomas. These lymphomas may be linked to infection with Epstein-Barr virus.

Other Neurologic Complications

Other complications affecting the nervous system can be classified as follows:

1. Complications arising from the underlying diseases
2. Problems resulting from the transplant procedure
3. Side effects of immunosuppression
4. Post-transplantation disorder peculiar to the specific type of transplant

The complications include compressive neuropathies, plexopathies, and radiculopathies; encephalopathy (especially with renal, liver, and heart transplants), and cerebral infarctions (with bone marrow and heart transplants). Chronic graft versus host disease (especially with bone marrow transplant) involves the peripheral nervous system (but not the CNS), for example, polymyositis, myasthenia gravis, and peripheral neuropathy, including CIDP. A complication associated with liver transplantation is central pontine myelinolysis, which is manifested as altered mental status or coma, pseudobulbar palsy, and quadriplegia.

QUESTIONS

Multiple Choice (choose the one best answer)

1. A 42-year-old woman presents with acute onset of headache, vertigo, nausea, and vomiting. Examination reveals left horizontal nystagmus, left Horner syndrome, absence of left gag reflex, left appendicular ataxia, and anesthesia to pinprick on the left side of the face and the right upper extremity. What is the most likely diagnosis?
   a. Complicated migraine
   b. Vertebral artery dissection
   c. Subarachnoid hemorrhage
   d. Acute multiple sclerosis
   e. Transverse sinus thrombosis

2. A 56-year-old woman is evaluated for a 5-month history of numbness and tingling in the feet and bilateral leg weakness. Examination reveals weakness in the iliopsoas, hamstrings, and foot dorsiflexors bilaterally and brisk knee and ankle muscle stretch reflexes. She has loss of vibratory and position sense in the toes and fingers bilaterally. Which of the following would be most likely to reveal an abnormality?
   a. Electromyography
   b. Lumbar myelography
   c. Cervical magnetic resonance imaging
   d. Computed tomography of the head
   e. Magnetic resonance angiography

3. A patient is brought to the emergency department in a coma. He has no response to verbal or painful stimuli; decreased muscle tone in all limbs, with bilateral extensor plantar response; absence of corneal and oculovestibular responses; and miotic and reactive pupils. He had

hypotension and bradycardia. What is the most likely diagnosis?

a. Mesencephalic hemorrhage
b. Nonconvulsive status epilepticus
c. Uncal herniation
d. Drug overdose
e. Basilar artery occlusion

4. A 65-year-old woman has a 3-month history of progressive upper and lower extremity weakness. Examination reveals weakness and mild atrophy in the deltoid, triceps, biceps, and quadriceps muscles. The stretch reflexes are normal and there are no fasciculations or sensory loss. What is the most likely diagnosis?

a. Cervical spondylotic myelopathy
b. Motor neuron disease
c. Chronic inflammatory demyelinating polyradiculopathy
d. Lambert-Eaton myasthenic syndrome
e. Inflammatory myopathy

5. A 32-year-old woman is evaluated for diplopia. Neurologic examination demonstrated inability to adduct the left eye on attempting to look to the right but the ability to adduct both eyes on looking to her nose was preserved. The right eye abducts but develops nystagmus in this position. What is the most likely diagnosis?

a. Multiple sclerosis
b. Posterior communicating artery aneurysm
c. Cavernous sinus meningioma
d. Myasthenia gravis
e. Graves ophthalmopathy

6. A 62-year-old man is evaluated for a recent episode of diplopia, dysarthria, and dysphagia that resolved in 3 hours. Neurologic examination revealed mild bilateral esophoria and facial weakness. When he attempted to count vigorously to 150, his voice became increasingly breathy, hoarse, and hypernasal. What study would most likely provide the diagnosis?

a. Magnetic resonance imaging of the head, focusing on the brain stem
b. Vertebrobasilar angiography
c. Cerebrospinal fluid analysis
d. Acetylcholine receptor antibodies
e. Serum level of creatine kinase

7. A 52-year-old woman is evaluated for a 1-month history of progressive numbness in the hands and feet and gait instability. Neurologic examination demonstrated that she walked with a broad-based gait, was unable to maintain an erect posture with her eyes closed, and had no vibratory or joint position sense in the fingers and toes. Strength was normal, but muscle stretch reflexes were absent. What laboratory test is most likely to provide the diagnosis?

a. Antineuronal nuclear antibodies (ANNA-1) (anti-Hu)
b. Porphyrins
c. Magnetic resonance imaging of the head
d. Cervical myelography
e. Electronystagmography

8. A 58-year-old woman has a 2-week history of progressive weakness and numbness in the lower extremities and difficulty urinating. Neurologic examination demonstrated bilateral weakness in the iliopsoas, hamstrings, and foot dorsiflexors; absence of knee stretch reflex; ankle clonus; extensor plantar responses; and decreased joint position and vibratory sense in the toes. The anal reflex was normal. What should you consider in the early evaluation?

a. Magnetic resonance imaging of the head
b. Magnetic resonance imaging of the spine
c. Cerebrospinal fluid analysis
d. Electromyography
e. Somatosensory evoked potentials

9. A 45-year-old woman was admitted to the emergency department because of an acute onset of headache, vomiting, diplopia, and blurred vision. Neurologic examination demonstrated decreased visual acuity bilaterally, a bitemporal field defect, and weakness of the lateral and medial rectus muscles bilaterally. What is the most likely diagnosis?

a. Ruptured posterior communicating artery aneurysm
b. Cavernous sinus thrombophlebitis
c. Complicated migraine
d. Pituitary apoplexy
e. Basilar artery thrombosis

10. A 32-year-old woman has a 3-day history of progressive leg weakness. Neurologic examination demonstrated bilateral weakness in the orbicularis oculi, orbicularis ori, neck extensors, deltoid, biceps, triceps, intrinsic hand muscles, iliopsoas, quadriceps, anterior tibialis, and gastrocnemius muscles. Muscle stretch reflexes were absent in the upper and lower extremities. Which of the following is most likely to be abnormal?

a. Magnetic resonance imaging of the head and spine
b. Antineuronal nuclear antibody
c. Cerebrospinal fluid protein
d. Acetylcholine receptor antibodies
e. Creatine kinase

11. A 65-year-old man with shuffling gait and rest tremor is treated with carbidopa/levodopa 25/100 4 times daily with good response for 6 months. Because of recent incomplete benefit, an anticholinergic drug was added. One week into treatment with this drug combination, he developed agitated behavior and visual hallucinations. What is the most appropriate step in evaluation and management?
    a. Add clozapine
    b. Add pergolide
    c. Discontinue anticholinergic drug
    d. Load with phenytoin
    e. Add selegiline

12. A 25-year-old woman was admitted because of a 5-day history of severe abdominal pain, bizarre behavior, and two generalized tonic-clonic seizures. Laboratory studies revealed low levels of porphobilinogen deaminase. What is the safest treatment for her seizures in this setting?
    a. Phenytoin
    b. Carbamazepine
    c. Phenobarbital
    d. Primidone
    e. Gabapentin

13. A 45-year-old woman has a 2-week history of progressive numbness in the hands and feet and gait instability. Neurologic examination demonstrated a broad-based gait and a tendency to fall backward, which was markedly worse when she closed her eyes. She had an absence of joint position and vibratory sensation in the fingers, wrists, toes, and ankles. Stretch reflexes were absent, but muscle strength and pinprick sensation were normal. What drug is most likely to produce these findings?
    a. Phenytoin
    b. Cisplatin
    c. Cyclosporine
    d. Isoniazid
    e. Nitrofurantoin

14. A 58-year-old man is evaluated because of a 3-day history of severe muscle pain and weakness, associated with red decoloration of his urine. The serum level of creatinine kinase is 6,000. Which of the following drugs is most likely to produce these findings?
    a. Prednisone
    b. Amiodarone
    c. Lovastatin
    d. Spironolactone
    e. Zidovudine

15. A 52-year-old woman with a history of diabetes mellitus and hypertension is evaluated for dizziness. On neurologic examination, she had postural instability with a tendency to fall forward. Blood pressure was 160/90 mm Hg in the supine position (with a heart rate of 85 beats/min). On standing, blood pressure was 100/70 mm Hg (with a heart rate of 88 beats/min), and she complained of a "spinning sensation" associated with neck and shoulder pain. What is the most appropriate first step in her management?
    a. Fludrocortisone
    b. Magnetic resonance angiography
    c. Discontinue antihypertensive drugs
    d. Vestibular evaluation
    e. Magnetic resonance imaging of the cervical spine

16. A 73-year-old woman has had headache and malaise for 1 week and a few hours before evaluation, an episode of transient monocular blindness in the right eye. Which next step would be the most appropriate in her evaluation?
    a. Carotid ultrasonography
    b. Lumbar puncture
    c. Computed tomography of the head
    d. Erythrocyte sedimentation rate
    e. Magnetic resonance angiography

17. A 35-year-old woman with a 5-year history of complex partial seizures well controlled with carbamazepine developed headache, fever, and a cough. Treatment was started with erythromycin and codeine. On the next day she was brought to the emergency department because of drowsiness, diplopia, and myoclonic jerks. Neurologic examination findings were otherwise normal. Which next step is most appropriate for further diagnosis or treatment?
    a. Perform lumbar puncture
    b. Determine carbamazepine levels
    c. Add clonazepam
    d. Obtain blood cultures
    e. Administer naloxone

18. A 43-year-old woman was evaluated because of a 3-month history of episodes of severe throbbing left retro-orbital headaches that last 10 to 15 minutes and recur up to 10 times a day. Neurologic examination findings were normal. What would be the most appropriate treatment?
    a. Prednisone
    b. Carbamazepine
    c. Sumatriptan
    d. Indomethacin
    e. Amitriptyline

19. A 62-year-old man was evaluated because of a 6-month history of progressive gait difficulty and hand weakness. Neurologic examination demonstrated weakness, atrophy, and fasciculations in the left deltoid, right biceps, both interossei, left quadriceps, and right gastrocnemius muscles. Stretch reflexes were normal in the upper and lower extremities, and the Babinski sign was present bilaterally. The sensory examination was normal. Magnetic resonance imaging of the entire spine and examination of the cerebrospinal fluid showed no abnormality. What treatment could be considered in this condition?
    a. Methylprednisolone
    b. Vitamin B_{12}
    c. Riluzole
    d. Plasma exchange
    e. Methotrexate

20. A 65-year-old woman is evaluated because of a 2-year history of progressive cognitive decline. Neurologic examination demonstrated an inability to remember four words that were given to her 5 minutes earlier, but digit span, calculation, and naming abilities were relatively preserved. Gait, motor, and sensory examination findings were unremarkable. Laboratory test results were normal, including vitamin B_{12} levels, thyroid function tests, and serologic testing for syphilis. Magnetic resonance imaging of the head demonstrated bilateral atrophy in the hippocampus and mild hydrocephalus. What would be the most appropriate treatment?
    a. Ventriculoperitoneal shunt
    b. Gabapentin
    c. Vitamin C
    d. Amitriptyline
    e. Donepezil

ANSWERS

1. Answer b.

The combination of vertigo, nystagmus, left Horner syndrome, left cerebellar ataxia, left palatal weakness, and dissociated anesthesia (left face and right body) indicates involvement of the left vestibular nucleus, cerebellum, sympathetic pathway, nucleus ambiguus, descending trigeminal nucleus and tract, and spinothalamic tract at the level of the lateral medulla. Lateral medullary syndrome occurs with infarction in the territory of the vertebral artery or the posterior inferior cerebellar artery and may be a manifestation of vertebral artery dissection. Complicated migraine, subarachnoid hemorrhage, acute multiple sclerosis, and transverse sinus thrombosis do not typically produce a lateral medullary syndrome.

2. Answer c.

The combination of upper and lower extremity signs of involvement of the dorsal columns and corticospinal tract indicates a lesion at the level of the cervical spinal cord. Common causes include cervical spondylosis, demyelinating disease, vitamin B_{12} deficiency, and neoplasm. Cervical magnetic resonance imaging and serum levels of vitamin B_{12} should be obtained in this setting. Electromyography is not indicated in the absence of lower motor neuron findings. In the absence

of signs suggesting a posterior fossa or supratentorial lesion, computed tomography of the head or magnetic resonance angiography are not indicated.

3. Answer d.

In a comatose patient, the preservation of pupillary responses in the absence of oculocephalic, oculovestibular, and corneal responses suggests a "metabolic" cause of coma. An important cause is intoxication with benzodiazepines, barbiturates, or opioids. In general, these are associated with hypotension, bradycardia, and hypoventilation. Pinpoint reactive pupils may occur with pontine hemorrhage or basilar artery occlusion, but these are associated with decerebrate rigidity instead of hypotonia and with central hyperventilation and sympathoexcitation. A mesencephalic hemorrhage is likely to produce dilated unreactive pupils because of involvement of the third nerve nucleus. Uncal herniation produces ipsilateral third nerve palsy. Neither these two conditions nor nonconvulsive status epilepticus should impair the oculovestibular reflexes, which are integrated at the level of the pontomedullary junction.

4. Answer e.

The presence of proximal symmetrical muscle weakness with or without atrophy, absence of fasciculations, and normal reflexes and sensation are characteristic of myopathy. The differential diagnosis includes inflammatory, toxic, metabolic, and hereditary (dystrophy) forms. Cervical myelopathy generally produces long-tract sensory loss, hyperreflexia, and extensor plantar responses. Motor neuron disease produces atrophy and fasciculations. Lambert-Eaton myasthenic syndrome is characterized by fluctuating weakness, areflexia, and autonomic dysfunction. Chronic inflammatory demyelinating neuropathy produces loss of sensation and muscle stretch reflexes in a predominantly distal distribution.

5. Answer a.

Inability to adduct one eye on attempting lateral gaze, but normal adduction during convergence, is characteristic of involvement of the ipsilateral medial longitudinal fasciculus at the level of the dorsal pons. In a young patient, the most common cause is multiple sclerosis. The preservation of adduction during accommodation is not consistent with a third nerve palsy, as may occur with a posterior communicating artery aneurysm or cavernous sinus meningioma. Myasthenia gravis, Graves ophthalmopathy, and Wernicke encephalopathy should always be considered in the differential diagnosis of diplopia, but they rarely, if ever, produce true internuclear ophthalmoplegia.

6. Answer d.

The presence of fluctuating weakness and muscle fatigue is the hallmark of a defect in neuromuscular transmission. Myasthenia gravis is the most common of these disorders and is due to antibodies directed against the muscle nicotinic acetylcholine receptors. It frequently affects the cranial musculature, producing fluctuating ptosis, diplopia, dysarthria, and dysphagia. Brain stem lesions produce nonfluctuating symptoms generally associated with long-tract findings (such as hyperreflexia and the Babinski sign). The fatigability and reversibility with resting of the muscle are not consistent with a transient ischemic attack. Myopathies such as mitochondrial disorders may produce external ophthalmoplegia, but dysphagia is unusual. Oculopharyngeal myopathies produce slowly progressive muscle weakness.

7. Answer a.

The presence of gait ataxia that worsens with the eyes closed and the absence of vibratory and joint position sense and muscle stretch reflexes are suggestive of a large fiber peripheral neuropathy or neuronopathy. One important cause is a paraneoplastic disorder generally associated with lung carcinoma and detected with antineuronal nuclear (anti-Hu) antibodies. Other causes include Sjögren syndrome, vitamin B_6 or cisplatin toxicity, and some monoclonal gammopathies. This clinical syndrome does not occur with intracranial lesions,

cervical myelopathy, predominantly motor neuropathies (such as porphyria), or vestibular dysfunction.

8. Answer b.

The combination of sensory and motor symptoms in the lower extremities and bladder dysfunction indicates a lesion at the level of the spinal cord. The combination of absent knee stretch reflex, ankle clonus, extensor plantar responses, and preserved anal reflex indicates a lesion at the L3-4 level, producing a neurogenic bladder. This is a neurologic emergency that is evaluated best with magnetic resonance imaging of the spine.

9. Answer d.

The presence of an abrupt onset headache, bitemporal visual field loss, and bilateral oculomotor palsy should immediately raise the possibility of pituitary apoplexy, with involvement of the optic chiasm and cavernous sinus. This is a medical emergency, because of both visual loss and acute adrenal insufficiency. The differential diagnosis includes cerebral aneurysm, carotid sinus thrombophlebitis, ophthalmoplegic migraine, diabetic ophthalmoparesis, and temporal arteritis, but these conditions do not produce bitemporal hemianopia.

10. Answer c.

The subacute development of ascending weakness in the lower and upper extremities, bilateral facial nerve palsy, and areflexia should raise the suspicion of an acute inflammatory demyelinating neuropathy (Guillain-Barré syndrome). In this disorder, the cerebrospinal fluid typically shows increased protein levels with little or no increase in cells. The presence of cerebrospinal fluid pleocytosis in this setting suggests an alternative cause, such as Lyme disease or meningeal carcinomatosis. Myasthenia gravis (detectable with acetylcholine receptor antibodies) and inflammatory myopathies (detectable by increased levels of creatine kinase) can also produce subacute weakness, but in these conditions the muscle stretch reflexes are normal. Areflexia is also inconsistent with a central nervous system lesion, such as multiple sclerosis.

11. Answer c.

In a patient with acute confusional state or other change in mental status, a careful history and examination are important to detect potential triggering factors. A common cause of delirium in the elderly is drug intoxication, particularly by drugs with anticholinergic side effects. Therefore, anticholinergic drugs are contraindicated in elderly patients with Parkinson disease. Levodopa/carbidopa and direct dopaminergic agents can also produce hallucinations, and this risk may increase with the addition of a monoamino-oxidase B inhibitor such as selegiline. Clozapine, a mixed $D_2/5-HT_1$ antagonist, lacks extrapyramidal side effects and is the drug of choice for treatment of hallucinations in these patients. However, it poses the risks of granulocytopenia, orthostatic hypotension, and seizures.

12. Answer e.

In a patient with seizures, the presence of psychosis and abdominal pain should raise the suspicion of acute intermittent porphyria. The episodes generally are triggered by use of drugs that induce liver enzymes, such as estrogens, corticosteroids, and many anticonvulsants, including phenobarbital, phenytoin, carbamazepine, and primidone. Because gabapentin does not undergo liver metabolism and does not induce liver enzyme activity, it is likely the safest anticonvulsant for patients with hepatic porphyria.

13. Answer b.

Several drugs may produce peripheral neuropathies. Cisplatin and amiodarone produce a predominantly large fiber sensory neuropathy with severe loss of joint position and vibratory sense. Phenytoin and isoniazid generally produce a distal sensorimotor peripheral neuropathy. Nitrofurantoin produces a predominantly motor neuropathy.

14. Answer c.

The presence of muscle pain, weakness, myoglobinuria, and marked increase in muscle creatine kinase are typical of a necrotizing myopathy. An important cause is the use of HMG-CoA inhibitors such as lovastatin. The risk of developing this complication increases with the concomitant use of other lipid-lowering drugs such as clofibrate and with the use of cyclosporine. Prednisone, zidovudine, and amiodarone can produce myopathy by different mechanisms.

15. Answer c.

Orthostatic hypotension is an important cause of dizziness, particularly in patients at risk for developing autonomic failure, such as those with diabetic neuropathy or parkinsonism. The hallmark of orthostatic hypotension due to autonomic failure is an inability to increase heart rate in the setting of a profound decrease in blood pressure on standing. The first step in managing orthostatic hypotension is to correct potentially reversible causes, particularly the use of vasodilator, diuretic, and anticholinergic agents. Simple maneuvers, such as increasing salt and water intake, elevating the head of the bed, and postural maneuvers should be tried before pharmacologic management.

16. Answer d.

Recent onset headache, transient visual symptoms, and malaise in an elderly patient raise the suspicion of giant cell arteritis. Other suggestive features are jaw claudication and scalp tenderness. An erythrocyte sedimentation rate should be the first test, because it is markedly increased in more than 90% of these patients. Urgent treatment with prednisone (60 mg/day) should then be started to prevent visual loss due to ischemic optic neuropathy. The diagnosis can be confirmed in equivocal cases with temporal artery biopsy.

17. Answer b.

Somnolence, diplopia, and myoclonus are some of the neurologic manifestations of carbamazepine toxicity. Several frequently used drugs, including erythromycin, may interfere with liver metabolism of carbamazepine and increase its level or those of its active epoxide derivative, producing neurologic toxicity. Drug interaction should be suspected in every patient receiving long-term antiepileptic drug treatment who develops new neurologic symptoms, and this is one of the indications for measuring antiepileptic drug levels.

18. Answer d.

Episodes of unilateral throbbing retro-orbital headache of sudden onset and short duration (10-20 min) recurring several times a day are typical of chronic paroxysmal hemicrania. This type of vascular headache is typically controlled with indomethacin. This pattern is atypical for trigeminal neuralgia, which responds to carbamazepine, or for migraine or cluster headaches, which respond to sumatriptan. Prednisone is indicated in temporal arteritis or to control an episode of cluster headache. Amitriptyline is used for prophylaxis of migraine or tension headache.

19. Answer c.

The combination of lower motor neuron findings (weakness, atrophy, and fasciculations) in cranial musculature and/or more than one limb in association with upper motor neuron findings (hyperreflexia, Babinski sign) and in the absence of sensory or sphincter disturbance is typical of amyotrophic lateral sclerosis. Clinical trials indicate that riluzole, a drug that blocks sodium channels and decreases the release of glutamate, produces a slight but significant slowing of disease progression. Given the inexorable progression of the disease, other treatable causes should be investigated. Electromyography is indicated not only for diagnosis but also to look for evidence of demyelination of conduction block. Magnetic resonance imaging of the cervical spine should be performed in some cases to exclude a structural lesion such as cervical spondylosis or neoplasm. Other potentially useful tests are special protein electrophoresis to look for monoclonal gammopathy and cerebrospinal fluid examination. The absence of sensory findings, the upper motor neuron findings, and normal cerebrospinal fluid protein would not be consistent with chronic inflammatory demyelinating neuropathy, a condition that responds to methylprednisolone or plasma exchange. The presence of atrophy and fasciculations would be atypical for vitamin B_{12} deficiency.

20. Answer e.

Progressive cognitive decline involving primarily memory, with relative preservation of attention, and interfering with the patient's activities indicates the possibility of a degenerative dementia. Alzheimer disease is the most common degenerative dementia and should be suspected in patients with a deficit in attention, language, and other high cortical functions who otherwise have a normal neurologic examination, family history of dementia, and bilateral atrophy of the hippocampus and surrounding areas. Donepezil, an anticholinesterase drug, has been shown in clinical trials to improve some cognitive indices in patients with Alzheimer disease. Pseudodementia of depression should be considered in all patients with progressive cognitive decline, and a trial with an antidepressant drug may be indicated. However, tricyclic antidepressants with central anticholinergic side effects, such as amitriptyline, should be avoided.

CHAPTER 18

ONCOLOGY

Scott H. Okuno, M.D.
Henry C. Pitot, M.D.

BREAST CANCER

Magnitude of the Problem

In the United States, 180,000 new cases of breast cancer are diagnosed annually. Breast cancer will develop in approximately 1 in 10 women who achieve a normal life expectancy. Breast cancer is the second most common cause of cancer death among women in the United States (lung cancer is the most common).

- Breast cancer will develop in 1 in 10 American women.
- Incidence is increasing (largely due to screening).
- It is the second most common cause of cancer death in American women.

Risk Factors

The risk factors for breast cancer are outlined in Table 18-1. In addition those women with breast cancer-associated genes (*BRCA1* and *BRCA2*) have up to an 80% chance of developing breast cancer in their lifetime. It should be noted that less than 25% of women with breast cancer have known high-risk factors.

- Less than 25% of women with breast cancer have known high-risk factors.

Screening

The use of screening mammography in the age group 50 years or older has decreased mortality by 20% to 30%. The use of screening mammography in the age group 40 to 50 years is controversial. There is general consensus that women 50 years or older should be screened with annual clinical examination and mammography. For women deemed at high risk for breast cancer, screening should be instituted at an appropriate earlier age, generally taken as 5 to 10 years before the earliest diagnosis of breast cancer in the family. Currently, mammography will miss about 10% of breast cancers detectable on physical examination. Thus, a biopsy specimen should be obtained of any suspicious palpable lump despite a negative mammogram.

- Screening for breast cancer can reduce mortality.
- Women ≥50 years old need annual examinations and mammography.
- There is controversy about screening normal women 40 to 50 years old.
- Ten percent of breast cancers found on physical examination are missed by mammography.
- Biopsy is recommended for suspicious palpable lump, even if mammogram is negative.

Table 18-1.—Risk Factors for Breast Cancer

High risk: relative risk >4.0	Moderate risk: relative risk 2-4	Low risk: relative risk 1-2
Older age	Any first-degree relative with breast cancer	Menarche before age 12 years
Personal history of breast cancer		Menopause after age 55 years
Family history of premenopausal bilateral breast cancer or familial cancer syndrome	Personal history of ovarian or endometrial cancer	Caucasian race
Breast biopsy showing proliferative disease with atypia	Age at first full-term pregnancy >30 years	Moderate alcohol intake
	Nulliparous	Long-duration (≥15 years) estrogen replacement therapy
	Obesity in postmenopausal women	
	Upper socioeconomic class	

Pathology

Breast cancers are classified as ductal or lobular, corresponding to the ducts and lobules of the normal breast (Fig. 18-1). Invasive, or infiltrating, breast cancer has the potential for systemic spread, as opposed to carcinoma in situ, which does not have the metastatic potential because by definition it has not invaded through the basement membrane. Infiltrating ductal carcinoma is the most common histologic type (70% of breast cancers), and lobular cancer is more frequently multifocal and bilateral.

- Infiltrating ductal carcinoma is the most common histologic type of breast cancer.
- Lobular disease is more frequently multifocal and bilateral.
- Ductal carcinoma in situ is noninvasive, does not have the potential for systemic spread, and is treated with local therapy only.

Staging

The staging system of the American Joint Committee on Cancer is shown in Table 18-2.

Natural History and Prognostic Factors

Nodal Status

The number of involved axillary nodes remains the single best predictor of outcome (Fig. 18-2).

Tumor Size

After nodal status, tumor size is generally the most important prognostic factor (Table 18-3).

Hormone Receptor Status

In general, patients with estrogen-receptor-positive tumors have a better prognosis. However, the difference in recurrence rates at 5 years is only 8% to 10%.

Table 18-2.—Staging of Breast Cancer

Primary tumor (T)	
TIS	Carcinoma in situ
T1	T = ≤2 cm
T2	T = 2.1-5 cm
T3	T = >5 cm
T4	T of any size with direct extension to chest wall or skin

Regional nodes (N)
N0	No involved nodes
N1	Movable ipsilateral axillary nodes
N2	Matted or fixed nodes

Distant metastasis (M)
M0	None detected
M1	Distant metastasis present (includes ipsilateral supraclavicular nodes)

Stage grouping

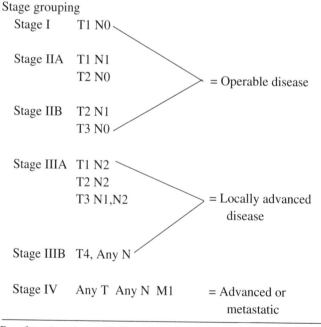

Stage I   T1 N0

Stage IIA   T1 N1
            T2 N0   = Operable disease

Stage IIB   T2 N1
            T3 N0

Stage IIIA T1 N2
            T2 N2
            T3 N1,N2   = Locally advanced
                                       disease

Stage IIIB T4, Any N

Stage IV   Any T Any N M1   = Advanced or
                                       metastatic

Data from American Joint Committee on Cancer: Breast. *In* Manual for Staging of Cancer. Fourth edition. Edited by OH Beahrs, DE Henson, RVP Hutter, BJ Kennedy. Philadelphia, JB Lippincott Company, 1992, pp 149-154.

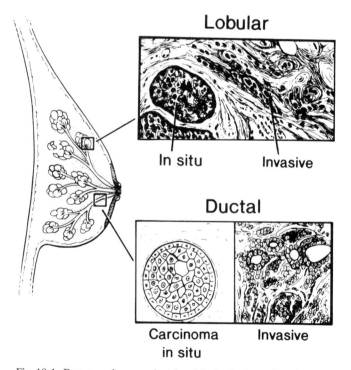

Lobular

In situ   Invasive

Ductal

Carcinoma   Invasive
in situ

Fig. 18-1. Breast carcinomas: ductal vs. lobular, in situ vs. invasive.

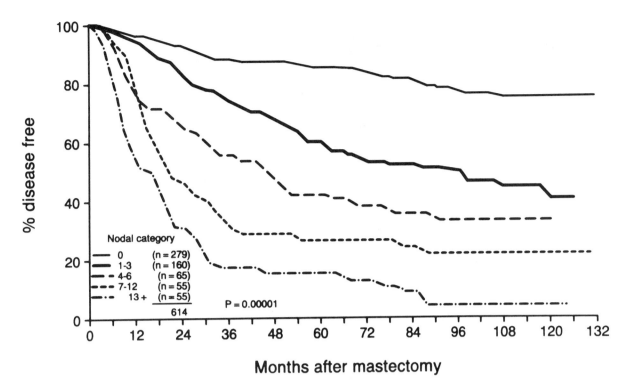

Fig. 18-2. Relation of disease-free survival to numbers of nodal metastases in more than 600 women with breast cancer treated with radical mastectomy alone in the early 1970s. (From Fisher ER, Sass R, Fisher B, and Collaborating NSABP Investigators: Pathologic findings from the National Surgical Adjuvant Project for Breast Cancers [protocol no. 4]. X. Discriminants for tenth year treatment failure. Cancer 53:712-723, 1984. By permission of Wiley-Liss.)

Grade

Most breast cancers are high-grade. Patients with low-grade tumors have fewer recurrences and longer survival.

- Number of involved axillary nodes is best predictor of outcome.
- After nodal status, tumor size is most important prognostic factor.
- Patients with receptor-positive tumors have better prognosis.
- Patients with low-grade tumors have better prognosis.

Treatment

Primary or Local-Regional Therapy

Primary local treatment for invasive breast cancer is either breast conservation (lumpectomy with axillary lymph node dissection and breast radiation) or mastectomy. Several randomized controlled clinical trials have shown therapeutic equivalence for breast conservation versus mastectomy. The outcome for women with invasive breast cancer depends on the presence of distant microscopic metastatic disease rather than the treatment of local disease.

- Breast conservation and mastectomy have demonstrated therapeutic equivalence.

Adjuvant Treatment

After primary treatment of the breast, additional systemic treatment (adjuvant) may be offered to women to help eradicate the microscopic metastatic disease and ultimately improve overall survival. The number of involved axillary lymph nodes is the single best predictor of outcome. All women with metastatically involved axillary lymph nodes should be offered adjuvant treatment (Table 18-4). Women with negative lymph nodes have only a 25% chance of microscopic metastatic disease, and their risk of recurrence can be further estimated by using Table 18-5. Adjuvant systemic treatment should be offered to women in the intermediate- and high-risk groups.

- Women with node-positive disease are at high risk of systemic disease and should be offered adjuvant treatment.
- Women with node-negative disease have only a 25% chance of systemic disease and adjuvant treatment should be given for intermediate- and high-risk groups.

Treatment of Advanced Disease

We currently lack curative therapy for recurrent or metastatic breast cancer. The median duration of survival for recurrent disease is 2.5 years. Survival is longer with bone or soft tissue recurrence than with visceral recurrence. Because

Table 18-3.—Long-Term Results[*] in Patients With Node-Negative Breast Cancer Treated Surgically

Tumor size, cm	No. of patients	% free of recurrence	% dead of disease
<1	171	88	10
1.1-2.0	303	74	24
2.1-3.0	188	72	24
3.1-5.0	105	61	36

[*]Median duration of follow-up was 18 years.
Data from Rosen PP, Groshen S, Kinne DW: Survival and prognostic factors in node-negative breast cancer: results of long-term follow-up studies. Monogr Natl Cancer Inst 11:159-162, 1992.

Table 18-4.—Adjuvant Therapy: Node-Positive Breast Cancer

	Estrogen-receptor status	
	Positive	Negative
Premenopausal	Chemo + Tam	Chemo
Postmenopausal	Tam + Chemo	Chemo

Chemo, combination chemotherapy; Tam, tamoxifen.

Table 18-5.—Adjuvant Therapy: Node-Negative Breast Cancer[*]

	Risk		
	Low	Intermediate	High
Tumor size, cm	<1	1-2	>2
ER or PR	+	+	-
Grade	1	1-2	2-3

[*]Most oncologists would not treat tumors less than 1 cm.
ER, estrogen receptor; PR, progesterone receptor.

treatment is not curative, the initial systemic treatment for patients with estrogen-receptor–positive advanced disease is usually hormonal. Chemotherapy is used once women have progressed on hormonal therapy or in women with estrogen-receptor–negative breast cancer.

- There is no curative therapy for recurrent or metastatic breast cancer.
- The average survival with recurrent breast cancer is 2.5 years.

Chemotherapy

Active drugs against breast cancer include doxorubicin (Adriamycin, A), cyclophosphamide (C), methotrexate (M), 5-fluorouracil (F), paclitaxel (Taxol), docetaxel (Taxotere), capecitabine (Xeloda), vincristine/vinblastine, mitomycin-C, etoposide, and cisplatin. Common combination regimens are CMF, CAF, and AC. The side effects of chemotherapy include reversible lowering of the blood counts and reversible hair loss. After 20 years of follow-up, there has been no increased risk of second malignancies for women who received adjuvant chemotherapy.

Hormonal Agents

Tamoxifen is the most widely used hormonal agent in the treatment of patients with breast cancer. Tamoxifen is a nonsteroidal compound that on selected tissue acts like an antiestrogen (breast tissue) but on other tissue acts like an estrogen (bones, lipids, uterus). Its beneficial effects include 1) antitumor effects on breast cancer cells, 2) decreased risk (by 40%) of contralateral breast cancer for women taking adjuvant tamoxifen, 3) improved bone density, and 4) favorable effects on lipid profiles. Tamoxifen also has some side effects, including 1) vaginal dryness and hot flashes, 2) thromboembolic risk (1%-2%), and 3) increased risk of endometrial cancer.

- Tamoxifen has both antiestrogen and estrogen-like activity.
- Beneficial effects of tamoxifen: antitumor effects, increased bone density, improved lipid profile, and decreased risk of contralateral breast cancer.
- Side effects of tamoxifen: hot flashes, vaginal dryness, thromboembolic risk, and increased risk of endometrial cancer.

Other hormonal agents include megestrol acetate (Megace), a progestational agent; fluoxymesterone (Halotestin), an androgen; and the new nonsteroidal aromatase inhibitors anastrozole (Arimidex) and letrozole (Femara).

Other Agents

Herceptin

About 25% of breast cancers over-express the growth factor HER2. A monoclonal antibody directed against HER2 (herceptin) has been shown to have activity against refractory breast cancer and is synergistic with certain chemotherapy agents.

Pamidronate

The use of the bisphosphonate pamidronate has reduced the need for radiation, bone fixation, and pain medicine in women with lytic bone metastases.

CERVICAL CANCER

Background

The incidence of and mortality from cervical cancer have decreased by 30% to 40% in recent decades, attributed to widespread use of Papanicolaou smear screening. Currently, 16,000 new cases of cervical cancer are diagnosed in U.S. women each year, and there are 5,000 deaths annually. In addition, more than 50,000 cases of carcinoma in situ of the cervix are diagnosed annually. Risk factors for cervical cancer include first intercourse at an early age, a greater number of sexual partners, smoking, history of sexually transmitted disease, especially herpes or human papillomavirus (HPV) lesions, and lower socioeconomic class. It is now understood that HPV is an etiologic agent for cervical carcinogenesis.

If a cytologic smear shows dysplasia or malignant cells, colposcopy with directed biopsy should be done. The Papanicolaou smear has limited sensitivity; false-negative rates of 20% frequently are quoted. The American Cancer Society recommends that asymptomatic, low-risk women 20 years of age or older, and those younger than 20 years who are sexually active, have a Papanicolaou smear annually for 2 consecutive years and, if those are negative, at least one every 3 years.

Treatment

Treatment for carcinoma in situ of the cervix is usually a total hysterectomy. If additional childbearing is desired, a more conservative approach, such as a therapeutic conization, is another option. Early invasive carcinoma of the cervix is usually treated with total hysterectomy. For patients with higher-stage disease, radiation therapy is used.

COLORECTAL CANCER

Background

Colorectal cancer is diagnosed in approximately 135,000 Americans each year and causes 56,000 deaths. Colorectal cancer is most common in North America and Europe. It is associated with high-fat, low-fiber diets. Population screening with fecal occult blood testing remains problematic. Although one study showed a reduction in mortality from colorectal cancer with fecal occult blood screening (N Engl J Med 328:1365-1371, 1993), it should be noted that any participants who had positive results went on to have colonoscopy. Another study showed that fecal occult blood tests failed to detect 70% of colorectal cancers and 80% of large (≥2 cm) polyps (JAMA 269:1262-1267, 1993). For high-risk patients, such as those with a family history of colorectal cancer or a prior colorectal cancer, structural studies of the entire large bowel, such as colonoscopy or proctoscopy plus barium enema, should be performed at appropriate intervals (such as every 1-3 years).

- Colorectal cancer is associated with high-fat, low-fiber diets.
- Screening for colorectal cancer remains controversial.
- For high-risk patients, the entire large bowel should be studied at appropriate intervals.

Risk Factors

High-risk groups include persons with 1) familial polyposis syndromes (familial adenomatous polyposis—gene recently identified on chromosome 5—and Gardner syndrome—gut polyps plus desmoid tumors, lipomas, sebaceous cysts, and other abnormalities); 2) familial cancer syndromes without polyps (hereditary nonpolyposis colorectal cancer or Lynch syndromes, which are marked by colon cancer with or without endometrial, breast, and other cancers); and 3) inflammatory bowel disease (incidence 12% after 25 years).

- High-risk factors are familial polyposis syndromes, including familial adenomatous polyposis and Gardner syndrome, both inherited as autosomal dominant trait; select familial cancer syndromes without polyps; and inflammatory bowel disease.

Treatment

Surgery

Surgical resection is the preferred method of curative treatment for carcinomas of the colon or rectum. Surgical exploration and resection allows for pathologic determination of tumor depth of penetration through the bowel wall and assessment of regional lymph nodes. Prognosis is directly related to the stage of disease (Table 18-6), although rectal tumors tend to have a worse prognosis than colon carcinomas. Five-year survival rates for locoregional disease have improved in recent decades as a result of many factors, including improvements in preoperative staging, surgical technique, and adjuvant therapy.

- Surgical resection is the preferred treatment for colorectal cancer.
- Prognosis is directly related to the stage of disease.
- Five-year survival rates are improving.

Adjuvant Therapy

For *colon cancers*, adjuvant 5-fluorouracil (5-FU) and leucovorin, given for 6 months, are recommended for node-positive (stage III) disease. Controversy exists on standard recommendations for deeply invasive (stage II) colon carcinomas. For *rectal cancers*, combined chemotherapy (5-FU–based) and pelvic irradiation are standard for stage II and III disease.

Table 18-6.—Staging of Colorectal Cancer and Survival

Dukes stage	AJCC stage	Depth of penetration	Nodal status	5-Year survival, %
A	I	Submucosa or muscularis	Negative	90
B	II	Through muscularis or to other organs	Negative	60-80
C	III	Any	Positive	30-60

AJCC, American Joint Committee on Cancer.

- For stage III colon cancers, adjuvant chemotherapy includes 5-FU and leucovorin.
- For rectal cancer, combined chemotherapy (5-FU–based) and radiotherapy are the standard recommendations.

Metastatic Disease

Certain patients with locally recurrent or advanced colorectal cancer may be candidates for an attempt at curative resection. Of carefully selected patients with limited metastatic disease to the liver or lung, approximately 25% survive beyond 5 years without further evidence of disease recurrence (Ann Intern Med 129:27-35, 1998).

Palliative chemotherapy is the only option for the vast majority of patients with advanced metastatic colorectal cancer. The median survival for patients treated with chemotherapy is 10 to 14 months. Combined 5-FU and leucovorin (a modulator of 5-FU) is the initial standard approach. Significant tumor response is observed in approximately 30% of patients. The principal toxic effects include stomatitis, diarrhea, and leukopenia. Irinotecan (CPT-11) was recently approved for treatment of advanced colorectal cancer that is refractory to 5-FU. Responses are observed in approximately 15% of patients, and diarrhea and neutropenia are the common side effects. A recent trial comparing irinotecan to best supportive care in patients refractory to 5-FU demonstrated a prolonged median survival and better quality of life (Lancet 352:1413-1418, 1998).

- Surgical resection of metastatic disease can result in long-term disease-free survival.
- Standard palliative chemotherapy for advanced colorectal carcinoma is 5-FU plus leucovorin.
- Irinotecan (CPT-11) is an option for 5-FU patients refractory to 5-FU; diarrhea is a common side effect.

Carcinoembryonic Antigen (CEA)

Proponents of CEA monitoring after operation for colorectal cancer argue that early recurrences, curable surgically, can be detected. However, CEA monitoring lacks sensitivity and specificity. It is estimated that cancer cures attributable to CEA monitoring occur in less than 1% of patients monitored (JAMA 270:943-947, 1993).

LUNG CANCER

Magnitude of the Problem

Approximately 170,000 new cases of lung cancer are diagnosed in the United States annually, resulting in 150,000 deaths. Thus, only approximately 10% of patients diagnosed with lung cancer survive their disease. Lung cancer is the leading cause of cancer mortality in American men and women.

Risk Factors

About 95% of lung cancers in men and about 80% of lung cancers in women result from cigarette smoking. Men who smoke 1 to 2 packs per day have up to a 25-fold increase in lung cancer compared with those who have never smoked. The risk of lung cancer in an ex-smoker declines with time. Passive smoking is associated with an increased risk of lung cancer. Certain occupations (smelter workers, iron workers), chemicals (arsenic, methyl ethyl ether), and exposure to radioactive agents (radon, uranium) and asbestos have been associated with increased risks for development of lung cancer.

- 95% of lung cancers in men and 80% in women result from cigarette smoking.
- Men who smoke 1 to 2 packs a day have 25-fold increase in lung cancer compared with those who never smoked.
- Passive smoking is associated with increased risk of lung cancer.

Screening

Several large, randomized trials have tested the utility of chest radiography and sputum cytology in screening for lung cancer. None of these studies have shown that either sputum cytology or regular chest radiography improves survival from lung cancer. Thus, screening is not standard at the present time. However, there are recognized methodologic problems with these studies, and some believe that there is benefit to screening for this disease (Chest 107 Suppl:270S-279S, 1995).

- Randomized trials have not demonstrated an advantage to screening for lung cancer.

Histologic Types and Characteristics

Lung cancer is divided into small-cell and non–small-cell types. Small-cell lung cancer occurs almost exclusively in smokers. The primary tumors are often small but are associated with bulky mediastinal adenopathy. They may be associated with paraneoplastic syndromes, including the syndrome of inappropriate secretion of antidiuretic hormone and various neurologic abnormalities. Non–small-cell lung cancers can be divided into squamous, adenocarcinoma, and large-cell types. Squamous cell carcinomas may be associated with hypercalcemia due to the secretion of a parathyroid hormone-like peptide. Squamous carcinomas tend to occur centrally, whereas large-cell and adenocarcinoma types tend to be more peripheral. Adenocarcinoma is the most frequent histologic subtype in non-smokers. Bronchoalveolar carcinoma is a low-grade non-small-cell carcinoma that frequently presents as a patchy infiltrate. It may be multifocal.

Staging

The "classic *T*umor-*N*ode-*M*etastasis" system is simplified in Table 18-7.

Natural History

The natural history of surgically treated lung cancer, by stage, is shown in Figure 18-3.

Treatment

Non–Small-Cell Lung Cancer (NSCLC)

Surgery is the treatment of choice for clinical stage I, II, and selected IIIa disease. The use of adjuvant chemotherapy has not been shown to improve survival compared with surgery alone. The use of adjuvant radiation does not improve survival in resected stage II and III disease, but it is able to decrease the likelihood of local recurrence. In patients with locally advanced unresectable NSCLC, the use of chemotherapy before radiation therapy improves the long-term survival compared with radiation alone. Although patients with metastatic disease are not cured, the use of chemotherapy has improved the overall survival and the quality of life compared with best supportive care.

- Surgery is the treatment of choice for stages I and II NSCLC.

Table 18-7.—Staging of Lung Cancer

Non-small cell	
Stage I	Primary tumor >2 cm from carina; node negative
Stage II	Primary tumor >2 cm from carina; hilar nodes positive
Stage IIIA	Tumor <2 cm from carina, or invading a resectable structure, or ipsilateral mediastinal nodes positive
Stage IIIB	Tumor invading an unresectable structure, supraclavicular or contralateral mediastinal nodes positive or cytologically positive pleural effusion
Stage IV	Metastatic disease
Small cell	
Limited	Limited to one hemithorax less supraclavicular lymph nodes. Can be encompassed within a tolerable radiation port
Extensive	All other disease (metastatic disease)

- There is no improvement in survival with adjuvant chemotherapy or radiation therapy.
- Chemotherapy is not curative for metastatic NSCLC.
- Chemotherapy improves the overall survival and quality of life for patients with metastatic NSCLC.

Chemotherapy for NSCLC

Active chemotherapy agents for NSCLC include etoposide, cisplatin, carboplatin, cyclophosphamide, mitomycin-C, ifosfamide, gemcitabine, irinotecan, docetaxel, and paclitaxel.

Small-Cell Lung Cancer

Treatment of limited-stage small-cell lung cancer consists of both chemotherapy and chest irradiation. Operation has not been shown to improve survival. For patients who have a complete response to chemotherapy and chest radiation therapy, prophylactic cranial irradiation is sometimes used to decrease the frequency of failure in the central nervous system. However, even though prophylactic cranial irradiation decreases the rate of relapse in the brain, it does not affect survival. It is associated with the risk of a delayed leukoencephalopathy, but this risk can be reduced by the administration of radiation in small-dose fractions without concomitant chemotherapy. For limited-stage small-cell disease, the median duration of survival is approximately 18 months; 30% to 40% of patients survive 2 years, and 10% to 20% survive 5 years.

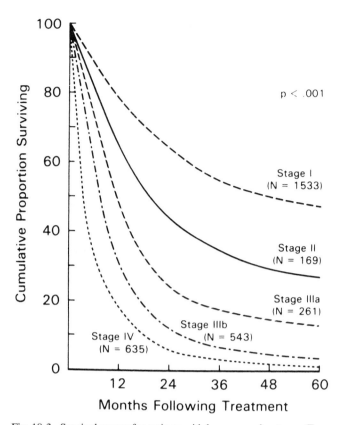

Fig. 18-3. Survival curves for patients with lung cancer by stage. (From Mountain CF: A new international staging system for lung cancer. Chest 89:225S-233S, 1986. By permission of American College of Chest Physicians.)

- For small-cell lung cancer, treatment of limited-stage disease consists of both chemotherapy and chest irradiation.
- Prophylactic cranial irradiation decreases the risk of relapse in the brain but does not affect overall survival.
- Median survival is 18 months with limited-stage disease.

Treatment of extensive stage (stage IV) small-cell lung cancer is with chemotherapy. Combination chemotherapy is favored over single-agent therapy. Active drugs include etoposide, cisplatin, cyclophosphamide, doxorubicin, and vincristine. High-dose chemotherapy with or without autologous bone marrow transplantation or marrow colony-stimulating factors has not yet been proved superior, on a consistent basis, to standard chemotherapy. The median duration of survival is approximately 9 months; about 10% of patients survive 2 years, and 1% or less survive 5 years.

- For extensive stage small-cell lung cancer, treatment is chemotherapy.
- High-dose chemotherapy has not yet been proved superior to standard chemotherapy.
- Median survival is 9 months.

MELANOMA

Background
Malignant melanoma is increasing at a rapid rate. If current trends continue, by the year 2000 the lifetime risk for malignant melanoma to develop in an American will be 1 in 75. Fortunately, the 5-year survival rate has doubled from approximately 40% in the 1940s to approximately 80% now, a change attributed to earlier detection. Melanoma is more common among fair-skinned people, persons with multiple atypical nevi, patients with freckling tendency, and certain families (first-degree relatives or dysplastic nevus syndrome).

- Incidence of malignant melanoma is increasing rapidly.
- 5-year survival rate has improved as a result of earlier detection.
- High-risk populations are identifiable.

Diagnosis ("ABCD") and Prognosis
Keys to the early diagnosis include the following:
A: Asymmetry, especially a changing lesion
B: Borders are irregular
C: Color is variable, especially with blues, blacks, and tans dispersed throughout the lesion
D: Diameter 6 mm or more

The Breslow microstaging method measures the thickness (i.e., depth of penetration of the tumor from the epidermis into the dermis/subcutis) of a malignant melanoma and is the best independent predictor of survival (Table 18-8).

Management
Surgical excision to achieve a 1- to 3-cm margin around the lesion remains the principal treatment for primary malignant melanoma. In the absence of palpable adenopathy, an elective lymph node dissection is not routinely performed. With clinically palpable regional nodes, a node dissection is performed for curative intent and to achieve maximal local tumor control. For patients with deep primary tumors (>1.5 mm) or resected node-positive disease, recent clinical trials support the use of adjuvant interferon-α, although the exact dose and schedule remain controversial (Lancet 351:1905-1910, 1998).

Treatment for metastatic melanoma is primarily palliative. Surgical resection in selected patients (those with a long disease-free interval and limited disease at recurrence) can be considered. Systemic treatments commonly include immunotherapy (interleukin-2 or interferon), chemotherapy (dacarbazine or nitrosoureas), or various combinations.

OVARIAN CANCER
This disease is diagnosed annually in 25,000 American women. It is the leading cause of death due to gynecologic

Table 18-8.—Ten-Year Survival in Melanoma, by Depth of Tumor

Depth, mm	% alive
<0.85	96
0.85-1.69	87
1.7-3.6	66.5
>3.6	46

Data from Friedman RJ, Rigel DS, Silverman MK, Kopf AW, Vossaert KA: Malignant melanoma in the 1990s: the continued importance of early detection and the role of physician examination and self-examination of the skin. CA Cancer J Clin 41:201-226, July/Aug 1991.

cancer. There are no early warning signs; most patients present with vague gastrointestinal complaints such as bloating. Most patients (75%) present with advanced disease (i.e., stages III and IV, disease spread beyond the pelvis). The term "ovarian cancer" refers to tumors derived from the ovarian surface epithelium, not germ cell tumors.

- Ovarian cancer is the leading cause of death due to gynecologic cancer.
- There are no early warning signs.
- Most patients (75%) present with advanced disease.

Staging

Stage I is confined to the ovary, stage II is confined to the pelvis, stage III includes spread to the upper abdomen, and stage IV includes spread to distant sites.

CA-125

The tumor antigen, CA-125, is expressed by approximately 85% of epithelial ovarian tumors and released into the circulation. However, it is detectable in only 50% of patients with stage I disease. The highest serum levels of CA-125 are found in patients with ovarian cancer, but the serum CA-125 level may also be increased in other malignancies, as well as in pregnancy, endometriosis, and menstruation. CA-125 is clearly of value for monitoring the course of ovarian cancer.

- CA-125 is expressed by about 85% of epithelial ovarian tumors.
- CA-125 level may also be increased in other malignancies and in pregnancy, endometriosis, and menstruation.
- CA-125 is useful for monitoring course of disease.

Screening

The tools evaluated thus far, namely, pelvic ultrasonography and determination of serum cancer antigen CA-125, are inadequate for screening the general female population.

Screening for this disease is difficult for several reasons. The incidence of ovarian cancer is relatively low, and there are no recognized pre-invasive lesions. Moreover, pelvic ultrasonography and CA-125 lack sufficient sensitivity and specificity. However, it seems reasonable to apply these techniques on a periodic basis to women at particularly high risk of ovarian cancer, for example, those with a significant family history of the disease (two or more affected relatives). The cause of epithelial ovarian cancer is unknown. A small subset of patients (<5%) has an inherited predisposition to this disease. Generally, this occurs in families with both breast and ovarian cancer.

- Population screening for ovarian cancer is not recommended.
- Pelvic ultrasonography and CA-125 lack sufficient sensitivity and specificity.
- A small subset of patients (<5%) has an inherited predisposition to ovarian cancer and should be screened.

Treatment

The initial management of patients with epithelial ovarian cancer includes a thorough surgical staging and debulking procedure. Outcome in this disease depends on the amount of tumor tissue removed at initial operation. Subsequently, patients are treated with six cycles of platinum- and paclitaxel-based chemotherapy.

- Management of ovarian cancer includes thorough surgical staging and debulking followed by chemotherapy.
- Outcome depends on the amount of tumor tissue removed at initial operation.
- Subsequent chemotherapy consists of a platinum compound and paclitaxel (Taxol).

Outcome

Outcome depends on stage. Ninety percent of patients with stage I disease are alive at 5 years, versus 80% for stage II disease. Unfortunately, survival with advanced disease is poor; 15% to 20% of patients with stage III disease are alive at 5 years and only 5% of patients with stage IV disease are alive.

PROSTATE CANCER

Background

There are approximately 190,000 new cases of prostate cancer annually in the United States. It is the most common cancer in men in the United States and is the second leading cause of death from cancer in men in the United States (40,000 deaths annually). Identified risk factors for the development of prostatic cancer include older age, race (African-American), family history (first-degree relative), and possibly dietary fat. The American Cancer Society recommends a digital rectal examination in men aged 40 years or older and determination of the prostate-specific antigen (PSA) value in men 50 years or older. Use of the PSA value for prostate cancer screening is a controversial issue and has not been shown to reduce mortality.

- Prostate cancer is the most common cancer among U.S. males (190,000 cases annually) and the second leading cause of death from cancer (40,000 cases annually).
- Risk factors include older age, African-American males, family history, and a high-fat diet.

Prostate-Specific Antigen (PSA)

PSA is a serine protease produced by normal and neoplastic prostatic ductal epithelium. Its concentration is proportional to the total prostatic mass. The inability to differentiate benign prostatic hyperplasia from carcinoma on the basis of the PSA level renders it inadequate as the sole screening method for prostate cancer. PSA is useful for monitoring response to therapy in cases of known prostate cancer, particularly after radical prostatectomy, when PSA should be undetectable.

- Concentration of PSA is proportional to total prostatic mass.
- The PSA test is inadequate as sole screening test for prostate cancer.
- PSA is useful for monitoring response to therapy.

Prognostic factors for prostate cancer include stage of disease, grade of tumor, and pretreatment PSA level. Table 18-9 simplifies the staging of prostate cancer, including the TNM classification. Grading of tumors is performed by the pathologist with the Gleason scoring system. The surgical specimen is graded by the most predominant pattern of differentiation added to the secondary architectural pattern (e.g., $3 + 5 = 8$). Gleason grades 2 through 6 are associated with a better prognosis. Recent retrospective results indicate that the pretreatment PSA value is a strong predictor of disease outcome after operation or radiotherapy.

- Prognostic factors for the outcome of prostate cancer include tumor stage, grade, and pretreatment PSA value.
- Gleason grades 2 through 6 have a better prognosis.

Management

Management of Specific Stages

Significant controversy surrounds the primary treatment of prostate cancer in nearly all stages of the disease. In general, patients with T1A prostate tumors are observed without treatment.

Table 18-9.—Staging of Prostate Cancer

Whitmore	TNM*	Criteria
A1	T1A	Incidental focus of tumor in ≤5% of resected tissue
A2	T1B	Incidental tumor in >5% of resected tissue
B0	T1C	Tumor identified by needle biopsy (performed on basis of increased PSA value)
B1	T2A	Tumor ≤1/2 of one lobe
B2	T2B	Tumor >1/2 of one lobe but not both lobes
	T2C	Tumor involvement both lobes
C	T3 or T4	Extracapsular local disease or local invasion
D1	N1	Pelvic node involvement
D2	M1	Distant disease

*Tumor-Node-Metastasis system.

For organ-confined prostate cancer (T1B, T1C, and T2 tumors), both radiation therapy and radical prostatectomy are equally viable options. Recently, some investigators have proposed observation alone and treatment with hormonal agents at the time of progression because the rate of death from prostate cancer is low for well-differentiated early-stage disease. A large trial is currently under way in the United States to test the value of operation compared with observation for organ-confined prostate cancer.

For stage C (T3 or T4) disease (locally advanced), radiotherapy is generally used. A recent trial combining androgen deprivation with local radiation therapy showed improved local control and overall survival in this patient cohort (N Engl J Med 337:295-300, 1997). Some centers use androgen deprivation to downstage tumors before an aggressive surgical approach.

For stage D1 disease (positive pelvic nodes), the management is controversial. Divergent approaches include androgen deprivation alone, x-ray therapy with or without androgen deprivation, close observation with androgen deprivation at progression, or infrequently prostatectomy with androgen deprivation. For advanced (D2) disease, androgen deprivation is the treatment of choice.

Prostatectomy

This is reserved for patients with localized disease. The

15-year disease-specific survival rate after prostatectomy is 85% to 90% for stage A2 or B disease. Impotence occurs in most patients, especially older individuals. Total urinary incontinence is rare (<2% of patients).

- Prostatectomy used for localized disease.
- 15-year survival rate is 85%-90% for stage A2 or B disease.

Radiation Therapy

External beam radiotherapy is considered the equivalent of prostatectomy. It is preferred for stage C disease at most centers. Impotence can occur, but less often than with prostatectomy. A concern related to radiotherapy is that repeat biopsies after treatment have shown apparently viable tumor in more than 35% of patients. The clinical importance of this residual tumor is unclear, but there may be a correlation with the subsequent appearance of distant metastasis, especially with a persistent, palpable abnormality in the gland.

- External beam radiotherapy is considered the equivalent of prostatectomy at most centers.
- Impotence is less frequent with radiotherapy than prostatectomy.

Androgen Deprivation

For advanced (D2) disease, bone is the most frequent site of metastatic disease. Hormonal therapy, although it is very effective and produces a response in most patients, is noncurative. The average duration of response to initial hormonal maneuver is 18 months. The average duration of survival is 2 to 3 years. Once the disease progresses after the initial hormonal maneuver, it is typically very refractory to secondary treatment attempts (such as hormonal or chemotherapy).

- Bone is the most frequent site of metastatic disease from prostate.
- Hormonal therapy is effective and produces a response, but it is noncurative.
- Average duration of survival with advanced prostatic cancer is 2-3 years.

The two sources of androgens in men are the testes (testosterone, 95%) and adrenal glands (5%). Androgen deprivation can be accomplished surgically with orchiectomy or medically. Potential agents include luteinizing hormone-releasing hormone (LHRH) agonists such as leuprolide, buserelin, and goserelin. They decrease androgen levels through continuous binding of the LHRH receptor and subsequent decrease of LH and thus testosterone. They are administered as a monthly injection of a depot preparation. A 3-month depot preparation is also available. LHRH agonists, on initial binding of the LHRH receptor, transiently stimulate LH release and thus cause an initial increase in the testosterone level. This explains the transient flare of prostate cancer that can occur in men with advanced disease when therapy with an LHRH agonist is initiated. This possibility must be considered in patients with impending spinal cord compression or urinary obstruction.

- Androgen deprivation is accomplished with orchiectomy or medically.
- Luteinizing hormone-releasing hormone agonists depress androgen levels.
- These agonists initially stimulate a transient release of luteinizing hormone and testosterone.

Antiandrogens compete with androgens at the receptor level. These include flutamide, nilutamide, and bicalutamide. To effect total androgen blockade, an antiandrogen is added to therapy in patients who have had orchiectomy or who are receiving an LHRH agonist (these block testicular testosterone production but not adrenal androgen production). A prospective U.S. study combining an LHRH analog with flutamide versus placebo suggested an advantage for the addition of flutamide. However, other studies of total blockade have failed to show an advantage. Studies comparing orchiectomy alone with orchiectomy plus flutamide are under way in the United States. The antiandrogens may also block the "flare" induced by LHRH agonists.

- Some physicians believe an antiandrogen should be used in combination with orchiectomy or LHRH agonist.
- Antiandrogens block the "flare" induced by LHRH agonists.

TESTICULAR CANCER

Background

This cancer is diagnosed in 7,500 men annually. It is the most common carcinoma in males aged 15 to 35 years. It is highly curable, even when metastatic. At high risk are males with cryptorchid testes (40-fold relative risk) or Klinefelter syndrome (also increased risk of breast cancer). Two broad categories are seminomas (40%) and nonseminomas. Types of nonseminomas include embryonal carcinoma, mature and immature teratoma, choriocarcinoma, yolk sac, and endodermal sinus tumors. There is often an admixture of several cell types within nonseminomas. Any nonseminomatous component plus seminoma is treated as a nonseminoma.

- Testicular cancer is the most common carcinoma in males 15-35 years old.
- Testicular cancer is highly curable, even when metastatic.

- High-risk factors: cryptorchid testes, Klinefelter syndrome.
- Two categories: seminomas (40%) and nonseminomas.

Evaluation includes determination of β-human chorionic gonadotropin (hCG) and α-fetoprotein values and computed tomography of the abdomen (retroperitoneal nodes) and chest (mediastinal nodes or pulmonary nodules).

Staging

Stage I disease is confined to the testis, stage II includes infradiaphragmatic nodal metastases, and stage III is spread beyond retroperitoneal nodes. About 85% of nonseminomas have elevated β-hCG or α-fetoprotein value. Approximately 10% of seminomas have increased β-hCG level. α-Fetoprotein value is never increased in pure seminoma; if it is increased, the tumor is nonseminoma and should be treated as such.

- 85% of nonseminomas have elevated β-hCG or α-fetoprotein value.
- 10% of seminomas have increased β-hCG.
- α-Fetoprotein value is never increased in pure seminoma.

Management

Radical (inguinal) orchiectomy is the definitive procedure for both pathologic diagnosis and local control. Scrotal orchiectomy or biopsy is associated with a high incidence of local recurrence or spread to inguinal nodes. After orchiectomy, the management depends on cell type (Table 18-10). Seminomas are radiosensitive. For stage I and nonbulky stage II seminoma, infradiaphragmatic lymphatic irradiation is used. The 5-year disease-free survival rate is more than 95%. For bulky stage II disease and stage III, platinum-based chemotherapy is used. Approximately 85% of patients are cured. For stage I nonseminoma, close follow-up is often used rather than immediate retroperitoneal node dissection (a controversial issue). For stages II and III, platinum-based chemotherapy is given. Cure rates are more than 95% for minimal metastatic disease, 90% for moderate bulk disease, and about 50% for bulky disease (multiple pulmonary metastases, bulky abdominal masses, liver, bone, or central nervous system metastases).

- Radical orchiectomy is the definitive initial procedure for testicular cancer.
- Early-stage seminoma is treated with x-ray therapy.
- Stage I nonseminoma may require no treatment after orchiectomy.
- Platinum-based chemotherapy is used for all other patients and results in high cure rates.

Extragonadal Germ Cell Tumor

This is uncommon. Patients present with elevated hCG or

Table 18-10.—Management of Testicular Cancer

| Stage | Treatment, by cell type | |
	Seminoma	Nonseminoma
I	XRT	? Observe
II	XRT	Chemo
III	Chemo	Chemo

Chemo, chemotherapy; XRT, x-ray therapy.

α-fetoprotein values with midline mass lesions (retroperitoneum, mediastinum, or pineal gland). No gonadal primary tumor is identifiable on examination or ultrasonography. Cisplatin-based chemotherapy is frequently effective.

UNKNOWN PRIMARY

Background

Patients presenting with metastatic carcinoma with unknown primary make up 5% to 10% of general oncologic practice. The first principle of management is to establish the diagnosis with a sufficient histologic specimen. In general, open biopsy is preferable to fine needle aspiration, because a larger specimen allows optimal histologic and immunohistochemical analysis. All patients should have a careful history and complete physical examination, including pelvic and rectal examinations. Most patients, approximately 60%, have an adenocarcinoma. In 35% of patients, a diagnosis of poorly differentiated carcinoma will be made. Once a pathologic diagnosis is established, additional evaluation should be tailored according to the patient's symptoms and signs, sites of metastasis, and the histologic diagnosis. Special consideration should be given to rule out possible treatable malignancies, such as germ cell tumors, breast or ovarian carcinoma, or prostate cancer. Women presenting with axillary adenocarcinomas, with no clear breast primary, should receive treatment for breast cancer. Women with peritoneal carcinomatosis are generally taken for exploratory laparotomy with surgical cytoreduction, as for ovarian carcinoma. Men presenting with bone metastases, particularly osteoblastic metastases, should have a prostate-specific antigen measured and their tumor material stained for prostate-specific antigen expression.

Treatment

If a potentially treatable neoplasm is ruled out, most patients with metastatic cancer of unknown primary have a very poor prognosis, with expected survival of 4 to 6 months. Some may benefit from palliative treatment (radiation or chemotherapy); many are managed with best supportive care.

PARANEOPLASTIC SYNDROMES

General
These conditions are the effects of a cancer occurring at a distance from the tumor; they are called "remote effects." They do not indicate metastatic disease. Common paraneoplastic syndromes and associated tumor types are listed in Table 18-11.

Carcinoid Syndrome
This is caused by peptide mediators secreted by carcinoid tumors of the small intestine which have metastasized extensively to the liver. It is less frequent with primary carcinoids arising from other sites such as lung, thymus, or ovary. The most common symptoms are episodic flushing and diarrhea; bronchospasm may occur. Flushing and diarrhea may occur spontaneously or be precipitated by emotional factors or ingestion of food or alcohol. Carcinoid heart disease (right-sided valvular disease) is a potential late complication.

Lambert-Eaton Syndrome
This consists of muscle weakness (proximal) and gait disturbance. Strength is increased with exercise. It is associated with small-cell lung cancer.

Dermatomyositis
The female:male ratio is 2:1. Findings include muscle weakness (proximal), inflammatory myopathy, and increased creatine kinase values. Skin changes are variable and include heliotrope rash, periorbital edema, and Gottron papules. Underlying malignancy (lung, breast, gastrointestinal) is common in patients older than 50 years.

Table 18-11.—Classification of Paraneoplastic Syndromes

Syndrome	Mediator	Tumor type
Endocrine		
Cushing syndrome[*]	ACTH	Small-cell lung cancer
SIADH[*]	ADH	Lung, especially small cell
Hypercalcemia[*]	PTH-like peptide	Lung, especially squamous; breast; myeloma
Carcinoid syndrome	? serotonin ? substance P	Gut neuroendocrine tumors
Hypoglycemia	Insulin Insulin-like growth factors	Gut neuroendocrine tumors; other
Neuromuscular		
Cerebellar degeneration	Anti-Purkinje cell antibodies	Lung, especially small cell; ovarian; breast
Dementia	?	Lung
Peripheral neuropathy[*]	Autoantibodies	Lung, gastrointestinal, breast
Lambert-Eaton	Antibodies to cholinergic receptor	Small-cell lung cancer
Dermatomyositis	?	Lung, breast
Skin		
Dermatomyositis	?	Lung, breast
Acanthosis nigricans	? TGF-α	Intra-abdominal cancer, usually gastric
Hematologic		
Venous thrombosis[*]	Activators of clotting cascade and platelets	Various adenocarcinomas, especially pancreatic and gastric
Nonbacterial thrombotic endocarditis	Activators of clotting cascade and platelets	Various adenocarcinomas, especially pancreatic and gastric

[*]Most common types.
ACTH, adrenocorticotropic hormone; ADH, antidiuretic hormone; PTH, parathyroid hormone; SIADH, syndrome of inappropriate secretion of antidiuretic hormone; TGF-α, transforming growth factor-α.

CHEMOTHERAPY

Basic Concepts

Currently, approximately 40 cytotoxic agents are available for use in North America. Taken generally, chemotherapeutic agents impair the process of cell division. Their selectivity for tumor cells is based primarily on a higher replicative rate in neoplastic cells. This selectivity for rapidly dividing cells explains the typical patterns of toxicity that occur with chemotherapy (that is, bone marrow, gastrointestinal mucosa, and hair follicles). The general classes and mechanisms of chemotherapeutics are shown in Figure 18-4.

Applications

Chemotherapy can be used in the following settings: 1) advanced disease, 2) as adjuvant therapy after definitive local treatment, and 3) as primary or "neo-adjuvant" therapy. The last application refers to situations in which patients present with a locally advanced malignancy and initial tumor reduction is needed before a primary treatment (such as operation or radiation) can be applied.

Solid Tumors Sensitive to Chemotherapy

Germ cell tumors of the testis and ovary, choriocarcinomas, breast cancer, ovarian cancer, and small-cell lung cancer are in this category. In recent years, combination chemotherapy regimens have also produced impressive tumor reductions in transitional cell carcinomas of the bladder, head and neck cancer, and cervical cancer.

Why Chemotherapy Fails to Cure Most Advanced Solid Tumors

The reasons for failure are 1) tumor cell heterogeneity, including populations of cells resistant to cytotoxic agents; 2) large numbers of noncycling or resting cells; and 3) pharmacologic sanctuaries—blood-tissue barriers and blood supply-tumor barriers.

Side Effects

The most common side effects of various chemotherapeutic agents are outlined in Table 18-12.

Mechanisms of Tumor Cell Drug Resistance

Mechanisms include decreased drug uptake, increased drug efflux, decreased drug activation, increased drug inactivation, and increased production of a target enzyme.

Tumor cells may be resistant to a specific drug or they can have broad cross-resistance to structurally dissimilar drugs. This latter phenomenon is referred to as "multidrug resistance." This seems to be mediated by a large plasma membrane glycoprotein, termed the "p-glycoprotein," that functions as an energy-dependent drug-efflux pump.

- Tumor cells may be resistant to structurally dissimilar chemotherapy drugs ("multidrug resistance").

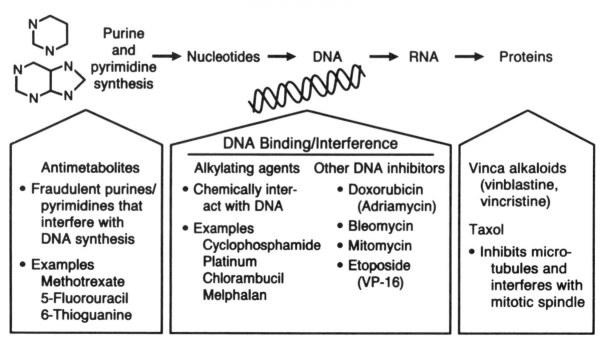

Fig. 18-4. General classes of chemotherapeutic agents.

Colony-Stimulating Factors

In recent years, bone marrow colony-stimulating factors have been isolated and are now available for clinical use. These naturally occurring glycoproteins stimulate the proliferation, differentiation, and function of specific cells in the bone marrow. They may act at the level of the earliest stem cell or at later mature functional cells. They differ in their specificity.

Granulocyte colony-stimulating factor (G-CSF), for example, acts fairly specifically to stimulate production of mature neutrophils; granulocyte-macrophage CSF (GM-CSF) acts more generally, stimulating several cell lineages, including monocytes, eosinophils, and neutrophils. Both CSFs have been used to stimulate white cell recovery after chemotherapy-induced myelosuppression. As a general rule, CSFs do not affect the depth of the leukocyte nadir but shorten the duration of neutropenia. Unfortunately, no currently available CSF reliably protects against thrombocytopenia. To be effective, a CSF should be initiated shortly after completion of chemotherapy (1-2 days) and delivered through the expected neutrophil nadir. Placebo-controlled studies examining the efficacy of G-CSF initiated at documentation of chemotherapy-induced neutropenia have failed to demonstrate clinical benefit.

ONCOLOGIC COMPLICATIONS AND EMERGENCIES

Hypercalcemia

The most common underlying causes are malignancies and primary hyperparathyroidism. Patients with primary hyperparathyroidism have elevated serum parathyroid hormone (PTH) values, but PTH is suppressed in cancer-associated hypercalcemia. Cancer-related hypercalcemia is often mediated by a PTH-related protein secreted by the tumor. This PTH-related protein can be detected with current assays. Tumors can also cause hypercalcemia by secreting other bone-resorbing substances or by enhancing conversion of 25-hydroxyvitamin D to 1,25-dihydroxyvitamin D. Another mechanism is due to the local effects of osteolytic bone metastases.

Effects on bone and kidney contribute to hypercalcemia. Accelerated bone resorption is due to activation of osteoclasts

Table 18-12.—Side Effects of Chemotherapy

Class or agent	Side effects	
	Acute	Chronic
Alkylating agents	Nausea, vomiting	Marrow: secondary leukemias
	Marrow: cytopenias	Pulmonary
		Gonads: decreased fertility, premature menopause
Cisplatin	Nausea, vomiting	
	Renal: ↓ GFR; tubular damage leads to electrolyte losses, especially cations	Renal: ↓ GFR; tubular damage and electrolyte losses, especially cations
	Peripheral neuropathy	Peripheral neuropathy
	Tinnitus, hearing loss	Tinnitus, hearing loss
Doxorubicin	Nausea, vomiting	Cardiac
	Marrow	Congestive heart failure
	Cardiac	Cumulative, dose-dependent, occurs in
	Pump or conduction	1%-10% of patients receiving 550 mg/m^2
	Stomatitis	
Bleomycin	Pulmonary	Pulmonary (may be aggravated by high FiO$_2$, as
	Skin (hyperpigmentation)	in perioperative period)
	Fever	
Antimetabolites	Mucositis/diarrhea	
	Marrow	
Microtubule inhibitors Vincristine	Neuropathy	Neuropathy
Taxol	Cardiac: conduction	

FiO$_2$, fraction of inspired oxygen; GFR, glomerular filtration rate.

by various mediators, primarily the PTH-like peptide. The same factors that induce osteoclast-mediated bone resorption also stimulate renal tubular reabsorption of calcium. The hypercalcemic state interferes with renal resorption of sodium and water, leading to polyuria and eventual depletion of extracellular fluid volume. This reduces the glomerular filtration rate, further increasing the serum calcium level. Immobilization tips the balance toward bone resorption, worsening the hypercalcemia.

- PTH is suppressed in cancer-associated hypercalcemia.
- Malignancy-associated hypercalcemia is often mediated by PTH-related protein secreted by a tumor.
- Bone and kidney pathophysiology lead to elevated calcium level.

Symptoms of hypercalcemia include gastrointestinal (anorexia, nausea, vomiting, constipation), renal (polyuria, polydipsia, dehydration), central nervous system (cognitive difficulties, apathy, somnolence, or even coma), and cardiovascular (hypertension, shortened QT, enhanced sensitivity to digitalis).

Cancers associated with hypercalcemia include lung (squamous cell), renal, myeloma, lymphoma, breast, and head and neck. Patients with breast cancer and those with myeloma are more likely to have bony involvement with their disease.

For treatment of hypercalcemia, the magnitude of the hypercalcemia and the degree of symptoms are key considerations. Generally, patients with a serum calcium value more than 14 mg/dL should be hospitalized for immediate treatment. The serum calcium value should be adjusted if the serum albumin value is abnormal. The conversion formula is 0.8 mg/dL of serum total calcium for every 1 g of serum albumin more or less than 4 g/dL. If the serum albumin value is elevated (as with dehydration), the total calcium value should be adjusted downward; if the serum albumin value is reduced (as in chronic illness), the total calcium value should be adjusted upward.

For hydration, intravenously administered normal saline (200-400 mL/hr) is initially given. Loop diuretics are used *after* volume expansion. Furosemide facilitates urinary excretion of calcium by inhibiting calcium resorption in the thick ascending loop of Henle. A loop diuretic will help correct for volume overload once the patient has been rehydrated. Specific agents are listed below:

1. Bisphosphonates (pamidronate or etidronate) are given intravenously (gastrointestinal absorption is poor). They bind to hydroxyapatite and inhibit osteoclasts.
2. Gallium nitrate (200 mg/m^2 per day) is given as continuous intravenous infusion for 5 days (unless normocalcemia is achieved earlier). It is a highly effective inhibitor of bone resorption.
3. Mithramycin (25 μg/kg) is given intravenously over 4

hours; this treatment can be repeated if necessary. Maximal hypocalcemic effect is reached at 48 to 72 hours. It is associated with hepatic and renal side effects.
4. Glucocorticoids have an antitumor effect on neoplastic lymphoid tissue.
5. Calcitonin is given subcutaneously or intramuscularly. It has a rapid onset of action; thus, it is useful in immediate life-threatening situations. It is a relatively weak agent with short-lived effect. Allergic reactions to salmon calcitonin are unusual, but an initial skin test with 1 unit is recommended before a full dose is given.

- Volume expansion must precede administration of furosemide.
- Furosemide inhibits calcium resorption in thick ascending loop of Henle.
- Bisphosphonates bind to hydroxyapatite and inhibit osteoclasts.
- Mithramycin has hepatic and renal side effects.
- Calcitonin is a relatively weak agent with rapid, short-lived effect.

Tumor Lysis Syndrome

This syndrome occurs as a result of the overwhelming release of tumor cell contents into the bloodstream such that concentrations of certain substances become life-threatening. It most commonly occurs in cancers with large tumor burdens and high proliferation rates which are exquisitely sensitive to chemotherapy. Examples include high-grade lymphomas, leukemia, and, much less commonly, solid tumors. The syndrome is characterized by increased uric acid, which leads to renal complications; acidosis; increased potassium, which can cause lethal cardiac arrhythmias; increased phosphate, which leads to acute renal failure; and decreased calcium, which causes muscle cramps, cardiac arrhythmias, and tetany. The syndrome can be prevented with adequate hydration, alkalinization, and administration of allopurinol before chemotherapy.

- Tumor lysis syndrome is a result of overwhelming release of tumor cell contents into bloodstream.
- It is most common in cancers with large tumor burdens and high proliferation rates exquisitely sensitive to chemotherapy.
- It is characterized by increased uric acid, increased potassium, increased phosphate, acidosis, and decreased calcium.

Febrile Neutropenia

This is defined as a temperature of 38.5°C or more on one occasion or three episodes of 38.0°C or more plus an absolute neutrophil count of 500 x 10^9/L or less (or leukocyte count of 1,000 x 10^9/L or less). Management involves immediate hospitalization and institution of parenteral, broad-spectrum antibiotics. Patients usually have no infection documented, but appropriate cultures should be rapidly obtained before antibiotics are given. Use of colony-stimulating factors at the time of documentation of febrile neutropenia has not been shown to have clinical utility.

Spinal Cord Compression

Acute cord compression is a neurologic emergency. It results most commonly from epidural compression by metastatic tumor (lung, breast, prostate, myeloma, kidney). Occasionally, compression can occur from neighboring nodal involvement and tumor infiltration through intervertebral foramina (lymphoma). The locations are cervical in 10% of cases, thoracic in 70%, and lumbar in 20%. Multiple noncontiguous levels are involved in 10% to 40%.

More than 90% of patients present with pain. Cervical pain may radiate down the arm. Thoracic pain radiates around the rib cage or abdominal wall; it may be described as a compressing band bilaterally around the chest or abdomen. Lumbar pain may radiate into the groin or down the leg. Pain may be aggravated by coughing, sneezing, or straight-leg raising. Focal neurologic signs depend on the level affected. Paresthesias (tingling, numbness), weakness, and altered reflexes also can be present (Table 18-13). Tenderness over the spine may help localize the level. Autonomic changes of urinary or fecal retention or incontinence may be present.

Imaging studies include bone scanning or plain radiography, which reveal vertebral metastases in approximately 85% of patients with epidural compression. Myelography or magnetic resonance imaging of the entire spine is generally recommended.

Treatment usually includes an initial bolus of 10 to 100 mg of dexamethasone intravenously, depending on the severity of block. Thereafter, dexamethasone is given (4 mg four times a day), although some physicians favor higher doses for a few days followed by a rapid taper. Radiation therapy is applied to the involved area(s). Operation is used in select circumstances:

if no previous diagnosis of malignancy, spine instability, prior radiation to cord tolerance, and progressive neurologic decline despite radiation.

Outcome depends on the patient's neurologic function at presentation (Table 18-14).

PALLIATIVE CARE

Background

More than 70% of patients with cancer have significant pain during the course of their disease. Multiple studies have shown that patients with cancer-related pain are not given adequate analgesic therapy (42% of patients are not given adequate pain relief, Ann Intern Med 119:121-126, 1993). Primary barriers to optimal management of cancer pain include inadequate pain assessment by health care professionals; physician reluctance to prescribe opioids; and patient reluctance to take opioids. Physician reluctance to prescribe opioids stems from concern about addiction, lack of familiarity with the agents, and problems with management of side effects of opioids. Of note, psychological addiction to opioids in cancer patients is very rare, occurring in less than 1% of such patients.

Evaluation

Evaluation should include 1) a history regarding onset, quality, severity, and location of pain; exacerbating and relieving factors; associated symptoms; and 2) physical examination, which should include a complete neurologic examination. Diagnostic studies are determined by the results of the history and physical examination.

Treatment

Three-Tiered Approach

Step 1: For mild pain, administer acetaminophen or a nonsteroidal anti-inflammatory drug around-the-clock. Of note, studies of nonsteroidal anti-inflammatory drugs for cancer pain have shown that these agents are only 1.5 to 2 times more effective than placebo.

Table 18-13.—Reflexes and Their Corresponding Roots and Muscles

Reflex	Root(s)	Muscle
Biceps	C5-6	Biceps
Triceps	C7-8	Triceps
Knee jerk	L2-4	Quadriceps
Ankle jerk	S1	Gastrocnemius

Table 18-14.—Outcome of Patients With Spinal Cord Compression, by Neurologic Status

Status at presentation	% ambulatory after radiation
Ambulatory	>80
Paraparetic	<50
Paraplegic	<10

Step 2: When step 1 fails to provide adequate analgesia, or for moderate pain, add codeine or oxycodone.

Step 3: For severe pain or inadequate pain relief with steps 1 and 2, agents include morphine, hydromorphone, levorphanol, methadone, and fentanyl (Table 18-15).

General Principles

For most cancer pain, opioids are the main treatment approach. Orally administered immediate-release morphine is the usual first-line drug selected for severe pain from cancer. The average starting oral dose is 10 to 30 mg every 4 hours. Remember, there is no "standard dose." The dose should be increased until analgesia is achieved. Use around-the-clock, NOT as-needed dosing. When the patient's total daily morphine requirements are defined, convert that total daily dose to a long-acting morphine product that can be given every 8 or every 12 hours. Provide rescue doses of morphine (usually 5%-10% of the total daily dose should be available every 1-2 hours as needed). Adverse effects of opioids include sedation, nausea, constipation, respiratory depression, and myoclonus. Tolerance to opioid-induced sedation and nausea usually develops within a few days. For opioid-induced constipation, initiate use of docusate sodium and senna with opioids. Respiratory depression typically follows sedation; if a patient is somnolent, doses should be held. No narcotic is more or less likely to result in a particular side-effect profile. However, one narcotic may produce an adverse effect in a patient whereas another will not. Thus, sequential trials of different opioids may be needed to determine the one best suited for a patient. The fentanyl patch (a transdermal formulation) delivers drug continuously over 72 hours. It is especially useful for patients with poor tolerance of orally administered opioids or those unable to take medications orally.

ACKNOWLEDGMENT

We gratefully acknowledge Lynn Hartmann, M.D., for her extensive work on previous chapters. We also appreciate review and revisions in previous years by Richard M. Goldberg, M.D., Patrick A. Burch, M.D., and Randolph S. Marks, M.D.

Table 18-15.—Doses of Narcotics That Provide Equal Analgesia

Drug	Doses of equal analgesia	Half-life, hr	Peak effect, hr	Duration of effect, hr
Morphine	10 mg i.m./i.v.	2-4	0.5-1	4-6
	20-60 mg p.o.*	2-4	2	4-6
Slow-release morphine	20-60 mg p.o.*	3-4	4-6	8-12
Hydromorphone	1.5 mg i.m.	2-3	0.5-1	4-6
	7.5 mg p.o.	2-3	1-2	4-6
Levorphanol	2.0 mg i.m.	12-16	0.5-1	4-6
	4.0 mg p.o.	12-16	1	4-6
Methadone	10 mg i.m.	15-150+	0.5-1.5	4-6
	20 mg p.o.	15-150+	0.5-1.5	4-6
Codeine	130 mg i.m.	2-4	1	4-6
	200 mg p.o.	2-4	1-2	4-6
Oxycodone	30 mg p.o.	2-3	1	3-6
Meperidine	75 mg i.m.	3-4	0.5-1	3-5
	300 mg p.o.	3-4	1-2	4-6
Fentanyl	0.1 mg i.v.	3-4	0.25	0.5-2
	Transdermal patch	See text	See text	72

*Relative potency of intramuscular:oral morphine changes from 1:6 to 1:2-3 with chronic dosing.

i.m., intramuscular; i.v., intravenous; p.o., oral dose.

Modified from Foley KM: The treatment of cancer pain. N Engl J Med 313:84-95, 1985. By permission of the journal.

QUESTIONS

Multiple Choice (choose the one best answer)
1. Which one of the following statements is false with respect to lung cancer in the United States?
   a. Lung cancer is the leading cause of cancer mortality for both men and women
   b. Lung cancer is the second most commonly diagnosed cancer in women each year
   c. Lung cancer is the most commonly diagnosed cancer in men each year
   d. Lung cancer deaths attributed to smoking approach 80% for men

2. A 56-year-old woman presents to her local physician complaining of left breast irritation. She has no previous history of breast lesions and has never had a mammogram. On examination she has no palpable adenopathy. The left breast shows significant redness throughout with thickening in the left upper outer quadrant. The remainder of the physical examination is unremarkable. The hematology and blood chemistry group results are normal. The mammogram shows an edematous left breast with a 2-cm mass. The right breast is normal. A bone scan is normal. A general surgeon is asked to do a biopsy, and this shows grade 4 adenocarcinoma with dermal invasion. The estrogen and progesterone receptors are markedly positive. The most appropriate management at this point would be:
   a. Consult a surgeon for left radical mastectomy
   b. Consult a radiation therapist for initiation of combined radiation therapy and chemotherapy
   c. Consult a surgeon for left simple palliative mastectomy
   d. Initiate a combination of chemotherapy and an anthracycline-based regimen
   e. Initiate hormonal therapy with tamoxifen followed by radiation therapy

3. A 58-year-old woman presents with increasing abdominal girth and bloating. Her past medical history is unremarkable. On physical examination there is dullness to percussion at the right lung base, ascites, and no appreciable pelvic or adnexal masses. The initial laboratory studies reveal a normal hematology group and a serum creatinine value of 1.3 mg/dL (normal, 0.6-0.9 mg/dL). Chest radiography shows a moderate right pleural effusion. Computed tomography demonstrates ascites and a thickened omentum and a left ovarian lesion. The right effusion was tapped, and cytologic evaluation reveals adenocarcinoma cells. The most appropriate evaluation at this time would be:

   a. Tap ascites for cytologic examination
   b. Referral to a medical oncologist for immediate chemotherapy
   c. Radiotherapy consult for intraperitoneal radioactive phosphorus
   d. Consult a gynecologic surgeon for debulking surgery

4. Small-cell lung cancer (SCLC) is associated with several different paraneoplastic syndromes causing unusual metabolic disorders. When compared with other lung carcinomas, SCLC is diagnosed more frequently with all of the following syndromes *except*:
   a. Hypercalcemia
   b. Syndrome of inappropriate secretion of antidiuretic hormone (SIADH)
   c. Cerebellar degeneration
   d. Ectopic Cushing syndrome
   e. Eaton-Lambert syndrome

5. A 46-year-old woman presents to your office very nervous because her sister (age 49) was recently diagnosed with adenocarcinoma of the breast. Her mother died of breast cancer at age 58. She insists on a test to know whether she will get breast cancer. Your patient has been performing monthly self breast examinations and has had yearly medical breast examinations and annual/biannual mammograms (most recently done 6 months ago). After a complete history and physical examination, the most appropriate next step in management is:
   a. Test blood for *BRCA*1 (breast cancer-associated gene)
   b. Recommend rechecking mammogram immediately
   c. Recommend checking mammograms yearly
   d. Consider medical genetics consult
   e. Start tamoxifen therapy for breast cancer prevention

6. A 72-year-old man presents with complaints of progressive low back pain. The patient has known degenerative arthritis and is currently receiving ibuprofen, 400 milligrams three times per day. On physical examination there is tenderness to percussion over the lumbar spine. The prostate is enlarged with a firm nodule in the right lobe. A neurologic examination is normal. On laboratory studies, the hemoglobin level is 12.8 g/dL (normal, 13-15 g/dL) with a normal mean corpuscular volume. The blood chemistry group shows an alkaline phosphatase level of 450 U/L (normal, 90-250 U/L). The serum creatinine value is only mildy increased. The prostate specific antigen level is markedly increased at 250 ng/mL (normal, 0-5 ng/mL). A bone scan shows multiple metastatic lesions, including many vertebral levels. The most appropriate step in treatment management of this patient is:

a. Systemic chemotherapy with mitoxantrone and prednisone
b. Bilateral orchiectomy
c. Use of nonsteroidal antiandrogen followed by radiation therapy to symptomatic areas
d. LHRH agonist followed 2 weeks later by nonsteroidal antiandrogens (maximal androgen blockade)

7. Tumor lysis syndrome is a life-threatening complication of patients with large tumor burdens and high proliferative rates that are sensitive to cytotoxic chemotherapy. The syndrome is characterized by all of the following *except*:
a. Hypercalcemia
b. Hyperuricemia
c. Hyperkalemia
d. Hyperphosphatemia
e. Renal insufficiency

8. A 27-year-old man is seen in your office complaining of left testicular swelling. Initial antibiotic therapy was not beneficial. Ultrasonography of the testicle shows a solid mass. Further laboratory tests show increases of the β-human chorionic gonadotropin (β-hCG) value to 1,050 IU/L (normal, <2.5 IU/L) and the α-fetoprotein (AFP) level to 330 ng/mL (normal, <6 ng/mL). Chest radiography is negative, and computed tomography of the abdomen and pelvis is negative. The patient undergoes a left inguinal

orchiectomy. He is seen 5 days postoperatively and tumor marker tests are repeated. What levels of tumor markers would be expected at this time if the patient is cancer free?
a. The β-hCG will remain increased until the AFP is normal
b. An AFP level of 80 and a β-hCG level of 100
c. An AFP level of 80 and a β-hCG level of 30
d. An AFP level of 160 and a β-hCG level of 30

9. All of the following chemotherapeutic agents inhibit microtubules or interfere with mitotic spindle *except*:
a. Paclitaxel (Taxol)
b. Vinblastine
c. Vincristine
d. Docetaxel (Taxotere)
e. Cyclophosphamide

10. Colorectal cancer is the second most common cause of cancer-related deaths in the United States. Screening recommendations are controversial *except* for certain high-risk groups. Patients with all of the following are considered at high risk for development of colorectal carcinoma *except*:
a. Familial adenomatous polyposis
b. Long-standing inflammatory bowel disease
c. Lynch syndrome
d. Prior history of colon cancer
e. Previous gastric surgery

ANSWERS

1. Answer c.

The most commonly diagnosed cancer in men and women each year is prostate and breast cancer, respectively. In 1987, lung cancer surpassed breast cancer as the leading cause of cancer death in women and will account for 25% of all cancer deaths for women in 1999. The percentage of lung cancer deaths attributed to smoking for men and women is approximately 75% to 80%, and more than 90,000 deaths occur per year.

2. Answer d.

Nearly all patients with inflammatory breast cancer are dead within 5 years in the absence of systemic chemotherapy. Preoperative chemotherapy in this patient subgroup can

produce a response rate of about 80%. These patients can then go on to surgical resection with clear margins. Initial operation is not feasible in this patient with extensive inflammatory breast carcinoma. Radiation therapy is used in combined-modality therapy of locally advanced breast cancer. After initial response to chemotherapy, consultation with a surgeon and radiation therapist is most appropriate to decide on the timing of subsequent therapy. Hormonal therapy is also used after combined-modality treatment for receptor-positive patients. Long-term disease-free survival is feasible in 25% to 30% of patients with locally advanced breast carcinoma.

3. Answer d.

Patients with cytologically positive effusions with ovarian cancer have stage IV disease. Pleural effusions are not a contraindication to surgical resection of abdominal disease. Further cytologic evaluation of the ascites can be performed at operation. Neoadjuvant chemotherapy given before attempted surgical debulking has not proved beneficial in this patient population. Intraperitoneal radioactive phosphorus can be used in earlier-stage ovarian cancer.

4. Answer a.

Hypercalcemia is more frequently associated with squamous cell carcinoma of the lung. The frequency of SIADH associated with SCLC varies according to the definition of the syndrome but may be present in 10% of patients. Only approximately one-fourth of patients fulfilling diagnostic criteria for SIADH are symptomatic from the hyponatremia. Ectopic Cushing syndrome with clinically recognizable hypercortisolism is present in 2% to 3% of patients and is associated with shorter survival and more frequent complications from chemotherapy. The Eaton-Lambert syndrome and cerebellar degeneration are caused by autoantibody directed against presynaptic nerve terminals and Purkinje cells, respectively. In general, the endocrinologic paraneoplastic syndromes are ameliorated by response to chemotherapy, but this is not often the case with neurologic syndromes.

5. Answer d.

Anyone at increased risk of cancer who is referred for genetic testing must be provided with appropriate counseling. Although there is disagreement regarding the value of screening women aged 40 to 50 years, patients at high risk should be screened at an earlier age. Initiation of tamoxifen for breast cancer prevention may be appropriate; however, formal counseling would be the most appropriate referral for this young patient.

6. Answer b.

Hormonal therapy is the standard initial treatment for patients with metastatic prostate carcinoma. Mitoxantrone and prednisone therapy has shown clinical benefit in patients resistant to standard hormonal therapy. Use of single-agent nonsteroidal antiandrogen has proved less effective than orchiectomy or LHRH agonists. LHRH agonists can result in a tumor flare and therefore such therapy should be started after nonsteroidal antiandrogen medication.

7. Answer a.

Recognition of risk and prevention of tumor lysis syndrome are essential to management. Hypocalcemia and hyperkalemia can be evident, and cardiac monitoring should be done while these abnormalities are corrected. Hypocalcemia can be corrected by intravenous administration of calcium gluconate, and hyperkalemia treated with sodium polystyrene sulfonate (Kayexalate) or combined insulin-glucose therapy. With acutely worsening renal function in this syndrome, one should consider early initiation of renal dialysis to reverse the metabolic complications. Prevention of tumor lysis syndrome is key with use of allopurinol.

8. Answer d.

The AFP half-life is approximately 5 days. The β-hCG half-life is approximately 24 hours. Inappropriate levels of these tumor markers after several days indicate residual tumor. If appropriate levels are found, continued close observation with rechecking of markers is a reasonable option for clinical stage I disease.

9. Answer e.

Cyclophosphamide interacts with DNA and is classified as an alkylating agent. The other chemotherapeutic agents inhibit microtubules and interfere with mitotic spindles. Paclitaxel and docetaxel are both taxanes that shift the equilibrium between tubulin dimers toward polymerization and stabilize microtubules against depolymerization. The vinca alkaloids (vincristine and vinblastine) act via disruption of microtubules.

10. Answer e.

Prior gastric surgery for benign disease has been associated with development of gastric cancer. Some studies suggest patients who have undergone cholecystectomy are at increased risk for colorectal carcinoma. The cumulative incidence of colorectal carcinoma in patients with inflammatory bowel disease is 5% at 20 years and 12% at 25 years. Patients with a past history of large bowel adenocarcinoma are at threefold increased risk for development of a second primary bowel cancer. Patients with Lynch syndrome require frequent invasive screening beginning at a young age.

NOTES

CHAPTER 19

PREVENTIVE MEDICINE

Sally J. Trippel, M.D., M.P.H.
Philip T. Hagen, M.D.

DEFINITIONS

Preventive medicine is the practice of medicine that detects and alters or ameliorates 1) host susceptibility in a premorbid state (e.g., immunization), 2) risk factors for disease in a predisease state (e.g., increased cholesterol level), and 3) disease in the presymptomatic state (e.g., in situ cervical cancer). Not all disease is preventable because 1) not all risk factors (or all individuals at risk) are known, 2) the cost of screening everyone is not feasible, 3) barriers to medical access exist, 4) interval disease occurs, 5) characteristics of the target disease vary, 6) screening tests are imperfect, and 7) treatments are imperfect.

Primary prevention is the prevention of disease occurrence (e.g., immunization to prevent infection and blood pressure control to prevent stroke). *Secondary prevention* is the detection and amelioration of disease in a presymptomatic or preclinical stage (e.g., mammography detects small foci of cancer and Pap smear detects in situ cancer). *Tertiary prevention* is the prevention of future negative health effects of existing clinical disease (e.g., use of aspirin and β-blockers after myocardial infarction to prevent recurrence).

Efficacy is the potential or maximal benefit derived from applying a test or procedure under ideal circumstances (e.g., research studies with compliant patients, with ideal testing conditions, techniques, etc.). *Effectiveness* is the actual benefit that is derived from a test or procedure that is applied under usual—less than ideal—circumstances. Randomized trials in which results are analyzed by the "intention to treat" principle, that is, all members of a group are included in the analysis whether they complied or not, give a measure of effectiveness in a population. *Cost-effectiveness* is the unit of cost incurred to achieve a given level of effectiveness. It is often expressed as the dollars spent per year of life saved. Often, the most cost-effective method of testing is not the most effective. For example, performing Pap smears every 5 or 10 years is more cost-effective, but performing them every year is more effective.

- Cost-effectiveness: cost incurred to achieve a given level of effectiveness.
- The most cost-effective test may not be the most effective test or treatment.

Years of potential life lost is one measure of the relative impact of a disease on society. This term usually refers to the years lost due to death from a disease before age 65 years (or sometimes 70). For example, colon cancer kills approximately 55,000 men and women annually and breast cancer kills approximately 44,000 women. However, on average, breast cancer kills at a younger age and so has nearly 3x as many "years of potential life lost."

- Years of potential life lost: the years lost due to death from a disease before age 65 (or sometimes 70) years.

Incidence (rate) refers to the number of new events (deaths, diagnoses) that occur in a population in a given time (e.g., 170 cancer deaths per 100,000 people in the U.S. annually). *Prevalence* refers to the number of cases of a condition existing at a point in time in a population (e.g., currently, 1,200,000 people in the U.S. are infected with the human immunodeficiency virus [HIV]).

PRINCIPLES OF SCREENING FOR DISEASE

The term *mass screening* is generally applied to the relatively indiscriminate testing of a population with the intent to improve the aggregate health of the population but not necessarily of every person in the population. An example is blood pressure or cholesterol testing in a public setting such as a shopping mall.

- Mass screening: indiscriminate testing of a population to improve the aggregate health of the population.

Case finding is the technical term often used for screening conducted in the office setting. The intent is to detect asymptomatic disease and to improve the health of the person. In testing asymptomatic persons, it is important to bear in mind the dictum of "first do no harm."

- Case finding: screening conducted in the office setting to detect asymptomatic disease and to improve the health of a person.

Desirable Screening Characteristics

1. Disease characteristics: the diseases screened should be common, cause significant morbidity and mortality, have a long preclinical phase (which is curable/modifiable), have an effective treatment that is available to those screened, and have an acceptable treatment (i.e., one that is not excessively painful or disfiguring).
2. Test characteristics: the tests should be inexpensive, safe, acceptable, easy to administer, technically easy to perform, highly sensitive, and have a complementary, highly specific confirmatory test.
3. Host characteristics: the person should be at risk, have access to testing, be likely to comply with follow-up testing, and have adequate overall life expectancy/functional life expectancy.

Burden of U.S. Disease

Diseases that cause the most morbidity and mortality in the U.S. may or may not be amenable to screening or case finding. Heart disease and cancer are clearly the leading causes of death in the U.S. (Tables 19-1 and 19-2). The most recent year for which all actual statistics exist is 1995.

Cancer Screening

Lung Cancer

Lung cancer is a highly lethal form of cancer (it kills most of the people it afflicts) and is the leading cause of cancer death for men and women. Burden of disease (1999 estimates from the American Cancer Society): 171,600 new cases and 158,900 deaths. Peak incidence is 470/100,000 in 75-year-old men and 155/100,000 in 70-year-old women. Risk factors include 1) smoking—10x increased risk over nonsmoker; 2) age—70 years old, 10x greater risk than for 40 years old; 3) sex—male-to-female ratio is 2:1 and is primarily related to duration and intensity of smoking; 4) environmental, industrial, occupational, carcinogen exposure—radon, asbestos, hydrocarbons, and uranium. Screening tests include chest radiography and sputum cytology. Screening probably is not effective. Although the Mayo Clinic Lung Project detected more cancers, mortality was not altered in approximately 12 years of follow-up study. This may have been because of "overdiagnosis" of clinically irrelevant lesions or lead-time bias. Annual chest radiography (or sputum cytology) solely to look for treatable stage lung cancer should not be performed. Smoking is the leading preventable cause of cancer in the U.S. (and a leading cause of heart disease and stroke).

- Lung cancer: the leading cause of cancer death for men and women.
- Risk factors for lung cancer: smoking, age, sex (2:1 male-to-female ratio), and environmental exposure.
- Annual chest radiography or sputum cytology solely to look for treatable stage lung cancer should not be performed.
- Smoking is the leading preventable cause of cancer in the U.S.
- Physician advice to quit smoking and referral to smoking cessation programs are the most cost-effective preventive measures available.

Breast Cancer

Breast cancer is the second leading cause of cancer death for women. The lifetime risk is estimated at 1 in 8 women. Burden of disease (1999 estimates from the American Cancer Society):

Table 19-1.—Leading Causes of Mortality in the U.S., 1995

	No. of deaths	Death rate (per 100,000 population)	% of total deaths
Heart diseases	737,563	205.4	31.9
Cancer	538,455	169.1	23.3
Cerebrovascular diseases	157,991	42.0	6.8
Chronic obstructive lung disease	102,899	30.0	4.5
Accidents	93,320	31.6	4.0

From Landis SH, Murray T, Bolden S, Wingo PA: Cancer Statistics, 1999. CA Cancer J Clin 49:8-31 Jan/Feb, 1999.

Table 19-2.—Cancer Mortality for Women and Men, 1995 (U.S. Vital Statistics)

Age (years)					
40-59		60-79		80+	
Women					
Breast	12,202	Lung	37,426	Colon and rectum	11,720
Lung	9,937	Breast	20,083	Lung	11,463
Colon and rectum	3,297	Colon and rectum	13,855	Breast	9,793
Ovary	2,757	Pancreas	7,595	Pancreas	4,730
Uterine cervix	1,720	Ovary	7,237	Non-Hodgkin lymphoma	3,501
Men					
Lung	15,606	Lung	60,721	Prostate	15,657
Colon and rectum	4,275	Prostate	17,773	Lung	14,892
Non-Hodgkin lymphoma	2,370	Colon and rectum	16,306	Colon and rectum	7,416
Pancreas	2,347	Pancreas	7,715	Urinary bladder	2,752
Brain and other nervous system	1,949	Non-Hodgkin lymphoma	6,012	Leukemia	2,725

From Landis SH, Murray T, Bolden S, Wingo PA: Cancer statistics, 1999. CA Cancer J Clin 49:8-31 Jan/Feb, 1999. By permission of American Cancer Society.

176,300 new cases and 43,700 deaths. Thus, breast cancer is moderately lethal (it kills many but not most of the people it afflicts). The risk factors include 1) age—the risk increases throughout life, and the risk for an 80-year-old woman is 12x that for a 30-year-old woman; 2) family history—one first-degree relative with breast cancer, 2x-3x risk and two first-degree relatives, 4x-6x risk; 3) socioeconomic status—high, increases risk 2x; 4) nulliparity or age at first full-term pregnancy >30 years old, risk is increased 2x; 5) history of proliferative breast disease, history of breast cancer, and high-dose radiation exposure all increase risk approximately 2x.

- Breast cancer: the second leading cause of cancer death for women.
- Lifetime risk: 1 in 8 women.
- One first-degree relative with breast cancer, 2x-3x risk; two first-degree relatives, 4x-6x risk.

Screening procedures include:
1. Breast self-examination: recommended but no demonstrated effectiveness.
2. Clinical breast examination: sensitivity of about 50%-70% and specificity >90%.
3. Screen film mammography: sensitivity of 75%-95% for women ≥50 years old and 60%-80% for women <50 years. Specificity is 95%-99%. Positive predictive values (PPV) are about 5%-10%, with 20%-50% of

biopsies revealing cancer, depending on age (higher percentages in older women).
4. Randomized controlled trials worldwide have examined the effectiveness of mammography. They showed an approximate 30% decrease in mortality, but only two trials showed statistical significance. Data are conflicting or inconclusive in women younger than 50 or older than 70 years.

- Breast physical examination has a sensitivity of 50%-70% and a specificity of >90%.
- Mammography has a sensitivity of 75%-95% and a specificity of 95%-99%.
- Studies are inconclusive about the benefit of mammography for women younger than 50 or older than 70 years.

Screening risks—Radiation is estimated to produce 60 additional breast cancers in 1,000,000 women screened compared with the 93,000 cases expected to be detected. The Breast Cancer Detection and Demonstration Project showed that 2% of women were referred for surgical evaluation/aspiration, and of the 50-65-year-old women referred for biopsy, half were found to have cancer. About 3% of women 40-49 years old were referred for biopsy, with a smaller percentage yielding cancer.

- Radiation: 60 additional breast cancers in 1,000,000 women screened.

- Approximately 2% of screened women 50-65 years old will have biopsy and 3% of women 40-49 years old.

Cost-effectiveness: if 25% of women 40-75 years old in the U.S. were screened annually, 11,000,000/year would be screened at a cost of $1.3 billion annually for physical examination and mammography. The cost of screening and the work-up would be 100x as expensive as the costs saved by reduced treatment. Cost per year of life saved ranges from about $9,000 to $12,000, with lower cost in the 50-69-year-old group and higher costs in both younger and older age group.

- Cost of screening and work-up would be 100x as expensive as the costs saved by reduced treatment.
- Cost per year of life saved is $9,000-$12,000.

Recommendations:
1. General agreement—Clinical breast examination and mammography every 1-2 years for women 50-69 years old. Otherwise, recommendations vary.
2. American Cancer Society and several other groups— Clinical breast examination yearly for women ≥40 years old and mammography every 1-2 years. For women ≥50 years old, annual clinical breast examination and mammography.
3. United States Preventive Services Task Force (USP-STF)—Mammography alone or clinical breast examination and mammography every 1-2 years for women 50-69 years old. Screening may begin sooner for women at high risk.
4. American College of Physicians—Mammography every 2 years for women 50-74 years old.

Colon and Rectal Cancer

Colon cancer is the second leading cause of cancer death in the U.S. Burden of disease (1999 estimates from the American Cancer Society): 129,400 new cases of colorectal cancer and 56,600 deaths due to colorectal cancer. The lifetime risk of developing colon cancer is approximately 6%. Less than 2% of colon cancers occur in people <40 years old and 90% occur in those >50 years old. The risk of developing colon cancer is approximately 2.5x greater than the risk of dying of it (which reflects potential survivability of colon cancer and the age of the population involved, i.e., there are competing causes of mortality). Colon cancer is now the second cancer for which randomized controlled trial evidence has demonstrated decreased mortality due to screening.

- Colon cancer is the second leading cause of cancer death.
- Lifetime risk is 6%.
- 90% of colon cancers are in people > 50 years old.

Natural history: cancers may develop de novo in the colon, but most of them probably develop from adenomatous polyps. The risk of a polyp becoming malignant appears to be related to time and size. Clinically significant polyps are those larger than 7 mm. The average time from formation to malignant transformation for a polyp is 7-10 years. Ten-year survival for Dukes A or B cancer is 74%, 36% for Dukes C, and 5% for Dukes D.

- The risk of a polyp becoming malignant appears to be related to time and size.
- Clinically significant polyps: ones larger than 7 mm.
- The time from polyp formation to malignant transformation is 7-10 years.

The risk factors include 1) age—risk doubles every 7 years over age 50; 2) family history—if a first-degree relative has disease, the risk increases 2x-3x; 3) previous adenomatous polyps increase risk 2x-4x; 4) history of endometrial, ovarian, or breast cancer increases risk 2x; 5) familial polyposis, Gardner syndrome—approximately 100% risk by age 40; 6) ulcerative colitis—approximately 50% risk with a 30-year history of disease; and 7) cancer family syndrome (adenocarcinoma at various locations at an early age in multiple sibs)—approximately a 50% risk.

- Risk for colon/rectal cancer doubles every 7 years over age 50.
- If first-degree relative has colon/rectal cancer, risk increases 2x-4x.
- Previous adenomatous polyps, risk increases 2x-3x.
- History of endometrial, ovarian, or breast cancer, risk increases 2x.
- Familial polyposis (Gardner syndrome), risk is nearly 100% by age 40.
- Ulcerative colitis, about a 50% risk with a 30-year history of disease.

Tests: 1) fecal occult blood test is 26%-92% sensitive and does not detect polyps well; 2) proctoscopy is more than 90% sensitive for the bowel visualized and could detect about 30% of cancers; 3) flexible sigmoidoscopy is also more than 90% sensitive for the bowel visualized and could detect about 60% of cancers; 4) barium enema and colonoscopy usually visualize the entire colon and are 85%-95% sensitive.

- Fecal occult blood test is 20%-30% sensitive.
- Proctoscopy and flexible sigmoidoscopy are more than 90% sensitive for the area of the colon visualized.
- Barium enema and colonoscopy visualize the entire colon and are 85%-95% sensitive.

Recommendations—Randomized controlled trial data that are available show about a 30% decrease in mortality for persons >50 years with annual fecal occult blood testing. Yet, there is little consensus about whether to screen and how to screen for colorectal cancer. Mathematical modeling suggests that annual screening with barium enema or colonoscopy might reduce mortality by 85%, but the cost would be prohibitive. The American Cancer Society recommends 1) digital rectal examination (for prostate examination) yearly for men >40 years old and yearly for women (as part of pelvic examination) >40, 2) fecal occult blood test yearly over age 50, and 3) sigmoidoscopy every 3-5 years over age 50. The USPSTF recommends screening for all persons ≥50 years old with annual fecal occult blood test or sigmoidoscopy (periodicity unspecified) or both. The task force guidelines also recommend that persons with a family history of hereditary syndromes associated with a high risk of colon cancer should be referred for diagnosis and management. The American College of Physicians' (ACP) guidelines (revised in 1995) recommend offering various screening options to persons 50-70 years old, depending on resources and patient preference, including flexible sigmoidoscopy, colonoscopy, or air-contrast barium enema. The test(s) should be repeated at 10-year intervals with fecal occult blood test offered to persons who decline these screening tests.

- Fecal occult blood test screening annually decreases mortality by 30% for persons >50 years.
- Annual screening with barium enema or colonoscopy might reduce mortality by 85%, but the cost would be prohibitive.

Prostate Cancer

For the purposes of screening, prostate cancer is a troublesome disease, primarily because of the great difference between the "burden" of prevalent disease and the "burden" of clinical disease. The 1999 estimates from the American Cancer Society are 179,300 new cases of prostate cancer and 38,000 deaths due to it. Pathologic studies show that a small focus of prostate cancer can be found in 30%-40% of 60-year-old men. Yet in only 8%-9% of the men will prostate cancer be diagnosed, with many cases diagnosed incidentally at transurethral resection of the prostate. Currently, 80% of diagnoses are made in men older than 65 years. Relatively few men with prostate cancer die of the disease, only 3%-4% of U.S. men.

- 8%-9% of U.S. males will have the diagnosis of prostate cancer in their lifetime.
- 3%-4% of U.S. males die of prostate cancer.
- 80% of the diagnoses are made in men older than 65 years.

Natural history—Prostate cancer is a hormonally induced cancer that is generally slow growing. In most host males, it does not alter the life span or lifestyle. Growth of a tiny nidus of cancerous cells into a clinically important cancer takes 10-15 years. In elderly hosts, this process is usually halted by intervening causes of mortality. Aggressiveness and morbidity are related to size, grade, and ploidy. TA1 NxM0: Usually follow age-based mortality curve, normal survival. Mortality due to prostatic cancer is <5%. TA2 NxM0: near normal 10-year survival. TB2 or 3 NxM0: 5-year survival is about 50%.

- Prostate cancer is a hormonally induced cancer.
- It does not alter the life span or lifestyle of most host males.
- Growth into a clinically important cancer takes 10-15 years.

The risk factors include: 1) age—the risk increases exponentially after age 50; 2) race—in the U.S., African-American men have 2x the risk of whites, and whites have 2x the risk of Asians; 3) family history—a first-degree relative increases the risk 3x, a brother with cancer before age 63 increases the risk 4x, and a sister with breast cancer increases the risk 2x.

- For prostate cancer in the U.S., African-American men have twice the risk of whites, who have twice the risk of Asians.

Tests: 1) digital rectal examination has a PPV of 6%-33%; 2) transrectal ultrasonography has a PPV of about 10%-20% (values vary depending on population and previous screening); and 3) prostate-specific antigen (PSA) has a PPV of 10%-35% (values vary depending on population and prior screening). Note: because there is much undetected disease, PPV values do not have the usual meaning.

Recommendations: no good data are available from randomized controlled trials on the impact of early detection and treatment on survival. There is little agreement on recommendations for screening. Aggressive screening for prostate cancer will uncover many new cases (causing a surge in incidence) and result in many additional treatments. However, because of the natural history of the disease, screening may have minimal effect in decreasing mortality, the desired benefit. The American Cancer Society recommends digital rectal examination yearly for men >40 years old and this examination plus PSA for men ≥50 years and for men ≥40 years at high risk (African-American men and those with a family history). The USPSTF recommends no routine screening.

- There is little agreement on recommendations for prostate cancer screening.

Several authorities have recommended *against* any form of screening—rectal examination, ultrasonography, or

PSA—primarily because of concern that the impact on survival will be minimal and that the costs in detection and follow-up treatment and in deaths due to treatment (perioperative deaths) will be significant. The risk that the harm outweighs the good from detection of early stage disease exists. Screening, if performed, should be done in men likely to have a 10-year survival (the average life expectancy for a 50-year-old man is about 25 years and >10 years for a 70-year-old man).

Cervical Cancer

The 1999 estimates from the American Cancer Society are for 12,800 new cases of cervical cancer and 4,800 deaths. Cervical cancer has a bimodal risk curve divided between in situ carcinoma and invasive carcinoma. This cancer has a long preclinical phase, and progression from dysplasia to invasive cancer may take 10-15 years or more. A strong association exists between human papillomavirus infection (types 16, 18, and others) and cervical cancer. Cervical cancer may largely be a sexually transmitted disease.

- Cervical cancer: bimodal risk curve divided between in situ carcinoma and invasive carcinoma.
- It has a long preclinical phase.
- Cervical cancer is strongly associated with human papillomavirus infection.

The risk factors include: 1) age—the risk of invasive carcinoma increases throughout life; 2) sexual activity—early age at onset; 3) multiple sexual partners; 4) a history of sexually transmitted disease, especially HIV infection; and 5) smoking.

- Cervical cancer risk factors: early age at onset of sexual activity, multiple sexual partners, a history of sexually transmitted disease, and smoking.

Test: Pap smear has a sensitivity of 55%-80% and a specificity of 90%-99%. Experienced cytologists and pathologists as well as clinician sampling technique are important to test effectiveness.

- Pap smear has a 55%-80% sensitivity and a 90%-99% specificity.

Screening effectiveness—No randomized controlled trial of screening has been conducted in a general population. However, a significant body of evidence from case control studies and observational studies suggests effectiveness. Estimated overall effect of Pap smear: every 10 years, 64% reduction in invasive cancer; every 5 years, 84% reduction;

every 3 years, 91% reduction; every 2 years, 92.5% reduction; and every year, 93.5% reduction.

Recommendations—The general agreement is to recommend screening starting at the onset of sexual activity and every 1-3 years thereafter, depending on risk. The USPSTF recommends routine screening for all women who are or have been sexually active and who have a cervix. Screening should begin with the onset of sexual activity and should be repeated at least every 3 years. Consider discontinuing regular testing after age 65 in women who have had regular previous screening with consistently normal results. A consensus recommendation from the American Cancer Society, National Cancer Institute, and others advises all women who are or have been sexually active or who have reached age 18 to have annual Pap smears. The recommendation permits less frequent testing after three or more annual smears have been normal, at the discretion of the physician.

- General recommendation: screen at the onset of sexual activity and every 1-3 years thereafter, depending on risk.

Ovarian Cancer

Ovarian cancer is the fifth leading cause of cancer death in women. Burden of disease (1999 estimates from the American Cancer Society): 25,200 new cases of ovarian cancer and 14,500 deaths. Ovarian cancer is the leading cause of gynecologic cancer death. Age-adjusted death rates have been increasing slowly in the last 25 years.

- Ovarian cancer is the fifth leading cause of cancer death in women.
- Age-adjusted death rates have been increasing slowly.

Risk factors: 1) Lower risk—history of at least one term pregnancy has a relative risk of 0.64. The use of oral contraceptives for 3-6 months has a relative risk of 0.6; if used ≥10 years, the relative risk is 0.2. 2) Higher risk—family history as a risk is not well quantified, but it is an important factor if a first-degree relative had disease (only 1%-5% of ovarian cancers are familial). High fat diet and long duration of ovulatory years (i.e., late menopause) are possible risk factors.

- 1%-5% of ovarian cancers are familial.

Screening tests: 1) bimanual examination is insensitive; 2) ultrasonography, transvaginal or transabdominal, is more sensitive than bimanual examination but has a poor PPV; 3) CA-125 (blood test) is more sensitive than bimanual examination but also has a poor PPV. Ultrasonography and CA-125 have a significant false-positive rate. It is estimated that 10-60 abdominal operations would have to be performed for every one cancer detected, at a cost of more than $13 billion annually to screen the 43 million women >45 years old. An adequate study of efficacy, even with a highly sensitive and specific test, would require tens of thousands of participants.

- For ovarian cancer, bimanual examination is insensitive.
- Ultrasonography and CA-125 both are more sensitive than bimanual examination but both have a poor PPV.
- For every one ovarian cancer detected, 10-60 abdominal operations would have to be performed.

Recommendations: USPSTF recommends against screening for ovarian cancer. The American Cancer Society recommends bimanual palpation every 1-3 years for women age 20-40 and every year for women >40.

A 1994 NIH Consensus Conference recommended that women with presumed hereditary cancer syndrome should undergo annual pelvic examination, CA-125 measurement, and transvaginal ultrasonography until childbearing is completed or at age 35, at which time prophylactic bilateral oophorectomy was recommended.

Tuberculosis Prevention

Burden of disease: the worldwide prevalence of tuberculosis (TB) infection (past or active) is greater than 1 billion cases, with an annual incidence rate of about 8 million. Approximately 3,000,000 people worldwide die annually of TB. The U.S. incidence is approximately 20,000 cases per year, with 2,000 deaths per year. The incidence decreased from 1953 to 1985, but since then TB has made a resurgence because of immigration from endemic areas, HIV infection, and increased use of immunosuppressive drugs.

- TB: the U.S. incidence is approximately 20,000 cases and 2,000 deaths annually.

Natural history: infection occurs through inhalation of *Mycobacterium tuberculosis*-bearing droplets. After being infected, healthy persons are usually asymptomatic. However, it is believed that the tubercle bacillus remains viable in granulomata for many years. The risk of reactivation after asymptomatic infection (PPD conversion) is 2%/year for the first 2-3 years. A second reactivation peak occurs in the elderly with debility and disease.

- The tubercle bacillus remains viable in granulomata for many years.
- The risk of reactivation (after PPD conversion) is 2%/year for first 2-3 years after infection.
- A second reactivation peak occurs in the elderly with debility and disease.

Risk factors include: 1) foreign-born, with recent immigration; 2) institutionalization, e.g., in a nursing home; 3) prisoners; and 4) HIV/acquired immunodeficiency syndrome (AIDS) infection. If a person is HIV-positive and has a positive PPD, the 2-year risk of developing active infection is 15%. If TB occurs in a young person, check his or her HIV status.

- If a person is HIV-positive and has a positive PPD, the 2-year risk is 15%.
- If TB occurs in a young person, check his or her HIV status.

Test: the PPD (Mantoux) skin test—5-tuberculin units intradermal skin test. Measure the area of induration (not erythema) at 48-72 hours. In low-risk persons, consider the reaction positive if it is >15 mm. A 10-mm reaction is considered positive if the person is in a high-incidence group (foreign born, medically underserved low-income population, or resident of a long-term care facility). If there has been recent contact with an infected person, 5 mm is considered positive. HIV-infected persons may be anergic and 5 mm should be considered positive. Elderly persons may be relatively anergic but the response can be boosted by repeating the test (two-step PPD testing procedure). Previous BCG vaccination will produce skin reactivity, but positive reactors should be considered to have true infection and given appropriate follow-up care. Recent MMR and OPV vaccination (6 weeks) may diminish skin reactivity, and testing should be avoided during this interval. Chest radiography and sputum are not useful screening tests for conversion but may detect active disease in high-risk persons.

- Chest radiography and sputum are not useful screening tests for TB.

Persons with a positive PPD test should have chest radiography and clinical evaluation for TB.

Preventive measures: 1) Primary prevention is with BCG vaccine, an attenuated species of *Mycobacterium bovis*. It may be up to 80% effective when used properly. It is appropriate in high-risk areas because it is inexpensive, requires a single dose, and has a low risk (only 100 fatalities in 2 billion administrations). BCG vaccine is not indicated in low-prevalence areas because it confuses interpretation of PPD response. Another primary preventive measure is environmental controls, especially in a health care environment, with respiratory isolation, high-efficiency filter masks, and special venting of rooms/wards with TB cases.

- BCG vaccine is 80% effective when used properly.
- Its use is not indicated in low-prevalence areas.

2) Secondary prevention is with isoniazid (INH) treatment. Its use is indicated for recent converters (<2 years), contacts of infected persons with >5 mm PPD, history of TB with inadequate treatment, positive skin test with abnormal but stable chest radiographic findings, and positive PPD (of any duration) if <35 years old. The dosage is 5-10 mg/kg daily, up to a maximum of 300 mg daily (the usual adult dose) given as a single oral dose. Treatment should continue for 6-12 months (the longer the treatment, the greater the efficacy). Primary side effects are liver toxicity and peripheral neuropathy. Peak toxicity is in persons >50 years (2%-3%). Side-effect monitoring is generally through symptoms only, except in older persons (because of higher risk for toxicity) in whom serum levels of AST or ALT (liver function testing) should be determined every 4-6 weeks.

- Isoniazid: 5-10 mg/kg daily up to maximum of 300 mg daily.
- Treatment should continue for 6-12 months.
- Peak toxicity is in persons older than 50 years (2%-3%).

IMMUNIZATIONS

One of the greatest successes of modern medicine for preventing disease and for extending life has been immunization. Adults have continuing immunization needs throughout life. Physicians who administer vaccines are required by law to keep permanent vaccine records (National Childhood Vaccine Act of 1986) and to report adverse events through the Vaccine Adverse Event Reporting System (VAERS). Service in the U.S. military may be considered verification of vaccination for measles, rubella, tetanus, diphtheria, and polio. Providers are now required to give patients "vaccine information pamphlets" before vaccination as a mechanism for informed consent.

Immunity may be of two types. Passive immunity—preformed antibodies are provided in large quantities to prevent or to diminish the impact of infection or associated toxins (e.g., tetanus immune globulin [TIG] and hepatitis B immune globulin [HBIG]). Passive immunity lasts for up to 3 months. Active immunity—an antigen is presented to the host immune system that in turn develops antibodies (e.g., hepatitis or tetanus) or specific immune cells (e.g., BCG). Active immunity generally lasts from years to a lifetime. Active immunity may be induced by live virus vaccines (e.g., measles), killed virus vaccines (e.g., influenza), or refined antigen vaccines (e.g., pneumococcal).

Live virus vaccines are contraindicated in some persons. In general, pregnant women, people with immune-deficiency diseases, leukemia, lymphoma, generalized malignancy, or those who are immune-suppressed because of therapy with corticosteroids, alkylating drugs, antimetabolites, or radiation should *not* be given live virus vaccines. HIV-infected persons who are immune-competent and leukemia patients who have been in remission for ≥3 months after chemotherapy generally may be vaccinated with live virus vaccines. Live virus vaccines include measles, mumps, rubella, varicella, yellow fever, and polio (OPV).

Inactivated virus vaccines include enhanced inactivated polio (eIPV), hepatitis A, hepatitis B, influenza, and rabies. Inactivated bacterial vaccines include cholera, hemophilus influenza B, meningococcal, plague, and pneumococcal.

An adult immunization schedule has been developed and endorsed by several groups (Table 19-3).

Specific Vaccines/Chemo-Prevention

Diphtheria

Diphtheria is a rare disease primarily because of vaccination.

Table 19-3.—Recommended Adult Immunization Schedule

Vaccine	Age, yr	
	19-64	65+
Diphtheria, tetanus	Booster every 10 yr	
Hepatitis A	2 doses for those at increased risk of HAV infection and others wishing immunity	
Hepatitis B	3 doses for those with risk factors	
Influenza	Annually if at risk or wishing immunity	Annually
Measles, mumps, rubella	1-2 doses if born after 1956	
Pneumococcal	1-2 doses for those with risk factors	1-2 doses
Varicella	2-dose series for selected groups	

From Advisory Committee on Immunization Practices, American College of Physicians, Immunization Practices Task Force of the Minnesota Department of Health (MDH): Recommended adult immunization schedule. Minnesota Department of Health, April 1997.

However, up to 40% of adults lack protective antibody levels. Recommendation: vaccination in combination with tetanus toxoid (see tetanus), as Td. The DTP preparation recommended for children should not be used for adults.

Tetanus

Approximately 50 cases of tetanus are reported each year; most are in adults who are either unvaccinated or inadequately vaccinated. Vaccination is nearly 100% effective. Recommendations: primary series, a three-dose series, should be completed before adulthood, usually in early childhood. Primary series consists of Td (DTP in childhood). The last childhood dose is usually a booster at age 15. For adults who have had a primary series, vaccinate every 10 years (e.g., mid-decade is easy to remember; if last childhood dose at 15, vaccinate at ages 25, 35, 45, etc.). Clean, minor wounds received in the 10-year interval require no further vaccination. However, for a contaminated wound, the patient should get a Td booster if it has been more than 5 years since the last booster. If immune status is unknown or lacking (specifically, no primary series) both toxoid and TIG should be given (250 units intramuscularly). Td is the preferred toxoid in an emergency setting as well as for routine vaccination. Td and TIG when given in the emergency setting should be given in separate syringes at separate locations, but they may be given at the same time.

- Tetanus vaccination: the primary series is a three-dose series.
- Adults who have had a primary series should receive a booster every 10 years.
- For a contaminated wound, the patient should get a booster if it has been more than 5 years since the last booster.

Side effects: Td may be given in pregnancy, although it is desirable to wait until the second trimester. Maternal antibodies are passed to the infant transplacentally and confer passive immunity for a few months after birth.

- Maternal antibodies are passed to the infant transplacentally.

A history of neurologic reaction, urticaria, anaphylaxis, or other severe hypersensitivity reaction is a contraindication to the readministration of toxoids. Skin testing may be performed if necessary. In the emergency setting, if other than a clean minor wound is sustained, TIG may be used when T or Td is contraindicated. Arthus-type hypersensitivity, a severe local reaction starting 2-8 hours after injection, often with fever and malaise, may occur in persons who have received multiple boosters. These people have very high levels of antitoxin and do not need boosters, even in the emergency room setting, more frequently than every 10 years.

Measles

Vaccination has reduced the number of cases of measles from 500,000 yearly (with 500 deaths) to 3,600 yearly in the mid-1980s. A disease resurgence has occurred, and in 1990, there were 27,000 cases. The risk of encephalitis with measles infection in an adult is approximately 1 in 1,000. Infection in pregnancy may induce abortion, premature labor, and low birth weight. Malformation does not appear to be as much of a problem as with rubella.

- A resurgence of measles has occurred.
- The risk of encephalitis with measles infection in an adult is approximately 1 in 1,000.

Target: Adults born after 1956 who have no medical contraindication and who have no dated documentation of at least one dose of live measles vaccination on or after their first birthday, physician-documented disease, or documented immune titers should receive vaccination. Persons with expected exposure to measles should consider revaccination or titer measurement because 10% of persons born before 1957 are not immune. Persons at risk include travelers to endemic areas, those in school settings, and health care workers. They should have two doses of measles vaccine documented on or after their first birthday. MMR is the preferred vaccine. If they have never been vaccinated, they should receive two doses given at least 1 month apart.

Exposure precautions: If an exposed person is unvaccinated, vaccinate within 72 hours if possible and give immune globulin if the person is not a vaccine candidate (0.25-0.5 mL/kg body weight, up to 15 mL—dose depends on immune competence). Health care workers should remain away from work for days 5-21 after exposure if they are not immune.

Side effects: 1) fever, temperature >103°F usually occurs on day 5-12 in 5%-15% of those vaccinated; 2) rash occurs in 5%; 3) encephalitis is rare (1 case per 1 million immunizations). No apparent increase in side effects occurs with a second vaccination. Contraindications are immune globulin or blood products given within the previous 3 months, pregnancy, egg or neomycin allergy, and others as noted above for live virus vaccines.

Mumps

A highly effective vaccination program has decreased the number of cases of mumps from approximately 200,000 yearly to 3,000-5,000 yearly. Vaccine side effects of rash, pruritus, and purpura are uncommon, and central nervous system problems and parotitis are rare. There is no increased risk with revaccination. The contraindications are the same as for measles.

Rubella

Infection with rubella in the first trimester results in congenital rubella syndrome in up to 85% of infected fetuses. The goal of vaccination is to prevent the occurrence of this disease. Vaccination is highly effective, and there is no evidence of transmission of vaccine virus to close household contacts. The target population includes all women of childbearing age, all health care workers, and travelers to endemic areas. The side effects include arthralgias in 25% and transient arthritis in 10%, usually 1-3 weeks after vaccination. Vaccination rarely causes chronic joint problems, certainly much less frequently than natural infection. Contraindications are immune globulin given within the previous 3 months (but not blood products, e.g., $Rh_O(D)$ immune globulin [RhoGAM]), pregnant women or women likely to become pregnant within 3 months (although there are no documented cases of congenital rubella syndrome in vaccinated pregnant women), and allergy to neomycin but not to egg (as prepared in a diploid cell culture).

Influenza

Since 1957, 19 influenza epidemics, with more than 10,000 excess deaths each, have occurred, and 80%-90% of the deaths occurred in persons ≥65 years old. Incidence peaks occur in mid to late winter, earlier in recent years. Influenza A is classified by two surface antigens: hemagglutinin (subtypes H1, H2, H3) and neuraminidase (subtypes N1, N2). Because of differing subtypes and antigenic drift, infection or vaccination more than 1 year previously may not give protection the following year. Influenza B is antigenically more stable but still has moderate drift. Control is with vaccination (both influenza A and B) and/or chemoprophylaxis (for influenza A only).

The vaccine is an inactivated (killed) virus vaccine (virus grown in egg culture). Each year it contains three viruses, two A-type viruses and one B-type virus. Vaccines may contain whole virus or split virus (subvirion). Split-virus vaccines are used in children to decrease febrile reaction. All forms may be used in adults. Ideally, vaccination should be given in October and November.

The side effects include 1) local soreness (occurs in <1/3); 2) fever, malaise, myalgia (occurs 6-12 hours postvaccination and may last 1-2 days); and 3) anaphylactic reaction (probably due to egg protein). The target populations include 1) persons ≥65 years old, especially those who reside in a nursing home or chronic care facility; 2) persons with chronic pulmonary or cardiovascular disease, including asthma, chronic metabolic diseases such as diabetes mellitus, renal dysfunction, immunosuppression; and 3) health care workers. Consideration may be given to persons in vital roles, institutional settings, or who travel to the southern hemisphere between April and September. Contraindications are 1) first trimester of pregnancy, except

for those at high risk because of underlying disease, and 2) egg allergy.

Chemoprophylaxis for type A influenza is currently available in two forms, amantadine hydrochloride and rimantadine hydrochloride. These drugs interfere with the replication cycle of influenza A. In healthy populations, they are 70%-90% effective if given daily throughout the epidemic. For treatment of disease, they decrease fever and other symptoms if given within 48 hours of disease onset. These agents are used to control influenza outbreaks, usually in institutions, and are given to all unvaccinated workers and residents. They may be given regardless of vaccination status to persons at high risk. Workers should continue taking the medication until 2 weeks after vaccination or indefinitely during the period of risk if the vaccine is contraindicated. The dosage in healthy adults is 200 mg daily.

- Amantadine and rimantadine are used for influenza A only.
- They are 70%-90% effective.
- They are used to control influenza outbreaks, usually in institutions, and are given to all unvaccinated workers and residents.

The side effects are usually minor, occurring in 5%-10% of recipients, and may abate with continued use. Rimantadine has less frequent central nervous system side effects than amantadine. Central nervous system side effects are nervousness, anxiety, insomnia, and decreased concentration, and those of the gastrointestinal system include anorexia and nausea. Serious side effects are seizure and confusion, usually seen in the elderly or in those with renal or hepatic disease. In these groups, the dose should be decreased in accordance with the recommendations made in the package inserts.

Hepatitis A

Approximately 140,000 cases of hepatitis A infection occur in the U.S. each year. More than 70% of infected older children and adults develop clinical disease. Also, more than 10,000 infected persons are hospitalized yearly, and approximately 80 deaths are due to fulminant hepatitis. Signs and symptoms usually last <2 months. However, 10%-15% of patients have prolonged or relapsing illness, which may last up to 6 months.

Spread of hepatitis A virus (HAV) occurs by the fecal-oral route, most commonly within households. Common source outbreaks due to contaminated food and water supplies have occurred. Blood-borne transmission is uncommon but can occur through blood transfusion and contaminated blood products and from needles shared with an infected viremic person. Sexual transmission has also been reported.

Hepatitis A vaccination provides an opportunity to lower

disease incidence and ultimately to eradicate infection, because humans are the only natural reservoir of the virus. A single dose of hepatitis A vaccine induces a protective antibody level within 4 weeks after vaccination. A second dose of vaccine 6-18 months later induces long-lasting immunity. Target groups for immunization include 1) persons traveling to or working in countries that have high or intermediate HAV endemicity; 2) homosexual males; 3) illegal drug users; 4) persons who have an occupational risk of infection (those who work with HAV-infected primates or with HAV in a research laboratory); 5) persons who have chronic liver disease; 6) persons who have clotting-factor disorders; and 7) some food handlers. Hepatitis A vaccination of children has been used effectively to control outbreaks in communities that have high rates of hepatitis A.

Travelers who are allergic to a vaccine component or who elect not to receive vaccine should be encouraged to get immune globulin (0.02–0.06 mL/kg provides protection for 3-5 months). Immune globulin should also be given to travelers leaving on short notice, and it can be given concomitantly with vaccine, using separate sites and syringes.

Prevaccination serologic testing may be cost-effective for adults who were born or lived for extended periods in areas of high HAV endemicity and homosexual males. Postvaccination testing is not necessary because of the high rate of vaccine response.

Hepatitis B

The lifetime risk of acquiring hepatitis B is 5% for the general population; 150,000 cases occur annually in the U.S., resulting in 8,000 hospitalizations and 200 deaths. Of the patients affected, 90% are ≥20 years old; 5%-10% become carriers, and one-quarter of these have chronic active hepatitis. Annually, 4,000 persons die of hepatitis B virus-related cirrhosis and 1,500 die of hepatitis B virus-related liver cancer.

- The lifetime risk of acquiring hepatitis B is 5% for the general population.
- 5%-10% become carriers.
- Annually, 4,000 persons die of hepatitis B virus-related cirrhosis and 1,500 die of hepatitis B virus-related liver cancer.

The current vaccine is yeast recombinant, developed from the insertion of a plasmid into *Saccharomyces cerevisiae*, which produces the copies of the surface antigen. Human-purified vaccine is no longer made. The target population includes 1) adults at increased risk, that is, homosexual males, intravenous drug users, heterosexual persons with multiple sexual partners, and those with a history of other sexually transmitted diseases; 2) household and sexual contacts of hepatitis B virus carriers; 3) workers in health-related and

public safety occupations involving exposure to blood or body fluids; 4) hemodialysis patients; 5) recipients of concentrates of clotting factors VIII and IX; 6) morticians and their assistants; and 7) travelers who will be living for extended periods in high-prevalence areas or who are likely to have sexual contacts or contact with blood in the endemic areas (especially in eastern Asia and sub-Saharan Africa).

Vaccination—Normally, vaccination consists of three doses at 0, 1 month, and 6 months. An alternative dosing schedule to induce immunity more rapidly, for example, after exposure, involves 4 doses, the first three given 1 month apart and a fourth dose at 12 months. Postexposure prophylaxis consists of HBIG given in a single dose of 0.06 mL/kg or 5 mL for adults. It should be administered along with the vaccine in separate syringes at separate sites, but they may be administered at the same time. Current evidence suggests that for most vaccinees the vaccination has a duration of ≥7 years. Currently, revaccination is not routinely recommended. For persons who receive the vaccine in the buttock or whose management depends on knowledge of immune status (e.g., surgeons or venipuncturists), periodic serologic testing may be valuable. Those with titers <10 mIU should be revaccinated. Revaccination with a single dose is usually effective.

- Currently, revaccination for hepatitis B is not routinely recommended.

The most common side effect of hepatitis B vaccination is localized soreness. Guillain-Barré syndrome (0.5 per 100,000) was associated with human-derived hepatitis B vaccines. Comparable information is not available for the recombinant vaccination. Vaccination in pregnancy is considered advisable for women who are at risk for hepatitis B infection. The risk of hepatitis B virus infection in pregnancy far outweighs the risk of vaccine-associated problems.

- Guillain-Barré syndrome (0.5 per 100,000) was associated with human-derived hepatitis B vaccines.

Pneumococcal Disease

Two-thirds of persons with serious pneumococcal disease have been hospitalized in the previous 5 years (a missed opportunity to vaccinate). The risk of bacteremia for persons ≥65 years old is 50 per 100,000. The current vaccine contains purified capsular material of 23 different serotypes of streptococcus pneumonia. In most healthy adults, titers persist for ≥5 years. Persons who have received a 14-valent vaccine need not be routinely revaccinated. However, persons at highest risk for pneumococcal infections, such as asplenic patients, should be revaccinated with the 23-valent vaccine if it has been >6 years since the previous dose. Patients with nephrotic syndrome and renal failure and transplant patients should be revaccinated every 3-5 years because of waning immunity.

The target population is persons ≥65 years old, adults with chronic disease states such as cardiovascular or pulmonary disease, or persons at higher risk for pneumococcal infection, for example, because of alcoholism or cerebrospinal fluid leak. The target population also includes immunocompromised persons (such as those who are asplenic) and patients with Hodgkin disease, lymphoma, multiple myeloma, chronic renal failure, nephrotic syndrome, HIV infection, or organ transplant. The side effects are erythema and localized pain, which occur in about 50% of all vaccinees. Other side effects such as fever, myalgia, and severe local reactions occur in <1%. Five per 1,000,000 of those vaccinated develop anaphylaxis. Revaccination within approximately 1 year is associated with increased local reaction.

- The target population is persons ≥65 years old or adults with chronic disease.

Smallpox (Vaccinia)

In May 1980, WHO declared the world free of smallpox. Vaccination is no longer indicated except for persons working directly with the orthopoxviruses.

- Smallpox vaccination is no longer indicated except for persons working directly with the orthopoxviruses.

Polio

Polio has now been eradicated from the entire western hemisphere. The few cases that occur in the U.S. each year are due to the oral vaccine virus strain. There are OPV (live virus) and eIPV (killed virus) vaccines. A primary series with either one has >95% effectiveness. Polio vaccination is not recommended for persons >18 years old unless they plan to travel to an endemic area and have no history of a previous primary series. For these persons, eIPV is recommended because of the lower risk of paralysis. The primary series consists of eIPV followed in 4-8 weeks by eIPV, followed in 6-12 months by eIPV. If it is <4 weeks before travel, give a single dose of either OPV or eIPV. If the primary series is incomplete, complete it despite the interval since the last dose. If the person previously received IPV, give one dose of OPV or eIPV. For OPV, the risk of paralysis is approximately 1 in 1,000,000 after the first dose, and for susceptible household contacts, it is approximately 1 in 2,000,000.

- Polio vaccination is not recommended for persons >18 years old unless they plan to travel to an endemic area.

Rabies

Preexposure prophylactic vaccination is recommended for animal handlers, lab workers, persons traveling to endemic areas for >1 month, or those with vocations/avocations with exposure to skunks, raccoons, and bats as well as other animals. The reservoir of infection includes carniverous animals, particularly skunks, raccoons, foxes, and bats in the U.S. Except for woodchucks, rodents are rarely infected.

Varicella

Primary infection with varicella zoster virus (VZV) results in chickenpox and recurrent infection produces herpes zoster or shingles. Factors associated with recurrent disease include aging, immunosuppression, and intrauterine exposure to VZV and varicella at a young age (<18 months).

Complications of VZV infection, which occur more commonly in older children and adults, include bacterial infection of lesions, viral or secondary bacterial pneumonia, central nervous system manifestations (aseptic meningitis and encephalitis), hospitalization, and death.

Varicella vaccination is recommended for all children between 12 and 18 months old. It is also recommended for nonimmune adolescents and adults who are at highest risk of exposure and those most likely to transmit varicella to others. These groups include 1) health care workers, 2) family members of immunocompromised persons, 3) teachers of young children, 4) women of childbearing age, 5) military personnel, 6) persons working in institutional settings, and 7) international travelers.

Persons ≥13 years old should receive two doses of varicella vaccine separated by 4-8 weeks. Vaccine contraindications include severe allergy to neomycin, moderate or severe illness, immunosuppression, pregnancy, and recent receipt of a blood product. Adverse events following vaccination include injection site lesions, swelling, or pain; generalized varicella-like rash; and systemic reaction with fever. There is a risk of transmission of vaccine virus from a vaccinated person, especially with vaccine-associated rash, to a susceptible contact. However, this potential risk is low, and the benefits of vaccinating susceptible health care workers are thought to outweigh this risk.

Prevaccination serologic testing of adolescents and adults is probably cost-effective. Postvaccination testing is not necessary because of the high rate of seropositivity after two doses of vaccine (>99%).

QUESTIONS

Multiple Choice (choose the one best answer)

1. The use of daily aspirin prophylaxis, β-blocker therapy, postmenopausal hormone replacement therapy, or a combination of these in a 60-year-old woman following myocardial infarction (successfully treated with thrombolytic agent) represents:
   a. Primary prevention
   b. Secondary prevention
   c. Tertiary prevention
   d. None of the above

2. A 37-year-old nulliparous woman comes in for a periodic examination. She is healthy, a nonsmoker, has no complaints. She is sexually active with a single male partner (her spouse) and uses oral contraception. Her Pap smears have always been normal; the last one was completed 3 years ago. Her mother's identical twin sister had breast cancer diagnosed at age 42 years. Her maternal grandmother also had breast cancer in her 40s. There is no other family history of breast or female genital cancer. You recommend:
   a. Periodic pelvic examination and screening cervical/endocervical Pap smear
   b. Periodic breast and pelvic examinations; screening cervical/endocervical Pap smear
   c. Periodic breast and pelvic examinations; screening cervical/endocervical Pap smear; Chlamydia antigen testing (endocervical swab specimen)
   d. Periodic breast and pelvic examinations; screening cervical/endocervical Pap smear; bilateral screening mammography
   e. Periodic breast and pelvic examinations; screening cervical/endocervical Pap smear; bilateral screening mammography; measurement of CA-125 and pelvic ultrasonography

3. For which of the following patients would you recommend tuberculin testing using PPD?
   a. A 50-year-old Somali refugee who arrived in the U.S. 1 year ago and previously had BCG vaccination in childhood
   b. 22-year-old pregnant woman who is a crack cocaine user
   c. A 75-year-old woman undergoing nursing home placement
   d. A 38-year-old healthy man who was recently found to be HIV-positive
   e. All the above

4. A 26-year-old man comes to your office with fever and extensive swelling and erythema of his entire left arm. The swelling started within a day after he received a tetanus-diphtheria (Td) booster at a local emergency department after he sustained a minor cut on his hand from a kitchen knife. Physical examination reveals no evidence of neurovascular compromise of the left upper extremity. Immunization records indicate that he received a primary series of DTP in childhood as well as booster doses of DTP at age 5 and Td at age 13 years. He also received additional doses of Td at the time of injuries when he was 18 and 22 years old. You recommend:
   a. High-dose steroid therapy for the arm swelling and avoid tetanus-diphtheria boosters for the rest of his life
   b. Conservative therapy for the arm swelling and avoid tetanus-diphtheria boosters (even after tetanus-prone injury) more frequently than every 10 years
   c. Avoid use of tetanus immune globulin and tetanus-diphtheria boosters for the rest of his life
   d. Conservative therapy for the arm swelling and use only tetanus toxoid booster injections (without diphtheria toxoid) after injuries and for routine booster doses in the future
   e. Use tetanus immune globulin, rather than tetanus diphtheria booster, after tetanus-prone injury in the future

5. Currently, tobacco is the most important carcinogen in the U.S. It causes or contributes to development of about one-third of all cancers, including all the following *except*:
   a. Non-Hodgkin lymphoma
   b. Esophageal
   c. Lung
   d. Bladder
   e. Head and neck

6. A 48-year-old healthy male emergency department nurse was recently found to have a positive PPD, showing 22 mm of induration. His PPD was negative 1 year ago. He has no symptoms or physical examination findings suggestive of active TB. Chest radiographic findings are negative. He does not use alcohol or take any medications. You recommend isoniazid (INH) therapy for 6 months. You counsel him about potential adverse reactions of this medication, which include all the following *except*:
   a. Drug fever or rash
   b. Peripheral neuritis
   c. Hypersensitivity reactions
   d. Diarrhea
   e. Hepatitis

7. A 33-year-old woman comes for medical evaluation. She is married and has two children (10 and 12 years old). Her last evaluation was 5 years ago, and her general health has been good since then. While showering, she recently noted a small, painless lump in the left breast. She is not certain how long the lump has been present, because she does not routinely check her breasts. She has never had a mammogram. There is no family history of cancer. Physical examination reveals a rubbery, lobulated 2.0-cm lump in the upper outer quadrant of the left breast that feels benign. You recommend:
    a. Monthly breast self-examination with recheck if the lump changes
    b. Baseline screening bilateral mammography
    c. Repeat clinical breast examination in 1 year
    d. Diagnostic bilateral mammography and/or ultrasonographic scan of left breast nodule

8. A 55-year-old salesman smokes one pack of cigarettes per day (40-pack-year history) and has 12 to 14 alcoholic drinks per week. He rarely exercises and infrequently uses a seat belt. His blood pressure is 144/88 mm Hg and total cholesterol is 209 mg/dL. You should counsel him about the health behavior that is most likely to reduce his risk of dying in the next 10 years, which is:
    a. Exercise three times per week
    b. Stop smoking
    c. Stop drinking
    d. Avoid driving after drinking alcohol
    e. Follow a low cholesterol diet

9. A 33-year-old woman is planning a 10-day vacation in Belize, Central America, with her spouse. They plan to stay at a beach resort and visit prehistoric ruins in rural forested areas. She has no health problems. She will be early in the second trimester of pregnancy at the time of the planned trip. All routine immunizations are up to date (Td, MMR, and polio) and she had hepatitis A vaccination (2 doses) at the time of a previous trip to Mexico and Peru. You advise her that malaria is endemic in Belize and recommend which of the following regimens for prevention:
    a. Personal protective measures (bed nets/screened quarters, protective clothing, insect repellent) only
    b. Personal protective measures and doxycycline (100 mg daily)
    c. Personal protective measures and chloroquine phosphate (500 mg once weekly)
    d. Personal protective measures and mefloquine (250 mg once weekly)
    e. No malaria preventive measures necessary

10. When the vaccine becomes available in the fall, routine influenza vaccination would be recommended for all the following patients *except*:
    a. 68-year-old woman with chronic obstructive pulmonary disease, coronary heart disease, and history of egg allergy (urticaria, wheezing)
    b. 32-year-old woman with known rheumatic heart disease (moderate mitral stenosis) in first trimester of pregnancy
    c. 24-year-old man receiving insulin therapy for diabetes mellitus
    d. 28-year-old female outpatient clinic nurse in third trimester of pregnancy
    e. 40-year-old man with AIDS and moderate immunosuppression (CD4 cell count 300)

ANSWERS

1. Answer c.

Tertiary prevention is done after the diagnosis and initial treatment of clinical disease. It involves prevention of future negative health effects of existing clinical disease, that is, preventing recurrent myocardial infarction in the patient described. Primary prevention is done before the existence of disease and secondary prevention is after disease occurs but before it is symptomatic.

2. Answer d.

Periodic pelvic examination and screening cervical/endocervical Pap smear would be appropriate because the patient is sexually active and has not had a Pap smear for 3 years. Clinical breast examination and screening mammography would also be appropriate because of the family history of breast cancer in two relatives at an early age. In general, screening should start at least 5 years before the earliest age of onset in an affected relative. Routine screening with the tumor marker CA-125 and pelvic ultrasonography has not been shown to decrease mortality from ovarian cancer and, currently, is not recommended. The Centers for Disease Control currently suggests routine screening for *Chlamydia* only among sexually active women, 20 to 24 years old, especially those who do not consistently use barrier contraception and who have new or multiple partners.

3. Answer e.

In the U.S., control of tuberculosis involves screening high-risk populations and providing preventive therapy to persons who are most likely to develop active disease. High-risk populations include 1) foreign born, with recent immigration; 2) institutionalization, for example nursing home, mental institution; 3) prisoners; 4) persons infected with HIV; 5) high-risk substance abusers (injecting illicit drugs, crack cocaine users); 6) health care workers; 7) close contacts of persons known or suspected to have TB. Hence, all the patients listed are in a high-risk group.

4. Answer b.

The patient has developed an arthus-type hypersensitivity reaction soon after receiving a tetanus-diphtheria booster injection. The reaction typically occurs after receiving multiple booster doses of Td at less than 10-year intervals. Those affected have high levels of antitoxin and do not need boosters, even in an emergency department setting, more frequently than every 10 years. Conservative therapy is generally adequate for treatment of the arm swelling. Note: an adult who has received a primary series of DTP or Td would never need tetanus immune globulin, even after sustaining a tetanus-prone injury.

5. Answer a.

Smoking is the leading cause of numerous cancers, including those of the lung, oral cavity, larynx, and esophagus. It also contributes to cancer of the stomach, pancreas, bladder, kidney, cervix, and leukemia. The exact cause of non-Hodgkin lymphoma is unclear, although there is an association with oncogenic viruses (EBV, HTLV-1), ionizing radiation, congenital or acquired immunodeficiency, and exposure to pesticides.

6. Answer d.

Isoniazid is generally well tolerated, although there is an associated small risk of drug fever or rash and other hypersensitivity reactions. Neuropathy is more common among patients with diabetes, uremia, alcoholism, and malnutrition. Supplementation with pyridoxine/vitamin B_6 (25-50 mg once daily) may help prevent the neuropathy. The most serious potential side effect is hepatitis. Mild isoniazid-related liver function test abnormalities occur in 10% to 20% of adults older than 35 years and more severe hepatitis occurs in 2% to 3%. Diarrhea is not a side effect of isoniazid therapy.

7. Answer d.

Even though this patient's mass feels benign further evaluation is necessary to confirm its benign nature. Further evaluation would include diagnostic mammography and/or ultrasonography of the breast nodule. Alternatively, if the lump feels cystic, in-office diagnostic aspiration might be completed. Screening in the office setting, that is, case finding, is used to detect asymptomatic disease. Because the patient presents with disease, a breast lump, she is not a candidate for "screening" mammography (answer b) She has admitted that she does not check her breasts on a regular basis. Therefore, you would not want further evaluation to include only monthly self-breast examination (answer a).

8. Answer b.

Heart disease and cancer are the leading causes of death in the U.S. for males 55 to 74 years old. Smoking is a major modifiable risk factor for coronary heart disease, along with hypertension, hyperlipidemia, diabetes mellitus, obesity, and physical inactivity. Smoking is the leading modifiable cause of numerous cancers, including lung cancer, which is the leading cause of cancer deaths among males 55 to 74 years old. Hence, smoking cessation is likely to have the greatest effect in decreasing the risk of mortality during the next decade for a man of this age.

9. Answer c.

Malaria is endemic in Belize and is known to be chloroquine-sensitive. There is an increased risk of morbidity and mortality associated with malaria infection during pregnancy, especially *Plasmodium falciparum* infection. Hence, you would not want to recommend use of personal protective measures only (answer a). Chloroquine phosphate, in doses used for malaria prevention, is known to be safe for use throughout pregnancy. Mefloquine would be effective in preventing malaria, but safety of this medication during pregnancy has not been well established (answer d). Doxycycline and all tetracycline-related medications are contraindicated during pregnancy (answer b).

10. Answer a.

Influenza vaccine is contraindicated in persons who have anaphylactic hypersensitivity to eggs with a history of reactions, including urticaria, swelling of the lips and tongue, acute respiratory distress, or collapse. The vaccine is not recommended for use during the first trimester of pregnancy *except* for those at high risk because of underlying disease. In general, influenza vaccination is recommended for all persons who are at increased risk for influenza-related complications and those who can transmit influenza to high-risk persons.

CHAPTER 20

PSYCHIATRY

Deborah C. Newman, M.D.

Many psychiatric symptoms are as nonspecific as fever. Some signify problems of severe magnitude, whereas others are much less significant. Generally, the symptoms can be and should be investigated further before simply recommending symptomatic relief. The current paradigm of psychiatric assessment is the biopsychosocial model in which the biologic, psychologic, and social factors contributing to the patient's clinical presentation are evaluated.

Psychiatric disorders are divided into major diagnostic groups. A simplified way to conceptualize these groups is to look at the major symptomatic features of the patient's presentation: 1) mood—depression or mania; 2) anxiety—situational stress, panic disorder, generalized anxiety, others; 3) thought—psychotic process, acute (drug-induced, metabolic/toxic) versus chronic (schizophrenic process).

Any of the above diagnostic groups can be altered by alcohol or substance abuse/dependence, delirium, or dementia. The common psychiatric disorders seen by general physicians in outpatient settings are anxiety disorders, mood disorders, substance abuse, psychophysiologic disorders, and adjustment disorders. In the general hospital setting, the common psychiatric groups are mood disorders, adjustment disorders, substance abuse, delirium, and dementia. (The term "organic mental disorders" has been removed from the latest edition of *The Diagnostic and Statistical Manual* [DSM IV] *of the American Psychiatric Association 1994* and replaced by a category called "delirium, dementia, amnestic and other cognitive disorders.") The descriptions of the psychiatric disorders in this syllabus are based on the criteria described in DSM IV.

- Common psychiatric disorders seen by general physicians in an outpatient setting: anxiety disorders, mood disorders, substance abuse, psychophysiologic disorders, and adjustment disorders.
- Common psychiatric groups in a general hospital setting: mood disorders, adjustment disorders, substance abuse, delirium, and dementia.

MOOD DISORDERS

The prevalence of mood disorders in the general population of the U.S. is estimated at 5% to 8%; however, in the general medical setting, the rate may be as high as 5% to 15%.

Although the essential feature of mood disorders is a disturbance of mood, it is accompanied by related cognitive, psychomotor, vegetative (sleep, appetite, etc.), and interpersonal difficulties. Fluctuations in mood are a normal occurrence. It is only when the frequency or intensity (or both) of these changes is extreme and accompanied by the other features described that a formal mood disorder is diagnosed. The five major groups of mood disorders cover the range from mild to severe depression to the opposite extreme of mania. Three groups relate to depression: adjustment disorder with depressed mood, dysthymia, and major depression. Two groups relate to problems with mood fluctuations between various degrees of depression and mania: cyclothymia and bipolar disorder. Each of these five major groups has several subgroups. Another important group includes mood disorders due to a general medical condition and mood disorders that are substance-induced. The clinical presentation may be similar to that of a depressive or manic episode, but the cause may be related more specifically to a general medical condition or a particular substance(s) that then can be listed. The clinical phenomenology is similar to that of a manic or depressive episode.

- Mood disorders: the essential feature is disturbance of mood.
- They are accompanied by related cognitive, psychomotor, vegetative, and interpersonal difficulties.
- Mood disorders may also be related to a general medical condition or be substance-induced.

Adjustment Disorder With Depressed Mood

Adjustment disorder with depressed mood is a reaction that develops in response to an identifiable psychosocial stressor(s), for example, divorce, job loss, or family or marital problems.

It can occur any time in anyone if the psychosocial stressors are severe. The severity of the adjustment disorder (degree of impairment) does not always parallel the intensity of the precipitating event. The critical factor appears to be the relevance of the event or stressor to the individual and his or her ability to cope with the stress. In general, these reactions are relatively transient. Although they generally can be managed by an empathic primary care physician, the development of extreme withdrawal, suicidal ideation, or failure to improve as the circumstances improve may prompt psychiatric referral. Treatment includes supportive psychotherapy, psychosocial interventions, and, sometimes, use of antidepressant agents.

Dysthymia

Dysthymia is a form of chronic depression that may have either an early or late onset, as defined by onset before or after, respectively, age 21 years. It can be disabling for the person because the depressed mood is present most of the time during at least a 2-year period. Many of the patients have some associated vegetative signs such as disturbance of sleep and appetite, but they also often feel inadequate, have low self-esteem, and struggle with interpersonal relationships. If onset is in late adolescence, the dysthymia may become intertwined with the person's personality, behavior, and general attitude toward life. Treatment is usually a combination of psychotherapy (insight-oriented, cognitive, or interpersonal), behavioral therapy, and pharmacotherapy. Psychopharmacotherapy may be particularly useful in patients with a family history of mood disorders or in those who have the early onset form of dysthymia. In patients with dysthymia, major depressive episodes may develop. Also, some are prone to turn to alcohol or other substance abuse to "treat" their dysphoria.

- Dysthymia: a form of chronic depression.
- Depressed mood is present most of the time during at least a 2-year period.
- Treatment is usually a combination of psychotherapy and pharmacotherapy.
- Major depressive episodes may develop in patients with dysthymia.

Major Depression

Major depression is a serious psychiatric disorder that is set apart from adjustment disorder and dysthymia by the severity of the mood and cognitive disturbances and the presence of significant somatic symptoms. The primary symptoms of major depression include depressed mood, diminished interest or pleasure in all or almost all activities, significant weight loss or weight gain (>5% of body weight in a month), decrease or increase in appetite, insomnia or hypersomnia, psychomotor agitation or retardation, fatigue or loss of energy, feelings of worthlessness or of excessive or inappropriate guilt, diminished ability to concentrate, recurrent thoughts of death or suicidal ideation, or a suicide attempt. If delusions or hallucinations are also present, it would be classified as "major depression with psychotic features." Another severe form of major depression is the melancholic type. In addition to the symptoms listed above, this form is characterized by the lack of reactivity to pleasurable stimuli (does not feel better even temporarily if involved in what is usually a pleasurable activity), diurnal mood variation (depression regularly worse in the morning), and early morning awakening (at least 2 hours before usual time of awakening).

- Major depression: symptoms are depressed mood, diminished interest or pleasure in all or almost all activities, and significant weight loss or weight gain.
- Melancholic type: characterized by lack of reactivity to pleasurable stimuli, diurnal mood variation, early morning awakening.

Every year about 10 million Americans have a depressive episode but about only 20% usually seek treatment. Of those who seek treatment from a physician, as many as one-third are not diagnosed or are sometimes misdiagnosed because they often present with somatic complaints. As our population ages and more elderly patients seek medical care, diagnosing and treating their mood disorders are becoming more complicated because these patients often have overlapping medical and neurologic problems. Sometimes they present with the combination of a dementing process and depression, which if treated can help manage some of the other problems. The prevalence of depression in women is twice as high as in men. The peak age of onset of depression in women is 33 to 45 years and in men, older than 55 years.

- Of persons seeking treatment for major depression, as many as one-third are not diagnosed or are misdiagnosed.
- In elderly patients, diagnosing and treating mood disorders are becoming more complicated.
- Prevalence of depression in women is twice as high as in men.

Seasonal Affective Disorder

Seasonal affective disorder is a form of depression usually characterized by the onset of depression in the autumn or winter. It occurs twice as commonly in women as in men and is associated with psychomotor retardation, hypersomnia, overeating (carbohydrate craving), and weight gain. To make the diagnosis, this has to be a recurrent pattern for 2 to 3 consecutive years. Treatment has relied primarily on phototherapy, using a full-spectrum light source of 2,500 lux for 2 hr/day at a distance of 30 inches from the eyes or 10,000 lux sources, which can be used for 30 min/day. Newer sources of lights are being investigated, as are more specific details about the cause of this disorder. It appears that the antidepressant agents that selectively block serotonin reuptake may also be helpful in treating this disorder.

- Seasonal affective disorder: onset of depression in the autumn and winter.
- It is twice as common in women as in men.
- It is associated with psychomotor retardation, hypersomnia, and overeating.
- Treatment: primarily phototherapy.

Depressions are heterogeneous in their clinical presentation and so probably do not have a single etiologic agent. It appears that depression is more related to alterations of several neurotransmitter systems and neuropeptides, effects on presynaptic and postsynaptic receptors, neurohormonal alterations, and, in general, an alteration in the overall balance of these systems that are so interdependent on one another.

Treatment of Depression

There are four major groups of treatment modalities for depression: psychotherapy, pharmacotherapy, electroconvulsive therapy, and circadian rhythm manipulation such as sleep deprivation or phototherapy. Generally, they are used in some combination.

Psychotherapy—There are multiple forms of psychotherapy, many of which can be used in the treatment of depression. However, the two forms that have been used extensively for treating depression are cognitive therapy and interpersonal therapy. Cognitive therapy strives to help patients have a better integration of cognition (thoughts), emotion, and behavior. This therapy is based on the premise that our thoughts have a profound effect on our emotions, which have an effect on our behavior. If we can learn more adaptive ways of thinking, it may improve our general outlook and ultimately our behavior, with an increase in a sense of worth and improved self-esteem. Interpersonal therapy focuses on current interpersonal functioning. It is based on the concept that depression is associated with impaired social relationships that either precipitate or perpetuate the disorder.

- Cognitive therapy: to help patients have a better integration of cognition (thoughts), emotion, and behavior.
- Interpersonal therapy: focuses on current interpersonal functioning.

Pharmacotherapy—The selection of medication is based on the side-effect profile of the medication and the clinical profile of the patient. Dose: Start slowly and titrate to a therapeutic dose based on clinical judgment and blood levels (when available). Duration of treatment: Usually a minimum of 6 months, counting from the time the patient attained significant improvement. Often, patients may benefit from extended use of antidepressant agents, especially if they have had multiple episodes of depression. Antidepressant agents generally should be tapered rather than abruptly stopped when their use is discontinued. If the response to the first antidepressant agent is minimal or none, consider the addition of lithium carbonate or synthetic thyroid (T_3 or T_4), change to a different class of drug, or use electroconvulsive therapy, which is still probably the most consistently effective treatment for severe depression.

Cyclothymia

Cyclothymia can be thought of as a less severe form of bipolar disorder. By definition, it is a chronic disorder that usually appears in the late teens or early twenties and involves multiple hypomanic and depressive episodes that are not severe enough to meet criteria for mania or depression and do not generally cause significant impairment of occupational or social functioning. About 20% of patients with cyclothymia have a family history of bipolar disorder. About half of the patients report improvement while taking lithium.

- Cyclothymia: a less severe form of bipolar disorder.
- It is a chronic disorder that usually appears in the late teens to early twenties.
- It generally does not cause significant impairment of occupational or social functioning.

Mania and Bipolar Disorder

The essential features of a manic episode are the presence of an abnormally euphoric, expansive, or irritable mood associated with some of the following: inflated self-esteem or grandiosity, decreased need for sleep, pressured speech, flight of ideas, distractibility, increase in goal-directed activity or psychomotor agitation, and excessive involvement in pleasurable activities that have a high potential for painful consequences (e.g., unrestrained buying sprees, sexual indiscretions, or inappropriate financial investments). To make the diagnosis of a bipolar disorder, the patient must have had episodes of both depression and mania.

- Mania: the essential feature is an abnormally euphoric, expansive, or irritable mood.
- The prevalence of bipolar disorder is estimated to be about 1%.
- Bipolar disorder seems to occur at about the same frequency in women and men.
- The usual age at onset is from the teens to age 30.
- Patients generally have a family history of bipolar or other mood disorder.

Treatment is aimed at mood stabilization and improved social and occupational functioning. The primary pharmacologic treatment is lithium carbonate (see below). Other agents that are helpful include carbamazepine and valproic acid. Lithium may take up to 5 to 10 days to be effective. During this waiting period, the judicious use of antipsychotic agents or clonazepam is helpful in controlling the acute symptoms.

- Treatment of mania and bipolar disorder: aimed at mood stabilization and improved social and occupational functioning.
- Primary pharmacologic treatment: lithium carbonate.

Mood Disorders Due to a General Medical Condition

The essential feature of mood disorders due to a general medical condition is a disturbance of mood that is attributable to the physiologic effects of a specific medical condition. The clinical presentation may resemble that of a major depressive or manic episode, but the full criteria for one of these episodes need not be met. Medical conditions that may cause mood symptoms include endocrinopathies (Cushing syndrome, Addison disease, hyper- and hypothyroidism, and hyper- and hypoparathyroidism), certain malignancies (occult cancers, lymphomas, pancreatic carcinoma, gliomas), neurologic conditions (Parkinson disease, Huntington disease), autoimmune conditions (systemic lupus erythematosus), and infections (hepatitis, encephalitis, mononucleosis, human immunodeficiency virus [HIV]).

- Mood disorders due to a general medical condition: the essential feature is a disturbance of mood attributable to the physiologic effects of a specific medical condition.
- Many medical conditions can induce mood changes.

Substance-Induced Mood Disorders

The essential feature of a substance-induced mood disorder is a disturbance of mood that is judged to be due to the direct physiologic effects of a substance. Many substances can induce mood changes, including medications, toxin exposure, and substances of abuse. The mood symptoms may occur during the use of or exposure to the substance or during withdrawal from the substance. Medications that have been implicated in inducing mood disturbances include steroids, reserpine, methyldopa, propranolol, carbonic anhydrase inhibitors, stimulants, sedative-hypnotics, benzodiazepines, and narcotics and the chronic use or abuse of alcohol or hallucinogens.

- Substance-induced mood disorders: the essential feature is a disturbance of mood due to the physiologic effects of a substance.
- Many medications and drugs of abuse may induce mood changes.

PSYCHOTIC DISORDERS

"Psychosis" is a generic term used to describe behavior marked by a break from reality. Psychotic symptoms can occur in various medical, neurologic, and psychiatric disorders. Many psychotic reactions seen in medical settings are associated with the use of recreational or prescription drugs (Table 20-1). Some of these drug-induced psychotic reactions are nearly indistinguishable from schizophrenia (e.g., amphetamine and phencyclidine [PCP] psychoses). Other reactions may manifest as more nonspecific psychotic syndromes. Many brain regions may be involved with the production of psychotic symptoms, but abnormalities in the frontal, temporal, and limbic regions are more likely than others to produce psychotic features.

- Psychosis: a generic term describing behavior marked by a break from reality.
- Many psychotic reactions may be associated with use of recreational or prescription drugs.
- Some drug-induced psychotic reactions are nearly indistinguishable from schizophrenia.

There are disorders throughout the lifespan that may be associated with schizophrenia-like psychoses. These include genetic abnormalities, intrauterine events, neonatal brain injury, childhood neurologic insults, adolescent neuroendocrine changes, adult neurologic disorders, medical and metabolic diseases (e.g., infections, inflammatory disorders, endocrinopathies, nutritional deficiencies, uremia, hepatic encephalopathy), drug abuse, and psychologic stressors.

Schizophrenia in particular may also have a multifactorial cause. Current diagnostic criteria are divided into inclusion and exclusion criteria. Inclusion criteria include 1) presence of delusions and hallucinations; 2) marked decrement in functional level in areas such as work, school, social relations, and self-care; and 3) continuous signs of the disturbance for at least 6 months. Exclusion criteria

Table 20-1.—Classes of Drugs That Can Produce Psychotic Symptoms

Stimulants
Hallucinogens
Phencyclidine (PCP)
Catecholaminergic drugs
Anticholinergic drugs
Central nervous system depressants
Glucocorticoids
Heavy metals (lead, mercury, manganese, arsenic, thallium)
Others (digitalis, disulfiram, cimetidine, bromide)

include 1) absence of a consistent mood disorder component and 2) lack of evidence of an organic factor that produces the symptoms.

- Schizophrenia may have a multifactorial cause.

The five subtypes of schizophrenia are catatonic, disorganized, paranoid, undifferentiated, and residual.

ANXIETY DISORDERS

This group of disorders includes some of the ones seen most frequently in the outpatient setting. Anxiety symptoms may be misinterpreted as those of medical illness because many of the symptoms overlap, for example, tachycardia, diaphoresis, tremor, shortness of breath, nausea, abdominal pain, and chest pain. Autonomic arousal and anxious agitation in a medically ill patient can also be quickly attributed to stress or anxiety when it may represent pulmonary embolus or cardiac arrhythmia. Common sources of anxiety in the medical setting relate to fears of death, abandonment, loss of function, loss of a body part, pain, dependency, and loss of control. When to treat or to seek psychiatric consultation depends on the assessment of the degree of anxiety—is it at a level "expected" under the circumstances or is it unrealistic.

- Anxiety symptoms may be misinterpreted as those of medical illness.
- Common sources of anxiety in the medical setting relate to fears of death, abandonment, loss of function, loss of a body part, and pain.

Adjustment Disorder With Anxious Mood

Adjustment disorder with anxious mood is a maladaptive reaction to an identifiable environmental or psychosocial stress, accompanied primarily by symptoms of anxiety that interfere with the patient's usual functioning. Treatment may include supportive counseling and help with identifying the stressor. However, in some cases the anxiety may be so severe as to require short-term use of anxiolytic agents. However, they should be used with caution to avoid problems of long-term use and possible dependence.

- Adjustment disorder with anxious mood: a maladaptive reaction to an identifiable environmental or psychosocial stress accompanied by symptoms of stress.
- It may require short-term use of anxiolytic agents.

Panic Disorder With or Without Agoraphobia

Panic disorder is recurrent, discrete episodes of extreme anxiety accompanied by various somatic symptoms such as dyspnea, unsteady feelings, palpitations, paresthesias, hyperventilation, trembling, diaphoresis, chest pain or discomfort, or abdominal distress. Agoraphobia refers to extreme fear of being in places or situations from which escape may be difficult (or embarrassing). This may lead to avoidance of such situations as driving, travel in general, being in a crowded place, and many other situations, ultimately causing severe limitations in daily functioning for the person. Panic disorder is more common in women than in men; the usual age at onset is from the late teens to the early thirties. A history of childhood separation anxiety is reported in 20% to 50% of patients. The incidence is higher in first- and second-degree relatives. Most patients (78%) describe their first panic attack as spontaneous. They generally go to an emergency department after the first attack, believing they are having a heart attack or some severe medical problem.

- Panic disorder: recurrent, discrete episodes of extreme anxiety accompanied by various somatic symptoms.
- Agoraphobia: extreme fear of being in places or situations from which escape may be difficult.
- Agoraphobia is more common in women than in men.
- Patients generally go to an emergency department after their first panic attack, believing they are having a heart attack or some severe medical problem.

Some medical diagnostic groups to consider are 1) endocrine disturbances: hyperthyroidism, pheochromocytoma, and hypoglycemia; 2) gastrointestinal disturbances: colitis and irritable bowel syndrome; 3) cardiopulmonary disturbances: pulmonary embolism, exacerbation of chronic obstructive pulmonary disease, and acute allergic reactions; and 4) neurologic conditions: those associated with paresthesias, faintness, or dizziness.

Patients with panic attacks may also be prone to major episodes of depression. Alcohol use may temporarily reduce some of the distress of the panic attack and the interim anticipatory anxiety but may soon yield to rebound symptoms and potentially lead to alcohol overuse. Benzodiazepines may similarly be abused.

- Patients with panic attacks may be prone to episodes of major depression.
- Alcohol: may reduce distress of panic attacks but symptoms may rebound, potentially leading to alcohol abuse.
- Benzodiazepines may similarly be abused.

Post-Traumatic Stress Disorder

Post-traumatic stress disorder can be a brief reaction that soon follows an extremely traumatic, overwhelming, or catastrophic experience or it may be a chronic condition that produces severe disability. The syndrome is characterized by intrusive memories, flashbacks, nightmares, avoidance of reminders of the event, and often a restricted range of affect. It may occur in children. There is increased comorbidity with substance abuse, depression, and other anxiety disorders. Patients may be more prone to impulsivity, including suicide. As for other anxiety disorders, treatment is usually a combination of behavioral, psychotherapeutic, and, if necessary, pharmacologic interventions.

- Post-traumatic stress disorder: may be a brief reaction or a chronic condition that produces severe disability.
- Patients may be prone to impulsivity, including suicide.

Generalized Anxiety Disorder

Generalized anxiety disorder is characterized by chronic excessive anxiety and apprehension about life circumstances accompanied by somatic symptoms of anxiety, such as trembling, restlessness, autonomic hyperactivity, and hypervigilance. Treatment is usually a mixture of behavioral, progressive muscle relaxation, psychotherapeutic, and adjunctive psychopharmacologic modalities.

Obsessive-Compulsive Disorder

Obsessive-compulsive disorder is characterized by recurrent obsessions or compulsions that are severe enough to disrupt daily life. The obsessions are distressing thoughts, ideas, or impulses experienced as unwanted. Compulsions are repetitive, intentional behaviors usually performed in response to an obsession. The obsessions cause marked anxiety or distress, and the compulsions serve to neutralize the anxiety. Prevalence rates are about 2% to 3% and occur about equally in men and women. The onset of this disorder is usually in adolescence or early adulthood. Obsessive traits are often present before onset of the disorder. The predominant neurobiologic theory for the cause of obsessive-compulsive disorder involves dysfunction of brain serotonin systems. Pharmacologic treatment of this disorder uses antidepressants that are more selective for effects on the serotonin transmission system. These include clomipramine, selective serotonin reuptake inhibitors (fluvoxamine, fluoxetine, and sertraline), monoamine oxidase inhibitors (especially for patients who may also have panic attacks), and occasionally lithium augmentation of any of the preceding agents. In very severe, debilitating cases for which other treatments have failed, psychosurgery such as cingulotomy, stereotactic limbic leukotomy, or anterior capsulotomy may be of some benefit. The effectiveness of these procedures is thought to be related to disruption of the efferent pathways from the frontal cortex to the basal ganglia. Behavioral therapies and some forms of psychotherapy can also be helpful adjunctive therapies. As with the treatment of

many psychiatric disorders, it is a combination of treatments that is most often used. With obsessive-compulsive disorder, the pharmacologic treatments are generally not as effective as with major depressive episodes. Also, higher doses of the antidepressants may be needed for longer trial periods to see effectiveness in reducing symptoms of the obsessive-compulsive disorder.

- Obsessive-compulsive disorder is characterized by recurrent obsessions (distressing thoughts) and compulsions (repetitive behaviors) that are recognized as unreasonable but irresistible.
- Treatment consists primarily of antidepressants (with serotonergic activity) and behavioral therapy.

SOMATOFORM DISORDERS, FACTITIOUS DISORDERS, AND MALINGERING

Each of these disorders represents illness behaviors but differ with regard to whether the symptoms and motivations for their persistence are conscious or unconscious.

Somatoform Disorders

These include somatization disorder, conversion disorder, hypochondriasis, somatoform pain disorder (chronic pain syndromes), and body dysmorphic disorder.

Somatization Disorder

Somatization disorder is a polysymptomatic disorder that begins in early life and is characterized by recurrent multiple somatic complaints and an overwhelmingly positive review of symptoms. It mostly affects women. This disorder is often best managed with collaborative work with an empathic primary care physician and mental health professional. Regularly scheduled appointments with the primary care physician seem to lessen "doctor shopping" and frequent visits to an emergency department.

- Somatization disorder: begins in early life; characterized by recurrent multiple somatic complaints.
- It mostly affects women.
- "Doctor shopping" and frequent emergency room visits.

Conversion Disorder

Conversion disorder is a loss or alteration of physical functioning suggestive of a medical/neurologic disorder, but it cannot be explained on the basis of known physiologic mechanisms. The person is not conscious of intentionally producing the symptom. The disorder is not limited to pain or sexual dysfunction. It is seen most often in the outpatient setting. Patients frequently respond to any of several therapeutic modalities that suggest hope of a cure. If it becomes more of a chronic conversion disorder, it carries a poorer prognosis and is difficult to treat. Treatment focuses on management of the symptom rather than cure, much as in somatization or somatoform pain disorders.

- Conversion disorder: loss or alteration of physical functioning.
- It cannot be explained by known physiologic mechanisms.
- It is usually seen in the outpatient setting.
- Treatment focuses on management of the symptoms.

Somatoform Pain Disorder

Somatoform pain disorder (chronic pain syndromes) may occur at any age but most often starts in the 30s or 40s. It is diagnosed twice as often in women as in men and is characterized by preoccupation with pain for at least 6 months. No organic lesion is found to account for the pain, or if there is a related organic lesion, the complaint of pain or resulting interference with usual life activities is in excess of what would be expected from the physical findings. Treatment is usually multidisciplinary and focused on helping the patient manage or live with the pain rather than continuing with the expectation of "cure." Avoidance of long-term dependence on addictive substances is a general goal.

- Somatoform pain disorder: chronic pain syndromes that occur at any age but usually start in the 30s or 40s.
- It is diagnosed twice as often in women as in men.
- It is characterized by preoccupation with pain for at least 6 months.
- Treatment: usually multidisciplinary.

Hypochondriasis

Hypochondriasis is an intense preoccupation with the fear of having or the belief that one has a serious disease despite the lack of physical evidence to support the concern. It tends to be a chronic problem for the patient.

Factitious Disorders

Factitious disorders are characterized by the voluntary production of signs or symptoms of disease. The diagnosis of these disorders requires that the physician be highly suspicious. The most extreme form of the disorder is Munchausen syndrome, which is characterized by the triad of simulating disease, pathologic lying, and wandering. These cases have frequently involved men of lower socioeconomic class who have had a lifelong pattern of poor social adjustment. However, the common form generally occurs among "socially conforming young women of a higher socioeconomic class who are intelligent, educated, and frequently employed in a medically related field." The possibility of a coexisting medical disorder or intercurrent illness needs to be appreciated in the diagnostic and therapeutic management of these difficult cases. Factitious disorders are often found in patients with a history of childhood emotional traumas. These patients through their illness may be seeking to compensate for childhood traumas and secondarily to escape from and make up for stressful life situations.

- Factitious disorders: voluntary production of signs or symptoms of disease in order to assume the sick role.
- Munchausen syndrome: the most extreme form of factitious disorder; characteristic triad of simulating disease, pathologic lying, wandering.
- Common form: occurs among socially conforming young women of a higher socioeconomic class.
- Factitious disorders: often in patients with a history of childhood emotional traumas.

Malingering

The essential feature of malingering is the intentional production of false or exaggerated physical or psychologic symptoms. It is motivated by external incentives such as avoiding military service or work, obtaining financial compensation or drugs, evading criminal prosecution, or securing better living conditions. Malingering should be suspected in cases in which 1) a medicolegal context overshadows the clinical presentation, 2) a marked discrepancy exists between the person's claimed stress or disability and the objective findings, 3) there is lack of cooperation during the diagnostic evaluation and in compliance with prescribed treatments, and 4) there is presence of an antisocial personality disorder. The person who is malingering is much less likely to present his or her symptoms in the context of emotional conflict, and the presenting symptoms are less likely to be symbolically related to an underlying emotional conflict.

- Malingering: intentional production of false or exaggerated physical or psychologic symptoms.
- It is motivated by external incentives.

DELIRIUM AND DEMENTIA

The primary distinguishing feature between dementia and delirium is the retention and stability of alertness in dementia.

Delirium

Delirium is characterized by a fluctuating course of an altered state of awareness and consciousness. Although the onset usually is abrupt, it occasionally may be insidious. It may be accompanied by hallucinations (tactile, auditory, visual, or olfactory), illusions (misperceptions of sensory stimuli), delusions, emotional lability, paranoia, alterations in the sleep-wake cycle, and psychomotor slowing or hyperactivity. Delirium is usually reversible with correction of the underlying cause. It often is related to an external toxic agent, medication side effect, metabolic abnormalities, central nervous system abnormality, or withdrawal of a medication or drug. Delirium is relatively common (range, 10%-30%) in medical/surgical inpatients older than 65 years. The diagnosis is made primarily by clinical assessment and changes in the patient's mental status examination. High-risk groups include 1) elderly patients with medical illnesses (especially congestive heart failure, urinary tract infections, hyperkalemia, hyponatremia, malnutrition, dehydration, strokes); 2) postcardiotomy patients; 3) patients with brain damage; 4) patients in drug withdrawal; 5) burn patients; and 6) patients with acquired immunodeficiency syndrome (AIDS).

- Delirium: fluctuating course of an altered state of awareness and consciousness.
- It usually is reversible with correction of the underlying cause.
- It often is related to an external toxic agent, medication side effect, metabolic abnormality, central nervous system abnormality, or withdrawal of a medication or drug.
- Delirium is relatively common in medical/surgical patients older than 65 years.

The commonest cause of delirium in the elderly probably is intoxication with psychotropic drugs, especially drugs with sedative and anticholinergic side effects. Treatment initially can be separated by whether the cause is known. If it is, treating the underlying cause is most beneficial. If the cause is unknown and the patient's behavior interferes with his or her safety and medical care, several categories of intervention can be considered. Management aspects include 1) medical: monitor vital signs, electrolytes, fluid balance, and so forth; 2) pharmacologic: neuroleptic agents in parenteral form are helpful, such as haloperidol given intravenously; 3) environmental supports: to help with orientation, use calendars, clock, windows (family and others with orientation information are also helpful); and 4) psychosocial supports: family or other care providers can be helpful.

- The commonest cause of delirium in the elderly: intoxication with psychotropic drugs.

Dementia

Dementia is a syndrome of acquired persistent impairment of mental function involving at least three of the following five domains: memory, language, visuospatial skills, personality or mood, and cognition (including abstraction, judgment, calculations, and executive function). Some of the more common types of dementia are the following:

1. Cortical dementia—The common form is Alzheimer disease; other types include Pick disease and Creutzfeldt-Jakob disease. The overall prevalence is estimated at 2% to 10% of the population older than 65 years and 15% to 20% of those older than 85.
2. Subcortical dementia—Patients with this type of dementia often have an associated gait disturbance. The common type is multi-infarct dementia; other forms include normal-pressure hydrocephalus, Huntington disease, and Parkinson disease.
3. HIV-related dementia.
4. Dementias associated with multiple sclerosis, amyotrophic lateral sclerosis, vitamin B_{12} deficiency, hypothyroidism, and Wilson disease.

- Cortical dementia: the common form is Alzheimer type.
- Subcortical dementia: the common type is multi-infarct dementia.

Dementia is distinguished from delirium by intact arousal, more preserved attention, and persistence of the cognitive changes. Some forms may be reversible, as in dementia related to hypothyroidism, and some may be "treatable" without reversing the intellectual deficits, for example, preventing further ischemic injury in patients with vascular dementia. The dementia may be a chronic progressive form in which treatment is generally related to improved control of the behavioral disturbances.

PSYCHOLOGIC ASPECTS OF AIDS

From the early to the terminal phases of AIDS and its sequelae, many psychiatric symptoms and complications are possible. The organic mental disorders associated with this process can be primary (directly induced by HIV infection), secondary (related to the effects of the HIV infection leading to immunodeficiency and opportunistic infections or tumors systemically or within the central nervous system), or iatrogenic (resulting from the treatment of HIV or its sequelae). The delirium of AIDS often has a multifactorial cause, similar to delirium in general, that is, electrolyte imbalance, encephalopathy from intracranial or systemic infections, hypoxemia, or medication side effects. HIV itself causes encephalopathy. The dementia of AIDS can result from the chronic sequelae of most of the causes of delirium. However, direct cerebral infection with HIV probably causes much of the dementia.

Other psychiatric symptoms are more nonspecific, such as anger, depression, mania, psychosis, and the general problems of dealing with a terminal illness. Also, all these might be complicated by undiagnosed and, thus, untreated alcohol or drug dependence, especially in the early phases of the disease.

- AIDS: many possible psychiatric symptoms and complications.
- Organic mental disorders can be primary (due to HIV infection), secondary (due to immunodeficiency and opportunistic infections), or iatrogenic.
- Delirium in AIDS is multifactorial.
- Dementia in AIDS: can result from the chronic sequelae of most of the causes of delirium.

THE SUICIDAL PATIENT

Suicide is not an uncommon consequence of mental illness. It occurs in all psychiatric diagnostic categories. Emergency medicine physicians are often the first to deal with patients who have either completed suicide, attempted suicide, or have suicidal ideation. The recognition of risk factors for suicide and the acute medical management of the patient are important. Although the person who overdoses with a benzodiazepine may be more serious about the intent, the person who overdoses on aspirin may be at more risk for serious medical complications.

- Suicide: occurs in all psychiatric diagnostic categories.
- Recognition of the risk factors for suicide is important.

Recognition of a suicidal gesture is important in evaluating a patient in an emergency department. Although drug overdoses are the commonest form, alcohol intoxication, single vehicle accidents, and falls from heights at times merit further investigation. Many suicidal patients saw a physician the week before the attempt. Some of the risk factors to be aware of include older divorced or widowed men, caucasians, unemployment, poor physical health, past suicide attempts, family history of suicide (especially if parent), psychosis, alcoholism or drug abuse, chronic painful disease, sudden life changes, living alone, and anniversary of significant loss. Almost without exception, patients who come to an emergency department with intense suicidal ideation or gestures should not be sent home alone.

- In evaluating patients in an emergency department, the recognition of a suicidal gesture is important.
- Many suicidal patients saw a physician the week before the attempt.

- Patients who come to an emergency department with intense suicidal ideation or gestures should not be sent home alone.

EATING DISORDERS

The two common eating disorders are anorexia nervosa and bulimia. Both are more prevalent in women than in men. The onset is usually in the teenage or young adult years but can start prepubertally or after age 40. These disorders are now found across all income, racial, and ethnic groups. Both disorders have a primary symptom of preoccupation with weight and a desire to be thinner. The disorders are not mutually exclusive, and about 50% of patients with anorexia nervosa also have bulimia. Many patients with bulimia previously had at least a subclinical case of anorexia nervosa.

- The two common eating disorders: anorexia nervosa and bulimia.
- They are more prevalent in women than in men.
- Primary symptom: preoccupation with weight and a desire to be thinner.

Anorexia Nervosa

To meet the diagnostic criteria of anorexia nervosa, weight loss must be 15% below that expected for age and height. However, weight loss of 30% to 40% below normal is not uncommon and leads to the medical complications of starvation, such as depletion of fat, muscle wasting (including cardiac muscle in severe cases), bradycardia and other arrhythmias, ventricular tachycardia and sudden death, constipation, abdominal pain, leukopenia, hypercortisolemia, osteoporosis, and, in extreme cases, development of lanugo (fine hair of the body), and metabolic alterations to conserve energy (thyroid—low levels of T_3, cold intolerance, and difficulty maintaining core body temperature; reproductive—marked decrease or cessation of LH and FSH secretion and secondary amenorrhea).

Bulimia

The patients always feel as though their eating is out of control; many patients may have a concurrent depressive or anxiety disorder. Physical complications of the binge-purge cycle may include fluid and electrolyte abnormalities, hypochloremic-hypokalemic metabolic alkalosis, esophageal and gastric irritation and bleeding, large-bowel abnormalities due to laxative abuse, marked erosion of dental enamel with associated decay, parotid and salivary gland hypertrophy, and hyperamylasemia (25%-40% more than normal). If bulimia is untreated, it often becomes chronic. Some patients have a gradual spontaneous remission of some symptoms.

- Patients with bulimia may have a concurrent depressive or anxiety disorder.
- The binge-purge cycle causes physical complications.

ALCOHOLISM AND SUBSTANCE ABUSE DISORDERS

Alcoholism and substance abuse disorders are a major concern in all age groups and across all ethnic, socioeconomic, and racial groups. Despite national and international efforts to curb the problem and to make treatment more readily available, many people go undiagnosed and fewer than 10% of addicted people are involved in some form of treatment, either self-help groups or with professional supervision. The lifetime incidence of alcohol and drug abuse approaches 20% of the population. These disorders have devastating effects on families and significant others and contribute to other social problems such as motor vehicle accidents and fatalities, domestic violence, suicide, and increasing health care costs. Untreated alcoholics have been estimated to generate twice the general health care costs of nonalcoholics. Patients with addictive disorders are a heterogeneous group. They may present in many different ways. What may be most critical is improvement in the diagnostic skill in recognizing addictive disorders. The current definition of alcoholism approved by the National Council on Alcoholism and Drug Dependence may also be applicable to other drugs of abuse: alcoholism is a primary, chronic disease with genetic, psychosocial, and environmental factors influencing its development and manifestations. The disease is often progressive and fatal. It is characterized by continuous or periodic impaired control over drinking, preoccupation with the drug alcohol, use despite adverse consequences, and distortions in thinking, most notably denial.

- Fewer than 10% of addicted people are involved in some form of treatment.
- Lifetime incidence of alcohol and drug abuse approaches 20% of the population.
- Untreated alcoholics generate twice the general health care costs of nonalcoholics.
- Patients with addictive disorders are a heterogeneous group.

The adverse consequences of alcoholism and substance abuse disorders cross over into several domains:

1. Physical health—Alcohol withdrawal syndromes, liver disease, gastritis, anemia, and neurologic disorders.
2. Psychologic functioning—Impaired cognition and changes in mood and behavior.
3. Interpersonal functioning—Marital problems and child abuse and impaired social relationships.

4. Occupational functioning—Scholastic or job problems.
5. Legal, financial, and spiritual problems.

The substance abuse disorders are divided into ten major groups: alcohol; amphetamine; cannabis; cocaine; hallucinogens; inhalants; nicotine; opioids; phencyclidine; and benzodiazepines, sedative hypnotics, and anxiolytics. Some things are specific to each of these groups, but what may be surprising is that they probably have more similarities than differences when it comes to diagnosing a problem of abuse and/or dependence. In Table 20-2, these drugs are grouped according to their perceived effects. The descriptive titles of the groups give an idea of the physiologic and psychologic activity of the drug when taken. If one thinks of the converse of these states, the withdrawal states can be partly determined. As an example, if in the group of "downers," heart rate, blood pressure, and general autonomic functions slow down when the drugs are used, the opposite reaction would be expected with withdrawal from the substance. Another significant point is that within the group of "downers" there is considerable potential for crossover addictions.

- Within the group of "downers," there is considerable potential for crossover addictions.

Alcoholism

Medical data from physical examination and laboratory tests can be helpful. However, most of the pertinent findings are not apparent until after several years (often up to 5 years) of alcohol use and so are more reflective of middle-to-late stages of the disease. Two of the earlier detectable signs are increases of serum γ-glutamyltransferase and increased mean corpuscular volume. In both men and women, the combination of increased γ-glutamyltransferase levels and mean corpuscular volume can identify up to 90% of alcoholics. Other abnormal laboratory findings include increased levels of alkaline phosphatase, bilirubin, uric acid, and triglycerides. However, because of the number of false-negative results, it is not practical to rely on laboratory data alone for

Table 20-2.—Drugs Grouped According to Their Perceived Effects

Uppers	Downers	"All arounders"
Cocaine	Alcohol	Cannabis
Amphetamine	Opioids	Hallucinogens
Caffeine	Benzodiazepines	Inhalants
Nicotine	Sedative-hypnotics	Phencyclidine
	Barbiturates	

the diagnosis of alcoholism. Alcohol withdrawal can range from mild to quite severe, with the occurrence of withdrawal seizures and/or delirium tremens. The medical complications of alcoholism can affect nearly every organ system, but the central nervous system, liver, gastrointestinal tract, pancreas, and cardiovascular system are particularly sensitive to the effects of alcohol.

- Increased γ-glutamyltransferase levels and mean corpuscular volume can identify up to 90% of alcoholics.
- It is not practical to rely on laboratory data alone to make the diagnosis of alcoholism.
- Medical complications of alcoholism can affect nearly every organ system.

Benzodiazepines, Sedative-Hypnotics, and Anxiolytics

In contrast to many of the other groups, benzodiazepines, sedative-hypnotics, and anxiolytics are widely used in many areas of medicine, so the addictions that are often seen are iatrogenic. However, five characteristics may help distinguish medical use from nonmedical use: 1) Intent—What is the purpose of the use? 2) Effect—What is the effect on the user's life? 3) Control—Is the use controlled by the user only or does a physician share in the control? 4) Legality—Is the use of the drug legal or illegal? Medical drug use is legal. 5) Pattern—In what settings is the drug used?

These same characteristics can also be used to distinguish medical from nonmedical use of opioids. Withdrawal from use of benzodiazepines and barbiturates, in particular, can be serious because of the increased risk of withdrawal seizures.

- Withdrawal of use of benzodiazepines and barbiturates, in particular, can be serious because of the increased risk of withdrawal seizures.

PSYCHOPHARMACOLOGY

The use of a pharmacologic treatment for a psychiatric disorder or the use of psychoactive medications in other disorders is a decision that generally is made after considering multiple factors in the case. Medication alone is rarely the sole treatment for a psychiatric disorder but rather a component of a broader treatment plan. Because psychoactive medications are used in various circumstances for many different indications, the major groups of these medications—antidepressants, antipsychotics, antimanic agents, anxiolytics, and sedative drugs—are discussed below in general terms rather than for treatment of specific disorders. The choice of a medication generally is based on its side-effect profile and the clinical profile of the patient. There are many effective drugs in each

of the major groups, but they differ in terms of pharmacokinetics, side effects, and available routes of administration.

- Medication alone is rarely the sole treatment for a psychiatric disorder.
- The choice of a medication generally is based on its side-effect profile and the clinical profile of the patient.

Antipsychotic Agents

The several classes of antipsychotic agents can be categorized by chemical structure: phenothiazines (including their derivatives and piperidines and piperazines), thioxanthenes, butyrophenones, dibenzoxazepine, indole derivatives, pimozide, and dibenzodiazepine (Clozaril). Clinically, antipsychotic agents are now discussed as "standard antipsychotics" versus "atypical" or "new-generation antipsychotic agents." The currently available new-generation antipsychotics include clozapine, olanzapine, quetiapine, and resperidone. Others may be available soon.

The choice of medication is based on the patient's clinical situation, side-effect profile of the chosen agent, history of previous response, and issues related to compliance. The prevailing theory about the mechanism of action of these agents is that they cause blockade of postsynaptic dopamine receptors. This relates to both the antipsychotic activity and other side effects, depending on which dopamine pathways in the brain are affected and which of the several types of dopamine receptor is preferentially affected. If the nigrostriatal dopaminergic system (involved with motor activity) is affected, extrapyramidal symptoms may result. Blockade of the dopamine pathways in the pituitary and hypothalamus causes the increased release of prolactin and changes in appetite and temperature regulation. The effects of these drugs on the limbic system, midbrain tegmentum, septal nuclei, and mesocortical dopaminergic projections are thought to be responsible for their antipsychotic action.

- The theory about the mechanism of action of antipsychotic agents is that they cause blockade of postsynaptic dopamine receptors.
- The antipsychotic effects of these agents are due to their action on the limbic system, midbrain tegmentum, septal nuclei, and mesocortical dopaminergic projections.

Side Effects: Extrapyramidal Reactions

Acute dystonic reactions occur within hours or days after initiating treatment with antipsychotic drugs. These reactions are characterized by uncontrollable tightening of the face and neck muscles with spasms. The effect on the eyes may cause an oculogyric crisis, and the effect on the laryngeal muscles may cause respiratory or ventilatory difficulties. Treatment is usually with intravenous or intramuscular administration of an anticholinergic agent, followed by the use of an oral anticholinergic agent for a few days (antipsychotic agents have long half-lives).

- Acute dystonic reactions: occur within hours or days after initiating treatment with antipsychotic drugs.
- Reactions: uncontrollable tightening of the face and neck muscles with spasms.
- Treatment: intravenous or intramuscular administration of an anticholinergic agent.

Parkinsonian syndrome has a more gradual onset and can be treated with oral anticholinergic agents and/or decreased doses of the antipsychotic agent. *Akathisia* is an unpleasant feeling of restlessness and the inability to sit still. It often occurs within days after initiating treatment with antipsychotic agents. Akathisia is sometimes mistaken for exacerbation of the psychosis. Treatment, if possible, is to decrease the dose of the antipsychotic agent or to try using a β-adrenergic blocking agent such as propranolol, if not contraindicated. *Akinesia* is characterized by diminished spontaneity, few gestures, and apathy. It may be mistaken for a depressive reaction. This condition usually can be treated with an anticholinergic agent.

- Akathisia: unpleasant feeling of restlessness and the inability to sit still.

Tardive dyskinesia consists of involuntary movements of the face, trunk, or extremities. The most consistent risk factor for its development is older age. Prevention is the most important aspect of management, because no reliable treatment is available. It is best if treatment with the antipsychotic agent can be discontinued, although there may be a temporary increase in the symptoms of tardive dyskinesia.

- Tardive dyskinesia: involuntary movements of the face, trunk, or extremities.
- Prevention: the most important aspect of management.

Neuroleptic malignant syndrome is a potentially life-threatening disorder that may occur after the use of any antipsychotic agent, although it is generally more common with the high-potency antipsychotic agents. Its clinical presentation is characterized by severe rigidity, fever, leukocytosis, tachycardia, tachypnea, diaphoresis, blood pressure fluctuations, and marked increase in creatine phosphokinase levels due to muscle breakdown. Treatment consists of discontinuing the use of the antipsychotic agent and providing life-support measures (ventilation, cooling, etc.). Pharmacologic interventions may include the use of dantrolene sodium, which is a direct-acting

muscle relaxant, and/or bromocriptine, which is a centrally acting dopamine agonist. Often, one of the most effective treatments is electroconvulsive therapy.

- Neuroleptic malignant syndrome: potentially life-threatening.
- It may occur after the use of any antipsychotic agent.
- Characteristics: severe rigidity, fever, leukocytosis, tachycardia, tachypnea, diaphoresis, blood pressure fluctuations, marked increase in creatine phosphokinase levels (muscle breakdown).

Other, non-extrapyramidal side effects of antipsychotic agents are listed in Table 20-3.

Newer Antipsychotics

The newer antipsychotic agents now available are clozapine, risperidone, olanzapine, and quetiapine. They are significantly different from their predecessors in terms of potential mechanisms of action and their side-effect profiles. These agents are less likely to cause bothersome extrapyramidal side effects, and their potential for causing tardive dyskinesia may be less. The evidence for the latter will take time to establish because the onset of the symptoms is delayed and the drugs have not been widely used long enough to determine the risk of tardive dyskinesia. Neuroleptic malignant syndrome has been reported to occur with clozapine and risperidone. Clozapine has a 1% to 2% risk of producing agranulocytosis, which is reversible if use of the medication is withdrawn. Because of this serious potential side effect, there is a specific requirement for performing regular blood cell counts (weekly in the first 6-18 months and then possibly less often). No other serious side effects have been reported to occur frequently, but similar to their predecessors, increased levels of prolactin

Table 20-3.—Side Effects of Antipsychotic Agents Aside From Extrapyramidal Effects

Anticholinergic
Orthostatic hypotension—related to α-adrenergic receptor blockade
Hyperprolactinemia—gynecomastia possible in men and women, galactorrhea (rare), amenorrhea, weight gain, breast tenderness, decreased libido
Sexual dysfunction
Dermatologic—pigmentary changes in the skin and photosensitivity
Decreased seizure threshold—caused by most antipsychotic agents

and weight gain can occur with some of these agents. These agents have not been in use long enough for us to be aware of the degree of drug interactions with other prescribed medications. These new-generation antipsychotic agents are also significantly more expensive than their predecessors.

Antianxiety Medications

These drugs are used most appropriately to treat time-limited anxiety or insomnia related to an identifiable stress or change in sleep cycle. If used long term (>2-3 months), benzodiazepines and related substances should be tapered rather than be discontinued abruptly to avoid any of the three "discontinuation syndromes."

1. Relapse—Return of the original anxiety symptoms, often after weeks to months.
2. Rebound—Intensification of the original symptoms; it usually lasts several days and appears within hours to days after abrupt cessation of drug use.
3. Withdrawal—May be mild to severe and includes autonomic and central nervous system symptoms that are different from the original presenting symptoms of the disorder.

Benzodiazepines are well-absorbed orally but have unpredictable availability with intramuscular use, except for lorazepam. There is great variability among the benzodiazepines in terms of their pharmacokinetics. Many of these drugs have metabolites with very long half-lives. Therefore, much smaller doses need to be used in the elderly, in patients with brain damage, and in children—all these patient groups are prone to the paradoxical reactions (anxiety, irritability, aggression, agitation, insomnia), especially patients with known brain damage.

- Benzodiazepines: great variability in terms of their pharmacokinetics.

Buspirone is a non-benzodiazepine anxiolytic drug whose mechanism of action is not known. However, the drug has effects on many neurotransmitter systems, especially the serotonergic and dopaminergic systems. Cross-tolerance does not exist between the benzodiazepines and buspirone. It generally takes 2 to 3 weeks for the drug to become effective.

- Buspirone: a non-benzodiazepine anxiolytic drug.
- It takes 2-3 weeks for the drug to become effective.

Antidepressant Agents

More than 20 antidepressant agents are available in the U.S. to treat depression, and there are at least two other drugs that are antidepressants but are approved for use in this country primarily for the treatment of obsessive-compulsive disorder

(clomipramine and fluvoxamine). The first-generation antidepressant agents included the tricyclics and monoamine oxidase inhibitors. The newer generation antidepressant agents are not easily grouped by their chemical structure or function but rather are a diverse group of compounds. Currently, the most widely used of this group of agents are the selective serotonin reuptake inhibitors.

Although the early generation antidepressant agents were effective in treating depression, they were associated with significant side effects, which limited their use in certain groups of patients, especially those with other medical problems. In particular, tricyclics are associated with orthostatic hypotension, anticholinergic side effects, and cardiac conduction defects. Monoamine oxidase inhibitors are effective antidepressants but require special dietary restrictions and special attention to interactions with other medications. Because the newer generation antidepressants have fewer potential side effects and drug interactions, they are prescribed more widely, but they are not effective for everyone.

1. Tricyclics—Tertiary amines, including imipramine, amitriptyline, doxepin, and trimipramine, and secondary amines, including desipramine, nortriptyline, and protriptyline.
2. Monoamine oxidase inhibitors—Phenelzine, isocarboxazid, tranylcypromine, and pargyline.
3. Newer generation antidepressants—Maprotiline, amoxapine, trazodone, bupropion, fluoxetine, sertraline, paroxetine, fluvoxamine, citalopram, venlafaxine, and nefazadone.

The mechanism of action is their effect on the catecholaminergic and serotonergic systems of the central nervous system. The various cyclic antidepressant agents block the reuptake of norepinephrine or serotonin (or both), increasing the amount of these neurotransmitters at the synapse. Monoamine oxidase inhibitors block the catabolism of several biogenic amines (norepinephrine, serotonin, tyramine, phenylephrine, and dopamine), thereby increasing the amount of these neurotransmitters available for synaptic release.

- Antidepressant agents affect the catecholaminergic and serotonergic systems of the central nervous system.
- Monoamine oxidase inhibitors block the catabolism of several biogenic amines.

Antidepressant agents are primarily approved for use in the treatment of depression. However, they are useful in several other disorders, including panic disorder, obsessive-compulsive disorder, enuresis, chronic pain, migraine headache, bulimia, and attention-deficit disorder. Because they are so widely used, familiarity with the basics of their use, side effects, and drug interactions may be helpful. The choice of which antidepressant agent to use is often based on the side-effect profile of the drug and the clinical presentation of the patient. The side effects of the major groups of antidepressant agents are listed in Table 20-4.

A complete trial of antidepressant medication consists of 6 weeks of therapeutic doses before considering refractoriness. If some improvement has occurred with the initial trial, but the condition is not yet back to baseline, it may be worthwhile to try augmenting therapy with lithium carbonate before changing the medication to another class of antidepressant. Another alternative is a trial of thyroid hormone (T_3) supplementation before switching use of antidepressant medications. After clinical improvement has been noted, the medication may need to be maintained for an extended period.

- A complete trial of antidepressant medication: 6 weeks of therapeutic doses.
- Augmenting therapy with lithium carbonate may be worthwhile before changing the medication to another class of antidepressant.

Monoamine Oxidase Inhibitors

Most clinical concerns about the use of monoamine oxidase inhibitors relate to reactions from the ingestion of tyramine, which is not metabolized because of the inhibition of intestinal monoamine oxidase. Tyramine may act as a false transmitter and displace norepinephrine from synaptic vesicles. Patients should be instructed in a tyramine-restricted diet, especially

Table 20-4.—Side Effects of the Major Groups of Antidepressant Agents

Orthostatic hypotension—The cardiovascular side effect that most commonly results in serious morbidity, especially in the elderly
Anticholinergic effects—Dry mouth, blurred vision, urinary retention, etc.; beware of these side effects in patients with prostatic hypertrophy and narrow-angle glaucoma. Drugs with more anticholinergic side effects also seem to be the more sedating, e.g., tertiary amine tricyclics
Cardiac conduction effects—Most of the tricyclics prolong PR and QRS intervals. Therefore, these drugs need to be used with caution in patients with preexisting heart block, such as second-degree heart block or markedly prolonged QRS and QT intervals. The tricyclics are potent antiarrhythmic agents because of their quinidine-like effect. Newer generation antidepressants have considerably fewer cardiac interactions
Sedating types—Tertiary amine tricyclics and trazadone
Potentially more stimulating types—Secondary amine tricyclics, bupropion, fluoxetine, sertraline, and paroxetine

to avoid aged cheeses, smoked meats, pickled herring, beer and red wine (generally all alcohol should be restricted), yeast extracts, fava beans, and overripe bananas and avocadoes. Certain general anesthetics and drugs with sympathomimetic activity should be avoided; especially beware of over-the-counter cough and cold preparations, decongestants, and appetite suppressants. Meperidine (Demerol) is absolutely contraindicated because of its potentially lethal interaction with monoamine oxidase inhibitors.

- Clinical concerns about monoamine oxidase inhibitors: reactions due to ingestion of tyramine, which is not metabolized.
- Tyramine: a false neurotransmitter that displaces norepinephrine from synaptic vesicles.
- Meperidine (Demerol): absolutely contraindicated because of its potentially lethal interaction with monoamine oxidase inhibitors.

Treatment of hypertensive reactions relies on administering drugs with α-adrenergic blocking properties, such as intravenous administration of phentolamine. This should be done in an emergency department. Patients may take nifedipine (10 mg sublingually) before reaching an emergency department if they have a moderate-to-severe occipital headache while taking a monoamine oxidase inhibitor.

LITHIUM

For many years, lithium carbonate has been the drug of choice for treating bipolar disorders. It can also be effective in patients with recurrent unipolar depressions and as an adjunct for maintenance of remission of depression after electroconvulsive therapy. Acute manic symptoms usually respond to treatment with lithium within 7 to 10 days. While waiting for this effect, the adjunctive use of antipsychotic agents and benzodiazepines may be helpful. Lithium is well absorbed from the gastrointestinal tract, with peak levels in 1 to 2 hours. Its half-life is about 24 hours. Levels are generally checked 10 to 12 hours after the last dose. Relatively common side effects include fine hand tremor, diarrhea, polyuria, polydipsia, thirst, and nausea, which is often improved by taking the medication on a full stomach. Lithium is contraindicated in the first trimester of pregnancy, because of its potential for causing defects in the developing cardiac system. Renal effects generally can be reversed with discontinuation of treatment with lithium. The most noticeable renal effect is the vasopressin-resistant effect leading to impaired concentrating ability and nephrogenic diabetes insipidus with polyuria and polydipsia. Most patients who take lithium develop some polyuria but not all develop more severe manifestations of nephrogenic diabetes insipidus. Renal function should be followed in all patients receiving maintenance lithium therapy. However, whether lithium has significant nephrotoxic effects is a matter of controversy. A hematologic side effect is a benign leukocytosis. Hypothyroidism may occur in as many as 20% of patients taking lithium, because of the direct inhibitory effects on thyroid hormone production or increased antithyroid antibodies.

- Lithium carbonate: the drug of choice for treating bipolar disorders.
- Common side effects: hand tremor, diarrhea, polyuria, polydipsia, thirst, and nausea.
- Renal effects generally can be reversed with discontinuation of treatment with lithium.
- Most noticeable renal effect: impaired concentrating ability.
- Hypothyroidism occurs in as many as 20% of patients taking lithium.

Because the range between the therapeutic and toxic levels of lithium in the plasma is narrow, patients and physicians should be familiar with conditions that may increase or decrease lithium levels and with the signs and symptoms of lithium toxicity so it can be recognized and treated promptly (Tables 20-5 and 20-6).

Other Mood Stabilizers

The anticonvulsants carbamazepine and valproic acid are effective in the treatment of acute manic episodes and for prophylactic maintenance therapy of bipolar disorders. The mechanism of action for their mood-stabilizing effects is not clear. Carbamazepine has a chemical structure similar to that of the tricyclic antidepressants and has a quinidine-like effect. The side effect of most concern with valproic acid is hepatotoxicity, which has occurred mostly in children receiving treatment with multiple anticonvulsants.

Table 20-5.—Conditions That Increase or Decrease Lithium Levels in the Plasma

Increase levels	Decrease levels
Dehydration	Increased caffeine consumption
Overheating and increased perspiration with exercise and/or hot weather	Theophylline
Nonsteroidal anti-inflammatory drugs	
Thiazide diuretics	
Angiotensin-converting enzyme inhibitors	
Certain antibiotics—tetracycline, spectinomycin, and metronidazole	

Table 20-6.—Signs and Symptoms of Lithium Toxicity

Mild-to-moderate toxicity (plasma levels, 1.5-2.0 mEq/L)	Moderate-to-severe toxicity (plasma levels, 2.0-2.5 mEq/L)	Severe toxicity (plasma levels, >2.5 mEq/L)
Vomiting	Persistent nausea and vomiting	Generalized seizures
Abdominal pain	Anorexia	Oliguria and renal failure
Dry mouth	Blurred vision	Death
Ataxia	Muscle fasciculations	
Slurred speech	Hyperactive deep tendon reflexes	
Nystagmus	Delirium	
Muscle weakness	Convulsions	
	Electroencephalographic changes	
	Stupor and coma	
	Circulatory system failure	
	Decreased blood pressure	
	Cardiac arrhythmias	
	Conduction abnormalities	

Modified from Silver JM, Hales RE, Yudofsky SC: Biological therapies for mental disorders. *In* Clinical Psychiatry for Medical Students. Edited by A Stoudemire. Philadelphia, JB Lippincott Company, 1990, pp 459-496. By permission of publisher.

Other anticonvulsants are also being investigated as mood-stabilizing agents.

- The anticonvulsants carbamazepine and valproic acid are effective for the treatment of acute mania and maintenance treatment of bipolar disorders.

ELECTROCONVULSIVE THERAPY

Electroconvulsive therapy is the most effective treatment for severely depressed patients, especially those with psychotic features. It is also helpful in treating catatonia and mania and may be used in children and adults. Also, electroconvulsive therapy can be administered to pregnant women. It may be effective in patients with overlapping depression and Parkinson disease and/or dementia. Electroconvulsive therapy is administered with the patient under barbiturate anesthesia, with succinylcholine or a similar muscle relaxant to minimize peripheral manifestations of the seizure. An anticholinergic agent such as atropine is generally given to decrease secretions and to prevent bradycardia caused by central stimulation of the vagus nerve. A usual course of treatment is 6 to 12 sessions given over a 2- to 4-week period. Therapy is often initiated with unilateral, nondominant electrode placement to minimize memory loss. If satisfactory results cannot be obtained with this method, bilateral electrode placement is used.

- Electroconvulsive therapy: the most effective treatment for severely depressed patients, especially those with psychotic features.
- It is also helpful in treating catatonia and mania.
- It can be given to pregnant women.
- It may be helpful in cases of overlapping depression and Parkinson disease and/or dementia.

Mechanism of action—Electroconvulsive therapy induces changes in several transmitter-receptor systems, particularly acetylcholine, norepinephrine, dopamine, and serotonin. It downregulates β-adrenergic receptors and may decrease calcium levels in the cerebrospinal fluid. It may also affect neuropeptides and electrical conduction systems (similar to those studied by cardiac electrophysiologists).

- Electroconvulsive therapy induces changes in acetylcholine, norepinephrine, dopamine, and serotonin transmitter-receptor systems.
- It downregulates β-adrenergic receptors.
- It may decrease calcium levels in the cerebrospinal fluid.

No longer are there any absolute contraindications to electroconvulsive therapy, although there are several relative contraindications. Previously, the only absolute contraindication was the presence of an intracranial space-occupying lesion and increased intracranial pressure. Serious complications or mortality is generally reported as less than 1 per 10,000, which makes this therapy one of the safest interventions that uses general anesthesia. Morbidity and mortality usually are due to cardiovascular complications, such as arrhythmia, myocardial infarction, or hypotension. The major risks are those associated with the brief general anesthesia. Medical evaluations performed before giving the therapy should pay particular attention to cardiovascular function, pulmonary function (because positive pressure respiration is used during anesthesia), electrolyte balance, and the patient's previous experiences with anesthesia.

- Electroconvulsive therapy: no longer any absolute contraindications.
- There are several relative contraindications.
- Morbidity and mortality are usually due to cardiovascular complications.

QUESTIONS

Multiple Choice (choose the one best answer)

1. A 20-year-old man with a history of alcohol and poly-substance dependence and a recent serious suicide attempt came to the urgent care clinic because he does not have a regular physician. He states that he is feeling more depressed and anxious and his psychologist thinks he needs a medicine to help him. He tells you that he is not thinking of suicide now, he just needs help to feel better. Your options would include all the following *except*:
   a. Get permission to call the referring psychologist and get more history
   b. Review any previous trials of antidepressants
   c. Consider prescribing a selective serotonin reuptake inhibitor
   d. Give him a refillable prescription for alprazolam, because it may take him some time to find a regular physician
   e. Inquire about his current alcohol and drug use

2. You are following a 44-year-old woman with a difficult-to-treat major depression with psychotic features. She has recently been prescribed a combination of medications that seem to help her. These include verapamil for tachycardia, sertraline and lithium for depression, risperidone for psychotic symptoms, benztropine for side effects of the risperidone, and trazodone for help with sleep. Her psychiatrist is away, and the family calls you, explaining that the patient has become confused and disoriented, her sleep is disrupted, her gait is unstable, and she has fallen twice. She also has started to see bugs crawling around her. Possible causes of these symptoms would include all the following *except*:
   a. Dehydration
   b. Lithium toxicity
   c. Worsening of her depression
   d. Neuroleptic malignant syndrome
   e. Delirium related to the interactions of her medications

3. A 20-year-old single woman with a long history of severe anorexia nervosa is sent to you for a general medical evaluation as she has not had one in several years. She is gaunt, has lanugo hair on her back, and has never menstruated regularly. Which of the following laboratory studies would be helpful in the evaluation of this patient?
   a. Electrocardiography
   b. TSH, LH, and FSH
   c. Complete blood count
   d. Electrolytes
   e. All the above

4. The newer antipsychotic agents offer all the following advantages *except*:
   a. Lower incidence of extrapyramidal symptoms
   b. More effect on the negative symptoms of schizophrenia
   c. More cost-effective
   d. Decreased incidence of increased prolactin levels
   e. Potential of improved patient compliance

5. Which of the following statements about alcohol and drug use is false?
   a. Alcoholics often use denial as a primary defense
   b. Although tolerance to the effects of cannabis may develop with chronic use, cessation does not produce significant withdrawal phenomenon
   c. Cocaine addiction often occurs in the presence of another substance addiction
   d. Laboratory studies are very helpful in the definitive diagnosis of alcohol dependence
   e. Combined alcohol and drug abuse problems are becoming increasingly common

6. The newer antidepressants are safer in terms of overdose fatalities because:
   a. They cost so much that most people cannot afford to have a large enough supply to take an overdose
   b. They cause fewer cardiac arrhythmias and fewer seizures in high doses
   c. They have a lower threshold for toxic doses
   d. They more easily potentiate the effect of alcohol and other central nervous system depressants
   e. All the above

7. Neuroleptic malignant syndrome can be fatal. The best laboratory variable to check for the presence of the disorder and the response to treatment is:
   a. Serum level of magnesium
   b. Electrocardiography
   c. White blood cell count
   d. Creatine phosphokinase level
   e. Urine myoglobin concentration

8. Patients receiving long-term lithium treatment should have which of the following laboratory studies checked at regular intervals?
   a. Creatinine
   b. Lithium level
   c. TSH
   d. White blood cell count
   e. All the above

9. A 28-year-old single woman with an acute exacerbation of asthma is admitted to your hospital service by a colleague who is going out of town. She is otherwise in good health. However, she appears somewhat depressed. She explains to the nursing staff that she wishes to have her code status listed as "do not resuscitate." On further questioning by nurses she confides that she has been having suicidal ideation. The nurses call you with this information and ask you whether her code status may be listed as she has requested. All the following options would seem reasonable *except*:
    a. Tell the patient that this is not acceptable
    b. Ask for a psychiatric consultation to help with the situation
    c. Express your concerns to the patient that this seems to be an unusual request on her part considering that her medical status is serious but not critical
    d. Ask the patient for permission to speak with other family members whom she trusts
    e. Inquire whether the patient has ever had these thoughts of suicide before and has ever attempted suicide in the past

10. Delirium, dementia, and depression are not uncommon in the nursing home population. These three phenomena can occur independently or in some combination with each other. Which of the following statements is false regarding these conditions?
    a. The most common cause of delirium in elderly patients is medication side effects
    b. Depression and dementia may overlap, but in this case the depression is generally refractory to treatment
    c. Although the electroencephalogram in dementia may be normal, it is almost always positive in delirium
    d. Using electroconvulsive therapy to treat depression in the face of dementia may help improve the behavioral dyscontrol of the dementia
    e. Antipsychotic medications in low doses may be indicated as part of the treatment for each of these conditions

ANSWERS

1. Answer d.

With his chemical-dependence history, one needs to be cautious about prescribing anxiolytics. Alprazolam is very short acting and, thus, has a high potential for abuse and addiction. However, anxiolytics are safer in overdose than the antidepressants. If anxiolytics are prescribed for such a person, they should be prescribed in controlled amounts with regular follow-up.

2. Answer d.

The symptoms of the acute change are not indicative of neuroleptic malignant syndrome. Although all the other choices are potential explanations, lithium toxicity is likely the primary factor.

3. Answer e.

All the mentioned tests can be abnormal in anorexia nervosa and should be monitored, although not all need specific treatment other than helping the patient regain a healthy weight.

4. Answer c.

The newer antipsychotic agents offer many advantages, but at this point they are very expensive.

5. Answer d.

Laboratory abnormalities usually occur fairly late in the course of alcohol dependence and are not usually the most conclusive part of the diagnosis.

6. Answer b.

The newer antidepressants, especially the selective serotonin reuptake inhibitors (SSRIs) do not inhibit fast sodium channels as the tricyclic antidepressants do. They do not have the impact on intracardiac conduction. Also, they do not affect the seizure threshold. Furthermore, SSRIs do not readily potentiate the effect of alcohol and other central nervous system depressants, which are often taken in combination with antidepressants in overdoses.

7. Answer d.

An increased level of creatine phosphokinase (CPK) in

conjunction with the other physical symptoms of neuroleptic malignant syndrome is the hallmark of the disorder. Following the levels of CPK can also help determine the course of recovery. The other laboratory tests mentioned with the exception of magnesium (which is irrelevant to this discussion) are generally abnormal but not as specific as CPK.

8. Answer e.

All of these laboratory studies merit follow-up. Lithium has a very narrow therapeutic index and is cleared by the kidneys; it can cause hypothyroidism and leukocytosis. The leukocytosis is usually benign and reversible with discontinuation of the lithium, but the hypothyroidism needs to be treated.

9. Answer a.

This clearly presents an ethical dilemma with a person who is hospitalized, has suicidal ideation, and asks to be a "no code." Is this really an informed decision? This requires further discussion and exploration with the patient and cannot just be ignored or handled by disregarding the patient's statement.

10. Answer b.

When depression occurs with dementia, cognitive functioning and general psychosocial functioning of the patient can be much worse and interfere significantly with the care of the patient. The positive part is that the depression is often amenable to treatment, which can improve some aspects of the patient's level of functioning such as improving the sleep pattern, appetite, and behavior control. Electroconvulsive therapy can be very helpful in this case. Although electroconvulsive therapy can cause more temporary confusion, the longer term benefit of treating the underlying depressive symptoms can improve the overall management of the patient.

NOTES

CHAPTER 21

PULMONARY DISEASES

Udaya B. S. Prakash, M.D.

SYMPTOMS AND SIGNS

Cough

A cough can be a voluntary act or a reflex. The afferent limb of the cough reflex includes the sensory branches of the trigeminal, glossopharyngeal, superior laryngeal, and vagus nerves. The efferent limb includes the recurrent laryngeal and spinal nerves. Lesions in the nose, ears, pharynx, larynx, bronchi, lungs, pleura, and abdominal viscera can cause cough.

- Inflammatory, mechanical, chemical, or thermal injury to the afferent limb of the cough reflex can cause cough.
- Healthy women have a more sensitive cough reflex than do healthy men.
- Cough can be the presenting or only manifestation of asthma.

Chronic cough is cough that lasts 3 weeks without an obvious cause. Neutrophils and cytokines associated with neutrophil chemotaxis and activation may contribute to the pathogenesis of nonasthmatic, chronic dry cough. Evaluation may require an ear-nose-throat examination, esophagography or acid reflux test (or both), pH monitoring, and methacholine inhalation challenge to exclude asthma. About one-half of the patients with persistent cough evaluated by a general practitioner have asthma or chronic obstructive pulmonary disease (COPD) (BMJ 316:1286-1290, 1998). Nonpulmonary diseases (temporal arteritis, rheumatoid bronchiolitis, Sjögren syndrome, and reflux esophagitis) may present with cough. Bronchoscopy in the absence of chest radiographic (CXR) abnormalities carries a low (4%) diagnostic yield. Cough is a complication in up to 10% of patients who take angiotensin-converting enzyme (ACE) inhibitors. ACE receptor blockers are not associated with cough. Cough syncope: hard cough produces increased intrathoracic pressure, which causes a decrease in cardiac output and cerebral perfusion. Chronic cough is reported to be associated with increased risk of myocardial infarction (Am J Med 106:279-284, 1999).

- Postnasal drip, asthma, reflux, and recent infection are responsible for >90% of chronic coughs.
- Complications of cough: cough syncope, rib fracture, pneumothorax.
- Bronchoscopy: low diagnostic yield if CXR is normal.
- Nonpulmonary diseases can present with cough.
- ACE inhibitors cause cough in 6% of patients (more common in women).
- Chronic cough is more common in women.

Sputum

Purulent sputum occurs in bronchiectasis and lung abscess. The sputum is frothy pink in pulmonary edema. Expectoration of bronchial casts, mucous plugs, or thin strings occurs in asthma, bronchopulmonary aspergillosis, and mucoid impaction syndrome, and expectoration of stone (lithoptysis) occurs in broncholithiasis. Plastic bronchitis is the formation of thick bronchial casts in asthma, bronchopulmonary aspergillosis, and other conditions. Bronchorrhea (expectoration of thin serous fluid >100 mL/day) occurs in 20% of patients with diffuse alveolar cell carcinoma.

- Bronchorrhea occurs in diffuse alveolar cell carcinoma.
- The most common cause of broncholithiasis: histoplasmosis.
- Sputum microscopy to identify eosinophils, Charcot-Leyden crystals, Curschmann spirals in asthmatics.

Hemoptysis

Hemoptysis is the expectoration of blood or blood-streaked sputum that originates below the level of the larynx. Bronchial arterial bleeding occurs in chronic bronchitis, bronchiectasis, malignancies, and broncholithiasis and with the presence of foreign bodies. Pulmonary arterial bleeding occurs in pulmonary arteriovenous malformations, fungus ball, tumors, vasculitis, pulmonary hypertension, and lung abscess. Pulmonary capillary bleeding occurs in mitral stenosis, left ventricular failure, pulmonary infarction, vasculitis, Goodpasture syndrome, and idiopathic pulmonary hemosiderosis. Airway-vessel fistula (e.g., tracheoinnominate) can cause massive hemoptysis (>200 mL/24 hr). Pseudohemoptysis is expectoration of blood previously aspirated into the airways or lungs from the gastrointestinal tract, nose, or supraglottic areas.

- History, examination, and CXR are important in diagnosis.
- Common causes of streaky hemoptysis: chronic bronchitis or postinfectious.
- Bronchoscopy is indicated in almost all patients.
- The cause of death in massive hemoptysis is asphyxiation, not exsanguination.

Dyspnea

Dyspnea is the awareness of breathlessness. Its causes include disorders of the pulmonary, cardiac, skeletal (kyphoscoliosis, etc.), endocrine, metabolic, neurologic, and hematologic systems. Other causes are physiologic dyspnea of pregnancy, drugs, psychogenic, deconditioning, and obesity. The grades of severity are grade 0, no dyspnea except with strenuous exercise; grade 1, slight dyspnea on hurrying on a level surface or walking up a hill; grade 2, dyspnea while walking on a level surface and being unable to keep up with peers and having to stop to catch breath; grade 3, dyspnea on walking 100 yards or after a few minutes and the need to stop for breath; grade 4, dyspnea on dressing or undressing or minimal exertion; and grade 5, dyspnea at rest.

- Disease in any organ can cause dyspnea.
- The most common cause: cardiopulmonary disease.
- Clinical grades are based on the New York Heart Association classification.

Dyspnea usually is the result of increased work of breathing. Other mechanisms include abnormal activation of respiratory centers, voluntary hyperventilation, and Cheyne-Stokes breathing. A medical history, physical examination, CXR, and pulmonary function tests are required in most patients. Blood gases and cardiopulmonary physiologic testing also may be required. *Orthopnea* is dyspnea in the supine posture, as in congestive heart failure, bilateral diaphragmatic paralysis, severe COPD, asthma, sleep apnea, or severe reflux. *Trepopnea* is dyspnea in the lateral decubitus position, as in tumors of main-stem bronchi, unilateral pleural effusion, or after pneumonectomy. *Platypnea* is dyspnea in the upright posture and is due to an in increased right-to-left shunt in lung bases; it is seen in liver disease, severe lung fibrosis, or after pneumonectomy. *Paroxysmal nocturnal dyspnea* is nocturnal episodes of dyspnea, resulting in frequent waking up (associated with pulmonary edema and asthma).

- Tachypnea >20 breaths/min and bradypnea <10 breaths/min.
- Trepopnea: dyspnea in the lateral decubitus position.
- Platypnea: dyspnea in the upright posture.
- Orthodeoxia: oxygen desaturation in the upright position (seen with platypnea).

Chest Pain

Pulmonary causes of chest pain are often difficult to distinguish from cardiac and other causes. Tightness of chest and dyspnea are also described as "chest pain" by patients. Pleuritic pain is encountered in pleuritis, pleuropericarditis, pericarditis, pneumothorax, pleural effusion, mediastinitis, pulmonary embolism/infarction, esophageal disease, aortic dissection, and chest wall trauma. Subdiaphragmatic diseases that produce chest pain include pancreatitis, cholecystitis, and colonic distention.

Cyanosis

Cyanosis is the bluish discoloration of the skin and mucous membranes that occurs when the capillary content of reduced hemoglobin is greater than 5 g/dL. Clinically, it may be difficult to detect. Cyanosis may occur when arterial hemoglobin is unsaturated or when tissue extraction is high. The causes of central cyanosis are severe hypoxia (PaO_2 is usually <55 mm Hg), anatomical shunt, mild hypoxia with polycythemia, shock, and abnormal hemoglobin. Methemoglobinemia and sulfhemoglobinemia, argyria (from silver nitrate), and hemochromatosis cause pseudocyanosis. Anemia does not cause cyanosis. Peripheral cyanosis results from decreased peripheral perfusion with increased oxygen extraction.

- Cyanosis occurs when reduced hemoglobin is >5 g/dL.
- Central cyanosis should be distinguished from peripheral cyanosis.
- Polycythemia vera causes "red cyanosis."
- Methemoglobinemia: "pseudocyanosis."
- Cherry-red flush (not cyanosis) is caused by carboxyhemoglobinemia.

Clubbing

Clubbing is the bulbous enlargement of the distal segment of a digit (fingers or toes) caused by increased soft tissue mass. Its mechanisms are neurogenic, humoral/hormonal, hereditary, and idiopathic. A vagally mediated efferent reflex is perhaps the most common mechanism. CLUBBING can be caused by: **C** (cyanotic heart diseases), **L** (lung cancer, lung abscess, lung fibrosis), **U** (ulcerative colitis), **B** (bronchiectasis), **B** (benign mesothelioma), **I** (infective endocarditis, idiopathic, inherited), **N** (neurogenic tumors), and **G** (gastrointestinal diseases, e.g., cirrhosis, regional enteritis).

Clubbing can be the presenting manifestation of any of above entities.

- Clubbing may precede other clinical features of lung cancer.
- Common causes: pulmonary fibrosis, congenital heart disease with right-to-left shunt, cystic fibrosis, and idiopathic.
- Differential diagnosis: "CLUBBING" (see above) and hypertrophic pulmonary osteoarthropathy.

Hypertrophic Pulmonary Osteoarthropathy

Hypertrophic pulmonary osteoarthropathy (HPO): clubbing, painful periosteal hypertrophy of long bones, and symmetrical arthralgias of large joints (usually knees, elbows, and wrists). Other features include gynecomastia, fever, and an increased erythrocyte sedimentation rate (ESR). Mechanisms of HPO include neurogenic (vagal afferents), hormonal, and idiopathic. The commonest cause is bronchogenic carcinoma, usually adenocarcinoma or large cell carcinoma. HPO is an early sign of pulmonary metastasis from nasopharyngeal carcinoma. Clubbing is present in 30% of patients with non-small cell lung cancer; it is more common in women than in men (40% vs 19%). Radiographs of long bones reveal thickened and raised periosteum. Bone scans show increased uptake of radionuclide by the affected periosteum. If HPO does not resolve after tumor resection, treatment options include the administration of a somatostatin analog or ipsilateral vagotomy.

- Common causes of HPO: adenocarcinoma and large cell carcinoma of the lung and idiopathic.
- Radionuclide bone scans show characteristic changes.
- Therapy: resection of the tumor, somatostatin analog, or ipsilateral vagotomy.

Horner Syndrome

Horner syndrome consists of ipsilateral miosis, anhidrosis, and ptosis on the side of the lesion. It is a complication of a superior sulcus tumor (Pancoast tumor) of the lung.

- Horner syndrome: ipsilateral miosis, anhidrosis, and ptosis.
- Superior sulcus tumor (Pancoast tumor).

Superior Vena Cava Syndrome

Superior vena cava syndrome is caused by obstruction of blood flow through the superior vena cava. Common causes are lung cancer (particularly small cell cancer), Hodgkin lymphoma, and other tumors. Other causes include mediastinal fibrosis, radiation fibrosis, and large tumors in the upper anterior mediastinum. Facial edema, fullness of the head, and prominent venous channels over the chest are often noted.

- Common causes of superior vena cava syndrome: small cell carcinoma, Hodgkin lymphoma, mediastinal fibrosis.

Other Signs and Symptoms

Conjunctival suffusion is seen in severe hypercarbia, superior vena cava syndrome, and conjunctival sarcoid. Asterixis is seen in severe acute or subacute hypercarbia. Telangiectasia of the skin and mucous membranes occurs in patients with pulmonary arteriovenous malformation. Skin lesions of various types can be seen in patients with pulmonary involvement by Langerhans cell granuloma (eosinophilic granuloma or histiocytosis X), tuberous sclerosis, sarcoidosis, and lung cancer.

- Asterixis is seen in severe acute or subacute hypercarbia.
- Mental obtundation is seen with hypercarbia.

HISTORY AND EXAMINATION

An approach to history taking and physical examination in patients with pulmonary disease is outlined in Table 21-1. Percussion and auscultation findings associated with various pulmonary conditions are listed in Table 21-1.

DIAGNOSTIC TESTS

Radiology

CXR, plain tomography, computed tomography (CT), magnetic resonance imaging (MRI), bronchography, pulmonary angiography, and bronchial angiography are among the tests used in the diagnosis of chest diseases.

Plain Chest Radiography

Every internist should become familiar with the interpretation of common abnormalities on a plain CXR. Even normal CXRs should be viewed so that reading CXRs becomes routine. Many of the "radiographic" diagnoses such as pneumothorax, pleural effusion, and lung nodule can be established by CXR, but it is essential to correlate clinical and other laboratory data with CXR findings.

It is important to compare the present film with previous films, particularly in assessing the seriousness of a "newly" identified abnormality. It is unlikely that a normal CXR will be shown on the American Board of Internal Medicine (ABIM) examination. Subtle abnormalities, if shown, will be easy to identify, if the candidate knows how to detect an abnormality. A lateral CXR is of great help in identifying retrocardiac and retrodiaphragmatic abnormalities.

- Develop the habit of reading CXRs.
- Obtain earlier CXRs for comparison.

Table 21-1.—History and Physical Examination in Patients With Pulmonary Disease

History
  Smoking
  Occupational exposure
  Exposure to infected persons or animals
  Hobbies and pets
  Family history of diseases of lung and other organs
  Past malignancy
  Systemic (nonpulmonary) diseases
  Immune status (corticosteroid therapy, chemotherapy, cancer)
  History of trauma
  Previous chest radiography
Examination
  Inspection
    Respiratory rate, hoarseness of voice
    Respiratory rhythm (abnormal breathing pattern)
    Accessory muscles in action (FEV_1 <30%)
    Postural dyspnea (orthopnea, platypnea, trepopnea)
    Intercostal retraction
    Paradoxical motions of abdomen/diaphragm
    Cough (type, sputum, blood)
    Wheeze (audible with or without stethoscope)
    Pursed lip breathing/glottic wheeze (patients with chronic obstructive pulmonary disease)
    Cyanosis (central vs. peripheral)
    Conjunctival suffusion (CO_2 retention)
    Clubbing
    Thoracic cage (anteroposterior diameter, kyphoscoliosis, pectus, etc.)
    Trachea, deviation
    Superior vena cava syndrome
    Asterixis, central nervous system status
    Cardiac impulse, jugular venous pressure, pedal edema (signs of cor pulmonale)
  Palpation
    Clubbing
    Lymphadenopathy
    Tibial tenderness (hypertrophic pulmonary osteoarthropathy)
    Motion of thoracic cage (hand or tape measure)
    Chest wall tenderness (costochondritis, rib fracture, pulmonary embolism)
    Tracheal deviation, tenderness
    Tactile (vocal) fremitus
    Subcutaneous emphysema
    Succussion splash (effusion, air-fluid level in thorax)
  Percussion
    Thoracic cage (dullness, resonance)
    Diaphragmatic motion (normal, 5-7 cm)
    Upper abdomen (liver)
  Auscultation
    Tracheal auscultation
    Normal breath sounds
    Bronchial breath sounds
    Expiratory slowing
    Crackles
    Wheezes
    Pleural rub
    Mediastinal noises (mediastinal crunch)
    Heart sounds
    Miscellaneous (muscle tremor, etc.; see section on Other Signs and Symptoms)

Percussion/auscultation finding	Chest expansion	Fremitus	Resonance	Breath sounds	Egophony	Bronchophony
Pleural effusion	Decreased	Reduced	Reduced	Decreased	Absent>>present	Absent>>present
Consolidation	Decreased	Increased	Reduced	Bronchial	Present	Present
Atelectasis	Decreased	Reduced	Reduced	Decreased	Absent>present	Absent>present
Pneumothorax	Variable	Reduced	Increased	Decreased	Absent	Absent

Note: Trachea is shifted ipsilaterally in atelectasis and contralaterally in effusion. Whispered pectoriloquy is present in consolidation. FEV_1, forced expiratory volume in 1 second.

- Lateral CXRs are important in visualizing retrocardiac and retrodiaphragmatic abnormalities.

The ability to identify normal radiographic anatomy is essential. A "routine" step-by-step method of interpretation should be developed so that subtle abnormalities are not missed. Initially, the CXR should be "eyeballed," without focusing on any one area or abnormality. This is to ensure that the technical aspects are adequate and the patient identification markers and orientation of CXR (identification of left and right sides) are proper. Next, the extrapulmonary structures are viewed. For instance, destructive arthritis of a shoulder joint seen on a CXR may be the result of rheumatoid arthritis and may prompt the CXR reader to look for pulmonary manifestations of this disease. The absence of a breast shadow on the CXR of a female is a good hint to look for signs of pulmonary metastases. The visualization of a tracheostomy stoma and/or cannula on the CXR may indicate previous laryngeal cancer and, thus, provide a hint to complications such as aspiration pneumonia and lung metastases. Infradiaphragmatic abnormalities such as calcifications in the spleen, displacement of the gastric bubble and the colon, and signs of upper abdominal surgery (metal sutures, feeding tubes, etc.) may indicate the cause of a pleuropulmonary process.

- Initially look at the entire CXR as a single picture.
- Look for absent breast shadow, infradiaphragmatic abnormalities, and extrapulmonary skeletal abnormalities.

The skeletal thorax should be viewed to exclude rib fracture, osteolytic and other lesions of the ribs, rib notching, missing ribs, and vertebral abnormalities. Changes due to a previous thoracic surgical procedure such as coronary artery bypass, thoracotomy, lung resection, or esophageal surgery may provide clues to the pulmonary disease. Next, the intrathoracic but extrapulmonary structures such as the mediastinum (great vessels, esophagus, heart, lymph nodes, and thymus) should be assessed. The superior mediastinum should be viewed to see whether the thyroid gland extends into the thoracic cage. A calcified mass in the region of thyroid almost always indicates a goiter. The esophagus can produce significant abnormalities in the CXR. A large esophagus, as in achalasia, may mimic a mass or a large hiatal hernia with an air-fluid level may mimic a lung abscess. The aortopulmonary window (a notch below the aortic knob on the left, just above the pulmonary artery), if obliterated, may indicate a tumor or lymphadenopathy. Right paratracheal and paramediastinal lymphadenopathy can be subtle. Hilar regions are difficult to interpret. Lymphadenopathy, vascular prominence, and tumor may make the hila appear larger. The retrocardiac region may show hiatal hernia with an air-fluid level; this may be helpful in the diagnosis of reflux or aspiration. A lateral CXR is important to assess the retrocardiac and retrodiaphragmatic recesses.

- Rib lesions: osteolytic, expansile, notching, or absence of a rib.
- Note changes due to previous surgical procedures.
- Assess the mediastinum: the esophagus, thyroid, thymus, great vessels.

The pleural regions should be examined for pleural effusion, pleural thickening (particularly in the apices), blunting of costophrenic angles, pleural-based lesions such as pleural plaques or masses, and pneumothorax. A lateral decubitus film may be necessary to confirm the presence of free fluid in the pleural space. An air bronchogram depicting the major airways may indicate a large tumor (cut off of air bronchogram), deviation of airways, signs of compression or stenosis, and the relationship of major airways to the esophagus. Finally, the lung parenchyma should be evaluated. Nearly 15% of the pulmonary parenchyma is located behind the heart and diaphragm; a lateral CXR is helpful in examining this region. It is important *not* to overinterpret increased interstitial lung markings. Oligemia of the lung fields is difficult to assess because the clarity of the film depends on the duration of the exposure of the film. Generally, bronchovascular markings should be visible throughout the lung parenchyma. The complete absence of any markings within the lung parenchyma should suggest bulla or an air-containing cyst. Apical areas should be evaluated carefully for the presence of pleural thickening, pneumothorax, small nodules, and subtle infiltrates. If the apices cannot be visualized properly with a standard CXR, a lordotic view should be obtained.

- Look for small pneumothorax, nodules, and large airway lesions.
- Examine the apices for thickening, pneumothorax, nodules, and subtle infiltrates.
- Examine the lung parenchyma behind the heart and diaphragm.

Some of the common CXR abnormalities are depicted in Figures 21-1 to 21-20.

Tomography

Plain tomography is useful in evaluating solitary lung nodules. Calcification, location of the lesion, the margins of the nodule, cavitation, and the presence of adjacent nodules (satellite lesions) can be discerned with tomography (Fig. 21-21 to 21-26). CT is now the preferred technique to assess lung nodules.

Fluoroscopy

Fluoroscopy is useful in localizing lesions during biopsy and aspiration procedures. It also is valuable in assessing diaphragmatic motion and in diagnosing diaphragmatic paralysis by the sniff test. Paradoxic motion of the diaphragm suggests diaphragmatic paralysis.

- Up to 6% of normal subjects exhibit paradoxic diaphragmatic motion.

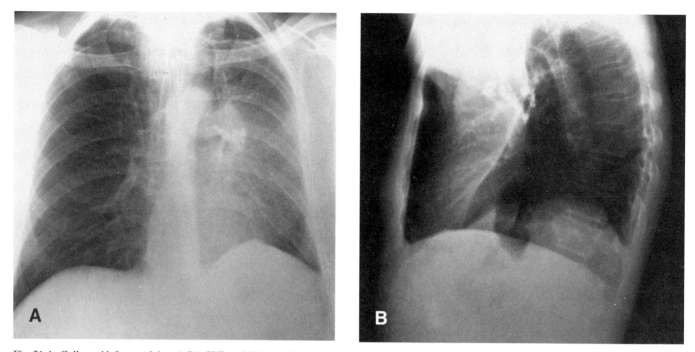

Fig. 21-1. Collapsed left upper lobe. *A*, PA CXR and *B*, lateral CXR. The ground-glass haze over the left hemithorax is typical of a partially collapsed left upper lobe. In >50% of patients with collapsed lobes, loss of volume is evidenced by left hemidiaphragmatic elevation, mediastinum is shifted to left, and left hilus is pulled cranially. Also, left mainstem bronchus deviates cranially. The calcification in the left hilar mass represents an unrelated old granulomatous infection. In *B*, the density from the left hilus down toward the anterior portion of the chest represents the partially collapsed left upper lobe. The radiolucency substernally is the right lung.

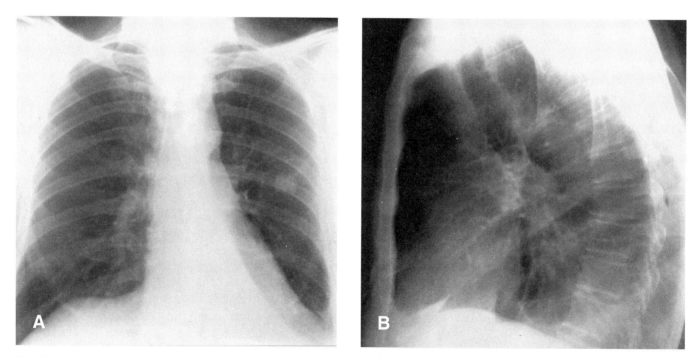

Fig. 21-2. Collapsed left lower lobe. *A*, PA CXR and *B*, lateral CXR. Nodule in the left mid-lung field plus collapsed left lower lobe, seen as a density behind the heart. This entity represents two separate primary lung cancers, viz., synchronous bronchogenic carcinomas. Do not stop with the first evident abnormality, such as nodule in mid-lung field, without carefully looking at all other areas. *B* demonstrates an increased density over the lower thoracic vertebrae without any obvious wedge-shaped infiltrate. Over the anterior portion of the hemidiaphragm, the small wedge-shaped infiltrate is not fluid in the left major fissure, because left major fissure is pulled away posteriorly. Instead, it is an incidental normal variant of fat pushed up into the right major fissure.

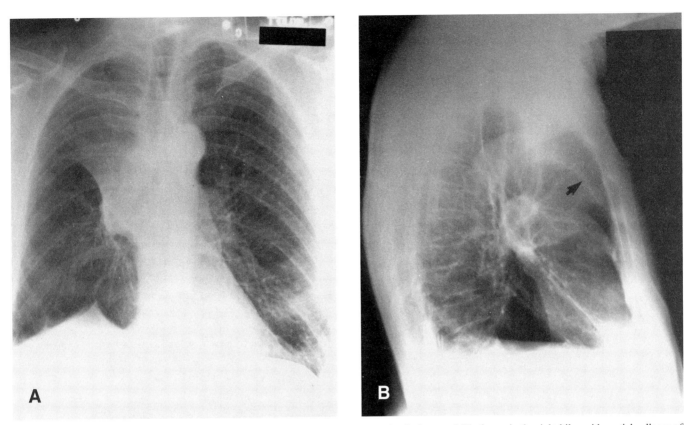

Fig. 21-3. Collapsed right upper lobe. *A*, PA CXR and *B*, lateral CXR. *A*, This is a classic "reversed S" of mass in the right hilus with partial collapse of the right upper lobe. Loss of volume is evident with the elevation of the right hemidiaphragm. In *B*, the partially collapsed right upper lobe is faintly seen in the upper anterior portion of the hemithorax (*arrow*).

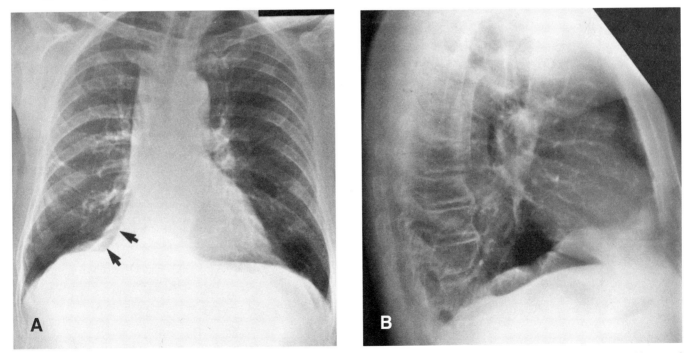

Fig. 21-4. Collapsed right lower lobe. *A*, PA CXR and *B*, lateral CXR. *A*, This 75-year-old smoker had hemoptysis for 1 1/2 years; his CXR had been read as "normal" on several occasions. Note the linear density (*arrows*) projecting downward and laterally along the right border of the heart. It projects below the diaphragm and is not a normal line. Also, the right hilus is not evident; it has been pulled centrally and downward because of carcinoma obstructing the bronchus of the right lower lobe. Note the very slight shift in mediastinum to the right, indicative of some loss of volume. In the lateral view, in spite of significant collapse of right lower lobe, only subtle increased density over lower thoracic vertebrae represents this collapse.

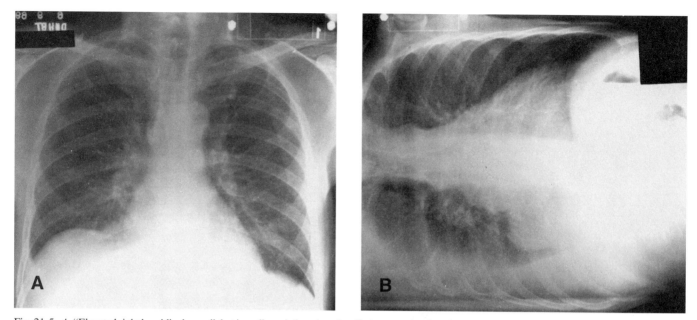

Fig. 21-5. *A,* "Elevated right hemidiaphragm" that is really an infrapulmonic effusion, or subpulmonic, as seen on the decubitus film. *B,* For unknown reasons, a meniscus is not formed in some people with infrapulmonic pleural effusion. Thus, any seemingly elevated hemidiaphragm should be examined with the suspicion that it could be an infrapulmonic effusion. Subpulmonic effusions occur more frequently in patients with nephrotic syndrome. Decubitus CXR or ultrasonography would disclose the free fluid.

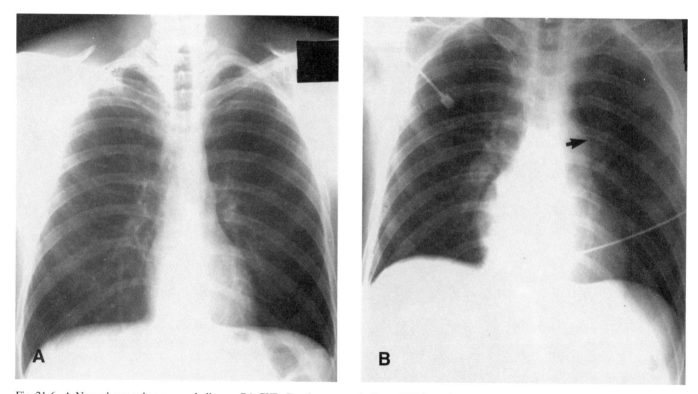

Fig. 21-6. *A,* Normal, pre-pulmonary embolism on PA CXR; *B,* pulmonary embolism. CXR is read as normal in up to 30% of patients with angiographically proven pulmonary embolism. In comparison with *A, B* shows a subtle elevation of the right hemidiaphragm. In *A,* right and left hemidiaphragms are equal. Elevated hemidiaphragm is the most common finding with acute pulmonary embolism in some series. Also, note the plumpness of the right pulmonary artery, prominent pulmonary outflow tract on left (*arrow*), and subtle change in cardiac diameter. This 28-year-old man was in shock at the time of CXR from massive pulmonary emboli as a result of major soft tissue trauma produced by a motorcycle accident 7 days earlier.

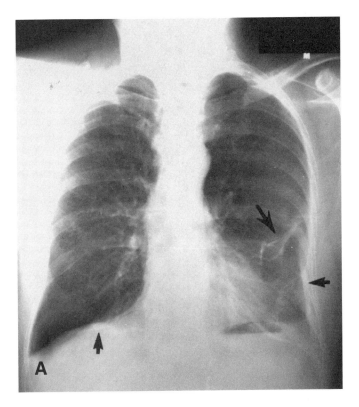

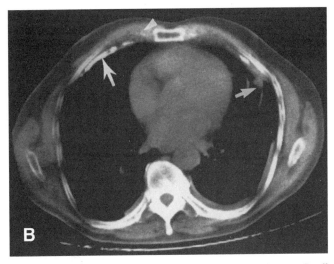

Fig. 21-7. Abnormal CXR, *A*, in a 68-year-old asymptomatic man. *Small arrows* outline areas of pleural calcification, particularly on the right hemidiaphragm. This is a tip-off to previous asbestos exposure. The process in the left mid-lung was worrisome (*large arrow*), perhaps indicating a new process such as bronchogenic carcinoma in this smoker. However, CT, *B*, disclosed rounded atelectasis (*small arrow*). The "comma" extending from this mass is characteristic of rounded atelectasis, which is the result of subacute-to-chronic pleural effusion resolving and trapping some lung as it heals. Also note pleural calcification in *B* (*large arrow*).

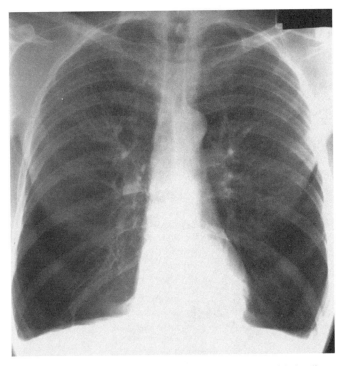

Fig. 21-8. Panlobular emphysema at the bases consistent with the diagnosis of alpha₁-antitrypsin deficiency. Emphysema should not be read into CXR, because all it usually represents is hyperinflation that can occur with severe asthma as well. However, in this setting, there are markedly diminished interstitial markings at the bases, with radiolucency. Also, there is increased blood flow to the upper lobes because that is where most of the viable lung tissue is. Note flattening of the hemidiaphragms from hyperinflation.

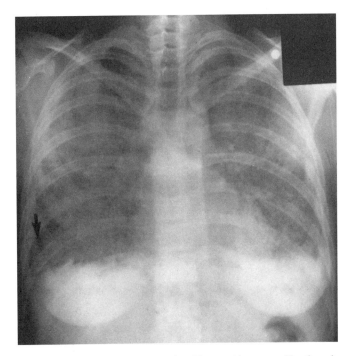

Fig. 21-9. Lymphangitic carcinoma in a 27-year-old woman with a 6-week history of progressive dyspnea and weight loss. Because of her young age, neoplasm was not considered. Yet, features present on this CXR should have suggested it, viz., bilateral pleural effusions, Kerley B lines as evident in the right base (*arrow*), and mediastinal and hilar lymphadenopathy in addition to diffuse parenchymal infiltrate.

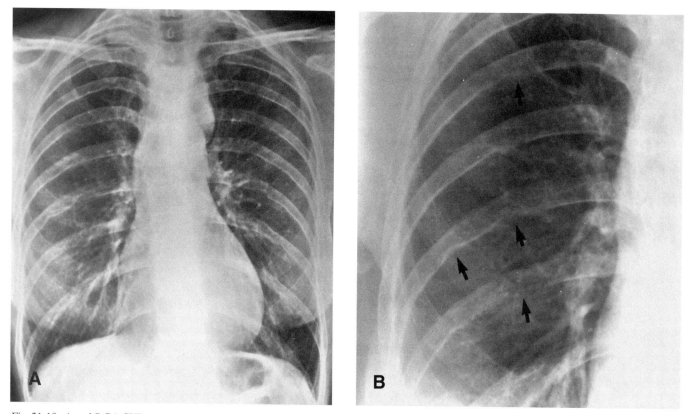

Fig. 21-10. *A* and *B*, PA CXR. *A* and *B*, Coarctation with tortuous aorta, mimicking a mediastinal mass. This occurs in about 1/3 of patients with coarctation. Rib notching is indicated by *arrows* in *B*.

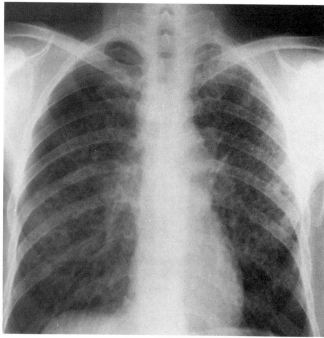

Fig. 21-11. Histiocytosis X, or eosinophilic granuloma, shows extensive change but predominantly in the upper two-thirds of the lung fields. Eventually 25% of these patients have pneumothorax, as seen on this CXR. The honeycombing, also described as microcysts, is characteristic of advanced histiocytosis X.

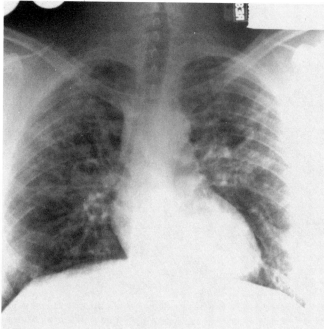

Fig. 21-12. Sarcoidosis in a 35-year-old patient. This CXR shows the predominant upper 2/3 parenchymal pattern seen in many patients with stage II or III sarcoidosis. The pattern can be interstitial, alveolar (which this one is predominantly), or a combination. There probably is some residual adenopathy in the hila and right paratracheal area.

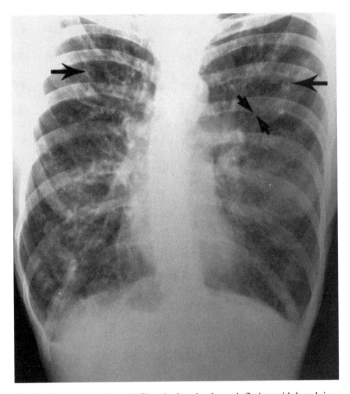

Fig. 21-13. Advanced cystic fibrosis showing hyperinflation with low-lying hemidiaphragms, bronchiectasis (*small arrows* on parallel lines), and microabscesses (*large arrows*) representing small areas of pneumonitis distal to the mucous plug that has been coughed out. Cystic fibrosis almost always begins in the upper lobes.

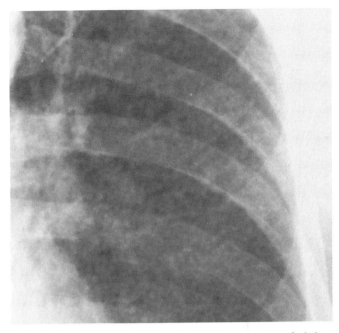

Fig. 21-14. Miliary tuberculosis. CXR shows a miliary pattern of relatively discrete micronodules, with little interstitial (linear or reticular) markings. Disseminated fungal disease has a similar appearance, as does bronchioalveolar cell carcinoma; however, these patients do not usually have the systemic manifestations of miliary tuberculosis. Other, less common differential diagnoses include lymphoma, lymphocytic interstitial pneumonitis, and pulmonary edema. *Pneumocystis carinii* pneumonia usually has more interstitial reaction.

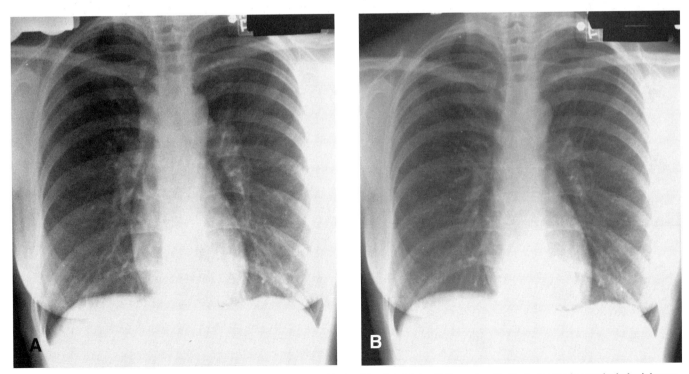

Fig. 21-15. *A*, CXR of 30-year-old woman with stage I pulmonary sarcoidosis with subtle bilateral hilar and mediastinal adenopathy, particularly right paratracheal and left infra-aortic adenopathy. *B*, CXR 1 year later, after spontaneous regression of sarcoidosis.

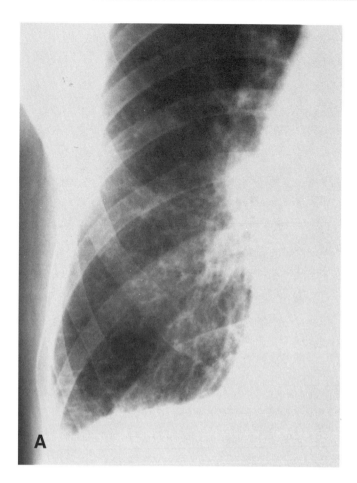

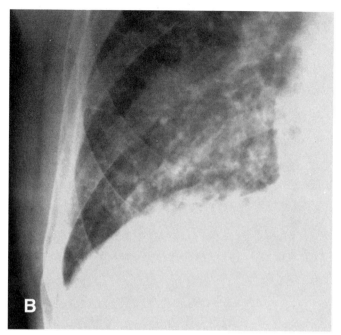

Fig. 21-16. *A* and *B*, Two examples of Kerley B lines that can be helpful in interpreting CXRs. *A*, Kerley B lines in a 75-year-old man with colon cancer. *B*, Kerley B lines are from metastatic adenocarcinoma of the colon and were a tip-off that the parenchymal process in this patient was due to metastatic carcinoma and not to a primary pulmonary process such as pulmonary fibrosis, which was the working diagnosis.

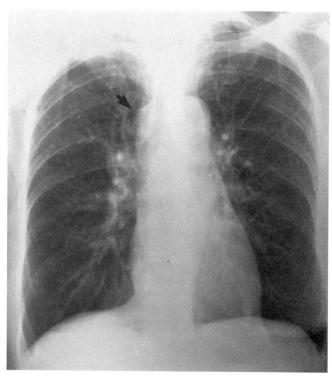

Fig. 21-17. CXR of a 55-year-old woman who had had a right mastectomy for breast carcinoma now shows subtle but definite right paratracheal (*arrow*) and right hilar adenopathy from metastatic carcinoma of the breast.

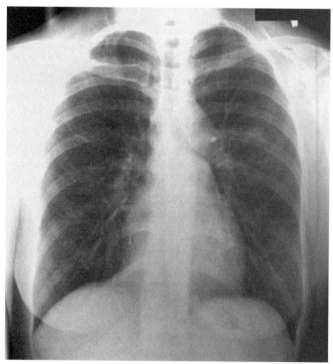

Fig. 21-18. The nodule in the left mid-lung field is technically not a "solitary pulmonary nodule" because of another abnormality in the thorax that might be related to it, left infra-aortic adenopathy. The differential would be bronchogenic carcinoma with hilar nodal metastasis or, as in this case, acute primary pulmonary histoplasmosis. Had this patient been in an area with coccidioidomycosis, it would also be in differential diagnosis.

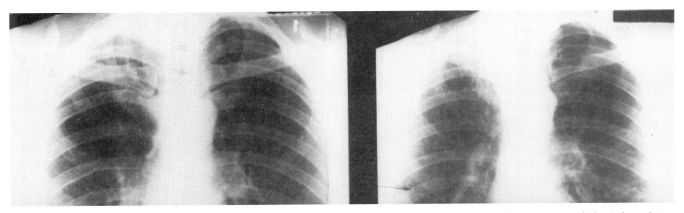

Fig. 21-19. Pancoast tumor. Subtle asymmetry at the apex of the right lung was more obvious 3 1/2 years later, at the time the Pancoast lesion (primary bronchogenic carcinoma) was diagnosed. The patient was symptomatic at time of initial CXR, with symptoms attributed to a cervical disk.

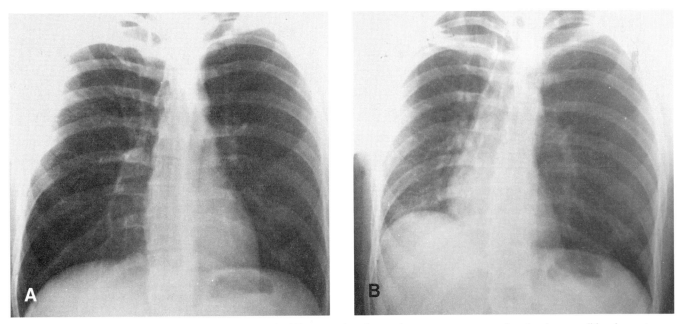

Fig. 21-20. The adage that "not all that wheezes is asthma" should be remembered every time you encounter an asthmatic whose condition does not seem to improve. In the case shown here, *A*, wheezes were predominant over the left hemithorax. A forced expiration film, *B*, showed air trapping in the left lung. Bronchial carcinoid of the left main bronchus was diagnosed at bronchoscopy.

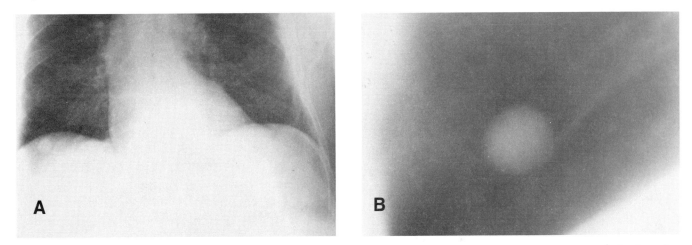

Fig. 21-21. *A*, Solitary pulmonary nodule evident below the right hemidiaphragm, where at least 15% of the lung is obscured. *B*, Tomography shows that the nodule has a discrete border but is noncalcified. It was not present 18 months earlier. This is an adenocarcinoma.

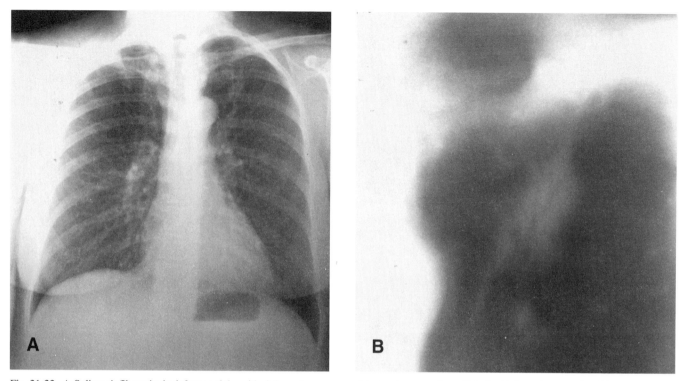

Fig. 21-22. *A*, Solitary infiltrate in the left upper lobe with air bronchogram, as evident on tomography or CT. *B*, Air bronchogram should be considered a sign of bronchoalveolar cell carcinoma or lymphoma until proved otherwise.

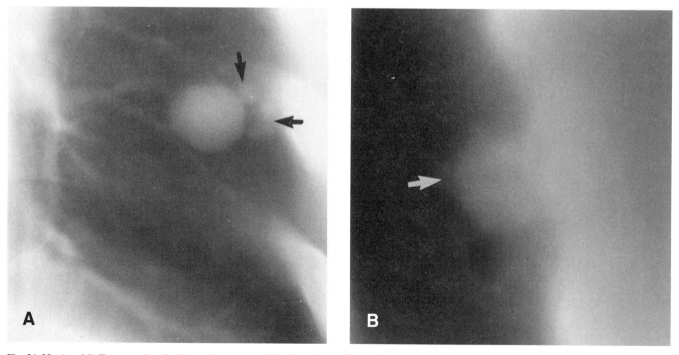

Fig. 21-23. *A* and *B*, Tomography of solitary pulmonary nodules showing satellite nodules (*arrows*). This is characteristic of granulomas.

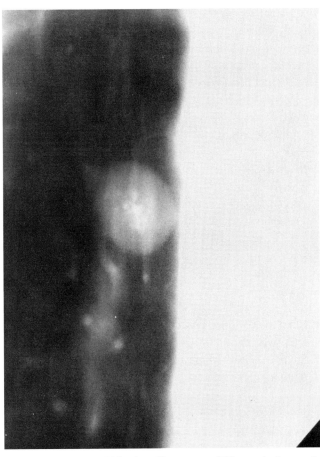

Fig. 21-24. Popcorn calcification of hamartoma. This can also be seen in granuloma and represents a benign process.

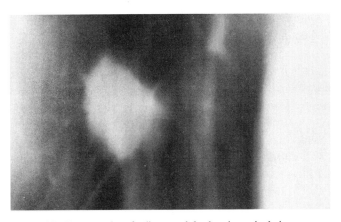

Fig. 21-25. Tomography of solitary nodule showing spiculation, or sunburst effect, characteristic of primary bronchogenic carcinoma. Spicules represent extension of tumor into septa. CT shows a similar appearance.

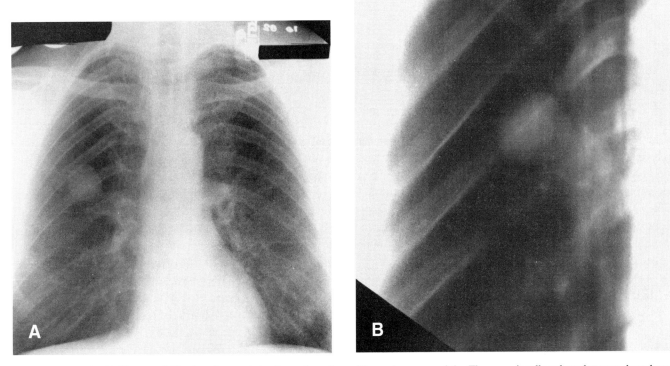

Fig. 21-26. *A* and *B*, Bull's-eye calcification characteristic of granuloma in a solitary pulmonary nodule. They occasionally enlarge but even then almost never warrant removal.

Computed Tomography

Standard CT is useful in the staging of lung cancer and in assessing mediastinal and hilar lesions, diffuse lung disease, and pleural processes. High-resolution CT (HRCT) reveals characteristic findings in pulmonary Langerhans cell granuloma (nodular-cystic spaces in the upper lung fields), lymphangitic pulmonary metastasis (interlobular septal enlargement and nodularity), lymphangioleiomyomatosis (well-defined cystic spaces in lung parenchyma), and idiopathic pulmonary fibrosis (subpleural honeycombing). HRCT findings in pulmonary fibrotic diseases are more than 90% accurate; honeycombing is seen in 90% of patients, as compared with 30% on traditional CXR. HRCT is also helpful in diagnosing certain granulomatous lung diseases (sarcoidosis and mycobacterial infections), asbestosis, sarcoidosis, pulmonary alveolar phospholipoproteinosis, chronic eosinophilic pneumonia, and bronchiolitis obliterans. Ultrafast CT is better than ventilation-perfusion (V/Q) scan in detecting pulmonary emboli in the main and lobar arteries. The role of CT in the diagnosis of peripheral pulmonary emboli has not been established.

- Characteristic HRCT features in pulmonary Langerhans cell granuloma, lymphangioleiomyomatosis, idiopathic pulmonary fibrosis, and lymphangitic pulmonary metastasis.
- CT is helpful in the staging of lung cancer.
- CT is useful in evaluating the presence of multiple lung nodules (metastatic) and calcification in the nodule(s).
- Ultrafast CT is better than V/Q scan for diagnosing pulmonary emboli.

Magnetic Resonance Imaging

MRI is recommended for the initial evaluation of superior sulcus tumor (Pancoast tumor), lesions of the brachial plexus, and paraspinal masses that on CXR appear most consistent with neurogenic tumors. MRI is superior to CT in the evaluation of chest wall masses and in the search for small occult mediastinal neoplasms (e.g., ectopic parathyroid adenoma). MRI is useful when CT with contrast media is contraindicated in patients with renal failure or contrast allergy. MRI may be superior to CT in evaluating pulmonary sequestration, arteriovenous malformation, vascular structures, and tumor recurrence in patients with total pneumonectomy.

- MRI: useful for evaluation of superior sulcus tumor.
- MRI: useful for evaluation of neurogenic tumors.

Bronchography

Bronchography has been replaced by HRCT for the detection of bronchiectasis. Bronchography is indicated 1) if HRCT findings are nonspecific in the presence of clinical bronchiectasis, 2) if better mapping of bronchiectatic areas is needed before lung resection for the disease, 3) in certain cases of bronchial strictures, and 4) in very young children in whom HRCT is not possible.

- HRCT has replaced bronchography for diagnosing bronchiectasis.

Pulmonary Angiography

The main indication for pulmonary angiography is to detect pulmonary emboli. The detection of proximal (up to lobar arteries) is excellent. However, small peripheral emboli may not be seen. Pulmonary angiography is also useful in the diagnosis of pulmonary arteriovenous fistulas and malformations, and it is usually a prerequisite if embolotherapy is planned.

- Main indications: pulmonary embolism and pulmonary arteriovenous malformations and fistulas.
- Pulmonary angiography may not detect a peripheral or tiny pulmonary embolism.

Bronchial Angiography

Bronchial angiography is used to determine whether the bronchial arteries are causing massive pulmonary hemorrhage or massive hemoptysis. It is a prerequisite if bronchial arterial embolotherapy is planned.

- Main indication: suspected bronchial arterial bleed in massive hemoptysis.
- Both pulmonary and bronchial angiography may be needed for some patients with massive hemoptysis.

Radionuclide Lung Scans

The V/Q scan is commonly used in diagnosing pulmonary embolism. The likelihood of pulmonary embolism in a V/Q scan that shows "high probability" and a scan that shows "low probability" is greater than 90% and less than 5%, respectively. An "intermediate probability" scan usually is an indication for pulmonary angiography. However, clinical suspicion should guide the decision. The quantitative V/Q scan is used to assess unilateral and regional pulmonary function by measuring V/Q relationships in different regions of the lungs. It is indicated for patients who are poor surgical candidates for lung resection because of their underlying pulmonary dysfunction. If the lung region to be resected shows minimal or no lung function by the quantitative V/Q scan, the resection is unlikely to impair further the patient's pulmonary reserve. The gallium scan is of minimal or no use in the diagnosis of diffuse lung diseases. The [99]technetium scan is useful in detecting diffuse pulmonary calcification associated with chronic hemodialysis.

- Quantitative V/Q scan is used to assess unilateral or regional pulmonary function.
- Gallium scan has no role in the diagnosis of diffuse lung disease.
- ^{99}Technetium lung scan detects diffuse pulmonary calcification.

Sputum Microscopy

Simple microscopy with a "wet" slide preparation of sputum is helpful in assessing the degree of sputum eosinophilia and detecting the presence of Charcot-Leyden crystals. Gram staining of sputum should be used to evaluate suspected bacterial infections. However, routine examination with Gram stain is unnecessary in all patients with COPD who present with acute exacerbations. Induced sputum is helpful in identifying mycobacteria, fungi, *Pneumocystis carinii*, and malignant cells. Gastric washings are used to identify mycobacteria and fungi. Hemosiderin-laden macrophages in sputum do not always indicate alveolar hemorrhage; smokers can have a significant number of hemosiderin-laden macrophages in their sputum.

- Sputum "wet prep" detects eosinophilia and Charcot-Leyden crystals.
- Induced sputum is excellent for identification of *Pneumocystis carinii*.

Pulmonary Function Tests

The major indication for pulmonary function tests (PFTs) is dyspnea. PFTs do not diagnose lung disease. They assess the mechanical function of the respiratory system and quantitate the loss of lung function. PFTs can separate obstructive from restrictive phenomena. They also can detect bronchospastic disease when used with provocation inhalation challenge (e.g., methacholine). Results of previous PFTs are helpful in following the course of lung disease.

- Obstructive dysfunction: indicates obstruction to flow of air through the airways, as in asthma, bronchitis, and emphysema.
- Asthma causes obstruction to airflow during inspiration and expiration.
- An increase (>20%) in flow rates after bronchodilator therapy suggests reversible airway disease.
- Restrictive dysfunction: limitation to full expansion of the lungs because of disease in the lung parenchyma, chest wall, or diaphragm; volumes are diminished but flow rates are normal.

- A combination of obstructive and restrictive patterns is also possible (e.g., COPD with pulmonary fibrosis).

Provocation Inhalation Challenge

The provocation inhalation challenge test is useful when the diagnosis of asthma or hyperactive airway disease is uncertain. The test uses agents that elicit a bronchospastic response. These agents include methacholine, carbachol, histamine, industrial irritants, exercise, isocapneic hyperventilation, and cold air. A 20% decrease in forced expiratory volume in 1 second (FEV_1) from baseline is considered a positive test result. Many normal subjects exhibit a positive response to provocation challenge without symptoms of asthma.

- A 20% decline in FEV_1 from baseline is considered positive.
- Up to 10% of normal subjects exhibit positive inhalational challenge.

Interpretation of Pulmonary Function Tests

A simplified step-by-step approach is as follows:

1. Evaluate volumes and flows separately.
2. Total lung capacity (TLC), functional residual capacity (FRC), and residual volume (RV) indicate volumes. TLC = VC (vital capacity) + RV. Increases in TLC and RV suggest hyperinflation (asthma, COPD). If TLC and VC are decreased, consider restrictive lung disease (fibrosis) or loss of lung volume (surgery, diaphragmatic paralysis, skeletal problems).
3. VC measured during a slow (not forced) expiration is not affected by airway collapse in COPD. Forced VC may be low with forced expiration because of airway collapse. In normal subjects, VC equals forced VC (i.e., VC = FVC).
4. FEV_1 and forced expiratory flow between 25% and 75% of VC (FEF_{25-75}) indicate flow rates. Flow rates are diminished in COPD, but smaller decreases in flows can be seen if lung volumes are low. Decreased FEV_1/FVC indicates obstruction to airflow.
5. The maximal voluntary ventilation (MVV) test requires rapid inspiratory and expiratory maneuvers and, thus, tests airflow through major airways and muscle strength. Patients with severe COPD may have low MVV, whereas those with restrictive lung diseases have normal MVV (because there is no obstruction to airflow). MVV also tests muscle strength. Neuromuscular diseases may lead to decreased MVV.

- MVV is decreased in obstructive disease (i.e., MVV = FEV_1 x 33).

- If MVV is low and flow rates are normal (i.e., no airway obstruction), consider weakness of the respiratory muscles, especially the diaphragm.
- MVV is also significantly decreased in major airway lesions.
- Respiratory muscle weakness can be assessed by Pi_{max} and Pe_{max}.
- Clinical features should be correlated with the results of PFTs.

6. Diffusing capacity (DLCO) is dependent on the thickness of the alveolocapillary membrane (DM), hemoglobin level (θ), and pulmonary capillary volume (Vc). DLCO is represented by $\left(\frac{1}{DLCO} = \frac{1}{DM} + \frac{1}{\theta Vc}\right)$. DLCO is low in anatomical emphysema ($\downarrow$Vc), anemia ($\downarrow\theta$), restrictive lung diseases ($\uparrow$DM), pneumonectomy ($\downarrow$Vc), pulmonary hypertension, and recurrent pulmonary emboli ($\downarrow$Vc). DLCO is increased in the supine posture ($\uparrow$Vc), after exercise ($\uparrow$Vc), in polycythemia ($\uparrow\theta$), obesity ($\uparrow$Vc), left-to-right shunt ($\uparrow$Vc), and in some asthmatics. Isolated low DLCO (with normal results on PFTs) is seen in pulmonary hypertension, multiple pulmonary emboli, and anemia.

- DLCO is decreased in anatomical emphysema.
- Isolated decrease in DLCO (normal volumes and flows) may occur in pulmonary hypertension, multiple pulmonary emboli, and severe anemia.
- Decrease in hemoglobin by 1 g diminishes DLCO by 7%.

- Flow-volume curves are helpful to separate intrathoracic and extrathoracic major airway obstructions.

Explanations of Table 21-2

Patient 1. Typical features of hyperinflation (high TLC and RV). VC is low because of high RV (TLC - RV = VC). Flow rates are very low, and MVV is moderately reduced. The very low DLCO suggests parenchymal damage. Without inhalation challenge, it is not possible to discern a bronchospastic component. Clinical diagnosis: moderately severe obstructive disease with severe anatomical emphysema.

Patient 2. Young nonsmoker with hyperinflation (high TLC and RV). Flow rates and MVV are also severely decreased. These suggest obstructive lung disease. The low DLCO suggests parenchymal damage (emphysema). Clinical diagnosis: severe emphysema caused by familial deficiency of α_1-antitrypsin.

Patient 3. Flow rates and lung volumes are decreased only slightly but are within normal limits. MVV is severely decreased. In this patient, Pi_{max} and Pe_{max} are severely decreased, suggesting muscle weakness. Clinical diagnosis: severe thyrotoxicosis with proximal muscle weakness (thyrotoxic myopathy). This pattern of results on PFTs can also occur in neuromuscular diseases such as amyotrophic lateral sclerosis and myasthenia gravis.

Patient 4. Slightly increased but normal TLC and slightly diminished VC. Flow rates are moderately decreased. This patient has a mild-to-moderate obstructive phenomenon.

Table 21-2.—Try to Interpret These Results of Pulmonary Function Tests Before Reading the Explanations*

Patient	1	2	3	4	5	6	7	8	9	10
Age (yr) and sex	73 M	43 M	53 F	43 M	50 M	20 M	58 F	40 M	28 F	44 M
Weight, kg	52	53	50	63	73	80	59	75	52	148
Tobacco	63PY	NS	NS	NS	20PY	NS	NS	NS	NS	NS
Total lung capacity, %	140	128	84	118	110	100	56	68	108	90
Vital capacity, %	52	75	86	78	82	95	62	58	106	86
Residual volume, %	160	140	90	110	112	90	65	80	98	90
FEV_1, %	35	38	82	48	80	90	85	42	112	96
FEV_1/FVC, %	40	34	80	40	60	85	88	50	85	78
FEF_{25-75}	18	14	80	35	75	88	82	24	102	88
Maximal voluntary ventilation, %	62	48	40	60	105	120	108	62	88	90
Diffusing capacity (normal)	9 (22)	10 (28)	20 (20)	28 (28)	26 (27)	32 (34)	8 (26)	8 (28)	6 (32)	40 (28)

*Values of 80%-120% of predicted are considered normal.

FEF_{25-75}, forced expiratory flow between 25%-75% of vital capacity; FEV_1, forced expiratory volume in 1 second; FVC, forced vital capacity; NS, nonsmoker; PY, pack-years of smoking.

Normal DLCO excludes anatomical emphysema or other parenchymal problems. Bronchodilator testing elicited improved lung volumes and flow rates. Clinical diagnosis: typical asthma.

Patient 5. Mild hyperinflation (increased TLC and RV). Because these are within normal limits (80%-120% of predicted), true hyperinflation is not present. Flow rates show slight reductions, and MVV and DLCO are normal. Bronchodilator inhalation showed no improvement. Note the slightly diminished FEV_1/FVC ratio. This together with slightly diminished FEF_{25-75} suggests a mild obstructive lung disease of a nonasthmatic type. Because of normal DLCO, significant anatomical emphysema can be excluded. Clinical diagnosis: nonasthmatic bronchitis.

Patient 6. Normal lung volumes and flows (80%-120% of predicted normal). A former "super athlete," he recently noted cough and chest tightness after exertion. Previous PFTs were unavailable. Important points: 1) In a young, otherwise healthy patient, the lung volumes and flow rates are usually above normal, more so in an athlete. 2) This patient may have had very high volumes and flow rates in the past, but without previous PFTs, no comparison can be made (if earlier PFT results were available, the new results might represent a severe decrease in pulmonary function). 3) The history suggests the possibility of exercise-induced asthma; spirometry after an exercise test showed 28% reduction in flow rates 5 to 10 minutes after termination of exercise. 4) Note the relatively high DLCO in this patient, a phenomenon seen in asthmatic patients. Clinical diagnosis: exercise-induced asthma.

Patient 7. Moderately severe decrease in lung volumes and normal flow rates. MVV is normal, but DLCO is severely diminished. These suggest severe restrictive lung disease. The slightly diminished flow rates are the result of decreased lung volumes. Clinical diagnosis: biopsy-proved idiopathic pulmonary fibrosis. Patients who have had lung resection also show low lung volumes and decreased DLCO.

Patient 8. Moderately decreased lung volumes. Flow rates are also diminished more than expected from the decreases in lung volumes. Reduction in the FEV_1/FVC ratio suggests the presence of obstructive dysfunction. MVV is also reduced, and DLCO is severely decreased. Compared with patient 7, this patient has obstructive disease plus severe restrictive lung disease. A very low DLCO suggests parenchymal disease. CXR shows bilaterally diffuse nodular interstitial changes, especially in the upper two-thirds of the lungs. Biopsy of bronchial mucosa and lung revealed extensive endobronchial sarcoidosis. Clinical diagnosis: severe restrictive lung disease from parenchymal sarcoidosis and obstructive dysfunction caused by endobronchial sarcoidosis.

Patient 9. Normal lung volumes and flow rates. MVV is slightly reduced but within normal limits. DLCO is very low.

PaO_2 is 56 mm Hg. Clinical diagnosis: primary pulmonary hypertension.

Patient 10. Normal lung volumes and flow rates. Previous PFT results were not available. DLCO is abnormally high. This patient was extremely obese, and all the abnormal results on PFTs can be explained on the basis of this. Obese patients show diminished lung volumes because of poor effort made during testing. Abnormally high DLCO is reported to be a result of increased Vc. Clinical diagnosis: obesity-related pulmonary dysfunction.

Preoperative Evaluation of Lung Functions

If patients scheduled to undergo lung resection have suspected or documented lung disease, PFTs should be performed preoperatively. A patient can tolerate pneumonectomy if the values are more than 50% of predicted for FEV_1, MVV, RV/TLC, and DLCO. If the values are less than 50% of predicted, quantitative V/Q scan will help assess regional lung functions. Preoperative bronchodilators, chest physiotherapy, incentive spirometry, and physical conditioning decrease the risk of postoperative pulmonary complications. Increased morbidity and mortality are associated with severe COPD and $PaCO_2$ >45 mm Hg (hypoxemia is not a reliable indicator). Upper abdominal operations (gallbladder and abdominal aortic aneurysm repair) carry higher rates of pulmonary complications than lower abdominal procedures.

Exercise Testing

Exercise testing can assess cardiopulmonary function. Indications for exercise testing include unexplained dyspnea or effort intolerance, ability/disability evaluation, quantitation of severity of pulmonary dysfunction, separation of cardiac from pulmonary causes of disability, evaluation of progression of a disease process, estimation of operative risks before cardiopulmonary surgery (lung resection, heart-lung or lung transplantation), rehabilitation, and evaluation of need for supplemental oxygen. Special equipment and expertise are required to perform an optimal exercise study.

Blood Gases and Oximetry

The interpretation of blood gas abnormalities is discussed in Chapter 5.

Bronchoscopy

Common diagnostic indications for bronchoscopy include persistent cough, hemoptysis, suspected cancer, lung nodule, atelectasis, diffuse lung disease, and lung infections. Therapeutic indications include atelectasis, retained secretions, tracheobronchial foreign bodies, airway stenosis (dilatation), and obstructive lesions (laser therapy, stent placement). Bronchoscopy is valuable in the staging of lung cancer.

Complications from bronchoscopy are minimal and include bleeding from mucosal or lung biopsy, pneumothorax (from lung biopsy), and hypoxemia. The risk of bleeding is increased in patients with renal failure, thrombocytopenia, and other bleeding diatheses.

- Bronchoscopy is safe in most patients.
- Low diagnostic yield in pleural effusion.
- Useful in the diagnosis and staging of lung cancer.

Bronchoalveolar Lavage

Bronchoalveolar lavage (BAL) is performed by instilling 100 to 150 mL of normal saline into the diseased segment(s) of the lung. The instilled saline is aspirated back via the bronchoscope. The aspirated effluent can be analyzed for cells, chemical constituents, and cultures for infectious agents. BAL in normal subjects shows alveolar macrophages (93% ± 3%) and lymphocytes (7% ± 1%). Other types of leukocytes are rarely found in normal subjects.

- BAL can quantify and identify cell morphology at the alveolar level.
- Normal subjects: macrophages (93%), lymphocytes (7%), and neutrophils (<1%).

BAL has no clinical value in the diagnosis of sarcoidosis or idiopathic pulmonary fibrosis. However, it may be helpful in diagnosing alveolar proteinosis, pulmonary Langerhans cell granuloma, and lymphangitic pulmonary metastasis. The CD4/CD8 ratio in BAL effluent is reversed in patients with acquired immunodeficiency syndrome (AIDS) complicated by lymphocytic interstitial pneumonitis and in many patients with hypersensitivity pneumonitis. BAL is extremely helpful in the diagnosis of *Pneumocystis carinii*, tuberculosis, mycoses, and other infections.

- BAL is helpful in diagnosing opportunistic lung infections.
- BAL has a limited role in the diagnosis of sarcoidosis and idiopathic pulmonary fibrosis.
- BAL is diagnostic in >60% of patients with lymphangitic carcinomatosis of the lungs.

Lung Biopsy

Lung biopsy can be performed via bronchoscopy, thoracoscopy, or thoracotomy. The indications for lung biopsy in diffuse lung disease should be based on the clinical features, treatment planned, and risks from biopsy and risk from treatment without a pathologic diagnosis. Bronchoscopic lung biopsy provides a 70% to 80% yield in sarcoidosis, pulmonary Langerhans cell granuloma, eosinophilic pneumonitis, lymphangioleiomyomatosis, infections, pulmonary alveolar proteinosis, lymphangitic carcinomatosis, drug-induced lung disease, and hypersensitivity pneumonitis. The major complications after bronchoscopic lung biopsy are pneumothorax (<2%) and hemorrhage (<3%).

OBSTRUCTIVE LUNG DISEASES

A common pathophysiologic feature of obstructive lung diseases is the obstruction to flow of air. Under this heading are included emphysema, bronchitis, asthma, bronchiectasis, cystic fibrosis, bronchiolitis, bullous lung disease, and airway stenosis. The term "chronic obstructive pulmonary disease" (COPD) is used to describe the common obstructive lung diseases, that is, emphysema, bronchitis, and asthma. Nearly 80% of patients with COPD have features of all three diseases. Nevertheless, it is important to differentiate the salient features of each disease (Table 21-3).

Etiology

Tobacco smoking is the major cause of COPD. Nearly 10% of smokers exhibit an accelerated rate of decline in FEV_1. This decline is proportional to the number of pack years of smoking. Smokers have 10 times the risk of nonsmokers of dying of chronic bronchitis and emphysema. Pipe and cigar smokers have between 1.5 and 3 times the risk of nonsmokers. Smoking increases the risk of developing COPD in people with α_1-antitrypsin deficiency. Smokers have an increased incidence of COPD, atherosclerosis, abdominal aortic aneurysm, and carcinoma of the lung, larynx, esophagus, and bladder. Diseases associated with or aggravated by smoking include asthma, lung fibrosis, calcification of pleural plaques in asbestosis, pulmonary alveolar phospholipoproteinosis, pulmonary Langerhans cell granuloma, and lung hemorrhage in Goodpasture syndrome. Passive smoking (second-hand smoke) is also carcinogenic. Other increased risks (particularly in children) include infections of the lower respiratory tract, fluid collection in the middle ear, decreased lung function, increased severity of preexistent asthma, and increased risk of developing asthma.

- Nearly 10% of smokers exhibit an accelerated rate of decline in FEV_1.
- Pulmonary Langerhans cell granuloma and pulmonary alveolar proteinosis are more common in smokers.
- Passive smoking is also carcinogenic.

Air pollution caused by oxidants, oxides of nitrogen, hydrocarbons, and sulphur dioxide has a significant role in exacerbations of COPD. Occupational exposures, heredity (α_1-antitrypsin deficiency), infections, allergy (in asthma), and other factors are also involved in the etiology of COPD.

Table 21-3.—Salient Differential Features of Bronchial Asthma, Chronic Bronchitis, and Emphysema*

Differential feature	Bronchial asthma	Chronic bronchitis	Emphysema
Onset	70% <30 yr old	≥50 yr old	≥60 yr old
Cigarette smoking	0	++++	++++
Pattern	Paroxysmal	Chronic, progressive	Chronic, progressive
Dyspnea	0 to ++++	+ to ++++	+++ to ++++
Cough	0 to +++	++ to ++++	+ to +++
Sputum	0 to ++	+++	+, ++
Atopy	50% (adult)	15%	15%
Infections	↑ Symptoms	↑↑↑ Symptoms	↑ Symptoms
Chest roentgenogram	Usually normal	↑ Marking	Hyperinflation
$Paco_2$	Normal or ↓ in attack	Increased	Normal or increased
Pao_2	Normal or ↓ in attack	Low	Low
DLCO	Normal	Normal or slight decrease	Decreased
FEV_1,%	↓↓ in attack or normal	↓↓	↓↓
Total lung capacity	Normal or ↑ in attack	Normal or slight ↑	↑↑↑
Residual volume	Normal or ↑ in attack	Normal or slight ↑	↑↑↑
Cor pulmonale	Rare	Common	Rare
Hematocrit	Normal	Normal or increased	Normal or increased

*↑ indicates increase; ↓, decrease; ↑↑, increased more; ↓↓, decreased more; ↑↑↑, increased greatly; ↓↓↓, decreased greatly; +, present; ++, bothersome; +++, major problem; ++++, significant problem; $Paco_2$, partial arterial carbon dioxide pressure; Pao_2, partial arterial oxygen pressure; DLCO, diffusion capacity:total lung capacity ratio; and FEV_1,%, percentage of vital capacity expired in 1 second.
From Kaliner M, Lemanske R: Rhinitis and asthma. JAMA 268:2807-2829, 1992. By permission of the American Medical Association.

Pathology

Obstruction to airflow in COPD can result from airway collapse during expiration (COPD), bronchospasm (many causes), mucosal inflammation and edema (bronchitis, asthma, etc.), and mucous gland hypertrophy (bronchitis, asthma, etc.). The airway collapse occurs because of greatly increased intrathoracic pressure during expiration and the loss of elastic recoil of the lung (which normally prevents excessive collapse of the airways during expiration). The airway collapse during expiration typically occurs in emphysema, bullous lung disease, chronic bronchitis, long-standing asthma, and other obstructive lung diseases. The premature collapse of airways leads to air-trapping and hyperinflation of the lungs (barrel chest). Bronchospasm in susceptible persons occurs as a result of increased bronchomotor tone in the smooth muscles of the airways. Bronchospasm can occur as a result of many underlying complex mechanisms mediated by the vagus nerve, extrinsic allergens, release of intrinsic chemicals, external physical and chemical injury, hypothermia of airways, and other factors. Mucous gland hypertrophy occurs in chronic bronchitis, asthma, and other airway diseases as a result of direct or indirect stimulation of mucous glands. Increased bronchomotor tone can be elicited by using provocation inhalation challenge tests (see above). Histologically, centrilobular emphysema is the most common type and usually starts in the upper lobes;

most patients with COPD have this. The panlobular type usually starts in the lower lobes. It is seen in panlobular emphysema associated with α_1-antitrypsin deficiency.

- Causes of airway obstruction: expiratory collapse of airways, bronchospasm, mucosal inflammation, and mucous gland hypertrophy.
- Centrilobular emphysema is more common than the panlobular type.
- Panlobular emphysema is caused by α_1-antitrypsin deficiency.

Physiology

Decreased flow rates are characteristic of COPD. Lung compliance is increased in emphysema, and elastic recoil of the lung is decreased (the opposite occurs in restrictive lung disease). DLCO is diminished in emphysema (as well as in most restrictive lung diseases). Hyperexpansion is manifested by increased total lung capacity and residual volume. Retention of carbon dioxide (hypercarbia) is more common in bronchitic than in emphysematous patients.

- Normal lung compliance = 0.2 L/cm H_2O.
- Lung compliance is increased in emphysema (decreased in restrictive lung disease).

Chronic Bronchitis

Chronic bronchitis is defined as cough with sputum for 3 months or more per year for 2 or more consecutive years. Pathologically, the Reid index (i.e., the ratio of bronchial mucous glands to bronchial wall thickness) is increased. Cigarette smoking is the most common cause of chronic bronchitis. Occupational exposure and air pollution also contribute to the exacerbations. Patients exhibit productive cough, have a tendency to retain carbon dioxide, have a lower PaO_2, show cyanosis ("blue bloaters"), and tend to be slightly overweight.

- Chronic bronchitic patients ("blue bloaters") tend to retain carbon dioxide, cough, and develop cor pulmonale sooner than emphysematous patients ("pink puffers") do.

Emphysema

Emphysema is characterized by enlargement of the airspaces distal to the terminal bronchioles and destruction of the alveolar walls. CT of the lungs is excellent for documentation of emphysema and bullous lung disease. Pure anatomical emphysema is less common than chronic bronchitis. Emphysematous patients are thin, maintain near normal PaO_2 by increasing the work of breathing, and look adequately oxygenated ("pink puffers"). Severe weight loss is a relatively common finding in severe emphysema. Carbon dioxide retention is not seen until late in the disease.

- Emphysematous patients are "pink puffers."

Bullous Lung Disease

Small apical bullae are present in many normal persons. Bullous lung disease can be congenital or acquired. Lack of communication with bronchi may cause air-trapping. Complications include pneumothorax, COPD, infection and formation of lung abscess, bleeding into a bulla, and compression of adjacent normal lung. Surgical therapy may improve lung function by 5% to 10% in 10% to 15% of patients. The incidence of lung cancer is increased in patients with bullous emphysema.

- Panlobular emphysema may look like a bulla.
- Bullous changes may be seen in Marfan and Ehlers-Danlos syndromes, burnt-out sarcoidosis, and cadmium exposure.
- Bullous lung disease is associated with an increased risk of lung cancer.

α_1-Antitrypsin Deficiency

Synthesis of α_1-antitrypsin, a secretory glycoprotein, by hepatocytes is determined by the α_1-antitrypsin gene on chromosome 14. α_1-Antitrypsin inhibits many proteolytic enzymes

and, thus, protects the lungs from destructive emphysema. It is an autosomal recessive disease. Phenotypes: normals (P_IMM), heterozygote (P_IMZ), homozygote (P_IZZ), and null (P_INull). The threshold for disease is set at less than 11 $\mu mol/L$. The prevalence of P_IZZ in the U.S. is 1:1,670 to 1:3,000. Up to 10% of patients with P_IZZ α_1-antitrypsin deficiency do not develop lung disease. In nonsmoking P_IZZ persons, lung function decreases with increasing age, especially after age 50 years. Men are at greater risk of lung function deterioration than women. Smoking hastens the onset of emphysema. Signs and symptoms appear during the 3rd or 4th decade of life. α_1-Antitrypsin deficiency is associated with neonatal liver disease (hepatitis, cryptogenic cirrhosis, periportal fibrosis) and respiratory distress syndrome. A lack of α_1-antitrypsin seems to increase the propensity to develop asthma. α_1-Antitrypsin derived from human plasma has been used as replacement therapy; minimal decreases in the rate of decline of FEV_1 (~27 mL/yr) have been observed in patients with severe emphysema.

- Smoking hastens the onset of emphysema.
- Basal emphysema on CXR, absence of α_1-globulin on protein electrophoresis, patient with COPD, and family history of COPD.
- Hepatic cirrhosis develops in up to 3% of patients.
- In young patients with clinical features of COPD, consider asthma, α_1-antitrypsin deficiency, cystic fibrosis, ciliary dyskinesia, and bronchiectasis.

Asthma

Asthma or asthmatic bronchitis is an acute or chronic disease characterized by recurrent episodes of reversible bronchospasm (wheezing) leading to paroxysmal obstruction of the airways. Asthma is primarily an inflammatory disease. Therefore, inhaled corticosteroids are considered the first line of therapy by many physicians. Cough can be the only presenting symptom of bronchial asthma. Exercise-induced asthma (EIA) is more common in younger people and is manifested as chest tightness or cough (without wheeze) after termination of exercise. EIA occurs in 10% to 50% of recreational and elite athletes. Most subjects with EIA have normal PFTs during the asymptomatic period. A more detailed discussion of asthma is given in Chapter 2.

- All that wheezes is not asthma and not all asthmatics wheeze.
- Drug-induced bronchospasm: β-blockers, prostaglandin inhibitors (acetylsalicylic acid, indomethacin), ultrasonic nebulizers, acetylcysteine, *Ascaris* antigen, and occupational exposures.
- Provocation inhalation challenge is used to detect latent asthma.

Treatment of COPD

The therapeutic approach to COPD consists of identifying the type of COPD, quantification of pulmonary dysfunction and response to bronchodilator therapy, selection of appropriate bronchodilators, anticipation and appropriate treatment of complications, and initial as well as continued education of the patient and family about long-term therapy. Pulmonary rehabilitation reduces disability and improves handicap, but PFTs show minimal improvement.

Bronchodilators

Bronchodilator drugs are administered to reverse bronchoconstriction (bronchospasm). They can be classified into adrenergic agonists (sympathomimetics), β-adrenergic agonists (β$_2$-selective agonists), phosphodiesterase inhibitor (theophylline), anticholinergics (ipratropium, etc.), mast cell inhibitors (cromolyn sodium, etc.), leukotriene receptor antagonist, antihistamines, anti-inflammatory agents (corticosteroids and methotrexate), and other agents (troleandomycin, γ-globulin, mucolytics, etc.).

Adrenergic Agonists (Sympathomimetics)

These include epinephrine, isoproterenol, ephedrine, and isoetharine. Epinephrine acts on both α and β receptors of effector cells. It is used in the treatment of acute asthma. In adults, a dose of 0.1 to 0.3 mg (0.1-0.3 mL of a 1:1,000 dilution) by injection is commonly used. The maximal dose is 3 (each 15 minutes apart). Isoproterenol (Isuprel) has a rapid onset of action (<5 minutes) and a duration of action of 2 hours. Isoetharine (Bronkosol) is administered as an aerosol (0.5 mL diluted with 2.5 mL saline). Currently, ephedrine is rarely used in the treatment of asthma. Adverse reactions associated with adrenergic agonists include anxiety, headache, palpitations, cardiac arrhythmias, skin flushing, tremor, diaphoresis, and paradoxic bronchospasm. In current practice, adrenergic agonists have been replaced by β-adrenergic (selective) agonists.

- Sympathomimetics are used to treat acute bronchospasm.

Short-Acting β-Adrenergic (β$_2$-Selective) Agonists

These are the most commonly used bronchodilators. They include albuterol, terbutaline, metaproterenol, pirbuterol, and bitolterol. These agents bring about bronchodilatation by stimulation of cyclic adenosine monophosphate (AMP) production through activation of adenyl cyclase in the cell membrane. In most patients, single doses of these agents produce clinically significant bronchodilatation within 5 minutes, a peak effect 30 to 60 minutes after inhalation, and a beneficial effect that lasts for 3 to 4 hours. Many of these agents are available in inhaled form (metered dose inhalers) as well as tablet, powder, syrup, and injection forms. The standard dose for inhalation therapy is two inhalations four times daily. It is essential to tailor the dosages on the basis of the clinical features and the potential side effects. Adverse effects include tremor, anxiety, restlessness, tachycardia, palpitations, increased blood pressure, and cardiac arrhythmias. Prostatism may become exacerbated. Side effects are more likely in the elderly and in the presence of cardiovascular, liver, or neurologic disorders and in those taking other medications for nonpulmonary diseases (β-blockers for cardiac disease, etc.). Normal therapeutic dosages of theophylline and β-agonists used in combination usually are not associated with serious side effects. Paradoxic bronchospasm may rarely result from tachyphylaxis (a rapidly decreasing response to a drug after a few doses) or from exposure to preservatives and propellants. A newer single-isomer β-agonist, levalbuterol, binds to β-adrenergic receptors with 100-fold greater affinity than albuterol.

- β-Adrenergic agonists stimulate cyclic AMP.
- Standard dose: 2 inhalations 4 times a day.
- Side effects: tremor, anxiety, tachycardia, palpitations, increased blood pressure, cardiac arrhythmias, exacerbated prostatism.

Long-Acting β-Adrenergic (β$_2$-Selective) Agonists

These include salmeterol, fenoterol, and formoterol. Currently, in the U.S., only salmeterol is available. Salmeterol is more β$_2$-adrenoreceptors-selective than isoproterenol, a short-acting bronchodilator, which has approximately equal agonist activity on β$_1$- and β$_2$-adrenoreceptors. Albuterol has a β$_2$- to β$_1$-adrenoreceptor selectivity ratio of 1:1,400. Salmeterol is at least 50 times more selective for β$_2$-adrenoreceptors than albuterol. Salmeterol is highly lipophilic (albuterol is hydrophilic), hence the depot effect in tissues. Salmeterol has a prolonged duration of action (10-12 hours) and inhibits the release of proinflammatory and spasmogenic mediators from respiratory cells. It has a persistent effect in inhibiting histamine release for up to 20 hours, as compared with the short duration of action of isoproterenol, albuterol, and formoterol. Salmeterol is also effective in preventing EIA, methacholine-induced bronchospasm, and allergen challenge. The dosage of salmeterol is two inhalations (100 µg) twice daily. The longer duration of action may aid in the management of nocturnal asthma. The side effects are similar to those of other β-adrenergic agents. However, tachyphylaxis is distinctly uncommon. Salmeterol and other β-adrenergic bronchodilators may potentiate the actions of monoamine oxidase inhibitors and tricyclic antidepressants.

- Salmeterol is lipophilic (albuterol is hydrophilic).
- Long-acting bronchodilator (>12 hours).
- Dose: 2 inhalations (100 µg) 2 times a day.

Phosphodiesterase Inhibitor

Theophylline (methylxanthine) is the main drug in this group. Proposed mechanisms of action include inhibition of cyclic guanosine monophosphate (GMP), augmentation of adrenergic terminal output to airway smooth muscle, adenosine receptor antagonism, and stimulation of endogenous catecholamine. The result is a decrease in free calcium levels in smooth muscle. Overall, the use of theophylline has diminished, with β-agonists being used more often in its place. Theophylline is effective in combination with $β_2$-agonists in the management of moderate and severe asthma. Theophylline increases respiratory muscle contractility in a dose-related fashion. The clearance of theophylline is shown in Table 21-4.

- The exact mechanism of action of theophylline is unclear.
- Theophylline is effective in combination with $β_2$-agonists.

The recommended blood level of theophylline is 10 to 15 µg/mL. The loading dose is 6 mg/kg (range, 5-7 mg); the maintenance dose is 0.5 mg/kg per hour or 1.15 g/24 hours. The normal adult dose is usually less than 1,000 mg/day. Longer acting preparations may be given in a single dose of 300 to 600 mg. The dosage should be decreased by 50% if the patient has received theophylline in the preceding 24 hours or has heart failure, severe hypoxemia, hepatic insufficiency, or seizures. Each dosage should be increased by 50 to 100 mg if the therapeutic effect is suboptimal and in smokers who can tolerate the increased dose. Each dose should be decreased by 50-100 mg if toxic effects develop or if progressive cardiac or liver failure develops. Tobacco smoke decreases the efficacy (half-life) of theophylline. The main side effects are tremors, aggravation of prostatism, tachycardia, and arrhythmias.

Table 21-4.—Theophylline Clearance

Increased by	Decreased by
β-Agonists	Allopurinol
Carbamazepine	Antibiotics (macrolides)—
Dilantin	ciprofloxacin, norfloxacin,
Furosemide	isoniazid
Hyperthyroidism	β-Blocker—propranolol
Ketoconazole	Caffeine
Marijuana	Cirrhosis
Phenobarbital	Congestive cardiac failure
Rifampin	H_2 blocker—cimetidine
Tobacco smoke	Mexiletine
	Oral contraceptives
	Viral infection

- Tobacco smoking decreases the half-life of theophylline.
- The recommended blood level is 10-15 µg/mL.
- Frequently measuring serum theophylline levels is unnecessary in clinical practice.

Anticholinergic Agents

Anticholinergic agents (ipratropium, atropine, etc.) prevent the increase in intracellular concentration of cyclic GMP caused by the muscarinic receptors in bronchial smooth muscle. They also inhibit vagally mediated reflexes by blocking the effects of acetylcholine. They are useful in patients with chronic bronchitis or asthmatic bronchitis, but they are not beneficial in pure emphysema. Ipratropium is a synthetic quaternary ammonium congener of atropine. As a single agent, ipratropium is not effective in the management of acute or chronic airway disease. It is efficacious if used with β-adrenergic agents and theophylline in the treatment of mild-to-moderate asthma. Ipratropium prevents bronchoconstriction caused by cholinergic agents such as methacholine and carbachol. It does not protect against bronchoconstriction produced by tobacco smoke, citric acid, sulfur dioxide, or carbon dust. Allergen-induced bronchospasm also responds poorly to ipratropium therapy. Ipratropium has no effect on mucus production, mucus transport, or ciliary activities. The usual dose is two inhalations four times daily. The duration of action is 3 to 5 hours. No more than 12 inhalations should be permitted in 24 hours. Side effects include nervousness, headache, gastrointestinal upset, dry mouth, and cough. The drug may aggravate narrow-angle glaucoma, prostatic hypertrophy, and bladder neck obstruction.

- Ipratropium inhibits vagally mediated reflexes by blocking the effects of acetylcholine.
- It has minimal or no benefit in pure emphysema.
- It is not very effective if used alone.

Mast Cell Inhibitors

Cromolyn and nedocromil (pyranoquinoline) block the release of IgE-mediated mast cell mediators, histamine, and other mediators of bronchoconstriction. Nedocromil is 4 to 10 times more potent than cromolyn. These are "preventive" drugs and should not be used to reverse a full-blown asthmatic attack. They are available as powdered preparations (Spinhaler) or liquids for aerosolization. They are excellent drugs for EIA and for asthmatics with known allergens. The duration of action is 4 to 6 hours. The dosage is two inhalations three or four times daily. For EIA, treatment is given 15 to 20 minutes before exercise. The side effects include irritation of the throat, hoarseness, and dryness of the mouth.

- Not true bronchodilators (they prevent bronchospasm).

- Mast cell inhibitors should be used to prevent extrinsic asthma.
- Excellent for EIA and allergen-induced asthma.

Antileukotrienes

Leukotrienes are formed by the breakdown of arachidonic acid (membrane component) via the 5-lipoxygenase pathway. By occupying the receptor sites, leukotrienes cause airway edema, bronchial smooth muscle contraction, and altered airway cellular activity in patients with asthma. There are several leukotrienes (LTC_4, LTD_4, LTE_4, etc.). Asthmatic persons are up to 100 times more sensitive to the bronchoconstrictor effects of LTD_4 than nonasthmatic subjects. Leukotriene receptor antagonists available in the U.S. include zafirlukast and montelukast. Zileuton is an inhibitor of leukotriene synthesis (5-lipoxygenase inhibitor). These agents improve FEV_1 by 8% to 20% but are effective in only 50% to 70% of asthmatic patients. Antileukotrienes are not true bronchodilators; they prevent bronchospasm. The standard dosages are zafirlukast 20 mg orally twice daily and zileuton 600 mg orally four times daily. The most common side effects associated with zafirlukast are headache in 13% of patients, respiratory infection in 3.5% (in those >55 years), nausea in 3%, and diarrhea in 2%. Patients taking warfarin should have the prothrombin time (PT) checked and dose altered as necessary (mean PT increases by 35% by inhibiting cytochrome P450). The simultaneous use of zafirlukast with theophylline, terfenadine, or erythromycin results in decreased mean plasma levels of zafirlukast. Use with aspirin also decreases the mean plasma level of zafirlukast. Zileuton may cause dyspepsia, nausea, myalgia, abdominal discomfort, and increased serum levels of alanine aminotransferase (ALT). Corticosteroid withdrawal in asthmatic patients treated with zafirlukast has resulted in the development of Churg-Strauss syndrome.

- Leukotrienes cause bronchoconstriction in asthmatic persons.
- Antileukotrienes block receptor occupation by leukotrienes.
- Antileukotrienes can be used in the prevention and chronic therapy of asthma.

Corticosteroids

Corticosteroid is the most effective anti-inflammatory drug available for the treatment of asthma. The mechanism of action of corticosteroids (inhaled and systemic) is unclear. Because inflammation is a main feature of asthma, inhaled corticosteroid is considered by many to be the first-line drug in the treatment of mild asthma. The dosages of oral or injectable corticosteroids depend on the severity and duration of the asthma. Corticosteroids have no bronchodilating effect in emphysematous patients. Bronchitic patients, however, may benefit from the anti-inflammatory action. Short- or long-term systemic corticosteroid therapy is an important aspect of treating moderate-to-severe asthma. Systemic corticosteroid therapy in nonasthmatic COPD has a limited role; only about 15% of patients show improvement. Inhaled corticosteroids can be used in conjunction with systemic (oral) corticosteroids, especially during the weaning period of long-term or high-dose systemic (oral) corticosteroids. All inhaled corticosteroids, when used in higher doses, are associated with greater side effects and fewer benefits. The most common side effect with aerosolized corticosteroids is oral candidiasis. Inhaled corticosteroids in doses greater than 1.5 mg/d (0.75 mg/d for fluticasone propionate) may lead to slowing of linear growth velocity in children, reduction in bone density (particularly in perimenopausal women), posterior subcapsular cataracts, or glaucoma.

- Corticosteroid is considered by many to be the first-line drug in the treatment of asthma.
- Oropharyngeal candidiasis is a complication of aerosolized corticosteroids.
- Systemic corticosteroid therapy is important in the treatment of refractory asthma.

Nonsteroidal Anti-Inflammatory ("Steroid-Sparing") Agents

The efficacy and safety of methotrexate as a steroid-sparing agent is controversial, and the beneficial responses are not consistent. Therefore, methotrexate should not be considered a standard anti-asthma drug. Gold salts have been used as anti-inflammatory agents in asthmatic patients. The bronchodilator effect may not be apparent until a daily dose of 1,500 mg has been administered for 6 to 12 months. Troleandomycin, a macrolide antibiotic, has shown a steroid-minimizing effect by decreasing the elimination of steroid. It works best with methylprednisolone rather than with prednisone or prednisolone. The normal dose is 250 mg four times daily. Other agents in this group include cyclosporine, hydroxychloroquine, and dapsone. High-dose immunoglobulin therapy has been tried in some refractory cases.

- Steroid-sparing agents have a limited role in the management of asthma.
- Some steroid-sparing agents (methotrexate and gold) can produce lung toxicity.

Antihistamines

Because asthma is provoked in many patients by the release of histamine and histamine analogues, antihistamines have been used to treat asthma. Astemizole (10 mg once daily) and terfenadine (60 mg twice daily) are effective in preventing pollen-induced asthma. Histamine (H_1) antagonists produce bronchodilatation without inducing sedation. These drugs can produce prolongation of the QT_c interval on electrocardiography (ECG). This may lead to ventricular tachycardia. This serious side effect is more likely in patients with liver or heart disease and if the patient is taking ketoconazole or macrolide antibiotics.

- Antihistamines are not standard anti-asthmatic drugs.
- Astemizole: prolongation of the QT_c interval on ECG.

Adjuvant Therapy

Expectorants and mucolytics (acetylcysteine, guaifenesin, iodinated glycerol, and potassium iodide) are used to treat symptoms rather than the underlying bronchospasm. They are not considered standard drugs for asthma. Antibiotic therapy is helpful in patients with symptoms suggestive of bacterial infection. Desensitization therapy in patients with proven extrinsic allergies may prevent acute asthmatic attacks on exposure to known allergens. Maintenance of good oral hydration, avoidance of tobacco smoking and other respiratory irritants, annual influenza vaccination, and prompt treatment of respiratory infections are equally important.

Asthma in a pregnant female should be treated as aggressively as asthma in a nonpregnant female. Fetal growth and development and maternal lung function should be monitored. Therapy for asthma during pregnancy should include a short-acting symptom reliever medication (usually an inhaled short-acting beta$_2$-agonist) and long-term daily medication to control intermittent disease.

Oxygen

Nocturnal low-flow oxygen (<2 L/min) therapy is recommended when the PaO_2 is ≤55 mm Hg, PaO_2 is ≤59 mm Hg with polycythemia or clinical evidence of cor pulmonale, or SaO_2 is ≤88%. The lack of carbon dioxide retention should be assured before recommending oxygen. Continuous oxygen therapy is more useful than nocturnal-only treatment. Oxygen therapy is indicated for patients with persistent polycythemia, recurrent episodes of cor pulmonale, severe hypoxemia, and central nervous system symptoms induced by hypoxemia. The need for chronic or indefinite oxygen therapy should be reassessed after 3 months of treatment. For each liter of oxygen administered, the fraction of inhaled oxygen (FIO_2) increases by 3%. Exercise therapy improves exercise tolerance and maximal oxygen uptake but does not improve the results of PFTs.

- Oxygen therapy is recommended if the PaO_2 ≤55 mm Hg and/or SaO_2 ≤88%.
- FIO_2 increases by 3% for each liter of supplemental oxygen.
- An exercise program does not improve PFT results.

The practical aspects of managing COPD are outlined in Table 21-5.

Complications and Causes for Exacerbation of COPD

The complications and causes for exacerbation of COPD include viral and bacterial respiratory infections (commonly *Haemophilus influenzae, Moraxella catarrhalis,* and *Streptococcus pneumoniae*), cor pulmonale, myocardial infarction, cardiac arrhythmias, pneumothorax, pulmonary emboli, bronchogenic carcinoma, environmental exposure, oversedation, neglect of therapy, excessive oxygen use (suppression of hypoxemic drive), and excessive use of β$_2$-agonist (tachyphylaxis). Nocturnal oxygen desaturation is common in "blue bloaters," as are premature ventricular contractions and episodic pulmonary hypertension. A decrease in SaO_2 correlates with an increase in pulmonary artery pressure. Severe weight loss, sometimes more than 50 kg, is noted in 30% of patients with severe COPD.

- Bacterial infections in COPD are caused by *H. influenzae, M. catarrhalis,* and *S. pneumoniae.*
- Nocturnal oxygen desaturation is more common in "blue bloaters."
- A decrease in SaO_2 correlates with an increase in pulmonary artery pressure.
- Severe weight loss is seen in 30% of COPD (emphysema) patients.

Table 21-5.—Practical Aspects of Managing Chronic Obstructive Pulmonary Disease (COPD)

Steps in management
    Identify the type of COPD
    Identify pathophysiology
    Assess lung dysfunction
    Eliminate causative/exacerbating factors
    Aim drug therapy at underlying pathophysiology
    Anticipate and treat complications
    Rehabilitation program
    Education of patient and family
Stepped care approach (especially in asthma)
    Mild asthma (FEV$_1$ >65% of predicted): inhaled steroids; β$_2$-agonists as needed
    Moderate asthma (FEV$_1$ 36%-65% of predicted): inhaled steroids and theophylline; β$_2$-agonist as needed
    Severe asthma (FEV$_1$ <35% of predicted): inhaled steroids, theophylline, β$_2$-agonist regularly and as needed, and oral (or parenteral) steroids

FEV$_1$, forced expiratory volume in 1 second.

Other Topics in COPD

Nicotine gum and patch help maintain nicotine blood levels while a smoker tries to cope with the psychologic and other aspects of nicotine addiction. Nearly 25% of smokers require treatment for more than 12 months to remain tobacco-free. Nicotine from gum is absorbed more slowly from the buccal mucosa and stomach than from the airways with inhaled smoke. Side effects include mucosal burning, light-headedness, nausea, stomachache, and hiccups. The patch causes a rash in a significant number of patients. Use of the nicotine patch with continued smoking aggravates cardiac problems.

- Nicotine gum and patch are important aspects of a tobacco cessation program.
- Simultaneous use of cigarette and nicotine products aggravates cardiac problems.

Lung volume reduction surgery (resection of 20%-30% of peripheral lung parenchyma) in emphysematous patients appears to improve pulmonary functions at least during short-term follow-up. The benefit is thought to be the result of regaining normal or near-normal mechanical function (of the thoracic cage) that was compromised by the severe hyperinflation of the lungs. The procedure is of benefit to some but not all patients. Lung transplantion is used to treat various end-stage pulmonary diseases. It does not confer a survival advantage for patients with advanced emphysema, but it does confer a survival advantage for patients with cystic fibrosis as well as for those with idiopathic pulmonary fibrosis. Regardless of the underlying disease for which a transplant is performed, the procedure improves the quality of life.

- Lung volume reduction surgery is experimental.

Cystic Fibrosis

Cystic fibrosis is the most common lethal autosomal recessive disease among whites in the U.S. The locus of the responsible gene is on the long arm of chromosome 7. Cystic fibrosis develops in 1 in 2,000 to 3,500 live births among whites; about 1 in 20 (2%-5%) whites is a heterozygous carrier. There is no sex predominance. Occurrence in blacks is 1 in 17,000 and 1 in 90,000 in Asians. Both parents of a child with cystic fibrosis must be heterozygotes; siblings of such a child have a 50% to 65% chance of being heterozygotes. The diagnosis is made in 80% of patients before the age of 10 years; in 10%, the diagnosis is not made until adolescent years. Obstruction of exocrine glands, with the exception of sweat glands, by viscous secretions causes almost all the clinical manifestations. Mucociliary clearance is normal in patients with minimal pulmonary dysfunction and is decreased in those with obstructive phenomena.

- Cystic fibrosis: the most common lethal autosomal recessive disease among whites.
- In 10% of patients, the diagnosis is not made until adolescent years.
- Siblings of children with cystic fibrosis have a 50%-65% chance of being heterozygotes.
- All exocrine glands, except sweat glands, are affected.

Up to 10% of patients with cystic fibrosis and heterozygous carriers demonstrate nonspecific airway hyperactivity and an increased susceptibility to asthma and atopy. There is an increased risk of allergic bronchopulmonary aspergillosis developing in atopic cystic fibrosis patients. Many patients exhibit type I and type III hypersensitivity reactions to antigens. Positive serologic reactions to *Aspergillus* species and *Candida albicans* occur with higher frequency in patients with cystic fibrosis than in those with asthma. Allergic bronchopulmonary aspergillosis occurs in up to 10% of patients with cystic fibrosis.

- Up to 10% of patients with cystic fibrosis and carriers exhibit increased airway response.
- Up to 10% of patients show increased susceptibility to asthma and atopy.
- Allergic bronchopulmonary aspergillosis occurs in up to 10% of patients.

There is no evidence for a primary defect in sodium transport. However, the epithelial cells in cystic fibrosis are poorly permeable to chloride ions. The normally negative potential difference across the cell membrane becomes more negative (because of chloride impermeability) in cystic fibrosis.

- No evidence for a primary defect in sodium transport.
- Epithelial cells are poorly permeable to chloride ions.
- Marked increase in the electrical potential difference across the nasal and tracheobronchial epithelium compared with that of normal subjects and heterozygote relatives.

Quantitative pilocarpine iontophoresis is helpful in diagnosis; abnormal results on at least two tests are necessary for the diagnosis. Abnormal sweat chloride: adult, greater than 80 mEq/L; child, greater than 60 mEq/L. Note that normal sweat chloride values do not exclude cystic fibrosis. Conditions associated with high levels of sodium/chloride in sweat include smoking, chronic bronchitis, malnutrition, hereditary nephrogenic diabetes insipidus, adrenal insufficiency, and ectodermal dysplasia. The concentration of sweat sodium/chloride increases with age. Heterozygotes may have normal sweat sodium/chloride values. False-negative test results are common in edematous states. When sweat chloride levels are normal in a patient in whom cystic fibrosis is highly suspected, alternative diagnostic tests (nasal transepithelial voltage measurements, genotyping, etc.) should be considered.

- Diagnosis in adults requires at least three of the following: clinical features of cystic fibrosis, positive family history, sweat chloride ≥80 mEq/L, and pancreatic insufficiency.
- Respiratory manifestations: sinusitis, nasal polyps, progressive cystic bronchiectasis, purulent sputum, atelectasis, hemoptysis, and pneumothorax.
- *Pseudomonas aeruginosa* is the dominant organism and is impossible to eradicate.
- Increased incidence of *Pseudomonas cepacia* respiratory infection; the presence of *P. cepacia* is associated with rapid deterioration in lung function.

Cystic fibrosis is the most common cause of COPD and pancreatic deficiency in the first 3 decades of life in the U.S. Males constitute 55% of the adult patients. The diagnosis is made after the age of 15 years in 17% to 25% of patients. In adults (≥17 years), COPD is the major cause of morbidity and mortality. Adults with cystic fibrosis have a higher incidence of minor hemoptysis (60% of patients), major hemoptysis (71%), pneumothorax (16%), and sinusitis and nasal polyposis (48%). Pancreatic insufficiency is present in 95% of patients, but it is seldom symptomatic. Intussusception and fecal impaction (similar to meconium ileus) are more frequent (21%) in adults than in children. Hyperinflation of lungs on CXR and lobar atelectasis are both less frequent in adults than in children. The mean age at onset of massive hemoptysis is 19 years, and median survival from the initial episode of hemoptysis is about 3.5 years. Mean age at occurrence of pneumothorax in adults is 22 years. Azoospermia occurs in 95% of patients.

- COPD is present in 97% of adults with cystic fibrosis; COPD is the major cause of morbidity and mortality.
- Adults with cystic fibrosis: minor hemoptysis (60%), major hemoptysis (71%), pneumothorax (16%), and sinusitis and nasal polyposis (48%).
- Pancreatic insufficiency in 95%; it is seldom symptomatic.

Respiratory therapy of cystic fibrosis includes management of obstructive lung disease, chest physiotherapy, postural drainage, immunization against influenza, and hydration. Chronic or intermittent intravenous antipseudomonal antibiotic therapy is an option. Lung transplantation is an option for advanced cases. Sputum in cystic fibrosis patients contains high concentrations of extracellular DNA, a viscous material released by leukocytes. Aerosolized recombinant human DNase I (dornase alfa) reduces sputum viscosity by degrading the DNA. Results of DNase I therapy have shown reduced risk of lung infections, improvement in FEV_1, and reduced antibiotic requirement. The usual dose is 2.5 mg once a day via nebulizer; patients older than 21 years may benefit from 2.5 mg twice a day. Serum antibodies to dornase alfa develop in about 2% to 4% of patients, but anaphylaxis has not been noted. Side effects of dornase alfa have included voice alteration, hoarseness, rash, chest pain, pharyngitis, and conjunctivitis. Other forms of therapy include nebulized antibiotics and domiciliary long-term intravenous antibiotics. Intermittent administration of inhaled tobramycin has been shown to improve pulmonary function, decrease the density of *P. aeruginosa* in sputum, and decrease the risk of hospitalization. Systemic corticosteroids, anti-inflammatory agents such as high doses of ibuprofen, and aerosolized DNase reduce sputum viscosity attributable to DNA from recruited neutrophils. Aerosolized amiloride has been administered to try to inhibit excessive sodium absorption, repeated sputum culture, hospitalization for acute exacerbation, and frequent bronchoscopy to clear the airways. The risk of death from cystic fibrosis is 38% to 56% within 2 years when FEV_1 has reached 20% to 30% of predicted. Patients younger than 18 years have worse survival rates once these deteriorations in FEV_1 have occurred.

- Nearly 50% of patients with cystic fibrosis survive to age 25.
- The overall survival rate for cystic fibrosis patients older than 17 years is closer to 50%.
- Poor prognostic factors: female sex, residence in a non-northern climate, pneumothorax, hemoptysis, recurrent bacterial infections, presence of *P. cepacia*, and systemic complications.

Bronchiectasis

Bronchiectasis is ectasia, or dilatation, of the bronchi due to irreversible destruction of bronchial walls. Airway inflammation in bronchiectasis is characterized by tissue neutrophilia, a mononuclear cell infiltrate composed mainly of CD4+ T cells and CD68+ macrophages, and increased IL-8 expression. Bronchiectasis is reversible when it results from severe bronchitis, acute pneumonia, or allergic bronchopulmonary aspergillosis. Bronchiectasis most commonly occurs in the lower lung fields. Mild cylindrical bronchiectasis seen in many heavy smokers with chronic bronchitis may be diffuse. Distal bronchial segments are involved in most cases of bronchiectasis. An exception is proximal bronchial involvement in allergic bronchopulmonary aspergillosis. In most cases of bronchiectasis, second- to fourth-order bronchi are involved. Disease is bilateral in 30% of patients.

- Reversible bronchiectasis in allergic bronchopulmonary aspergillosis, acute pneumonia, and chronic bronchitis.
- Upper lobe involvement in cystic fibrosis, allergic bronchopulmonary aspergillosis, and chronic mycotic and mycobacterial infections.

Most cases are diagnosed on clinical grounds (chronic cough with purulent sputum expectoration). Some patients with "dry bronchiectasis" caused by tuberculosis do not have productive cough, but episodes of significant hemoptysis may develop. Many mildly symptomatic or asymptomatic patients with atelectatic segments of the right middle lobe (right middle lobe syndrome) and lingular segments of the left upper lobe have minor degrees of bronchiectasis. CXR shows increased markings in the bases, crowding of bronchi, segmental atelectasis, honeycombing with cystic spaces less than 2.0 cm, loss of lung volume, and air-fluid levels (if cystic bronchiectasis is present). HRCT findings include signet-ring shadows (a dilated bronchus with bronchial artery forming the "stone"), bronchial wall thickening, dilated bronchi extending to the periphery, bronchial obstruction due to inspissated purulent secretions, loss of volume, and air-fluid levels if cystic or saccular changes are present. HRCT diagnosis of "nodular bronchiectasis" usually indicates peribronchial granulomatous infiltration caused by secondary infection by *Myobacterium avium* complex. High seroprevalence of *Helicobacter pylori* has been reported in active bronchiectasis, but the clinical implications are unclear.

- Nonpulmonary symptoms: fetor oris, anorexia, weight loss, arthralgia, clubbing, and HPO.
- HRCT of the chest has replaced bronchography (in most cases) in the diagnosis.
- PFTs usually show obstructive phenomena.

Causes and Associations of Bronchiectasis

Infections

Most cases of bronchiectasis in adults are related to adenoviral and/or bacterial infections (measles, influenza, or pertussis) in childhood. Tuberculosis is a common cause of bronchiectasis, particularly in the upper lobes. Occasionally, chronic histoplasmosis and coccidioidomycosis can cause bronchiectasis. However, in patients with chronic stable bronchiectasis, *P. aeruginosa* is the predominant organism in respiratory secretions.

- "Dry bronchiectasis" with episodes of significant hemoptysis without sputum is usually due to bronchiectasis in an area of old tuberculous damage.
- Bronchiectasis may result from chronic mycoses.

Ciliary Dyskinesia (Immotile Cilia) Syndrome

Cilia normally are present in many organs, and their absence or abnormality may cause clinical problems (listed in parentheses): nasal mucosa (nasal polyps), paranasal sinuses (chronic sinusitis), eustachian tube (inner ear infection, deafness), tracheobronchial tree (chronic bronchitis, bronchiectasis). Many types of ciliary abnormalities (loss of radial spokes, eccentric tubules, absent tubules, adhesion of multiple cilia, etc.) occur. Although the term "immotile cilia" is commonly used, the cilia do move, but their motion is abnormal and dyssynchronous.

- Many forms of ciliary abnormalities can occur.
- Ciliary dyskinesia, not ciliary immotility, is the major abnormality.

The immotile cilia syndrome (Kartagener syndrome) is an autosomal recessive disorder. Loss of the dynein arm—the fundamental defect—is an inherited abnormality involving a single protein. The prevalence of the disorder is 1 in 20,000 to 40,000 persons. Up to 50% of patients with ciliary dyskinesia exhibit the triad of situs inversus, sinusitis, and bronchiectasis or at least bronchitis. Loss of the dynein arm results in sinusitis and otitis (less common in adults), nasal polyposis, bronchiectasis (in 75% of adults), situs inversus, and infertility in males. Infertility is not a universal phenomenon, and, in fact, women with immotile cilia syndrome are often fertile. Kartagener syndrome accounts for 0.5% of the cases of bronchiectasis and 15% of the cases of dextrocardia.

- Ciliary dyskinesia (Kartagener syndrome) is an autosomal recessive disorder.
- Loss of the dynein arm is the fundamental defect.
- Situs inversus, sinusitis, and bronchiectasis are seen in 50% of cases.

Deficiency of radial spokes may result in sinusitis, nasal polyposis, otitis, mastoiditis, recurrent bronchitis, and infertility in both sexes. The diagnosis depends on the clinical features and documentation of ciliary abnormalities by electron microscopic examination of nasal mucosa, bronchial mucosa, or semen. At least 20 types of axonemal defects have been described. Ciliary defects are not always inherited; acquired forms of ciliary dyskinesia are seen in smokers and patients with bronchitis, viral infections, or other pulmonary diseases.

- Ciliary defects are not always inherited.
- Acquired ciliary defects occur in smokers, in patients with bronchitis, and after viral infections.

Hypogammaglobulinemia

Congenital (or Bruton X-linked) agammaglobulinemia predisposes to recurrent bacterial infections and bronchiectasis. The bacteria that are isolated include *H. influenzae, S. aureus,* and *S. pneumoniae.* Acquired agammaglobulinemia (common variable) may be manifested as sinopulmonary infections in the 2nd or 3rd decade. Selective IgA deficiency is the most common immunoglobulin deficiency; most of these patients are asymptomatic. IgA deficiency is frequently associated with IgG subclass (IgG2 and IgG4) deficiency. Despite the inability to form antibody, most patients have a normal number of circulating B cells, which fail to dedifferentiate into plasma cells that make immunoglobulins. Pulmonary disease occurs more commonly and is more severe than in patients with X-linked agammaglobulinemia. Infections caused by encapsulated bacteria are more common. Bronchiectasis and obstructive airway disease occur in up to 40% of patients. Hyperimmunoglobulinemia E (Job syndrome) is a rare disorder characterized by phagocyte dysfunction, high serum levels of IgE and IgD, and normal IgG, IgA, and IgM. Respiratory complications include sinusitis, pneumonia, and bronchiectasis caused by *S. aureus, S. pneumoniae,* gram-negative bacilli, *Candida albicans,* and *Aspergillus* species, pneumatoceles, and chronic dermatitis.

- The overall incidence of bronchiectasis in hypo/agammaglobulinemia is about 10%.
- Selective IgA deficiency is the most common immunoglobulin deficiency; most of these patients are asymptomatic or minimally symptomatic.
- IgA deficiency is frequently associated with IgG subclass (IgG2 and IgG4) deficiency.

Right Middle Lobe Syndrome

Right middle lobe syndrome is recurrent atelectasis associated with localized bronchiectasis of the right middle lobe. Mechanisms include compression of the middle lobe bronchus by lymph nodes, acute angulation of the origin, narrow opening of the bronchus, lengthy bronchus, and lack of collateral ventilation. CXR usually points to the diagnosis, although many patients are asymptomatic.

- Right middle lobe syndrome: chronic atelectasis and volume loss in the right middle lobe.
- The diagnosis is frequently made as an incidental CXR finding.
- Most patients are asymptomatic.

Allergic Bronchopulmonary Aspergillosis

Central bronchiectasis is present in 85% of patients with this disease at the time of the initial diagnosis and has been used as a diagnostic criterion of the disease. Allergic bronchopulmonary aspergillosis is discussed below with eosinophilic pulmonary diseases.

Yellow Nail Syndrome

This syndrome consists of the triad of 1) yellow to yellow-green discoloration of the nails, with a thickened and curved appearance in all extremities; 2) lymphedema of the lower extremities; and 3) lymphocyte-predominant pleural effusion. Bronchiectasis is seen in about 20% of patients. Some patients have sinusitis. Lymphedema may affect the breasts. Raynaud phenomenon is noted in some patients. Patients may present with chronic and insidious edema of the extremities. Lymphatic hypoplasia or atresia has been proposed as the factor(s). Pleural effusions occur in 35% to 40% of patients, and recurrent pleural effusions are noted in about one-third. Pleural effusions may appear years after the nail changes occur and tend to be bilateral and small-to-moderate in amount. Both exudates and transudates have been described.

- Triad of yellow discoloration of the nails, lymphedema of the lower extremities, and pleural effusion.

Obstructive Azoospermia (Young Syndrome)

Obstructive azoospermia denotes primary infertility in males who have normal spermatozoa in the epididymis but none in the ejaculate. The reason for the relationship between obstructive azoospermia and lung disease is unknown. The following pulmonary abnormalities have been noted: grossly abnormal sinus radiograph (59% of patients), sinusitis (56%), repeated otitis media (32%), chronic bronchitis (35%), abnormal CXR findings (53%), and bronchiectasis (29%).

- Obstructive azoospermia and bronchiectasis.
- Pulmonary and ears-nose-throat symptoms in 30% of patients.

Unilateral Hyperlucent Lung Syndrome (Swyer-James or Macleod Syndrome)

Normally, the diagnosis of this syndrome is an incidental CXR finding. Hyperlucency and hyperinflation of the lung (usually left) are found in conjunction with a small pulmonary artery. Bronchiectasis is seen in 25% of patients, but most patients are asymptomatic. The cause is unknown, but congenital atresia of the pulmonary artery or acquired bronchiolitis soon after birth is postulated.

- Unilateral hyperlucency of the lung, with small ipsilateral pulmonary artery.
- Bronchiectasis in 25%; most patients are asymptomatic.

Miscellaneous Causes and Associations

Nearly 10% of bronchiectatic patients may demonstrate an abnormal α_1-antitrypsin phenotype, with serum levels less than 66% of normal. Other causes and associations include rheumatoid arthritis (Felty syndrome), toxic chemicals, recurrent aspiration, heroin, inflammatory bowel disease, foreign body, sequestrated lung, relapsing polychondritis, chronic tracheoesophageal fistula, heart-lung transplantation, chronic granulomatous disease of childhood, and postobstructive (tumors, long-standing foreign body, stenosis, etc.).

- Uncommon causes of bronchiectasis include α_1-antitrypsin deficiency, Felty syndrome, toxic inhalation, chronic tracheobronchial stenosis.

Complications of Bronchiectasis

Complications include hemoptysis (in 50% of patients), progressive respiratory failure with hypoxemia and cor pulmonale, and secondary infections by fungi and noninfectious mycobacterioses. The presence of these organisms usually represents a saprophytic state, but active infection has to be excluded. The most commonly isolated bacterium in bronchiectasis is *P. aeruginosa*. As in cystic fibrosis, it is impossible to eradicate this bacterium. Patients with bronchiectasis infected by *P. aeruginosa* have more extensive bronchiectasis than those without this infection. Routine culture of respiratory secretions is not warranted for all patients.

- The source of bleeding in bronchiectasis is the bronchial (systemic) circulation; hence, it can be brisk.
- The presence of mycobacteria and fungi may represent saprophytic growth.

Treatment

Treatment of bronchiectasis is aimed at controlling the symptoms and preventing complications. Predisposing conditions should be sought and treated aggressively (gamma globulin injections, removal of foreign body or tumor, control of aspiration, and treatment of infections of paranasal sinuses, gums, and teeth). Postural drainage, chest physiotherapy, humidification, bronchodilators, and cyclic antibiotic therapy are effective in many patients. Surgical treatment is reserved for patients with troublesome symptoms, localized disease, and severe hemoptysis. High-dose inhaled steroid therapy (fluticasone) is reportedly effective in reducing the sputum inflammatory indices in bronchiectasis.

Broncholithiasis

Broncholithiasis results when calcified granulomas within the lung parenchyma (pulmoliths or pneumoliths) erode into the lumen of the tracheobronchial tree. Histoplasma infection is the most common cause of broncholithiasis in the U.S. Symptoms include cough, hemoptysis, wheezing, and postobstructive pneumonia with signs of lung infection. The broncholiths can erode into the esophagus and cause tracheoesophageal fistula. Bronchoscopy is valuable in the diagnosis. Surgery may be necessary to remove the broncholiths.

- Broncholithiasis results from calcified granulomas.
- The most common cause is earlier infection with histoplasma.
- Symptoms: cough, hemoptysis, and wheeze.

Bronchiolitis Obliterans With Organizing Pneumonia

Bronchiolitis obliterans with organizing pneumonia (BOOP) is a nonspecific histologic diagnosis. The main abnormality is the presence of intraluminal fibrosis in the distal airways, alveolar ducts, and perialveolar spaces. This condition is seen in patients with rheumatoid arthritis, systemic lupus erythematosus, polymyositis-dermatomyositis, mixed connective tissue disease, and silo filler's lung and after exposure to noxious gases, bleomycin, amiodarone, cytomegalovirus, influenza virus, bacteria (*Legionella*, *Nocardia*), *Mycoplasma*, *Cryptococcus,* and *Pneumocystis carinii.* BOOP also occurs after heart and bone marrow transplants and in chronic eosinophilic pneumonia and is observed as a secondary phenomenon in Wegener granulomatosis, infarcts, granulomas, and neoplasms. CXR usually shows a patchy and diffuse ground-glass infiltrate or features similar to idiopathic pulmonary fibrosis and chronic eosinophilic pneumonia (peripheral alveolar infiltrate). HRCT may show a "mosaic" pattern (ground-glass infiltrates alternating with areas of hyperinflation). The diagnosis of idiopathic BOOP is one of exclusion. Treatment consists of excluding offending agents and high doses of systemic corticosteroids. Erythromycin can resolve certain types of BOOP.

- BOOP is a nonspecific histologic diagnosis.
- BOOP has many causes.

Sleep Apnea

Apnea is defined as cessation of all airflow at the nose and mouth for 10 seconds or longer. Hypopnea denotes 10 seconds or more of a 50% decrease or greater in airflow with 3% to 4% oxygen desaturation and/or EEG arousal. Sleep apnea syndrome is present if at least 30 episodes of apnea occur during a 7-hour sleep period. *Central sleep apnea* is the cessation of airflow accompanied by an absence of respiratory effort. *Obstructive sleep apnea* is the cessation of airflow with continued respiratory effort. *Mixed apnea* is the cessation of airflow that typically begins with no respiratory effort but ends with increasing respiratory effort. Although most patients referred for evaluation of sleep apnea syndrome have a predominantly obstructive pattern, the mixed type is the most common form. In obstructive sleep apnea, the upper airway obstruction occurs either at the level of the soft palate or posterior to the base of the tongue. The occlusion is exaggerated by a large neck circumference, increased size of the uvula, and pharyngeal mucosal edema (from long-term snoring).

- Central sleep apnea: cessation of airflow accompanied by an absence of respiratory effort.
- Obstructive sleep apnea: cessation of airflow with continued respiratory effort.
- Mixed sleep apnea: cessation of airflow that typically begins with no respiratory effort but ends with increasing respiratory effort.

Obstructive sleep apnea is present in 1% to 2% of the population. Clinical features include sonorous snoring, abnormal motor behavior during sleep, daytime somnolence, personality changes, intellectual deterioration, systemic hypertension, loss of libido, abnormal behavioral outbursts, morning headaches, nightmares, hypnogogic hallucinations/automatic behavior, memory deficit, depression, and nocturnal enuresis. Male sex, older age, obesity, genetic factors, COPD, and use of sedative drugs or alcohol may contribute to or exacerbate obstructive sleep apnea syndrome. It is important to obtain a sleep history from the patient's spouse or relatives. Polysomnography (Fig. 21-27) establishes the diagnosis and is necessary to detect and quantitate obstructive sleep apnea. In obstructive apnea, there is apnea but the thoracoabdominal muscles contract. In comparison, there is no contraction of respiratory muscles in central apnea. Severe oxygen desaturation develops during sleep. Sinus arrhythmia is seen in 90% of patients. Other forms of cardiac arrhythmias include second-degree block, premature ventricular contractions (threefold increase when SaO_2 is <60%), and ventricular tachycardia.

Sleep-disordered breathing in women 70 years or younger is associated with the risk of coronary artery disease (odds ratio 4). The incidence of cerebrovascular disease/accidents is increased in chronic obstructive sleep apnea. There is also a strong association between sleep apnea, as measured by the apnea-hypopnea index, and the risk of traffic accidents.

- Clinical features: sonorous snoring, apneic episodes, and abnormal motor behavior during sleep.
- It is important to obtain a sleep history from a sleep observer.
- Polysomnography is helpful in making the diagnosis and in identifying different types of sleep disorders.

Pulmonary hypertension is episodic in the early stages of significant sleep apnea but can be sustained later on. The site of airway obstruction in obstructive sleep apnea is the oropharynx; here, the tone of the genioglossus muscle and pharyngeal abductors (geniohyoid) decreases, and the resulting pharyngeal collapse produces obstruction. Before polysomnography is performed, patients should have an ears-nose-throat (ENT) examination, thyroid function testing, and PFTs, because similar symptoms are seen in patients with myxedema, ENT abnormalities, and COPD. Sleep apnea is also seen in retrognathia, cordotomy, poliomyelitis, Shy-Drager syndrome, sudden infant death syndrome, adenotonsillar hypertrophy, and severe altitude-related polycythemia.

- The site of airway obstruction in obstructive sleep apnea is the oropharynx.
- Exclude hypothyroidism, ENT causes, narcolepsy, and severe COPD before performing polysomnography.
- COPD can produce disordered breathing, apnea, hypopnea, and periodic breathing.

The treatment of obstructive sleep apnea includes weight loss (in obese patients), nasal constant positive airway pressure

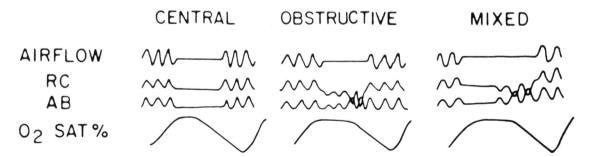

Fig. 21-27. Polysomnography in sleep apnea; airflow is absent in all forms of sleep apnea. Rib cage (RC) and abdominal (AB) movements are absent in central apnea but present in obstructive apnea. (From Strohl KP, Cherniack NS, Gothe B: Physiologic basis of therapy for sleep apnea. Am Rev Respir Dis 134:791-802, 1986. By permission of American Lung Association.)

(CPAP) ventilation, tracheostomy, and uvulopalatopharyngo-plasty. The treatment of choice is nasal CPAP, which produces a pneumatic splinting of the upper airway and increases airway volume and cross-sectional area. Compliance rate with nasal CPAP is 75% to 90%. For patients with predominantly central sleep apnea, respiratory stimulants such as medroxyprogesterone acetate are used. Other drugs used in both obstructive and central sleep apnea include methylphenidate (Ritalin), protriptyline, clonidine (α_2-adrenoreceptor antagonist), and fluoxetine (serotonin antagonist). In severe cases of obstructive apnea with congestive heart failure, polycythemia, bizarre behavior, and cardiac arrhythmias, treatment should include weight loss, treatment of the congestive heart failure, oxygen therapy, and consideration of tracheostomy (if nasal CPAP is ineffective or cannot be used).

- Nasal CPAP is the treatment of choice for obstructive sleep apnea.
- Respiratory stimulants may relieve central sleep apnea.

The pickwickian syndrome accounts for only 5% of all sleep apnea cases. Patients are usually morbidly obese, hypersomnolent, cyanotic, plethoric, and polycythemic. In late stages, right ventricular failure is followed by left ventricular failure. Hypoxemia and hypercarbia are common. The efficiency of respiratory muscles is reduced to 60% to 70% of normal. The upper airway resistance syndrome is a form of sleep-disordered breathing in which repetitive increases in resistance to airflow within the upper airway lead to brief arousals and daytime somnolence.

The upper airway resistance syndrome is a form of sleep-disordered breathing in which repetitive increases in resistance to airflow within the upper airway lead to brief arousals and daytime somnolence. Polysomnographic findings are normal.

- Pickwickian syndrome accounts for only 5% of all sleep apnea cases.

DIFFUSE LUNG DISEASE

Diffuse lung disease usually refers to an infiltrative process affecting most of the segments of both lungs. The term "diffuse lung disease" usually implies interstitial and/or alveolar filling defects. It is the result of injury to structures in the alveolar space, interstitial space, or both. The interstitial space is located between the alveolar lining cells and the capillary endothelium. The interstitium contains reticular and elastic fibers, alveolar interstitial cells (alveolar cells and histiocytes), small lymphocytes, arterioles, and a capillary network.

Pathology

Alveolar cell injury is associated with altered permeability in the alveolocapillary interphase and resultant alveolar exudation, followed by invasion of the alveolar spaces by various cells. This alveolitis produces an "alveolar" infiltrate on CXR. Infiltration of interstitial spaces by mononuclear cells, neutrophils, and other cells (interstitial inflammation) increases the thickness of the pulmonary interstitium. Capillary damage causes increased permeability and edema formation within interstitial spaces or alveolar spaces or both. In chronic cases, deposition of fibrous tissue in the interstitium (interstitial fibrosis) contributes to the interstitial infiltrate seen on CXR.

- Diffuse lung disease can be alveolar or interstitial.

Physiology

Lung volumes generally are decreased in most diffuse lung diseases. TLC, VC, and RV decrease with disease progression. This is commonly referred to as a "restrictive defect." The loss of lung volumes is best correlated with interstitial fibrosis, although it can be markedly low in many alveolar diseases. Early in the disease, lung volumes may be normal. Airflow rates are usually normal until late in the course of the disease, when marked reduction in the volumes can be associated with mildly to moderately reduced flow rates. The static compliance is decreased, but airway resistance is normal. The "stiff lung" increases the work of breathing, and to overcome this, patients typically exhibit rapid, shallow breathing. Exercise-induced hypoxemia and decreased DLCO are the earliest changes to occur. Hypocarbia is common and is due to rapid, shallow breathing. Carbon dioxide retention does not occur until late stages of the disease and is due to "respiratory exhaustion." Carbon dioxide retention is a poor prognostic sign.

- Decreased lung volumes (restrictive pattern).
- Flow rates are near normal.
- Lung compliance is decreased, and elastic recoil is increased.
- DLCO is decreased early in the course.
- Exercise-induced hypoxemia.
- Hypocarbia in early stages; hypercarbia in late disease.

RADIOLOGY

Typical CT findings in diffuse lung diseases are described above. The main abnormalities seen on CXR can be classified into alveolar (air space) and interstitial patterns. Many diseases demonstrate both patterns. The alveolar pattern is limited to a smaller number of diseases, for example, pulmonary edema (cardiogenic and noncardiogenic), alveolar sarcoidosis, uremic lung, intra-alveolar hemorrhage, aspiration pneumonia, pulmonary alveolar (phospholipo)proteinosis, certain bacterial pneumonias, desquamative pneumonia, certain viral and protozoal pneumonias, diffuse alveolar cell carcinoma, and diffuse pulmonary lymphoma.

● The alveolar pattern is seen in most entities that include the word "alveolar."

Alveolar infiltrates are seen in pulmonary edema, hematogenous metastases, acute respiratory distress syndrome, noxious gas exposure, alveolar hemorrhage syndromes, diffuse alveolar cell carcinoma, pulmonary alveolar phospholipoproteinosis, desquamative interstitial pneumonitis, early rheumatoid lung disease, amyloidosis, and alveolar microlithiasis.

● Pulmonary edema is the most common cause of the alveolar pattern.

Because the interstitial pattern includes many diseases, it is convenient to group them into the following categories: idiopathic pulmonary fibrosis, systemic diseases (e.g., rheumatologic diseases), occupational lung diseases (including pneumoconioses and toxic exposures), drug-induced lung diseases (including radiation pneumonitis), granulomatous lung diseases (sarcoidosis, etc.), lymphangitic pulmonary metastasis, chronic mycotic and mycobacterial infections, unusual diseases (pulmonary Langerhans cell granuloma, lymphangioleiomyomatosis, and tuberous sclerosis), and others (chronic bronchiectasis, cystic fibrosis, etc.).

● Grouping of interstitial pattern diseases is helpful in considering the differential diagnosis.
● Lymphangitic lung metastasis is an important cause of interstitial lung disease.

The combination of alveolar-interstitial patterns and diffuse micronodular changes is also common. The anatomical distribution of the infiltrates is an important clinical consideration because certain diseases predominantly affect the upper lung zones. Other diseases may involve lower zones. These entities may produce an interstitial, alveolar, or a combination alveolar-interstitial pattern on CXR.

● Bilateral upper lobe process: silicosis, coal workers' pneumoconiosis, sarcoidosis, mycoses, mycobacterioses, cystic fibrosis, pulmonary Langerhans cell granuloma (histiocytosis X), and pulmonary lymphangioleiomyomatosis.

Classification of Diffuse Pulmonary Diseases

Many of the diffuse pulmonary processes are classified on the basis of morphological features. Many of the diffuse pulmonary diseases have identical clinical and pathophysiologic features; yet, they are classified by different terms and abbreviations. The number of abbreviations used to describe these (see below) has resulted in significant confusion for practicing physicians; the abbreviations are listed in Table 21-6.

Idiopathic Pulmonary Fibrosis

Idiopathic pulmonary fibrosis is the most common cause of chronic diffuse interstitial lung disease. Hepatitis C virus infection, silent gastroesophageal reflux, and environmental exposures have been implicated in the etiology. The diagnosis is based on clinical features, namely, a gradually progressive interstitial process (CXR typically shows a bibasilar interstitial process that eventually spreads upward), progressive dyspnea, clubbing (>70% of patients; clubbing is more common in men than in women [54% vs 40%]), Velcro crackles, positive rheumatoid factor (30% of patients), antinuclear antibody (35%), or polyclonal gammopathy (>50%). HRCT shows

Table 21-6.—Abbreviations Used in the Literature to Describe Diffuse Pulmonary Diseases

BIP	Bronchiolitis-interstitial pneumonitis (a form of bronchiolitis obliterans with organizing pneumonia)
BOOP*	Bronchiolitis obliterans with organizing pneumonia
CIPF	Classic interstitial pneumonitis-fibrosis
DAD*	Diffuse alveolar damage (as in adult respiratory distress syndrome)
DIP	Desquamative interstitial pneumonitis (thought to predispose to idiopathic pulmonary fibrosis)
GIP	Giant cell interstitial pneumonitis (very rare)
HRS	Hamman-Rich syndrome
IAF	Idiopathic alveolar fibrosis (same as idiopathic pulmonary fibrosis)
IPF*	Idiopathic pulmonary fibrosis
LIP*	Lymphocytic interstitial pneumonitis (many causes)
NSIP*	Nonspecific interstitial pneumonitis
PIP	Plasma cell interstitial pneumonitis (uncommon)
RAD	Regional alveolar damage
UIP	Usual interstitial pneumonitis (an earlier term for idiopathic pulmonary fibrosis)

*For clinical purposes, these entities are important because they constitute >90% of all the above.

subpleural honeycombing and an interstitial process in the basal areas. Mild mediastinal and hilar lymphadenopathy can be seen. PFTs show restrictive pulmonary dysfunction, low diffusing capacity, hypoxemia worsened by exercise, and hypocapnia. Other causes (see below) of an interstitial process should be excluded. Lung biopsy shows nonspecific interstitial fibrosis without granuloma formation. The response is poor to corticosteroids, colchicine, and immunosuppressive drugs (<20% of patients show measurable improvement). A preliminary study has observed substantial improvements after 12 months of treatment with interferon beta-1b plus prednisolone in patients who had no response to glucocorticoids alone (NEJM 341:1264-1269, 1999). Hypoxemic patients benefit from supplemental oxygen. Lung transplantation is an option. Gradual progression leads to cor pulmonale. Idiopathic pulmonary fibrosis is predominantly a disease of elderly patients and has a poor prognosis. The 5-year survival rate is less than 30%.

- Idiopathic pulmonary fibrosis: clubbing, Velcro crackles, and abnormal immunologic findings (rheumatoid factor, antinuclear antibody).
- Restrictive lung dysfunction.
- Hypoxemia, low diffusing capacity, and hypocapnia.
- Poor response to corticosteroids and other agents.

Differential Diagnosis of Idiopathic Pulmonary Fibrosis

Many disease entities can produce nonspecific lung fibrosis, and at times, it is difficult to differentiate idiopathic pulmonary fibrosis from these diseases. Important ones to consider in this group are rheumatoid lung, scleroderma lung, late stages of sarcoidosis, certain drug-induced lung diseases (e.g., nitrofurantoin), radiation pneumonitis, end-stage hypersensitivity pneumonitis, certain pneumoconioses (asbestos), noxious gases, paraquat, recurrent pulmonary edema, end-stage pulmonary Langerhans cell granuloma, end-stage cystic fibrosis and bronchiectasis, chronic aspiration pneumonia, and recurrent intra-alveolar hemorrhage (e.g., mitral stenosis, pulmonary hemosiderosis, and Goodpasture syndrome). Nonspecific interstitial pneumonia/fibrosis is a subclass of idiopathic interstitial lung diseases. Radiologically, patchy areas of interstitial infiltrates distinct from usual, desquamative, and acute interstitial pneumonia are seen. Nonspecific interstitial pneumonia/fibrosis can be caused by many disorders, including collagen diseases.

- Rheumatoid lung and scleroderma lung can mimic idiopathic pulmonary fibrosis.
- Any end-stage diffuse lung disease can mimic idiopathic pulmonary fibrosis.

Sarcoidosis

Sarcoidosis is a multisystemic granulomatous disease of unknown cause that affects persons in the 25- to 45-year age group. It is characterized by widespread noncaseous epithelioid cell granulomas, depression of delayed type hypersensitivity and a decreased number of T lymphocytes, and proliferation of B lymphocytes. IL-2 receptor concentrations (CD25+) are increased in peripheral blood and bronchoalveolar lavage specimens. Granulomas contain CD4+ T lymphocytes, with few CD8+ T lymphocytes present. The epithelioid cells in the granulomas synthesize ACE. Interleukin 1, tumor necrosis factor (TNF)-alpha, and interferon gamma (IFN-gamma) are present in bronchoalveolar lavage and lung parenchyma, but their role in the disease is unknown.

- Sarcoidosis: multisystemic disease.
- Diminished number of T lymphocytes and increased number of B lymphocytes.

Other granulomatous diseases with noncaseous granulomas are mycobacterioses (noncaseous in early stages), leprosy, mycoses, syphilis, mononucleosis, carcinoma, silicosis, hypersensitivity pneumonitis, zirconium, berylliosis, talcosis, Bakelite exposure, Crohn ileitis, primary biliary cirrhosis, cat-scratch disease, foreign-body granulomas, hypogammaglobulinemia, and granulomatous arteritis.

- The presence of noncaseous granuloma by itself is not diagnostic of sarcoidosis.

Clinical Staging

Clinical staging of sarcoidosis is based on CXR findings rather than clinical severity, even though the CXR changes roughly parallel the clinical disease. Five types (formerly known as stages) of disease are seen. Type 0: normal CXR findings, with noncaseous granulomas in other sites (e.g., conjunctiva, liver, lymphoid tissue). Type I: bilateral hilar and paratracheal lymphadenopathy (40%-50% of all patients, erythema nodosum in 3%-30%, iridocyclitis in 5%-8%). Type II: bilateral hilar and paratracheal lymphadenopathy, with pulmonary parenchymal involvement (40%-50% of patients). Type III: diffuse pulmonary parenchymal disease without lymphadenopathy (14%-16% of patients). Type IV: end-stage pulmonary fibrosis with bullous changes (<5% of patients).

- Bilateral hilar lymphadenopathy is seen in sarcoidosis, Hodgkin and non-Hodgkin lymphoma, metastatic carcinoma, histoplasmosis, coccidioidomycosis, tuberculosis, berylliosis, etc.
- Most diseases that produce noncaseous granulomas also produce hilar lymphadenopathy.

Clinical Features

Intrathoracic disease is present in 90% of patients, but almost all organs can be involved. Initial complaints are lymphadenopathy (8%-70% of patients), cough (30%), dyspnea (28%), weight loss (20%-28%), fatigue (20%-27%), skin lesions (14%-25%), visual complaints (10%-21%), and fever (10%-15%). Asymptomatic disease is seen in 12% to 34% of the patients. Generalized lymphadenopathy occurs in 25% of patients, skin (lupus pernio, nodules) excluding erythema nodosum in 25%, eyes (lacrimal enlargement, corneal band opacities, iridocyclitis, glaucoma, and choroidoretinitis) in 25%, liver involvement in 25%, splenomegaly in 14%, endobronchial involvement in 11% (occurs in >50% of blacks), central nervous system involvement (paralysis of seventh cranial nerve, chronic meningitis, hypopituitarism) in 7%, bone cysts in 6%, and kidney involvement in 5%. Other manifestations include salivary gland involvement (uveoparotid fever, or Heerfordt syndrome) in 6%, nasal mucosal lesions, keloid in areas of surgical scars, diffuse arthralgias of small joints, heart (arrhythmias) in 5%, persistent violaceous skin plaques, transient vesicular eruptions on fingers, and persistent scars of old trauma on the knees.

- Almost any organ can be affected by sarcoidosis.
- Band keratopathy, lupus pernio.
- Cystic bone lesions in terminal phalanges.
- Cranial nerve VII involvement.

Laboratory Tests

Complete or partial anergy to skin tests (PPD and others) is seen in 60% of patients. Increased CD4/CD8 ratio, high serum level of antibodies to viruses (Epstein-Barr virus, rubella, parainfluenza, herpes simplex), autoantibodies to rheumatoid factor, and antinuclear antibody are the other findings. Hypercalcemia results from increased sensitivity to vitamin D and increased gastrointestinal tract absorption of calcium (15% of patients). Other findings include hypercalciuria in 40% of patients and increased IgG (50%), IgA (25%), IgM (12%), and alkaline phosphatase (15%). Serum levels of ACE are applicable only to adults (>20 years), because children and teenagers have high and widely variable levels. Nearly 80% of patients with active sarcoidosis have increased serum levels of ACE (in comparison, serum levels of ACE are increased in 5% of normal subjects). Changes in levels may correspond to the activity of sarcoidosis. Some physicians use serum levels of ACE to monitor disease activity. Increased serum ACE levels occur in primary biliary cirrhosis, Gaucher disease, leprosy, atypical mycobacteriosis, miliary tuberculosis, acute histoplasmosis, silicosis, and histiocytic lymphoma.

- Negative PPD in 60% of patients (suppression of T lymphocytes).

- Increased antibodies to viruses and hyperglobulinemia (increase in B lymphocytes).
- Serum levels of ACE are increased in 70%-80% of patients.
- Increased ACE levels do not establish the diagnosis of sarcoidosis.
- ACE serum levels are also increased in other diseases.

Biopsy

Noncaseous granulomas can be identified in nearly 100% of biopsy specimens from mediastinal nodes, lung, nasal mucosal lesions, and subcutaneous nodules. Diagnostic rates of 80% to 90% can be obtained from biopsy specimens of skin lesions, palpable scalene nodes, bronchial lesions, conjunctival lesions, and liver. Diagnostic accuracy decreases to less than 65% with biopsy specimens from bone marrow, scalene fat pad, and normal-appearing bronchial mucosa.

- Biopsy of involved organs provides a high diagnostic rate.
- Common areas for biopsy: mediastinal nodes, lung, and tracheobronchial mucosa.
- Noncaseous granuloma is not diagnostic of sarcoidosis.
- It is important to culture biopsy specimens to exclude infectious causes of noncaseous granuloma.

Treatment

Systemic corticosteroids (prednisone 1 mg/kg daily initially; alternate days later on for 9-12 months) are indicated in progressive or symptomatic type II and type III disease, ocular sarcoidosis, persistent hypercalcemia or calciuria, progressive or disfiguring skin lesions, neurosarcoidosis, myocardial sarcoidosis, and progressive systemic disease. Second-line medications have included azathioprine, methotrexate, cyclosporine, and pentoxifylline. Patients with sarcoidosis are sensitive to vitamin D (increased absorption of calcium from the small intestine). The active form of vitamin D is produced at sites of sarcoid granulomas.

- Systemic corticosteroids for progressive or symptomatic type II and type III disease.
- Avoid vitamin D and calcium supplements.

Lymphocytic Interstitial Pneumonitis

The diagnosis of lymphocytic interstitial pneumonitis is based on the demonstration of diffuse interstitial infiltration by lymphocytes in lung biopsy specimens. Lymphocytic interstitial pneumonitis may result from Hodgkin lymphoma, non-Hodgkin lymphoma, early lymphomatoid granulomatosis, chronic lymphocytic leukemia, Waldenström macroglobulinemia, angioimmunoblastic lymphadenopathy, Sézary syndrome, pseudolymphoma, AIDS, graft-versus-host disease, and congenital agammaglobulinemia. Idiopathic lymphocytic interstitial pneumonitis is a diagnosis of exclusion, although the current understanding is that almost all cases of the disease represent low-grade B-cell lymphoma.

- Most lymphoproliferative diseases can produce lymphocytic interstitial pneumonitis.
- Lymphocytic interstitial pneumonitis is a complication in AIDS.
- Most cases of lymphocytic interstitial pneumonitis represent low-grade B-cell lymphoma.

Eosinophilic Pulmonary Diseases (PIE Syndromes)

Eosinophilic pulmonary diseases, also known as "pulmonary infiltrates with eosinophilia (PIE) syndromes," are a heterogeneous group of disorders, except for the presence of CXR abnormality and peripheral blood eosinophilia. The presence of eosinophils in the peripheral blood may provide a clue to the diagnosis if clinical circumstances are suggestive of a PIE syndrome. Lung biopsy or bronchoalveolar lavage are seldom needed to document the diagnosis. Almost all entities under the classification of PIE syndrome require systemic corticosteroid therapy for prolonged periods. The following is a classification of PIE syndromes.

Asthma

Asthma is the most common cause of PIE syndrome. Eosinophilic bronchitis is characteristic of typical asthmatic episodes. The pulmonary infiltrate is usually caused by lung infection, and the eosinophilia results from exacerbation of asthma. The eosinophil count is usually 15% to 20%. Peripheral blood and bronchoalveolar lavage eosinophil counts correlate with the degree of airflow obstruction. Appropriate therapy for infection and asthma produces complete resolution. However, systemic corticosteroid therapy is indicated in many patients.

- Asthma is the most common cause of PIE syndrome.

Simple Pulmonary Eosinophilia

Simple pulmonary eosinophilia, also known as "Löffler syndrome," is characterized by migratory peripheral (subpleural) pulmonary infiltrates (alveolar or interstitial or combined), peripheral eosinophilia, and minimal or no respiratory symptoms. In the original series, most patients had parasitic infections. The diagnosis of Löffler syndrome requires the exclusion of parasitic infection and drug reaction. The prognosis is excellent.

- One-third of patients have no identifiable cause.
- Should exclude parasitic infection or drug reaction.

Allergic Bronchopulmonary Aspergillosis

Allergic bronchopulmonary aspergillosis is often difficult to distinguish from the above, but the eosinophilia is more severe (30%) and longer lasting. The overall prevalence is 6%. More than 95% of patients have extrinsic asthma, and the disease develops in 10% of patients with extrinsic asthma. Asthma previously under control that becomes refractory to treatment with nonsteroidal bronchodilators, expectoration of brownish mucus plugs, segmental atelectasis, and increasing eosinophilia and serum IgE are indicators of allergic bronchopulmonary aspergillosis. Allergic bronchopulmonary aspergillosis also occurs in about 10% of patients with cystic fibrosis. The disease is caused by both IgG- and IgE-mediated immune responses directed at *Aspergillus* species. Type I (bronchospasm), type III (pulmonary destructive changes), and type IV (parenchymal granuloma and mononuclear cell infiltrates) reactions are involved. The major criteria are asthma, blood eosinophilia greater than 1,000/mm^3, immediate skin reactivity (type I reaction—IgE dependent) to *Aspergillus* antigen, IgG antibodies (type III reaction) to *Aspergillus* antigens, high IgE titer (>1,000 ng/mL), transient or fixed pulmonary infiltrates, and central bronchiectasis (seen in 85% of patients). A normal IgE level in a symptomatic patient virtually excludes allergic bronchopulmonary aspergillosis. Minor criteria include the presence of *Aspergillus* in sputum, expectoration of brownish mucus plugs, and late-phase (Arthus) skin test reactivity to *Aspergillus* antigen. CXR shows fleeting infiltrates ("gloved finger" sign, "tramtrack line" lesions, and "toothpaste shadows") in 85% of patients, mucoid impaction in 15% to 40%, atelectasis, and central bronchiectasis. Although generally associated with *Aspergillus fumigatus*, allergic bronchopulmonary mycosis can be caused by *Candida albicans*, *Aspergillus terreus*, *Curvularia lunata*, *Helminthosporium* species, and *Stemphyllium lanuginosum*. Systemic corticosteroid therapy for more than 6 months is required for most patients.

- Allergic bronchopulmonary aspergillosis; almost always in patients with extrinsic asthma.
- May develop in 10% of patients with cystic fibrosis.
- Types I, III, and IV immune reactions may be involved.
- An increased IgE level is the most useful laboratory test.
- Presence of *A. fumigatus* is only a minor criterion for the diagnosis.
- Therapy consists of long-term systemic corticosteroids.

Acute Eosinophilic Pneumonia

Acute eosinophilic pneumonia is relatively uncommon and characterized by an acute febrile illness of less than 5 days' duration; hypoxemic respiratory failure; diffuse alveolar or mixed alveolar-interstitial infiltrates; bronchoalveolar lavage eosinophilia (>25% of patients); absence of parasitic, fungal, or other infection; and prompt and complete response to corticosteroid therapy. Many patients require mechanical ventilatory support. Bilateral pleural effusions are common. The cause is unknown. Treatment consists of systemic corticosteroids.

- Adult respiratory distress syndrome, with fever, diffuse infiltrates, and eosinophilia.
- No recurrence after corticosteroid therapy.

Chronic Eosinophilic Pneumonia

More than 50% of patients have asthma of less than 5 years' duration. The female-to-male ratio is 2:1, and the median age is 50 years. The onset is insidious, and the duration of symptoms before the diagnosis is made is 7 months. Symptoms include cough (90% of patients), fever (85%), dyspnea (60%), wheezing (35%), and weight loss (56%). Patients may present with severe respiratory distress, fever, and very high peripheral (>40%) and tissue eosinophilia. IgE levels are increased in 65% of patients. The ESR is high in most patients. CXR usually shows peripheral alveolar infiltrates ("negative image of pulmonary edema"). CT of the lungs shows groundglass type of peripheral infiltrates. The pathologic features include tissue eosinophilia and BOOP. Obstructive airways disease can occur in some patients. Biopsy is not required in most cases. Chronic eosinophilic pneumonia is a serious illness that requires long-term corticosteroid therapy. Recurrences are common if corticosteroid therapy is less than 6 months.

- Chronic eosinophilic pneumonia: chronic illness of middle-aged patients (female:male = 2:1).
- May present as adult respiratory distress syndrome, with fever and high ESR.
- CXR: "negative" image of pulmonary edema.

Churg-Strauss Syndrome

Churg-Strauss syndrome is an uncommon vasculitis that is also known as "allergic angiitis-granulomatosis." Most patients have significant asthma. The eosinophil count is high (>50%). (See discussion below.)

Parasitic Infections

Almost all parasitic infections encountered in the tropics are known to cause PIE. The PIE syndromes from parasites are considered distinct from the PIE syndromes caused by tropical eosinophilia (see below). In the U.S., the most commonly encountered parasites are *Ascaris lumbricoides, Ascaris suum, Strongyloides stercoralis, Necator americanus, Entamoeba histolytica,* and *Toxocara canis.* The clinical features of strongyloidosis include peripheral blood eosinophilia, skin rash, and transient lung infiltrates. Pulmonary infiltrates occur before ova can be detected in the stool. Chronic, recurrent strongyloidosis can last for several years. Ascariasis produces skin rash, nonproductive cough, chest pain, and, occasionally, hemoptysis. CXR shows bilateral discrete densities several centimeters large in perihilar regions. Respiratory symptoms resolve over 8 to 10 days. *Toxocara* causes visceral larva migrans.

- In the U.S.: strongyloidosis, ascariasis, and *Toxocara* infection are common causes of PIE syndrome.
- Skin rash, eosinophilia, and patchy lung infiltrates.

Drug Reactions

Many drugs can cause PIE syndrome. The important ones include sulfasalazine, nitrofurantoin, aspirin, ampicillin, cromolyn, ibuprofen, iodinated contrast dye, methotrexate, minocycline, naproxen, aminosalicylate (para-aminosalicylic acid), penicillin, inhaled pentamidine, phenytoin, sulindac, tamoxifen, tetracycline, desipramine, clofibrate, chlorpromazine, bleomycin, mesalazine, trazodone, and interleukin-2. Many other drugs also reportedly cause PIE syndrome.

- Drug-induced PIE syndromes are clinically important.

Neoplasms

Pulmonary neoplasms (adenocarcinoma, lymphoma, and other tumors) are associated with peripheral eosinophilia. The mechanism is unknown, although an eosinophilic chemotactic factor secreted by the tumors is thought to be responsible.

- Pulmonary neoplasms may be associated with peripheral eosinophilia.

Tropical Eosinophilia

The cause of tropical eosinophilia is unclear, although parasitic infestation (filariasis) from *Wuchereria bancrofti* and *Brugia malayi* most likely are responsible. Microfilariae have been identified in lung sections surrounded by eosinophils. Repeated laboratory examinations may be required to rule out parasitic infection as the cause of a PIE syndrome. Symptoms include nocturnal cough, dyspnea, wheezing, fever, weight loss, and malaise. An asthma-like illness develops in many patients. Eosinophil counts range from 20% to 50%. CXR may be normal or show diffuse reticulonodular infiltrates. Diethylcarbamazine citrate (Hetrazan) is the drug of choice.

- Tropical eosinophilia: very high eosinophilia.
- Diethylcarbamazine citrate is the drug of choice.

Hypereosinophilic Syndrome

Idiopathic hypereosinophilic syndrome is a rare and often fatal disease of unknown cause manifested by peripheral eosinophilia greater than 1,500/μL for more than 6 months, absence of obvious reasons for eosinophilia, and signs of end-organ damage related directly to the eosinophilia. Most patients are in their 3rd or 4th decade, and the male-to-female ratio is 7:1. Symptoms include cough, fever, weight loss, night sweats, anorexia, and pruritus. The leukocyte count is usually greater than 10,000/μL, with eosinophil counts of 30% to 70%. The lung is involved in 40% of patients, and CXR shows interstitial nodular infiltrates, with pleural effusions in 50% of patients. BAL may reveal more than 70% eosinophils. Pulmonary fibrosis may develop in chronic cases. Other serious complications include endomyocardial fibrosis, restrictive cardiomyopathy, mural thrombus formation, arterial thromboembolic disease, deep venous thrombosis, cerebrovascular lesions, and peripheral neuropathy.

- Hypereosinophilic syndrome: very high eosinophilia in men in their 3rd or 4th decade.
- Lung involvement in 40% of patients.
- Cardiac involvement is the most serious complication.

Bronchocentric Granulomatosis

Bronchocentric granulomatosis is not a well-defined syndrome. Surgical biopsy is required for diagnosis. Histologically, there is granulomatous and necrotizing replacement of the bronchial epithelium. It is a diagnosis of exclusion because similar pathologic features can be encountered in Wegener granulomatosis, fungal and mycobacterial infections, aspiration, and rheumatoid lung disease. One-third of patients have tissue eosinophilia and tend to have asthma, peripheral eosinophilia, and positive sputum cultures for *Aspergillus* species. CXR may show nodular masses (60%) or pneumonic infiltrates (20%). Upper lobe and unilateral involvement is more common. Corticosteroids and cyclophosphamide have been tried.

- Bronchocentric granulomatosis: an ill-defined clinical entity; a diagnosis of exclusion.
- One-third of patients have asthma and eosinophilia.

Pulmonary Langerhans Cell Granuloma

Pulmonary Langerhans cell granuloma (pulmonary eosinophilic granuloma, or histiocytosis X) results from an abnormal proliferation of histiocytes. Pulmonary Langerhans cell granuloma is uncommon, and only about 1,500 cases have been reported. Most (>95%) of the patients are smokers. It is more frequent in whites (it is rare in blacks). Nearly 30% of the patients have nonspecific symptoms: fatigue, fever, and weight loss. Dyspnea is observed in 40% of patients and may

result from a spontaneous pneumothorax or an osteolytic rib lesion. Physical findings are unhelpful in diagnosis. PFTs show a restrictive type defect, with decreased lung volumes, normal flow rates, and decreased diffusing capacity. It is usual to see good pulmonary function even when CXR reveals extensive abnormalities. HRCT of the chest shows characteristic cystic, nodular changes. As the disease progresses, fibrosis replaces the granulomatous process, with formation of characteristic honeycomb cysts. Typically, the involvement is diffuse, bilateral, and most pronounced in the upper two-thirds of the lung fields. Spontaneous resolution is seen in a significant number of patients. In progressive disease, corticosteroids and *Vinca* alkaloid derivatives have been used.

- Pulmonary Langerhans cell granuloma: more than 95% of the patients are smokers.
- It commonly is limited to the lungs or bones or both.
- Spontaneous pneumothorax (in 25%) may be the presenting symptom.
- Young patient with spontaneous pneumothorax and honeycomb changes on CXR.

Pulmonary Alveolar Phospholipoproteinosis

Pulmonary alveolar phospholipoproteinosis, a rare disease of unknown cause, affects mostly young adults. It is more common in smokers. The male-to-female ratio is 3:1. The alveoli contain a strongly periodic acid-Schiff (PAS)-positive granular eosinophilic material. The alveolar material is made up of dipalmitoyl lecithin (surfactant). Similar pathologic features are found in patients with silica exposure, mycobacterial infections, fungal infections, leukemia, or pneumocystis infection. The pathogenesis is likely related to excessive production of surfactant and/or diminished clearance of surfactant by alveolar macrophages. Clinically, an initial febrile episode is followed (after an interval of weeks to months) by progressive dyspnea with productive cough, low-grade fever, chest pain, and weight loss. CXR shows an alveolar filling defect in the lower two-thirds of the lung field. Infections by *Nocardia* occur with a higher frequency. A restrictive pattern seen on PFTs in combination with decreased diffusing capacity is typical. BAL and/or lung biopsy may be needed to make the diagnosis. CXR features resemble those of pulmonary edema, but the costophrenic angles are spared. Spontaneous resolution occurs in one-third of patients. Treatment of symptomatic patients consists of whole lung lavage to remove the intra-alveolar material. Granulocyte-macrophage colony stimulating factor has been used in isolated cases to treat pulmonary alveolar phospholipoproteinosis.

- Pulmonary alveolar phospholipoproteinosis: most patients are smokers.

- Bilateral alveolar infiltrates; costophrenic angles spared.
- Increased incidence of *Nocardia* lung infection.
- Treatment: therapeutic whole lung lavage.

Pulmonary Alveolar Microlithiasis

Pulmonary alveolar microlithiasis is a rare, often familial (autosomal recessive) disorder of unknown cause. Siblings are commonly affected in familial cases. CXR is characterized by fine, sand-like mottling distributed uniformly through both lungs and extensive intra-alveolar deposition of calcium bodies. Patients are relatively asymptomatic, but cor pulmonale may occur. Most patients are between 30 and 50 years old, with an equal male-to-female ratio. Dyspnea is a major complaint in advanced cases, but most patients are asymptomatic. There is no known therapy.

- Pulmonary alveolar microlithiasis: fine, well-defined, sand-like infiltrates (due to calcispherites) on CXR.
- No known cause or treatment.

Lymphangioleiomyomatosis

Lymphangioleiomyomatosis is an uncommon progressive disorder of women of childbearing age. It is characterized by nodular and diffuse interstitial proliferation of the smooth muscle in the lungs, lymph nodes, and thoracic duct. Dyspnea (in >80%) of patients, hemoptysis, and spontaneous pneumothorax (in >50%) are common. Common extrapulmonary features are retroperitoneal adenopathy (in >75%) and renal angiomyolipomas (in 60%). Two-thirds of the patients have chylous pleural effusion, and chylous ascites may develop in many of them because of obstruction of the thoracic duct. CXR may show diffuse nodular-interstitial infiltrates with multiple small cystic areas. HRCT of the chest is characteristic (cystic spaces). The most common abnormalities on PFTs are decreased DLCO (>80% of patients), hypoxemia (>50%), and airway obstruction (>50%). Rapidly progressive airway disease occurs in a significant number of patients. This condition is thought to be a forme fruste of tuberous sclerosis (see below). Treatment includes hormonal therapy, oophorectomy, and lung transplantation.

- Lymphangioleiomyomatosis: women of childbearing age with recurrent pneumothorax, chylous effusion, doughy abdomen, and hemoptysis.
- Obstructive pattern on PFTs, with low diffusing capacity, hypoxemia.
- Hyperinflated lungs with reticulonodular/nodular infiltrates.

Tuberous Sclerosis

Tuberous sclerosis, an inherited disease of mesodermal development, is characterized by epilepsy, mental retardation, congenital tumors, and malformations of the brain, skin, and viscera. Pulmonary involvement occurs in a small number (≤8%) of patients, most of whom are women. The onset of the respiratory symptoms is between the ages of 18 and 34 years. Pulmonary pathologic features, CXR findings, and pulmonary function abnormalities are similar to those in lymphangioleiomyomatosis. Spontaneous pneumothorax is common. Pulmonary tuberous sclerosis is usually accompanied by the involvement of other organs.

- Tuberous sclerosis is identical to lymphangioleiomyomatosis.

Several diseases reveal diffuse interstitial/alveolar/nodular changes on CXR, but PFTs show an obstructive pattern instead of a restrictive one. Examples include pulmonary lymphangioleiomyomatosis, pulmonary Langerhans cell granuloma, tuberous sclerosis, cystic fibrosis, bronchiectasis, sarcoidosis with endobronchial involvement, and rheumatoid lung.

Neurofibromatosis

Neurofibromatosis is a relatively common disease of dominant inheritance. It is manifested clinically by café-au-lait spots, freckling, and neurofibromas of the skin and internal organs. Pulmonary fibrosis is seen in ≤10% of patients. The interstitial fibrosis is usually seen in the basal areas of the lungs, whereas the bullous lesions occur in the apical areas. Clinical manifestations are mild, usually consisting of only exertional dyspnea, but a restrictive pattern on PFTs and decreased diffusing capacity may be observed. Intrathoracic neurofibromas and meningoceles may occur. Pulmonary manifestations become evident in adulthood.

- Neurofibromatosis: a common disease of dominant inheritance.
- Pulmonary fibrosis, bullous lung disease, and intrathoracic meningiomas.

Hereditary Hemorrhagic Telangiectasia (Osler-Weber-Rendu Disease)

Hereditary hemorrhagic telangiectasia is an inherited (autosomal dominant) disorder characterized by telangiectasia of the skin and mucous membranes and intermittent bleeding from vascular abnormalities. About 20% of the patients develop pulmonary arteriovenous malformations/fistulas, usually located in the lower lobes and multiple in one-third of the patients. Most arteriovenous malformations are diagnosed in the 3rd and 4th decades of life; the male-to-female ratio is 1:2. Dyspnea is present in nearly 60% of patients, but hemoptysis is the most common presenting symptom, noted in 15%. Clubbing and pulmonary bruit are present in 35% and 50% of patients, respectively, and cyanosis is observed in 30%. Catheterization studies show a decreased PaO_2 and SaO_2 but normal pulmonary artery pressure. On CXR, the arteriovenous malformations appear as oval or round homogeneous nodular lesions, from a few millimeters to several centimeters in diameter. Tomograms of the lesion usually disclose an artery entering the fistula and a vein leaving it. Pulmonary angiography confirms the diagnosis in virtually all patients. The symptoms depend on the degree of shunting. Paradoxic embolism is a potential complication. Central nervous system symptoms related to paradoxic embolic phenomenon are present in more than 30% of patients. In almost all cases, therapeutic embolization or surgical resection of the malformation is recommended.

- Hereditary hemorrhagic telangiectasia: pulmonary arteriovenous malformation is seen in 20% of patients.
- Symptoms depend on the degree of right-to-left shunt.
- Paradoxic embolism causes neurologic complications in 30% of patients.

Marfan Syndrome

Marfan syndrome is a heritable, generalized disorder of connective tissue. Pulmonary abnormalities are seen in about 10% of the patients in the form of emphysema, bullous disease, generalized honeycombing, spontaneous pneumothorax (most common pulmonary complication, seen in 5% of patients), upper lobe fibrosis, or bronchiectasis. Spontaneous pneumothorax and bullae are causally related to Marfan syndrome. Obstructive sleep apnea occurs with a higher prevalence in patients with Marfan syndrome than in the general population.

- Marfan syndrome: bullous lung disease.
- Spontaneous pneumothorax in 5% of patients.

OCCUPATIONAL LUNG DISEASES

Asbestos

Prolonged exposure to asbestos fibers may cause parietal pleural plaques, pleural thickening, pleural effusions, pulmonary fibrosis (asbestosis), malignant mesothelioma (both pleural and peritoneal), gastrointestinal cancer, or laryngeal carcinoma. The interval between exposure and increase in the number of deaths is 15 to 35 years for bronchogenic carcinoma and 30 to 40 years for malignant mesothelioma. The annual death rate from malignant mesothelioma is 1,200 (smoking has no effect on the death rate in this group) and 100 deaths from asbestosis (smokers have 3 times a higher death rate).

- The majority of asbestos-related deaths are due to bronchogenic carcinoma.
- Prolonged exposure is necessary to develop asbestos-induced malignant mesothelioma.

Pleural plaque (hyalinosis simplex) is the most common asbestos-related thoracic disorder. Anthophyllite appears to be the most potent form of asbestos in the etiology of plaques. It usually represents exposure that occurred more than 20 years earlier. It is not precancerous, but it tends to progress and to calcify over a long period (with 20-30 years' exposure, 10% of patients have calcification and with >40 years, 60% have calcification). The disease is bilateral and symmetrical and occurs along the path of the ribs. In one-third of patients, it is associated with asbestosis (see below).

- Pleural plaque is the most common asbestos-related disorder.
- It is not precancerous.
- Calcified diaphragmatic pleura on CXR is almost always diagnostic of asbestos (other causes include ankylosing spondylitis and old tuberculous pleurisy).

Thickened pleura (hyalinosis complicata) is an uncommon complication. Progressive calcification involves both the visceral and parietal pleurae, the lung apices, and the pericardium. A recurrent acute inflammatory phase is associated with fever and exudative pleural effusion. Restrictive disease can lead to cor pulmonale.

- Uncommon; painful.

Pleural effusion may occur with asbestosis, hyalinosis complicata, and malignant mesothelioma. It is always an exudate, unilateral or bilateral or recurrent, and bloody in 70% of patients. Malignant mesothelioma has to be excluded.

- Bloody effusion; recurrent, unilateral or bilateral.
- It is difficult to differentiate from malignant mesothelioma.

Asbestosis represents pulmonary fibrosis as well as fibrosis of the visceral pleura. Progressive fibrosis and honeycombing can lead to cor pulmonale. Progressive massive fibrosis is a complication. The pathogenesis is unknown, but many patients exhibit rheumatoid factor and antinuclear antibody in the sera, presumably the result of asbestos-induced immune mechanisms. Early massive exposure produces severe disease. Asbestosis is clinically similar to idiopathic pulmonary fibrosis and affects the lower lung zones.

- Asbestosis: similar to idiopathic pulmonary fibrosis.

- Antinuclear antibody and rheumatoid factor present in serum.

Carcinogenicity from asbestos exposure is not well understood, but tobacco smoking greatly compounds the risk. The lower lobes-to-upper lobes ratio is 2:1. Tumors are peripheral and frequently involve the pleura. Adenocarcinoma is more common than squamous cell carcinoma. Roentgenographic progression of asbestosis over a few years is reported to denote a higher risk of lung cancer.

- Tobacco smoking + asbestos exposure = synergistic effect on carcinogenicity.
- Peripheral adenocarcinoma in the lower lobes.

Malignant mesothelioma is not always related to asbestos. A possible viral connection has been postulated and in one study, 60% of mesotheliomas were demonstrated to contain and to express simian virus 40-like DNA (SV40) sequences. All types of asbestos fibers have been implicated in the etiology of mesothelioma. There is no correlation with smoking. Initial exposure is more than 40 years before the tumor is diagnosed; the incidence is 60 cases/million persons per year. It is more common in older patients, and insulation workers are at greatest risk. Common symptoms are chest pain and dyspnea. It presents as a painful exudative pleural effusion, followed by pleural nodules or masses.

- Malignant mesothelioma is not always related to asbestos exposure.
- It is not related to smoking.
- It is detected many years (>40 years) after exposure to asbestos.

Silicosis

Silicon dioxide exposure occurs, among other places, in mines, quarries, sandblasting areas, road building, stone finishing, and in foundry and ceramic work. Recent publications have shown an increased risk of lung cancer in patients with silicosis. Four clinical problems can be seen:

1. Acute silicosis is rare and has a progressively fatal course (months to years). Ceramic workers, silica workers, and tunneling operators are at risk. CXR shows ground-glass, alveolar (upper lung fields), or fibrotic-appearing infiltrates. The pathologic features are sometimes akin to those of pulmonary proteinosis (silicoproteinosis).
2. Chronic simple silicosis: silicotic nodules of varying size (from millimeters to <1.5 cm) occur predominantly in the upper lung zones. The nodules may enlarge, coalesce, and produce mass-like changes (progressive massive fibrosis). The number and size of nodules increase with increased exposure. Eggshell calcification of hilar nodes is common. PFT findings are normal or minimally abnormal.
3. Complicated silicosis, or progressive massive fibrosis: progressive massive fibrosis, less common than in coal workers' pneumoconiosis, is disabling and life-threatening. It starts as simple silicosis and gradually produces bilateral symmetrical pulmonary masses (>1 cm) in the upper lung fields. Compensatory emphysema with both obstructive and restrictive lung functions produces hypoxemia, which in turn causes cor pulmonale. An autoimmune mechanism is postulated because of the high prevalence of abnormal immunologic laboratory data (antinuclear antibody, rheumatoid factor, etc.). Caplan syndrome (rheumatoid lung nodules with silicosis) may be a more benign form of progressive massive fibrosis.
4. Silicotuberculosis: the risk of tuberculosis is 4 to 6 times higher in those with silicosis. CXR abnormalities are such that it is difficult to differentiate tuberculosis from silicosis-induced changes. The relapse rate of tuberculosis is high, and longer-than-usual antituberculous therapy may be needed. Mycobacteria involved include *M. tuberculosis*, *M. kansasii*, and *M. avium* complex. Patients with silicosis should be tested (PPD) annually. Patients with silicosis or an old fibrotic lesion on CXR who have a positive PPD should receive 4-month therapy with isoniazid and rifampin, although 12 months of isoniazid alone is an acceptable alternative.

- Silicosis does not increase the risk of developing lung cancer.
- Eggshell calcification of hilar lymph nodes is seen in silicosis and sarcoidosis.
- High prevalence of positive rheumatoid factor and antinuclear antibody in progressive massive fibrosis.
- In a patient with silicosis and fever with or without weight loss, consider silicotuberculosis.

Coal Workers' Pneumoconiosis

A coal macule is usually smaller than 4 mm and consists of macrophages, fibroblasts, and reticulin and collagen fibers. Collections of these macules around small airways cause bronchiolar dilatation and focal spongy emphysema. CXR shows tiny nodular infiltrates in the upper lung zones; these become profuse and may lead to progressive massive fibrosis. Radiographically, nodules are classified into micronodules (<7 mm diameter) and macronodules (>7 mm diameter). Simple coal workers' pneumoconiosis is a contributor to decrements in pulmonary function and to an increased risk of respiratory symptoms. However, significant pulmonary dysfunction is uncommon in the absence of smoking. Nonspecific bronchitis may occur with the inhalation of large amounts of coal dust. Melanoptysis (the expectoration of black sputum) is sometimes seen in coal workers' pneumoconiosis.

- PFT abnormalities are usually caused by smoking.
- Coal workers' pneumoconiosis does not increase the risk of malignancy or tuberculosis.

Byssinosis

Byssinosis is an occupational lung disease caused by the inhalation of cotton, flax, or hemp dust. In cotton mills, carding rooms provide the greatest exposure. The mechanism of the lung injury is unknown; IgE is not involved. The persons affected complain of cough, paroxysmal wheezing, dyspnea, and chest tightness on the first day of work, with gradual resolution of symptoms as the work-week progresses. A decline in FEV_1 occurs on the first day, and lung functions improve during the week. Persistent exposure results in clinical disease indistinguishable from COPD. Workers in a cotton environment are significantly more likely to suffer from chronic bronchitis and this is most marked in workers older than 45 years. Treatment includes prevention of exposure and cessation of smoking.

- Byssinosis: the mechanism of lung injury is unknown; IgE is not involved.
- Symptoms are worse on the first day of exposure.

Berylliosis

Acute beryllium exposure (ceramic workers, beryllium processors, and some aerospace workers) by inhalation may cause tracheobronchitis and chemical pneumonitis. Chronic berylliosis is the result of a delayed-type hypersensitivity reaction that results in the formation of sarcoid-like granulomatous disease. The ACE genotype is thought to be important in the immune response to beryllium and in the progression to beryllium disease. Clinically, physiologically, and radiographically, chronic berylliosis resembles sarcoidosis. In suspected cases, the diagnosis can be established by performing the beryllium lymphocyte transformation test. Symptomatic patients should be treated with corticosteroids. Beryllium exposure does not increase the risk of lung cancer.

- Berylliosis resembles sarcoidosis.

Hypersensitivity Pneumonitis

Hypersensitivity pneumonitis, also known as "extrinsic allergic alveolitis," is an immune-mediated lung disease. Many fungal precipitins and several avian proteins (pigeon-breeder's lung), animal proteins, chemicals (isocyanates), and metals (trimellitic anhydride and phthalic anhydride) cause this condition. Studies have shown the presence of viruses (influenza A) in the lower airways of patients with acute hypersensitivity pneumonitis.

- Hypersensitivity pneumonitis: also known as extrinsic allergic alveolitis.

Acute (classic) and chronic forms of hypersensitivity pneumonitis occur. Acute farmer's lung is the prototype of the acute form. *Micropolyspora faeni* and *Thermoactinomyces vulgaris* are usually responsible. Symptoms appear 4 to 6 hours after exposure and include fever, chills, sweats, dry cough, and dyspnea. Examination reveals tachypnea and basal crackles without wheezing. Leukocytosis, hyperglobulinemia, and precipitating antibody can be detected. Symptoms resolve rapidly (within 18-24 hours) and recur on reexposure. CXR may show increased bronchovascular markings and fine reticular and nodular defects. Biopsy (rarely indicated) may show BOOP.

- Symptoms start 4-6 hours after exposure to causative precipitin.
- Respiratory distress of varying intensity; wheezing is not a feature.
- Symptoms resolve within 18-24 hours and recur on reexposure.

Chronic farmer's lung follows repeated exposure to precipitins. Obtaining a good history is important in establishing the diagnosis of chronic hypersensitivity pneumonitis because symptoms are insidious in onset, eventually resulting in progressive fibrosis. A decrease in lung volumes, compliance, and diffusing capacity and exercise-induced hypoxemia are typical in late stages. Clinically, this disease is identical to idiopathic pulmonary fibrosis. BAL may show reversal of the CD4/CD8 ratio. Lung biopsy usually reveals a granulomatous reaction with round cell infiltrates, epithelioid cells, and septal swelling with lymphocytes and plasma cells. Hypersensitivity pneumonitis has occurred from exposure to *M. avium* complex contaminating hot water tubs.

- Most cases are due to fungal precipitins.
- Typically restrictive lung dysfunction.
- Hot water tubs contaminated by *M. avium* complex can cause hypersensitivity pneumonitis.

The points to remember about occupational lung diseases are summarized in Table 21-7.

In pigeon-breeder's lung disease, the histologic features consist of foamy macrophages and interstitial granulomas.

Table 21-7.—Pulmonary Diseases: Causes and Associations

Pulmonary disease	Causes and associations
Progressive massive fibrosis	Silicosis, coal, hematite, kaolin, graphite, asbestosis
Autoimmune mechanism	Silicosis, asbestosis, berylliosis
Monday morning sickness	Byssinosis, bagassosis, metal fume fever
Metals and fumes producing asthma	Bakers' asthma, meat wrappers' asthma, printers' asthma, nickel, platinum, toluene diisocyanate, cigarette cutters' asthma
Increased incidence of tuberculosis	Silicosis, hematite lung
Increased incidence of carcinoma	Asbestos, hematite, arsenic, nickel, uranium, chromate
Welder's lung	Siderosis, pulmonary edema, bronchitis, emphysema
Centrilobar emphysema	Coal, hematite
Generalized emphysema	Cadmium
Silo filler's lung	Nitrogen dioxide
Farmer's lung	*Thermoactinomyces, Micropolyspora*
Asbestos exposure	Mesothelioma, bronchogenic cancer, gastrointestinal tract cancer
Eggshell calcification	Silicosis, sarcoid
Sarcoid-like disease	Berylliosis
Diaphragmatic calcification	Asbestosis (also ankylosing spondylitis)
Nonfibrogenic pneumoconioses	Tin, emery, antimony, titanium, barium
Minimal abnormality in lungs	Siderosis, baritosis, stannosis
Bullous emphysema	Bauxite lung
Occupational asthma	Toluene diisocyanate, laboratory animals, grain dust, biologic enzymes, gum acacia, tragacanth, silkworm, anhydrides, wood dust, platinum, nickel, formaldehyde, Freon, drugs

Positive serologic findings are not diagnostic because 20% of asymptomatic farmers and 40% of asymptomatic pigeon breeders have positive precipitins, and 10% of symptomatic farmers have negative precipitins. Digital clubbing is frequent (51% of patients) in pigeon breeder's disease and may help to predict clinical deterioration. The treatment for symptomatic patients is to avoid exposure to the causative precipitins and the use of corticosteroids.

● Pigeon-breeder's lung disease is due to avian proteins.

DRUG-INDUCED LUNG DISEASE

Mechanisms of drug-induced lung disease include hypersensitivity, direct damage from toxic metabolites and oxygen radicals, alkylation of pulmonary tissue macromolecules, antigen-antibody reaction (type III), and type I immune reactions. The different types of pulmonary problems caused by various drugs are listed in Table 21-8.

Drug-Induced Systemic Lupus Erythematosus

Older white persons are particularly prone to drug-induced systemic lupus erythematosus. The clinical features include arthralgias and arthritis (90% of patients), fever and malaise (40%), abnormal test results for antinuclear antibody (100% of patients), lupus erythematosus cell clot (75%), rheumatoid factor (33%), and low complement level (70%). Commonly implicated agents include cardiac drugs (procainamide, quinidine, and practolol), antibiotics (nitrofurantoin, penicillin, griseofulvin, sulpha, and tetracycline), anticonvulsant agents (phenytoin, mephenytoin, and carbamazepine), antihypertensive drugs (hydralazine, methyldopa, and L-dopa), antituberculous drugs (isoniazid, streptomycin, and para-aminosalicylic acid), phenothiazines (chlorpromazine and promethazine), and miscellaneous agents (D-penicillamine, methysergide, oral contraceptives, phenylbutazone, propylthiouracil, tolazamide, etc.).

● More common in older white persons.
● Drug-induced systemic lupus erythematosus: pleural effusion in 50% of patients and pulmonary infiltrates in 30%.

Narcotic Abuse

Heroin, morphine, methadone, and propoxyphene cause pulmonary edema, adult respiratory distress syndrome, pneumonia (in 30% of heroin addicts), bronchiectasis, and talc granulomas. Pulmonary edema is the most common complication

Table 21-8.—Drug-Induced Pulmonary Diseases

Interstitial pneumonitis/fibrosis

    Chemotherapeutic agents

    Nitrofurantoin (chronic)

    Drug-induced systemic lupus erythematosus

    Gold

    Talc (intravenous use)

    Aspirated oil

    D-Penicillamine

    Pituitary snuff

    Radiation

    Oxygen

    Sulfasalazine (Azulfidine)

    Cromolyn sodium

    Methysergide

    Hexamethonium, pentolinium, mecamylamine

Noncardiac pulmonary edema

    Heroin, methadone, morphine

    Acetylsalicylic acid

    Nitrofurantoin (acute)

    Chlordiazepoxide (Librium)

    Ethchlorvynol (Placidyl)

    Interleukin-2

Pleural effusion

    Nitrofurantoin (acute)

    Methysergide (chronic)

    Drug-induced systemic lupus erythematosus

    Chemotherapeutic drugs

    Radiation

    Dantrolene

Drug-induced pulmonary infiltrate with eosinophilia

    Sulfonamides

    Sulfasalazine (Azulfidine)

    Penicillin

    Isoniazid

    Aminosalicylate

    Nitrofurantoin (acute)

    Leukoagglutinin

    Methotrexate

    Procarbazine

    Carbamazepine (Tegretol)

    Imipramine (Tofranil)

    Salicylates

    Cromolyn sodium

    Methylphenidate (Ritalin)

    Dantrolene

Drug-induced hilar and mediastinal widening

    Corticosteroids

    Methotrexate

    Phenytoin (Dilantin)

Bronchospasm

    Propranolol, other β-blockers

    Acetylsalicylic acid

    Indomethacin

    Fenoprofen

    Mefenamate

    Isuprel

    Drugs that produce pulmonary infiltrate with eosinophilia

    Nebulized medications

Pulmonary hypertension

    Oral contraceptives

    Aminorex and other appetite suppressants

    15-Methyl-prostaglandin-F_2

Pulmonary granulomas

    Talc

    Mineral oil

    Methotrexate

    Cromolyn sodium

    Cotton fibers (intravenous drug use)

of heroin and morphine overdose; it usually is seen within hours after consumption and resolves within 24 to 48 hours. Pneumonia may be secondary to the aspiration of gastric contents and septic emboli from endocarditis. Methadone produces similar pulmonary complications. Talc granuloma is the result of the intravenous use of crushed analgesic tablets, talc contamination, and cotton fibers used as filters. Cornstarch (used as an adulterant) also causes granulomas.

- Noncardiogenic pulmonary edema is due to capillary damage.
- Narcotic abuse: adult respiratory distress syndrome, pneumonia, endocarditis, and talc granulomas.

Nitrofurantoin

Nitrofurantoin is the drug most commonly reported to produce pulmonary abnormalities. The acute reaction (from 3

hours to 3 months) includes dyspnea (90% of patients), cough (66%), fever (70%), crackles (65%), wheezes (40%), eosinophilia (30%), patchy process (30%), and effusions (10%-20%). Chronic cases (6 months to 7 years) are uncommon but show similar features, although a diffuse process is more common. The average dose is 150 mg/day. Pulmonary functions in acute reactions may reveal obstructive phenomena, whereas chronic cases usually show a restrictive type of pulmonary dysfunction. Most patients recover after the drug is withdrawn.

- Acute reaction within 3 hours to 3 months; average dose, 150 mg/day.
- Cough, wheeze, pleural effusion, and eosinophilia.

Chemotherapeutic Agents

Many chemotherapeutic drugs produce cytotoxic changes characterized by "bizarre-appearing" type II pneumocytes. However, nonspecific changes are common. Fever occurs in most patients and may precede the onset of cough, dyspnea, or CXR abnormalities. PFTs reveal a restrictive pattern. Arterial oxygen desaturation is common. Busulfan (Myleran) causes "busulfan lung" in about 8% of patients. The findings on PFTs may be abnormal without clinical or CXR evidence of disease. A pulmonary reaction is usually seen after 6 months of therapy. CXR shows diffuse interstitial and alveolar infiltrates. Death may occur despite stopping the drug and the use of steroids. Cyclophosphamide (Cytoxan) produces (but less commonly) similar reactions. However, changes are seen earlier than with busulfan. Bleomycin has a 10% incidence of pulmonary toxicity, which increases with increasing age (>70 years) and increasing dosage (>450 units). The simultaneous use of a high concentration of inhaled oxygen increases the risk of bleomycin lung toxicity. Acute hypersensitivity reaction with eosinophilia has been reported in some patients receiving bleomycin treatment. Chlorambucil (uncommonly) produces complications similar to those caused by busulfan, cyclophosphamide, and bleomycin. Carmustine produces pulmonary reactions in 1% of patients within 8 months after therapy, similar to the reactions seen with other chemotherapeutic agents. A higher incidence of pneumothorax has been noted. Methotrexate is the only antimetabolite known to produce pulmonary disease that is self-limiting and is frequently associated with peripheral eosinophilia. Most methotrexate-induced pulmonary reactions have been seen in children treated for acute lymphatic leukemia; symptoms begin within a few days to several weeks after the initiation of therapy. CXR shows diffuse fine interstitial infiltrates, hilar adenopathy, or pleural effusion in 10% of patients.

- Chemotherapeutic agents: bizarre type II pneumocytes seen in lung tissue (except in those treated with methotrexate).

- "Busulfan lung" occurs in 8%-10% of patients, usually after 6 months of therapy.
- Bleomycin lung toxicity occurs in 10% of patients; dose- (>450 units) and age- (>70 yr) related, and if high FIO_2 is used.
- Methotrexate produces eosinophilia, hilar adenopathy, and pleural effusion.

Radiation

The effects of radiation on lung tissue tend to be cumulative. However, the rate at which it is given is most important. A second or third course of radiation to the lung is more likely to result in a pneumonitis that can occur earlier and be devastating. Radiation initially affects pulmonary capillary endothelial cells and type II pneumocytes. Lymphocytic stimulation can lead to BOOP. The lymphocyte-mediated response can cause BOOP in nonradiated lung. In the chronic stage, nonspecific fibrosis is common. Symptoms of radiation pneumonitis begin insidiously 1 to 3 months after completion of radiation treatment. Cough, fever, and dyspnea may precede the onset of CXR changes. The late phase begins 6 months after radiation therapy. Dyspnea is usually out of proportion to the CXR changes. Corticosteroid therapy produces varying responses.

- The concomitant use of bleomycin and cyclophosphamide and the withdrawal of corticosteroid therapy increase the risk of radiation pneumonitis.
- The acute phase occurs about 1-3 months after radiation, and the chronic phase is seen after 6 months.
- The earlier the onset, the worse the prognosis.

Corticosteroids

Patients receiving high doses (>1 mg/kg per day) of corticosteroids are more likely to have opportunistic infections from *Nocardia asteroides*, *Cytomegalovirus*, *Mycobacterium tuberculosis*, *Aspergillus fumigatus*, *Candida albicans*, and *Cryptococcus neoformans*. Mediastinal lipomatosis in the mid and anterior mediastinum results from excessive deposition of fat in these areas. CT of the mediastinum is diagnostic. To prevent *Pneumocystis carinii* lung infection in patients taking more than 20 mg of prednisone daily, some recommend prophylactic treatment with trimethoprim-sulfamethoxazole.

- Chronic corticosteroid therapy can cause mediastinal lipomatosis.

Analgesic Agents

Pulmonary complications of salicylate therapy include bronchospasm in aspirin-sensitive patients, pulmonary infiltrates with eosinophilia, and noncardiogenic and pulmonary edema

(when the blood salicylate level is >50 mg/dL). Salicylate overdose initially causes respiratory alkalosis (respiratory stimulation), followed by metabolic alkalosis. Pulmonary edema occurs within 1 to 2 hours after ingestion; CXR changes may persist for a week or longer. Gold sodium thiomalate and aurothioglucose produce pulmonary toxicity in 3% to 5% of patients. With gold therapy, the lung reaction can be acute or insidious and is usually dose-related, with most patients having received more than 300 mg. CXR shows a diffuse interstitial process caused by lymphocytic and plasma cell infiltrates. Symptoms include cough, fever, and dyspnea. Bronchospasm has resulted from naproxen, indomethacin, ibuprofen, and mefenamate, and pulmonary edema has occurred after treatment with phenylbutazone or oxyphenbutazone.

- Bronchospasm occurs with acetylsalicylic acid, but not all salicylates cause bronchospasm.
- Respiratory alkalosis is followed by metabolic acidosis in salicylate overdose.

Oxygen

Oxygen toxicity can be avoided if the FIO_2 is kept below 0.5. If the duration of FIO_2 of 1.0 exceeds 24 hours or if FIO_2 of 0.6 exceeds 72 hours, the risk of pulmonary damage increases. Oxygen-induced adult respiratory distress syndrome is not amenable to any treatment, and patients usually succumb to lung failure. Histologic features include an early exudative phase, followed by an irreversible proliferative and fibrotic phase.

Oil Aspiration

With the aspiration of oil, abnormalities range from solitary nodules to various types of infiltrates, especially in the dependent lower lung fields. Mineral oil for softening stools, oily nose drops, ophthalmic drops, and other oily preparations are used frequently. Bronchographic medium has the potential to induce bronchospasm and transient changes in pulmonary function. Nontuberculous mycobacterial infection is a complication of lipoid pneumonia.

- Aspiration of oil: common but frequently overlooked by clinicians.

Inhaled Medications

Inhaled medications cause bronchospasm, irritation of the upper airways, and cough in some patients. Cromolyn sodium, used by asthmatic patients, can produce bronchospasm, pulmonary infiltrates with eosinophilia, and nonspecific upper airway irritation.

- Cromolyn can produce bronchospasm, eosinophilia, and lung infiltrates.

- Ultrafine nebulized aerosols can cause cough and bronchospasm.

Blood Products

Leukoagglutinins in the blood may produce acute pulmonary edema. The exact mechanism is unknown, but a hypersensitivity reaction has been postulated. There is acute onset of fever, chills, cough, and dyspnea. Pulmonary infiltrates may persist for several days. Eosinophilia is seen in some patients. CXR shows a varying picture of pulmonary edema.

- Blood products: pulmonary edema, eosinophilia, lung infiltrates, and human immunodeficiency virus transmission.

Miscellaneous

β-Blockers (propranolol, metoprolol, nadolol, and timolol) may aggravate asthma. Amiodarone causes interstitial pneumonitis in 1% to 4% of patients; lung reaction is dose-related and is seen usually with a dose greater than 400 mg/day. Dyspnea and cough are noted 2 to 3 months after starting therapy with the drug. ACE inhibitors cause cough in 6% of patients. D-Penicillamine provokes four types of pulmonary reaction: bronchiolitis obliterans, Goodpasture syndrome-like illness, diffuse alveolitis, and drug-induced systemic lupus erythematosus. Paraquat is a potent weed killer, and most cases of illness induced by it are due to accidental ingestion; bronchiolitis, adult respiratory distress syndrome, and severe pulmonary fibrosis are common. L-Tryptophan-induced eosinophilia-myalgia syndrome is related to a contaminant in the manufacturing process. Iodized contrast media produce pulmonary infiltrates, restrictive dysfunction, and low diffusing capacity. Lymphangiography can produce a "stippling" type of CXR changes. Methysergide has caused pleuropulmonary fibrosis; pleural effusion is seen in nearly 50% of patients. Mesalamine has been associated with eosinophilia and lung infiltrates. The use of abciximab has resulted in alveolar hemorrhage. Retinoic acid syndrome induces fever, respiratory distress, weight gain, pleural or pericardial effusions, alveolar hemorrhage (due to pulmonary capillaritis), peripheral edema, thromboembolic events, and intermittent hypotension. Zafirlukast therapy in asthmatic patients taking steroids has resulted in Churg-Strauss syndrome after steroid therapy was withdrawn. Mycophenolate mofetil, an immunosuppressive drug, has caused acute respiratory failure and pulmonary fibrosis.

- β-Blockers aggravate asthma and COPD.
- Amiodarone causes diffuse lung infiltrates; dose usually >400 mg/day.
- ACE inhibitors cause cough in 4%-6% of patients.
- Penicillamine can cause bronchiolitis and drug-induced systemic lupus erythematosus.

EFFECTS OF ALTITUDE, DIVING, AND DROWNING

Effects of High Altitude

Acute Mountain Sickness

Physiologic changes at high altitude are the result of reduced barometric pressure. PIO_2 decreases by 4 to 5 mm Hg for each 1,000 feet of elevation. The ventilatory response varies with time. Acute high altitude-induced hypoxia increases minute ventilation and reduces $PaCO_2$. This reaction is mediated by peripheral chemoreceptors. It can be reversed rapidly by oxygen inhalation. After 5 to 10 days, there is a further increase in ventilation and a greater decrease in $PaCO_2$, which an ambient PO_2 fails to correct. Acute ascent to high altitude increases hemoglobin concentration because of diuresis; a transient increase in the serum level of erythropoietin occurs. Acute mountain sickness affects 25% to 50% of lowlanders 6 to 90 hours after ascent to more than 7,000 ft, producing lethargy, insomnia, headache, nausea, vomiting, and dyspnea. It is exacerbated by alcohol, sedatives, or overexertion soon after ascent. Cyanosis and signs of cerebral edema can occur. Prophylactic diuretic (acetazolamide is the drug of choice) therapy (before ascent) prevents acute mountain sickness. Acetazolamide plus low-dose dexamethasone has been shown to be better than acetazolamide alone to treat symptoms of acute mountain sickness.

- Acute mountain sickness: affects lowlanders 6-90 hours after ascent.
- Lethargy, insomnia, headache, nausea, vomiting, and dyspnea.
- Preventive diuretic therapy before ascent is recommended.
- Cerebral edema occurs in severe acute mountain sickness.

High-Altitude Pulmonary Edema

High-altitude pulmonary edema is noncardiogenic in origin and occurs after rapid ascent to more than 14,000 ft. It is thought to result from hypoxic pulmonary vasoconstriction. The incidence among mountaineers is 0.5% to 10%, but susceptible persons have a 60% incidence on reexposure to high altitude. Cold weather and exertion contribute to this condition. A time lag from 24 to 36 hours is common. Typically, symptoms appear after 36 hours and consist of dyspnea, cough, fatigue, altered mental status, and somnolence. Clinically, high-altitude pulmonary edema is similar to acute pulmonary edema from other causes, but left ventricular failure is not a feature. CXR shows patchy infiltrates. These disappear 6 to 48 hours after return to sea level or after therapy with high doses of oxygen.

- High-altitude pulmonary edema is a type of noncardiogenic pulmonary edema.
- Individual susceptibility increases the risk of the condition on reexposure to high altitude.

Chronic Mountain Sickness

Highlanders adapt to physiologic changes and ventilate less than acclimatized lowlanders and maintain a higher $PaCO_2$ and a lower PaO_2. The respiratory drive is lost and primary alveolar hypoventilation develops. Chronic mountain sickness (Monge disease) is the result of the progressive loss of acclimatization to high altitude. Susceptible highlanders develop chronic malaise, headache, dizziness, easy fatigability, paresthesias, somnolence, and diminished mental activity. Marked cyanosis, clubbing of the fingers, polycythemia, oxygen desaturation, and cardiac enlargement occur, but the lung fields appear normal on CXR. Pulmonary arterial pressure is twice as high as that of a nonsusceptible highlander.

- Chronic mountain sickness: due to progressive loss of acclimatization to high altitude.
- The most serious complication is irreversible pulmonary hypertension.

Air Travel

Because most commercial aircraft (pressurized) cruise at high altitudes (10,000-55,000 ft), the reduced FIO_2 within the aircraft is similar to that at an altitude of 6,000 ft to 8,500 ft. As a result, patients with underlying hypoxemic pulmonary diseases may experience exacerbation of their symptoms. Long flights, reduced humidity, undue exertion on board, and smoking (by other passengers) in the cabin add to the problems. If the PaO_2 is less than 50 mm Hg (SaO_2 <85%) at rest, supplemental oxygen should be prescribed.

- Supplemental O_2 is recommended if PaO_2 is <50 mm Hg (SaO_2 <85%) at rest.

Drowning and Barotrauma

Drowning

Drowning is the fourth leading cause of accidental deaths in the U.S. Most drowning accidents occur in children (<5 years), young adults (15-29 years old), males and blacks, and in southern states. Two-thirds of drownings occur in fresh water. The greatest risk factor for drowning in adults and teenagers is alcohol consumption (in 45% of adult victims). Although hypothermia by itself is rarely the actual cause of death, it can have a significant effect on the prognosis of near-drowning victims. Aspiration occurs in about 85% of drowning or near-drowning victims; the other 15% have laryngospasm

and, thus, do not have signs of aspiration. The duration of hypoxemia caused by drowning is more important in predicting mortality rather than fresh water versus salt water drowning or the electrolyte imbalance. Adult respiratory distress syndrome and aspiration pneumonia are more common in those who aspirate. Other complications include metabolic and respiratory acidosis, secondary arrhythmias, cerebral edema, shock-induced acute tubular necrosis, and hypothermia.

- Alcohol consumption is a major risk factor for drowning in adults.
- Pulmonary complications are more common in those who aspirate.

Barotrauma

Pulmonary barotrauma is manifested by arterial gas embolism, mediastinal emphysema, and pneumothorax. Barotrauma is more common in divers. It is caused by the contraction or expansion of gas that occurs because of changes in barometric pressure after a descent or ascent, respectively. Barotrauma sustained during ascent can be life-threatening. Arterial gas embolism is an important cause of death among scuba divers. Within minutes after surfacing, an afflicted diver will have neurologic symptoms ranging from focal motor, sensory, or visual deficits to unconsciousness and death. Characteristic marbling over the upper torso and focal pallor of the tongue may be seen. Pulmonary complications from overdistention include pneumothorax (in 10% of barotrauma victims), pneumomediastinum, hemoptysis, chest pain, and interstitial emphysema. Divers with preexisting small lung cysts and/or end-expiratory flow limitation may be at risk for pulmonary barotrauma.

- Arterial gas embolism is an important cause of death among scuba divers.
- Interstitial emphysema is more common than pneumothorax in deep sea divers.

PULMONARY NEOPLASMS

Solitary Pulmonary Nodule

A solitary pulmonary nodule is defined as a solitary lesion seen on plain CXR. It is less than 4 cm and is round, ovoid, or slightly lobulated. The lesion is located in lung parenchyma, is at least moderately circumscribed, and uncalcified on plain CXR. It is not associated with satellite lesions or other abnormalities on plain CXR. Common causes include carcinoma of the lung (15%-50% of patients), mycoses (5%-50%), tuberculosis, unidentified granulomas, resolving pneumonia, hamartoma, and metastatic lesions. Uncommon causes include carcinoid, bronchogenic cyst, resolving infarction, rheumatoid and vasculitic nodules, and arteriovenous malformation.

- Granulomas and hamartomas make up 40%-60% of all solitary pulmonary nodules and 90% of nonmalignant solitary pulmonary nodules.
- Hamartomas alone comprise <10% of nonmalignant nodules.

Clinical Evaluation

The following are important in the evaluation of solitary pulmonary nodules: age of patient, availability of previous CXR, smoking history, previous malignancy, exposure to tuberculous patients, travel to areas endemic for mycoses, recent respiratory infection, recent pulmonary infarction, recent trauma to chest, asthma, mucoid impaction, systemic diseases (congestive heart failure, rheumatoid arthritis, etc.), ear-nose-throat symptoms (Wegener vasculitis), mineral oil, oily nose drops, immune defense mechanisms, and family history (arteriovenous malformation).

- History: old CXR, age, smoking history, previous malignancy, and exposure history are important.

Diagnosis

Physical examination, routine blood tests, chemistry group, and the exclusion of obvious causes (congestive heart failure, vasculitis, rheumatoid arthritis, etc.) are important for making the diagnosis. Obtain earlier CXR for comparison. Generally, sputum cytology, skin tests, serologic studies, and cultures on a routine basis are unrewarding in asymptomatic patients. Localized tomograms identify the location of a solitary pulmonary nodule, calcification, cavitation, satellite lesions, and margins. Chest CT is helpful in assessing calcification, density, multiple nodules (particularly in evaluating metastatic malignancy), and staging of lung cancer. Contrast enhancement of a nodule on CT is more likely if the nodule is malignant. Dynamic positron emission tomography (PET) with F-18 fluorodeoxyglucose (FDG) imaging is reported to differentiate malignant from benign pulmonary lesions more accurately than CT scan. In asymptomatic patients with a single lung nodule, extensive studies (gastrointestinal tract series, intravenous pyelography, and scans of bone, brain, liver, bone marrow, etc.) are not indicated because of the low diagnostic yield (<3%).

- CT detects 30% more nodules than CXR.
- Contrast enhancement on CT is more likely if the nodule is malignant.
- Bronchoscopy has a 60% diagnostic yield in cancer.

- Transthoracic needle aspiration (CT- or fluoroscopy-guided) has an 85% diagnostic yield in cancer and a 20% risk of pneumothorax.

Decision Making

General guidelines for decision making are given in Table 21-9. If a benign cause cannot be firmly established after complete clinical, imaging, culture, and biopsy evaluations, the following clinical decisions advocate surgical resection: 1) the solitary pulmonary nodule is probably malignant, because little or no other clinical information is available to indicate a benign diagnosis or 2) the nodule may be benign but must be resected now because the benign nature cannot be established. If the clinical information firmly indicates a benign cause, follow-up CXR is recommended.

- If there is no change in the size or shape of the nodule for over 2 years, repeat CXR every 6-12 months.
- If the patient is a poor surgical risk or the surgeon or patient refuses the operation, repeat CXR every 3 months (enlargement of lesion may convince patient/surgeon to consider resection).

Primary Lung Cancer

Lung cancer is the most common malignant disease and the most common cause of cancer death in the U.S. The estimated incidence of new lung cancer cases in 2000 is 14% (of all cancers) for both men and women. It is estimated that more than 190,000 new cases will be diagnosed and more than 160,000 deaths will be attributable to lung cancer. The risk factors include cigarette smoking (25% of cancers may result from passive smoking), other carcinogens, cocarcinogens, radon daughters (uranium mining), arsenic (glass workers, smelters, and pesticides), asbestos (insulation, textile, and asbestos mining), coal dust (coke oven, road work, and roofer), chromium (leather, ceramic, and metal), vinyl chloride (plastic), chloromethyl ether (chemical), and chronic lung injury (idiopathic pulmonary fibrosis and COPD). Genetic and nutritional factors (perhaps deficiency of vitamin A) have been implicated.

The World Health Organization (WHO) classification of pathologic types of pulmonary neoplasms is given in Table 21-10 and the TNM classification for staging of non-small cell lung cancer, in Table 21-11.

Small cell cancer is staged as follows:

1. Limited: single hemithorax, mediastinum, ipsilateral supraclavicular nodes.
2. Extensive: anything beyond limited stage.

Overall Survival

The overall survival for all stages of lung cancer is 14%. The overall survival rate for patients with occult and in situ cancers is greater than 70%. The overall survival for other stages is as follows: stage I, 50%; stage II, less than 20%; stage III, less than 10%. One-year survival for stage I cancer is greater than 80%. In small cell cancer, the median survival is less than 12 months; the 5-year survival for limited stage cancer is 15% to 20% and for extensive disease, 1% to 5%.

- The overall 5-year survival for all lung cancers is 14%.

Cell Types

Primary lung cancer is broadly divided into non-small cell (adenocarcinoma, 35%; squamous cell carcinoma, 30%; and large cell carcinoma, 1%-15%), small cell carcinoma (20%-25%), mixed (small and large cell), and others (metastatic lesions).

- Small cell and non-small cell types.

Clinical Features

Most patients are older than 50 years. Only 5% of lung cancer patients are asymptomatic. The presentation is highly variable and depends on the cell type, location, rate of growth, paraneoplastic syndromes, systemic symptoms, and other factors. Cough is the most frequent symptom and is more likely in squamous cell carcinoma and small cell cancer than in other types of lung cancer. Hemoptysis occurs in 35% to 50% of patients and is more common with squamous cell,

Table 21-9.—Likelihood of Benign or Malignant Single Pulmonary Nodule According to Clinical and Radiographic Variables

Clinical factor, radiographic result	More likely benign	More likely malignant
Age	<35 yr	>35 yr
Sex	Female	Male
Smoking	No	Yes
Symptoms	No	Yes
Exposure to tuberculosis, cocci, etc.	Yes	No
Previous malignancy	No	Yes
Nodule size	<2.0 cm	>2.0 cm
Nodule age	>2 yr	<2 yr
Doubling time	<30 days	>30 days
Nodule margins	Smooth	Irregular
Calcification	Yes	No
Satellite lesions	Yes	No

Table 21-10.—World Health Organization Classification of Pulmonary Neoplasms

Type	Histologic type
I	Squamous cell carcinoma
II	Small cell carcinoma
	Oat cell carcinoma
	Intermediate cell carcinoma
	Combined oat cell carcinoma
III	Adenocarcinoma
	Acinar adenocarcinoma
	Papillary adenocarcinoma
	Bronchoalveolar carcinoma
	Solid carcinoma with mucus formation
IV	Large cell carcinoma
	Giant cell carcinoma
	Clear cell carcinoma
V	Combined cell types
VI	Carcinoid tumors
VII	Bronchial gland tumors
	Cylindroma
	Mucoepidermoid
VIII	Papillary tumors

small cell, carcinoid, and endobronchial metastases than with other types of tumors. Wheezing is due to intraluminal tumor or extrinsic compression. Dyspnea depends on the extensiveness of the tumor, COPD, degree of bronchial obstruction, and other factors. Persistent chest pain may suggest rib metastasis, local extension, or pleural involvement. Superior vena cava syndrome may suggest small cell carcinoma, lymphoma, squamous cell carcinoma, or Pancoast tumor. Horner syndrome is indicative of Pancoast tumor. Fever, postobstructive pneumonitis, nonthoracic skeletal pains, central nervous system symptoms, and abdominal pain/discomfort and hepatomegaly are indicative of possible distant metastases. Central nervous system metastasis is found in 15% of patients with squamous cell carcinoma, in 25% with adenocarcinoma, in 28% with large cell carcinoma, and in 30% with small cell carcinoma.

- Cough and hemoptysis are more common in squamous cell carcinoma and carcinoid.
- Chest pain may indicate pleural effusion, pleural metastasis, or rib lesion.
- Nonpulmonary symptoms may indicate distant metastases or paraneoplastic syndromes.
- Central nervous system metastasis is more common with small cell carcinoma.

Squamous Cell Carcinoma

More than 65% of squamous cell carcinomas arise in the proximal tracheobronchial tree (first four subdivisions). They also may arise in the upper airway and esophagus. Symptoms appear early in the course of the disease because of proximal bronchial involvement and consist of cough, hemoptysis, and lobar/segmental collapse with postobstructive pneumonia. CXR findings include atelectasis (23% of patients), obstructive pneumonitis (13%), hilar adenopathy (38%), and cavitation (5%). One-third of cases present as peripheral masses. Sputum cytology and bronchoscopy are indicated in almost all patients. One-third of squamous cell carcinomas have thick-walled irregular cavities. Treatment is with resection, radiation, and chemotherapy. Laser bronchoscopy and endobronchial brachytherapy are palliative measures.

- Squamous cell carcinoma: proximal airway disease in 66% of cases, peripheral mass in 33%, and cavitation in 35%.
- Sputum cytology and bronchoscopy are important tests.

Adenocarcinoma

Most adenocarcinomas arise in the periphery and, thus, remain asymptomatic and undetected until they have spread locally or distally. This means that the chance of dissemination to extrapulmonary sites is higher for these tumors. However, incidentally detected peripheral carcinomas tend to be in an early stage. Adenocarcinoma is the most common type of peripheral primary lung cancer. Sputum cytology has a low diagnostic yield. The most common presentation is as a solitary peripheral nodule. A small number cavitate. Clubbing and hypertrophic pulmonary osteoarthropathy are more common than in other kinds of primary lung cancer. The response to radiation and chemotherapy is generally poor.

- Adenocarcinoma: may arise as a solitary pulmonary nodule in the periphery.
- The symptomatic stage usually denotes advanced disease.
- Sputum cytology has a low diagnostic yield.
- Clubbing and hypertrophic pulmonary osteoarthropathy are more common than in squamous cell carcinoma.

Bronchoalveolar Cell Carcinoma

Bronchoalveolar cell carcinoma is thought to arise from alveolar type II pneumocytes and/or Clara cells. The tumor presents in two forms: as a localized solitary nodular lesion and as a diffuse alveolar process. More than 60% of patients are asymptomatic. The cancer presents as a solitary nodule in 85% of patients and as lobar pneumonitis or diffuse infiltrate in 15%. The solitary form has the best prognosis of all types of lung cancer, with a 1-year survival rate greater than 80%. The diffuse variety has a mean survival rate of less than 6 months. Bronchorrhea (>100

Table 21-11.—Staging of Lung Cancer: TNM Classification

T, primary tumor

T0	No evidence of primary tumor
TX	Cancer cells in respiratory secretions; no tumor on chest radiographs or at bronchoscopy
Tis	Carcinoma in situ
T1	Tumor ≤3 cm in greatest dimension, surrounded by lung tissue; no bronchoscopic evidence of tumor proximal to lobar bronchus
T2	Tumor >3 cm in diameter, or tumor of any size that involves visceral pleura, or associated with atelectasis extending to hilum (but not involving entire lung); must be ≥2 cm from main carina
T3	Tumor involves chest wall, diaphragm, mediastinal pleura, or pericardium, or is <2 cm from main carina (but does not involve it)
T4	Tumor involves main carina or trachea, or invades mediastinum, heart, great vessels, esophagus, or vertebra, or malignant pleural effusion

N, nodal involvement

NX	Regional lymph nodes cannot be assessed
N0	No demonstrable lymph node involvement
N1	Ipsilateral peribronchial or hilar lymph nodes involved
N2	Metastasis to ipsilateral mediastinal lymph nodes, or to subcarinal lymph nodes
N3	Metastasis to contralateral mediastinal and/or hilar lymph nodes, or to scalene and/or supraclavicular lymph nodes

M, metastasis

MX	Presence of distant metastasis cannot be assessed
M0	No known distant metastasis
M1	Distant metastasis present (specify site or sites)

Stage Grouping—TNM Subsets[*]

Stage 0	Carcinoma in situ	Stage IIIB	T4N0M0
			T4N1M0
Stage IA	T1N0M0		T4N2M0
Stage IB	T2N0M0		T1N3M0
			T2N3M0
Stage IIA	T1N1M0		T3N3M0
Stage IIB	T2N1M0		T4N3M0
	T3N0M0		
		Stage IV	Any T Any N M1
Stage IIIA	T3N1M0		
	T1N2M0		
	T2N2M0		
	T3N2M0		

[*]Staging is not relevant for occult carcinoma, designated TXN0M0.

mL of thin serous mucus secretion/24 hours) is seen in 20% of patients. CXR shows a solitary nodule, localized infiltrate with vacuoles on tomography, or pneumonic lesions. Both forms of bronchoalveolar cell carcinoma can mimic ordinary pneumonia. Because of the slow growth, the chronic course of the disease may suggest a benign process; thus, close surveillance is imperative. The treatment for a solitary lesion is resection. The response to radiation and chemotherapy is poor, although bronchorrhea seems to respond to radiation in some patients.

- Bronchoalveolar cell carcinoma: unrelated to tobacco smoking.
- The solitary form grows slowly and may mimic a benign lung nodule.

- The solitary (localized) form has >80% 1-year survival rate after resection.
- The diffuse form has a mean survival rate of <6 months.
- Bronchorrhea occurs in 20% of patients (usually diffuse form).

Large Cell Carcinoma

Large cells are seen on histologic examination, and CXR shows large masses. Large cell carcinoma grows more rapidly than adenocarcinoma. Cavitation is seen in 20% to 25% of patients. Clubbing and hypertrophic pulmonary osteoarthropathy are more common than in other tumors except for adenocarcinoma. The treatment is surgical. The response to radiation and chemotherapy is poor.

- Large cell carcinoma: a large, rapidly growing lung mass; cavitation in 25% of patients.
- Clubbing and hypertrophic pulmonary osteoarthropathy are common.

Small Cell Carcinoma

Small cell carcinoma (oat cell carcinoma) accounts for 25% of all bronchogenic carcinomas. The tumor originates from neuroendocrine cells and invades the tracheobronchial tree and spreads submucosally. Later, it breaks through the mucosa and produces changes similar to those seen in squamous cell carcinoma. CXR shows a unilateral, rapidly enlarging hilar or perihilar mass or widening of the hila/mediastinum. Less than 20% of these tumors are peripheral. Bronchoscopy may show heaped-up or thickened mucosa. This tumor responds better to radiation and chemotherapy than do other lung tumors. Brain metastasis is common. Prophylactic brain radiation is standard at many medical centers; this decreases the frequency of brain metastasis but does not prolong survival. Peripheral nodules that are found, after resection, to be small cell carcinoma should be treated as any small cell carcinoma.

- Small cell carcinoma: smokers and uranium miners are at high risk.
- It may be associated with many paraneoplastic syndromes: syndrome of inappropriate antidiuretic hormone, ACTH production, and myasthenic syndrome.
- Surgical treatment is not a standard therapeutic option; radiation and chemotherapy are.

Carcinoid

Carcinoid arises from the same cells as small cell carcinoma, but its clinical behavior is different. Typically, carcinoid presents with cough, with or without hemoptysis, in young adults. CXR may show a solitary nodule or segmental atelectasis. Paraneoplastic syndromes develop from hormonal secretion (ACTH and PTH). Treatment is surgical resection of the tumor without lung resection. The diagnosis of malignant carcinoid is based on the extent of spread noted at resection or clinical behavior.

- Carcinoid: a young adult with cough and hemoptysis.
- The symptoms may be related to the production of ACTH (Cushing syndrome, hypertension) and PTH (hypercalcemia).
- Carcinoid "syndrome" is rare, occurring in <1% of patients with bronchial carcinoid.

Bronchial Gland Tumors

Cylindroma (adenoid cystic carcinoma) and mucoepidermoid tumors usually are located centrally and cause cough, hemoptysis, and obstructive pneumonia. Distant metastasis is unusual. Surgical treatment is used for major airway obstructive lesions. The response to radiation and chemotherapy is poor.

- Cylindroma arising in salivary glands can metastasize to the lungs after many years.

Mesenchymal Tumors

This group of tumors includes lymphoma, lymphosarcoma, carcinosarcoma, fibrosarcoma, mesothelioma (discussed above), and soft tissue sarcomas. Many of these present as large peripheral masses, homogeneous densities, and cavitated lesions.

Lymphoma

Pulmonary involvement occurs in 65% and 45% of patients with Hodgkin and non-Hodgkin lymphoma, respectively. CXR findings include bilateral hilar adenopathy, chylous pleural effusion, segmental atelectasis from endobronchial lesions, diffuse nodular process, fluffy infiltrates, and diffuse interstitial/alveolar infiltrates. Pseudolymphoma is a collection of abnormal lymphocytes and presents as a slow-growing lung mass; currently, it is considered a low-grade lymphoma. Almost all cases of lymphocytic interstitial pneumonitis represent low-grade lymphomas that originate from the mucosa-associated lymphoid tissue ("maltoma"); they show a good response to chemotherapy.

- Intrathoracic involvement is common in Hodgkin lymphoma.
- Bilateral hilar lymphadenopathy and chylous pleural effusion occur in young adults.
- Hodgkin lymphoma can produce any type of CXR abnormality.

Diagnostic Tests

Sputum cytology is positive in 60% of patients with squamous cell carcinoma, in 21% with small cell carcinoma, in 16% with adenocarcinoma, and in 13% with large cell carcinoma. CXR diagnoses more tumors than sputum cytology, but CXR is not recommended as a surveillance tool for all patients. Bronchoscopy is helpful in diagnosing the cell type, in assessing staging and resectability, in using laser treatment for large airway tumors, and in brachytherapy. Transthoracic needle aspiration has an 85% to 90% yield, but the incidence of pneumothorax is 25%, with most patients requiring chest tube drainage. CT is helpful in assessing the number of nodules in patients with pulmonary metastasis and in examination of the hila and mediastinum. Positive results on pleural fluid cytology establish stage IIIB disease. Mediastinoscopy and mediastinotomy (Chamberlain procedure) are staging procedures that are often used before thoracotomy is performed.

- CXR helps diagnose more lung tumors than sputum cytology.
- Sputum cytology findings are positive in 60% of patients with squamous cell cancer.
- Routine surveillance of all susceptible persons (heavy smokers) with CXR and sputum cytology is not recommended.

Paraneoplastic Syndromes

As a group, primary lung tumors are the most common cause of paraneoplastic syndromes. The presence of a paraneoplastic syndrome does not indicate metastatic spread of lung cancer. It is more helpful to consider paraneoplastic manifestations based on each organ system (see below).

- Primary lung tumors cause most of the paraneoplastic manifestations.
- A paraneoplastic syndrome does not indicate metastatic spread of lung cancer.

Endocrine

Small cell carcinoma is associated with the syndrome of inappropriate antidiuretic hormone and ACTH production. Hypokalemia, muscle weakness, and CXR abnormality should suggest ACTH production. These patients do not live long enough to develop typical Cushing syndrome. The ACTH levels are high and not suppressed by dexamethasone. Hypercalcemia is not associated with small cell carcinoma. The overall frequency of hypercalcemia is 13%, with squamous cell cancer causing it in 25% of patients, large cell carcinoma in 13%, and adenocarcinoma in 3%. Bony metastasis can also cause hypercalcemia. Hyperpigmentation from MSH occurs in small cell carcinoma. Calcitonin is secreted in 70% of patients with small cell carcinoma and in adenocarcinoma. The syndrome of inappropriate antidiuretic hormone is also seen in some patients with alveolar cell carcinoma and adenocarcinoma. Hypoglycemia with insulin-like polypeptide is found in patients with squamous cell carcinoma and mesothelioma. The hCG, LH, and FSH secreted by adenocarcinoma and large cell carcinoma may be responsible for gynecomastia.

- Abnormal CXR, hypokalemia, and muscle weakness: small cell carcinoma (ACTH).
- ACTH is also produced by bronchial carcinoid.
- Hypercalcemia: squamous cell carcinoma and carcinoid.

Central Nervous System

The mechanisms for encephalopathy, myelopathy, sensory-motor neuropathies, and polymyositis are unknown but may include toxic, nutritional, autoimmune, and infectious causes. Cerebellar ataxia is similar to alcohol-induced ataxia and is more common with squamous cell carcinoma. Myasthenic syndrome (Lambert-Eaton syndrome) is closely associated with small cell carcinoma; the proximal muscles are initially weak, but strength returns to normal with repeated stimulation. Focal neurologic signs should suggest central nervous system metastasis. Acute and rapidly progressive lower extremity signs should indicate spinal cord compression by tumor. Antineuronal nuclear antibody (ANNA-1) is positive in many patients with small cell carcinoma.

- Myasthenic syndrome may precede clinical detection of small cell carcinoma.
- Cerebellar ataxia (similar to alcohol-induced ataxia) is more common in squamous cell carcinoma.

Skeletal

HPO indicates periosteal bone formation and is associated with clubbing and symmetrical arthralgias. Other features include fever, gynecomastia, and an increased ESR. The proposed mechanisms include neural (vagal afferents), hormonal, and others. HPO is more common in adenocarcinoma and large cell carcinoma than in squamous cell and small cell lung cancers and may precede detection of the tumor by months. Clubbing alone can be the only feature. Removal of the tumor relieves the HPO. Octreotide appears to be effective in treating HPO.

- HPO is more common in adenocarcinoma and large cell carcinoma.
- Octreotide (somatostatin analogue) or ipsilateral vagotomy if the HPO persists after resection of tumor.

Others

Other paraneoplastic manifestations include malignant cachexia, marantic endocarditis, increased incidence of thrombophlebitis, fever, erythrocytosis, leukocytosis, lymphocytopenia, eosinophilia, thrombocytosis, leukemoid reaction, disseminated intravascular coagulation, dysproteinemia, fever, acanthosis nigricans (adenocarcinoma), epidermolysis bullosa (squamous cell carcinoma), and nephrotic syndrome.

Pulmonary Metastases

Nearly 30% of all cases of malignant disease from extrapulmonary sites metastasize to the lung. More than 75% present with multiple lesions, and the rest may present as a solitary pulmonary nodule, a diffuse process, lymphangitic spread (breast, stomach, thyroid, pancreas, and the lung itself), and endobronchial metastases (kidney, colon, Hodgkin lymphoma, and breast). Solitary metastases are more common with carcinoma of the colon, kidneys, testis, breast, and with sarcoma and melanoma. The estimated occurrence of pulmonary metastasis by primary tumor is as follows: choriocarcinoma, 80%; osteosarcoma, 75%; kidney, 70%; thyroid, 65%; melanoma, 60%; breast, 55%; prostate, 45%; nasopharyngeal, 20%; gastrointestinal malignancies, 20%; and gynecologic malignancies, 20%.

PLEURA

Pleural Effusion

The normal volume of pleural fluid is 0.1 to 0.2 mL/kg of body weight. Excess pleural fluid collects in the pleural space when fluid collection exceeds normal removal mechanisms. Hydrostatic, oncotic, and intrapleural pressures regulate fluid movement in the pleural space. Any of the following mechanisms can produce pleural effusion: changes in capillary permeability (inflammation), increased hydrostatic pressure, decreased plasma oncotic pressure, impaired lymphatic drainage, increased negative intrapleural pressure, and movement of fluid (through diaphragmatic pores and lymphatic vessels) from the peritoneum. The principal causes of pleural effusion are listed in Table 21-12.

Transudate Versus Exudate

The effusion is a *transudate* if the protein content is less than 3 g, the specific gravity is less than 1.016, fluid lactic dehydrogenase is less than 60% of serum (fluid/serum <0.6), and the serum-effusion albumin gradient (serum minus effusion albumin) is greater than 1.2 g/dL. It is an *exudate* if the protein content is greater than 3 g, fluid/serum protein is greater than 0.5, the specific gravity is greater than 1.016, and fluid lactic dehydrogenase is greater than 60% of serum lactic dehy-

Table 21-12.—Principal Causes of Pleural Effusion

Osmotic-hydraulic*
    Congestive cardiac failure
    Superior vena caval obstruction
    Constrictive pericarditis
    Cirrhosis with ascites
    Hypoalbuminemia
    Salt-retaining syndromes
    Peritoneal dialysis
    Hydronephrosis
    Nephrotic syndrome
Infections[†]
    Parapneumonic (bacterial) effusions
    Bacterial empyema
    Tuberculosis
    Fungi
    Parasites
    Viruses and mycoplasma
Neoplasms[†]
    Primary and metastatic lung tumors
    Lymphoma and leukemia
    Benign and malignant tumors of pleura
    Intra-abdominal tumors with ascites
Vascular disease[†]
    Pulmonary embolism
    Wegener granulomatosis
Intra-abdominal diseases[†]
    Pancreatitis and pancreatic pseudocyst
    Subdiaphragmatic abscess
    Malignancy with ascites
    Meigs syndrome*
    Hepatic cirrhosis with ascites*
Trauma[†]
    Hemothorax
    Chylothorax
    Esophageal rupture
    Intra-abdominal surgery
Miscellaneous
    Drug-induced effusions[†]
    Uremic pleuritis[†]
    Myxedema*
    Yellow nail syndrome[†]
    Dressler syndrome[†]
    Familial Mediterranean fever[†]

*Usually a transudate.
[†]Usually an exudate.

drogenase or fluid lactic dehydrogenase is greater than 200 units. Increased lactic dehydrogenase in fluid is nonspecific, but it is increased in pulmonary embolism, rheumatoid effusion, and most exudative effusions.

- It is not necessary to perform all the above tests to differentiate a transudate from an exudate.
- Clinically, it is more useful to classify cause by considering the source (organ system) of the fluid (Table 21-12).
- The classification of pleural fluid into transudates and exudates does not permit consideration of all causes.
- The most common cause of a transudate is congestive heart failure (pulmonary artery wedge pressure >25 mm Hg).
- The most common cause of an exudate is pneumonia (parapneumonic effusion).

Glucose and pH

Pleural fluid hypoglycemia (<60 mg/dL or fluid/plasma glucose <0.6) is seen in rheumatoid effusion, malignant mesothelioma, empyema, systemic lupus erythematosus, esophageal rupture, and yellow nail syndrome. The pH of pleural fluid is less than 7.20 in empyema, esophageal rupture, rheumatoid effusion, tuberculosis, carcinoma, and trauma. If the pH is low (<7.20) and clinical suspicion is high for infection, drainage with a chest tube should be considered. Empyema caused by *Proteus* species produces a pH greater than 7.8 (because of ammonia production).

- The pleural fluid glucose concentration and pH usually go together (i.e., if glucose is low, so is pH).
- Low glucose levels in rheumatoid effusion, malignant mesothelioma, and empyema.

Amylase

Pleural fluid amylase concentration increases in pancreatitis, pseudocyst of the pancreas, rupture of abdominal viscera, and esophageal rupture. The amylase level in the fluid remains higher for longer periods than that in the serum.

- Increased concentration of pleural fluid amylase in esophageal rupture is due to leakage of salivary amylase.
- In any unexplained left-sided effusion, consider pancreatitis and measure the amylase level in the pleural fluid.

Chylous Effusion

Chylous effusion cannot be diagnosed on the basis of the color or appearance of the fluid. More than 90% of true chylous effusions contain triglyceride levels greater than 100 mg/dL, and a triglyceride level less than 50 mg/dL is less likely to be chylous. Clinicians should ascertain that the serum level of triglyceride is normal. Chylous effusions can occur in conditions listed below as well as in Kaposi sarcoma with mediastinal adenopathy, after Valsalva maneuver during childbirth, esophagectomy, esophageal sclerotherapy, and thrombosis of the superior vena cava or the innominate or subclavian vein. Cholesterol effusions (fluid cholesterol >250 mg/dL) are not true chylous effusions. They are seen in old tuberculous effusions and rheumatoid effusions and in some cases of nephrotic syndrome.

- Chylous effusion is seen in the "5 Ts": **T**horacic duct **T**rauma, **T**umor (lymphoma), **T**uberculosis, **T**uberous sclerosis (lymphangiomyomatosis).
- True chylous effusion contains chylomicrons.
- Cholesterol effusions are not true chylous effusions.

Complement

Total, C3, and C4 components in the pleural fluid are decreased in systemic lupus erythematosus (80% of patients), rheumatoid arthritis (40%-60% of patients), carcinoma, pneumonia, and tuberculosis. Increased pleural fluid antinuclear antibody (>1:160) is strongly suggestive of lupus erythematosus. Rheumatoid factor is greater than 1:320 in rheumatoid pleural effusion.

- Low pleural fluid complement: systemic lupus erythematosus (including in drug-induced form).
- Presence of lupus erythematosus cells in the pleural fluid is diagnostic of systemic lupus erythematosus.

Cell Counts

An erythrocyte count greater than 100,000/dL in the pleural fluid produces a "bloody effusion." This is seen in trauma, tumor, asbestos effusion, pancreatitis (60%), pulmonary embolism with infarctions, and other conditions. A leukocyte count greater than 20,000/dL is seen in parapneumonic effusions, empyema, and leukemic effusions (rare). Pleural fluid eosinophilia is nonspecific and occurs in trauma, pulmonary infarction, psittacosis, drug-induced effusion, pulmonary infiltrate with eosinophilia-associated effusions, and pneumothorax. Pleural fluid lymphocytosis occurs in tuberculosis, chronic effusions, lymphoma, and some collagenoses.

- Bloody effusion in lung cancer, even if cytologic results are negative, usually denotes pleural metastasis.
- Eosinophilia in pleural fluid is nonspecific.
- Differential leukocyte count in pleural fluid is generally unhelpful.

Cytology

Cytologic examination should be performed on most effusions in adults if the clinical features do not suggest an obvious benign cause. Cytologic findings are positive in 60% and pleural biopsy results in less than 50% of all malignant effusions. Cytologic examination and biopsy give a slightly higher yield than either one alone. Cytologic examination is less helpful in malignant mesothelioma, and an open biopsy is often necessary. Positive fluid cytologic findings in primary lung carcinoma mean unresectability (stage IIIB).

- Cytologic examination is an important test in most adults with an "unknown" effusion.
- The overall yield from a cytologic examination is 60%; less in cases of mesothelioma and lymphoma.

Cultures

Tuberculous effusions (fluid alone) yield positive cultures in fewer than 15% of cases. Pleural biopsy (histology and culture) has a higher (>75%) diagnostic yield. Culture is of value in effusions due to actinomycosis and *Nocardia* infection but is less helpful in other mycoses. However, if fungal infection of the pleural space is suspected, cultures should be performed. Cultures for viruses (influenza A, ornithosis, coxsackievirus B, and mycoplasma) are often negative. Paragonimiasis causes pleural effusion. The diagnosis of tuberculous pleuritis is strongly suggested by a high adenosine deaminase (ADA) level in the pleural fluid. Another relatively sensitive test for the diagnosis of tuberculous pleuritis is the level of interferon-gamma in the pleural fluid.

- In tuberculosis, it is important to culture pleural biopsy specimens.
- ADA level is elevated in tuberculous pleural effusion.
- Poor yield in viral infections.

Pleural Biopsy

Pleural biopsy is indicated if tuberculous involvement of the pleural space is suspected. The diagnostic rate from pleural biopsy in tuberculosis is greater than 75%, whereas pleural fluid alone has a much lower yield (<15%). The overall diagnostic yield in malignant pleural effusions is about 50%. Diagnostic rates are low (<30%) in malignant pleural mesothelioma.

- Pleural biopsy is indicated if tuberculous pleural disease is suspected.

Miscellaneous

At least 350 to 400 mL of fluid has to be present to be seen on CXR. Look for subpulmonic effusions, elevated hemidiaphragms, and blunting of the costophrenic angle. When in doubt, obtain a lateral decubitus CXR. Ultrasonography is helpful in tapping small amounts of fluid and loculated fluid collections. Look for signs of trauma (rib fracture), abdominal surgery, acute abdomen, pancreatitis, and cirrhosis. Asbestos-induced effusions frequently mimic malignant pleural mesothelioma, with pain, bloody fluid, and recurrence. Mesothelioma should be excluded by repeated thoracentesis, pleural biopsy, or thoracotomy.

- Small effusions are common after abdominal operations and the normal labor of pregnancy; almost all resolve spontaneously.
- Drug-induced pleural effusion: nitrofurantoin, methysergide, drug-induced systemic lupus erythematosus, and busulfan.
- Nearly 20% of all effusions are undiagnosed despite extensive studies, including open pleural biopsy.

Complications

Complications of thoracentesis include pneumothorax (in 3%-20% of patients), hemothorax, pulmonary edema, intrapulmonary hemorrhage, hemoptysis, vagal inhibition, air embolism, subcutaneous emphysema, bronchopleural fistula, empyema, and puncture of the liver or spleen.

Pneumothorax

Spontaneous pneumothorax occurs more commonly in young, previously healthy adults. The incidence of primary spontaneous pneumothorax is 9 cases/100,000 persons per year, with a male-to-female ratio of 6:1. Many are caused by the rupture of apical bullae. Smoking increases the risk of spontaneous pneumothorax. Secondary spontaneous pneumothorax occurs most frequently in COPD, with an annual incidence of 4 cases/100,000 patients and a male-to-female ratio of 3:1. Other causes of spontaneous secondary pneumothorax include pulmonary Langerhans cell granuloma, asthma, emphysema, bullous lung disease, cystic fibrosis, lung tumors, end-stage fibrosis and honeycombing of the lungs, Marfan disease, and, in young females, during the menses (catamenial pneumothorax). Iatrogenic pneumothorax may be seen after thoracentesis, trauma, esophageal rupture, tracheal fracture, subclavian needle sticks, high positive end-expiratory pressure, transtracheal aspiration, severe Valsalva maneuver, and secondary to pneumoperitoneum. The treatment of spontaneous pneumothorax includes chest tube drainage, chemical pleurodesis (tetracycline or other chemicals), talc pleurodesis, and, occasionally, surgical decortication.

- Spontaneous pneumothorax: Langerhans cell granuloma, peripheral lung tumors, lymphangioleiomyomatosis, bullous lung disease, and COPD.
- In younger females with pleuritic chest pain during menses, consider catamenial pneumothorax.
- An end-expiratory CXR is better for identifying a small pneumothorax.

Pleurodesis

Pleurodesis is indicated in the treatment of recurrent pneumothorax or pleural effusion. If repeated therapeutic thoracentesis fails to relieve symptoms, then chemical pleurodesis with pleural instillation of tetracycline (15 mg/kg in 30 mL of saline), doxycycline (10 mg/kg), minocycline (5 mg/kg), or talc (2.5-10 g) is done through a chest tube. Talc pleurodesis is more than 90% effective, whereas other chemicals are 65% effective. Surgical pleurodesis may be indicated if these agents do not produce closure of the pleural space.

- Antibiotic pleurodesis is 65% effective.
- Talc pleurodesis is >90% effective.

Empyema

Empyema is the collection of pus in the pleural space. For clinical purposes, the presence of bacteria in the pleural fluid is also considered empyema. Empyema is caused by bacterial pneumonia in more than 50% of patients (empyema develops in about 2% of patients with pneumonia), bacteremia in less than 10%, compromised host in less than 10%, trauma in 5% to 15%, thoracic surgery in 10% to 25%, esophageal perforation, lung abscess, and infarction. Bacteria that commonly are isolated are *S. aureus* (25%-35% of patients), anaerobes (15%-35%), gram-negative bacilli (15%-30%), and *S. pneumoniae* and other streptococci (12%-15%). In one-third of the cases of anaerobic empyema, cultures of the fluid are positive, whereas less than 5% of the cases of parapneumonic effusion due to *S. pneumoniae* are positive on culture. Treatment consists of systemic antibiotics, chest tube drainage, thoracostomy, and decortication. The success rate for conventional tube thoracostomy drainage to treat empyema is 32% to 71%. Intrapleural thrombolysis for the treatment of thoracic empyema has success rates of 44% to 100%. Video-assisted thoracic surgery is a safe and effective operative strategy for the treatment of complicated empyema. Mortality from empyema is higher in older patients and in those with multiple bacterial isolates, gram-negative bacilli, serious illnesses, and hospital-acquired empyema.

- A chest tube is indicated if purulent effusion, positive gram stain, pH <7.00 or glucose <40 mg and LDH >1,000 U/L.

MEDIASTINUM

Mediastinal Lesions

Clinically, it is useful to divide mediastinal lesions into their location, namely, anterior, middle, and posterior mediastinum. The anterior compartment contains the thymus, thyroid, ascending aorta, innominate artery and vein, superior vena cava, fat, and lymph nodes. More than 50% of mediastinal tumors are located in this compartment, and 60% of them are thymic tumors, lymphomas, and germ cell tumors. The middle mediastinum contains the cardiac chambers, pericardium, aortic arch and its branches, trachea and bronchi, esophagus, and mediastinal nodes. Most of the tumors in this compartment are cystic and 25% are metastatic malignancies. The posterior compartment contains the lower esophagus, descending aorta, sympathetic chain, and intercostal nerves. Nearly 25% of all mediastinal tumors are in the posterior compartment, and 70% of them are neurogenic tumors.

- Nearly 30% of mediastinal masses are malignant.
- Anterior mediastinum: the "6 Ts"—**T**hymoma, **T**eratoma, **T**umor (lymphoma and carcinomas), **T**horacic aortic aneurysm, **T**rauma (hematoma or aneurysm), and **T**hyroid.
- Posterior mediastinum: neurogenic tumors make up 70% of the tumors.
- Middle mediastinum: one-fourth are metastatic tumors.

Thymoma is the most common tumor in the anterior mediastinum and is associated with myasthenia gravis, red cell aplasia, and collagenoses. Neurilemoma and neurofibroma are the most common tumors in the posterior mediastinum. In adults, fewer than 4% of these tumors are malignant. Up to 40% of patients with neurofibromas have von Recklinghausen disease. MRI may be required to exclude intraspinal extension of a mediastinal neurogenic tumor.

- Thymoma: 15%-45% are associated with myasthenia gravis.
- 10%-15% of patients with myasthenia gravis have thymoma.
- Thymoma is also associated with red cell aplasia, hypogammaglobulinemia, and Cushing syndrome (ACTH from thymic carcinoid).
- Malignant changes are uncommon in posterior mediastinal tumors in adults.

Mediastinitis

An acute infection of the mediastinal space usually produces mediastinitis. Acute mediastinitis is an acute medical/surgical emergency. One of the most common causes is esophageal rupture produced by iatrogenic trauma (instrumentation) or tumor necrosis in the mediastinum. Fever, dyspnea, neck and thoracic paraspinal pain, dysphagia, and odynophagia are frequent. CXR almost always reveals pleural effusion and may show air in the neck or mediastinum (pneumomediastinum). Contrast imaging of the esophagus may be necessary to document the process. Immediate surgical drainage and intensive antibiotic therapy are required in all patients. Mortality is high (>50%) if the diagnosis is delayed for more than 24 hours.

- Acute mediastinitis is caused most commonly by esophageal perforation.

- High mortality if it is not diagnosed and treated within 24 hours.

Mediastinal Fibrosis/Granuloma

Mediastinal fibrosis, or fibrosing mediastinitis, represents an exuberant fibrotic reaction in the mediastinum. In the U.S., it is caused most commonly by histoplasmosis. Other causes include tuberculosis, autoimmune process, drugs (methysergide), and idiopathic. It most likely represents a delayed hypersensitivity reaction to fungal, mycobacterial, or other antigens. Most patients with mediastinal fibrosis do not have active histoplasmosis at the time of the diagnosis. Special stains of fibrotic tissue may show nonviable histoplasma organisms. Granuloma formation may also be seen. Extensive calcification of hilar and mediastinal lymph nodes may be seen in some patients. Calcified tissue may erode into the bronchial lumen, causing broncholithiasis. The excessive fibrotic process may encircle the airways, esophagus, major veins, and arteries in the hilar region and cause compression and, sometimes, occlusion of these structures. The clinical features depend on the extent of involvement of intrathoracic organs.

- Mediastinal fibrosis/granuloma is caused most often by histoplasmosis.
- Active infection is not present in patients with mediastinal fibrosis.
- The fibrotic process encircles mediastinal organs and causes symptoms.

VASCULAR DISEASES

Pulmonary Embolism

Pulmonary embolism (PE) is the cause of death in 5% to 15% of patients dying in hospitals in the U.S. A multicenter study of PE observed that the mortality rate at 3 months was 15%, and significant prognostic factors include age older than 70 years, cancer, congestive heart failure, COPD, systolic arterial hypotension, tachypnea, and right ventricular hypokinesis. It is detected in 25% to 30% of routine autopsies. Antemortem diagnosis is made in less than 30% of cases. Among hospitalized patients, the prevalence of PE is 1%. In about 90% of patients who die of PE, death occurs within 1 to 2 hours. The risk of fatal PE is greater among patients with severe deep venous thrombosis (DVT).

- PE is a common problem; consider PE in all patients with lung problems.
- Antemortem diagnosis is made in <30%.
- The risk of death from untreated PE = 8%.

Etiology

The factor responsible for most PEs is DVT of the lower extremities. Among patients with fatal PE, DVT has been identified clinically in only 50%. In those with large angiographically diagnosed PE, DVT is detected in about 35%. About 60% of patients with PE have lower extremity DVT that is asymptomatic. Approximately 45% of femoral and iliac DVTs embolize to the lungs. Other sources of emboli include thrombi in the upper extremities, right ventricle, and indwelling catheters. In up to 20% of patients, the DVTs from the calves propagate to the thigh and iliac veins, and up to 10% of cases of superficial thrombophlebitis are complicated by DVT. The risk of recurrent DVT is similar among carriers of factor V Leiden and patients without this mutation (NEJM 341:801, 1999). The primary and secondary coagulation abnormalities that predispose to the development of DVT and PE are listed in Table 21-13.

- DVT is detected in only 40% of cases of pulmonary embolism.
- Consider deficiencies of antithrombin III, proteins S and C, and the presence of lupus anticoagulant among predisposing factors for DVT and PE.
- Idiopathic, recurrent DVT: look for an occult neoplasm.

The incidence of DVT in various clinical circumstances is as follows: major abdominal surgery, 14% to 33% (odds 1:20 without prophylaxis and 1:50 with prophylaxis); thoracic surgery, 25% to 60%; gynecologic surgery, less than 3% (40 years and younger) and 10% to 40% (40 years and older) and 40% to 70% (older than 40 years with other added risks); urologic surgery, 10% to 40%; hip surgery, 50% to 75%; post-myocardial infarction, 20% to 40%; congestive heart failure, 70%; stroke with paralysis, 50% to 70%; postpartum, 3%; and trauma, 20% to 40%. Idiopathic DVT, particularly when recurrent, may indicate the presence of neoplasm in 10% to 20% of patients. The presence of varicose veins does not increase the risk of developing DVT.

- Risk of DVT: thoracic surgery, 25%-60%; hip surgery, 50%-75%; post-myocardial infarction, 20%-40%; congestive heart failure, 70%; and stroke with paralysis, 50%-70%.

DVT is diagnosed in only 50% of clinical cases. A diagnosis based on physical examination findings is unreliable. Homans sign (pain and tenderness on dorsiflexion of the ankle) is elicited in less than 40% of cases of DVT, and a false-positive Homans sign occurs in 30% of high-risk patients. Impedance plethysmography (IPG) and duplex ultrasonography (US) together are the most commonly used noninvasive tests and

Table 21-13.—Coagulation Disorders Predisposing to the Development of Deep Venous Thrombosis and Pulmonary Embolism

Primary hypercoagulable states	Secondary hypercoagulable states
Activated protein C resistance* (factor V Leiden carriers)	Cancer
Antithrombin III deficiency†	Postoperative states (stasis)
Protein C deficiency†	Lupus anticoagulant syndrome
Protein S deficiency†	Increased factor VII and fibrinogen
Fibrinolytic abnormalities	Pregnancy
Hypoplasminogenemia	Nephrotic syndrome
Dysplasminogenemia	Myeloproliferative disorders
tPA release deficiency	Disseminated intravascular coagulation
Increased tPA inhibitor	Acute stroke
Dysfibrinogenemia	Hyperlipidemias
Homocystinuria	Diabetes mellitus
Heparin cofactor deficiency	Paroxysmal nocturnal hemoglobinuria
Increased histidine-rich glycoprotein	Behçet disease and vasculitides
	Anticancer drugs (chemotherapy)
	Heparin-induced thrombocytopenia
	Oral contraceptives
	Obesity

tPA, tissue plasminogen activator.

*Prevalence of factor V Leiden in patients with deep venous thrombosis is 16%; presence of factor V Leiden is associated with a 40% risk of recurrent deep venous thrombosis (*N Engl J Med* 336:399-403, 1997).

†Prevalence of these protein deficiencies in patients with deep venous thrombosis is 5% to 10%.

From Prakash UBS: Pulmonary embolism. *In* Mayo Clinic Cardiology Review. 2nd Ed. Edited by JG Murphy. Philadelphia, Lippincott Williams & Wilkins, 2000, pp 379-406. By permission of Mayo Foundation for Medical Education and Research.

have a diagnostic accuracy of 90% to 95% in detecting iliac and femoral DVTs. Their accuracy in the diagnosis of calf vein thrombosis is clinically unreliable. Serial (daily) IPG or US (or both) is recommended in high-risk patients because of a 15% detection rate of DVT after the initial negative study. Currently, IPG is used less commonly than US. US is less accurate for the diagnosis of chronic DVT and less useful in pelvic DVT than in the diagnosis of acute femoral DVT. Venography is considered nearly 100% sensitive and specific. Venography should be performed when other tests are nondiagnostic or impossible to perform. MRI has a high sensitivity and specificity for the diagnosis of pelvic DVT.

- DVT is diagnosed in only 50% of clinical cases.
- IPG + duplex US are up to 95% accurate for detecting iliac and femoral DVTs.
- Serial IPG is important in chronically hospitalized patients.

Clinical Features

PE has no typical clinical symptoms and signs. Tachypnea and tachycardia are observed in nearly all patients. Other symptoms include dyspnea in 80%, pleuritic pain in up to 75%, hemoptysis in fewer than 25%, pleural friction rub in 20%, and wheezing in 15%. The differential diagnosis of PE includes myocardial infarction, pneumonia, congestive heart failure, pericarditis, esophageal spasm, asthma, exacerbation of COPD, intrathoracic malignancy, rib fracture, pneumothorax, pleurisy from any cause, pleurodynia, and nonspecific skeletal pains. Acute cor pulmonale occurs if more than 65% of the pulmonary circulation is obstructed by emboli. PE should be suspected in the setting of syncope or acute hypotension.

- PE has no typical signs or symptoms.
- Acute cor pulmonale occurs when >65% of the vasculature is obstructed by PE.

Diagnostic Tests

Clinical examination, ECG, CXR, blood gas abnormalities, and increased plasma D-dimer test have a low specificity and sensitivity for the diagnosis of PE. Clinical suspicion is the most important factor in steering a clinician toward the appropriate diagnostic tests to diagnose PE. CXR may show diaphragmatic elevation in 60% of patients, infiltrates in 30%, focal oligemia in 10% to 50%, effusion in 20%, an enlarged pulmonary artery in 20%, and normal findings in 30%. Nonspecific ECG changes are noted in 80%, ST and T changes in 65%, T inversion in 40%, S_1Q_3 pattern in fewer than 25%, right bundle branch block in 12%, and left axis deviation in 12%. Early echocardiography is recommended in critical patients to assess right ventricular hypokinesia/dysfunction. The recommendations of the American Thoracic Society for the diagnosis of PE are listed in Figure 21-28.

- Normal CXR in 30% of patients with PE.
- The classic S_1Q_3 pattern is seen in only 15% of patients.

Both the PaO_2 and $P(A-a)O_2$ gradient may be normal in 15% to 20% of patients. The $(A-a)O_2$ gradient shows a linear correlation with the severity of the PE. A normal $(A-a)O_2$ gradient does not exclude PE. Indeed, in the PIOPED study, about 20% of patients with angiographically documented PE had a normal $P(A-a)O_2$ gradient ($\leq$20 mm Hg). Most patients with acute PE demonstrate hypocapnia.

- The $P(A-a)O_2$ gradient correlates linearly with the severity of the PE.

- 20% of patients with PE show a normal $P(A-a)O_2$ gradient ($\leq$20 mm Hg).

The levels of D-dimer (a specific fibrin degradation product) are increased in DVT and PE. However, high levels themselves have no positive predictive value for PE. A normal level of D-dimer does not exclude PE but makes it unlikely in patients with a low pretest probability of PE. Age and pregnancy are associated with increased levels. Levels less than 300 µg/L (by ELISA) or less than 500 µg/L (by latex agglutination) are considered to reliably exclude PE in patients with an abnormal but not high-probability V/Q lung scan. A plasma D-dimer concentration less than 500 µg/L allows the exclusion of PE in fewer than 30% of patients suspected of having PE. Currently, the D-dimer test cannot be recommended as a standard part of the PE or DVT diagnostic algorithm (Am J Resp Crit Care Med 160:1043, 1999).

- Increased D-dimer levels have no positive predictive value for PE.

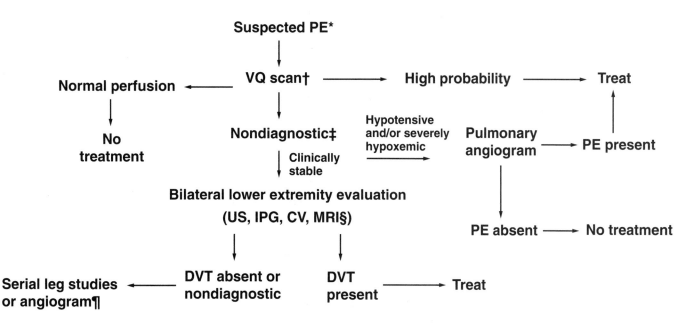

Fig. 21-28. Diagnostic algorithm, recommended by the American Thoracic Society, for patients with symptoms suggesting acute pulmonary embolism (PE). DVT, deep venous thrombosis.

*When PE is suspected and the risk of bleeding is deemed low, it is appropriate to begin anticoagulation while diagnostic testing is under way.

†A perfusion scan alone may suffice. Diagnostic alternatives to the ventilation-perfusion (VQ) scan include spiral computed tomography (CT) and magnetic resonance imaging (MRI).

‡Patients with low probability VQ scans and low clinical suspicion are unlikely to have PE. Others require further evaluation. There are several options when the VQ scan (or spiral CT or lung MRI) is nondiagnostic. Pulmonary angiography is the appropriate approach if the patient is unstable. Otherwise, leg studies can be performed. If spiral CT or lung MRI is performed, a negative result should be interpreted together with the level of clinical suspicion. Although these techniques appear to be sensitive, additional studies (pulmonary angiography or leg studies) should be performed as deemed appropriate.

§A positive test is useful. The sensitivity for compression ultrasound (US) and impedance plethysmography (IPG) is low in asymptomatic patients, and negative or nondiagnostic studies require additional data.

¶Negative serial IPG in this setting has been associated with excellent outcome without anticoagulation at certain centers.

Modified from American Thoracic Society: The diagnostic approach to acute venous thromboembolism. Clinical practice guidelines. Am J Respir Crit Care Med 160:1043-1066, 1999. By permission of American Thoracic Society.

● Normal (<500 µg/L) D-dimer levels exclude PE in fewer than 30% of cases.

Echocardiography can identify right-sided heart thrombi in up to 15% of patients with PE. Dysfunction of the right ventricle, frequently seen in massive as well as recurrent PE, can be detected by echocardiography. Although the echocardiographic findings are abnormal in more than 80% of patients with documented PE, the findings are nonspecific. The presence of associated abnormalities (intracardiac tumors, myxoma, etc.) poses a difficulty in distinguishing among the lesions. A highly mobile intracavitary thrombus-in-transit has a 98% risk of acute PE and a 1-week mortality of 50%. Transesophageal echocardiography is reportedly 97% sensitive and 86% specific for the diagnosis of centrally located pulmonary arterial thrombi. Currently, the role of echocardiography in the diagnosis of acute PE is undefined (Am J Resp Crit Care Med 160:1043, 1999).

The V/Q scan is commonly used in the diagnosis of PE. A high-probability lung scan has a sensitivity of 41% and a specificity of 97%. A "low-probability" lung scan excludes the diagnosis of PE in more than 85% of patients. A normal lung scan excludes PE in 100%. An "intermediate- or indeterminate-probability" scan is associated with PE in 21% to 30% of patients. Therefore, patients with an "intermediate-probability" lung scan usually require pulmonary angiography. A negative or normal perfusion-only scan (excluding ventilation scan) rules out PE with a very high probability.

● High-probability scan = 90% probability of PE.
● Intermediate-probability scan = 30% probability of PE.
● Low-probability scan = 15% probability of PE.
● Normal scan excludes PE in 100%.

CT permits ultrafast scanning of pulmonary arteries during contrast injection. Spiral (helical) CT is used more frequently to detect PE. Sensitivity and specificity rates greater than 95% have been reported. Spiral CT has the greatest sensitivity in the diagnosis of PE in the main, lobar, or segmental arteries. Lymph node enlargement may result in false-positive studies. MRI may have the advantage of detecting both DVT and PE.

● Ultrafast CT is better than V/Q scan for the diagnosis of PE.

Pulmonary angiography is the best diagnostic test. It should be performed within 24 to 48 hours after the diagnosis has been considered. However, it is nondiagnostic in 3% of cases. Major and minor complications following pulmonary angiography occur in 1% and 2% of patients, respectively, and mortality from the procedure is 0.5%. Pulmonary angiography

followed by therapy with tissue plasminogen activator (tPA) is associated with a 14% risk of major hemorrhage.

● Major and minor complications from pulmonary angiography = 1% and 2%, respectively.

Treatment

The therapy for uncomplicated DVT is identical to that for PE. For acute disease, treatment can begin simultaneously with both heparin and warfarin unless warfarin is contraindicated. When treatment with both drugs is begun simultaneously, an overlap for 4 to 5 days is recommended. For patients with acute disease, heparin (80 U/kg) is administered as a bolus, followed by the maintenance dose of 18 U/kg per hour intravenously. The dose should be adjusted to maintain an activated partial thromboplastin time (APTT) above 1.5 times the control value. Nonweight-based heparin dosage in acute DVT and acute PE consists of initial intravenous boluses of 5,000 units and 15,000 to 20,000 units, respectively; the maintenance dosage is more than 1,200 U/hr intravenously or 15,000 to 20,000 units subcutaneously to maintain an APTT greater than 1.5 times control. Low-molecular-weight heparin (LMWH) is better than unfractionated heparin, according to recent studies, and can be used to treat patients at home.

● In acute DVT/PE, heparin and warfarin treatment can begin simultaneously.
● Heparin dose: bolus = 80 U/kg; maintenance = 18 U/kg per hour.

Long-term anticoagulant therapy can be maintained with either heparin or warfarin. Heparin is indicated when warfarin is contraindicated or not tolerated. The usual dose of heparin is 5,000 to 10,000 units subcutaneously twice daily. However, the dose should be adjusted based on the APTT, as noted above. The weight-based heparin dosage is not reliable for maintenance therapy by the subcutaneous route. Low-molecular-weight heparin, 30 mg twice daily subcutaneously, has been used in patients who have difficulty monitoring the APTT. Warfarin at a dosage to achieve a PT of 1.3 to 1.5 times control or an International Normalized Ratio (INR) of 2 to 3 is recommended. The loading dose of warfarin usually is 10 mg/day for 1 or 2 days, followed by adjustment of the dosage to maintain an INR of 2.0 to 3.0. Recurrent and complicated cases (coagulopathies, etc.) may require lifelong anticoagulation, maintenance of higher APTT or PT levels, and other measures such as plication of the inferior vena cava.

● APTT in uncomplicated cases: 1.5x-2.0x normal.
● PT in uncomplicated cases: 1.3x-1.5x normal (INR of 2-3).
● Treatment for uncomplicated DVT/PE: 6 months.

Thrombolytic agents (streptokinase, urokinase, and tPA) are used in massive PE and massive iliofemoral thrombosis. The indications are debated, although these drugs generally are indicated in patients with massive DVT and/or PE. One-year mortality among those treated with heparin alone and those treated with thrombolytic agents is 19% and 9%, respectively. The rate of recurrent PE in heparin-alone therapy versus thrombolytic therapy is 11% and 5.5%, respectively. Ideally, thrombolytic agents are administered within 24 hours after PE. The dosages for different agents are as follows: streptokinase, loading dose of 250,000 IU infused over 30 minutes, followed by a maintenance dose of 100,000 IU/hr for up to 24 hours; urokinase, loading dose of 4,400 IU/kg infused over 10 minutes, followed by continuous infusion of 4,400 IU/kg per hour, for 12 hours; and for tPA, a total dose of 100 mg intravenously over a 2-hour period. The adequacy of thrombolytic therapy is monitored with thrombin time. Heparin infusion is begun or resumed if the APTT is less than 80 seconds after thrombolytic therapy. Contraindications to thrombolytic agents include recent (within 10 days) surgery, intra-arterial procedures, renal or liver biopsies within the preceding 14 days, ulcer disease, recent cerebrovascular accident, hemorrhagic diathesis, or pregnancy.

- Thrombolytic agents should be given within 24 hours after PE.
- Heparin therapy is necessary after thrombolytic therapy.

Bleeding complications from heparin are 3% to 8% and for warfarin, 4%. Among patients receiving chronic warfarin therapy, the cumulative incidence of fatal bleeding is 1% at 1 year and 2% at 3 years. A greater risk of major hemorrhage exists when anticoagulation is continued indefinitely. The presence of malignant disease at the initiation of warfarin therapy is significantly associated with major hemorrhage. Age, reason for anticoagulation, use of interfering drugs, and hypertension are not associated with bleeding in those receiving chronic warfarin therapy. Hemorrhagic risk does not appear to be related to heparin dosage or APTT values. Among patients with PE treated with thrombolytic drugs, the risk of intracranial bleeding is about 1%.

- Hemorrhagic complications for heparin are 3%-8% and 4% for warfarin.
- Thrombolytic therapy: 1% risk of intracranial bleeding.

Drugs that prolong the effect of warfarin include among others salicylate, heparin, estrogen, antibiotics, clofibrate, quinidine, and cimetidine. Drugs that decrease the effect of warfarin include glutethimide, rifampin, barbiturates, and ethchlorvynol. This is only a partial list of drugs that interfere with warfarin metabolism. Therefore, the physician recommending warfarin therapy should ascertain the drug-drug interaction or consult a pharmacist.

- Knowledge of the interaction of warfarin with other drugs is important.

Inferior Vena Caval Interruption

Inferior vena caval interruption is aimed at preventing PE while maintaining blood flow through the inferior vena cava. Inferior vena caval interruption is indicated when anticoagulant therapy is contraindicated, complications result from anticoagulant therapy, anticoagulant therapy fails, a bleeding disorder is present, chronic recurrent PE and secondary pulmonary hypertension occur, or surgical pulmonary thromboendarterectomy has been or is intended to be performed. Inferior vena cava plication does not replace anticoagulant therapy; many patients require both. Anticoagulant therapy after filter insertion is aimed at preventing DVT at the insertion site, inferior vena cava thrombosis, cephalad propagation of a clot from an occluded filter, or propagation or recurrence of lower extremity DVT.

- Inferior vena cava plication does not replace chronic anticoagulant therapy.
- PE occurs in 2.5% of patients despite vena caval interruption.

Prophylaxis

Prophylaxis against DVT and PE includes early ambulation after surgery or immobilization, intermittent pneumatic compression of the lower extremities, active and passive leg exercises, and a low dose of heparin given subcutaneously (10,000-15,000 U/day). A low dose of heparin reduces the incidence of DVT from 25% to 8%; 5,000 units are given preoperatively and then every 8 to 12 hours postoperatively. Prophylactic enoxaparin, 40 mg/d subcutaneously, safely reduces the risk of DVT in patients with acute medical illnesses (NEJM 341:793, 1999). LMWH has been approved in the U.S. for prophylaxis against DVT and PE after total hip arthroplasty and total knee arthroplasty. A postoperative, fixed-dose LMWH (enoxaparin, 30 mg subcutaneously every 12 hours) is more effective than adjusted-dose warfarin (INR 2-3) in preventing total DVT after total hip or knee arthroplasty. LMWH has a rapid onset of action and, in the future, may supersede standard heparin. LMWH is safe and approximately 50% more effective than standard heparin. Because of a more predictable dose response to LMWH, it is not as important to monitor the dose and APTT.

- LMWH has been approved (in U.S.) for DVT and PE prophylaxis after total hip arthroplasty.

- LMWH therapy does not require APTT measurement.
- Heparin-induced thrombocytopenia is reduced with LMWH.

Complications of PE

Pulmonary infarction occurs in less than 10% of patients with PE. Pulmonary infarction and hemorrhage occur more frequently in patients with disseminated intravascular coagulation. Complications of pulmonary infarction include secondary infection, cavitation, pneumothorax, and hemothorax. Recurrent PE is a common cause of secondary pulmonary hypertension. Mechanical obstruction of one-half to two-thirds of the pulmonary vascular bed by emboli is necessary for this complication to develop.

- Pulmonary infarction in <10% of patients.
- Recurrent PE in 8%.
- Secondary pulmonary hypertension occurs in 0.5%.

Pulmonary Hypertension

Pulmonary hypertension has been defined by WHO as a mean pulmonary arterial pressure greater than 25 mm Hg at rest or greater than 30 mm Hg during exercise. The normal ranges for adults at sea level for important factors are the following: 1) pulmonary arterial pressure—systolic, 18 to 25 mm Hg; diastolic, 6 to 10 mm Hg; and mean, 12 to 16 mm Hg; 2) pulmonary vascular resistance, 60 to 120 dynes·s·cm^{-5}; 3) pulmonary capillary wedge pressure, 6 to 10 mm Hg; and 4) cardiac index, 2.6-4.2 L/min per m^2. The extreme distensibility of the pulmonary vascular bed dictates that at least 50% of the vascular bed must be occluded to produce pulmonary hypertension.

- Pulmonary hypertension: mean pulmonary arterial pressure >25 mm Hg at rest or >30 mm Hg during exercise.
- At least 50% of the vascular bed must be occluded to produce clinical pulmonary hypertension.
- Pulmonary artery catheterization is necessary to obtain an accurate measurement of pulmonary arterial pressure.

Primary Pulmonary Hypertension

Primary pulmonary hypertension is rare. Of all patients with pulmonary hypertension, fewer than 5% have the primary form. Between 1981 and 1985, the national registry for primary pulmonary hypertension in the U.S. was able to collect only 187 patients. The diagnosis should be considered only after all the secondary causes of pulmonary hypertension have been excluded. The pathologic changes start with endothelial damage caused by one or more of the following: shear forces, viruses, drugs, hypoxia, acidosis, and toxins. Histologically, both plexogenic and thrombotic (in situ) lesions are seen. The national registry included 187 patients, with a mean age of 36.4 years (but 20% were 50 years or older and 10% were older than 65 years) and a female:male ratio of 1.7:1 (4:1 in blacks [3:1 in other series] and 1:1 in children); 12% were blacks and 7% had familial primary pulmonary hypertension. An autoimmune mechanism may be involved; up to 6% of patients exhibit positive antinuclear antibody titers greater than 1:80. Many autoimmune diseases, including AIDS, Raynaud phenomenon, and several collagen diseases, are complicated by pulmonary hypertension.

- Of all patients with pulmonary hypertension, <5% have the primary form.
- About 10% of patients are >65 years old.
- Positive antinuclear antibodies in 40% of patients.

The clinical course is highly variable. Most patients present with advanced stages of the disease. Symptoms include gradually progressive exertional dyspnea (in 90% of patients), dizziness, syncope (10%), anterior chest discomfort or pain (20%) (right-sided angina from a relatively underperfused right ventricle), and fatigue (25%). Less frequently, patients have hemoptysis (10%), cough (30%), hoarseness, or Raynaud phenomenon (10%). Examination may show a loud P$_2$, right ventricular heave (82% of patients), palpable systolic impulse of the pulmonary artery (80%), pulmonary ejection murmur (70%), tricuspid regurgitation (70%), RV-S$_4$/RV-S$_3$ (50%), pulmonary regurgitation (20%), hepatomegaly (20%), peripheral edema, ascites, or cyanosis. The lungs usually are clear. CXR shows enlarged main pulmonary arteries (90% of patients), pruning of peripheral vessels (50%), and clear lung fields. CXR is normal in 6% of patients. ECG usually demonstrates right-axis deviation, tall R waves in V$_1$-V$_2$, ST-segment depression, and T-wave inversion. A right bundle branch block pattern and tall and peaked P waves are also seen. A V/Q scan is performed to exclude multiple PEs.

- Dyspnea (90% of patients), syncope (10%), chest pain (20%), and fatigue (25%).
- Cough (30% of patients), hemoptysis (10%), and Raynaud phenomenon (10%).
- CXR is normal in 6% of patients.

Chronic therapy with anticoagulants and vasodilators and oxygen in hypoxemic patients are the options. Vasodilator therapy should be initiated in the hospital under hemodynamic monitoring. Only patients who have a 20% or greater decrease in both pulmonary vascular resistance and pulmonary arterial pressure should be considered "responders" to acute tests. Only 20% to 30% of patients have a response to vasodilators. The short-term response to vasodilator trials has indicated a favorable prognosis, independent of long-term therapy.

Calcium channel blockers are the most commonly used drugs. Prostacyclin (epoprostenol) administered intravenously has been shown to reduce pulmonary arterial pressure and vascular resistance during long-term follow-up. Currently, epoprostenol is the therapy of choice for primary pulmonary hypertension. Digoxin has no beneficial effect in right ventricular failure caused by pulmonary hypertension. Heart-lung or single lung transplantations are performed for primary pulmonary hypertension.

- Chronic anticoagulant and vasodilator therapy is the mainstay of therapy.
- Vasodilator therapy should be initiated under hemodynamic monitoring.
- Responders: pulmonary vascular resistance decreases ≥20% and pulmonary arterial pressure decreases ≥20%; only 20%-30% of patients are "responders."

Thromboembolic Pulmonary Hypertension

Recurrent PE is a relatively common cause of secondary pulmonary hypertension. Mechanical obstruction of one-half to two-thirds of the pulmonary vascular bed by emboli is necessary for pulmonary hypertension to develop. It is often difficult to distinguish secondary pulmonary hypertension caused by recurrent PE from primary pulmonary hypertension. A significant number (10%) of patients have underlying coagulopathies (deficiencies of antithrombin III and proteins S and C and presence of lupus anticoagulant). The gradual onset of dyspnea and signs of pulmonary hypertension and right ventricular strain are the presenting symptoms. Exercise-induced hypoxemia is common. Perfusion scans may not be entirely reliable if the emboli are small and peripheral. Even pulmonary angiography may not provide definite clues. Clinical suspicion, hemodynamic measurements, perfusion scan, pulmonary angiography, pulmonary angioscopy, and lung biopsy may be needed for documentation. In progressive disease, surgical therapy (pulmonary thromboendarterectomy) may be indicated. Palliative therapy includes life-long anticoagulant therapy, calcium channel blockers, and supplemental oxygen.

- It is difficult to distinguish secondary pulmonary hypertension caused by PE from primary pulmonary hypertension.
- High incidence (10%) of underlying coagulopathies.
- Surgical thromboendarterectomy is indicated in selected patients.
- Life-long anticoagulation after inferior vena caval interruption is required in most patients.

Pulmonary Veno-Occlusive Disease

Pulmonary veno-occlusive disease, an uncommon disease of young adults (male:female = 6:1), is the result of in situ thrombosis of pulmonary veins and venules. Nearly 250 cases have been described worldwide. The proposed causes include viral and mycoplasma infection, toxic reaction to drugs and chemicals (bleomycin, etc.), and hilar/mediastinal processes (fibrosis, tumors, etc.). The clinical findings are similar to those of primary pulmonary hypertension. CXR may show Kerley B lines. Pulmonary capillary wedge pressure is usually normal. Vasodilator therapy does not seem to benefit. The median survival is less than 3 months.

- Pulmonary veno-occlusive disease is the result of pulmonary venous thrombosis.
- Proposed causes: viruses, mycoplasma, familial, toxins (bleomycin, etc.).
- Median survival: <3 months.

Hypoxemic Pulmonary Hypertension

Hypoxemic pulmonary hypertension is perhaps the most common cause of pulmonary hypertension worldwide. Clinically, it is overdiagnosed as cor pulmonale or "congestive heart failure" in patients with COPD and underdiagnosed in non-COPD patients with hypoxemic pulmonary diseases. The mean pulmonary arterial pressure is from 25 to 40 mm Hg. Hypoxemic pulmonary hypertension is the result of chronic hypoxemia, chronic acidosis, and persistent increase in carbon dioxide, attenuation of pulmonary vessels, and increased blood viscosity (polycythemia). Increasing hypoxemia during exacerbations of COPD and during exercise in these patients may lead to significant increases in pulmonary arterial pressure. Long-term administration of supplemental oxygen is beneficial.

- Mechanism(s): hypoxemia, acidosis, hypercarbia, attenuation of vessels, and polycythemia.
- Mean pulmonary arterial pressure: usually 25-40 mm Hg; cardiac index is usually normal.
- Long-term administration of oxygen is recommended.

Miscellaneous Forms of Pulmonary Hypertension

Scleroderma and the CREST (**C**alcinosis, **R**aynaud, **E**sophageal involvement, **S**clerodactyly, and **T**elangiectasia) variant of scleroderma are associated with pulmonary hypertension in more than 50% of patients: 80% are females, and many exhibit positive Raynaud phenomenon, antinuclear and anticentromere antibodies, and rheumatoid factor. Systemic lupus erythematosus, mixed connective tissue disease, and Sjögren syndrome are also associated with pulmonary hypertension.

- Pulmonary hypertension occurs in >50% of patients with scleroderma.

- Pulmonary hypertension: much more common in CREST.

Aminorex fumarate (a sympathomimetic used in the 1970s), L-tryptophan (used in the 1980s for health reasons), and fenfluramine, phentermine, and dexfenfluramine (used as appetite suppressants) cause toxic pulmonary hypertension. Pulmonary hypertension caused by anorexigens is identical to idiopathic (primary) pulmonary hypertension. Other drugs and toxins implicated in causing toxic pulmonary hypertension include indomethacin, phenformin (metabolic acidosis), H_2 inhibitors, *Crotalaria* (*fulva, retusa*, and *spectabilis*), bush tea, oral contraceptives, and ragwort (*Senecio jacobae*).

- Endothelial damage by toxins leads to pulmonary hypertension.
- Dexfenfluramine, fenfluramine, aminorex, L-tryptophan, toxic oil, phentermine, indomethacin, phenformin, H_2 inhibitors, *Crotalaria*, bush tea, oral contraceptives, and ragwort can cause pulmonary hypertension.

Patients with AIDS develop a form of pulmonary hypertension indistinguishable from primary pulmonary hypertension. Most patients have been young men (mean age, 35 years). HIV may initiate endothelial damage that in turn leads to pulmonary hypertension. Patients with HIV-associated pulmonary hypertension exhibit a significantly increased frequency of HLA-DR6 histocompatibility alleles.

- Clinically, physiologically, and histologically similar to primary pulmonary hypertension.
- Most patients have been males (mean age 35 years).
- Lung biopsy samples show plexiform lesions but no pulmonary veno-occlusive disease.

Recurrent subacute tumor emboli to the pulmonary arterial tree can lead to pulmonary hypertension. Tumor emboli are clumps of malignant cells within the lumen of the pulmonary artery. When more than 50% of the pulmonary vascular bed is occluded by tumor emboli, clinical features of pulmonary hypertension appear. Rapidly progressive dyspnea is out of proportion to the underlying malignancy.

- Malignant cells obstruct the pulmonary arterial lumen.
- Rapidly progressive dyspnea is out of proportion to the underlying malignancy.
- Source: tumors of right heart chambers, kidney, colon, prostate, liver, pancreas, lung, and breast.

Worldwide, the most common cause of pulmonary vascular obstruction is schistosomiasis. The ova as well as the worms can occlude the pulmonary arteries. All *Schistosoma* species can produce significant embolic lesions. Other causes of pulmonary hypertension include intravenous drug abuse, intravenous injection of lipids, certain chemotherapeutic drugs, long-standing hepatic cirrhosis, portal hypertension, primary amyloidosis, and obstruction of the pulmonary artery or venous trunks by extrinsic physical compression of these vessels by tumor. Radiation-induced fibrosis, mediastinal granuloma, mediastinal fibrosis, and other processes have the same result as long-term banding.

- Worldwide, schistosomiasis is the most common cause of pulmonary vascular obstruction.
- Intravenous drug abuse, injection of lipids, and certain chemotherapeutic drugs.
- Pulmonary hypertension occurs in 0.26% (0.02% in normal population) of patients with long-standing cirrhosis.

Pulmonary Vasculitides

The vasculitides are a heterogeneous group of disorders of unknown cause characterized by varying degrees of inflammation and necrosis of the arteries and, sometimes, veins. Immunologic factors, the absence or deficiency of certain chemical mediators in the body, and infectious processes caused by mycoses, particularly *Aspergillus* and *Mucor*, are associated with vasculitis. The common vasculitides and their incidence in North America are as follows: giant cell (temporal) arteritis, 26.5%; polyarteritis nodosa, 14.6%; Wegener granulomatosis, 10.5%; Schönlein-Henoch purpura, 10.5%; Takayasu arteritis, 7.8%; and Churg-Strauss syndrome, 2.5%. The other vasculitides are due to collagen diseases and nonspecific causes.

Wegener Granulomatosis

Wegener granulomatosis is a systemic vasculitis of arteries and veins characterized by necrotizing granulomatous vasculitis of the upper and lower respiratory tract, glomerulonephritis, and variable degrees of small vessel vasculitis. The Wegener triad consists of necrotizing granulomas of the upper and/or lower respiratory tract, generalized focal necrotizing vasculitis of arteries and veins in the lungs, and glomerulonephritis. BOOP, bronchocentric inflammation, a marked eosinophilic infiltrate, and alveolar hemorrhage are atypical features. Pulmonary capillaritis is present in up to 40% of patients. Eosinophilic infiltrates are seen in tissue samples, but peripheral blood eosinophilia is *not* a feature of Wegener granulomatosis. The term "limited Wegener granulomatosis" is used to describe the disease involving the lungs only.

- Wegener granulomatosis is a systemic disease with major respiratory manifestations.
- Renal involvement with focal segmental glomerulonephritis is characteristic.

The cause of Wegener granulomatosis is unknown. Occupational exposure has been suggested as an etiologic factor; a sevenfold risk for development of Wegener granulomatosis was observed in persons with a history of inhalation of silica-containing compounds and grain dust. Heterozygotes for the P_I*Z variant of the *a$_1$-antitrypsin* gene are reported to have a sixfold greater risk of developing the disease than the general population. The prevalence of Wegener granulomatosis in the U.S. is approximately 3.0 per 100,000 persons. Some have noted associations between disease exacerbations during the winter months and during pregnancy.

● The cause is unclear but environmental, seasonal, and genetic factors have been proposed.

The mean age at the onset of symptoms is 45.2 years (male:female = 2:1); 91% of the patients are white. The initial symptoms are nonspecific: fever, malaise, weight loss, arthralgias, and myalgias. The organs affected are the ear-nose-throat (initial complaints in 90% of patients: rhinorrhea, purulent or bloody nasal discharge, sinus pain, nasal mucosal drying and crust formation, epistaxis, and otitis media), the skin (40%-50% of patients), eyes (43%), and central nervous system (25%). Arthralgias occur in 58% of patients and frank arthritis in 28%. Patients older than 60 years show a relatively low incidence of upper respiratory tract complaints but a high incidence (4.5-fold) of neurologic involvement.

● Major organs affected: "ELKS," i.e., **E**NT, **L**ungs, **K**idney, and **S**kin.
● Ear-nose-throat symptoms are the initial complaints in 90% of patients.
● Nasal septal perforation and ulceration of the vomer bone are two important signs.
● Differential diagnosis of "saddle-nose" deformity: Wegener granulomatosis, relapsing polychondritis, and leprosy.

Ulcerated lesions of the larynx and trachea occur in 30% of untreated patients and subglottic stenosis in 8% to 18% of treated patients. The pulmonary parenchyma is affected in more than 60% of patients. Symptoms include cough, hemoptysis, and dyspnea. The clinical manifestations can range from subacute to rapidly progressive respiratory failure. Most patients with pulmonary symptoms have associated nodular infiltrates on CXR. Hemoptysis is seen in 98% of patients and CXR abnormalities in 65%, including unilateral (55% of patients), bilateral (45%), infiltrates (63%), nodules (31%), infiltrates with cavitation (8%), and nodules with cavitation (10%). CXR shows rounded opacities (from a few millimeters to several centimeters large). The nodules are usually bilateral and one-third cavitate. Solitary nodules occur in 30% to 40% of patients.

Pneumonic infiltrates, lobar consolidation, and pleural effusions are also seen. Massive pulmonary alveolar hemorrhage is occasionally a life-threatening emergency. Benign stenoses of the tracheobronchial tree are more likely in chronic cases and in patients whose disease is stable.

● Hemoptysis occurs in almost all patients.
● CXR: multiple nodules or masses with cavitation in 35% of patients.
● Diffuse alveolar infiltrates indicate alveolar hemorrhage.
● Tracheobronchial stenosis occurs in 15% of patients.

Laboratory tests reveal mild-to-moderate normochromic normocytic anemia, mild leukocytosis, mild thrombocytosis, positive rheumatoid factor, and elevations of immunoglobulins IgG and IgA and circulating immune complexes. A highly increased ESR (often >100 mm/hr) is a consistent finding. Peripheral blood eosinophilia is *not* a feature. All these abnormalities are nonspecific. Urinalysis is an important test because hematuria, proteinuria, and red cell casts are found in 80% of patients.

● Increased ESR.
● Hematuria, proteinuria, and red cell casts in 80% of patients.

The antineutrophil cytoplasmic antibodies (ANCA) are used to corroborate the diagnosis of Wegener granulomatosis. The two main patterns of ANCA are cytoplasmic ANCA (c-ANCA) and perinuclear ANCA (p-ANCA). Almost all c-ANCA are directed to proteinase 3 (Pr3), whereas myeloperoxidase (mpo) is the major target antigen of p-ANCA. c-ANCA is highly specific and sensitive for Wegener granulomatosis and is present in more than 90% of patients with systemic Wegener granulomatosis. In active disease, the sensitivity and specificity are 91% and 98%, respectively, whereas in inactive disease, the values are 63% and 99.5%. The following points are important: a positive c-ANCA without clinical evidence of disease does not establish the diagnosis; some patients with active disease show negative c-ANCA; some patients show persistently positive c-ANCA results despite inactive disease or disease in remission; c-ANCA titers may increase without evidence of an increase in disease activity; and c-ANCA is present in other diseases such as hepatitis C virus infection, some cases of microscopic polyangiitis, ulcerative colitis, and as a manifestation of sulfasalazine toxicity.

● c-ANCA is generally considered specific for Wegener granulomatosis.
● Positive c-ANCA without clinical evidence of disease does not establish the diagnosis.
● c-ANCA can be positive in other diseases.

p-ANCA is positive in various diseases, including inflammatory bowel disease, autoimmune liver disease, rheumatoid arthritis, and many other vasculitides. p-ANCA with specificity against mpo reportedly is closely associated with microscopic polyangiitis, mononeuritis multiplex, leukocytoclastic vasculitis of the skin, pauci-immune necrotizing-crescentic glomerulonephritis, and other vasculitides affecting small vessels. Some cases of Churg-Strauss syndrome may demonstrate p-ANCA with specificity for mpo.

● p-ANCA has been noted in other vasculitides and collagen diseases.
● p-ANCA with specificity for mpo should suggest small vessel vasculitis (microscopic polyangiitis).

The combination of corticosteroids and cyclophosphamide produces complete remission in more than 90% of patients. The usual dosage of each drug is up to 2 mg/kg daily orally. In milder cases, corticosteroids alone may be sufficient. Because of immunosuppression, the overall incidence of *Pneumocystis carinii* pneumonia in these patients is approximately 6%. Respiratory infection, particularly from *Staphylococcus aureus*, is more common. The nasal carriage rate for this bacteria is higher in patients with Wegener granulomatosis. Disease relapse usually is associated with viral or bacterial infections. A combination of trimethoprim, 160 mg/day, and sulfamethoxazole, 800 mg/day, is an effective prophylactic regimen to prevent disease relapse; 82% of treated patients remain in remission for 24 months compared with 60% who do not receive prophylaxis. Stenosis of large airways may require bronchoscopic interventions, including dilation by rigid bronchoscope, YAG-laser treatment, and placement of silicone airway stents.

● Cyclophosphamide and corticosteroids are effective.
● Trimethoprim/sulfamethoxazole is effective in preventing relapse.

Giant Cell (Temporal) Arteritis

Giant cell arteritis, also known as "temporal arteritis," "cranial arteritis," and "granulomatous arteritis," is a vasculitis of unknown cause. Giant cell arteritis usually affects middle-aged or older persons. Pulmonary complications may present with cough, sore throat, and hoarseness. Nearly 10% of patients with giant cell arteritis have prominent respiratory symptoms, and the respiratory symptoms are the initial manifestation in 4%. Giant cell arteritis should be considered in older patients who have a new cough or throat pain without obvious cause. Pulmonary nodules, interstitial infiltrations, pulmonary artery occlusion, and aneurysms have been described. Virtually all patients have a favorable response to systemic corticosteroid therapy.

● Giant cell arteritis: nearly 10% of patients have prominent respiratory symptoms.
● Cough, sore throat, and hoarseness may be the presenting features.

Churg-Strauss Syndrome

Churg-Strauss syndrome, also called "allergic granulomatosis" and "angiitis," is among the least common vasculitides. It is characterized by pulmonary and systemic vasculitis, extravascular granulomas, and eosinophilia, which occur exclusively in patients with asthma or a history of allergy. Allergic rhinitis, nasal polyps, nasal mucosal crusting, and septal perforation occur in more than 70% of patients. Nasal polyposis is a major clinical finding. The chief pulmonary manifestation is asthma, which is noted in almost all patients. CXR abnormalities are noted in more than 60% of patients: patchy and occasionally diffuse alveolar-interstitial infiltrates in the perihilar area, with a predilection for the upper two-thirds of the lung fields. Up to one-third of patients with Churg-Strauss vasculitis develop pleural effusions. A dramatic response can be expected with high doses of systemic corticosteroids.

● Churg-Strauss syndrome: refractory asthma and progressive respiratory distress.
● Allergic rhinitis, nasal polyps, nasal mucosal crusting, and septal perforation occur in >70% of patients.
● Tissue and blood hypereosinophilia and elevation of IgE.

Behçet Disease

Behçet disease is a chronic relapsing multisystemic inflammatory disorder characterized by aphthous stomatitis along with two or more of the following: aphthous orogenital ulcerations (in >65% of patients), uveitis, cutaneous nodules or pustules, synovitis, and meningoencephalitis. Superficial venous thrombosis and DVT of the upper and lower extremities and thrombosis of the inferior and superior venae cavae occur in 7% to 37% of patients. Pulmonary vascular involvement produces major hemoptysis. Serious hemoptysis, initially responsive to therapy with corticosteroids, tends to recur; death is due to hemoptysis in 39% of patients. CXR may show lung infiltrates, pleural effusions, prominent pulmonary arteries, and pulmonary artery aneurysms. Aneurysms of the pulmonary artery communicating with the bronchial tree (bronchovascular anastomosis) should be considered in patients with Behçet disease and massive hemoptysis. Because of the high incidence of DVT of the extremities and the venae cavae, PE commonly occurs in these patients. Corticosteroids and chemotherapeutic agents have been used to treat Behçet disease. The prognosis is poor for those who develop significant hemoptysis.

- Behçet disease: major hemoptysis is the cause of death in 39% of patients.
- Fistula between the airway and vascular structures is common.
- High incidence of DVT and PE.

Takayasu Arteritis

Takayasu arteritis, also known as "pulseless disease," "aortic arch syndrome," and "reversed coarctation," is a chronic inflammatory disease of unknown cause that affects primarily the aorta and its major branches, including the proximal coronary arteries and renal arteries and the elastic pulmonary arteries. Pulmonary artery involvement occurs in more than 50% of patients, with lesions in the medium- and large-sized arteries. Early abnormalities occur in the upper lobes, whereas the middle and lower lobes are involved in later stages of the disease. Perfusion lung scans have shown abnormalities in more than 75% of patients; pulmonary angiography reveals arterial occlusions in 86%. Corticosteroid therapy has produced symptomatic remission within days to weeks. Pulmonary involvement signifies a poor prognosis.

- Takayasu arteritis: pulmonary artery involvement in >50% of patients.

Urticarial Vasculitis

Urticarial vasculitis is manifested by urticarial lesions, pruritus, and arthralgias in 60% of patients, arthritis in 28%, abdominal pain in 25%, and glomerulonephritis in 15%. Many of the pulmonary complications described have been in patients with the hypocomplementemic variety of the disease. Pulmonary vasculitis has not been demonstrated in patients with urticarial vasculitis. However, up to 62% of those with hypocomplementemic urticarial vasculitis acquire COPD. Many of these patients have been smokers.

- Higher incidence of COPD in patients who have hypocomplementemic urticarial vasculitis.

Eosinophilia-Myalgia Syndrome

The eosinophilia-myalgia syndrome is a multisystem inflammatory disease with features characteristic of myalgia and eosinophilia. An epidemic of eosinophilia-myalgia syndrome in 1989 was linked to dietary ingestion of L-tryptophan tablets. Clinical manifestations of this syndrome included myalgias, fatigue, muscle weakness, arthralgias, edema of the extremities, skin rash, oral and vaginal ulcers, scleroderma-like changes, ascending neuropathy, and peripheral blood eosinophilia. About 60% of the patients had pulmonary complications: pulmonary infiltrates associated with severe pulmonary distress and progressive hypoxemia, pleural effusion, diffuse bilateral reticulonodular infiltrates, and pulmonary hypertension.

- Eosinophilia-myalgia syndrome: caused by a contaminant in L-tryptophan preparations.
- Pulmonary hypertension, interstitial granulomas, and respiratory distress.
- Similar features observed in Spanish toxic oil syndrome.

Mixed Cryoglobulinemia

This disease is characterized by recurrent episodes of purpura, arthralgias, weakness, and multiorgan involvement. Frequently, cryoglobulin and rheumatoid factor are increased. Biopsy findings of vascular structures are similar to those in leukocytoclastic vasculitis. The most serious complication is glomerulonephritis caused by deposition of immune complexes. Pulmonary insufficiency, Sjögren syndrome-like illness with lung involvement, subclinical T-lymphocytic alveolitis, diffuse pulmonary vasculitis with alveolar hemorrhage, BOOP, and bronchiectasis have been described in isolated cases.

- Mixed cryoglobulinemia: lymphocytic alveolitis, BOOP, alveolar hemorrhage.

Polyarteritis Nodosa

Polyarteritis nodosa is characterized by a necrotizing arteritis of small- and medium-sized muscular arteries that involves multiple organ systems. Note that this disease seldom affects the lungs. Arteritis affecting bronchial arteries and producing diffuse alveolar damage has been reported. Lung involvement is rare also in Schönlein-Henoch purpura.

- Polyarteritis nodosa and Schönlein-Henoch purpura rarely affect the lungs.

Secondary Vasculitis

Many of the rheumatologic diseases (e.g., systemic lupus erythematosus, rheumatoid arthritis, and scleroderma) demonstrate secondary vasculitic processes in the tissues involved. Certain infectious processes, particularly mycoses, may cause secondary vasculitis. When confronted with vasculitic lesions, the well-known etiologic agents such as drugs and chemicals should be considered.

- Collagen diseases are common causes of secondary vasculitis.

Alveolar Hemorrhage Syndromes

Diffuse hemorrhage into the alveolar spaces is called "alveolar hemorrhage syndrome." Disruption of the pulmonary capillary lining may result from damage caused by different immunologic mechanisms (e.g., Goodpasture syndrome, renal-pulmonary syndromes, glomerulonephritis, and systemic lupus erythematosus), direct chemical/toxic injury (toxic or chemical inhalation, abciximab, all-*trans*-retinoic acid, trimellitic anhydride, smoked crack cocaine, etc.), physical trauma (pulmonary contusion), and increased vascular pressure within the capillaries (mitral stenosis, severe left ventricular failure). The severity of hemoptysis, anemia, and respiratory distress depends on the extent and rapidity with which bleeding occurs in the alveoli. More than 20% of hemosiderin-laden macrophages among the total alveolar macrophages recovered by BAL is reported to indicate alveolar hemorrhage. Pulmonary alveolar hemorrhage is significantly associated with thrombocytopenia ($<50,000/mm^3$), other abnormal coagulation variables, renal failure (creatinine ≥ 2.5 mg/dL), and a history of heavy smoking.

- Alveolar hemorrhage syndrome is caused by different mechanisms.
- Hemoptysis is not a consistent feature.
- Increased risk if: platelet $<50,000/mm^3$, other coagulopathy, creatinine ≥ 2.5 mg/dL, and heavy smoking.
- Drugs that cause alveolar hemorrhage: penicillamine, abciximab, all-*trans*-retinoic acid, mitomycin.

Goodpasture Syndrome

Goodpasture syndrome is a classic example of cytotoxic (type II) disease. The Goodpasture antigen (located in type IV collagen) is the primary target for the autoantibodies. The highest concentration of Goodpasture antigen is in the glomerular basement membrane (GBM). The alveolar basement membrane is affected by cross-reactivity with the GBM. Lung biopsy shows diffuse alveolar hemorrhage. Immunofluorescent microscopy shows linear deposition of IgG and complement along basement membranes. Anti-GBM antibody is positive in more than 90% of patients, but it is also present in persons exposed to influenza virus, hydrocarbons, and penicillamine and in some patients with systemic lupus erythematosus, polyarteritis nodosa, and Schönlein-Henoch purpura. The cause of Goodpasture syndrome is unknown, but influenza virus, hydrocarbon exposure, penicillamine, and unknown genetic factors are known to stimulate anti-GBM antibody production. Inadvertent exposure to hydrocarbons has resulted in the exacerbation of Goodpasture syndrome. The treatment of rheumatoid arthritis and other diseases with penicillamine and carbimazole has been associated with Goodpasture syndrome, circulating anti-GBM antibodies, and focal necrotizing glomerulonephritis with crescents. Azathioprine hypersensitivity may mimic pulmonary Goodpasture syndrome.

- Goodpasture syndrome: a classic example of cytotoxic (type II) disease.
- Anti-GBM antibody is positive in >90% of patients.
- Anti-GBM antibody is also present in persons exposed to influenza virus, hydrocarbons, and penicillamine and in some patients with collagen diseases.
- Exposure to hydrocarbons may exacerbate the disease.

Patients with anti-GBM antibody-mediated nephritis demonstrate two principal patterns of disease: 1) young men presenting in their twenties with Goodpasture syndrome (glomerulonephritis and lung hemorrhage) and 2) elderly patients, especially women, presenting in their sixties with glomerulonephritis alone. In the classic form (in younger patients) of Goodpasture syndrome, men are affected more often than women (male:female ratio = 7:1), and the average age at onset is approximately 27 years. Recurrent hemoptysis, pulmonary insufficiency, renal involvement with hematuria and renal failure, and anemia are the classic features. Pulmonary hemorrhage almost always precedes renal manifestations. Active cigarette smoking increases the risk of alveolar hemorrhage. Frequent initial clinical features include hemoptysis, hematuria, proteinuria, and an increased serum level of creatinine.

- Classic form: young men with glomerulonephritis and lung hemorrhage.
- Atypical form: elderly patients, especially women, with glomerulonephritis alone.
- Pulmonary hemorrhage almost always precedes renal manifestations.
- Active cigarette smoking increases the risk of alveolar hemorrhage.

CXR shows a diffuse alveolar filling process, with sparing of the costophrenic angles. One-third of the patients with anti-GBM disease (Goodpasture syndrome) test positive for p-ANCA-mpo. These patients are more prone to develop fulminant pulmonary hemorrhage than those who are p-ANCA negative. Plasmapheresis is the treatment of choice for Goodpasture syndrome. Although complete recovery can be expected in most patients treated with systemic corticosteroids, immunosuppressive agents, or plasmapheresis, relapse occurs in up to 7% of them. A previous history of pulmonary hemorrhage significantly reduces DLCO without affecting other variables of pulmonary function.

- One-third of the patients with anti-GBM disease test positive for p-ANCA-mpo.
- Patients with positive p-ANCA-mpo are more likely to develop fulminant pulmonary hemorrhage.
- Plasmapheresis is the treatment of choice.

Glomerulonephritis

Rapidly progressive glomerulonephritis, in the absence of anti-GBM antibody, is a major cause of pulmonary alveolar hemorrhage. Nearly 50% of the patients with alveolar hemorrhage syndromes caused by a renal mechanism do not have anti-GBM antibody. Alveolar hemorrhage is mediated by immune-complex disease. Several vasculitic syndromes, including Wegener granulomatosis and microscopic polyangiitis, belong to this group. ANCAs have been detected in patients with idiopathic crescentic glomerulonephritis and alveolar hemorrhage syndrome. The alveolar hemorrhage syndrome in systemic lupus erythematosus and other vasculitides is discussed elsewhere.

- Glomerulonephritis: a major cause of pulmonary alveolar hemorrhage.
- Alveolar hemorrhage is mediated by immune-complex disease.

Vasculitides

Diffuse alveolar hemorrhage is seen sometimes in patients with vasculitides. Alveolar hemorrhage is rare as an initial symptom of Wegener granulomatosis and is more common in Churg-Strauss syndrome and Schönlein-Henoch purpura. Alveolar hemorrhage is much more common in Behçet disease than in other vasculitides. Pulmonary capillaritis is a distinct histologic lesion characterized by extensive neutrophilic infiltration of the alveolar interstitium. Subclinical alveolar hemorrhage may occur in patients with this disease. This pathologic lesion can be seen in various vasculitides such as Wegener granulomatosis, microscopic polyarteritis, systemic lupus erythematosus, and other collagen diseases.

Microscopic Polyangiitis

Microscopic polyangiitis is distinct from classic polyarteritis nodosa, which typically affects medium-sized arteries. Pulmonary capillaritis is the most common lesion in microscopic polyangiitis but absent in classic polyarteritis nodosa. Microscopic polyangiitis is a systemic vasculitis associated with renal involvement in 80% of patients, characterized by rapidly progressive glomerulonephritis. Other features include weight loss (70% of patients), skin involvement (60%), fever (55%), mononeuritis multiplex (58%), arthralgias (50%), myalgias (48%), and hypertension (34%). Males are affected more frequently than females; the median age at onset is 50 years. Pulmonary alveolar hemorrhage is observed in 12% to 29% of patients and is an important contributory factor to morbidity and mortality. ANCAs are detected in 75% of patients with microscopic polyangiitis, and the majority are the p-ANCA-mpo type.

- Microscopic polyangiitis: progressive glomerulonephritis is a major feature.
- Pulmonary alveolar hemorrhage is observed in 12%-29% of patients.
- p-ANCA (mpo) positive in 75% of patients.

Mitral Valve Disease

Diffuse alveolar hemorrhage is a well-known feature of mitral stenosis, even though the possibility is rarely considered in clinical practice. Severe mitral insufficiency can also produce alveolar hemorrhage. Hemoptysis can be the presenting feature. It is caused either by the rupture of dilated and varicose bronchial veins early in the course of mitral stenosis or as a result of stress failure of pulmonary capillaries. In surgically untreated patients, recurrent episodes of alveolar hemorrhage may lead to chronic hemosiderosis of the lungs, fibrosis, and punctate calcification/ossification of the lung parenchyma.

- Mitral stenosis is an important cause of alveolar hemorrhage syndrome.

Idiopathic Pulmonary Hemosiderosis

Idiopathic pulmonary hemosiderosis is a rare disorder of unknown cause. The term "idiopathic pulmonary hemorrhage" has been suggested instead of the traditional name. Idiopathic pulmonary hemosiderosis is a diagnosis of exclusion. It is manifested as recurrent intra-alveolar hemorrhage, hemoptysis, transient infiltrates on CXR, and secondary iron deficiency anemia. The cause is unknown, but many factors have been implicated: heritable defect, an immunologic mechanism based on the presence of antibodies to cow's milk (Heiner syndrome), cold agglutinins, and increased serum IgA, viral infections, a primary disorder of airway epithelial cells, and a structural defect of pulmonary capillaries. Idiopathic pulmonary hemosiderosis has been described in association with idiopathic thrombocytopenic purpura, autoimmune hemolytic anemia, and nontropical sprue (celiac disease). A pediatric form of pulmonary hemosiderosis, presumed to be caused by the toxins of a spore growing in humid basements, has been described.

- Idiopathic pulmonary hemosiderosis: a diagnosis of exclusion.
- It is also called "idiopathic pulmonary hemorrhage."

Most cases begin in childhood. Although this disease is often fatal, a prolonged course is common. In childhood, the male:female ratio is 1:1 and in adults, 3:1. Pathologic features include hemosiderin-laden macrophages. No autoimmune phenomena are noted. Some patients have cold agglutinins.

The iron content in the lung depends on the duration of the disease. Clinical features are chronic cough with intermittent hemoptysis, iron deficiency anemia, fever, and weight loss. CXR shows transient, blotchy, perihilar alveolar infiltrates in the mid and lower lung fields. Small nodules, fibrosis, and cor pulmonale may also be found. Intrathoracic lymphadenopathy occurs in up to 25% of patients. Treatment is repeated blood transfusions, iron therapy, corticosteroids, and, possibly, cytotoxic agents. A 30% mortality rate within 5 years after disease onset has been reported.

- Generalized lymphadenopathy in 25% of patients, hepatosplenomegaly in 20%, and clubbing in 15%.
- The kidneys are not involved.
- Eosinophilia in 10% of patients.

Toxic Alveolar Hemorrhage

Dust or fumes of trimellitic anhydride (a component of certain plastics, paints, and epoxy resins) cause acute rhinitis and asthmatic symptoms if exposure is minor. With greater exposure, alveolar hemorrhage occurs. The trimellitic anhydride-hemoptysis anemia syndrome occurs after "high-dose exposure" to fumes. Antibodies to trimellitic anhydride, human proteins, and erythrocytes have been found in these patients. Isocyanates have caused lung hemorrhage. Other toxins known to cause alveolar hemorrhage syndromes are penicillamine and mitomycin C. Lymphangiography has been complicated by pulmonary alveolar hemorrhage. Pulmonary lymphangioleiomyomatosis is an uncommon cause of alveolar hemorrhage syndrome. Alveolar hemorrhage occurs in a significant number of patients with pulmonary veno-occlusive disease. Anticardiolipin antibody syndrome is another cause of alveolar hemorrhage.

- Alveolar hemorrhage occurs with penicillamine and mitomycin C.
- Trimellitic anhydride can cause pulmonary hemorrhage-anemia syndrome.
- Alveolar hemorrhage occurs with tumor emboli and after bone marrow transplant.

LUNGS IN NONPULMONARY DISEASES

Rheumatoid Arthritis

Pleuropulmonary involvement occurs in up to 45% of patients with rheumatoid arthritis. Even though rheumatoid arthritis occurs more frequently in females, the respiratory complications are more common in middle-aged men. Thoracic complications may precede the onset of arthritic symptoms.

- Pleuropulmonary complications are more common in those with active disease.
- Pleuropulmonary complications are more common in males.
- Pleuropulmonary complications may precede arthritic features.

Rheumatoid pleurisy is the most common thoracic manifestation of rheumatoid arthritis. In clinical practice, its incidence is 8% in males and 1.6% in females with rheumatoid arthritis. One-third of the patients with rheumatoid pleurisy remain asymptomatic. Pleural effusion may precede the onset of arthritic symptoms by months. The effusions are usually unilateral, small, persistent, or recurrent. Pleural fluid analysis shows that the effusion is typically an exudate, usually yellow and rarely bloody. Chronic effusions appear opalescent green because of a high cholesterol content ("pseudochylothorax"). The glucose level is low (<30 mg/dL) in more than 80% of patients. Total complement levels in pleural fluid are low in 40% of patients.

- Pleural involvement occurs in up to 10% of patients.
- Pleural fluid has low glucose levels and high cholesterol levels.

Rheumatoid lung, which indicates diffuse interstitial pneumonitis and fibrosis, occurs in up to 5% of patients and is the most serious pleuropulmonary complication of the disease. Smoking and the presence of secondary Sjögren syndrome might be important in the development of lung disease. CXR shows an interstitial process in up to 4.5% of patients, whereas PFTs suggest a restrictive lung process in more than 30%. Clinical, physiologic, and histologic features mimic those of idiopathic pulmonary fibrosis. The earliest physiologic abnormality is diminished DLCO. CXR reveals a bibasilar interstitial process, micronodules, or (in late stages of the disease) honeycombing. Systemic corticosteroid therapy in the early stages of the condition may reverse the lung process.

- Rheumatoid lung mimics idiopathic pulmonary fibrosis.

Rheumatoid (necrobiotic) nodules occur in the lung parenchyma. These are more common in those with seropositive rheumatoid arthritis. The nodules may precede the arthritic symptoms. Rheumatoid nodules produce minimal symptoms. They are from a few millimeters to several centimeters in size, are usually bilateral, and occur near pleuropulmonary surfaces. Two-thirds of them cavitate. Rheumatoid pneumoconiosis (Caplan syndrome) is pneumoconiosis associated with rheumatoid nodules. It occurs in persons with silicosis, asbestosis, aluminosis, or other conditions. This syndrome is characterized by pulmonary nodules (1-5 cm in diameter) that evolve rapidly and may undergo cavitation.

- Rheumatoid nodules occur in active disease.
- Caplan syndrome: pneumoconiosis associated with rheumatoid nodules.

Obstructive airway disease is seen in one-third of patients with rheumatoid arthritis. Histologic findings include follicular bronchiolitis and bronchitis. The combination of rheumatoid arthritis and smoking is associated with a much higher prevalence of obstructive lung disease than either of these conditions alone. A genetic predisposition to obstructive lung disease may be a contributing factor. Patients with rheumatoid airway disease exhibit a 50% incidence of non-PiM (PiMZ and PiMS) phenotypes for alpha$_1$-antitrypsin. Penicillamine and gold salts, which are used to treat rheumatoid arthritis, are known to cause bronchiolitis obliterans.

- Obstructive airway disease is seen in 34% of patients with rheumatoid arthritis.
- Penicillamine and gold salts can cause bronchiolitis obliterans.

Miscellaneous complications include cricoarytenoid arthritis that leads to chronic persistent sore throat and hoarseness, rheumatoid nodules of the larynx, and pulmonary hypertension. HRCT of the chest has shown bronchiectasis or bronchiolectasis in 50% of patients with rheumatoid arthritis. Isolated pulmonary capillaritis and diffuse alveolar hemorrhage have been described in rheumatoid arthritis.

Systemic Lupus Erythematosus

Pleuropulmonary complications occur in up to 60% of patients with systemic lupus erythematosus. Pleural involvement is the most common and, often, the presenting feature of systemic lupus erythematosus in 50% to 83% of patients. Painful pleurisy is observed in 50% of patients, and pleural effusions are small to moderate and bilateral in 50%. The fluid is almost always an exudate, and the glucose level is normal or high. Levels of C50 as well as C3 and C4 in pleural fluid are decreased in 80% of patients. Lupus erythematosus cells have been found in as few as none and in as many as 85% of effusions. The presence of these cells is specific for lupus pleuritis. Diffuse interstitial pneumonitis is distinctly uncommon in systemic lupus erythematosus. Patchy and irregular areas of interstitial pneumonitis and fibrosis develop in 15% to 45% of patients; plate-like or discoid atelectasis is more common and occurs in the lower two-thirds of the lung fields. Infectious processes, particularly in patients receiving immunosuppressive therapy, are the most common cause of pulmonary parenchymal infiltrates. PFTs usually show restrictive dysfunction.

- Systemic lupus erythematosus: pleural involvement is common.
- Pleural effusion is more common with procainamide- and hydralazine-induced systemic lupus erythematosus than with other drug-induced forms of the disease.
- Complement level in pleural fluid is low.

Pulmonary hemorrhage is an important complication noted in up to 10% of patients. It can be the presenting feature of the disease and be subclinical or massive. The presence of uremia, bleeding diathesis, oxygen toxicity, and infection increase the risk of pulmonary hemorrhage. Pulmonary hemorrhage may range from subclinical to massive. Significant hemoptysis is observed in 8% to 15% of patients. CXR shows bibasal, patchy, alveolar infiltrates. The mortality from alveolar hemorrhage is greater than 50%, with patients dying within several days after the onset of hemoptysis.

- Alveolar hemorrhage is seen in 10% of patients.
- Significant hemoptysis occurs in up to 15% of patients.

PE is more common than in other collagenoses because of the lupus anticoagulant syndrome (manifested by a prolonged APTT, normal clotting and platelet counts, presence of anticardiolipin antibody, and false-positive results on the VDRL test). Long-term anticoagulation therapy is required to prevent venous thromboembolic phenomena.

- Pulmonary embolism is relatively common.

Lupus pneumonitis, a rare feature of systemic lupus erythematosus, is characterized by acute dyspnea, high temperature, and cough with occasional hemoptysis. Diaphragmatic dysfunction has been described in some patients, but its clinical significance is unclear, even though it may account for the "unexplained dyspnea." Acute reversible hypoxemia, a syndrome reported in a small group of acutely ill patients, is thought to be the result of the aggregation of circulating leukocytes in the pulmonary vasculature due to complement-mediated phenomena. Other thoracic complications include BOOP, bilateral hilar adenopathy, lymphocytic interstitial pneumonitis, and pulmonary amyloidosis.

- Diffuse pulmonary fibrosis is very uncommon.
- Lupus pneumonitis is rare.

Scleroderma (Progressive Systemic Sclerosis)

Lung involvement is common in scleroderma, with postmortem examinations showing abnormal histologic features in up to 80% of patients. However, most patients are minimally symptomatic during life. Risk factors for developing severe restrictive lung disease include black race, male sex, early onset of scleroderma, and primary cardiac involvement due to scleroderma. Antihistone antibodies in the serum are suspected to indicate more severe lung disease. All pulmonary complications are more severe in the CREST (**C**alcinosis, **R**aynaud phenomenon, **E**sophageal disease, **S**clerodactyly, **T**elangiectasia) variant of scleroderma.

- The lung is involved in 80% of patients with scleroderma.
- Pulmonary complications are more severe with CREST.

Diffuse pulmonary fibrosis is noted in up to 75% of patients at post mortem. Clinically, chronic progressive pulmonary fibrosis is seen in two-thirds of patients. The pathologic features are identical to those of idiopathic pulmonary fibrosis. One-third of patients have abnormal CXR findings, but more than 50% complain of exertional dyspnea and exhibit low diffusing capacity. The most common abnormality on PFTs is the slow but progressive restrictive dysfunction with low diffusing capacity. The earliest abnormality is decreased DLCO. Deterioration in lung function is an important predictor of mortality.

- Diffuse lung fibrosis (similar to that of idiopathic pulmonary fibrosis) is seen in most patients.

Aspiration pneumonia results from the esophageal dysfunction and reflux that are extremely common in scleroderma. Pulmonary hypertension is common in scleroderma, especially in the CREST variant, and is a major cause of mortality and morbidity. The pathogenic mechanisms include chronic hypoxemia due to pulmonary fibrosis and/or medial hypertrophy of the pulmonary arteries. The latter mechanism is responsible for pulmonary hypertension in 35% to 60% of patients. Pleural disease, pleural effusion, obstructive disease, and hemoptysis are uncommon in scleroderma.

- Aspiration pneumonia: due to esophageal dysfunction and reflux.
- Pulmonary hypertension: major cause of morbidity and mortality.
- Pleural involvement is rare.

Polymyositis-Dermatomyositis

Basal interstitial pneumonitis and fibrosis are the most common pulmonary abnormalities and occur in up to 10% of patients. Pulmonary disease caused by polymyositis may present as acute pneumonitis with alveolar or mixed alveolar-interstitial infiltrates. The severity and progression of the myositis and the severity of respiratory disease are not related. More than 50% of patients with anti-Jo-1 antibody exhibit interstitial pulmonary disease. Not all patients have this antibody in their serum. In 35% of patients, pulmonary disease precedes the skin and/or myopathic features by 1 to 24 months. Pulmonary disease presents as dyspnea, cough, and hypoxemia; symptoms related to gastroesophageal reflux may be the initial manifestation in some patients. Aspiration pneumonitis is a common feature because of esophageal involvement. A restrictive type of lung dysfunction is present in nearly 50% of patients. Poor cough strength due to weakness of respiratory muscles augments the progression of aspiration pneumonia, which is the cause of death in 10% of patients. Hypoventilation results from proximal myopathy. Progressive hypoventilation and respiratory failure manifested by increasing hypercarbia are poor prognostic signs. The paraneoplastic variant of polymyositis-dermatomyositis should be differentiated from the autoimmune type of the disease discussed here. When elderly patients present with polymyositis-dermatomyositis, an underlying malignancy must be excluded before considering the diagnosis of autoimmune polymyositis-dermatomyositis.

- Polymyositis-dermatomyositis: interstitial pneumonitis and fibrosis in up to 10% of patients.
- More than 50% of patients with anti-Jo-1 antibody have interstitial pulmonary disease.
- Aspiration pneumonia due to esophageal dysfunction is the cause of death in 10% of patients.
- Hypoventilation due to proximal myopathy is the leading cause of death.
- Weakness of proximal muscles and a characteristic skin rash (heliotrope hue).

Mixed Connective Tissue Disease

Patients with mixed connective tissue disease have the clinical features of systemic lupus erythematosus, scleroderma, and polymyositis-dermatomyositis and high titers of a specific circulating antibody to an extractable nuclear ribonucleoprotein antigen (ENA). Most of the patients are women, and the average age at diagnosis is 37 years. Renal disease occurs in 10% to 20% of patients and pulmonary involvement in 20% to 80%. Many of the clinical and pathophysiologic pleuropulmonary manifestations are similar to those in systemic lupus erythematosus, scleroderma, and polymyositis-dermatomyositis. Abnormal findings on PFTs and CXR have been observed in 69% of asymptomatic patients, impaired diffusing capacity in 67%, and restrictive lung volumes in 50%. Pleurisy is a common manifestation of the disease, with an incidence of 6% to 40%. Pleural fluid has the same characteristics as that in systemic lupus erythematosus. The effusions are usually small and resolve spontaneously. Pulmonary hypertension is the most serious complication of mixed connective tissue disease and is noted in up to 67% of patients.

- Mixed connective tissue disease: the clinical features of systemic lupus erythematosus, scleroderma, polymyositis-dermatomyositis, and positive ENA.
- Pulmonary fibrosis, pleural effusion, aspiration pneumonia, and pulmonary hypertension.

Ankylosing Spondylitis

Ankylosing spondylitis (rheumatoid spondylitis or Marie-Strümpell disease) is a chronic disorder of unknown cause characterized by progressive inflammatory disease involving the axial spine and adjacent soft tissues. The sacroiliac, hip, and shoulder joints are commonly affected. It is distinctly a disease of males. Pulmonary involvement is reported in 2% to 70% of the patients. However, only a small number (<5%) demonstrate clinically discernible pulmonary problems. Pulmonary problems include chest wall restriction due to ankylosis of the costovertebral joints, fibrosis of the lung apices, and, rarely, apical cavitations. The most common abnormality is the fibro-bullous apical lesion noted in 14% to 30% of patients. Bullous changes, mycetomas, parenchymal fibrosis, and bronchiectasis are other complications. The cavitated lesions may occasionally become infected by *Aspergillus*, *M. avium* complex, or *M. kansasii*. Pleural effusion is rare. Fixation of the cricoarytenoid with respiratory distress, calcification and ossification of cartilaginous structures in the upper airways, ankylosing hyperostosis of the bodies of cervical vertebrae, and bilateral vocal cord paralysis with airway obstruction have been described. Costovertebral ankylosis seldom produces pulmonary symptoms even though PFTs show diminished total lung capacity, vital capacity, and diffusing capacity. Increased residual volume and functional residual capacity are common findings.

- Less than 5% of patients have pulmonary problems.
- Fibrobullous lesions in the lung apices may become secondarily infected.
- Diaphragmatic calcification develops in a small number of patients.

Relapsing Polychondritis

Relapsing polychondritis, a rare disease of unknown cause, affects cartilage throughout the body. It is an autoimmune disease and has been described in association with Wegener granulomatosis, systemic lupus erythematosus, cryptogenic cirrhosis, and hydralazine therapy. Even though the involvement of the tracheobronchial cartilage is a late phenomenon, more than 50% of deaths are due to respiratory involvement. Involvement of the laryngotracheal region portends poor prognosis. Tracheobronchial stenosis and collapse and tracheobronchial wall thickening and/or calcifications are common. Other manifestations are iritis, episcleritis, hearing deficit, cataracts, aortic valvular insufficiency, anemia, increased ESR, and liver dysfunction.

- Relapsing polychondritis: expiratory collapse of the major airways.
- Recurrent lung infections and respiratory distress.

Sjögren Syndrome

Sjögren syndrome, or autoimmune epitheliitis, can be primary or secondary. Pulmonary complications are seen in both forms of the syndrome and occur in 1.5% to 75% of patients. Significant abnormalities in pulmonary function occur in about 24% of patients. Interstitial fibrosis has a prevalence rate of about 8%. Other complications include desiccation of the upper respiratory tract (xerotrachea), an obstructive process involving both large and small airways, localized infiltrates, bronchiectasis, pleurisy, and pleural effusion. The diffuse interstitial process in Sjögren syndrome usually represents lymphocytic interstitial pneumonitis. Both primary and secondary forms of Sjögren syndrome are associated with lymphoproliferative diseases in the respiratory system. Pulmonary involvement by lymphoma is associated with the syndrome in 15% to 20% of patients. Hilar lymphadenopathy or masses should also suggest the likelihood of lymphoma. Most of these lymphomas are of B-cell origin and respond favorably to therapy.

- Sjögren syndrome: a diffuse lung infiltrate usually represents lymphocytic interstitial pneumonitis.
- The most serious complication is lymphoma.
- Cough is common and caused by xerotrachea.

Angiocentric T-Cell Lymphoma

Angiocentric T-cell lymphoma (lymphomatoid granulomatosis, polymorphic reticulosis, midline malignant reticulosis, midline granuloma, or Stewart granuloma) is a lymphoproliferative disease. In the same patient, the histologic features form a spectrum from benign-appearing lymphocytic interstitial pneumonitis to frank lymphoma. Lymphoma develops in more than 50% of patients. Multisystem involvement is common. The mean age at diagnosis for males is 48 years; the male:female ratio is 1.7:1. Cough, dyspnea, hemoptysis, fever, weight loss, malaise, central nervous system symptoms, and peripheral neuropathy are common. Skin lesions occur in 30% of patients. CXR findings are similar to those in Wegener granulomatosis, with patchy ill-defined infiltrates and multiple nodules. Nearly one-third of the nodules cavitate. Pleural effusions occur in 25% of patients. The presence of hilar lymphadenopathy suggests lymphomatous changes. Airway involvement is unusual but can be extensive. Progressive respiratory involvement, usually due to lymphoma and related complications, is the most frequent cause of death.

- Angiocentric T-cell lymphoma = lymphomatoid granulomatosis.
- Clinical features may resemble those of Wegener granulomatosis.

Leukemia

The lungs are commonly involved in late leukemia. Infection is the most common cause of death. Mediastinal and hilar adenopathy are seen in 25% of patients (especially in chronic lymphocytic leukemia), parenchymal involvement in 25% (especially in acute monomyelocytic leukemia and chronic lymphocytic leukemia), pleural effusion in 20%, and pulmonary hemorrhage in 6%. Infectious pneumonia is a frequent and often fatal complication and is responsible for up to 75% of deaths. Gram-negative organisms are the most common cause of pneumonia. Fungal pneumonia occurs in up to 30% of patients. The risk for the development of invasive aspergillosis is directly proportional to the duration of granulocytopenia. Pulmonary alveolar hemorrhage is found at autopsy in up to 65% of leukemic patients. Pulmonary hemorrhage usually is associated with thrombocytopenia and may be extensive.

- Leukemic lung infiltrates are uncommon.
- The most common cause of infiltrates is infection.
- Patients who are receiving chemotherapy and develop prolonged (>3 weeks) granulocytopenia are most likely to have disseminated aspergillosis.

Plasma Cell Dyscrasia

Amyloidosis involving the lungs is common in the primary form of amyloidosis. The diffuse type has a poor prognosis. Tracheobronchial amyloidosis produces diffuse submucosal infiltration and hemoptysis. Solitary amyloidoma presents as a lung mass. Myeloma is seen as a direct extension of a rib lesion, plasmacytoma, parenchymal infiltrates (rare), or as a pleural effusion (rare). Waldenström macroglobulinemia produces pleural effusion in 50% of patients and may also produce parenchymal infiltrates.

- Tracheobronchial amyloidosis causes luminal obstruction.
- Amyloidosis is also associated with sleep apnea (macroglossia).

Transfusion Reactions

Transfusion-related acute lung injury is a form of noncardiogenic pulmonary edema. It is caused by the passive transfer of granulocyte or lymphocyte antibodies in the donor serum. HLA-specific antibodies are identified in the donor sera of 65% of patients who have this reaction. Typically, acute respiratory distress occurs within 4 hours (after 2 hours in most) after transfusion. Clinical manifestations include chills, fever, tachycardia, dry cough, and blood eosinophilia. CXR shows perihilar patchy opacities. Recovery is rapid and complete in almost all patients.

- Consider transfusion-related reaction if CXR findings suggest pulmonary edema.

Hemoglobinopathies

Sickle cell disease is associated with several pulmonary complications, and pulmonary infections are seen in more than 50% of patients. The factors that predispose these patients to infections include abnormal complement activity, poor splenic function, and a lack of type-specific pneumococcal antibody. Pneumonia caused by *Streptococcus pneumoniae* is a major cause of morbidity and mortality in children, whereas *Staphylococcus aureus* or *Haemophilus* species predominate in adults. The majority of pneumonias suspected in adults are due to PE; pulmonary infarctions are common in adults and recurrent PE and infarction may lead to pulmonary hypertension. The differentiation of infectious pneumonia from acute chest syndrome or PE is difficult. The acute chest syndrome (also called "sickle chest syndrome," "chest crisis," "pulmonary sickle crisis," and "pulmonary infarction") occurs in up to 35% of patients hospitalized with sickle cell disease and is associated with significant morbidity. It is the leading cause of death in patients with sickle cell disease. Acute chest syndrome is characterized by chest pain, fever, and prostration. Up to 40% of patients have hypoxemia (PaO_2 <50 mm Hg). Dense bilateral lower lung consolidations are common. Lung functions in chronic cases show a restrictive pattern. Pneumovax is indicated for all patients with sickle cell disease. Hydroxyurea significantly decreases the frequency of acute chest syndrome and other complications. Bone marrow fat embolism of the pulmonary vasculature is a common complication in patients with sickle cell disease and is responsible for many cases of severe acute chest syndrome.

- Recurrent lung infections; *S. pneumoniae* in children and *S. aureus* or *H. influenzae* in adults.
- Pneumovax is important (asplenia or hyposplenia).
- Acute chest syndrome: chest pain, fever, prostration, and CXR abnormalities.
- Recurrent pulmonary embolism and secondary pulmonary hypertension.

Methemoglobinemia

The methemoglobin content of normal red blood cells is less than 1%. Methemoglobinemia occurs when more than 1% of blood hemoglobin is oxidized to the ferric form. Both hereditary (congenital) and acquired forms of methemoglobinemia exist. When the methemoglobin concentration exceeds

1.5 g/dL (10% of total hemoglobin), cyanosis becomes clinically obvious. Acquired methemoglobinemia (toxic methemoglobinemia) results when drugs or toxins oxidize hemoglobin directly. Patients should be evaluated for asymptomatic cyanosis, normal PaO_2, low SaO_2, and a history of drug ingestion. Severe toxic methemoglobinemia should be treated with intravenous methylene blue (2 mg/kg).

- Methemoglobinemia: normal PaO_2, low SaO_2.

Renal Diseases

Uremic lung is a form of noncardiogenic pulmonary edema that occurs in acute and chronic renal failure. "Butterfly" shadows (alveolar infiltrates limited to the inner two-thirds of both lungs, with sparing of peripheral areas) seen on CXR should suggest this diagnosis. The CXR changes are proportional to the degree of azotemia and acidosis in acute renal failure. In chronic renal failure, pulmonary edema may develop without uremia, in part from sodium retention and increased blood volume. Pleural effusion is common in acute and chronic renal failure, uremia, and nephrotic syndrome and in patients receiving peritoneal and hemodialysis. In most cases, the fluid is a transudate. Pulmonary calcification occurs in chronic renal failure, especially in patients receiving chronic maintenance hemodialysis. It is due to "metastatic calcification" of the lungs. CXR shows soft infiltrates that resemble pulmonary edema. The diagnosis is made by demonstrating pulmonary uptake of [99]technetium diphosphonate in radionuclide scans. Hypoxemia during dialysis is the result of hypoventilation to compensate for the loss of carbon dioxide through the dialysis membrane. Hemodialysis is reported to increase the risk for developing sleep apnea. Pulmonary-renal syndromes, sometimes called "lung purpura," consist of those entities in which the lungs and kidneys are affected by the same pathologic process. Examples include Goodpasture syndrome, Wegener granulomatosis, Schönlein-Henoch purpura, Churg-Strauss syndrome, systemic lupus erythematosus, scleroderma, and drug-induced vasculitis.

- Uremic lung (pulmonary edema) is proportional to the degree of azotemia.
- "Butterfly" alveolar pattern is seen on CXR.
- Subdiaphragmatic pleural effusions are common.
- Pulmonary calcification occurs with chronic hemodialysis.
- Hypoventilation (thus, low PaO_2) during hemodialysis is due to the loss of carbon dioxide through the dialysis membrane.

Gastrointestinal Diseases

Acquired tracheoesophageal fistulas as a result of malignancy in the trachea, esophagus, and mediastinum account for approximately 60% of fistulas in adults. It is important to look on CXR for hiatal hernia and an air-fluid level behind the heart. Aspiration pneumonia should be considered in any patient with esophageal problems or symptoms. Gastrectomy patients have an increased incidence of pulmonary tuberculosis. Celiac sprue has been reported in association with pulmonary hemosiderosis and fibrosis. Chronic ulcerative colitis and Crohn ileitis are associated with an increased incidence of asthma, obstructive airway disease, bronchiectasis, and upper airway involvement. Whipple disease is associated with cough (50% of patients), hilar adenopathy, endobronchial lesions and large pulmonary nodules, and pleuropericardial effusions. Mycobacterial infections caused by rapidly growing mycobacteria (*M. fortuitum*, *M. chelonei*, and others) occur more frequently in patients with achalasia and other esophageal disorders. This complication is more likely if lipoid pneumonia develops because of recurrent aspiration.

- Hiatal hernia and other esophageal problems should be considered in determining the cause of aspiration pneumonia and other lung problems.
- Tuberculosis occurs in postgastrectomy patients.
- Nontuberculous mycobacterial infection in those with gastroesophageal reflux disease, lipoid pneumonia.

Liver Diseases

Pleural effusion occurs in 6% of patients with hepatic cirrhosis; it usually is right-sided and almost always associated with ascites. The fluid is identical in character to ascitic fluid. Uninfected fluid is usually a transudate. A large amount of peritoneal fluid may push both hemidiaphragms superiorly, causing respiratory distress. Unless ascites is treated adequately, pleural fluid continues to accumulate despite repeated thoracentesis. Arterial hypoxemia occurs in up to 50% of patients with hepatic cirrhosis. Orthodeoxia (desaturation in the upright posture) and platypnea (dyspnea in the upright posture) are due to increased right-to-left shunting from gravitational forces. The hepatopulmonary syndrome denotes the arterial hypoxemia in patients with cirrhosis. The pathogenic mechanism consists of low pulmonary vascular tone characterized by a poor or absent hypoxic pressor response, which results in a marked dilatation of the pulmonary vasculature. Alpha$_1$-antitrypsin deficiency may be associated with hepatic cirrhosis, especially in children. Pulmonary hypertension also occurs with greater frequency in hepatic cirrhosis. Hepatitis C virus infection has been suggested as a cause of idiopathic pulmonary fibrosis. The use of recombinant interferon alfa to treat hepatitis C virus infection has been associated with diffuse interstitial lung infiltration and acute respiratory failure.

- Ascites: right-sided pleural effusion; usually a transudate.

- Pleural effusion persists unless ascites is treated adequately.
- Dyspnea (platypnea) and hypoxemia (orthodeoxia) are made worse by standing.
- Alpha$_1$-antitrypsin deficiency is associated with cirrhosis.

Pancreatic Diseases

Acute pancreatitis can produce adult respiratory distress syndrome, pulmonary edema, left-sided pleural effusion, elevation of a hemidiaphragm, and basal atelectasis. Pleural fluid accumulates in up to 15% of patients. The effusion is left-sided in 95% of patients, almost always an exudate, and has high amylase levels. Pulmonary edema (adult respiratory distress syndrome) is seen in up to 50% of patients with acute pancreatitis. Pancreatitis-induced adult respiratory distress syndrome usually is attributed to the release of active enzymes and vasoactive substances from the pancreas, which leads to diminished production of lecithin, the main constituent of the surfactant dipalmitoyl lecithin. Massive effusions and pleuropancreatic fistulae can occur in chronic pancreatitis.

- Adult respiratory distress syndrome is the most serious pulmonary complication of pancreatitis.
- Pleural effusion (exudate) is left-sided in 95% of patients; bloody in 30%.

Endocrine Diseases

Acromegaly is associated with sleep apnea. Total lung capacity in acromegaly is significantly increased from predicted values. Thyroid goiter causes tracheal deviation and cough; stridor and superior vena cava syndrome are rare. Of intrathoracic goiters, 85% are anterior to the trachea and present as anterior mediastinal masses. The other 15% arise from the posterior aspect. Thyrotoxicosis is seen in some patients. Intrathoracic extension of goiter does not predispose to malignant changes. Calcification within the mass is common. Thyrotoxicosis commonly produces exertional dyspnea; this is related to myopathy, increased work of breathing, and increased oxygen uptake. Asthma is difficult to manage in thyrotoxicosis because of more sensitive bronchomotor tone and rapid metabolism of bronchodilators. Myxedema may be associated with small pleural effusions and transudates. Both central and obstructive sleep apnea occur in myxedema, and both resolve with treatment of myxedema. Diabetes mellitus is associated with an increased incidence of bronchitis, tuberculosis, and mucormycosis. Cushing syndrome and excessive steroid therapy may produce mediastinal lipomatosis and widening (chest CT is diagnostic). Electrolyte imbalances can affect respiratory function. Severe hypophosphatemia can cause respiratory muscle weakness and respiratory failure. Hypokalemia and hypomagnesemia can also cause respiratory weakness. Severe metabolic alkalosis can present as hypercarbic respiratory acidosis (due to compensatory hypoventilation).

- No increased risk of malignant transformation with intrathoracic goiters.
- Thyrotoxic dyspnea is common.
- Obstructive and central sleep apnea are seen in myxedema; both resolve with treatment of myxedema.

Pregnancy

Dyspnea occurs during the second (in 50% of pregnant women) and third (in 75%) trimesters. Increased resting ventilation is common. Hiatal hernia (moderately symptomatic) occurs in 60% of pregnant women. Pulmonary edema occurs in eclampsia, toxemia, and amniotic fluid embolism and with the use of tocolytics (β_2-agonists). Amniotic fluid embolism accounts for 5% of maternal deaths. Varicella pneumonia and coccidioidomycosis carry higher morbidity and mortality in pregnant women. Sarcoidosis resolves during pregnancy but recurs post partum. Molar pregnancy is associated with trophoblastic embolization into the lungs in 10% of women undergoing evacuation of a hydatidiform mole. Choriocarcinoma metastasizes to the lung in 65% of cases.

Gynecology

Catamenial (associated with menses) pneumothorax is responsible for 5% of the cases of spontaneous pneumothorax in women 50 years or younger. The cause is unclear, although diaphragmatic defects and endometriosis have been proposed. Almost all cases of pneumothorax are right-sided. Thoracic endometriosis may cause hemoptysis, atelectasis, and catamenial pneumothorax. In Meig-Salmon syndrome, ascites and pleural effusion occur in association with ovarian fibroma and other benign tumors. The effusions are frequently right-sided transudates. The effusion resolves with resection of the ovarian tumor.

Neurologic Diseases

Central (neurogenic) hypoventilation is usually acquired from causes such as narcotic overdose, cerebral edema, central nervous system infections, myxedema, syringomyelia, and, in some cases, Parkinson disease. Central hyperventilation is a regular, rapid breathing that keeps the rate of respiration 3 to 6 times the normal rate for hours or days. Although the arterial oxygen level of these patients is normal, they reportedly have a high mortality rate. Neurogenic pulmonary edema is a complication of catastrophic cerebrovascular accidents, trauma to the head, epileptic seizures, and acute trauma to the spinal cord. Coma and loss of consciousness result in loss of airway protection, which in turn may lead to aspiration pneumonia. In chronic cases, recurrent pulmonary infections and pulmonary thromboembolism are serious threats to life.

In patients with quadriplegia, lung volumes (total lung capacity and vital capacity) may be diminished by 33% to 55% of predicted normal values. Most deaths associated with quadriplegia are due to pulmonary complications, such as hypoventilation, aspiration, ineffective cough, recurrent infections, and PE. Neuromyopathies that affect the respiratory system include myasthenia gravis, myasthenic syndrome, amyotrophic lateral sclerosis, polymyositis, periodic paralysis, acid maltase deficiency, hypokalemia, and hypophosphatemia. In myasthenia gravis, the risk of respiratory failure is increased by surgical procedures, infections, corticosteroid therapy, and the use of aminoglycosides. In addition to decreased static lung volumes, patients with neuromyopathies may have decreased inspiratory and expiratory forces.

Testing of maximal inspiratory and expiratory pressures is a sensitive way to assess respiratory muscle weakness. Anterior horn cell disorders such as acute febrile polyneuritis (Guillain-Barré syndrome) and acute poliomyelitis produce hypoventilatory respiratory failure. Patients with myotonic dystrophy or progressive muscular dystrophy may have insidious chronic respiratory failure. Autonomic nervous system disorders such as familial dysautonomia can diminish the response to hypoxia and hypercapnia. Autonomic dysfunction due to diabetes mellitus, amyloidosis, and syringomyelia may progress to respiratory failure. Obstructive sleep apnea and central sleep apnea have been reported in autonomic disturbances.

- Neurogenic pulmonary edema is a form of noncardiogenic pulmonary edema.
- Comatose and unconscious patients: aspiration pneumonia, recurrent pulmonary infections, and pulmonary thromboembolism.
- Myasthenia gravis: risk of respiratory failure is increased by surgical procedures, infections, corticosteroid therapy, and the use of aminoglycosides.
- Maximal inspiratory and expiratory pressures assess respiratory muscle weakness.
- Obstructive sleep apnea and central sleep apnea occur in diseases of the autonomic nervous system.
- In middle-aged or elderly persons with progressive respiratory deterioration, hypercapnia, and aspiration (with or without fasciculations), look for amyotrophic lateral sclerosis.

Diaphragmatic Paralysis

Unilateral diaphragmatic paralysis decreases total lung capacity by 35% and vital capacity and maximal voluntary ventilation by 20%. Bilateral diaphragmatic paralysis diminishes vital capacity by 50% in the upright position and perhaps by 60% to 75% in the supine position. In patients with bilateral diaphragmatic paralysis, orthopnea is a major problem. Ipsilateral diaphragmatic dysfunction is frequently associated with hemiplegia. A sniff test (to demonstrate paradoxical motion) or diaphragmatic electromyography may be necessary to document diaphragmatic paralysis.

- Acute dyspnea in the supine posture is seen in bilateral diaphragmatic paralysis.
- Diaphragmatic fluoroscopy (sniff test) is useful, but 6% of normal subjects have positive findings on this test.
- Chronic diaphragmatic paralysis (>6 months) usually is idiopathic.
- Acute unilateral diaphragmatic paralysis should be evaluated; hilar mass should be excluded.

Skeletal Diseases

Kyphoscoliosis is the most common spinal deformity associated with pulmonary complications. The causes of scoliosis include congenital, neuropathic (poliomyelitis, cerebral palsy, and syringomyelia), myopathic (muscular dystrophy, amyotonia, and Friedreich ataxia), and traumatic causes. It also occurs in mesenchymal disorders and in association with neurofibromatosis. Idiopathic scoliosis is the most common variety. A familial type is also reported. The curvature or angulation of a scoliotic spine is best measured by the Cobb scoliotic angle. Pulmonary symptoms are noted when the angle is greater than 70 degrees. Angulation increases during younger life, and pulmonary symptoms appear during the fourth and fifth decades. The most common pulmonary abnormality is a decrease in static lung volumes: total lung capacity and vital capacity. There is an inverse correlation between the angle and vital capacity, total lung capacity, functional residual capacity, residual volume, and compliance. Although arterial hypoxemia is often present in symptomatic patients, $Paco_2$ is normal in most cases. Hypoventilation and mismatch are mainly responsible for hypoxia. Pulmonary hypertension and cor pulmonale are serious complications. Pectus excavatum ("funnel chest," caving in of the sternum and the anterior ends of the cartilages and ribs) is associated with pulmonary sequestration, Marfan syndrome, and *M. avium* complex infection. Pectus carinatum ("pigeon breast," bulging or protrusion of the sternum and anterior cartilages and ribs) is associated with congenital heart disease.

- Pulmonary symptoms begin when the scoliotic angle is >70 degrees.
- Respiratory symptoms appear during the fourth and fifth decades.
- Arterial hypoxemia is often present in symptomatic patients; $Paco_2$ is normal in most patients.

- Inverse relationship between scoliotic angle and lung volumes.
- Pectus deformities may be associated with congenital cardiac disorders.

PULMONARY INFECTIONS

Viral Infections

The common cold is caused by rhinovirus, parainfluenza virus, adenovirus, respiratory syncytial virus, and coxsackievirus A21. Coxsackieviruses are a more frequent cause of viral respiratory tract infections in the summer and autumn. Respiratory syncytial virus is an important cause of acute lower respiratory tract disease among the elderly. Viruses cannot be isolated in 40% of infections presumed to be caused by viruses. The temporary interference with mucociliary clearance caused by acute viral infection may increase the risk of other infections. Viral respiratory tract infections constitute 83% of all acute infections. Nearly one-half of the general population has a viral respiratory tract infection during December-February and only 20% in June-August. Coxsackievirus B causes pleurodynia (Bornholm disease or "devil's grip"): fever, headache, malaise, and severe pleuritic pain lasting from several days to weeks.

- Coxsackieviral infections are more frequent in the summer and autumn.

Viral Pneumonia

Viral pneumonia is caused by parainfluenza virus, adenovirus, and influenza virus A and B. Respiratory syncytial virus is the common cause of respiratory problems in children, and parainfluenza virus types 1 and 3 cause bronchiolitis. In adults, varicella (chickenpox) pneumonia is a severe illness, the resolution of which may be followed by nodular pulmonary calcification. In adults with chickenpox, cough (seen in 25%), profuse rash, fever for more than 1 week, and age older than 34 years are the most significant predictors of varicella pneumonia. Early aggressive therapy with intravenous acyclovir is recommended for patients at risk for pneumonia. Herpesvirus may cause pneumonia in an immunocompromised host or in patients with extensive burns. Cytomegalovirus, a member of the herpesvirus group, is found in almost all body secretions of infected patients. This virus is seen more commonly in immunocompromised and transplant patients and in cases of lymphoreticular malignancy, cardiopulmonary bypass, and multiple blood transfusions and in association with *Pneumocystis carinii* infection (AIDS). Cytomegalovirus is the second most common infection in patients with AIDS. Diffuse, small nodular, or hazy infiltrates are seen on CXR in 15% of patients with pneumonia caused by cytomegalovirus, but interstitial pneumonia due to cytomegalovirus is seen in 50% of bone marrow graft recipients. Findings of inclusion bodies and high titers of cytomegalovirus may help in making the diagnosis. Corticosteroids reportedly are of value in the treatment of previously well patients with life-threatening varicella pneumonia.

- Viral pneumonia in nonimmunocompromised adults is caused by influenza virus and adenovirus.
- Varicella (chickenpox) pneumonia is more common in adults than in children and results in diffuse pulmonary calcification.
- Cytomegalovirus infection is more common in immunocompromised patients and in patients with AIDS (CD4 count <50/μL).
- Isolation of cytomegalovirus from respiratory tract secretions does not always establish that infection is present.

Influenza

Influenza is responsible for more than 50% of cases of viral pneumonias diagnosed in adults. Influenza A pneumonia is a major cause of morbidity and mortality during the winter months in the U.S. Influenza B is more endemic than influenza A and is responsible for 20% to 30% of influenza infections. Parainfluenza viruses are responsible for 15% of all viral pneumonias. Nearly all patients with influenza A pneumonia have underlying heart disease, usually rheumatic valvular disease. The clinical features are high temperature, dyspnea, cyanosis, fluffy or nodular infiltrates in the mid lung fields, and respiratory failure. Annual (in the autumn) influenza vaccination is recommended for high-risk persons (COPD, heart disease, diabetes mellitus, kidney disease, chronic anemia, debilitated condition, >60 years old, and immunocompromised patients). Overall protection rates are 70%. Recently, antiviral agents have been approved to shorten the duration of illness from influenza.

- Secondary bacterial pneumonia is common.

Hantavirus Pulmonary Syndrome

Hantavirus pulmonary syndrome, first recognized in the southwestern U.S. in 1993, is caused by an RNA virus (family, Bunyaviridae; genus, *Hantavirus*). The rodent reservoir for this virus is the deer mouse (*Peromyscus maniculatus*). The infection is via inhalation of rodent excreta. No human-to-human transmission has been documented. The syndrome is more common in the southwestern U.S. The demographic features include the following: median age of patients, 32 years (range, 12-69 years), males (52%), and Native Americans (55%). The illness is characterized by a short prodrome of fever, myalgia, headache, abdominal pain, nausea or vomiting (or both), and cough, followed by the abrupt onset of respiratory distress. Bilateral pulmonary infiltrates (noncardiogenic pulmonary edema) that occur within 48 hours after the onset of illness have been reported in all patients. Pleural effusions are common and can be transudates or exudates. Hemoconcentration occurs in 71% of patients and thrombocytopenia in 71%. Fever, hypoxia, and hypotension occur after hospitalization. Autopsy has routinely revealed serous pleural effusions and heavy edematous lungs, with interstitial mononuclear cells in the alveolar septa, alveolar edema, focal hyaline membranes, and occasional alveolar hemorrhage. *Hantavirus* antigens are detected with immunohistochemistry. Serologic (*Hantavirus*-specific immunoglobulin M or increasing titers of IgG), polymerase chain reaction, and other studies are available. For those in shock and who have lactic acidosis, the prognosis is poor. No sequelae have been reported in survivors. The mortality rate has been 50% to 75%.

- The reservoir for *Hantavirus* is the deer mouse.
- Features: left-shift neutrophilia, hemoconcentration, thrombocytopenia, and circulating immunoblasts.
- Respiratory distress, bilateral pulmonary infiltrates, and pleural effusion.
- Shock and hypoxemia.

Mycoplasma

Because humans are the only reservoir for *Mycoplasma*, spread is from person to person. Thus, infections occur in epidemic and endemic form, and outbreaks occur in closed populations (e.g., military camps and colleges). Epidemics are more common in the summer and autumn. Illness is more common in school-aged children and young adults. The incubation period is 2 to 3 weeks. The predilection is for the respiratory tract. Clinical features include fever (85% of patients), coryza, pharyngitis (50%), bullous myringitis (20%), tracheobronchitis, cough (>95%), pleural effusion, hemolytic anemia, erythema multiforme, hepatitis, thrombocytopenia, and Guillain-Barré syndrome. Nearly 20% of all community-acquired pneumonias and 50% of all pneumonias in healthy young adults in close living quarters (e.g., military recruits and dormitory students) may be caused by *M. pneumoniae*. Pneumonia occurs in only 3% to 10% of infected persons and is more likely in younger adults (military recruits or summer camps); it causes interstitial pneumonia and acute bronchiolitis. CXR shows unilateral bronchopneumonia, lower lobe involvement (65% of patients), and pleural effusion (5%). Cold agglutinins (>1:64 in 50% of patients) appear during the 2nd or 3rd week after the onset of symptoms and the titer decreases to insignificant levels by 4 to 6 weeks. With complement fixation serology, a fourfold increase in titer is noted in 50% to 80% of patients. The

organism can be cultured from respiratory tract secretions, the middle ear, and the cerebrospinal fluid.

- Mycoplasma infections: epidemic and endemic forms in closed populations.
- Bullous myringitis, hemolytic anemia, erythema multiforme, and Guillain-Barré syndrome.
- Causes interstitial pneumonia and acute bronchiolitis.
- Cold agglutinins (>1:64 in 50% of patients) appear during 2nd-3rd week.

Bacterial Infections

Sinusitis

Most bacterial infections of sinuses occur after an acute viral infection of the nasal mucosa. Bacteria in acute (A) and chronic (C) sinusitis are pneumococci (A, 20%-35% of patients; C, 5%-15%), *H. influenzae* (A, 15%-30%; C, 3%-10%), *Streptococcus*, anaerobes and aerobes (A, 5%-35%; C, 10%-25%), *S. aureus* (A, 3%-6%; C, 5%-15%), and no growth (A, 2%-25%; C, 25%-60%). *M. catarrhalis* is also frequently involved. The maxillary sinus is commonly involved, and nearly 10% of the cases of maxillary sinusitis are related to odontogenic infections. Cultures of the nasal secretions from more than 90% of patients with chronic rhinosinusitis are positive for fungi. CT scans of the sinuses are better than traditional radiographs for detecting sinusitis.

- Sinus involvement is also seen in asthma, chronic bronchitis, bronchiectasis, cystic fibrosis, Kartagener syndrome, and Wegener granulomatosis.
- Fungal sinusitis is common in chronic rhinosinusitis.

Otitis Media

The relationship between otitis media and common viral infections is strong, especially in children. Nearly 10% of children with measles have otitis media. Bacteria are isolated from 70% to 80% of patients with otitis media and include pneumococci (25%-75% of patients), *H. influenzae* (15%-30%), anaerobes (peptococci and propionibacteria) (20%-30%), group A streptococci (2%-10%), and *S. aureus* (1%-5%). Ampicillin-resistant *H. influenzae* is found in 15% to 40% of patients.

- Otitis media in adults occurs in severe diabetes mellitus and cystic fibrosis.

Pharyngitis

Pharyngitis is caused by group *A S. pyogenes* (>30% of patients), *Neisseria gonorrhoeae*, *Corynebacterium diphtheriae*, and *M. pneumoniae* (5%). Sore throat is also caused by adenovirus, Epstein-Barr virus, and other viruses.

Pneumonia

Streptococcus pneumoniae

S. pneumoniae is responsible for 90% of cases of pneumonia in adults. It is most common in infants and the elderly. The incidence peaks in the winter and spring, when carrier rates in the general population may be as high as 70%. People at high risk include those with cardiopulmonary disease (especially pulmonary edema), viral respiratory infections, hemoglobinopathy, and hyposplenism and immune-suppressed patients. Many patients are elderly, alcoholic, or immunocompromised. The incidence of bacteremic pneumonia in hospitalized patients is 25% and carries a mortality rate of 20%. Bacteremic pneumonia in the elderly is not associated with fever in 30% but is associated with minimal respiratory symptoms in 50%, altered mental state in 50%, and volume depletion in 50%. Leukocytosis of 10,000 to 30,000/mm^3 is common. Sputum may be blood-streaked or rusty. Early in the disease, CXR findings may be normal, but later, they may show classic lobar pneumonia. Pleurisy/effusion is common, and cavitation is rare.

- *S. pneumoniae*: mortality rate of about 30% in bacteremic patients >50 years old.
- Mortality is associated with pneumococcal meningitis in 20%.

The pneumococcal vaccine consists of purified capsular polysaccharide from the 23 pneumococcal types, accounting for at least 90% of pneumococcal pneumonias. It offers as much protection against drug-resistant pneumococci as against drug-sensitive ones. Vaccination decreases serious complications of pneumococcal infection by about one-half and reduces the carrier state among the general population. Pneumococcal vaccination is recommended for elderly persons (>65 years) and for those with diabetes mellitus, significant heart and lung diseases, renal insufficiency, hepatic insufficiency, sickle cell anemia, asplenia or hyposplenia, hematologic and other malignancies, chemotherapy, alcoholism, cerebrospinal fluid leakage, immune deficiency states, organ transplants, or AIDS. Some recommend pneumococcal vaccination for all adults, especially health care workers. Some recommend repeat vaccination every 10 years. Patients with nephrotic syndrome and other protein-losing nephropathies rapidly lose pneumococcal antibody and, thus, should receive pneumovax every 5 or 6 years. Pneumococcal vaccination should be given to pregnant women only if clearly needed.

- Overall efficacy of the pneumococcal vaccine is 60%.
- Efficacy rates for certain diseases vary (diabetes mellitus, 84%; coronary artery disease, 73%; congestive heart failure, 69%; COPD, 65%; and anatomical asplenia, 77%).

- Pneumovax decreases the incidence of pneumonia by 79%-92%.

Staphylococcus aureus

S. aureus occurs in the nasal passages of 20% to 40% of normal adults, but pneumonia is uncommon. *S. aureus* pneumonia is more likely to occur in patients with severe diabetes mellitus or immunocompromised status, in patients receiving dialysis, in drug abusers, and in those with influenza or measles. In drug addicts, it may begin as septic emboli with right-sided endocarditis. It is one of the nosocomial types of pneumonia. Consolidation, bronchopneumonia, abscess with air-fluid level, pneumatocele, empyema, and a high mortality rate characterize staphylococcal pneumonia.

- *S. aureus*: present in the nasal passages of normal subjects.
- Immunocompromised, diabetics, and drug abusers.
- Lung abscess and pneumatoceles are more common.

Pseudomonas aeruginosa

P. aeruginosa is a ubiquitous organism commonly isolated from patients with cystic fibrosis and bronchiectasis. Pneumonia may occur in patients with COPD, congestive heart failure, diabetes mellitus, kidney disease, alcoholism, tracheostomy, prolonged ventilation, or postoperative status and in compromised hosts. *Pseudomonas* pneumonia results in microabscess, alveolar hemorrhage, and necrotic areas. CXR may show bilateral patchy infiltrates.

- *P. aeruginosa*: difficult to distinguish colonization from true infection.
- Important pathogenic organism in cystic fibrosis, bronchiectasis, malignant otitis media, and ventilator patients.

Klebsiella pneumoniae

Pneumonia due to *K. pneumoniae* is more likely in alcoholics, diabetics, and hospitalized patients. Also, it is more common in males. Dependent lobes are affected more frequently than nondependent ones. In lobar pneumonia caused by *K. pneumoniae*, CXR may show a "bulging fissure." Complications include abscess and empyema.

- *K. pneumoniae*: more likely to cause pneumonia in alcoholics, diabetics, and hospitalized patients.
- "Bulging fissure" sign.

Haemophilus influenzae

Unencapsulated strains of *H. influenzae* are present in the sputum of 30% to 60% of normal adults and in 58% to 80% of patients with COPD. In contrast, bacteremia is almost always associated with encapsulated strains. Both strains cause pulmonary infections and otitis, sinusitis, epiglottitis, and pneumonia. Most patients with pneumonia have underlying COPD or alcoholism, even though *H. influenzae* pneumonia develops in healthy military recruits. The amount of sputum production is significant. Pneumonia is seen in the lower lobes more often than in the upper lobes. CXR findings are typical for bronchopneumonia or lobar pneumonia. Pleural effusions occur in 30% of patients, and cavitation is rare.

- *H. influenzae* pneumonia: pleural effusion in 30% of patients with pneumonia; cavitation is rare.
- More common in those with COPD and alcoholism and in military recruits.

Moraxella catarrhalis

M. catarrhalis, a gram-negative diplococcus, is part of the normal flora. Colonization is more common in the winter. It causes sinusitis, otitis, and pneumonia. The latter is more likely in patients with COPD, alcoholism, diabetes mellitus, and immunocompromised status. Bacteremia is rare. Infection produces segmental patchy bronchopneumonia in the lower lobes. Cavitation and pleural effusion are rare. These bacteria produce β-lactamase, and most are resistant to penicillin and ampicillin.

- *M. catarrhalis* pneumonia: COPD, immunocompromised status, and alcoholics.
- Most strains produce β-lactamase.

Legionella pneumophila

Legionella is a gram-negative bacillus whose natural habitat is water. Disease results from inhalation of aerosolized organisms. Epidemics have occurred from contaminated air-conditioning cooling towers, construction or excavation in contaminated soil, and contaminated hospital showers. Most cases occur in the summer and early autumn. Risk factors include COPD, smoking, cancer, diabetes mellitus, immunosuppression, and chronic heart and kidney diseases. Almost all cases of pneumonia are caused by *L. pneumophila* (85% of patients) and *L. micdadei* (10%). Bacteria can be demonstrated in tissue with the Dieterle stain and fluorescent antibody staining. The incubation period is 2 to 10 days. Symptoms, in decreasing order of frequency, are abrupt onset of cough (hemoptysis in 30% of patients), chills, dyspnea, headache, myalgia, arthralgia, and diarrhea. Common signs include fever, relative bradycardia, and change in mental status. The diagnosis is established by fluorescent antibody stain (FA stain), which is positive in the sputum in 20% of serologically positive patients. Bacteria can be cultured from tissue or other samples. Serologic testing takes from 1 to 3 weeks before a titer of 1:64 is seen; peak titer is reached in 5 to 6 weeks. A titer of 1:128 is suspicious, and a fourfold increase in titer is diagnostic.

- Risk factors for *L. pneumophila* pneumonia: COPD, smoking, cancer, diabetes mellitus, immunosuppression, chronic heart and kidney diseases.
- Hyponatremia and hypophosphatemia in 50% of patients, lobar consolidations in 50%, leukocytosis (>10,000) in 60%, proteinuria in 20%, and increased SGOT in 60%.
- False-positive titer can be seen in plague, tularemia, leptospirosis, and adenovirus infections.
- *Legionella* serology titer of 1:128 is suspicious, and a fourfold increase in titer is diagnostic.

Anaerobic Bacteria

Bacteroides melaninogenicus, *Fusobacterium nucleatum*, anaerobic cocci, and anaerobic streptococci are responsible for most cases of anaerobic pneumonia. *Bacteroides fragilis* is recovered from 15% to 20% of patients with anaerobic pneumonia. Most of these anaerobes reside in the oropharynx as saprophytes. Common factors responsible for aspiration of anaerobes include altered consciousness, tooth extraction, poor dental hygiene, oropharyngeal infections, and drug overdose. Anaerobic bacterial infections may complicate underlying pulmonary problems (cancer, bronchiectasis, foreign body, etc.). More than 50% of patients have foul-smelling sputum. Patchy pneumonitis in dependent segments may progress to lung abscess and empyema.

- Aspiration of anaerobes is facilitated by altered consciousness, tooth extraction, poor dental hygiene, oropharyngeal infections, and drug overdose.
- Cavitated lung abscess in dependent lobes.

Community-Acquired "Atypical" Pneumonia

Organisms causing "atypical" community-acquired pneumonia include *Mycoplasma pneumoniae*, *Chlamydia psittaci*, *Chlamydia pneumoniae*, *Coxiella burnetii*, tularemia, and *Legionella* species. Mycoplasma pneumonia and legionellosis are discussed above. Community-acquired "typical" pneumonias are caused by *Streptococcus pneumoniae* (45% of patients), gram-negative bacilli (15%), and *Haemophilus influenzae* (15%). For patients not admitted to the hospital, the mortality from community-acquired pneumonia is less than 1%. However, the overall mortality for patients admitted to the hospital is 14%, and 18% for elderly patients and 20% for those with bacteremia. The mortality of patients with community-acquired pneumonia who are admitted to an intensive care unit is 37%.

- Community-acquired "atypical" pneumonia is caused by *M. pneumoniae*, *C. psittaci*, *C. pneumoniae*, *C. burnetii*, and *Legionella* species.

Chlamydia pneumoniae (TWAR strain)

C. pneumoniae is confined to the human respiratory tract; no reservoirs are known. Person-to-person spread occurs among schoolchildren, family members, and military recruits. The incubation period is 10 to 65 days (mean, 31 days). Reinfection is common, with cycles of disease every few years. *C. pneumoniae* is the cause of at least 10% of all cases of community-acquired pneumonia. About 15% of patients are symptomatic, and their clinical features include pharyngitis (90% of the patients), pneumonia (10%), bronchitis (5%), and sinusitis (5%). Pharyngeal erythema and wheezing are common. Among older adults, 40% of community-acquired cases of pneumonia are due to *C. psittaci*. CXR shows unilateral segmental patchy opacity. The complement fixation test is insensitive and nonspecific.

- *C. pneumoniae*: person-to-person spread among schoolchildren, family members, and military recruits.
- Pneumonia in 10% of patients, and bronchitis in 5% of symptomatic patients.
- *C. pneumoniae* is considered an etiologic agent in coronary artery disease.

Chlamydia psittaci

C. psittaci causes psittacosis (ornithosis) in humans. The organism is found in psittacine birds (parrots and lories), turkeys, pigeons, and other birds. Infected birds have anorexia, weight loss, diarrhea, ruffled feathers, conjunctivitis, and rhinitis and they are not able to fly. In humans, the incubation period is 1 to 6 weeks. Clinical features include myalgias, fever, headache, pharyngitis, lethargy, confusion, delirium, neutropenia (in 25% of patients), and splenomegaly (in 1%-10%). Pulmonary symptoms are late and mild. CXR shows patchy unilateral or bilateral lower lobe pneumonia and an occasional small pleural effusion. Laboratory findings include normal leukocyte count, increased CPK level, and a fourfold increase in complement fixation test over more than 2 weeks.

- Psittacosis: caused by exposure to sick birds that harbor *C. psittaci*.
- Clinical features: myalgias, fever, headache, lethargy, confusion, delirium, and splenomegaly.
- Note the differences: chlamydia pneumonia (human-to-human transmission of virus), psittacosis (birds-to-human transmission of virus), and pigeon-breeder's or bird fancier's lung (hypersensitivity pneumonitis caused by immune reaction to avian proteins).

Coxiella burnetii

It causes Q fever. *C. burnetii* is a rickettsia shed in the urine, feces, milk, and birth products of sheep, cattle, goats, and cats. However, epidemiologic factors such as contact with cats or farm animals are found in only 40% of patients. Humans are infected by inhalation of dried aerosolized material. The incubation period is 10 to 30 days. Clinical features include fever, myalgias, chills, chest pain, and cough (late). The leukocyte count is normal, and the ESR is increased. CXR may be normal or show unilateral bronchopneumonia and small pleural effusions. Lobar consolidation is seen in 25% of patients. Hepatitis and endocarditis can occur. Hyponatremia occurs in more than 25% of patients. Liver enzyme levels may increase; the complement fixation serologic test is positive.

- *C. burnetii*: rickettsial illness (Q fever).
- Inhalation of dried inoculum from urine, feces, milk, and birth products of sheep, cattle, goats, and cats.
- Bronchopneumonia and pleural effusion.

Francisella tularensis

F. tularensis is a gram-negative bacillus transmitted to man from wild animals and by bites of ticks or deer flies. The incubation period is 2 to 5 days. Cutaneous ulcer and lymphadenopathy are common features. Cough, fever, and chest pain are frequent, but many patients are asymptomatic. CXR shows unilateral lower lobe patchy infiltrates (bilateral in 30% of patients) and pleural effusion in 30% of patients. The leukocyte count is normal; the organism is not seen with Gram staining of the sputum. Serologic testing (agglutinins) shows a fourfold change (titer >1:160).

- *F. tularensis*: a gram-negative bacteria; causes tularemia.
- Transmitted from wild rabbits, squirrels, and other wild animals.
- Bronchopneumonia and pleural effusion.

Yersinia pestis

Y. pestis is a gram-negative bacillus that causes plague. It is more prevalent in New Mexico, Arizona, Colorado, and California than in other states. It is spread from wild rodents (occasionally, cats), either directly or by fleas, usually in May to September. The incubation period is 2 to 7 days. Clinical features are fever, headache, bubo (groin or axilla), cough, and tachypnea. Pneumonia occurs in 10% to 20% of patients. CXR shows bilateral lower lobe alveolar infiltrates. Pleural effusion is common, and nodules and cavities can occur. The leukocyte count is greater than 15,000/mL. The organism is seen with Giemsa staining and in cultures or direct fluorescent antibody from blood, lymph node, or sputum. Serologic testing gives positive results.

- *Y. pestis*: more prevalent in the southwestern U.S.
- Spread is from wild rodents, either directly or by fleas.

- Pneumonia in 10%-20% of patients; pleural effusions are common.

Pseudomonas pseudomallei

P. pseudomallei is a gram-negative rod responsible for melioidosis. The disease is more prevalent in parts of Southeast Asia; sporadic cases have been reported in the U.S. The organism is widely distributed in water and soil, and infection occurs after direct inoculation through the skin or, less commonly, by inhalation. Although the incubation period can be as short as 3 days, the disease remains latent and may become evident months to years later. Up to 2% of U.S. Army personnel stationed in Vietnam were seropositive for *P. pseudomallei* even though the majority of these were free of clinical disease. Clinical features include acute community-acquired pneumonia, pleurisy, subacute presentation with upper lobe lesions (sometimes with cavitation), or chronic cavitary lung disease that resembles tuberculosis. Diagnosis is by positive findings on culture.

- Melioidosis may resemble chronic cavitary tuberculosis.

Hospital-Acquired (Nosocomial) Pneumonia

About 60% of the cases are caused by gram-negative bacilli, 10% by *S. aureus*, 10% by *S. pneumoniae*, and the rest by anaerobes, *Legionella* species, and others. Risk factors include coma, hypotension, shock, acidosis, azotemia, prolonged treatment with antibiotics, major surgical operations, lengthy procedures, mechanical ventilation, and immunosuppressive therapy.

- About 60% of cases of nosocomial pneumonia are caused by gram-negative bacilli, 10% by *S. aureus*, 10% by *S. pneumoniae*.
- In hospital outbreaks involving a single type of organism, consider contaminated respiratory equipment.

Aspiration Pneumonitis

Two separate types of aspiration pneumonitides are acute and chronic. The acute type usually results from aspiration of a volume larger than 50 mL with a pH less than 2.4. It produces classic aspiration pneumonia. Predisposing factors include nasogastric tube, anesthesia, coma, seizures, central nervous system problems, diaphragmatic hernia with reflux, and tracheoesophageal fistula. Nosocomial aspiration pneumonia is caused by *E. coli*, *S. aureus*, *K. pneumoniae*, and *P. aeruginosa*. Community-acquired aspiration pneumonias are caused by infections due to anaerobes (*B. melaninogenicus*, *F. nucleatum*, and gram-positive cocci). Preventive measures are important. Chronic aspiration pneumonia results from recurrent aspiration of small volumes. Examples include patients with reflux aspiration who develop mineral oil granuloma. Symptoms include chronic cough, patchy lung infiltrates, and nocturnal wheeze.

- Acute aspiration pneumonia: from the aspiration of a volume >50 mL with a pH of <2.4.
- Chronic aspiration pneumonia: from the aspiration of small volumes on a chronic recurrent basis.

Lung Abscess

Lung abscess is a circumscribed collection of pus in the lung that leads to cavity formation and a CXR finding of an air-fluid level in the cavity. It usually is caused by bacteria, particularly anaerobic bacilli (30%-50% of cases), aerobic gram-positive cocci (25%), and aerobic gram-negative bacilli (5%-12%). Suppuration leading to lung abscess can result from primary, opportunistic, and hematogenous lung infection. Primary lung abscess is caused by oral sepsis; aspiration accounts for up to 90% of all abscesses. Alcohol abuse and dental caries also contribute. Lung abscesses caused by opportunistic infections are seen in elderly patients with blood dyscrasia and in patients with cancer of the lung or oropharynx. Hematogenous lung abscesses occur with septicemia, septic embolism, and sterile infarcts (3% of patients). A history of any of these conditions in association with fever, cough with purulent or blood sputum, weight loss, and leukocytosis suggests the diagnosis. CXR may show cavitated lesions. The abscess may rupture into the pleural space and cause empyema. Bronchoscopy may be necessary to obtain cultures, to drain the abscess, and to exclude obstructing lesions. High rates of morbidity and mortality (20%) are associated with lung abscess despite antibiotic therapy. The prognosis is worse for patients with a large abscess and for those infected with *S. aureus*, *K. pneumoniae*, and *P. aeruginosa*. Treatment includes drainage (physiotherapy, postural, and bronchoscopic), antibiotics for 4 to 6 weeks, and surgical treatment if medical therapy fails.

- Primary lung abscess: aspiration accounts for up to 90% of all abscesses.
- Opportunistic lung abscesses are more common in elderly patients and in patients with cancer of the lung or oropharynx and in association with steroid therapy, postoperative status, and nosocomial pneumonia.
- Hematogenous lung abscess is seen in septicemia and septic embolism.

Mycobacterioses

Mycobacterium tuberculosis

M. tuberculosis causes the most common type of human-to-human chronic infection by mycobacteria worldwide. HIV infection has been implicated in about 10% of deaths caused by tuberculosis. The number of cases of tuberculosis has declined in the 1990s. Drug-resistant tuberculosis continues to occur in sporadic outbreaks. The most common mode of transmission of infection is by inhalation of droplet nuclei from expectorated respiratory secretions. Patients who are smear-negative and culture-positive for tuberculosis also contribute significantly to the propagation of tuberculosis. Of those exposed to *M. tuberculosis*, 30% become infected, and among the latter group, less than 5% develop active primary disease and less than 5% develop active disease from reactivation.

Active infection is diagnosed by documenting the presence of *M. tuberculosis* in respiratory secretions or other body fluids or tissues. The diagnostic yields of various tests are sputum, 30%; induced sputum, 55%; laryngeal swab, 25%; and gastric washing, 34%. According to a large study from San Francisco, acid-fast bacilli smears identified the most infectious patients, but patients with smear-negative culture-positive tuberculosis were responsible for about 17% of tuberculosis transmission. Bronchoscopically obtained specimens have a 30% greater yield than induced sputum and gastric washing. Culture of pleural fluid alone yields the diagnosis in less than 20% of cases, but culture of pleural biopsy specimens has a 70% diagnostic yield. Faster culture results are available with the use of broth culture systems (1.5-2 weeks) and nucleic acid amplification (8 hours). Culture-positive pulmonary tuberculosis with normal CXR findings is not uncommon, and the incidence of this presentation is increasing.

- Purified protein derivative (PPD) skin test indicates exposure to mycobacteria and not active infection.
- Active infection should be confirmed by the growth of *M. tuberculosis* in respiratory secretions or other body fluids or tissues.
- Bronchoscopically obtained specimens have a higher diagnostic yield.
- CXR findings can be normal in active tuberculosis.

PPD tuberculin skin test positivity is an example of a delayed (T-cell-mediated) hypersensitivity reaction. PPD is negative in 25% of patients with active tuberculosis. A false-negative PPD is also seen in infections with viruses or bacteria, live virus vaccinations, chronic renal failure, nutritional deficiency, lymphoid malignancies, leukemias, steroids and immunosuppressive drugs, newborn or old age, recent or overwhelming infection with mycobacteria, and acute stress. The annual risk of active tuberculosis in those who are PPD-positive depends on the underlying medical condition (annual risk in parentheses): HIV-positive (8%-10%), recent converters (2%-5%), abnormal CXR (2%-4%), intravenous drug abuse (1%), end-stage renal disease (1%), and diabetes mellitus (0.3%).

PPD skin testing should use a 5-tuberculin unit (TU) preparation; the widest induration is read at 48 and 72 hours.

- PPD reaction is a delayed type of hypersensitivity reaction.
- PPD can become positive within 4 weeks after exposure to *M. tuberculosis*.
- PPD is negative in 25% of patients with active tuberculosis.

Indications for PPD include persons with signs and symptoms suggestive of current tuberculous infection, recent contacts with known or suspected cases of tuberculosis, abnormal CXR findings compatible with past tuberculosis, patients with diseases that increase the risk of tuberculosis (silicosis, gastrectomy, diabetes mellitus, immune suppression, and HIV infection), and groups at high risk for recent infection with *M. tuberculosis* (immigrants, long-time residents and workers in hospitals, nursing homes, prisons, and inner city or skid-row populations). The following criteria are used to determine a "positive" PPD skin test:

- ≥5 mm: adults and children with HIV infection, close contact with infectious cases, and those with fibrotic lesions on CXR.
- ≥10 mm: other at-risk adults and children, including infants and children <4 years old.
- ≥15 mm: any person without a defined risk factor for tuberculosis.
- Recent PPD skin test converters: ≥10 mm increase within a 2-year period for those <35 years old; ≥15 mm increase for those ≥35 years old; and infants and children <4 years old with ≥10 mm skin reaction.

Pleural tuberculosis used to be more common in younger (<40 years) patients; now, it is more common among the elderly. In the U.S., 4% of all tuberculous patients have pleural involvement, and pleural tuberculosis constitutes 23% of the cases with extrapulmonary tuberculosis. Effusions usually occur 3 to 6 months after primary infection. Acute presentation (cough, fever, and pleuritic chest pain) is more common in younger patients. Bilateral exudative effusions occur in up to 8% of patients, and the PPD is positive in more than 66%. Low levels of glucose (<50 mg/dL) in the pleural fluid and a low pH occur in 20% of patients. Pleural biopsy is positive for caseous granulomas in up to 80% of patients and cultures in more than 75%. Cultures of pleural fluid are positive in only 15% of patients and the sputum is positive in 40%. Bronchopleural fistula is a complication.

- Tuberculous pleuritis seen in younger (<40 years old) patients.

● Effusion occurs 3-6 months after primary infection.

Miliary tuberculosis constitutes 10% of extrapulmonary cases. It is characterized by the diffuse presence of small (<2 mm) nodules throughout the body. The spleen, liver, and lung are frequently involved. The disease can be acute and fatal or insidious in onset and slowly progressive. CXR shows typical miliary lesions in more than 65% of patients. Mortality is high (30%) even with therapy. Tuberculous lymphadenitis (scrofula) is the most common form of extrapulmonary tuberculosis. It is more common in children and young adults than in older persons. Cervical lymph nodes are affected most commonly; one or more nodes (painless, nontender, and rubbery) may be palpable. Abscess and sinus formation may occur. Skeletal tuberculosis is becoming less common; when seen, it is more common in young than in older adults. Any bone can be involved, but the vertebrae are involved in 50% of cases. Pott disease is tuberculous spondylitis and may produce severe kyphosis. Tuberculous meningitis is the most common form affecting the nervous system and is localized mainly to the base of the brain. It occurs more commonly in intravenous drug users who are HIV-positive and in immunocompromised patients. Tuberculous meningitis is often insidious in onset. Abdominal tuberculosis frequently affects the peritoneum. Ileocecal tuberculosis can lead to ulcerative enteritis, strictures, and fistulas. Genitourinary tuberculosis is responsible for up to 13% of extrapulmonary disease. It is usually a late manifestation of the infection and is more common in older patients. The renal cortex is affected initially, and the infection then can spread to the renal pelvis, ureter, bladder, and genitalia. Sterile pyuria is an important feature. Laryngeal tuberculosis is usually a complication of pulmonary tuberculosis. Pericardial tuberculosis is usually due to hematogenous spread. Pericardial constriction may begin subacutely and become a chronic problem.

● Miliary disease is responsible for 10% of extrapulmonary disease.
● Peripheral lymphadenitis is the most common extrapulmonary disease.
● Tuberculous meningitis is often insidious in onset.

HIV-positive persons are particularly prone to develop tuberculosis. In this group of patients, a CD4 count less than 200/μL and a PPD positive status increase the risk. Furthermore, there is an increased rate of reactivation, increased rate of progressive primary infection, increased incidence of multidrug resistance, atypical clinical features, and increased progression of HIV disease. Among those with HIV-positivity who are exposed to *M. tuberculosis*, nearly 40% develop primary tuberculosis, and the rate of reactivation is 8% to 10% per year.

Tuberculous pleurisy and hilar/mediastinal lymphadenopathy are more common in AIDS than in non-AIDS patients with tuberculosis. Treatment of tuberculosis is identical in HIV-negative and HIV-positive patients. Rifamycin-containing regimens are effective in curing tuberculosis in HIV-positive patients. Initiation of HIV protease inhibitor therapy in patients who are HIV-positive or have AIDS increases the symptoms and signs of the underlying mycobacterial infection. Rifampicin accelerates the metabolism of protease inhibitors (decreased plasma levels) and leads to HIV resistance. Isoniazid prophylaxis for 12 months decreases the incidence of tuberculosis and increases the life expectancy for HIV-infected patients (Ann Intern Med 129:779, 1998).

● HIV-positive persons are particularly prone to develop tuberculosis.
● The simultaneous presence of HIV and tuberculosis leads to increased severity of both infections.
● HIV protease inhibitor therapy may lead to worsening of symptoms and signs of tuberculosis.

Definitive therapy is indicated for all patients with culture-positive tuberculosis. Treatment usually should include multiple drug (>2 drugs) therapy for all patients with active tuberculosis (Tables 21-14–21-16). With rigidly administered 6-month regimens, more than 90% of patients are smear-negative after 2 months of therapy, more than 95% are cured, and less than 5% have a relapse. A 9-month regimen provides cure rate greater than 97% and relapse rate less than 2%. All treatment programs should be recommended and preferably undertaken by physicians and health care workers experienced in the management of mycobacterial diseases.

Extrapulmonary tuberculosis can be treated effectively with either a 6- or a 9-month regimen. However, miliary tuberculosis, bone/joint tuberculosis, and tuberculous meningitis in infants and children may require treatment for 12 or more months. Systemic corticosteroid therapy may be useful in the prevention of pleural fibrosis, pericardial constriction, neurologic complication from tuberculous meningitis, tuberculous bronchial stenosis, and adrenal insufficiency caused by tuberculosis. Extrapulmonary tuberculosis confined to lymph nodes has no effect on obstretrical outcomes, but tuberculosis at other sites adversely affects the outcome of pregnancy.

● Miliary, skeletal, and meningeal tuberculosis may require >12 months of therapy.
● Corticosteroids are helpful in extrapulmonary tuberculosis.

Drug-resistant tuberculosis is an iatrogenic disease. Drug resistance can develop against a single drug or multiple drugs.

Multiple-drug resistance is usually defined as *M. tuberculosis*-resistant to at least isoniazid and rifampin. Drug-resistant tuberculosis is a problem in many large cities; for example, a rate of 30% has been reported in New York City. Multiple-drug resistance is more likely in the following settings: nonadherence to treatment guidelines and treatment "errors" by physicians and health care workers, lack of compliance by patients, homelessness, drug addiction, and exposure to multiple-drug resistant tuberculosis in high-prevalence countries with inadequate tuberculosis control programs. Multiple-drug resistance occurs rapidly in HIV-infected persons. The American Thoracic Society (ATS) and the Centers for Disease Control and Prevention (CDC) recommend an intensive phase of therapy with four drugs if the local rate of resistance to isoniazid is greater than 4%. Even though the mortality from multiple-drug resistant tuberculosis is high in HIV-positive and HIV-negative patients, appropriate treatment produces a favorable outcome (>80%).

● Drug-resistant tuberculosis may require multidrug (4-6) therapy.

To prevent drug resistance and to effectively reduce the number of cases of tuberculosis, many health care organiza-

Table 21-14.—Regimen Options for Treatment of Tuberculosis (TB)*†

Option	Indication	Total duration, wk	Initial phase		Continuation phase		Comments
			Drugs	Interval and duration	Drugs	Interval and duration	
1	Pulmonary and extrapulmonary TB in adults and children	24	INH, RIF, PZA, and EMB or SM	Daily for 8 wk	INH, RIF	Daily or 2 or 3 times/wk‡ for 16 wk§	EMB or SM should be continued until susceptibility to INH and RIF is demonstrated. In areas where primary INH resistance <4%, EMB or SM may be unnecessary for patients with no individual risk factors for drug resistance
2	Pulmonary and extrapulmonary TB in adults and children	24	INH, RIF, PZA, and EMB or SM	Daily for 2 wk and then 2 times/wk‡ for 6 wk	INH, RIF	2 times/wk‡ for 16 wk§	Regimen should be directly observed. After the initial phase, continue EMB or SM until susceptibility to INH and RIF is demonstrated, unless drug resistance is unlikely
3	Pulmonary and extrapulmonary TB in adults and children	24	INH, RIF, PZA, and EMB or SM	3 times/wk‡ for 6 mo§	...	...	Regimen should be directly observed. Continue all four drugs for 6 mo.// This regimen has been shown to be effective for INH-resistant TB
4	Smear- and culture-negative pulmonary TB in adults	16	INH, RIF, PZA, and EMB or SM	Follow option 1, 2, or 3 for 8 wk	INH, RIF, PZA, and EMB or SM	Daily or 2 or 3 times/wk‡ for 8 wk	Continue all four drugs for 4 mo. If drug resistance is unlikely (primary INH resistance <4% and patient has no individual risk factors for drug resistance), EMB or SM may be unnecessary, and PZA may be discontinued after 2 mo

Table 21-14 (continued)*†

Option	Indication	Total duration, wk	Initial phase		Continuation phase		Comments
			Drugs	Interval and duration	Drugs	Interval and duration	
5	Pulmonary and extra-pulmonary TB in adults and children when PZA is contraindicated	36	INH, RIF, and EMB or SM¶	Daily for 4-8 wk	INH, RIF	Daily or 2 times/wk‡ for 24 wk§	EMB or SM should be continued until suscept-ibility to INH and RIF is demonstrated. In areas where primary INH re-sistance <4%, EMB or SM may be unnecessary for patients with no individual risk factors for drug resistance

EMB, ethambutol; INH, isoniazid; PZA, pyrazinamide; RIF, rifampin; SM, streptomycin.

*For all patients, if susceptibility results show resistance to any of the first-line drugs or if the patient remains symptomatic or smear or culture remains pos-itive after 3 mo, consult a TB medical expert.

†INH, RIF, PZA, and EMB are administered orally; SM is administered intramuscularly.

‡Directly observed therapy should be used with all regimens administered 2 or 3 times a week.

§For infants and children with miliary TB, bone and joint TB, or TB meningitis, treatment should be given for at least 12 mo. For adults with these types of extrapulmonary TB, response to therapy should be monitored closely. If response is slow or suboptimal, treatment may be prolonged, as judged on a case-by-case basis.

//Some evidence shows that SM may be discontinued after 4 mo if the isolate is susceptible to all drugs.

¶Avoid SM in pregnant women because of the risk of ototoxicity to the fetus.

From Centers for Disease Control and Prevention, Division of Tuberculosis Elimination: Core Curriculum on Tuberculosis. 3rd ed. 1994. Available at: http://www.cdc.gov/nchstp/tb/pubs/corecurr.htm.

tions recommend administration of antituberculous drugs by directly observed therapy (DOT) in which a health care provider monitors each patient as every dose of a 6-month regimen is taken. This approach makes a cure almost cer-tain in those with drug-sensitive tuberculosis. The DOT reg-imen is particularly important for the homeless, chronic alco-holics, intravenous drug abusers, patients with AIDS, and prison inmates. Even though fixed-dose combinations of antituberculous drugs (Rifamate and Rifater; Table 21-17) are available and have been strongly recommended by WHO, CDC, ATS, and IUATLD, less than 25% of rifampin-con-taining therapies use the fixed-dose regimen. Treatment completion rates for pulmonary tuberculosis are most likely to exceed 90% with DOT. However, DOT may not increase the cure rate in areas where the rate of cure is high (without DOT).

- DOT for 6 months is effective in preventing relapses and emergence of drug-resistant tuberculosis.
- DOT is also useful in the treatment of drug-resistant tuber-culosis and tuberculosis in immunocompromised patients.
- Fixed-dose combination should be considered in newly diagnosed cases.

Prophylactic therapy is indicated in various groups of sus-ceptible persons (Table 21-18). If an isoniazid-sensitive organism is suspected to have caused PPD-positivity, the prophylactic options include 1) isoniazid, 300 mg/day, with pyridoxine, 50 mg/day, or 2) isoniazid, 900 mg, and pyri-doxine, 50 mg, biweekly. Rifampin, 600 mg/day, is an alter-native option. If isoniazid resistance is suspected or known, the options include rifampin, 600 mg/day, or rifabutin, 300 mg/day. The recommended duration of prophylactic thera-py is outlined below:

- Isoniazid in HIV-positive adults and children: 12 months.
- Isoniazid in HIV-negative adults: at least 6 months.
- Isoniazid in HIV-negative children: 9 months.
- Rifampin or rifabutin: 12 months.
- Silicosis or old fibrotic lesion on CXR without active tuber-culosis: 4-month therapy with isoniazid and rifampin, although 12 months of isoniazid alone is an acceptable alter-native.

In the U.S., Bacille Calmette-Guérin (BCG) vaccine is rec-ommended for PPD-negative 1) infants and children who are at high risk for intimate and prolonged exposure to persistently

Table 21-15—First-Line Drugs for Tuberculosis (TB)*[†]

Drug	Dose, mg/kg						Adverse reactions	Monitoring
	Daily		2 times/wk[‡]		3 times/wk[‡]			
	Children[§]	Adults	Children[§]	Adults	Children[§]	Adults		
INH,[//] maximal dose, mg	10-20 (300)	5 (300)	20-40 (900)	15 (900)	20-40 (900)	15 (900)	Hepatic enzyme elevation, hepatitis, peripheral neuropathy, mild effects on central nervous system, drug interactions	Baseline measurements of hepatic enzymes for adults Repeat measurements if baseline results are abnormal, if patient is at high risk for adverse reactions, if patient has symptoms of adverse reactions
RIF,[¶] maximal dose, mg	10-20 (600)	10 (600)	10-20 (600)	10 (600)	10-20 (600)	10 (600)	GI upset, drug interactions, hepatitis, bleeding problems, influenza-like symptoms, rash	Baseline measurements for adults: complete blood cell count, platelets, hepatic enzymes Repeat measurements if baseline results are abnormal, if patient has symptoms of adverse reactions
PZA,[#] maximal dose, g	15-30 (2)	15-30 (2)	50-70 (4)	50-70 (4)	50-70 (3)	50-70 (3)	Hepatitis, rash, GI upset, joint aches, hyperuricemia, gout (rare)	Baseline measurements for adults: uric acid, hepatic enzymes Repeat measurements if baseline results are abnormal, if patient has symptoms of adverse reactions
EMB[**]	15-25	15-25	50	50	25-30	25-30	Optic neuritis	Baseline and monthly tests: visual acuity, color vision
SM,[††] maximal dose, g	20-40 (1)	15 (1)	25-30 (1.5)	25-30 (1.5)	25-30 (1.5)	25-30 (1.5)	Ototoxicity (hearing loss or vestibular dysfunction), renal toxicity	Baseline and repeat as needed: hearing, kidney function

EMB, ethambutol; GI, gastrointestinal; INH, isoniazid; PZA, pyrazinamide; RIF, rifampin; SM, streptomycin.
*Adjust weight-based dosages as weight changes.
[†]INH, RIF, PZA, and EMB are administered orally; SM is administered intramuscularly.
[‡]Directly observed therapy should be used with all regimens administered 2 or 3 times a week.
[§]Younger than 12 yr.
[//]Hepatitis risk increases with age and alcohol consumption. Pyridoxine can prevent peripheral neuropathy.
[¶]Severe interactions with methadone, oral contraceptives, and many other drugs. Drug colors body fluids orange and may permanently discolor soft contact lenses.
[#]Treat hyperuricemia only if patient has symptoms.
[**]Not recommended for children too young to be monitored for changes in vision unless TB is drug resistant.
[††]Avoid or reduce dose in adults >60 yr.
From Centers for Disease Control and Prevention, Division of Tuberculosis Elimination: Core Curriculum on Tuberculosis. 3rd ed. 1994. Available at: http://www.cdc.gov/nchstp/tb/pubs/corecurr.htm.

untreated or ineffectively treated patients with infectious pulmonary tuberculosis, cannot be removed from the source of exposure, and cannot be given long-term prophylactic therapy and 2) health care workers in settings in which the likelihood of transmission and subsequent infection with *M. tuberculosis* strains resistant to isoniazid and rifampin is high, provided comprehensive tuberculosis infection-control precautions have been implemented in the workplace and have not been successful. BCG is not recommended for HIV-positive children and adults.

Table 21-16.—Treatment Regimens for Patients With Tuberculosis, According to HIV Status*

| Drug resistance | Patients | | Antiretroviral therapy |
	Without HIV infection	With HIV infection	
None	IRPE for 2 mo, IR for 4 mo[†]	IRPE for 2 mo, IR for 4-7 mo[‡]	No protease inhibitors or NNRTIs can be used with rifampin[§]
		or	
		IPE plus rifabutin for 2 mo, I plus rifabutin for 4-7 mo	Rifabutin can be used with indinavir or nelfinavir but not with saquinavir, ritonavir, or NNRTIs
Isoniazid	RPE for 6 mo	RPE for 6-9 mo[¶]	No protease inhibitors or NNRTIs can be used with rifampin
		or	
		rifabutin plus PE for 6-9 mo	Rifabutin can be used with indinavir or nelfinavir but not with saquinavir, ritonavir, or NNRTIs
Rifampin	IPE for 18-24 mo	IPE for 18-24 mo	All antiretroviral drugs can be used
		or	
		IPSE for 2 mo, IPS for 7-10 mo	All antiretroviral drugs can be used

E, ethambutol; HIV, human immunodeficiency virus; I, isoniazid; NNRTI, non-nucleoside reverse-transcriptase inhibitor; P, pyrazinamide; R, rifampin; S, streptomycin.

*Recommendations are based on those of the American Thoracic Society, the Centers for Disease Control and Prevention, and expert opinion.

[†]Streptomycin may be substituted for ethambutol. Ethambutol may be omitted only if rates of isoniazid resistance in the community are documented to be less than 4%.

[‡]Therapy should be more prolonged in patients with a slow clinical or bacteriologic response to treatment. A total of 12 months of therapy is recommended for patients who have miliary or skeletal tuberculosis, with or without HIV infection

[§]Protease inhibitors and NNRTIs should not be given for at least 2 weeks after rifampin has been discontinued, because of persistent induction of the cytochrome P450 CYP3A.

[¶]The American Thoracic Society recommends 6 months of therapy; the CDC recommends 6 to 9 months.

- BCG is indicated for children who are at high risk for intimate and prolonged exposure to *M. tuberculosis.*
- BCG is not recommended for HIV-positive adults or children.

Nontuberculous Mycobacteria

The mycobacteria other than *M. tuberculosis* and *M. leprae* are commonly classified as nontuberculosis mycobacteria (NTM) even though tubercle formation occurs. The types of human disease and NTM responsible are listed in Table 21-19.

Most NTM have been isolated from natural water and soil. Human-to-human spread has not been documented. Natural waters are the source for most human infections caused by *M. avium* complex; some cases are likely acquired from hospital tap water. *M. kansasii* has not been cultured from soil or natural water even though it has been recovered from tap water. *M. xenopi*, an obligate thermophile, grows in hot water and hot water taps. Colonization or a saprophytic state of NTM is uncommon.

- Human-to-human spread has not been documented.
- NTM disease is not reportable in the U.S.
- Source of *M. avium* complex: natural waters and soil.
- Source of *M. kansasii*: tap water.

Chronic pulmonary disease is most frequently caused by *M. avium* complex and *M. kansasii*. *M. kansasii* is the second most common NTM lung disease in the U.S. Pulmonary disease is more common in older adults, those with underlying COPD, smokers, alcohol abusers, and some children with cystic fibrosis. CXR features include thin-walled cavities with minimal surrounding infiltrates and pleural thickening adjacent to areas of lung involvement. Another group of patients who develop pulmonary infection from *M. avium-avium* are Caucasian women in their 60s who are HIV-negative without preexisting lung disease. Most (>90%) of these patients demonstrate bronchiectasis or small nodules without predilection for any lobe. Bronchoscopy or open lung biopsy is required for diagnosis in nearly half the cases. Therapy fails in half the patients, more than 80% remain symptomatic, and 60% do not tolerate their initial multidrug regimen. Nearly 90% of patients with *M. kansasii* and most patients with *M. avium* complex disease show cavitation. HRCT may show associated multifocal bronchiectasis with small (<5 mm) nodular infiltrates. Bilateral nodular and/or interstitial lung disease or isolated disease in the right

Table 21-17.—Antituberculosis Drugs, Dosages, and Major Toxicities

Drug	Adult dosage (daily)	Pediatric dosage (daily)	Main adverse effects
Isoniazid (INH)*†	300 mg PO, IM	10-20 mg/kg (max. 300 mg)	Liver toxicity, peripheral neuropathy
Rifampin*‡ (Rifadin, Rimactane)	600 mg PO, IV	10-20 mg/kg (max. 600 mg)	Liver toxicity, flu-like syndrome
Pyrazinamide§	1.5 to 2.5 g PO	15-30 mg/kg (max. 2 g)	Arthralgias, hepatic toxicity, hyperuricemia
Ethambutol//(Myambutol)	15-25 mg/kg PO	15-25 mg/kg PO	Optic neuritis
Streptomycin¶	15 mg/kg IM	20-30 mg/kg	Vestibular toxicity, renal damage
Combinations			
Rifamate (isoniazid 150 mg, rifampin 300 mg)	2 tablets	Not recommended	
Rifater (isoniazid 50 mg, rifampin 120 mg, pyrazinamide 300 mg)	≤44 kg: 4 tablets 45-54 kg: 5 tablets ≥55 kg: 6 tablets	Not recommended	
Second-line drugs			
Capreomycin (Capastat)	15 mg/kg IM	15-30 mg/kg	Auditory and vestibular toxicity, kidney damage
Kanamycin (Kantrex, and others)	15 mg/kg IM, IV	15-30 mg/kg	Auditory toxicity, kidney damage
Amikacin (Amikin)	15 mg/kg IM, IV	15-30 mg/kg	Auditory toxicity, kidney damage
Cycloserine# (Seromycin, and others)	250-500 mg bid PO	10-20 mg/kg	Psychiatric symptoms, seizures
Ethionamide (Trecator-SC)	250-500 mg bid PO	15-20 mg/kg	Gastrointestinal and liver toxicity, hypothyroidism
Ciprofloxacin (Cipro)	500-750 mg bid PO	Not recommended	Nausea, abdominal pain, restlessness, confusion
Ofloxacin (Floxin)	300-400 mg bid or 600-800 mg/day PO	Not recommended	Nausea, abdominal pain, restlessness, confusion
Aminosalicylic acid (PAS; Teebacin)	4-6 g bid PO	75 mg/kg bid	Gastrointestinal disturbance

*Intravenous preparations of isoniazid and rifampin are available.

†For intermittent use after a few weeks to months of daily therapy, dosage is 15 mg/kg (max. 900 mg) twice/week for adults. Pyridoxine 10 to 25 mg should be given to prevent neuropathy in malnourished or pregnant patients and in those with HIV infection, alcoholism, or diabetes mellitus.

‡For intermittent use after a few weeks to months of daily therapy, dosage is 600 mg twice/week.

§For intermittent use after a few weeks to months of daily therapy, dosage is 2.5 to 3.5 g twice/week.

//Usually not recommended for children less than 6 years old because visual acuity cannot be monitored. Some clinicians use 25 mg/kg per day during first 1-2 months or longer if organism is isoniazid-resistant. Decrease dosage if renal function diminished. For intermittent use after a few weeks to months of daily therapy, dosage is 50 mg/kg twice/week.

¶Available from Pfizer (800-254-4445) free of charge to physicians, clinics, or hospitals. When oral drugs are given daily, streptomycin is generally given 5 times per week (15 mg/kg, or a maximum of 1 g per dose) for an initial 2 to 12 week period, and then (if needed) 2 to 3 times per week (20 to 30 mg/kg, or a maximum of 1.5 g per dose). For patients >40 years old, dosage is reduced to 500 to 750 mg 5 times per week and 20 mg/kg when given twice per week. Some clinicians change to lower dosage at 60 rather than 40 years old. Dosage should be decreased if renal function is diminished.

From Drugs for Tuberculosis. The Medical Letter 37:67-70, Aug 4, 1995. By permission of The Medical Letter.

middle lobe or lingular disease is more predominant in elderly nonsmoking women. Hypersensitivity pneumonitis caused by exposure to *M. avium* complex growing in a hot water tub has been reported. *M. avium* complex is responsible for 5% of the cases of mycobacterial lymphadenitis in adults and more than 90% of mycobacterial lymphadenitis in children. Lymphadenopathy is usually unilateral and nontender. Disseminated disease caused by NTM presents as a fever of unknown origin in immunocompromised patients without AIDS.

- *M. avium* complex infection occurs in bronchiectasis.
- Cavitation occurs in >90% of patients with *M. kansasii* infection.

HIV-infected persons are at high risk for developing NTM infections. More than 95% of NTM disease in HIV-infected subjects is caused by *M. avium* complex. In those with AIDS, disseminated and localized infection occur in up to 40% and 5% of patients, respectively. Dissemination is more likely in those with a CD4 cell count less than 50/μL. The risk of developing disseminated infection is 20% per year when the CD4 cell count is less than 100/μL. High temperature and sweats are common. Anemia and increased alkaline phosphatase levels are common in disseminated disease. Dissemination is usually documented with positive blood cultures.

Table 21-18.—Indications for Prophylactic Treatment of Tuberculosis (TB)

Prophylactic group description	PPD, mm
Persons with known or suspected HIV infection	≥5
Close contacts of person with infectious TB	≥5
Persons with chest radiographic findings suggestive of previous TB and inadequate or no treatment*	≥5
Persons who inject drugs and are known to be HIV negative	≥10
Persons with certain medical conditions or factors	≥10
Diabetes mellitus, silicosis, prolonged corticosteroid or other immunosuppressive therapy, cancer of the head and neck, hematologic and reticuloendothelial diseases (e.g., leukemia and Hodgkin disease), end-stage renal disease, intestinal bypass or gastrectomy, chronic malabsorption syndromes, low body weight (≥10% below ideal)	
Persons in whom PPD converted from negative to positive within the past 2 yr	†
Age <35 yr in the following high-prevalence groups	≥10
Foreign-born persons from areas of the world where TB is common (e.g., Asia, Africa, Caribbean, and Latin America)	
Medically underserved, low-income populations including high-risk racial and ethnic groups (e.g., Asians and Pacific Islanders, African Americans, Hispanics, and American Indians)	
Residents of long-term care facilities (e.g., correctional facilities and nursing homes)	
Children younger than 4 yr	
Other groups identified locally as having an increased prevalence of TB (e.g., migrant farm workers or homeless persons)	
Persons <35 yr with no known risk factors for TB	≥15
Occupational exposure to TB (e.g., health care workers and staff of nursing homes, drug treatment centers, or correctional facilities)	‡
Close contacts with an initial PPD of <5 mm and normal findings on chest radiography	<5
Circumstances suggest a high probability of infection	
Evaluation of other contacts with a similar degree of exposure demonstrates a high prevalence of infection	
Child or adolescent	
Immunosuppressed (e.g., HIV infection)	

HIV, human immunodeficiency virus; PPD, purified protein derivative of tubercle bacillus.

*Isolated calcified granulomas are excluded.

†10 mm or greater increase if person is younger than 35 yr or is a health care worker; 15 mm or greater increase if person is 35 yr or older.

‡Appropriate cutoff for defining a positive reaction depends on the employee's individual risk factors for TB and on the prevalence of TB in the facility.

From Van Scoy RE, Wilkowske CJ: Antimicrobial therapy. Mayo Clin Proc 74:1038-1048, 1999. By permission of Mayo Foundation.

Table 21-19.—Classification of the Nontuberculous Mycobacteria Recovered From Humans

Clinical disease	Common etiologic species	Features of the common species		Unusual etiologic species
		Geography	Morphologic features*	
Pulmonary disease	1. *M. avium* complex	Worldwide	Usually not pigmented; slow growth (>7 days)	1. *M simiae*
	2. *M. kansasii*	U.S., coal mining regions, Europe	Pigmented; often large and beaded on acid-fast stain	2. *M. szulgai*
				3. *M. fortuitum*
	3. *M. abscessus*	Worldwide, but mostly U.S.	Rapid growth (<7 days); not pigmented	4. *M. celatum*
	4. *M. xenopi*	Europe, Canada	Slow growth; pigmented	5. *M. asiaticum*
	5. *M. malmoense*	UK, northern Europe	Slow growth; not pigmented	6. *M. shimodii*
				7. *M. haemophilum*
				8. *M. smegmatis*
Lymphadenitis	1. *M. avium* complex	Worldwide	Usually not pigmented	1. *M. fortuitum*
	2. *M. scrofulaceum*	Worldwide	Pigmented	2. *M. chelonei*
	3. *M. malmoense*	UK, northern Europe (especially Scandinavia)	Slow growth	3. *M. abscessus*
				4. *M. kansasii*
				5. *M. haemophilum*
Cutaneous disease	1. *M. marinum*	Worldwide	Photochromogen; requires low temperatures (28-30°C) for isolation	1. *M. avium* complex
				2. *M. kansasii*
				3. *M. nonchromo-genicum*
	2. *M. fortuitum*	Worldwide, mostly U.S.	Rapid growth; not pigmented	4. *M. smegmatis*
	3. *M. chelonae*			5. *M. haemophilum*
	4. *M. abscessus*			
	5. *M. ulcerans*	Australia, tropics, Africa, SE Asia	Grows slowly; pigmented	
Disseminated disease	1. *M. avium* complex	Worldwide	Isolates from patients with AIDS; usually pigmented (80%)	1. *M. abscessus*
				2. *M. xenopi*
				3. *M. malmoense*
	2. *M. kansasii*	U.S.	Photochromogen	4. *M. genavense*
	3. *M. chelonae*	U.S.	Not pigmented	5. *M. simiae*
	4. *M. haemophilum*	U.S., Australia	Not pigmented; requires hemin, often low temperatures, and CO_2 to grow	6. *M. conspicuum*
				7. *M. marinum*
				8. *M. fortuitum*

AIDS, acquired immunodeficiency disease.

*Photochromogen: isolate is buff-colored in the dark but turns yellow with brief exposure to light.

From American Thoracic Society: Diagnosis and treatment of disease caused by nontuberculous mycobacteria. Am J Respir Crit Care Med 156:S1-S25, 1997. By permission of American Lung Association.

- Disseminated *M. avium* complex in AIDS is more likely when the CD4 count is <50/μL.
- A single blood culture in disseminated *M. avium* complex infection has a sensitivity of 90%.

Specific skin tests are not available for the diagnosis of NTM. Routine cultures of sputum, blood, or stool in asymptomatic patients are not recommended. All specimens positive for acid-fast bacilli must be considered to indicate *M.*

tuberculosis until final culture results are available. The current diagnostic criteria used in HIV-seropositive and HIV-seronegative hosts are shown below (adopted with permission from Am J Respir Crit Care Med 156:S1-S25, 1997). The criteria apply to symptomatic patients with infiltrate, nodular or cavitary disease or HRCT scan that shows multifocal bronchiectasis and/or multiple small nodules. Also, the criteria fit best with *M. avium* complex, *M. abscessus*, and *M. kansasii*.

A. If three sputum/bronchial wash results are available from the previous 12 months:
   1. Three positive cultures with negative acid-fast bacilli (AFB) smear results or
   2. Two positive cultures and one positive AFB smear
B. If only one bronchial wash is available:
   1. Positive culture with a 2+, 3+, or 4+ AFB smear or 2+, 3+, or 4+ growth on solid media
C. If sputum/bronchial wash evaluations are nondiagnostic or another disease cannot be excluded:
   1. Transbronchial or lung biopsy yielding an NTM or
   2. Biopsy showing mycobacterial histopathologic features (granulomatous inflammation and/or AFB) and one or more sputums or bronchial washings are positive for an NTM even in low numbers

Treatment of infections caused by NTM should be undertaken by a physician who specializes in infections caused by mycobacteria. It should be noted that isoniazid is no longer used in the treatment of infections caused by *M. avium* complex; the macrolides, azithromycin and clarithromycin, are more important in the treatment of *M. avium* complex. The following summarizes the therapeutic recommendations by the American Thoracic Society for the treatment of infections caused by NTM (adopted with permission from Am J Respir Crit Care Med 156:S1-S25, 1997).

1. Treatment of *M. kansasii* pulmonary disease. A regimen of daily isoniazid (300 mg), rifampin (600 mg), and ethambutol (25 mg/kg for 2 months, then 15 mg/kg for 18 months), with a minimum of 12-month culture negativity, is recommended for pulmonary disease in adults caused by *M. kansasii*. Clarithromycin or rifabutin needs to be substituted for rifampin in HIV-positive patients who take protease inhibitors.
2. Treatment of *M. avium*-complex pulmonary disease. A regimen of daily clarithromycin (500 mg twice a day) or azithromycin (250 mg), rifampin (600 mg) or rifabutin (300 mg), and ethambutol (25 mg/kg for 2 months, then 15 mg/kg) is recommended for therapy for adults not infected with the HIV virus. Streptomycin two to three times per week should be considered for the first 8 weeks

as tolerated. Patients should be treated until culture-negative with therapy for 1 year.
3. Treatment of disseminated *M. avium*-complex disease. Therapy in adults should include daily clarithromycin (500 mg twice a day) or azithromycin (250 to 500 mg), plus ethambutol (15 mg/kg per day). Consideration should be given to the addition of a third drug (preferably rifabutin at a dose of 300 mg/day). Therapy should be continued for life until more data become available.
4. Prophylaxis of disseminated *M. avium*-complex disease. Prophylaxis should be given to adults with AIDS with CD4 counts less than 50/μL cells, especially with a history of a previous opportunistic infection. Rifabutin (300 mg/day), clarithromycin (500 mg twice daily), azithromycin (1,200 mg once weekly), and azithromycin (1,200 mg once weekly) plus rifabutin (300 mg daily) are all proven effective regimens.
5. Treatment of NTM cervical lymphadenitis. NTM cervical lymphadenitis is still treated primarily by surgical excision alone, with a 95% cure rate. A clarithromycin-containing regimen should be considered for patients with extensive disease or a poor response to excision.
6. Treatment of nonpulmonary rapidly growing mycobacteria. Therapy of nonpulmonary disease caused by *M. fortuitum*, *M. abscessus*, and *M. chelonae* should include drugs such as amikacin and clarithromycin, based on in vitro susceptibility tests.

- Isoniazid is not used to treat infection with *M. avium* complex.
- Macrolides are important in the therapy of infections with *M. avium* complex.

Toxicity From Antituberculous Drugs

When streptomycin is not included in a 6- to 9-month regimen, the incidence of adverse reactions is about 3%. Streptomycin increases the frequency of side effects to 8%. Patient compliance improves, and the risk of monotherapy (emergence of resistant organisms) diminishes when fixed-dose drug combinations are used. In adults, it is important to perform a baseline assessment of liver function, creatinine, complete blood count, platelet count, uric acid (if pyrazinamide is used), and ophthalmic examination (if ethambutol is used) before antituberculous therapy is begun. All patients should be evaluated periodically for adverse reactions to the drugs (Tables 21-15 and 21-17).

Isoniazid

Hepatitis is the most serious side effect. The incidence of hepatitis is age-dependent: it is rare in patients younger than 20 years, 0.3% for those between 20 and 34 years, 1.2% for those between 35 and 49 years, and 2.3% for those older than 50 years. The overall incidence is less than 1%. Liver dysfunction develops in 46% of patients within the first 2 months, in 36% during the 2nd month, and in 54% after the 3rd month. Middle-aged and black females are at higher risk. Hepatitis is more likely in patients who are "rapid acetylators," and neuritis is more likely in those who are "slow acetylators." Isoniazid also causes skin rash, purpura, drug-induced systemic lupus erythematosus, and arthritis. The addition of pyridoxine is recommended for patients with neuropathy (diabetes mellitus, uremia, alcoholism, and malnutrition), pregnancy, and seizure disorder. Patients older than 35 years who are receiving preventive therapy with isoniazid should have their liver function monitored, with levels of transaminase measured at 1, 3, 6, and 9 months.

- The incidence of isoniazid-induced hepatitis increases with age.
- Isoniazid causes peripheral neuropathy.
- Stop therapy if aspartate aminotransferase (AST) >5x normal or 3x above baseline.

Rifampin

The overall incidence of serious side effects is 1%. Gastrointestinal upset is the most common reaction. A transient increase in serum glutamic-oxaloacetic transaminase (SGOT) is common; true hepatitis occurs in fewer than 4% of patients. Hepatitis is worse with isoniazid therapy. Larger and/or intermittent doses (>10 mg/kg) are associated with thrombocytopenia, flu-like syndrome, hemolytic anemia, and cholestatic jaundice. Harmless orange discoloration of body secretions occurs. Rifampin increases the metabolism of contraceptive pills, corticosteroids, warfarin, oral hypoglycemic agents, theophylline, anticonvulsant agents, ketoconazole, cyclosporine, methadone, and antiarrhythmic drugs (digitalis, quinidine, verapamil, and mexiletine); therefore, dosages of these drugs may have to be increased.

- Rifampin: gastrointestinal upset is the most common side effect.
- Hepatitis is worse with isoniazid therapy.
- Rifampin induces liver microsomal enzymes.

Pyrazinamide

The most serious adverse reaction is liver damage. Hyperuricemia is common but gout is not, although arthralgias are reported occasionally. Skin rash and gastrointestinal upset are sometimes encountered.

- Pyrazinamide: liver damage is the most serious adverse reaction.

Ethambutol

Ethambutol in doses greater than 25 mg/kg causes retrobulbar neuritis in fewer than 3% of patients; symptoms usually are observed 2 months after therapy is begun. Because ophthalmoscopic findings are normal in these patients, symptoms are important (blurred vision, central scotoma, and red-green color blindness). These symptoms precede changes in visual acuity.

- Ethambutol: retrobulbar neuritis (dose-related) is the most frequent and serious side effect.
- Renal failure prolongs the half-life of the drug and increases the frequency of ocular toxicity.

Streptomycin

Because streptomycin is excreted by the kidneys, the dosage should be decreased in renal insufficiency. The most common adverse side effect is vestibular toxicity, which causes vertigo. Hearing loss may also occur. These side effects are more likely in the elderly. Ototoxicity and nephrotoxicity are related to both the cumulative dose and the peak serum concentration.

- Streptomycin: nephrotoxicity and vestibular toxicity are more common in persons >60 years.
- Streptomycin should be avoided in pregnancy.

Pulmonary Mycoses

Serious fungal infections are found at autopsy in 2% of patients overall, in up to 10% of those with solid tumors, and in up to 40% of those dying of leukemia. Renal transplantation patients (15%) have a fungal infection at some time during their post-transplantation course. Almost all mycoses produce granulomas. The saprophytic state of fungi is a common problem, particularly with *Aspergillus* species. Pulmonary manifestations are described here. Diagnostic methods and treatment of the mycoses are discussed in Chapter 14.

Histoplasmosis

Histoplasma capsulatum causes histoplasmosis. This infection is more common in the Mississippi, Ohio, and St. Lawrence River valleys than elsewhere. Infection is by inhalation of fungal spores. Infectious spores are especially numerous in chicken coops, dusty areas, starling roosts, bat-infested caves, and decayed wood. Clinical forms include asymptomatic infection, symptomatic infection (similar to viral upper respiratory tract infection), disseminated (immunocompromised host), chronic cavitary (structural defects), mediastinal granuloma, mediastinal fibrosis, pulmonary nodules, and calcified lesions on CXR. Disseminated disease may occur in patients with AIDS. Hilar adenopathy may be seen.

- Histoplasmosis: exposure to chicken coops, dusty areas, starling roosts, bat-infested caves, and decayed wood.
- The chronic cavitary form clinically mimics chronic tuberculosis.
- Mediastinal fibrosis, pulmonary calcification, broncholithiasis, and superior vena cava syndrome.
- Histoplasmosis is the most common cause of mediastinal granuloma.

Coccidioidomycosis

Coccidioides immitis causes coccidioidomycosis. The endemic zone extends from northern California to Argentina. Infections are more common when dry windy conditions exist, with epidemics occurring in the dry hot months after the rainy season, often after the soil has been disturbed. Clinical forms include mildly symptomatic pulmonary infection (flu-like illness in 40% of patients), asymptomatic nodules or thin-walled cavities, coccidioidal pneumonia, chronic cavitary form, disseminated form, and "valley fever" (erythema nodosum, erythema multiforme, arthralgia, arthritis, and eosinophilia). CXR may show lobar infiltrates (70% of patients), scattered patchy areas, atelectasis, hilar adenopathy (25%), pleural effusion (3%), cavities (8%), nodules (5%), and normal findings (3%). Filipinos, African-Americans, and Mexicans are at greater risk for dissemination and death. Infection acquired late during pregnancy is associated with higher maternal and fetal mortality.

- Coccidioidomycosis: endemic to southwestern U.S.
- Asymptomatic nodules, thin-walled cavities, coccidioidal pneumonia, chronic cavitary form, and disseminated form.

Blastomycosis

Blastomyces dermatitidis causes blastomycosis. Mini-epidemics have occurred in North Carolina, Minnesota, and Illinois. Most cases occur in the southern, south central, and Great Lakes states. Persons in contact with soil are more likely to be infected. The male:female ratio is 10:1. Pulmonary forms are acute pneumonic form (resolution or progressive pulmonary involvement), asymptomatic, and insidious pulmonary or extrapulmonary dissemination. The most characteristic CXR finding is a perihilar mass that mimics carcinoma. Mass-like infiltrates are associated more with chronic than acute presentations. Air-space and mass-like infiltrate predominately involve the upper lobes. Sputum analysis is helpful in diagnosis. Pleural effusion is seen in fewer than 3% of patients with the pneumonic form. Laryngeal blastomycosis can resemble cancer. No skin test is available. Serologic testing is unreliable.

- Blastomycosis: contact with soil, manual laborers, and Great Lakes states.

- Most characteristic CXR finding: a perihilar mass mimicking carcinoma.

Cryptococcosis

Cryptococcus neoformans, the only fungus that is not dimorphic (no mycelia), causes cryptococcosis. The organism is widely distributed in the soil, foods, and excreta of pigeons and other animals. In humans, it may exist as a saprophyte in preexisting lung disease, but one-third to one-half of patients with cryptococcosis are immunosuppressed. The lung is the portal of entry, but the most common clinical presentation is subacute or chronic meningitis (the common cause of death). Diseases that predispose to cryptococcosis include an immunocompromised state, Hodgkin and non-Hodgkin lymphomas, leukemia, sarcoidosis, and diabetes mellitus. The onset of neurologic symptoms, fever, nausea, and anorexia is insidious. Pulmonary features include cough with scant sputum (15% of patients), chest pain (45%), dyspnea (25%), hemoptysis (7%), and night sweats (25%). Nodular infiltrates with cavitation, especially in the lower lobes, occasional hilar adenopathy, and a solitary mass may be found. In non-AIDS patients with pulmonary cryptococcosis, masses and air space consolidation are common and atelectasis, lymphadenopathy, and pleural effusion or empyema are relatively rare. The diagnosis can be established with positive sputum cultures (35% of patients), bronchoscopic specimens (35%), and open lung biopsy (100%). India ink preparations of the cerebrospinal fluid are positive in 30% to 60% of patients. In HIV-infected patients, serum cryptococcal antigen testing is highly sensitive. Serologic testing (detects polysaccharide antigen) of the cerebrospinal fluid is positive in 90% of cases of central nervous system infections and in 30% of cases of non-central nervous system infection. Serologic testing should be performed on blood, cerebrospinal fluid, and urine.

- *C. neoformans*: saprophytic or pathogenic state.
- More common in immunocompromised patients.
- Nodular, cavitary, and patchy infiltrates.
- The cerebrospinal fluid should be examined in almost all patients who have organisms in respiratory secretions.

Aspergillosis

Aspergillus fumigatus, *A. flavus*, and *A. niger* are responsible for several pulmonary manifestations. The clinical forms include 1) allergic bronchopulmonary aspergillosis (see above), 2) hypersensitivity pneumonitis in red cedarwood workers, 3) mycetoma or fungus ball in preexisting lung disease, 4) locally invasive (chronic necrotizing) aspergillosis of lung tissue, 5) tracheobronchial form in immunocompromised, HIV, and lung transplant recipients (at anastomotic site), 6) disseminated, 7) bronchocentric granulomatosis, and 8) saprophytic. The organism frequently colonizes the respiratory tract in patients with lung disease. Invasive aspergillosis in immunosuppressed hosts is the most serious form of infection and occurs mainly in granulocytopenic patients with hematologic malignancies. The occurrence of life-threatening complications in patients with invasive fungal pneumonia is closely related to rapid granulocyte recovery. *Aspergillus* is isolated at autopsy in 10% of patients with acute leukemia. Of all patients with invasive aspergillosis (diagnosed pre- or postmortem), 40% have acute lymphocytic leukemia, 20% have acute myelomonocytic leukemia, 10% have chronic myelogenous leukemia, 5% have Hodgkin disease, and 10% have other hematologic malignancies. The presence of the organism in respiratory secretions is not diagnostic; tissue invasion should be documented. Aspergilloma is a mass of fungal hyphae in preexisting lung cavities. The major symptoms include hemoptysis, cough, low-grade fever, and weight loss. Fungus ball can be caused by *Candida*, *Coccidioides*, *Nocardia*, and *Sporotrichum*. CXR and tomograms show a meniscus of air around the fungus ball (Monod sign), almost always in the upper lobes. Skin testing gives positive results in 20% of patients, and serologic findings are positive in more than 90%. Because surgical therapy of aspergilloma carries a high morbidity and mortality, another therapeutic option is to use intracavitary instillation of amphotericin.

- Granulocytopenia and lung infiltrates in hematologic malignancies almost always mean disseminated aspergillosis.
- Aspergillosis is frequently accompanied by *Pseudomonas* or *Candida*.
- Aspergilloma (fungus ball) occurs in previously damaged lung; hemoptysis is a serious complication.

Zygomycosis (Mucormycosis)

Zygomycosis is caused by Mucorales (Phycomycetes) species. Serious infections of the lungs, central nervous system, and skin occur in patients with severe diabetes mellitus, hematologic malignancies, skin or mucosal injuries, and in immunocompromised state. The organism invades blood vessels in the lungs and causes significant hemoptysis. CXR may show patchy infiltrates, consolidation, cavitation, and effusions. Bronchial stenosis is a peculiar complication of zygomycosis. The diagnosis must be established by biopsy, although sputum culture may suggest it. No serologic test is available.

- Zygomycosis: immunocompromised and diabetic patients.
- Propensity to invade blood vessels; hemoptysis is common.

Candidiasis

Candidiasis is caused by *Candida albicans* and is responsible for up to 75% of serious infections. *Candida* species are present in the oropharynx of 30% of normal persons, in the gastrointestinal tract in 65%, and in the vagina of up to 70% of women. Systemic candidiasis is found at autopsy in as many as 25% of patients with leukemia. Risk factors for developing candidiasis include diabetes mellitus, cancer, cirrhosis, renal failure, blood dyscrasia, cytotoxic therapy, intravenous or urinary catheters, antibiotics given intravenously, prostheses, cachexia, burns, and HIV infection. Lung involvement is relatively rare, and CXR shows patchy or diffuse infiltrates. *Candida* bronchitis, an occupational disease of tea tasters, is manifested by low-grade fever, cough, and patchy infiltrates.

- Candidiasis: more common in patients with hematologic malignancies.
- Prolonged granulocytopenia predisposes to disseminated infection.
- Lung involvement is uncommon; patchy or diffuse lung infiltrates.

Sporotrichosis

Sporotrichosis is caused by *Sporothrix schenckii*. The organism is a dimorphous fungus that exists as a saprophyte in the soil, plants, wood, straw, sphagnum moss, decaying vegetation, cats, dogs, and rodents. Sporotrichosis is an occupational hazard of farmers, florists, gardeners, horticulturists, and forestry workers. Infection is by cutaneous inoculation. Cutaneous nodules along lymphatic vessels may appear in 75% of patients. Hematogenous dissemination to the lungs is rare, but inhalation-induced pulmonary disease mimics cavitary tuberculosis.

- Sporotrichosis: occupational hazard of florists, horticulturists, and gardeners.
- Lymphangitis of the skin and subcutaneous nodules.
- Pulmonary infection mimics chronic tuberculosis.

Nocardiosis

Nocardiosis is caused by *Nocardia asteroides*, *N. brasiliensis*, and *N. caviae*. *N. asteroides* is a weakly acid-fast saprophyte present in the soil, dust, plants, and water. The lungs and central nervous system are involved. Infection is more common in immunosuppressed patients and in those with pulmonary alveolar proteinosis. Primary infection leads to necrotizing pneumonia with abscess formation. No inflammatory response or granuloma formation occurs. Infection may produce pleural effusion. Lymphohematogenous spread is seen in 20% of patients; nearly all such patients develop brain abscesses. The diagnosis is made at autopsy in 40% of cases. Isolation of the organism from respiratory secretions is not diagnostic of infection because the saprophytic state is well recognized.

- Nocardiosis: more common in immunocompromised patients.
- Patients with pulmonary alveolar proteinosis prone to nocardiosis.
- Necrotizing pneumonia and lung abscess.
- Central nervous system involvement is common in those with disseminated infection.

Actinomycosis

Actinomycosis is caused by *Actinomyces israelii* or *A. bovis*. The organism is not found in the soil or vegetation. It is easily isolated from scrapings around the teeth, gums, and tonsils in subjects with poor dental or oral hygiene. It is an opportunistic organism and becomes invasive with severe caries, tissue necrosis, and aspiration. In tissue, the organism grows into a "sulfur granule" caused by mycelial clumps in a matrix of calcium phosphate. The disease is more common in rural areas, with a male:female ratio of 2:1. Infection is always mixed with anaerobes. Skin abscesses, ulcers, sinus tracts, and cervicofacial node involvement are found in up to 40% of patients. Pulmonary involvement is seen in 20% of patients, with cough, fever, pulmonary consolidation, pleurisy with effusion, and, eventually, draining sinuses.

- Actinomycosis: more likely with severe dental caries, tissue necrosis, and aspiration.
- Sulfur granules from abscesses, fistulas, or wounds.
- Cough, fever, pulmonary lesions, pleural effusion, and fistula and sinus tracts.

Pneumocystis carinii

P. carinii is a fungus with trophozoite and cyst stages. The cyst stains best with methenamine silver nitrate. *P. carinii* infections occur in immunosuppressed patients and account for 40% of the cases of interstitial pneumonia in these patients. The frequency of infection increases in proportion to the intensity of immunosuppressive treatment. *P. carinii* infection is seen in 5% of patients receiving treatment with a single drug, in 30% of those receiving four drugs, and in 40% of those receiving polychemotherapy and irradiation. Patients with AIDS (CD4 <200/μL) are in the high-risk group for *P. carinii* infection. Infection causes alveolar and interstitial inflammation and edema with plasma cell infiltrates. The organisms are found in alveolar macrophages. Clinical features include the abrupt onset of fever, tachypnea, hypoxia, cyanosis, respiratory distress, relatively normal findings on lung examination, and a patchy or diffuse interstitial/alveolar process. The typical CT finding is ground-glass attenuation. However, this classic radiographic presentation is less frequent now and is being replaced by cystic lung disease, spontaneous pneumothorax, and an upper lobe distribution of parenchymal opacities. Routine laboratory data are unhelpful. The diagnosis can be made with induced sputum, BAL, or lung biopsy findings. Induced sputum and BAL are excellent methods for diagnosis. The number of organisms seen in tissue preparations from non-AIDS patients is smaller.

- *P. carinii* infection: respiratory symptoms and signs are more serious in non-AIDS patients.
- Upper lobe process seen on CXR in patients receiving pentamidine aerosol therapy.

Parasitic Diseases

Parasitic infections of the lung are less common in the U.S. than in other parts of the world. Travelers to regions that are endemic for parasitic infestations may become infected and, when they return to the U.S., present as difficult diagnostic problems. However, dirofilariasis is indigenous to the eastern and southeastern U.S. Other parasitic infections, including helminthic infestations, also occur in the U.S. Even though the respiratory system may be affected by many parasitic infections, the parasites more likely to cause chronic pulmonary manifestations include *Paragonimus westermani* (paragonimiasis), *Echinococcus granulosus* (echinococcosis or hydatid disease), *Dirofilaria immitis* (dirofilariasis), *Schistosoma japonicum* and *S. mansoni* (schistosomiasis), and *Entamoeba histolytica* (amebiasis). Protozoal infections are more likely in patients whose cellular immunity is suppressed.

- Dirofilariasis is endemic to certain regions of the U.S.

Dirofilariasis is caused by the "dog heartworm" and transmitted to humans by mosquitoes. The disease is endemic to the Mississippi River valley, the southeastern U.S., and the Gulf Coast. Characteristically, the infection presents in the form of well-defined solitary or multiple lung nodule(s) 1.5 to 2.5 cm in diameter. Eosinophilia occurs in fewer than 15% of patients. Serologic tests may aid in the diagnosis. Echinococcosis has occurred in Alaska and the southwestern U.S. Lung disease presents with CXR findings of well-defined round or oval cystic or solid lesions up to 15 cm in diameter. Rupture of the cysts can cause anaphylactic shock, hypersensitivity reactions, and seeding of adjacent anatomical areas. Hepatic involvement (in 40% with lung disease) and positive serologic findings are common. Paragonimiasis is more likely in immigrants from Southeast Asia, but sporadic cases occur in the U.S. It typically is transmitted through consumption of raw or undercooked crabs or crayfish. Respiratory features resemble those in chronic bronchitis, bronchiectasis, or tuberculosis. Profuse brown-colored sputum and hemoptysis can be seen. Pleural effusion is relatively common. Peripheral eosinophilia is common. Ova can be found in pleural fluid, bronchial wash, or sputum. Schistosomiasis is not acquired in the U.S. The infection leads to gradual development of secondary pulmonary hypertension caused by occlusion of the pulmonary arterial tree by the parasite. Cor pulmonale develops in 5% of patients. Amebiasis may present as lobar pneumonia or lung abscess. Rupture into the bronchial tree (hepatobronchial fistula) may be followed by expectoration of "anchovy paste" or "chocolate" sputum. Rupture of the liver abscess into the pleural space causes empyema along with respiratory distress in many patients. Pericardial involvement can also occur. Strongyloidiasis involving the lungs can mimic asthma. Risk factors include steroid use, age older than 65, chronic lung disease, and chronic debilitating illness. Pulmonary signs and symptoms include cough, shortness of breath, wheezing, and hemoptysis in more than 90% of patients. Adult respiratory distress syndrome has been observed in 45% of patients and pulmonary infiltrates in 90%. Preexisting chronic lung disease and adult respiratory distress syndrome are significant predictors of a poor prognosis.

- Dirofilariasis: exposure to dog; solitary or multiple lung nodule(s).
- Pleural effusion: paragonimiasis and amebiasis.
- Tuberculosis-like illness: paragonimiasis.
- Pulmonary hypertension: schistosomiasis.
- Amebiasis: pleuropulmonary complications are almost always right-sided.
- Strongyloidosis: mimics asthma with eosinophilia.

Noninfectious Pulmonary Complications in AIDS

Infectious pulmonary complications are discussed in Chapter 14. The noninfectious pulmonary complications in AIDS are discussed in the following paragraphs.

Nonspecific interstitial pneumonitis is a common occurrence in patients with chronic AIDS. It represents 30% to 40% of all episodes of lung infiltrates in these patients. More than 25% of patients with this problem have concurrent Kaposi sarcoma, previous experimental treatments, or a history of *P. carinii* pneumonia or drug abuse. The clinical features are similar to those of patients with *P. carinii* pneumonia. Histologic examination of the lung may reveal varying degrees of edema, fibrin deposition, and interstitial inflammation with lymphocytes and plasma cells. No specific therapy is known.

- Nonspecific interstitial pneumonitis occurs in up to 40% of patients with AIDS.
- *P. carinii* pneumonia should be excluded.

Lymphocytic interstitial pneumonitis is caused by pulmonary infiltration with mature polyclonal B lymphocytes and plasma cells. It occurs in children of mothers in groups at high risk for AIDS and patients with AIDS. Corticosteroids may result in significant improvement. Pulmonary lymphoid hyperplasia has been reported in 40% of children with AIDS.

- Lymphocytic interstitial pneumonitis is diagnostic of AIDS when it occurs in a child <13 years old with positive HIV serologic findings.

Cystic lung disease is more common in patients with *P. carinii* infections and in those receiving aerosolized pentamidine therapy. Cystic lesions are more common in the upper and mid lung zones. Chest CT identifies these small- to medium-sized cystic lesions.

- Cystic lung disease is more common in those with *P. carinii* pneumonia receiving aerosolized pentamidine therapy.

Pneumothorax occurs with increasing frequency in patients with *P. carinii* pneumonia and in those receiving pentamidine aerosol therapy. Other causes of pneumothorax include Kaposi sarcoma, tuberculosis, and other infections. Pneumothorax in patients with AIDS carries a poor prognosis.

- High incidence of bilateral synchronous pneumothoraces.

Pleural effusion is seen in 25% of hospitalized patients with AIDS. Nearly one-third of the pleural effusions are due to noninfectious causes. Hypoalbuminemia is the leading cause of these effusions. Other important noninfectious causes include Kaposi sarcoma and atelectasis. Among the infectious causes, bacterial pneumonias, *P. carinii* pneumonia, and *M. tuberculosis* are important. Fungal infections can also produce pleural effusion. Large effusions are caused by tuberculosis and Kaposi sarcoma.

- Pleural effusion is caused by infections in two-thirds of hospitalized patients with AIDS.
- Kaposi sarcoma and tuberculosis cause large effusions.

Pulmonary hypertension has been found in patients with AIDS. It is more common in those with HLA-DR6 alleles. The mechanism is not clear, but HIV is thought to affect the endothelium directly and to cause vascular changes. The clinical, physiologic, and pathologic features are identical to those seen in primary pulmonary hypertension.

- Pulmonary hypertension is identical clinically to idiopathic pulmonary hypertension.

Kaposi sarcoma occurs with greater frequency in homosexuals with AIDS. It is believed to be caused by human herpesvirus-8 (HHV-8). The incidence of its occurrence has diminished. Previous or concurrent pulmonary opportunistic infections have been noted in more than 70% of patients with Kaposi sarcoma. Kaposi sarcoma occurs in the lungs of up to 35% of patients who have this tumor. The lung may be the only site in about 15% of patients. In most patients, pulmonary Kaposi sarcoma is established only at autopsy. The diagnostic yield from bronchoscopy is 24% and from lung biopsy, 56%. Hemoptysis is an uncommon complication in Kaposi sarcoma, although endobronchial metastasis develops in 30% of patients. CXR may show typical nodular infiltrates in less than 10% of patients. Pleural effusion may be seen.

- Pulmonary Kaposi sarcoma is usually preceded by cutaneous lesions.
- Lung involvement due to Kaposi sarcoma occurs in up to 35% of patients with this neoplasm.
- Clinically, pulmonary Kaposi sarcoma is indistinguishable from *P. carinii* pneumonia or opportunistic pneumonia.
- Multiple, discrete, raised, violaceous, or bright red tracheobronchial lesions can be seen on bronchoscopy.

Non-Hodgkin lymphoma involving the lungs is seen in less than 10% of patients with AIDS who develop lymphoma. The lymphoma in these patients is usually extranodal non-Hodgkin B-cell lymphoma. Lung involvement is a late occurrence. Nodules, masses, and infiltrates can be seen on CXR. A 6.5-fold increased incidence of primary lung cancer has been noted in HIV-infected and AIDS patients.

Other complications include chronic bronchitis, bronchiectasis, and BOOP. The CD4 counts in those with bronchitis and bronchiectasis are usually less than $100/\mu L$. PFTs often show decreased DLCO in asymptomatic patients.

ACKNOWLEDGMENT

The contribution of chest roentgenographic figures by Edward C. Rosenow III, M.D., is gratefully acknowledged.

QUESTIONS

Multiple Choice (choose the one best answer)

1. A 57-year-old woman, a 10-pack-year smoker, complains of a 6-month history of dry cough. She has some mild dysphagia to solids. She complains of mild dyspnea and wheeze on exertion. For hypertension diagnosed 12 months earlier, she started taking an antihypertensive medication 5 months later. Chest radiographic findings are normal. Which of the following is the *least likely* cause of the cough?
   a. Antihypertensive medication
   b. Gastroesophageal reflux
   c. Pulmonary fibrosis
   d. Bronchial asthma
   e. Bronchogenic carcinoma

2. Which of the following is *least* appropriate in the patient described in Question 1?
   a. Empiric bronchodilator therapy
   b. Spirometry with inhalation provocation challenge
   c. Discontinuation of antihypertensive drug
   d. Contrast study of esophagus
   e. Sputum cytology

3. A 51-year-old man, a nonsmoker, has progressive dyspnea that began 3 months ago. Recently, he began to cough and to expectorate large amounts (>1 cup/d) of thin clear mucous. He has no fever, chills, or malaise. Chest radiography shows an alveolar process involving both lobes of the left lung. What is the most *likely* diagnosis?
   a. Small cell carcinoma of lung
   b. Pulmonary alveolar proteinosis
   c. Metastasis from nonpulmonary malignancy
   d. Streptococcal pneumonia
   e. Alveolar cell carcinoma of lung

4. A 68-year-old man, a 56-pack-year smoker, undergoes bronchoscopy under topical anesthesia for evaluation of streaky hemoptysis. One hour after bronchoscopy, he notices bluish discoloration of his fingers and lips. He has minimal dyspnea and his vital signs are normal and stable. He has no chest pain. No significant past medical history is elicited. Blood gas analysis shows PaO_2 86 mm Hg, $PaCO_2$ 46 mm Hg, pH 7.38, and SaO_2 56%. What is most *likely* to have caused the bluish discoloration?
   a. Polycythemia from chronic obstructive lung disease
   b. Methemoglobinemia
   c. Right-to-left anatomical shunt
   d. Shock
   e. Peripheral arterial occlusive disease

5. A 64-year-old man, a 38-pack-year smoker, presents with recent onset of pain in both knees and shins. Examination reveals clubbing of the fingernails, mild bilateral

gynecomastia, tenderness of both shins, and mild expiratory slowing of lung sounds. Which test is *not* indicated at this time?

a. Chest radiography
b. Bone scan
c. Sputum cytology
d. Bronchoscopy
e. Radiography of knees and legs

6. A 56-year-old woman has had progressive dyspnea and cough for 12 months. She also has significant chronic dyspeptic symptoms. Examination reveals mild clubbing of the fingernails and late inspiratory crackles in both lung bases. Chest radiography shows a bilateral basal interstitial process. Which diagnostic test is *least likely* to help in the diagnosis?

a. ^{67}Gallium-citrate lung scan
b. High-resolution computed tomography of chest
c. Pulmonary function tests
d. Blood gas analysis
e. Esophagoscopy

7. A 30-year-old man, a nonsmoker, has a history of progressive dyspnea over a 12-month period. He has no cough, wheeze, or chest pain. He complains of generalized weakness. Chest radiography shows an anterior mediastinal mass. Pulmonary function tests showed the following (% predicted normal): TLC 78%, VC 76%, FEV$_1$ 82%, MVV 40%, and DLCO 86%. What is the *most likely* diagnosis?

a. Small cell carcinoma
b. Thymoma
c. Bilateral diaphragmatic paralysis
d. Pulmonary hypertension
e. Carcinoid tumor with ACTH production

8. A 60-year-old man, previously a heavy smoker with severe chronic obstructive pulmonary disease (COPD), is referred for consideration of supplemental oxygen therapy. Detailed clinical evaluations reveal severe expiratory slowing of lung sounds. Pulmonary function tests confirm severe COPD. Routine blood tests and arterial blood gas analysis were performed to assess the need for supplemental oxygen therapy. Which of the following is *not* an indication for supplemental oxygen therapy in this patient?

a. Pao$_2$, 53 mm Hg
b. Hemoglobin, 19 g/dL; hematocrit, 55
c. Diffusing capacity of lung for CO, 35% predicted
d. Recurrent cor pulmonale
e. Neuropsychiatric symptoms reversed by trial of supplemental oxygen

9. A 37-year-old Minnesota farmer has gradually progressive dyspnea that he has observed over the last several months. Lung sounds are normal on examination. Chest radiography shows bilateral interstitial infiltrates in both upper and lower lung zones. Computed tomography shows no lymphadenopathy, but interstitial micronodular infiltrates are seen. A diagnostic bronchoalveolar lavage shows CD4/CD8 (helper/suppressor) ratio of 1/3. What is the *most* likely diagnosis?

a. Pulmonary Hodgkin lymphoma
b. Silo-filler's lung disease
c. Sarcoidosis, stage III
d. Hypersensitivity pneumonitis
e. Pulmonary aspergillosis

10. A 27-year-old woman, a nonsmoker, with a history of childhood asthma with recent asthmatic exacerbations is brought to the emergency department because of an acute asthmatic attack. She has been noncompliant with previously recommended treatments. Examination discloses a dyspneic patient with severe wheezing bilaterally. Chest radiography shows mildly hyperinflated lungs. Which of the following treatments is *least likely* to treat her asthmatic exacerbation?

a. Corticosteroid aerosol
b. Corticosteroids (intravenous)
c. β-Agonist bronchodilator (aerosol)
d. Theophylline (intravenous)
e. Leukotriene receptor antagonist (aerosol)

11. A 48-year-old woman, a nonsmoker, presents with the chief complaints of progressive dyspnea (12 months) and cough (8 months). Examination reveals mild clubbing of the fingernails, diffuse bibasilar end-inspiratory crackles, and prominent pulmonary component of the second heart sound. Chest radiography indicates a basal interstitial process. High-resolution computed tomography shows honeycomb changes in subpleural peripheral lower lung zones. Pulmonary function tests show moderately severe restrictive lung disease. Blood tests demonstrate moderately increased titers of antinuclear antibody and rheumatoid factor. What is the *most likely* diagnosis?

a. Sarcoidosis, stage III
b. Systemic lupus erythematosus
c. Lymphangioleiomyomatosis
d. Pulmonary Langerhans cell granuloma
e. Idiopathic pulmonary fibrosis

12. A 27-year-old man, a 1-pack-per-day smoker, has mild exertional dyspnea. Physical examination findings are normal except for localized point tenderness over the left

eighth rib posterolaterally. Chest radiography shows cystic, nodular changes and large honeycomb abnormalities in the upper lung zones bilaterally. A small osteolytic rib lesion is noted in the left eighth rib. What is the *most likely* diagnosis?

a. Acute histoplasmosis with bony involvement
b. Sarcoidosis with bone cyst
c. Langerhans cell granuloma (histiocytosis X)
d. Lung cancer with bony metastasis
e. Pulmonary lymphangioleiomyomatosis

13. Which *one* of the following "pairings" (association/complication) is *incorrect*?
a. Langerhans cell granuloma (histiocytosis X) and smoking
b. Sarcoidosis (end-stage) and aspergilloma
c. Lymphangioleiomyomatosis and chylous pleural effusion
d. Pulmonary fibrosis and atypical mycobacterial infections
e. Pulmonary alveolar proteinosis and *Nocardia* infection

14. A 76-year-old man, exsmoker (50 pack-years), complains of chest pain and dyspnea of 6 months' duration. He provides a history of heavy exposure to asbestos in the past and chronically abnormal chest radiographic findings. Basal crackles are noted on examination. Which one of the following is *least likely* to be found in this patient?
a. Bilateral apical fibrosis
b. Calcification of diaphragmatic pleura
c. Pleural thickening/mass
d. Lung mass
e. Pleural effusion

15. A 59-year-old man is evaluated for sonorous snoring, abnormal motor behavior during sleep, daytime somnolence, systemic hypertension, morning headaches, and excessive somnolence. Polysomnography demonstrates significant obstructive sleep apnea. The patient wants to know the complications of this problem. Which one of the following is *not* a complication of sleep apnea?
a. Cor pulmonale
b. Cardiac arrhythmias, including ventricular tachycardia
c. Increased risk of coronary artery disease
d. Increased risk of cerebrovascular disease/accidents
e. Pulmonary embolism

16. A 36-year-old woman is hospitalized because of the recent onset of progressive dyspnea and lung infiltrates.

Previously healthy, she now has diffuse myalgias and a skin rash over the back and face. The erythrocyte sedimentation rate is 86 mm/hr. Lung biopsy shows bronchiolitis obliterans with organizing pneumonia (BOOP). Which of the following disorders is *least likely* in this patient?
a. Rheumatoid arthritis
b. Polymyositis-dermatomyositis
c. Alpha$_1$-antitrypsin deficiency
d. Amiodarone lung toxicity
e. Eosinophilic pneumonia

17. A 48-year-old man with chronic asthma treated with β-agonists, theophylline, leukotriene antagonist, and aerosolized corticosteroids complains of refractory wheezing, dyspnea, and cough with expectoration of thick, dark brown-black sputum. A 1-week course of azithromycin has not helped. Chest radiography exhibits bilateral soft (fluffy) infiltrates in the upper lung zones. Which of the following is *not* a major criterion to document the new complication of this patient's asthma?
a. Central bronchiectasis
b. Immediate skin reactivity (type I) to aspergillus antigen
c. Positive serologic results for *Aspergillus fumigatus*
d. Sputum culture identification of *Aspergillus* species
e. Elevated immunoglobulin E (IgE)

18. During a routine examination, a 55-year-old man, nonsmoker, is found to have a 1.5-cm uncalcified nodule in the right upper lobe. He has no respiratory symptoms. No earlier chest radiographs are available for comparison. There is no past history of malignancy or other systemic disorders. Which of the following is the *best* recommendation for this patient?
a. Extensive testing to detect nonpulmonary malignancy
b. Thoracoscopic resection
c. Bronchoscopic brush and biopsy
d. Needle aspiration under computed tomographic guidance
e. Repeat chest radiography in 3 months

19. A 59-year-old man is referred because of a 3-week history of pleuritic chest pain and dyspnea. He also has low-grade fever (100.5°F), cough, and arthralgias. He has been taking procainamide for arrhythmias and an oral hypoglycemic agent for type 2 diabetes. Examination demonstrates a pleural friction rub in left base posteriorly. Chest radiography shows a small left pleural effusion and plate-like atelectasis in the left base. The erythrocyte sedimentation rate is 68 mm/hr. Which test is *least likely* to provide diagnostic

information in this patient?
a. Serum complement
b. Computed tomography of the chest
c. Pleural fluid complement level
d. Pleural fluid lupus erythematosus cell clot
e. Serum antinuclear antibody

20. A 53-year-old woman is referred for evaluation of pulmonary hypertension. She has experienced several episodes of deep venous thrombosis (DVT) of both lower extremities, documented by venography. Previous diagnostic evaluations and anticoagulant therapy have been inadequate. Now she has grade 2 dyspnea and subacute pleuritic chest pains. Examination reveals a loud P_2 and right ventricular heave. There is no evidence of DVT. Which test is *inappropriate* in the diagnostic evaluation?
a. Assessment of coagulation cascade
b. Ultrasonographic Doppler study of the legs
c. Ventilation-perfusion lung scan
d. Ultrafast (imatron) computed tomography of the chest
e. Pulmonary angiography and measurement of pulmonary artery pressures

21. A 36-year-old woman is referred with the chief complaints of gradually progressive exertional dyspnea over the last 12 months, exertional dizziness and occasional syncope, anterior chest tightness, and fatigue. She also has noted Raynaud phenomenon during the last 6 months. Examination demonstrates a loud P_2 and right ventricular heave. The lungs are clear to auscultation. Chest radiography shows enlarged main pulmonary arteries. Blood gases are PaO_2 52 mm Hg and SaO_2 85%. The antinuclear antibody titer is elevated. Which of the following long-term therapeutic considerations is *inappropriate* in this patient?
a. Anticoagulation
b. Vasodilator (calcium channel blocker)
c. Systemic high-dose corticosteroid
d. Supplemental oxygen
e. Prostacycline

22. A 65-year-old woman, a 100-pack-year smoker, develops progressive weakness. Chest radiography shows mediastinal widening, new since an examination 6 months earlier. The serum potassium level is 2.3 mEq/L. Which one of the following is *not true* about this patient?
a. Chest computed tomography is likely to show a mediastinal/hilar mass
b. Electromyography will show decreasing muscle strength to repetitive stimuli
c. Serum ACTH level may be increased

d. Hyponatremia is a potential complication
e. Surgery is not a therapeutic option

23. Which one of the following statements is *incorrect* about the cytoplasmic antineutrophil cytoplasmic antibodies (c-ANCA) in Wegener granulomatosis (WG)?
a. Positive c-ANCA without clinical disease is not diagnostic of WG
b. Patients with active WG can have negative c-ANCA
c. c-ANCA is not seen in diseases other than WG
d. c-ANCA titers may increase without evidence of active WG
e. Persistently positive c-ANCA occurs despite inactive WG

24. Which of the following is *least likely* to cause alveolar hemorrhage syndrome?
a. Systemic lupus erythematosus
b. Mitral stenosis
c. Antiglomerular basement membrane antibody disease
d. Rheumatoid lung disease
e. Idiopathic pulmonary hemosiderosis

25. A 23-year-old African-American man with a 24-hour history of increasing pleuritic chest pain, fever, and prostration is evaluated in the emergency department. Cough with rusty sputum has been observed. Examination suggests a consolidative process in the right lower lobe. Total leukocyte count is 21,500. Blood gas analysis shows PaO_2 52 mm Hg and SaO_2 78%. Chest radiography demonstrates dense bilateral lower lobe (R>>L) pneumonic consolidations. The patient is known to have sickle cell anemia (Hb SS). What diagnosis is *least likely* in this patient?
a. Acute chest syndrome (sickle chest syndrome)
b. Acute pulmonary embolism
c. Pneumonia caused by *Staphylococcus aureus*
d. Pneumonia caused by *Haemophilus influenzae*
e. Pneumonia caused by *Pseudomonas aeruginosa*

26. A 42-year-old man with chronic renal failure and chronic hemodialysis is referred because of an abnormal "chest x-ray." He has been noncompliant with the dialysis program and dietary restrictions. What complication is *least likely* to be encountered in this patient?
a. Pulmonary hypertension
b. Noncardiogenic pulmonary edema
c. Recurrent pleural effusions
d. Pulmonary parenchymal calcification
e. Hypoxemia during hemodialysis

27. A 56-year-old woman with primary biliary cirrhosis is on

the waiting list for a liver transplant. Recently, she has noted dyspnea on exertion and in the upright position. She is found to have an enlarging ascites. Paracentesis shows no evidence of peritonitis. Which one of the following is *incorrect* regarding this patient?
a. Pleural fluid is a transudate (protein <3.0 g/dL)
b. Pleural effusion is more common on the left
c. Dyspnea may be caused by a right-to-left shunt
d. Pleural effusion may recur if ascites is not treated
e. Pulmonary hypertension is a complication

28. A 36-year-old patient is transferred from the detoxification center to a medical ward for evaluation of acute abdominal pain. The patient has a history of chronic alcohol use. Examination demonstrates a tender and taut upper abdomen, and dullness and diminished lung sounds in the left lung base. The serum amylase level is increased fivefold. Which one of the following is *unlikely* to complicate this patient's abdominal process?
a. Adult respiratory distress syndrome (ARDS)
b. Pleural effusion
c. Granulomatous pneumonitis
d. Pulmonary edema
e. Elevation of left hemidiaphragm

29. In the patient Question 28, percussion dullness increased over the next 48 hours, and chest radiography now shows a large left pleural effusion. The serum amylase level has decreased (now, threefold increase). Thoracentesis is planned. Which one of the following results is *unlikely* from the pleural fluid analysis?
a. Increased protein level (>3.0 g/dL)
b. Increased levels of amylase and lipase
c. Bloody-appearing effusion
d. Growth of gram-negative bacteria
e. Increased total leukocyte count

30. A 53-year-old salesman complains of a 4-month history of dyspnea. It has been progressive, and now he has mild orthopnea. Examination demonstrates diminished motion of the left diaphragm. Lung function tests show a total lung capacity of 65% predicted, vital capacity of 75% predicted, and maximal voluntary ventilation of 76% predicted. What diagnostic test is *least likely* to help in this patient?
a. Chest radiography
b. Diaphragmatic fluoroscopy (sniff test)
c. Computed tomography of the chest
d. Diaphragmatic electromyography
e. Computed tomography of the abdomen

31. A 78-year-old man, ex-smoker, develops cough productive of yellow/green sputum, fever (38.5°C), chest aches, anorexia, and lethargy. He is brought to the hospital 7 days later. Examination demonstrates a listless elderly patient with a hoarse voice. Bronchial breath sounds are audible over the right midlung posteriorly. Chest radiography shows a large cavitated lesion in the superior segment of the right lower lobe and a right hilar prominence. The serum sodium level is decreased at 124 mEq/L. Which of the following initial steps is *least appropriate* in the initial management of this patient?
a. Culture of respiratory secretions
b. Bronchoscopy
c. Computed tomography of the chest
d. Video-assisted thoracoscopic aspiration
e. Laryngoscopy

32. Which *one* of the statements about pneumonia caused by *Streptococcus pneumoniae* is incorrect?
a. *S. pneumoniae* is responsible for <40% of cases of pneumonia in adults
b. Carrier rates in the general population may be as high as 70% in the spring and winter
c. Bacteremic pneumonia occurs in 25% of hospitalized patients
d. Lung cavitation is rare in pneumococcal pneumonia
e. Occurrence rate is higher in patients with hemoglobinopathy and hyposplenism

33. A 44-year-old previously healthy man from Iowa, a nonsmoker, presents with a 10-day history of low-grade fever, cough with minimal sputum, and resolved skin rashes over the lower extremities. He just returned from a 4-week holiday in Arizona. Examination demonstrates minimal redness and induration over the shins. Chest radiography shows a cavitated lesion measuring 3 x 2 cm with a wall thickness of 2.0 mm in the right upper lobe. Which one of the following is *least likely* in this patient?
a. The skin lesion most likely is erythema nodosum
b. Positive serologic findings for the infecting organism
c. Positive sputum cytologic findings for malignancy
d. Symptomatic therapy alone is recommended
e. Chronic disabling illness is unlikely

34. Which one of the following statements is *not true* about nontuberculous mycobacterial lung infections?
a. Natural waters and soil are the source for most infections caused by *M. avium* complex
b. The source of *M. kansasii* is tap water
c. Lung cavitation occurs in >90% of patients with *M. kansasii* infection

d. Exposure to *M. avium* complex can cause hypersensitivity pneumonitis

e. Human-to-human spread occurs

35. A 32-year-old man (medical volunteer for 18 months) returns from Western Africa because of acute onset of cough, fever, and right pleuritic chest pain. Examination reveals fever (38.4°C), dullness, and decreased breath sounds in the right lung base. Chest radiography shows a moderate-sized right pleural effusion. A tuberculin skin test, negative 7 months earlier, now elicits a 16-mm induration. Diagnostic thoracentesis without pleural biopsy is planned. Which one of the following is *not* true in this patient?

a. Pleural fluid will show a low glucose level

b. Pleural fluid culture has a high (>75%) likelihood of identifying the infective organism

c. Pleural biopsy will increase the diagnostic yield

d. The likelihood of sputum positivity is about 40%

e. Bronchopleural fistula is a potential complication

36. A 39-year-old woman who is receiving chronic systemic corticosteroid therapy for systemic lupus erythematosus develops fever (38°C), chills, night sweats, nausea, anorexia, and generalized headaches. She also has poorly controlled diabetes. Examination demonstrates a mildly lethargic patient with frequent coughing. Lung sounds are normal. Neurologic examination elicits mild nuchal rigidity and lethargy. Chest radiography shows a cavitated lesion in the right midlung with surrounding nodularity. Random plasma glucose is 368 mg/dL. Which one of the following steps is *inappropriate* at this time?

a. Cerebrospinal fluid analysis

b. Computed tomography of the chest

c. Bronchoscopy and bronchoalveolar lavage

d. Amphotericin B (intravenous)

e. Computed tomography of the head

37. Which one of the following "pairings" about antituberculous drugs and their associated toxicity is *incorrect*?

a. Pyrazinamide and hepatitis

b. Ethambutol and retrobulbar neuritis

c. Rifampin and peripheral neuropathy

d. Streptomycin and renal toxicity

e. Isoniazid and hepatotoxicity

38. Which one of the following "pairings" (association/complication) is *incorrect*?

a. HIV infection and pulmonary hypertension

b. HIV infection and lymphocytic interstitial pneumonitis

c. HIV infection and cystic lung disease

d. HIV infection and pneumothorax

e. CD4 count of >200/μL and disseminated *M. avium* complex infection in AIDS

39. A 28-year-old man with known HIV infection complicated by recurrent (3) episodes of *Pneumocystis carinii* pneumonia develops progressive dyspnea and lung infiltrates. The culture of diagnostic bronchoalveolar lavage effluent shows growth of *Mycobacterium avium* complex. Which one of the following drugs is *not* indicated in this patient?

a. Trimethoprim-sulfamethoxazole

b. Isoniazid

c. Clarithromycin or azithromycin

d. Rifampin

e. Ethambutol

40. A 32-year-old known to have HIV infection complains of a 6-month history of progressive dyspnea. Physical examination demonstrates a chronically ill-appearing man with signs of weight loss. Chest radiography shows bilateral hilar vascular prominence, confirmed by chest computed tomography. What is the *most likely* diagnosis?

a. Pulmonary hypertension

b. Pulmonary Kaposi sarcoma

c. Pulmonary embolism

d. Non-Hodgkin lymphoma

e. *Pneumocystis carinii* pneumonia

ANSWERS

1. Answer c.

This patient's clinical features are compatible with all the diagnoses except pulmonary fibrosis. Wheezing and normal chest radiographic findings are unlikely in pulmonary fibrosis. The antihypertensive drug most likely to cause cough is an angiotensin-converting enzyme (ACE) inhibitor; cough occurs in up to 6% of patients. Wheezing, however, is not caused or aggravated by an ACE inhibitor.

2. Answer a.

Empiric bronchodilator therapy without evaluating dysphagia is inappropriate. Her cough stopped after discontinuation of antihypertensive therapy and the wheezing and dysphagia stopped after a leiomyoma of the mid-esophagus was resected.

3. Answer e.

This patient has bronchorrhea, defined as expectoration of >100 mL/d of thin serous mucus and seen in 20% of patients with alveolar cell carcinoma.

4. Answer b.

This patient has drug-induced methemoglobinemia. This was the result of benzocaine used as a topical anesthetic. The discrepancy between PaO_2 and SaO_2 is suggestive. Other causes of cyanosis mentioned would require this patient to have had other chronic illnesses.

5. Answer d.

This patient has hypertrophic pulmonary osteoarthropathy. The most likely tumor responsible is either an adenocarcinoma or large cell carcinoma of the lung. Bronchoscopy is not appropriate until chest radiography shows an abnormality.

6. Answer a.

Gallium lung scan is of little value in the evaluation of diffuse lung disease. This patient was found to have scleroderma complicated by diffuse scleroderma lung (pulmonary fibrosis). Other tests are indicated in the evaluation of this patient.

7. Answer b.

This patient has significant muscle weakness as noted by the low MVV. Myasthenia gravis was responsible for the weakness. The anterior mediastinal mass was a thymoma; 15%-45% of thymomas are associated with myasthenia gravis and 10%-15% of patients with myasthenia gravis have thymoma.

8. Answer c.

Low DLCO is not an indication for supplemental oxygen therapy.

9. Answer d.

The CD4/CD8 ratio is reversed in this patient. This is a finding in hypersensitivity pneumonitis and in lymphocytic interstitial pneumonitis in patients with AIDS. In sarcoidosis, the CD4/CD8 ratio is high, sometimes as high as 20/1.

10. Answer e.

Leukotriene receptor antagonist therapy is aimed at preventing asthmatic attacks. It and cromolyn are not useful in reversing acute asthmatic episodes.

11. Answer e.

All the features described in this patient are typical of idiopathic interstitial pulmonary fibrosis. Diffuse lung fibrosis is distinctly uncommon in lupus. Scleroderma can mimic idiopathic pulmonary fibrosis.

12. Answer c.

Pulmonary Langerhans cell granuloma (histiocytosis X). Bone involvement occurs in 40% of patients.

13. Answer d.

Pulmonary fibrosis complicated by atypical mycobacterial infection is the least common of the choices. Other associations are well known.

14. Answer a.

Pulmonary involvement in asbestosis is almost always in the lower lung zones. Apical involvement does not occur unless the person is also exposed to coal or silica.

15. Answer e.

There is no evidence that the incidence of pulmonary embolism is increased because of sleep apnea.

16. Answer c.

Bronchiolitis obliterans with organizing pneumonia (BOOP) is a nonspecific pathologic diagnosis. Even though many diseases are known to exhibit this finding, alpha$_1$-antitrypsin deficiency does not cause BOOP.

17. Answer d.

This patient has allergic bronchopulmonary aspergillosis (ABPA) complicating his chronic asthma. Presence of *Aspergillus fumigatus* in the sputum is considered a minor criterion for the diagnosis of ABPA.

18. Answer e.

In an asymptomatic and otherwise healthy nonsmoker, it is reasonable to observe the nodule. If the nodule was >2.0 cm in diameter, surgical resection may be considered.

19. Answer b.

Drug-induced (procainamide) lupus erythematosus. Pleural fluid and serum blood tests may help support the diagnosis. Computed tomography of the chest will not provide diagnostic information.

20. Answer b.

Ultrasonographic Doppler studies are unlikely to provide useful information at this point.

21. Answer c.

In this patient with primary pulmonary hypertension, systemic corticosteroid therapy has no role.

22. Answer b.

Small cell carcinoma of the lung with myasthenic syndrome. Electromyography typically shows increasing muscle response/strength to repetitive electrical stimuli. ACTH production and syndrome of inappropriate antidiuretic hormone are also encountered in small cell carcinoma.

23. Answer c.

c-ANCA is present in other diseases such as hepatitis C virus infection, some cases of microscopic polyangiitis, ulcerative colitis, and as a manifestation of sulfasalazine toxicity.

24. Answer d.

Rheumatoid lung disease seldom causes alveolar hemorrhage syndrome.

25. Answer e.

In sickle cell anemia, *Streptococcus pneumoniae* is a major cause of morbidity and mortality in children, whereas in adults *Staphylococcus aureus* or *Haemophilus* species predominate.

26. Answer a.

Pulmonary hypertension is not a known complication of chronic renal failure or chronic hemodialysis.

27. Answer b.

More than 90% of pleural effusions complicating cirrhosis and ascites occur on the right side.

28. Answer c.

Granulomatous pneumonitis is not a complication of acute pancreatitis.

29. Answer d.

Infection of the uncomplicated pleural effusion is least likely in this patient.

30. Answer e.

The patient has unilateral diaphragmatic paralysis. Diaphragmatic fluoroscopy may help in documenting the paralysis, but 6% of normal people exhibit paradoxic motion of the diaphragm. CT of the abdomen is least likely to help.

31. Answer d.

Thoracoscopy is not indicated in the initial management of a lung abscess. If cancer is documented, then various surgical options can be considered. Laryngoscopy is indicated to exclude laryngeal paralysis, which is perhaps responsible for aspiration.

32. Answer a.

Streptococcus pneumoniae is responsible for 90% of cases of pneumonia in adults.

33. Answer c.

The clinical diagnosis is coccidioidomycosis. The skin lesion is erythema nodosum. Cavitary malignant lesions usually are thick-walled.

34. Answer e.

Human-to-human spread of nontuberculous mycobacteria has not been documented.

35. Answer b.

Pleural fluid culture is positive in only 15% of patients with documented pleural tuberculosis. Pleural biopsy is positive for caseous granulomas in up to 80% of patients and cultures in more than 75%.

36. Answer d.

This patient may have cryptococcosis, nocardiosis, tuberculosis, or another infection. Empiric therapy with amphotericin is not recommended. The final diagnosis was cryptococcosis with pulmonary and central nervous system involvement.

37. Answer c.

The most serious complication of rifampin is hepatotoxicity.

38. Answer e.

Disseminated *Mycobacterium avium* complex infection is more likely in those with CD4 counts <50/μL.

39. Answer b.

Isoniazid is not used to treat *Mycobacterium avium* complex infection.

40. Answer a.

Pulmonary hypertension is a well-known complication of HIV infection.

CHAPTER 22

RHEUMATOLOGY

Robert M. Valente, M.D.
Marc D. Cohen, M.D.

PART I

Robert M. Valente, M.D.

RHEUMATOID ARTHRITIS

Rheumatoid arthritis is a chronic systemic inflammatory disease characterized by joint destruction. It affects 0.03% to 1.5% of the population worldwide. Its incidence peaks between the ages of 35 and 45 years; however, the age-related prevalence continues to increase even after age 65. The presentation of an unknown antigen to immunologically susceptible persons is believed to trigger rheumatoid arthritis. Several viruses have been implicated in chronic arthritis, including Epstein-Barr virus, HTLV-1 virus, rubella virus, cytomegalovirus, herpes simplex virus, parvovirus, and arbovirus. Immune reactions to infection with *Borrelia*, Whipple bacillus, *Neisseria gonorrhoeae*, or *Staphylococcus* can cause characteristic arthropathies. Autoimmunity to such endogenous components as immunoglobulin, heat shock proteins, proteoglycans, and collagen is also implicated.

There is an immunogenetic predisposition to developing rheumatoid arthritis. Class II major histocompatibility complex (MHC) molecules on the surface of antigen-presenting cells are responsible for initiating cellular immune responses and for stimulating the differentiation of B lymphocytes into plasma cells that produce antibody. Most Caucasian patients with rheumatoid arthritis have class II MHC type HLA-DR4 or HLA-DR1 or both. HLA-DR4 can be divided into five subtypes, two of which independently promote susceptibility to rheumatoid arthritis. Compared with controls, patients with HLA-DR2 are less likely to have rheumatoid arthritis. Rheumatoid arthritis patients with HLA-DR3 may have low-titer rheumatoid factor and increased toxicity to gold and D-penicillamine.

- Rheumatoid arthritis affects 0.03%-1.5% of the population.
- Most Caucasian patients with rheumatoid arthritis have class II MHC type HLA-DR4 or HLA-DR1 or both.
- There is a 6x increase in concordance of rheumatoid factor-positive rheumatoid arthritis among dizygotic twins.
- There is a 30x increased risk of rheumatoid arthritis in a monozygotic twin when sibling has the disease.
- There is a 3x-5x increased risk of rheumatoid arthritis in white Americans with HLA-DR4.

Pathogenesis

The immune reaction begins in the synovial lining of the joint. The earliest pathologic changes in the disease are microvascular injury that leads to increased vascular permeability and the accumulation of inflammatory cells (CD4 lymphocytes, polymorphonuclear leukocytes, and plasma cells) in the perivascular space. Cytokines, in particular tumor necrosis factor-α (TNF-α), anaphylatoxins, and chemoattractants are released. Mediators of inflammation promote synovial angiogenesis and synovial cell proliferation, the accumulation of neutrophils in synovial fluid, and the maturation of B cells into plasma cells. Plasma cells in the joint locally synthesize rheumatoid factor and other antibodies that promote inflammation. Immune complexes activate the complement system, releasing chemotactic factors and promoting vascular permeability and opsonization. Phagocytosis releases lysosomal enzymes and fosters the digestion of collagen, cartilage matrix, and elastic tissues. The release of oxygen free radicals injures cells. Damaged cell membranes set free phospholipids that fuel the arachidonic acid cascade. The local inflammatory response becomes self-perpetuating. Proliferating synovium polarizes into a centripetally invasive pannus, destroying the weakened cartilage and subchondral bone. Chondrocytes, stimulated in the inflammatory milieu, release their own proteases and collagenases. Patients have swelling, pain, and joint stiffness with the onset of vascular injury of the synovial lining, angiogenesis, and cellular proliferation. Joint warmth, swelling, pain, and limitation of motion worsen as the synovial membrane proliferates and the inflammatory reaction builds.

- Swelling, pain, and joint stiffness occur with the onset of immune-mediated vascular injury of the synovial lining, angiogenesis, and cellular proliferation.
- Rheumatoid factor is an immunoglobulin (usually IgM) that binds other immunoglobulins (usually IgG) at their Fc components, forming immune complexes.
- Cytokines, in particular TNF-α, and immune complexes, including rheumatoid factor, are important components of the joint inflammatory reaction.

Clinical Features

The joints most commonly involved (more than 85% of patients) in rheumatoid arthritis are the metacarpophalangeal and proximal interphalangeal joints and the wrists (Fig. 22-1). The distribution of involvement is symmetrical; predominantly small joints are involved. Ultimately, the knees (80% of patients), ankles (80%), shoulders (60%), elbows (50%), hips (50%), acromioclavicular joints (50%), cervical spine (40%), and temporomandibular joints (30%) can be involved. The sternoclavicular joints, cricoarytenoid joints, and the ear ossicles are affected infrequently. Joints affected with rheumatoid arthritis are warm and swollen. The joint enlargement feels spongy and occurs with the thickening of the synovium. An associated joint effusion may make the joint feel fluctuant. Patients describe deep aching and soreness in the involved joints which are aggravated by use and can be present at rest. Prolonged morning joint stiffness and "gelling" throughout the body and recurrence of this stiffness after resting are some of the many constitutional features that complicate rheumatoid arthritis.

- The joints most commonly involved in rheumatoid arthritis are the metacarpophalangeal and proximal interphalangeal joints and the wrists (>85% of patients).
- The distribution of involvement is symmetrical.
- Hallmarks of joint inflammation: stiffness, heat, redness, soft tissue swelling, pain, and dysfunction

Constitutional Features

Fatigue initially affects up to 40% of patients. Weight loss, muscle pain, excessive sweating, or low-grade fever occurs in 20% of patients presenting with rheumatoid arthritis. Most patients with *active* arthritis have more than 1 hour of morning

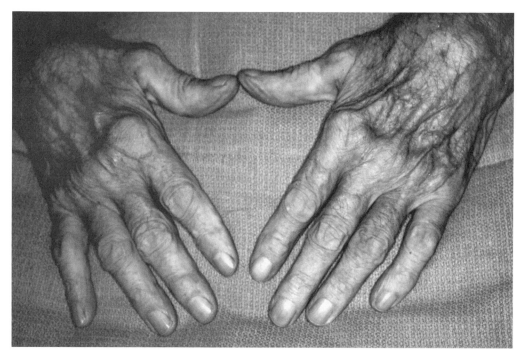

Fig. 22-1. Moderately active seropositive rheumatoid arthritis. The patient has soft-tissue swelling across the entire row of metatarsophalangeal joints and proximal interphalangeal joints bilaterally and soft tissue swelling mounding up over the wrists. Note the nearly complete lack of change at the distal interphalangeal joints.

stiffness. The musculoskeletal complications of rheumatoid arthritis are listed in Table 22-1.

Musculoskeletal Complications

Cervical Spine

One-half of all patients with rheumatoid arthritis have involvement of the cervical spine. It is diagnosed with cervical flexion and extension radiographs that demonstrate subluxation. One-half of these patients have subluxation at the atlantoaxial level, and the rest have subaxial subluxations, typically at two or more levels. The cervical instability is usually asymptomatic; however, patients may have pain and stiffness in the neck, occiput, shoulder, or interscapular areas. Patients may present with syncope, light-headedness, paresthesias of the face or limbs, or nystagmus. All patients with destructive rheumatoid arthritis should be managed with intubation precautions and the assumption that cervical instability is present. Occasionally, the first sign of cervical instability may be sudden ataxia, weakness of the limbs, or frank tetraplegia. Interference with blood flow in the vertebral arteries (vertebrobasilar insufficiency) explains some of the cranial nerve symptoms and the blackouts. New neurologic symptoms mandate urgent neurologic evaluation and consideration of surgical intervention. Indications for surgical treatment include neurologic or vascular compromise and intractable local symptoms. In active patients, prophylactic cervical spine

Table 22-1.—Musculoskeletal Complications of Rheumatoid Arthritis

---

Characteristic deformities include
  Boutonnière deformity of the finger, with hyperextension of the distal interphalangeal joint and flexion of the proximal interphalangeal joint
  Swan-neck deformity of the finger, with hyperextension at the proximal interphalangeal joint and flexion of the distal interphalangeal joint
  Ulnar deviation of the metacarpophalangeal joints; it can progress to complete volar subluxation of the proximal phalanx from the metacarpophalangeal head
  Compression of the carpal bones and radial deviation at the carpus
  Subluxation at the wrist
  Valgus of the ankle and hindfoot
  Pes planus
  Forefoot varus and hallux valgus
  Cock-up toes from subluxation at the metatarsophalangeal joints

---

stabilization is recommended when there is evidence of extreme (>8 mm) subluxation of C1 over C2. The probability of cervical involvement is predicted by the severity of peripheral arthritis.

- One-half of all patients with rheumatoid arthritis have involvement of the cervical spine.
- Patients with cervical spine involvement may present with syncope, light-headedness, paresthesias of face and limbs, nystagmus, ataxia, or acute myelopathy.
- Indications for surgical treatment: neurologic or vascular compromise and intractable local symptoms.
- The probability of cervical involvement is predicted by the severity of peripheral arthritis.

Popliteal Cyst

Flexion of the knee markedly increases the intra-articular pressure of a swollen joint. This pressure produces an outpouching of the posterior components of the joint space that is termed a "popliteal" or a "baker's" cyst. Ultrasonographic examination of the popliteal space can be diagnostic. A popliteal cyst should be distinguished from a popliteal artery aneurysm, lymphadenopathy, phlebitis and (more rarely) a benign or malignant tumor. The cyst can rupture down into the calf or, rarely, superiorly into the posterior thigh. Rupture of the popliteal cyst with dissection into the calf may resemble acute thrombophlebitis and is called "pseudophlebitis." Fever, leukocytosis, and ecchymosis around the ankle (crescent sign) can occur with the rupture. Treatment of an acute cyst rupture includes bed rest, elevation of the leg, ice massage or cryocompression, and an intra-articular injection of corticosteroid. Treatment of the popliteal cyst requires improvement in the knee arthritis.

- Popliteal cyst is also called "baker's" cyst.
- Rupture of a popliteal cyst may resemble acute thrombophlebitis ("pseudophlebitis").
- Ultrasonography can distinguish a cyst from a popliteal artery aneurysm, lymphadenopathy, phlebitis, and tumor.

Tenosynovitis

Tenosynovitis of the finger flexor and extensor tendon sheaths is common. It presents with diffuse swelling between the joints or a palpable grating within the flexor tendon sheaths in the palm with passive movement of the digit. Other tenosynovial syndromes in rheumatoid arthritis include de Quervain and wrist tenosynovitis. Persistent inflammation can produce stenosing tenosynovitis, loss of function, and, ultimately, rupture of tendons. Treatment of acute tenosynovitis includes immobilization, warm soaks, nonsteroidal anti-inflammatory drugs (NSAIDs), and local injections of corticosteroid in the tendon sheath.

- Tenosynovitis of the finger flexor and extensor tendon sheaths is common and can lead to tendon rupture.

Carpal Tunnel Syndrome

Rheumatoid arthritis is the second most common cause of carpal tunnel syndrome (pregnancy is the commonest cause). This syndrome is associated with paresthesias of the hand in a typical median nerve distribution. Discomfort may radiate up the forearm or into the upper arm. The symptoms worsen with prolonged flexion of the wrist and at night. Late complications include thenar muscle weakness and atrophy and permanent sensory loss. Other nerve entrapment syndromes, including tarsal tunnel syndrome, affect patients with rheumatoid arthritis. Treatment includes resting splints, control of inflammation, and local injection of glucocorticosteroids. Surgical release is recommended for persistent symptoms.

- Rheumatoid arthritis is the second most common cause of carpal tunnel syndrome.
- Carpal tunnel syndrome: paresthesias of the hand in a typical median nerve distribution.
- Other nerve entrapment syndromes, including tarsal tunnel syndrome, affect patients with rheumatoid arthritis.

Extra-Articular Complications of Rheumatoid Arthritis

Extra-articular complications occur almost exclusively in rheumatoid arthritis patients who have high titers of rheumatoid factor. In general, the number and severity of the extra-articular features vary with the duration and severity of disease.

Rheumatoid Nodules

From 20% to 35% of patients have rheumatoid nodules, which occur over extensor surfaces and at pressure points. They also occur in the lungs, heart, kidney, and dura mater. The nodules have characteristic histopathologic features. A central area of necrosis encircled by palisading fibroblasts is surrounded by a collagenous capsule and a perivascular collection of chronic inflammatory cells. Breakdown of the skin over rheumatoid nodules, with ulcers and infection, can be a major source of morbidity. The infection can spread to local bursae, infect bone, or spread hematogenously to joints.

- Extra-articular complications in rheumatoid arthritis occur almost exclusively in arthritis patients with positive rheumatoid factor.
- 20%-35% of patients have rheumatoid nodules.
- Rheumatoid nodules occur over extensor surfaces and at pressure points and are prone to ulceration and infection.

Rheumatoid Vasculitis

Rheumatoid vasculitis usually occurs in patients who have severe deforming arthritis and a high titer of rheumatoid factor. The vasculitis is mediated by the deposition of circulating immune complexes on the blood vessel wall, with or without activation of complement. At its most benign, it occurs as rheumatoid nodules, with small infarcts over the nodules and at the cuticles. Proliferation of the vascular intima and media causes this obliterative endarteropathy, which has little associated inflammation. It is best managed by controlling the underlying arthritis. Leukocytoclastic or small vessel vasculitis produces palpable purpura or cutaneous ulceration, particularly over the malleoli of the lower extremities. This vasculitis can cause pyoderma gangrenosum or peripheral sensory neuropathy. Secondary polyarteritis, which is clinically and histopathologically identical to polyarteritis nodosa, results in mononeuritis multiplex. Occasionally, the vasculitis appears after the joint disease appears "burned out." Glucocorticosteroid treatment does not promote rheumatoid vasculitis.

- Rheumatoid vasculitis usually occurs in patients who have severe deforming arthritis and a high titer of rheumatoid factor.
- Rheumatoid vasculitis is mediated by the deposition of circulating immune complexes on the blood vessel wall.
- Rheumatoid vasculitis comprises a spectrum of vascular disease, including rheumatoid nodules and obliterative endarteropathy, leukocytoclastic or small vessel vasculitis, and secondary polyarteritis (systemic necrotizing vasculitis).

Neurologic Manifestations

Neurologic manifestations of rheumatoid arthritis include mild peripheral sensory neuropathy. Sensory-motor neuropathy (mononeuropathy) suggests vasculitis or nerve entrapment (e.g., carpal tunnel syndrome). Cervical vertebral subluxation can cause myelopathy. Erosive changes may promote basilar invagination of the odontoid process of C2 into the underside of the brain, causing spinal cord compression and death.

Pulmonary Manifestations

The most common form of lung disease in patients with rheumatoid arthritis is mild obstructive pulmonary dysfunction. The prevalence of obstructive change increases with the duration of the disease. It is associated with keratoconjunctivitis sicca. Pleural disease has been noted in 40% of autopsies of cases of rheumatoid arthritis. Clinically significant pleural disease is less frequent. Characteristically, rheumatoid pleural effusions are asymptomatic until they become large enough to interfere mechanically with respiration. The pleural fluid is an exudate. The concentration of glucose in the pleural fluid is low (10-50 mg/dL) because of impaired transport of glucose into the pleural space. The pleural effusion in rheumatoid arthritis has a mononuclear cell predominance and usually fewer than 5,000 cells/μL. Pulmonary nodules appear singly or in clusters. Single nodules have the appearance of a coin lesion. Nodules typically are pleural-based and may cavitate and create a bronchopleural fistula. Pneumoconiosis complicating rheumatoid lung disease, or Caplan syndrome, results in a violent fibroblastic reaction and large nodules. Acute interstitial pneumonitis is a rare complication that may begin as alveolitis and progress to respiratory insufficiency and death. Interstitial fibrosis is a chronic slowly progressive process. It has physical findings of diffuse dry crackles on lung auscultation and a reticular nodular radiographic pattern affecting both lung fields, initially in the lung bases. A decrease in the diffusing capacity of the lung for carbon dioxide and a restrictive pattern on pulmonary function testing complicate symptomatic interstitial fibrosis. Interstitial changes are highly associated with smoking. Bronchiolitis obliterans with or without organizing pneumonia may occur with rheumatoid arthritis or its treatment. It produces an obstructive picture on pulmonary function testing and typically responds to corticosteroid treatment. High-resolution computed tomography (CT) is useful in distinguishing these different interstitial rheumatoid lung syndromes and predicting treatment response. Methotrexate treatment causes a lung reaction in 1% to 3% of treated rheumatoid arthritis patients. It can present insidiously with a dry cough or with life-threatening pneumonitis.

- Obstructive airway disease is found in 35% of patients with rheumatoid arthritis.
- Rheumatoid pleural disease is common but symptomatic. The pleural fluid is remarkable for low levels of glucose.
- Rheumatoid lung nodules are pleural-based and can cause a bronchopleural fistula.
- High-resolution CT distinguishes among rheumatoid-associated interstitial lung diseases, including interstitial pneumonitis, interstitial fibrosis, and bronchiolitis obliterans with or without organizing pneumonia.

Cardiac Complications

Pericarditis has been noted in 50% of autopsies of cases of rheumatoid arthritis. Rheumatoid nodules can occur in the pericardium. However, patients rarely present with pericardial symptoms. Effusive pericarditis uncommonly produces cardiac tamponade. Recurrent effusive pericarditis without symptoms occasionally evolves to chronic constrictive pericarditis. Untreated constrictive pericarditis has a 70% 1-year mortality. Rheumatoid arthritis carditis includes conduction abnormalities in the myocardium. Valve dysfunction and coronary vasculitis have also been described.

Granulomatous inflammation can spread to involve the base of the aorta.

- Patients rarely present with pericardial symptoms despite frequent serous pericarditis.
- Untreated constrictive pericarditis has a 70% 1-year mortality.
- Rheumatoid carditis includes conduction and valve abnormalities. Granulomatous rheumatoid inflammation can spread to the aortic root.

Liver Abnormalities

Patients with rheumatoid arthritis can have increased levels of liver enzymes, particularly alkaline phosphatase. Increased levels of aspartate aminotransferase, γ-glutamyltransferase, and acute-phase proteins and decreased levels of albumin also occur in active rheumatoid arthritis. Liver biopsy shows nonspecific changes of inflammation or nodular regenerative hyperplasia, which may cause portal hypertension and hypersplenism. Many medications used to treat rheumatoid arthritis increase liver enzyme levels.

- Increased levels of liver enzymes, particularly alkaline phosphatase, may occur in rheumatoid arthritis.
- Nodular hyperplasia of the liver can complicate rheumatoid arthritis and lead to portal hypertension and hypersplenism.
- Many medications used to treat rheumatoid arthritis increase the levels of liver enzymes.

Ophthalmic Abnormalities

Keratoconjunctivitis sicca, or secondary Sjögren syndrome, is the most common ophthalmic complication in rheumatoid arthritis. Episcleritis and scleritis also occur independently of the joint inflammation and are usually treated topically. Severe scleritis progressing to scleromalacia perforans causes blindness. Infrequent ocular complications of rheumatoid arthritis include episcleral nodules, palsy of the superior oblique muscle caused by tenosynovitis of its tendon sheath (Brown syndrome), and uveitis. Retinopathy is an infrequent complication of antimalarial drug treatment.

- Keratoconjunctivitis sicca, or secondary Sjögren syndrome, is the most common ophthalmic complication in rheumatoid arthritis.
- Severe scleritis progressing to scleromalacia perforans causes blindness.

Laboratory Findings

Nonspecific alterations in many laboratory values are common in patients with rheumatoid arthritis. Normocytic anemia (hemoglobin in the range of 10 g/dL), leukocytosis, thrombocytosis, hypoalbuminemia, and hypergammaglobu-linemia are common. Rheumatoid factor (IgM) occurs in 90% of patients, but its presence may not be detected for months to years after the initial joint symptoms are noted. Rheumatoid factor is a marker of immune stimulation and occurs in various connective tissue diseases and infections, including subacute bacterial endocarditis and lymphoprolifera-tive disorders. Diseases in bold type in Table 22-2 are most likely to have high titers of rheumatoid factor. Five percent of the normal population have a low titer of rheumatoid factor. Cryoglobulins and antinuclear antibodies are common. Eosinophilia occurs in up to 30% of patients with rheumatoid arthritis. It may be a marker for toxicity due to gold treatment or it may accompany rheumatoid vasculitis. C-reactive protein correlates with disease activity, but it is not more helpful than the erythrocyte sedimentation rate. Rheumatoid arthritis patients with active disease have low iron-binding capacity, low plasma levels of iron, and low erythropoietin levels, unless they are iron deficient.

Table 22-2.—Diseases That May Have Positive Rheumatoid Factor[*]

Rheumatoid arthritis
Sjögren syndrome
Systemic lupus erythematosus
Scleroderma
Sarcoidosis
Idiopathic pulmonary fibrosis
Mixed cryoglobulinemia
Hypergammaglobulinemic purpura
Asbestosis
Malignancies
Infectious mononucleosis
Influenza
Chronic active hepatitis
Vaccinations
Tuberculosis
Syphilis
Subacute bacterial endocarditis
Brucellosis
Leprosy
Salmonellosis
Malaria
Kala-azar
Schistosomiasis
Filariasis
Trypanosomiasis

---

[*]Diseases in boldface type are the most likely to have high-titer rheumatoid factor.

- Normocytic anemia and leukocytosis are common in rheumatoid arthritis.
- Rheumatoid factor is neither specific nor sensitive for the diagnosis of rheumatoid arthritis.
- Cryoglobulins and antinuclear antibodies are common in patients with seropositive rheumatoid arthritis.
- Eosinophilia may be a marker for rheumatoid vasculitis or toxicity due to gold treatment.
- C-reactive protein correlates with disease activity, but it is not more helpful than the erythrocyte sedimentation rate.

Synovial fluid is cloudy and light yellow, with poor viscosity, and typically contains 10,000 to 75,000 leukocytes/μL (60%-75% polymorphonuclear neutrophils). Synovial fluid levels of glucose are low. Microscopic crystals are absent. Ragocytes, phagocytic cells with intercellular immunoglobulin and cholesterol crystals, may be found.

Radiographic Findings

The radiographic findings in early rheumatoid arthritis are normal or show soft tissue swelling. Later, the characteristic changes of periarticular osteoporosis, symmetrical narrowing of the joint space, and marginal bony erosions become obvious. Radiographic changes at end-stage rheumatoid arthritis include subluxation and other deformities, joint destruction, fibrous ankylosis, and, rarely, bony ankylosis (Fig. 22-2).

- The characteristic radiologic changes in rheumatoid arthritis include periarticular osteoporosis, symmetrical narrowing of the joint space, and bony erosions of the joint margin.

Diagnosis of Rheumatoid Arthritis

To make the diagnosis of rheumatoid arthritis, symptoms must be present for more than 6 weeks in persons 16 years old or older. Four of the seven criteria of the American Rheumatism Association listed in Table 22-3 must be satisfied for the diagnosis to be made.

Natural History

More than one-half of patients with rheumatoid arthritis have insidious onset of the joint disease, occurring over weeks to months. However, in one-third of the patients, the onset is rapid, occurring in days or weeks. Early in the course of the disease, most patients have oligoarthritis. Their disease becomes polyarticular with time. From 10% to 20% of patients have relentlessly progressive arthritis. The course may be slow, fluctuating, or rapid, but the end point is the same: dis-abling, destructive arthritis. Seventy percent of the patients have polycyclic disease, with repeated flares interrupted by partial or complete remissions. Spontaneous remissions in the polycyclic or progressive group almost never occur after

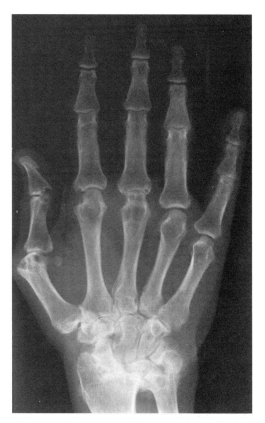

Fig. 22-2. Radiographic features of long-standing rheumatoid arthritis. Periarticular osteoporosis is marked by decreased cortical margins and reduction in trabecular textures in the periarticular areas. There is symmetrical narrowing of the joint space at the proximal interphalangeal joints and second and third metacarpophalangeal joints. Marginal erosions are best seen at the thumb interphalangeal and metacarpophalangeal joints and at the second and third metacarpophalangeal joints. Additional destructive changes have nearly obliterated the usual margins of the carpal bones, making it difficult to distinguish them individually.

Table 22-3.—American Rheumatism Association Criteria for Making the Diagnosis of Rheumatoid Arthritis[*]

One or more hours of morning stiffness in and around the joints

Arthritis of three or more joint areas involved simultaneously

Arthritis of at least one area in the wrist, metacarpophalangeal, or proximal interphalangeal joints

Symmetrical arthritis involving the same joint areas on both sides of the body

Rheumatoid nodules

Serum rheumatoid factor

Radiographic changes typical of rheumatoid arthritis, including periarticular osteoporosis, joint-space narrowing, and marginal erosions.

[*]1987 revision.

2 years of disease. Patients who meet the 1987 American Rheumatism Association modified criteria for rheumatoid arthritis, including wrist and metacarpophalangeal involvement, are at higher risk for progressive rheumatoid arthritis. Most of the disability is determined in the first several years of disease. The relationship between disease duration and inability to work is nearly linear. After 15 years of rheumatoid arthritis, 15% of patients are completely disabled. The life span of men and women with rheumatoid arthritis is decreased by 7.5 years and 3.5 years, respectively, in comparison with their normal counterparts. Mortality is predicted by age, disease severity, comorbid cardiovascular disease, and functional status. Mortality is also influenced by educational level and socioeconomic factors.

- In one-third of patients, the onset of rheumatoid arthritis is rapid (days or weeks).
- 70%-90% of patients have progressive arthritis.
- The relationship between disease duration and inability to work is nearly linear.
- With rheumatoid arthritis, life span is decreased by 7.5 years for men and 3.5 years for women.

Treatment of Rheumatoid Arthritis

The management of patients with rheumatoid arthritis requires making the correct diagnosis, determining the functional status of the patient, and selecting goals of management with the patient. Goals of management include relieving inflammation and pain and maintaining function. To anticipate or to attempt to achieve complete symptomatic relief in every patient is an unrealistic and impossible goal.

The principles emphasized by physical medicine include bed rest or rest periods, improving nonrestorative sleep, and joint protection (including modification of activities of daily life, range of motion exercises, orthotics, and splints, if they help the pain). Exercise should begin with range of motion and stretching to overcome contracture. Strengthening and conditioning exercises should be prescribed carefully, depending on the activity of the patient's disease.

Initial treatment is with an NSAID given at anti-inflammatory doses. If the response is inadequate after 3 or 4 weeks, a trial of a second nonchemically related NSAID is used. Glucocorticoids may be necessary to preserve function. Disease-modifying agents of rheumatic disease (DMARD) are also known as "second-line agents," "slow-acting antirheumatic drugs," or "remittive agents." Short-term studies with DMARD confirm improved quality of life. Traditionally, they have been used sequentially, although recent studies have shown an enhanced benefit with combination DMARD treatments that include methotrexate. The classic indications for adding disease-modifying, or second-line, agents include the correct diagnosis, failure of disease to respond to an NSAID, and as glucocorticoid-sparing agents. Six months of uninterrupted treatment with a disease-modifying agent is usually required to assess its efficacy. They augment the response to concomitantly used NSAIDs or corticosteroids given in low doses. Disease-modifying agents include the following:

- Methotrexate
- Hydroxychloroquine
- Penicillamine
- Sulfasalazine
- Intramuscular injections of gold salts
- Leflunomide
- Azathioprine
- Cyclophosphamide

Patients receiving one of these disease-modifying agents will take it, on average, for 3 to 5 years before the lack of efficacy or toxicity forces discontinuation of its use. A second disease-modifying regimen is substituted for the first one when a therapeutic or toxic roadblock is reached. No response to one DMARD does not predict a negative response or intolerance to the others. Evidence supporting the pivotal proinflammatory role of tumor necrosis factor alpha (TNF-α) in rheumatoid arthritis has been exploited clinically with the development of several effective TNF-α antagonists. One agent, soluble TNF receptor (p75) fused to the Fc portion of the human IgG immunoglobulin molecule (etanercept), has been approved for use in rheumatoid arthritis. It is an extremely effective and expensive anti-inflammatory treatment. (For information on individual drug indications and adverse effects, see the section on antirheumatic drugs at the end of Part I.)

- To anticipate or to attempt to achieve complete symptomatic relief in every patient is an unrealistic and impossible goal.
- Goals of management include relieving inflammation and pain and maintaining function.
- A disease-modifying regimen is added when symptoms are inadequately controlled with NSAIDs, to reduce dependence on glucocorticoids, and when disease activity justifies the risk of the drugs.
- Glucocorticosteroids may be necessary to preserve function.
- Disease-modifying agents: 6 months of uninterrupted treatment is usually required to assess efficacy.

Surgery in the Treatment of Rheumatoid Arthritis

Orthopedic surgery for resistant rheumatoid arthritis remains the most significant therapeutic option for preserving or enhancing patient function. Synovectomy of the wrist and nearby tendon sheaths is beneficial when medication alone fails to control the synovitis. The operation preserves joint function and prevents the lysis of extensor tendons that can result in a loss of function. Synovectomy of the knee, either open or through an arthroscope, can delay the progression of rheumatoid arthritis from 6 months to 3 years. Removal of nodules and treatment for local nerve entrapment syndromes are also important surgical treatments for rheumatoid arthritis. Arthroplasty is reserved for patients in whom medical management has failed and in whom intractable pain or compromise in function developed because of a destroyed joint. Arthroplasty, arthrodesis (wrist), and synovectomy are important components of well-balanced rheumatology treatment programs. Total joint arthroplasty has a slightly poorer long-term outcome in patients with rheumatoid arthritis than in those with osteoarthritis. Nevertheless, joint replacement surgery has had a major effect on patient disability.

- Orthopedic surgery is the most significant advance in the treatment of medically resistant rheumatoid arthritis.
- Total joint arthroplasty has a slightly poorer long-term outcome in patients with rheumatoid arthritis than in those with osteoarthritis.

CONDITIONS RELATED TO RHEUMATOID ARTHRITIS

Seronegative Rheumatoid Arthritis

Rheumatoid factor-negative (seronegative) rheumatoid arthritis is not associated with extra-articular manifestations. However, the arthritis usually is destructive, deforming, and otherwise indistinguishable from seropositive rheumatoid arthritis.

- Seronegative rheumatoid arthritis is not associated with extra-articular manifestations.

Seronegative Rheumatoid Arthritis of the Elderly

A subgroup of patients older than 60 years with seronegative rheumatoid arthritis may have milder arthritis. This subgroup suddenly develops polyarticular inflammation that is controlled best with low doses of prednisone. Minimal destructive changes and deformity occur. An additional group of elderly seronegative arthritis patients (men in their 70s) present with acute polyarthritis and pitting edema of the hands and feet. They have a prompt and gratifying response to low doses of prednisone.

- Patients >60 years who suddenly develop rheumatoid factor-negative polyarticular arthritis are best controlled initially with low doses of prednisone.

Adult Still Disease

Systemic *juvenile* rheumatoid arthritis is known as "Still disease." It has quotidian (fever spike with return to normal all in 1 day) high-spiking fevers, arthralgia, arthritis, seronegativity (negative rheumatoid factor and antinuclear antibody), leukocytosis, macular evanescent rash, serositis, lymphadenopathy, splenomegaly, and hepatomegaly. Fever, rash, and arthritis are the classic triad of Still disease.

Adult Still disease has a slight female predominance. Its onset commonly occurs between ages 16 and 35. Temperature greater than 39°C occurs in a quotidian or double quotidian pattern in 96% of the patients. The rash has a typical appearance: a macular salmon-colored eruption on the trunk and extremities. The transient rash is usually noticed at the time of increased temperature. Arthritis occurs in 95% of these patients, and in about one-third, the joint disease is progressive and destructive. Adult Still disease has a predilection for the wrist, shoulders, hips, and knees. Sixty percent of patients complain of sore throat, which can confuse the diagnosis with rheumatic fever. Weight loss is common. Lymphadenopathy occurs in two-thirds of the patients and hepatosplenomegaly in about one-half. Pleurisy, pneumonitis, and abdominal pain occur in fewer than one-third of the patients.

Treatment of adult Still disease includes high doses of aspirin or indomethacin. Corticosteroids may be needed to control the systemic symptoms. Half of the patients require methotrexate to control the systemic and articular features.

- Adult Still disease: classic triad of fever, rash, and arthritis.
- Rheumatoid factor and antinuclear antibodies are absent.
- There is a predilection for the wrist, shoulders, hips, and knees.
- 60% of patients complain of sore throat.

Felty Syndrome

Felty syndrome has the classic triad of rheumatoid arthritis, leukopenia, and splenomegaly. (Classic Felty syndrome usually occurs after 12 years or more of rheumatoid arthritis.) It occurs in fewer than 1% of patients with rheumatoid arthritis. Splenomegaly either may not be clinically apparent or may be manifested only after the arthritis and leukopenia have been present for some time. Other features of Felty syndrome are listed in Table 22-4. Patients with this syndrome frequently have bacterial infections, particularly of the skin and lungs. Infection related to the cytopenia is the major cause of mortality. High titers of rheumatoid factor are the rule, and a positive antinuclear antibody occurs in two-thirds of the patients. Hypocomplementemia often occurs with active vasculitis. Rarely, the hematologic abnormalities in Felty syndrome remit spontaneously. Shortened erythrocyte survival related to the splenomegaly aggravates inflammatory-block anemia. In 40%

Table 22-4.—Features of Felty Syndrome

Classic triad
Nodular, erosive polyarthritis
Leukopenia
Splenomegaly
Other features
Recurrent fevers with and without infection
Weight loss
Lymphadenopathy
Skin hyperpigmentation
Lower extremity ulcers
Vasculitis
Neuropathy
Keratoconjunctivitis sicca
Xerostomia
Other cytopenias

of patients, thrombocytopenia is caused by splenic sequestration. The leukocyte count typically is less than 3,500/μL. An absolute neutropenia occurs with granulocyte counts between 500 and 1,000/μL. Bone marrow studies usually document myeloid hyperplasia, with an excess of immature granulocyte precursors suggesting maturation arrest. The marrow is rarely hypocellular. Patients often die of sepsis despite vigorous antibacterial treatment.

Treatment can include corticosteroids, gold, methotrexate, lithium, granulocyte colony-stimulating factor, and splenectomy. There is considerable variability in the response to therapy. The increase in leukocytes seen with granulocyte colony-stimulating factor occasionally is accompanied by a flare in arthritis and vasculitis. The hematopoietic factors should be limited for use in patients with Felty syndrome who have repeated infections. Life-threatening infection or a life-threatening hemolytic anemia, despite treatment with hematopoietic factors, is an indication for splenectomy. Felty syndrome must be distinguished from a neoplastic disorder, large granular lymphocytosis, and nodular regenerative hyperplasia of the liver with portal hypertension and hypersplenism.

- Felty syndrome occurs in <1% of patients with rheumatoid arthritis.
- Felty syndrome has the classic triad of rheumatoid arthritis, leukopenia, and splenomegaly.
- High titers of rheumatoid factor are the rule.
- Patients with Felty syndrome frequently die of infection.

Sjögren Syndrome

Sjögren syndrome has a triad of clinical features: keratoconjunctivitis sicca (with or without lacrimal gland enlargement), xerostomia (with or without salivary gland enlargement), and connective tissue disease (usually rheumatoid arthritis). Idiopathic Sjögren syndrome is diagnosed predominantly in middle-aged women. Histologically, it is characterized by CD4 lymphocytic infiltration and destruction of lacrimal salivary glands. Clinically, it is manifested by dry eyes, dry mouth, and a waxing and waning polyarthritis. Additional features of primary Sjögren syndrome are listed in Table 22-5. Most patients with Sjögren syndrome have a polyclonal hypergammaglobulinemia. Autoantibodies typically are present, including rheumatoid factor, antinuclear antibodies, and antibodies to extractable nuclear antigens (SS-A and SS-B).

Patients can present with primary Sjögren syndrome without any additional connective tissue disease. The primary syndrome typically has an episodic and nondeforming arthritis. More commonly, rheumatoid arthritis, systemic lupus erythematosus, scleroderma, polyarteritis nodosa, or polymyositis accompanies Sjögren syndrome. There is no perfect definition for Sjögren syndrome, and no test is completely diagnostic. Simple dry eyes of the elderly must be distinguished from Sjögren syndrome. Patients with Sjögren syndrome have an increased risk of developing non-Hodgkin lymphoma.

Treatment of primary Sjögren syndrome is mainly symptomatic. Pilocarpine, 5 mg orally four times daily, improves salivary and lacrimal gland function in the majority of patients. Side effects, including flushing and sweating, limit its usefulness. In addition to hydration, systemic therapy is indicated if there is evidence of systemic inflammation. A Sjögren-like syndrome has been described in patients with human immunodeficiency virus (HIV) infection.

Table 22-5.—Features of Sjögren Syndrome

Classic triad
Arthritis: typically episodic polyarthritis
Dry eyes
Dry mouth (and other dry mucous membranes)
Other features
Constitutional features: fatigue, malaise, myalgia
Raynaud phenomenon
Cutaneous vasculitis
CNS abnormalities
Cerebritis, CNS vasculitis
Stroke
Multiple sclerosis-like illness
Peripheral neuropathy
Sensory
Autonomic
Interstitial lung disease
Pleurisy

CNS, central nervous system.

- Classic triad in Sjögren syndrome: dry eyes, dry mouth, and a connective tissue disorder (usually rheumatoid arthritis).
- Sjögren syndrome can exist by itself or with another formal connective tissue disease such as rheumatoid arthritis, systemic lupus erythematosus, scleroderma, or myositis.
- Treatment focuses on control of inflammation and symptoms of dryness.
- A Sjögren-like syndrome has been described in patients with HIV infection.

OSTEOARTHRITIS

Osteoarthritis is the failure of articular cartilage and subsequent degenerative changes in subchondral bone, bony joint margins, synovium, and para-articular fibrous and muscular structures. Osteoarthritis is the most common rheumatic disease; 80% of patients have some limitation of their activities, and 25% are unable to perform major activities of daily living. More than 10% of the population older than 60 years have osteoarthritis. Annually, half a million new patients develop symptomatic hip or knee osteoarthritis.

- Osteoarthritis is the most common rheumatic disease.
- More than 10% of the population older than 60 years have osteoarthritis.

Pathogenesis of Osteoarthritis

Two principal changes associated with osteoarthritis are the progressive focal degeneration of articular cartilage and the formation of new bone in the floor of the cartilage lesion at the joint margins (osteophytes). Not all the mechanisms causing osteoarthritis have been identified. Current theories include 1) mechanical process: cartilage injury, particularly after impact loading, and 2) biochemical process: failure of cartilage repair processes to adequately compensate for injury. A combination of mechanical and biochemical processes likely contribute in most cases of osteoarthritis. It must be emphasized that osteoarthritis is not just the consequence of "wear and tear."

- Osteoarthritis: progressive focal degeneration of articular cartilage, with subsequent degeneration of surrounding soft tissues and proliferation (osteophytosis) of bone.
- Osteoarthritis is not the consequence of normal use ("wear and tear").

Clinical Features of Osteoarthritis

The pain of an osteoarthritic joint is usually described as a deep ache. The pain occurs with use of the joint and is relieved with rest and cessation of weight bearing. As the disease progresses, the involved joint may be symptomatic with minimal activity or even at rest. The pain originates in the structures around the disintegrating cartilage (there are no nerves in cartilage). There may be stiffness in the joint with initial use, but this initial stiffness is not prolonged as it is in inflammatory arthritis, such as rheumatoid arthritis. Although the symptoms are related predominately to mechanical failure and motion limits, joint debris and the associated repair process promote mild inflammation, accumulation of synovial fluid, and mild hypertrophy of the synovial membrane. Acute inflammation can transiently occur at Heberden nodes (distal interphalangeal joints with prominent osteophytes as a consequence of osteoarthritis) or at the knee with tearing of a degenerative meniscal cartilage.

● Osteoarthritic pain is usually described as a deep ache with joint use, improved with rest.
● The stiffness with initial use of the joint is not prolonged in osteoarthritis as it is in inflammatory arthritis (rheumatoid arthritis).

Physical examination documents joint margin tenderness, fine crepitance, limits to motion, and enlargement of the joint. The enlargement is usually bony (proliferation of cartilage and bone to form osteophytes), but it can include effusions and mild synovial thickening. Deformity is a late consequence of the osteoarthritis and is associated with atrophy or derangement of the local soft tissues, ligaments, and muscles.

Radiographic or physical examination evidence of osteoarthritis severity does not reliably predict the patient's symptoms.

Clinical Subsets of Osteoarthritis

Primary Osteoarthritis

Primary osteoarthritis is cartilage failure without a known cause that would predispose to osteoarthritis. It almost never affects the shoulders, metacarpophalangeal joints, or ulnar side of the wrist. It is divided into several clinical patterns, as described below.

1. *Generalized osteoarthritis* involves the distal interphalangeal joints, proximal interphalangeal joints, first carpometacarpal joints, hips, knees, and spine (Fig. 22-3). It occurs most frequently in middle-aged postmenopausal women. Many of the patients have joint hypermobility. Mucous cysts are gelatinous cysts that form on the dorsolateral or dorsomedial aspect of the distal interphalangeal joints in osteoarthritis. Fluid aspirated from these cysts contains hyaluronic acid. A mucous cyst communicates with the distal interphalangeal joint space and can regress spontaneously or rupture. Joint sepsis can occur after cyst rupture. Surgical removal usually requires removal of the associated osteophyte; otherwise, the mucous cyst will recur.

2. *Isolated nodal osteoarthritis* is primary osteoarthritis that affects only the distal interphalangeal joints. It occurs predominantly in women and has a familial predisposition.

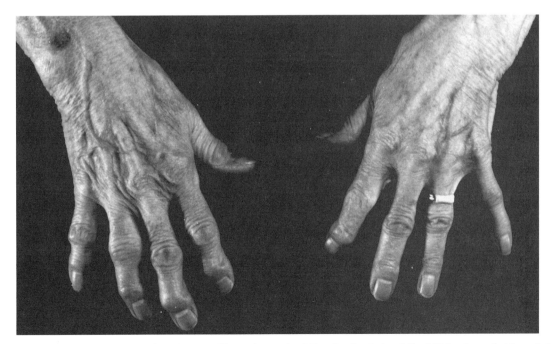

Fig. 22-3. Generalized osteoarthritis. Note prominent bony swelling at the proximal (Bouchard nodes) and distal (Heberden nodes) interphalangeal joints. The metacarpophalangeal joints are spared. Early hypertrophic changes are seen on profile at the first carpometacarpal joint, given a slight squaring of the hand deformity appreciated best on the left.

3. *Isolated hip osteoarthritis* is more common in men than in women. It has no clear association with obesity or activity.

4. *Erosive osteoarthritis* affects only the distal and proximal interphalangeal joints. Patients with erosive osteoarthritis have episodes of local inflammation. Mucous cyst formation is common. Painful flare-up of the disease recurs for years. Symptoms usually begin about the time of menopause. Bony erosions and collapse of the subchondral plate—features not usually seen in primary osteoarthritis—with osteophytes are markers of erosive osteoarthritis. Joint deformity can be severe. In many cases, bony ankylosis develops. Ankylosis is usually associated with relief of pain. The synovium is intensely infiltrated with mononuclear cells. This condition may be confused with rheumatoid arthritis. Up to 15% of the patients may later develop more classic features of rheumatoid arthritis.

5. *Diffuse idiopathic skeletal hyperostosis* is a variant of primary osteoarthritis. It occurs chiefly in men older than 50 years. It is also known as "Forestier disease," "ankylosing hyperostosis of the spine," "spondylitis ossificans ligamentosa," and "spondylosis hyperostotica." The diagnosis requires finding characteristic, exuberant, flowing osteophytosis that connects four or more vertebrae, with preservation of the disk space. Diffuse idiopathic skeletal hyperostosis must be distinguished from typical osteoarthritis of the spine with degenerative disk disease and from ankylosing spondylitis. Extraspinal sites of disease involvement include calcification of the pelvic ligaments, exuberant osteophytosis at the site of peripheral osteoarthritis, well-calcified bony spurs at the calcaneus, and heterotopic bone formation after total joint arthroplasty. Patients with diffuse idiopathic skeletal hyperostosis are often obese, and 60% have diabetes mellitus or glucose intolerance. Symptoms include mild back stiffness and, occasionally, back pain. Pathologically and radiologically, diffuse idiopathic skeletal hyperostosis is distinct from other forms of primary osteoarthritis.

- Primary osteoarthritis almost never affects the shoulders, metacarpophalangeal joints, or the ulnar side of the wrist.
- Generalized osteoarthritis involves the distal interphalangeal joints, proximal interphalangeal joints, first carpometacarpal joints, hips, knees, and spine.
- Isolated nodal osteoarthritis is primary osteoarthritis affecting only distal interphalangeal joints.
- Isolated hip osteoarthritis is more common in men than in women.
- Erosive osteoarthritis affects only the distal and proximal interphalangeal joints.
- Diffuse idiopathic skeletal hyperostosis is a variant of primary osteoarthritis.

Secondary Osteoarthritis

Secondary osteoarthritis is cartilage failure caused by some known disorder, trauma, or abnormality. Any patient with an unusual distribution of osteoarthritis or widespread chondrocalcinosis should be considered to have secondary osteoarthritis. Secondary osteoarthritis frequently complicates trauma and the damage caused by inflammatory arthritis. Inherited disorders of connective tissue, and several metabolic abnormalities, including ochronosis, hemochromatosis, Wilson disease, and acromegaly, are complicated by secondary osteoarthritis. Paget disease of bone, involving the femur or pelvis about the hip joint, can predispose to osteoarthritis.

- Osteoarthritis involving the shoulder, metacarpophalangeal joints, isolated large joints, or with chondrocalcinosis should prompt physicians to consider secondary causes of osteoarthritis.

Trauma. Trauma or injury to a joint and supporting periarticular tissues predisposes persons to the most common type of secondary osteoarthritis. Stress from repeated impact loading can weaken subchondral bone. Internal joint derangement with ligamentous laxity or meniscal damage alters the normal mechanical alignment of the joint. Isolated large joint involvement is a clue to post-traumatic osteoarthritis. Chronic rotator cuff tear with subsequent loss of shoulder joint cartilage (cuff arthropathy) and knee osteoarthritis that develops years after meniscal cartilage damage are examples of secondary osteoarthritis.

Congenital malformations of joints. Congenital hip dysplasia and epiphyseal dysplasia lead to premature osteoarthritis. Other developmental abnormalities, including slipped capital femoral epiphysis and Legg-Calvé-Perthes disease (idiopathic avascular necrosis of the femoral head), may first present as premature osteoarthritis years after they occur. Inherited disorders of connective tissue frequently predispose the afflicted person to premature osteoarthritis. Table 22-6 describes several inherited disorders, including their gene defects and characteristics.

- Injury to a joint or supporting periarticular tissues can predispose to osteoarthritis.
- Post-traumatic osteoarthritis is the most common form of secondary osteoarthritis.
- Isolated large joint involvement is a clue to post-traumatic osteoarthritis.

Alkaptonuria/ochronosis. This is a rare autosomal recessive disorder of tyrosine metabolism. Deficiency of the enzyme homogentisic acid oxidase leads to excretion of large amounts of homogentisic acid in the urine. Black, oxidized, polymerized

Table 22-6.—Inherited Disorders of Connective Tissue

Condition	Gene defect	Characteristics
Marfan syndrome (autosomal dominant)	Fibrillin gene	Hypermobile joints: osteoarthritis, arachnodactyly, kyphoscoliosis Lax skin, striae, ectopic ocular lens Aortic root dilatation (aortic insufficiency), mitral valve prolapse, aneurysms, and aortic dissection
Ehlers-Danlos syndrome (10 subtypes)	Type I and type III collagen gene defects	Joint hypermobility, friable skin, osteoarthritis Type III collagen defects associated with vascular aneurysms
Osteogenesis imperfecta (autosomal dominant and recessive variations; the most common heritable disorder of connective tissue: 1:20,000; 4 subtypes)	Type I collagen gene defects	Brittle bones, blue sclera, otosclerosis and deafness, joint hypermobility, and tooth malformation
Type II collagenopathies: Achondrogenesis type II Hypochondrogenesis Spondyloepiphyseal dysplasia Spondyloepimetaphyseal dysplasia Kniest dysplasia Stickler syndrome Familial precocious osteoarthropathy	Type II collagen gene defects	Spectrum from lethal (achondrogenesis) to premature osteoarthritis (Stickler syndrome)
Achondroplasia (autosomal dominant)	Fibroblast growth factor III receptor gene defect	Dwarfism, premature osteoarthritis
Pseudoachondroplasia Multiple epiphyseal dysplasia (autosomal dominant)	Cartilage oligomeric matrix protein (COMP) gene defect	Short stature, premature osteoarthritis

homogentisic acid pigment collects in connective tissues ("ochronosis"). The diagnosis may go unrecognized until middle life. The first manifestation can be secondary osteoarthritis. The patient's urine darkens when allowed to stand or with the addition of NaOH. Ochronotic arthritis affects the large joints (e.g., the hips, knees, and shoulders) and is associated with calcium pyrophosphate crystals in the synovial fluid. The radiographic finding of calcified intervertebral disks at multiple levels is characteristic of ochronosis. Other manifestations include grayish brown scleral pigment and generalized darkening of the ear pinnae.

- Alkaptonuria/ochronosis is a rare autosomal recessive disorder of tyrosine metabolism.
- Ochronosis: black, oxidized, polymerized homogentisic acid pigment collects in connective tissues.

- Ochronotic arthritis affects the large joints: the hips, knees, and shoulders.

Hemochromatosis. Hemochromatosis was formerly considered an unusual autosomal recessive disorder of white males. It is now considered the commonest inherited disease known. One in 10 Americans are heterozygous for the defective gene, *HLA-H*—a histocompatibility pseudogene—and carriers for the disease. One in 200 to 250 have the disease (1.5 million Americans), and prevalence rates are similar among blacks, hispanics, and women. The consequence of inheriting both copies of the flawed gene is influenced by diet and blood loss. One-third of the world's population still suffers from iron deficiency. The inheritance of one copy of the defective gene (*HLA-H*) would confer a hedge against nutritional deficiency, and the trait may be maintained through natural selection.

The full clinical spectrum of hemochromatosis includes hepatomegaly, bronze skin pigmentation, diabetes mellitus, the consequences of pituitary insufficiency, and degenerative arthritis. The arthropathy affects up to 50% of patients with hemochromatosis and generally resembles osteoarthritis; however, it involves the metacarpophalangeal joints and shoulders, joints not typically affected by generalized primary osteoarthritis. Attacks of acute pseudogout arthritis may occur in relation to deposition of calcium pyrophosphate dihydrate crystals. Chondrocalcinosis is commonly superimposed on chronic osteoarthritic change in hemochromatosis. The pathogenesis of joint degeneration in hemochromatosis is not clear. Screening for hemochromatosis should include the following: patients with a positive family history, new adult-onset diabetes mellitus, cardiomyopathy, hepatitis, impotence, osteoarthritis (particularly if the metacarpophalangeal joints or the shoulders are affected), or chondrocalcinosis. Serum iron saturation greater than 60% supports the diagnosis, which is confirmed by a quantitative iron determination in liver biopsy tissue. A genetic test is commercially available, is better than 90% sensitive, is quite expensive, and is not suitable for screening. Treatment for the arthritis is symptomatic; the underlying iron accumulation is also treated. Serum levels of ferritin are used to monitor treatment.

- Arthropathy affects up to 50% of patients with hemochromatosis.
- It involves the metacarpophalangeal joints and shoulders.

Wilson disease. Arthropathy occurs in 50% of adults with Wilson disease, a rare autosomal recessive disorder. This disease is suspected in anyone younger than 40 years with unexplained hepatitis, cirrhosis, or movement disorder. The diagnosis is suggested when the serum level of ceruloplasmin is less than 200 mg/L. Arthropathy is unusual in children with the disease. The radiologic appearance varies somewhat from that of primary osteoarthritis. There are more subchondral cysts, sclerosis, cortical irregularities, and radiodense lesions, which occur centrally and at the joint margins. Focal areas of bone fragmentation occur, but they are not related to neuropathy. Although chondrocalcinosis occurs, calcium pyrophosphate dihydrate crystals have not been observed in the synovial fluid.

- Arthropathy occurs in 50% of adults with Wilson disease.
- Arthropathy is unusual in children.

Apatite microcrystals. They are associated with degenerative arthritis and are found in patients with hypothyroidism, hyperparathyroidism, and acromegaly. They occur without an associated endocrinopathy. The role of microcrystalline disease in the progression of osteoarthritis is not clear, especially in the absence of acute recurrent flares of pseudogout.

Neuroarthropathy (Charcot joint). Neuroarthropathy commonly affects patients with diabetes mellitus. Men and women are equally affected. Patients with diabetic neuroarthropathy have had diabetes an average of 16 years. Frequently, the diabetes is poorly controlled. Diabetic peripheral neuropathy causes blunted pain perception and poor proprioception. Repeated microtrauma, overt trauma, small vessel occlusive disease (diabetes), and neuropathic dystrophic effects on bone contribute to neuroarthropathy. Patients can present with an acute arthritic condition that includes swelling, erythema, and warmth. The foot, particularly the tarsometatarsal joint, is involved most commonly in diabetics. Patients usually describe some milder pain than the condition would suggest, and they walk with an antalgic limp. Callus formation occurs over the weight-bearing site of bony damage, and the callus subsequently blisters and ulcerates. Infection can spread from skin ulcers to the bone. Osteomyelitis frequently complicates diabetic neuroarthropathy. Radiography shows disorganized normal joint architecture. Bone and cartilage fragments later coalesce to form characteristic sclerotic loose bodies. There is an attempt at reconstruction with new bone formation. This periosteal new bone is inhibited by small vessel ischemic change in some diabetics. Diabetic osteopathy is a second form of neuroarthropathy. Osteopenia of para-articular areas, particularly the distal metacarpals and proximal phalanges, results in rapidly progressive osteolysis and juxta-articular cortical defects. This can be associated with osteomyelitis. Initial treatment in diabetics includes good local foot care, treatment of infection, and protected weight bearing. Involvement of the knee, lumbar spine, and upper extremity is uncommon in diabetics. Classically, hip and spinal neuroarthropathy is caused by tertiary syphilis, and shoulder neuroarthropathy is associated with cervical syringomyelia.

- Neuroarthropathy (Charcot joints) most commonly affects the feet and ankles of patients with diabetes mellitus.
- Neuroarthropathy is a consequence of peripheral neuropathy and local injury.
- Osteomyelitis is caused by skin ulcers extending to the bone and should be suspected when an affected diabetic has sudden worsening of his or her glucose control.

Aseptic necrosis of the bone. Aseptic necrosis of the bone, also known as "avascular necrosis of bone," may lead to collapse of the articular surface and subsequent osteoarthritis. It usually is seen in the hip after femoral neck fracture. Systemic corticosteroid therapy increases the risk of aseptic necrosis. Aseptic necrosis of the bone has other causes, including alcoholism, sickle cell disease, and systemic lupus erythematosus

(Table 22-7). No underlying cause can be identified in 10% to 25% of patients. Aseptic necrosis of bone usually affects the hips, shoulders, knees, or ankles. Treatment is conservative, including reduced weight bearing and analgesics. Some investigators have treated patients successfully with vascularized bone grafts in the bed of necrotic trabecular bone, although controlled studies are not available. Core decompression may help with pain but does not influence progression to gonarthrosis. When there is evidence of cortical bone collapse, progression to advanced osteoarthritis is inevitable. The most sensitive test for aseptic necrosis is magnetic resonance imaging (MRI). Bone scans are positive in the affected bones that are symptomatic but may miss early asymptomatic disease. This is important because over time nontraumatic aseptic necrosis of the femoral head may occur bilaterally in up to 80% of patients, with one side becoming symptomatic long before the other side. Plain radiographs are insensitive to early aseptic necrosis.

- Aseptic necrosis usually is seen in the hip after femoral neck fracture and may lead to osteoarthritis.

Hypertrophic osteoarthropathy. Hypertrophic osteoarthropathy is characterized by clubbing of the fingernails and painful distal long bone periostitis. The patient may have a noninflammatory arthritis at the ankles, knees, or wrists. This condition complicates primary and metastatic pulmonary malignancies, chronic pulmonary infections, cystic fibrosis, and hypoxic congenital heart disease. Treatment is usually symptomatic.

Hemophilic arthropathy. Patients with hemophilia and recurrent hemarthroses are at risk for hemophilic arthropathy, a type of progressive degenerative arthropathy that is more destructive than primary osteoarthritis. Widening of the intercondylar notch of the knees is an early radiographic feature suggesting the diagnosis of this condition.

Table 22-7.—Pneumonic Device for Remembering Causes of Aseptic Necrosis of Bone

A	Alcohol, atherosclerotic vascular disease
S	Steroids, sickle cell anemia, storage disease (Gaucher disease)
E	Emboli (fat, cholesterol)
P	Postradiation necrosis
T	Trauma
I	Idiopathic
C	Connective tissue disease (especially SLE), caisson disease

SLE, systemic lupus erythematosus.

Radiographic Features of Osteoarthritis

The radiographic features of osteoarthritis do not always predict the amount of symptoms. Common radiographic features include osteophyte formation, asymmetrical joint-space narrowing, subchondral bony sclerosis, subchondral cysts, and buttressing of angle joints. Later bony changes include malalignment and deformity (Fig. 22-4). In the spine, the radiographic finding called "spondylosis" includes anterolateral spinous osteophytes, degenerative disk disease with disk-space narrowing, and facet sclerosis. A defect in the bony structure of the posterior neural arch produces spondylolysis. With bilateral spondylolysis, subluxation of one vertebra on another may occur, a condition called "spondylolisthesis." The causes of spondylolisthesis are trauma, osteoarthritis, and congenital. No laboratory studies of blood are useful in the diagnosis of osteoarthritis.

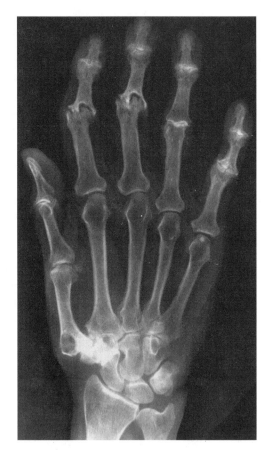

Fig. 22-4. Severe osteoarthritis. Hypertrophic changes, asymmetrical joint-space narrowing, and subchondral sclerosis are prominent at the interphalangeal joints and at the first carpometacarpal joint. Note that the metacarpophalangeal joints are completely spared, distinguishing this arthritis from rheumatoid arthritis. Also, there is joint-space narrowing and sclerosis at the base of the thumb at the first carpometacarpal joint and between the trapezium and the scaphoid. Osteoarthritis does not affect equally the entire wrist compartment. The involvement seen here is the most common. An additional interesting feature seen here is central erosions at the second and third proximal interphalangeal joints. This variant occasionally has been called "erosive osteoarthritis."

- Common radiographic features include: osteophyte formation, asymmetrical joint-space narrowing, subchondral bony sclerosis, subchondral cysts, and buttressing of angle joints.
- No laboratory studies of blood are useful in the diagnosis of osteoarthritis.

Therapy for Osteoarthritis

Therapeutic goals include relieving pain, preserving joint motion and function, and preventing further injury and wear of cartilage. Weight loss (important in knee osteoarthritis), use of canes or crutches, correction of postural abnormalities, and proper shoe support are helpful measures. Isometric or isotonic range of motion exercises and muscle strengthening provide para-articular structures with extra support and help reduce symptoms. Relief of muscle spasm with local application of heat or cold to decrease pain can help.

Initial drug therapy should be analgesics, such as acetaminophen (1 g four times daily as needed). NSAIDs are beneficial for inflammatory flares of osteoarthritis and usually do not need to be taken in anti-inflammatory doses every day. The imminent release of NSAIDs with specificity for inhibition of the COX-2 enzyme may increase the usefulness of this class of drugs for the treatment of osteoarthritis by increasing the ratio of benefit to toxic side effect. Tramadol is a unique centrally acting analgesic with weak opiate and antidepressant activities and little or no potential for addiction. Tramadol or other mild traditional narcotic analgesics frequently are better tolerated than currently available NSAIDs, particularly in the elderly population. Although the over-the-counter treatments glucosamine and chondroitin have not been shown to have cartilage-sparing effects, they relieve pain in some patients with symptomatic osteoarthritis. Rarely, depot corticosteroids offer some temporary relief. Injections of hyaluronic acid into the knee joint provide 3 to 12 months of improvement in symptomatic osteoarthritis in selected patients.

Joint arthroplasty may relieve pain, stabilize joints, and improve function. Total joint arthroplasty is very successful at the knee or hip. Table 22-8 describes the indications for total joint arthroplasty in patients with radiographically advanced osteoarthritis. Surgical treatment for osteoarthritis of the shoulder is usually reserved for patients with intractable pain. The functional outcome in total shoulder arthroplasty is less predictable. Tibial osteotomy redistributes knee-joint forces. Arthroscopy removes loose bodies and trims torn menisci to correct lockup or give way of the joint. Herniated disks or spinal stenosis may require decompression.

- Simple analgesics such as acetaminophen are the first choice for treating osteoarthritis.

Table 22-8.—Indications for Total Joint Arthroplasty

Radiographically advanced osteoarthritis
Night pain that cannot be modified by changing position
Lockup or give way of the weight-bearing joint associated with falls or near falls
Joint symptoms compromise activities of daily living

ARTHRITIS IN CHRONIC RENAL FAILURE

Up to 75% of patients undergoing chronic renal dialysis have musculoskeletal complaints after 4 years of dialysis. Renal failure arthritis affects the interphalangeal joints, metacarpophalangeal joints, wrists, shoulders, and knees. Symmetrical joint-space narrowing and para-articular osteoporosis, subchondral cysts, and erosions have been described. There is no osteophytosis to confuse this condition with osteoarthritis. The synovial fluid is noninflammatory, and the synovitis on biopsy is nonspecific. Possible causes of this arthritis include apatite microcrystal deposition, hyperparathyroidism, and renal failure amyloidosis. Aseptic necrosis occasionally affects large joints.

After 10 years of hemodialysis, 65% of patients have pathologic or radiologic evidence of amyloid deposition (renal failure amyloid arthropathy). The amyloid is composed of β_2-microglobulin, is arthrotropic, and results in complete joint-space loss that occurs over a 3- to 12-month period. Shoulder pain and stiffness syndrome and carpal tunnel syndrome are strongly related to this amyloid deposition. Currently, treatment is aimed at relieving the symptoms.

- Up to 75% of patients undergoing chronic renal dialysis develop musculoskeletal complaints after 4 years of dialysis.
- Destructive arthritis, shoulder pain, stiffness syndrome, and carpal tunnel syndrome are strongly related to amyloid deposition.

NONARTICULAR RHEUMATISM

Fibromyalgia

Fibromyalgia is a uniform syndrome characterized by chronic diffuse musculoskeletal pain. Other names for this condition are "fibrositis," "tension myalgias," "generalized nonarticular rheumatism," "psychogenic rheumatism," and "benign myalgic encephalomyelitis." For the diagnosis, the pain should be present for at least 3 months and should involve areas on both sides of the body above and below the waist and some part of the axial skeleton. Symptoms should not be explainable on the basis of other coexisting diseases or

conditions. A high tender point count is an additional obligatory criterion for classification of fibromyalgia. Fibromyalgia affects 2% to 10% of all populations studied and 15% of all general medical patients seen by internists; 75% to 95% of all the patients are women. It is unusual for the diagnosis to be made in a person younger than 12 years or for a first episode to occur after age 65. Of the patients (or their parents), 60% recall childhood growing pains or leg pains. Fibromyalgia is the second most common reason (after the common cold) for lost work days.

- Fibromyalgia: chronic diffuse musculoskeletal pain.
- Fibromyalgia affects 2%-10% of all populations studied; 75%-95% of patients are women.

Symptoms

The patients typically describe pain all over the body and use qualitatively different descriptions of the pain and discomfort than used by patients with rheumatoid arthritis. Patients localize the pain poorly, referring it to muscle attachment sites or muscles. The discomfort is worse in the morning and can be associated with stiffness. Physical activity or changes in the weather typically aggravate the symptoms. Most patients describe nonrestorative, nonrestful sleep. Anxiety is common. Active depression is not seen more commonly in these patients than in the general population. Patient complaints can include subjective joint swelling, hand and joint pain, prolonged morning stiffness, Raynaud-like vasospasm, and dry eyes. Headaches, paresthesias, numbness, and pseudosciatica-like pains are also common. About one-third of the patients have visceral symptoms, including urinary urgency, severe pelvic pain unexplainable as dysmenorrhea or endometriosis, and irritable bowel syndrome. The onset of fibromyalgia occurs after an acute illness, typically a viral syndrome, in more than half of the patients. In some patients, symptoms develop after trauma, such as injury on the job or motor vehicle accidents.

- Patients with fibromyalgia typically describe pain all over the body.
- Physical activity or weather changes typically aggravate the symptoms.
- Raynaud-like vasospasm, dry eyes, headaches, paresthesias, numbness, and pseudosciatica-like pains are common.
- The onset of fibromyalgia occurs after an acute illness, typically a viral syndrome, in more than half the patients.

Diagnosis

A detailed history and physical examination will exclude most inflammatory and neurologic diseases. The finding of painful points at muscle attachment sites supports the diagnosis of fibromyalgia. Laboratory evaluation includes performing a complete blood count, erythrocyte sedimentation rate, and thyroid function studies and determining levels of electrolytes, creatinine, calcium, and phosphorus. In selected cases, creatine kinase values and pelvic and spine radiographic findings are helpful in excluding other diseases. No diagnostic test confirms the diagnosis of fibromyalgia. Muscle biopsies, electromyographic and sleep studies, and MRI are not necessary for the diagnosis.

- The finding of painful points at muscle attachment sites supports the diagnosis of fibromyalgia.
- No laboratory test confirms the diagnosis of fibromyalgia.

Natural History

Fibromyalgia is a chronic waxing and waning problem. Patients have periods of pain and dysfunction alternating with variable periods of feeling reasonably well. Over a period of years, a patient's symptoms and concerns can shift considerably from musculoskeletal concerns to fatigue to headaches or to irritable bowel. There is no increased physical disability in patients who have had fibromyalgia for longer periods of time in comparison with those for whom the diagnosis is recent. Treatment includes reassurance and education, ensuring an adequate night's sleep, establishing a cardiovascular fitness program, and better flexibility and posture. NSAIDs have a slight synergistic effect with sedating medications. Chronic pain management techniques may be helpful for patients with impaired life skills.

- There is no progressive physical disability.

Low Back Pain

One-third of all people older than 50 years have episodes of acute low back pain. Chronic low back pain is the number one compensable work-related injury. The many causes of low back pain include mechanical, neurologic, inflammatory, infectious, neoplastic, and metabolic causes and referred pain from the viscera. Only 3% of patients presenting with acute low back pain have an organic cause not apparent after the initial interview and physical examination. More than 90% find relief on their own or with the help of a medical practitioner within the first 6 weeks after symptoms occur.

- Only 3% of patients presenting with acute low back pain have an organic cause not apparent after the initial interview and physical examination.

Diagnosis

The most important consideration during the initial evaluation of acute low back pain is the possibility of severe compromise of the spinal cord or cauda equina. In the absence of evidence for acute spinal cord compromise, spinal infection, or neoplastic involvement, immediate pursuit of a cause for the acute back pain is not appropriate. Objective leg weakness or bladder and bowel dysfunction is an indication for more extensive physical examination, consideration of urgent lumbar myelography, and possible surgical decompression. Significant weight loss or pain that increases with recumbency suggests a neoplastic or infectious process. Pain that worsens with coughing, straining, or sneezing suggests irritation of the dura mater. Radiating pain, weakness, or numbness in an extremity implicates irritation of a spinal nerve root. Exertional calf or thigh cramping but normal peripheral pulses suggests pseudoclaudication or symptomatic lumbar stenosis. Pseudoclaudication symptoms improve with leaning over a cart or with sitting (not standing still). Referred pain from an abdominal, pelvic, or hip area suggests an extra-axial cause. An insidious onset with prominent morning stiffness suggests an inflammatory axial arthropathy.

- Objective leg weakness or bladder or bowel dysfunction is an indication for more extensive examination.
- Significant weight loss or pain that interferes with sleep suggests a neoplastic or infectious process.
- Exertional calf or thigh cramping but normal peripheral pulses suggests pseudoclaudication.
- An insidious onset with prominent morning stiffness suggests an inflammatory axial arthropathy.

In the absence of specific historical or physical examination findings, laboratory or plain radiographic findings would not suggest malignancy, infection, systemic illness, or neurologic compromise. The radiographic findings of spondylosis, single disk degeneration, facet osteoarthritis, transitional lumbosacral segments, Schmorl nodes, spina bifida occulta, mild scoliosis, and increased lumbosacral angle are not relevant to a patient's complaints of acute back pain. The use of bone scans, electromyography, CT, or MRI is not necessary to evaluate routine acute low back pain. The indications for spinal radiography in patients with acute low back pain are listed in Table 22-9.

Treatment

The treatment of acute nonspecific low back pain begins with reassuring the patient, because 90% of all patients with acute low back pain have significant improvement in 6 weeks. Temporary modification of activities by empowering the patient to temporarily adjust lifestyle and demands works best. Bed rest should never be prescribed for more than 3 days to treat acute nonspecific low back pain. Short-term use of narcotic analgesics or tramadol can supplement the use of acetaminophen, NSAIDs, and muscle relaxants such as cyclobenzaprine.

Physical therapy measures include local heat and ice massage. Pelvic traction and transcutaneous electrical nerve stimulation (TENS) add little to the management of acute nonspecific low back pain. Epidural glucocorticosteroid injections are best suited to acute disk herniation, although their role is controversial. Injections into the facets are helpful occasionally, particularly if the patient describes a locking or catching as part of the pain syndrome.

- In 90% of patients, acute low back pain (local or sciatic presentations) remits within 4-6 weeks.
- Clinical suspicion of acute spinal cord compromise, spinal infection, or neoplasm requires immediate evaluation and prompt therapy.
- Pelvic traction and TENS add little to the management of acute nonspecific low back pain.

Bursitis

A bursa is a closed sac containing a small amount of synovial fluid and lined with a membrane similar to that surrounding a diarthrodial joint. Bursae are present in the areas where tendons and muscles move over bony prominences. Additional bursae form in response to irritative stimuli. Trauma or overuse, microcrystalline disease, chronic inflammatory arthritis, and infection cause bursitis. Treatment of aseptic bursitis involves strict immobilization, ice compresses, NSAIDs, bursal aspiration, corticosteroid injections, and, occasionally, physical therapy. Glucocorticosteroids should not be given if there is clinical suggestion of sepsis.

- Always consider infection or microcrystalline disease in the differential diagnosis of acute bursitis.

Septic bursitis may result from puncture wounds or cellulitis or occur after a local injection. Half of the time, there is no portal of entry for infection in septic superficial bursitis

Table 22-9.—Indications for Spinal Radiography in Patients With Acute Low Back Pain

First episode of acute back pain is after age 50
History of back disease
History of back surgery
History of neoplasm
Acute history of direct trauma to the back
Fever
Weight loss
Severe pain unrelieved in any position
Neurologic symptoms or signs

(olecranon and prepatellar bursae). The organisms frequently responsible for infection are staphylococci (*aureus* and *epidermidis*) and streptococci. Patients with septic superficial bursitis present with localized pain and swelling. Warmth about the area of the superficial bursa should raise the possibility of a septic bursa. If there is doubt, the bursa should be aspirated with strict aseptic technique. The needle should enter from the side through uninvolved skin—not at the point of maximal fluctuance—to avoid creating a chronic draining fistula. When infection is suspected, patients should be treated empirically with antistaphylococcal and antistreptococcal oral antibiotics, pending the microbiologic results. Gram stains are positive in only 40% to 60% of patients. The number of leukocytes in infected bursal fluid can be low compared with that in infected joint fluid. This may be due to the modest blood supply of the bursae compared with that of joints. Patients with more severe infections or with associated cellulitis frequently do not respond to outpatient management. They should be hospitalized and given antibiotics intravenously, and the affected part should be immobilized for 3 or 4 days. Repeated aspirations or percutaneous suction drainage may be necessary until the fluid stops accumulating. In chronic cases refractory to antibiotics, bursectomy is indicated.

- Septic bursitis frequently occurs without evidence of a portal of entry.
- Bursal warmth is the best predictor of infection.
- Gram stains are positive in only 40%-60% of patients.
- The number of leukocytes in infected bursal fluid can be low.
- Patients with more severe infections should be hospitalized.

Polymyalgia Rheumatica

Polymyalgia rheumatica is a clinical syndrome usually characterized by the sudden onset of aching and morning stiffness in the proximal musculature. The definition includes an increased erythrocyte sedimentation rate. Results of rheumatologic studies, including rheumatoid factor, antinuclear antibody, and complement levels, are negative or normal. In 1% to 3% of cases, patients can present with a normal erythrocyte sedimentation rate. The presence of other specific diseases such as rheumatoid arthritis, chronic infection, inflammatory myositis, or malignancy excludes the diagnosis of polymyalgia rheumatica. Some definitions of polymyalgia rheumatica require a rapid response to small doses of prednisone (10 to 15 mg daily). This condition is more common in whites and has a moderate female predominance. It almost never occurs in persons younger than 50 years. It is endemic in the population older than 50 years, with as many as 50 new cases annually per 100,000 population.

- Polymyalgia rheumatica: sudden onset of aching and morning stiffness in the proximal musculature and increased erythrocyte sedimentation rate.
- Negative rheumatoid factor, antinuclear antibody, and complement levels.
- The presence of other specific diseases excludes the diagnosis of polymyalgia rheumatica.
- It almost never occurs in persons <50 years old.

Features and Differential Diagnosis

Patients with polymyalgia rheumatica complain of stiffness more than pain. This stiffness is most prominent in the mornings and after prolonged sitting. They occasionally have mild constitutional symptoms, including sweats, fevers, anorexia, and weight loss. Prominent constitutional features or age older than 70 years should suggest associated giant cell arteritis. Extremity edema or oligoarticular synovitis can occur, particularly at the knees, wrists, and shoulders. Radionuclide joint scans in patients with active polymyalgia rheumatica confirm hip and shoulder synovitis. Polyarticular small joint arthritis is not a feature. Polymyalgia rheumatica patients without vasculitis may have granulomatous myocarditis and hepatitis. Muscles from these patients show normal tissue or mild type II muscle fiber atrophy. Table 22-10 summarizes the rheumatic syndromes and other diseases that occasionally present with a polymyalgia rheumatica-like syndrome. Depression must be considered in patients with atypical features. Clinical evaluation and screening laboratory tests usually distinguish polymyalgia rheumatica from these other conditions.

- Polymyalgia rheumatica: stiffness is more prolonged in the mornings and after prolonged sitting.
- Prominent constitutional features or age older than 70 years should suggest associated giant cell arteritis.
- Extremity edema or oligoarticular synovitis can occur.

Table 22-10.—Systemic Illnesses Presenting With a Polymyalgia-Like Syndrome

Rheumatic syndromes	Other systemic illnesses
Systemic vasculitis	Paraneoplastic syndromes
Myositis	Systemic amyloidosis
Systemic lupus erythematosus	Infectious endocarditis
Seronegative rheumatoid arthritis	Hyperthyroidism
Polyarticular osteoarthritis	Hypothyroidism
Fibromyalgia	Hyperparathyroidism
Remitting seronegative, symmetric synovitis and peripheral edema	Osteomalacia
	Depression

Pathogenesis and Relationship to Giant Cell Arteritis

The pathogenesis of polymyalgia rheumatica is unknown. Clinicians appreciate the close relationship between giant cell arteritis and polymyalgia rheumatica. Familial aggregation and increased incidence in patients of northern European background suggest a genetic predisposition. HLA-DR4 is associated with these conditions more commonly than would be expected by chance. Of patients with giant cell arteritis, 40% have symptoms of polymyalgia rheumatica during the course of their disease.

- Up to 15% of patients with polymyalgia rheumatica also have giant cell arteritis.
- 40% of patients with active giant cell arteritis have symptoms of polymyalgia rheumatica.
- Polymyalgia rheumatica can begin before, appear simultaneously with, or develop after the symptoms of giant cell arteritis.

Treatment

All patients with polymyalgia rheumatica should respond completely after 3 to 5 days of treatment with prednisone, 10 to 20 mg/day. After giant cell arteritis has been excluded, most patients can be managed initially with prednisone doses of 15 mg/day or less. Follow the patients clinically and, when necessary, determine the erythrocyte sedimentation rate to confirm the clinical suspicion of a disease flare. Polymyalgia rheumatica is thought to be a self-limited disease, although relapses occur. Prednisone treatment is discontinued in more than half the patients within 2 years.

- All patients should respond completely after 3-5 days of treatment with prednisone.
- Polymyalgia rheumatica is thought to be a self-limited disease although relapses occur.

VASCULITIC SYNDROMES

Introduction

Vasculitis, or angiitis, is an inflammatory disease of blood vessels. It often causes damage to the vessel wall and stenosis or occlusion of the vessel lumen by thrombosis and progressive intimal proliferation of the vessel. Vasculitic symptoms reflect the nonspecific systemic features of inflammation (constitutional features) and the ischemic consequences of vascular occlusion. The distribution of the vascular lesions and the size of the blood vessels involved vary considerably in different vasculitic syndromes and in different patients with the same syndrome. Vasculitis can be transient, chronic, self-limited, or progressive. It can be the primary abnormality or secondary to another systemic process. Histopathologic classification does not distinguish local from systemic illness or secondary from primary insult. The key clinical features suggestive of vasculitis are listed in Table 22-11. Vasculitis "look-alikes," or simulators, are listed in Table 22-12. These diseases and conditions should be considered whenever the patient's condition suggests vasculitis. A scheme for diagnosing vasculitis is outlined in Table 22-13. The ability to recognize characteristic clinical patterns of involvement is very helpful in making the diagnosis of systemic necrotizing vasculitis (Fig. 22-5).

- Vasculitic symptoms reflect the nonspecific systemic features of inflammation (constitutional features) and the ischemic consequences of vascular occlusion.

Specific Vasculitic Syndromes

Giant Cell Arteritis

Giant cell arteritis, also known as "temporal arteritis," predominantly affects persons older than 50 years. The prevalence exceeds 223 cases per 100,000 persons older than 50. It is most common in persons of northern European ancestry.

Table 22-11.—Clinical Features That Suggest Vasculitis

Constitutional features
  Fatigue, fever, weight loss, and anorexia
Skin lesions
  Palpable purpura, necrotic ulcers, livedo reticularis, urticaria, nodules, and digital infarcts
Arthralgia or arthritis
Myalgia or prominent fibrositis
  Polymyalgia rheumatica symptoms
Claudication or phlebitis
Headache
Cerebrovascular accident
Neuropathy
  Mononeuritis multiplex
Hypertension
Abnormal renal sediment
Pulmonary abnormalities
  Pulmonary hemorrhage, pulmonary nodules with cavities
Abdominal pain or intestinal hemorrhage
Nonspecific indicators of inflammation
  Anemia, thrombocytosis, low levels of albumin, elevated erythrocyte sedimentation rate, increased levels of liver enzymes, or eosinophilia

Table 22-12.—Syndromes That Mimic Vasculitis

Cardiac myxoma with embolization
Infective endocarditis
Thrombotic thrombocytopenic purpura
Atheroembolism: cholesterol or calcium emboli
Ergotism
Pseudoxanthoma elasticum
Ehlers-Danlos type 4
Neurovasculopathy secondary to antiphospholipid syndrome
Arterial coarctation or dysplasia
Infectious angiitis
    Lyme disease
    Rickettsial infection
    HIV infection

HIV, human immunodeficiency virus.

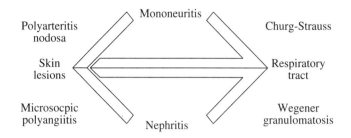

Fig. 22-5. Common organ involvement in systemic vasculitis.

Females outnumber males by 3:1. Polymyalgia rheumatica symptoms may develop in 40% to 50% of all patients with giant cell arteritis. Up to 15% of patients with polymyalgia rheumatica have temporal artery biopsy findings positive for giant cell arteritis. There is considerable morbidity with this disease; however, the rate of blindness is declining. The mortality rate for patients with giant cell arteritis is similar to that for the general population.

- Giant cell arteritis: most common in persons of northern European ancestry.
- Polymyalgia rheumatica develops in 40% of patients with giant cell arteritis.
- 15% of patients with polymyalgia rheumatica have temporal artery biopsies positive for giant cell arteritis.

Table 22-13.—The Diagnostic Approach to Vasculitis

Proper clinical suspicion for vasculitis[*]
Consider conditions that mimic vasculitis
Recognize clinical pattern of involvement
Define the extent and severity of disease
Narrow the diagnostic possibilities with laboratory tests
Select the confirmatory study
    Efficient (highest yield study)
    Safe as possible
Weigh urgency of diagnosis with risk of
    Diagnostics
    Therapeutics

[*]Table 22-11.

Pathology—Giant cell arteritis involves the primary and secondary branches of the aorta in a segmental or patchy fashion. However, any artery, and occasionally veins, can be affected. It is unusual for intracranial arteries to be involved. Histopathologically, all layers of the vessel wall are extensively disrupted, with intimal thickening and a prominent mononuclear and histiocytic infiltrate. Multinucleated giant cells infiltrate the vessel wall in 50% of cases. Fragmentation and disintegration of the internal elastic membrane, the other characteristic feature, is closely associated with the accumulation of giant cells and vascular occlusive symptoms.

- Giant cell arteritis affects primary and secondary branches of the aorta in a segmental or patchy fashion.

Clinical features—Early clinical features of giant cell arteritis include temporal headache, polymyalgia rheumatica symptoms, fatigue, and fever. The classic features of this disease are included in Table 22-14. Arteritis of the branches of the ophthalmic or posterior ciliary arteries causes ischemia of the optic nerve (ischemic optic neuritis) and blindness. Less often, retinal arterioles are occluded. Blindness occurs in fewer than 15% of untreated patients. Large peripheral artery involvement in giant cell arteritis occurs in about 10% of patients. Extremity claudication, Raynaud phenomenon, aortic dissection, decreased pulses, and vascular bruits suggest large peripheral artery involvement. Patients with large peripheral artery involvement do not differ from those with more classic giant cell arteritis, either histologically or with regard to laboratory findings. Late features include a markedly increased risk of thoracic aortic aneurysm.

- Early clinical features: temporal headache, polymyalgia rheumatica symptoms, fatigue, and fever.
- Blindness occurs in <15% of untreated patients.

Diagnosis—Positive temporal artery biopsy findings make a search for occult malignancy unnecessary and document the long-term need for corticosteroid therapy. The temporal artery

Table 22-16.—Clinical Features of Polyarteritis

Common features	Uncommon features
Fever, fatigue, weight loss	Coronary arteritis
Arthralgia, arthritis	Myocardial infarction
Myalgia	Congestive heart failure
Mononeuritis multiplex	Central nervous system abnormalities
Focal necrotizing glomerular nephritis	Seizures
Abnormal renal sediment	Cerebrovascular accident
Hypertension	Lung (interstitial pneumonitis)
Skin abnormalities	Eye (retinal hemorrhage)
Palpable purpura	Testicular pain
Livedo reticularis	
Cutaneous infarctions	
Abdominal pain/ischemic bowel	
Liver enzyme abnormalities	

Polyarteritis may be a manifestation or complication of other diseases. This secondary polyarteritis complicates hepatitis B infection, rheumatoid arthritis (RA), Sjögren syndrome, mixed cryoglobulinemia, hairy cell leukemia, myelodysplastic syndrome, and other hematologic malignancies. Secondary polyarteritis is suggested by complement consumption. Secondary polyarteritis is histopathologically and clinically indistinguishable from the primary forms of polyarteritis. However, some forms of secondary polyarteritis have favored clinical presentations. For instance, systemic rheumatoid vasculitis is most commonly manifest by constitutional symptoms, skin lesions, and neuropathy. It uncommonly causes a necrotizing glomerulonephritis.

- Polyarteritis is usually a systemic illness associated with prominent constitutional features, including fever, fatigue, weight loss, and, occasionally, myalgia or arthralgia along with manifestations of multisystem involvement, including kidney disease, lung lesions, skin rash, and neuropathy.
- Classic polyarteritis nodosa is distinguished from microscopic polyangiitis by aneurysms seen on visceral angiography and the absence of glomerulonephritis or a positive ANCA. In practice, this distinction can be difficult because of a substantial overlap in the symptoms and signs.
- Secondary polyarteritis may be a complication of other diseases.

Diagnosis—Abnormal laboratory findings include normocytic anemia, increased erythrocyte sedimentation rate, and thrombocytosis. MPA presents 90% of the time with positive c-ANCA or myeloperoxidase-specific p-ANCA. Complement consumption is not part of primary polyarteritis. Low complement may be evident if immune complexes such as cryoglobulins are part of the pathogenesis of secondary polyarteritis. Hepatitis B infection is found in a small proportion of patients with ANCA-negative (classic PAN) and should always be sought, because treatment is directed against the infection. Hepatitis C is associated with the secondary polyarteritis that complicates some cases of cryoglobulinemia. Evaluation should document the extent and severity of the condition. The confirmatory test typically is angiography or biopsy of involved tissue showing vasculitis. The biopsy should be of accessible symptomatic tissue. Visceral angiography, including views of the renal and mesenteric arteries, shows saccular or fusiform aneurysm formation coupled with smooth, tapered stenosis alternating with normal or dilated blood vessel (Fig. 22-6).

- MPA will present 90% of the time with positive c-ANCA or myeloperoxidase-specific p-ANCA.
- Hepatitis B infection is found in a small proportion of patients with ANCA-negative (classic PAN) and should always be sought, because treatment is directed against the infection. Hepatitis C is associated with the secondary polyarteritis that complicates some cases of cryoglobulinemia.
- Confirmatory test: typically, angiography or biopsy of involved tissue showing vasculitis.
- Visceral angiography shows saccular or fusiform aneurysm formation coupled with smooth, tapered stenosis.
- Consider visceral angiography to make the diagnosis when the patient has significant gastrointestinal symptoms or markedly elevated liver enzyme tests and no tissue or organ system (nerve, skin) is affected or easily sampled by biopsy. The angiogram is abnormal in classic PAN and in cases in which classic PAN and MPA overlap.

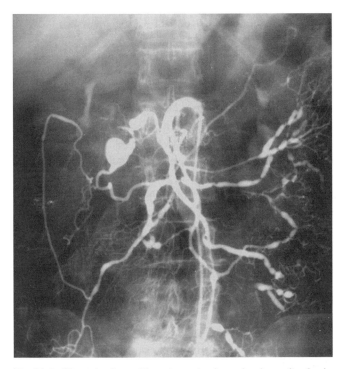

Fig. 22-6. Visceral polyarteritis nodosa. Angiography shows the classic features of smooth tapers followed by normal or dilated vessel. Note the large saccular aneurysm in the hepatic artery. (From Audiovisual Aids Subcommittee of the Education Committee of the American College of Rheumatology: Syllabus: Revised Clinical Slide Collection on the Rheumatic Diseases and 1985, 1988, and 1989 Slide Supplements. Atlanta, Georgia, American College of Rheumatology.)

Treatment—The cornerstone of treatment is early diagnosis and corticosteroid therapy. Cytotoxic and antimetabolite drugs such as cyclophosphamide, chlorambucil, methotrexate, and azathioprine are often used in combination with corticosteroids. These agents are added when the disease is rapidly progressive, particularly if polyarteritis involves an internal organ such as the kidney, gut, or heart. They also are useful as steroid-sparing agents. When confronted with deterioration of a patient's condition in the face of potent treatment, consider possible progression of disease, superimposed infection, or noninflammatory, proliferative, occlusive vasculopathy. Hepatitis-associated polyarteritis is treated best with anti-viral drugs.

● Cyclophosphamide, chlorambucil, methotrexate, and azathioprine are often used in conjunction with corticosteroids.

Outcome—In the first year after diagnosis of polyarteritis, deaths are related to the extent of disease activity, particularly gastrointestinal tract ischemia and renal insufficiency. Distinguishing classic PAN from MPA and type of organ involvement may influence treatment, complications, relapse rate, and mortality. After 1 year, complications of treatment, including infections in the immune-compromised patient, contribute most to mortality rates. MPA survival at 5 years with treatment is between 55% and 60%, and classic PAN survival at 5 years with treatment is between 75% and 90%.

● In the first year after diagnosis, deaths are related to the extent of disease activity, particularly gastrointestinal tract ischemia and renal insufficiency.
● Complications from treatment affect long-term mortality.

Churg-Strauss Vasculitis

Churg-Strauss vasculitis, or Churg-Strauss syndrome, is similar to polyarteritis and usually accounts for 6% to 30% of series that combine polyarteritis and Churg-Strauss syndrome. The median age at onset is about 38 years (range, 15 to 69 years). Churg-Strauss vasculitis is defined by 1) a history of or current symptoms of asthma, 2) peripheral eosinophilia ($>1.5 \times 10^9$ eosinophils/L), and 3) systemic vasculitis of at least two extrapulmonary organs. There is a slight male predominance. The histopathologic features of the disease include eosinophilic extravascular granulomas and granulomatous or nongranulomatous small vessel necrotizing vasculitis. It typically involves the small arteries, veins, arterioles, and venules.

● Churg-Strauss vasculitis: history of or current symptoms of asthma, peripheral eosinophilia ($>1.5 \times 10^9$ eosinophils/L), and systemic vasculitis of at least two extrapulmonary organs.
● It involves small arteries, veins, arterioles, and venules.

Clinical features—Churg-Strauss syndrome has three clinical stages. Patients need not progress in an orderly manner from one stage to another. There usually is a prodrome of allergic rhinitis, nasal polyposis, or asthma. In the second stage, peripheral blood and tissue eosinophilia develops, suggesting Löffler syndrome. Chronic eosinophilic pneumonia and gastroenteritis may remit or recur over years. The third stage is life-threatening vasculitis. Transient, patchy pulmonary infiltrates or nodules, pleural effusions, pulmonary angiitis and cardiomegaly, eosinophilic gastroenteritis, extravascular necrotizing granulomata of the skin, mononeuritis multiplex, and polyarthritis can complicate Churg-Strauss syndrome.

● Prodrome of allergic rhinitis, nasal polyposis, or asthma.
● Peripheral blood and tissue eosinophilia develops.
● Transient, patchy pulmonary infiltrates, extravascular necrotizing granulomata of the skin, and mononeuritis multiplex.

Treatment and outcome—One-year survival with treated Churg-Strauss syndrome is similar to that of polyarteritis. There is more cardiac involvement but fewer renal deaths than in polyarteritis. Treatment includes corticosteroids with or without the addition of cytotoxic agents. The eosinophilia resolves with treatment.

- Churg-Strauss syndrome: more cardiac involvement but fewer renal deaths than in polyarteritis.

Buerger Disease

Buerger disease, or thromboangiitis obliterans, occurs almost exclusively in young adult smokers who typically present with claudication of the instep and loss of digits from ischemic injury. They occasionally require amputation of an affected limb. Buerger disease affects the small- and medium-sized arteries and veins of the extremities. Acute vasculitis in Buerger disease is accompanied by characteristic intraluminal thrombus that contains microabscesses. Usually, the disease is arrested when smoking is stopped.

- Buerger disease occurs almost exclusively in young adult smokers.
- Claudication of the instep and loss of digits from ischemic injury.
- The disease is arrested when smoking is stopped.

Isolated (Primary) Angiitis of the Central Nervous System

Clinical features—Isolated, or primary, angiitis of the central nervous system, once thought to be rare, has a chronic fluctuating and progressive course. The average age of patients presenting with this disease is 45 years. Forty percent of the patients present with less than 4 weeks of symptoms, and another 40% present with symptoms that have been noted for more than 3 months. The most common symptom is headache (mild or severe) associated with nausea or vomiting. Nonfocal neurologic abnormalities (including confusion, dementia, drowsiness, or coma) may interrupt prolonged periods of apparent remission. Acute stroke-like focal neurologic presentations are increasingly described. Cerebral hemorrhage occurs in fewer than 4% of patients. Focal and nonfocal neurologic abnormalities coexist in half of the patients. Systemic features——fever, weight loss, arthralgia, and myalgia—are uncommon and occur in fewer than 20% of the patients; seizures occur in about 25%.

- Isolated angiitis of the central nervous system: a chronic fluctuating and progressive course, most commonly without evidence of systemic inflammation.
- Most common symptom is headache, with nausea or vomiting.
- Complicated by acute strokes, with or without nonfocal neurologic abnormalities (decreased consciousness or cognition), either at presentation or recurrently, interrupting prolonged periods of apparent remission.

- Cerebral hemorrhage occurs in <4% of patients.

Diagnosis—There are no reliable noninvasive tests for making the diagnosis. The mainstays of diagnosis are cerebral angiography and biopsy of central nervous system tissues, including the leptomeninges. The cerebrospinal fluid is abnormal in most of the patients with pathologically documented primary angiitis of the central nervous system. CT examinations of the head are not specific or sensitive for the condition. MRI examinations may be sensitive but do not distinguish this primary angiitis from other vasculopathic or demyelinating lesions of the brain, and they are not useful in following the condition. Patients with a chronic progressive course are more likely to have the diagnosis made pathologically and have abnormal results on examination of the cerebrospinal fluid.

- Mainstays of diagnosis: cerebral angiography and biopsy of central nervous system tissues, including the leptomeninges.

Rheumatologic syndromes that may produce a clinical picture similar to that of primary angiitis of the central nervous system include Cogan syndrome (nonsyphilitic keratitis and vestibular dysfunction), Behçet syndrome (uveitis, oral and genital ulcers, meningitis, and vasculitis), systemic lupus erythematosus, and polyarteritis. Drug-induced vasculopathy (particularly cocaine), demyelinating disease, HIV infection, Lyme disease, syphilis, carcinomatous meningitis, angiocentric immunoproliferative lesions, and antiphospholipid antibody syndrome are also part of the differential diagnosis of patients presenting with a syndrome suggesting primary angiitis of the central nervous system.

Treatment—The treatment for primary angiitis of the central nervous system may be influenced by the clinical subset. Younger patients with acute disease in whom the diagnosis was made with angiography may have a benign course and typically respond well to a short course of treatment with corticosteroids and calcium channel blockers to prevent vasospasm. Patients with a protracted course, abnormal cerebrospinal fluid, and diagnosis made with brain and leptomeningeal biopsy are best treated with combination therapy, including corticosteroids and cytotoxic agents. If untreated, this clinical subset has a high mortality rate.

- High mortality rate among patients with histopathologically confirmed or recurrent symptoms treated without cytotoxic agents.

Wegener Granulomatosis

Clinical features—Wegener granulomatosis is a well-recognized pathologic triad of upper and lower respiratory tract necrotizing granulomatous inflammation and focal segmental necrotizing glomerulonephritis. Wegener granulomatosis occurs in less than 1 person annually per 100,000 population. The peak incidence of the disease occurs in the fourth and fifth decades of life. There is a slight male predominance. Eighty-five percent of the patients have generalized disease, including glomerulonephritis; 15% can present with local inflammation involving only the upper respiratory tract or kidneys. The clinical features of this disease are summarized by the mnemonic ELKS: involvement of **E**ar/nose/throat, **L**ung, **K**idney, and **S**kin. Lung involvement most commonly includes thick-walled, centrally cavitating pulmonary nodules. Alveolitis and pulmonary hemorrhage occur in up to 20% of patients. Biopsy in the patients with renal involvement shows focal segmental necrotizing glomerulonephritis and, occasionally, granulomatous vasculitis. Skin involvement may include urticaria, petechiae, papules, vesicles, ulcers, pyoderma, and livedo reticularis. Inflammatory arthritis is usually oligoarticular and transient, occurring early in the clinical presentation. Nervous system involvement includes distal sensory neuropathy, mononeuritis multiplex, and cranial nerve palsies. Conjunctivitis, uveitis, and proptosis are not unusual. Neurosensory hearing loss has been described together with serous otitis and inner ear vasculitis. Wegener granulomatosis-associated subglottic tracheal stenosis due to chondritis should be distinguished from primary polychondritis.

- Wegener granulomatosis: triad of upper and lower respiratory tract necrotizing granulomatous inflammation and focal segmental necrotizing glomerulonephritis.
- ELKS: involvement of **E**ar/nose/throat, **L**ung, **K**idney, and **S**kin.
- Alveolitis and pulmonary hemorrhage occur in up to 20% of patients.
- Nervous system involvement: distal sensory neuropathy, mononeuritis multiplex, and cranial nerve palsies.

Pathologic diagnosis—The diagnosis of Wegener granulomatosis may require finding characteristic pathologic features in biopsy specimens. Biopsy of the upper respiratory tract suggests the diagnosis in 55% of patients, but only 20% show granulomata and/or vasculitis associated with necrosis. An open lung biopsy has a higher diagnostic yield than transbronchial biopsy. Renal biopsies usually document only a focal segmental necrotizing glomerulonephritis. Infrequently, renal biopsy shows vasculitis. Relevant laboratory findings in active Wegener granulomatosis include nonspecific increase in the erythrocyte sedimentation rate and platelet count, normocytic anemia, and low levels of albumin. Further refinement in the c-ANCA test may simplify diagnosis. The c-ANCA test alone is not adequate to make the diagnosis of Wegener granulomatosis unless the patient presents with a classic clinical picture.

- Diagnosis: may require finding characteristic pathologic features in biopsy specimens.
- Laboratory findings: nonspecific increase in erythrocyte sedimentation rate and platelet count and normocytic anemia.

ANCA—c-ANCA is directed against proteinase 3, a serine protease from azurophilic granules. c-ANCA occurs in more than 90% of active cases of generalized Wegener granulomatosis, in 75% of the cases without renal involvement, and in 10% to 50% of syndromes similar to Wegener granulomatosis. These syndromes include idiopathic crescentic glomerulonephritis (30% of cases), microscopic polyarteritis nodosa (50%), and Churg-Strauss syndrome (10%). However, in a patient with only sinusitis or a pulmonary infiltrate, a positive ANCA would have only a 5% positive predictive value for vasculitis. The antibody titer correlates loosely with disease activity, although the titers can remain increased despite clinical improvement. p-ANCA is directed against myeloperoxidase and other neutrophil cytoplasmic constituents. p-ANCA (anti-myeloperoxidase-specific) is found in idiopathic crescentic glomerulonephritis (70% of cases), microscopic polyarteritis nodosa (50%), Churg-Strauss syndrome (70%), Wegener granulomatosis (20%), and systemic lupus erythematosus. p-ANCA directed against leukocyte elastase, lactoferrin, and other antigens can occur in patients with various vasculitic syndromes, primary sclerosing cholangitis, ulcerative colitis, primary biliary cirrhosis, rheumatoid arthritis, and in 5% of normal subjects.

- c-ANCA occurs in >90% of active cases, in 75% of cases without renal involvement, and in 10%-50% of syndromes similar to Wegener granulomatosis.
- p-ANCA (myeloperoxidase) is found in idiopathic glomerulonephritis (70% of cases), microscopic polyarteritis nodosa (50%), Churg-Strauss syndrome (70%), Wegener granulomatosis (20%), and systemic lupus erythematosus.

Treatment and outcome—If untreated, generalized Wegener granulomatosis has a mean survival of 5 months and 95% mortality in 1 year. More than 95% of patients eventually have clinical remission with oral cyclophosphamide treatment. Corticosteroids are useful initially but can be tapered quickly after the disease is controlled. Mortality in the first year of disease is related primarily to the inflammatory process, with pulmonary hemorrhage or renal failure. In subsequent years, drug toxicity may dominate, with opportunistic infection and increasing risk of neoplasm and hemorrhagic cystitis related to the use of cyclophosphamide.

- If untreated, generalized Wegener granulomatosis has a mean survival of 5 months.
- Cyclophosphamide has revolutionized Wegener granulomatous treatment and dramatically altered the natural history.
- Corticosteroids are useful initially but can be tapered quickly after the disease is controlled.

Small Vessel Vasculitis/Cutaneous Vasculitis

Clinical features—Small vessel vasculitis occurs by itself or complicates many infectious, neoplastic, and connective tissue diseases. In the skin, it is manifest by urticaria, palpable purpura, livedo reticularis, or skin ulceration. It can be associated with peripheral neuropathy, arthralgia, or synovitis. Mononeuritis multiplex, diffuse pulmonary hemorrhage, and renal vasculitis are complications of systemic small vessel vasculitis as part of the formal primary or secondary vasculitis syndromes already mentioned. Small vessel vasculitis occurs with many illnesses; a partial listing is given in Table 22-17.

- Small vessel vasculitis: occurs by itself or complicates many infectious, neoplastic, and connective tissue diseases.
- In the skin, it is manifest by urticaria, palpable purpura, livedo reticularis, or skin ulceration.
- It can complicate most types of primary and secondary systemic vasculitis.

Histopathology—A neutrophilic- or (uncommonly) lymphocytic-predominant infiltrate surrounds small arteries, veins, arterioles, or venules. The histopathologic picture called "leukocytoclastic vasculitis" includes immune complexes deposited in vessel walls, along with fibrin deposition, endothelial cell swelling and necrosis, and a polymorphonuclear leukocytoclasis with scattering of nuclear fragment or nuclear dust. This is a pathologic diagnosis and does not predict the clinical condition. Palpable purpura is the classic clinical correlate of leukocytoclastic vasculitis. However, many other cutaneous presentations of leukocytoclastic vasculitis occur, including hives, infarcts, and ulcers.

- Classic clinical correlate of leukocytoclastic vasculitis: palpable purpura.

Diagnosis—The clinician must interpret small vessel/cutaneous vasculitis, which is a clinical finding and not a diagnosis. These various conditions are distinguished clinically and pathologically. For instance, Schönlein-Henoch vasculitis is suggested with the clinical features of abdominal pain or gastrointestinal hemorrhage in addition to the classic picture of lower extremity purpura, arthritis, and hematuria. Schönlein-Henoch vasculitis has IgA deposition in vessel walls and normal

Table 22-17.—Conditions With Small Vessel Vasculitis

Systemic small vessel vasculitis
  Systemic vasculitis
    Wegener granulomatosis
    Polyarteritis (primary and secondary)
    Churg-Strauss vasculitis
    Takayasu arteritis
    Schönlein-Henoch purpura/vasculitis
  Serum sickness
  Goodpasture syndrome
Nonsystemic small vessel vasculitis
  Hypocomplementemic vasculitis
  Leukocytoclastic vasculitis related to:
    Rheumatoid arthritis
    Sjögren syndrome
    Systemic lupus erythematosus
    Other connective tissue diseases
  Drug-induced and postinfectious angiitis
  Mixed cryoglobulinemia
  Malignancy-associated vasculitis
  Inflammatory bowel disease
  Organ transplant-associated vasculitis
  Hypergammaglobulinemic purpura of Waldenström

complement levels. Mixed cryoglobulinemia has circulating cryoglobulins and evidence of complement consumption. Complement levels, especially C4, may be low transiently in hypersensitivity vasculitis. Hypersensitivity vasculitis is almost always a nonsystemic small vessel vasculitis temporally related to infection, ingestion of drugs, or, less commonly, malignancy. The results of other laboratory studies are nonspecific. The leukocyte count and platelet count may be increased. Eosinophilia may be present. The erythrocyte sedimentation rate is usually increased.

- Complement levels may be low in mixed cryoglobulinemia and hypersensitivity vasculitis.
- Schönlein-Henoch vasculitis has four classic clinical features: lower extremity purpura, arthritis, gastrointestinal hemorrhage, and nephritis. Complement levels are normal in Schönlein-Henoch vasculitis.

Treatment and outcome—The outcome of nonsystemic small vessel vasculitis is good. Control of the infection or discontinuation of the offending drug may be all that is required. In other cases, corticosteroids or NSAIDs are beneficial. Hypersensitivity vasculitis is usually self-limited, but it may recur with repeated exposure to the antigen or drug.

- Nonsystemic small vessel vasculitis: the outcome is good.
- Hypersensitivity vasculitis may recur with repeated exposure to the antigen or drug.

Cryoglobulinemia

Cryoglobulins are immunoglobulins that reversibly precipitate at reduced temperatures. They are grouped into two major categories. *Type I cryoglobulins* are aggregates of a single monoclonal immunoglobulin and are generally associated with multiple myeloma, Waldenström macroglobulinemia, and lymphomas. They are usually found in high concentration (1-5 g/dL). Patients with type I cryoglobulins are often asymptomatic. Symptoms of type I cryoglobulinemia are usually related to increased viscosity and include headaches, visual disturbances, nosebleeds, Raynaud phenomenon, and ischemic ulceration from occlusion of arterioles and venules by precipitated immune complexes. Vasculitis is rare.

- Type I cryoglobulins are aggregates of a single monoclonal immunoglobulin.
- Patients with type I cryoglobulins are often asymptomatic.
- Symptoms are usually related to increased viscosity.
- Vasculitis is rare.

Type II cryoglobulins consist of more than one class of immunoglobulin. Type II cryoglobulinemia (or mixed cryoglobulinemia) can occur alone (primary) or secondary to another disease. Commonly, type II cryoglobulinemia involves an IgM molecule with anti-immunoglobulin specificity (rheumatoid factor). However, not all rheumatoid factors are cryoglobulins. Other components of the immune complexes formed include hepatitis C antigen, other infectious agents, cellular/nuclear antigens, and complement. These immune complexes precipitate slowly and are present in smaller quantities (50-500 mg/dL) than type I cryoglobulins. Type II cryoglobulins have been further divided into those complexes in which one immunoglobulin is a monoclonal protein (monoclonal-mixed cryoglobulinemia). This distinction appears to have little clinical or prognostic usefulness. Type II cryoglobulins are frequently associated with chronic infections (most commonly hepatitis C), autoimmune disorders, and, occasionally, lymphoma. The immune complexes that form precipitate on endothelial cells in peripheral blood vessels and fix complement, promoting vasculitic inflammation. The size of immune complexes, ability to fix complement, persistent IgM production, and many other factors may influence the clinical presentation of mixed cryoglobulinemia. The typical presentation is that of nonsystemic small vessel vasculitis with palpable purpura, urticaria, and cutaneous ulceration. Peripheral neuropathy, arthralgia, and arthritis are common. Less commonly, mixed cryoglobulinemia is complicated by hepatosplenomegaly, pneumonitis or pulmonary hemorrhage, focal segmental necrotizing glomerulonephritis, serositis (pleurisy, pericarditis), and thyroiditis.

- Type II cryoglobulins are frequently associated with chronic infections (most often hepatitis C) and immune disorders.
- Typical presentation: nonsystemic small vessel vasculitis with palpable purpura, urticaria, and cutaneous ulceration.
- Peripheral neuropathy, arthralgia, and arthritis are common.

Laboratory studies—Patients with type II cryoglobulinemia and small vessel vasculitis usually have an increased erythrocyte sedimentation rate, increased immunoglobulin levels, positive rheumatoid factor, and low levels of complement. Evidence of chronic hepatitis infection (particularly hepatitis C) is frequently identified. For cryoglobulin testing, it is important to draw blood into a warmed syringe and to keep it warm until transferred to a cryocrit tube. Cooled specimens must be kept for up to 3 days to identify type II cryoglobulins. Serum protein electrophoresis, immunoelectrophoresis, and quantitative immunoglobulin determinations can be helpful in some cases.

- Immunoglobulin levels and the erythrocyte sedimentation rate are increased, rheumatoid factor is positive, and complement levels are low.
- Evidence of chronic hepatitis infection (particularly hepatitis C) is frequently identified.

Outcome—The clinical course of nonsystemic vasculitis is mild and prolonged. In systemic small vessel vasculitis caused by mixed cryoglobulinemia, the course and prognosis depend on the organs involved. Progressive renal disease is the most common systemic complication. Pulmonary hemorrhage is life-threatening. Some patients with mixed cryoglobulinemia eventually develop cirrhosis or a lymphoproliferative disorder.

- Progressive renal disease is the most common systemic complication.

Vasculitis Associated With Connective Tissue Diseases

Obliterative endarteropathy—Vascular involvement in rheumatoid arthritis can have various presentations. A positive rheumatoid factor is invariably present in patients with vasculitis related to rheumatoid arthritis. Digital nail fold and nodule infarcts occur in some patients with active rheumatoid arthritis. Histopathologically, this is a bland, obliterative endarteropathy with intimal proliferation. Managing the rheumatoid arthritis itself is all that is needed, because these vasculopathic changes require no other therapy. A process similar to that

- NSAIDs decrease prostaglandin synthesis by inhibiting COX conversion of arachidonic acid to prostaglandin precursors, explaining most of their therapeutic effects.
- Prostaglandins mediate vasodilation and extravasation, pain sensation, potentiate inflammatory mediators, and influence cellular and humoral immunity.

Mechanisms of Toxicity of NSAIDs

Toxic reactions are due primarily to inhibition of COX and prostaglandin production. Recent investigation has uncovered two forms of COX: COX-1 and COX-2. COX-1 is constitutively expressed in most tissues and produces the prostaglandin precursors needed for "housekeeping function." Prostaglandins protect the gastric mucosal barrier from autodigestion. Patients with renal insufficiency or liver or cardiac disease may have prostaglandin-dependent renal blood flow. NSAIDs interfere with the synthesis of thromboxane via COX-1, which influences vascular tone, platelet aggregation, and hemostasis. COX-2 is not found in resting cells but is rapidly induced in activated fibroblasts, endothelial cells, and smooth muscle cells by cytokines, growth factors, and lipopolysaccharide. Currently available NSAIDs are all excellent inhibitors of COX-1 and COX-2 at reasonable therapeutic concentrations. Simply viewed, the acute anti-inflammatory effects of NSAIDs relate to their ability to inhibit COX-2. The side effects of NSAIDs reside mostly with their ability to inhibit COX-1 and the "housekeeping function" associated with the prostaglandins synthesized by COX-1. Selective COX-2 inhibitors now in development promise to change the current risk-and-benefit ratio of NSAIDs with an improved safety profile.

Blocking COX with currently available NSAIDs augments conversion of arachidonic acid to leukotrienes. Leukotrienes (previously known as "slow-reacting substance of anaphylaxis") aggravate asthma, rhinitis, hives, and nasal polyps.

- Acute anti-inflammatory action of NSAIDs is mediated by COX-2 inhibition.
- Toxic reactions are due primarily to inhibition of COX-1.
- Selective COX-2 inhibitors have the potential to significantly reduce NSAID side effects.
- NSAIDs interfere with the synthesis of thromboxane and influence platelet function.
- Leukotrienes aggravate asthma, rhinitis, hives, and nasal polyps. NSAIDs may increase production of leukotrienes.

NSAIDs are bound extensively to plasma proteins. Protein binding has obvious implications for other medications that are also protein bound. Phenylbutazone and aspirin inhibit the metabolism of oral hypoglycemic agents and increase the risk of hypoglycemia. Indomethacin, diclofenac, and piroxicam decrease lithium excretion. NSAIDs can also influence methotrexate toxicity at high doses (>50 mg/week) by interfering with the renal clearance of methotrexate.

- Phenylbutazone and aspirin inhibit the metabolism of oral hypoglycemic agents and increase the risk of hypoglycemia.
- Indomethacin, diclofenac, and piroxicam decrease lithium excretion.

Most NSAIDs attenuate the effects of antihypertensive medications. Diuretics, β-blockers, and angiotensin-converting enzyme inhibitors are the drugs affected most by the influence of NSAIDs on renal prostaglandins. Aspirin irreversibly inhibits COX. The effect of all the other NSAIDs on COX-1 is reversible. These drugs prolong bleeding time. The use of aspirin needs to be discontinued for up to 10 days before the bleeding time returns to normal. NSAIDs should be discontinued at least four-drug half-lives before invasive procedures in which bleeding is a concern. NSAIDs with a short half-life are best when an acute effect (e.g., treatment of acute gout) is required. The half-life is proportional to the onset of maximal clinical benefit. The common side effects of NSAIDs are listed in Table 22-20.

- Diuretics, β-blockers, and angiotensin-converting enzyme inhibitors are the drugs affected most by the influence of NSAIDs on renal prostaglandins.
- Aspirin irreversibly inhibits COX-1.
- NSAIDs usually prolong the bleeding time.
- Acetaminophen is not a potent prostaglandin inhibitor in peripheral tissue.

Gastrointestinal Side Effects

Twenty percent of chronic users of NSAIDs have gastric ulcer noted on endoscopy, and 15% to 35% report dyspepsia, but this complaint does not appear to be related to abnormal findings on endoscopy. Nausea and abdominal pain are described in up to 40% of users of NSAIDs. Stomach upset/pain forces discontinuation of these drugs in more than 10% of patients. Gastrointestinal blood loss related to these drugs is most often occult and can result in iron deficiency anemia. The true incidence of significant gastrointestinal bleeding requiring hospitalization or operation or resulting in death is unknown. However, the elderly, those with significant cardiovascular morbidity, and those with a previous history of NSAID-associated ulcer are at greatest risk for significant gastrointestinal toxicity related to NSAIDs. Alcohol, corticosteroid, and tobacco use also predisposes to the development of gastrointestinal toxicity.

- Of chronic users of NSAIDs, 20% have gastric ulcer and 15%-35% have dyspepsia.

Table 22-20.—Common Side Effects of Nonsteroidal Anti-Inflammatory Drugs

Gastrointestinal
  Nausea
  Abdominal pain
  Constipation or diarrhea
  Occult blood loss and iron deficiency anemia
  Peptic ulcer disease
  Colitis and colonic hemorrhage
Renal
  Reduced renal blood flow
  Reduced glomerular filtration rate
  Increased creatinine clearance
  Pyuria
  Interstitial nephritis
  Papillary necrosis
  Nephrotic syndrome
  Hyperkalemia and type IV renal tubular acidosis
  Fluid retention
Hematologic
  Bone marrow suppression
    Agranulocytosis
    Aplastic anemia
  Iron deficiency anemia
  Platelet aggregating defect
Neurologic
  Delirium/confusion
  Headache
  Dizziness
  Blurred vision
  Mood swings
  Aseptic meningitis
Dermatologic
  Urticaria
  Erythema multiforme
  Exfoliative syndromes (toxic epidermal necrolysis)
  Oral ulcers
  Dermatitis
Pulmonary
  Pulmonary infiltrates
  Noncardiac pulmonary edema (aspirin toxicity)
  Anaphylaxis and bronchospasm
  Nasal polyps
Drug interactions
  Augment hemostatic effect of warfarin
  Attenuate antihypertensive effect of diuretics, β-blockers, angiotensin converting enzyme inhibitors
  Influence drug metabolism
    Methotrexate (high doses only)
    Lithium
    Oral hypoglycemic agents

- Stomach upset/pain forces discontinuation of these drugs in >10% of patients.
- Gastrointestinal blood loss related to these drugs is most often occult.
- The elderly, those with significant cardiovascular morbidity, and those with a previous history of NSAID-associated ulcer are especially at risk for significant gastrointestinal toxicity related to NSAIDs.

Other Toxic Effects of NSAIDs

Bone marrow toxicity, including agranulocytosis and aplastic anemia, can occur with all NSAIDs, most frequently with phenylbutazone. Central nervous system symptoms such as headaches, dizziness, mood alterations, blurred vision, and confusion are reported most frequently with the use of indomethacin. Ibuprofen, tolmetin, and sulindac have been associated with aseptic meningitis in patients with systemic lupus erythematosus. All the central nervous system effects resolve when the use of NSAIDs is discontinued. Rashes, urticaria, exfoliative dermatitis, erythema multiforme, and scalded skin syndrome or toxic epidermal necrolysis all occur, albeit rarely, with the use of NSAIDs. Easy bruisability is a common complaint of chronic users of these drugs. Patients may develop dependent petechiae if their platelet function is already compromised. Pulmonary infiltrates, bronchospasm, and anaphylaxis may occur with all NSAIDs, including aspirin. Although it is not IgE-mediated, anaphylaxis is seen most commonly in patients who have the classic triad of asthma, nasal polyps, and aspirin sensitivity. Combination therapy with NSAIDs should be avoided. Whereas toxicity is additive, there is no evidence that the therapeutic effect is additive.

- Bone marrow toxicity, central nervous system effects, lung disease, and renal compromise can all occur with NSAIDs.
- Combination therapy with two different NSAIDs should be considered.

Nonacetylated Salicylates

Careful studies have not identified significant differences in efficacy of nonacetylated salicylates compared with NSAIDs. Nonacetylated salicylates minimally inhibit COX-1 and are about half as potent as aspirin as inhibitors of COX-2. Although their use decreases the incidence of gastrointestinal bleeding, they can cause many of the gastrointestinal symptoms that influence patient compliance. Tinnitus remains a potential problem. Nonacetylated salicylates do not interfere with renal blood flow, and they do not inhibit platelet function. They usually can be safely prescribed for patients with aspirin allergy.

- Nonacetylated salicylates minimally inhibit COX-1.

- Nonacetylated salicylates do not interfere with renal blood flow, and they do not inhibit platelet function.
- Nonacetylated salicylates can cause stomach upset or tinnitus.

Disease-Modifying Antirheumatic Drugs

Antimalarial Compounds (Hydroxychloroquine)

Open and randomized placebo-controlled studies have confirmed the benefit of hydroxychloroquine in the management of rheumatoid arthritis and systemic lupus erythematosus. The dose typically does not exceed 4.5 mg/kg daily. Retinopathy is the major toxic effect associated with the use of hydroxychloroquine. The risk of irreversible retinopathy is small (<3%) in patients taking less than 4.5 mg/kg daily. The elderly may be at somewhat increased risk. Regular eye examinations can identify the premaculopathy stage of the toxic reaction, which is reversible. Permanent symptomatic retinopathy is preventable when patients have eye examinations every 6 to 12 months.

- Retinopathy is the major toxic effect associated with the use of hydroxychloroquine.
- The risk of irreversible retinopathy is small (<3%) in patients taking <4.5 mg/kg daily.

The clinical response to hydroxychloroquine does not appear before 8 weeks. Improvement may not occur until 6 months of continuous therapy. Approximately 40% to 60% of patients with rheumatoid arthritis may respond (based on established criteria for response). It is used most commonly in combination with NSAIDs or low doses of corticosteroids in patients with early or mild polyarthritis.

- The clinical response to hydroxychloroquine does not appear before 8 weeks and may not occur until 6 months of continuous therapy.

Gold Salts

There are three preparations of gold salts: gold sodium thiomalate (Myochrysine, given intramuscularly), aurothioglucose (Solganal, given intramuscularly), and auranofin (Ridaura, given orally). Intramuscular injections of gold salts started in the first few years of rheumatoid arthritis can reduce the number of tender and swollen joints and improve grip strength. Gold treatment decreases the erythrocyte sedimentation rate and typically reduces the rheumatoid factor titer. Gold may work partly by influencing macrophage function. Gold given intramuscularly is also prescribed to patients with HLA-B27-associated peripheral arthritis. It has no effect on the axial (spinal) inflammatory arthritis. Intramuscular injections of gold may cause disease flares in systemic lupus erythematosus.

- Gold treatment decreases the erythrocyte sedimentation rate and typically reduces the rheumatoid factor titer.
- No effect on axial (spinal) inflammatory arthritis.
- There is a 60% chance that patients will respond to gold given intramuscularly.

It is unusual to see a clinical response until the patient has received at least 3 months of gold therapy. Gold therapy should be continued until at least 1,000 mg have been administered before a lack of response prompts discontinuation. It is important to check for any potential toxic reaction with each intramuscular injection. A complete blood count and urinalysis are usually performed before each injection. Adverse experiences in patients treated with injections of gold are responsible for 1-year toxicity dropout rates approaching 35%. Vasomotor responses (nitritoid reaction) occur more commonly with gold sodium thiomalate than with aurothioglucose. The nitritoid reaction occurs shortly after injection and is characterized by weakness, dizziness, nausea, vomiting, sweating, and facial flushing. Common reactions to intramuscular injections of gold include stomatitis and rashes. More than 50 types of rashes occur with gold injections. Often, the mucocutaneous reaction can be managed by changing the gold preparation or holding and later rechallenging with a lower dose. Gold therapy causes membranous glomerulonephropathy with proteinuria and nephrotic syndrome. Of the patients receiving intramuscular injections of gold, 40% have to discontinue use of the medication because of nephropathy. Hematologic disturbances occur in fewer than 2% of all patients receiving gold injections. Immune thrombocytopenia, agranulocytosis, and aplastic anemia can be life-threatening conditions.

- Gold therapy should be continued until at least 1,000 mg have been administered before a lack of response prompts discontinuation.
- Common reactions to intramuscular injections of gold include stomatitis and rashes and, less commonly, bone marrow suppression or membranous glomerulopathy.
- It is important to check for any potential toxic reaction with each intramuscular injection by questioning the patient and checking blood counts and a urinalysis.
- The nitritoid reaction (a vasomotor response) occurs shortly after a gold injection and is characterized by weakness, dizziness, nausea, vomiting, sweating, and facial flushing.

Auranofin is an orally administered gold compound. About 25% of the dose is absorbed rapidly; the majority of the medication is eliminated in the feces. The medication should be continued for at least 4 to 6 months to assess its therapeutic potential. Meta-analysis suggests auranofin is less effective than other disease-modifying antirheumatic drugs, including

gold given intramuscularly and methotrexate. The most frequent toxic effect is diarrhea.

- Auranofin is an orally administered gold compound.
- The most frequent toxic effect is diarrhea.

Penicillamine

Penicillamine is a treatment for systemic sclerosis (scleroderma) and rheumatoid arthritis. Penicillin allergy is not a contraindication to the use of penicillamine. The adage "go low, go slow" emphasizes dosing increments that decrease the toxic effects associated with penicillamine. It needs to be taken on an empty stomach, 1 hour before or 2 hours after meals. The medication should be tried for at least 6 months, if tolerated, to assess its potential for therapeutic benefit. Its toxicity profile is similar to that of intramuscular injections of gold, including the mucocutaneous reactions, nephropathy, and hematologic abnormalities. Several autoimmune phenomena have been described, including myasthenia gravis, polymyositis, systemic lupus erythematosus-like syndrome, and a Goodpasture-like syndrome. Penicillamine causes skin fragility and poor wound healing by inhibiting collagen synthesis.

- Penicillin allergy is not a contraindication to the use of penicillamine.
- Penicillamine needs to be taken on an empty stomach.
- Penicillamine can cause rashes, oral ulcers, nephropathy, and bone marrow suppression.
- Several autoimmune phenomena may occur secondary to treatment with penicillamine, including myasthenia gravis, polymyositis, a lupus-like illness, and Goodpasture syndrome.

Sulfasalazine

Enteric-coated tablets of sulfasalazine (Azulfidine-EN-tabs) have reduced some of the immediate gastrointestinal upset associated with this drug. The metabolites of sulfasalazine include 5-aminosalicylic acid and sulfapyridine. The results of short-term randomized trials indicate significant efficacy in mild-to-moderate rheumatoid arthritis. Rheumatologists also recommend treatment with sulfasalazine for seronegative spondyloarthropathies and psoriatic arthritis. The benefit of this drug in rheumatoid arthritis is equal to that of intramuscular injections of gold but with fewer toxic effects. Sulfasalazine treatment is usually reserved for milder cases of inflammatory polyarthritis. Although the onset of efficacy occurs as early as 8 weeks, the effect may not be documented for as many as 6 months. The toxic effects include nausea, vomiting, gastric ulcers, and, more rarely, hepatitis or cholestasis. Ten percent of patients complain of headache or sense of fatigue. Recently, a combination of sulfasalazine, hydroxychloroquine, and methotrexate was found superior to single

drug therapy in rheumatoid arthritis patients in whom treatment with at least one DMARD has failed.

- Sulfasalazine treatment: usually reserved for milder cases of inflammatory polyarthritis.
- The benefit of this drug in selected cases of rheumatoid arthritis may be equal to that of intramuscular injections of gold.

Methotrexate

Methotrexate is a structural analogue of folic acid and is considered an antimetabolite rather than a cytotoxic agent. It is used extensively in rheumatoid arthritis and also has a place in the treatment of psoriatic arthritis and peripheral arthritis of seronegative spondyloarthropathies. Methotrexate may have a role in the treatment of arthritis in systemic lupus erythematosus and scleroderma. Its mechanism of action includes inhibition of folate metabolism (critical in nucleotide production), inhibition of leukotriene B_4, and increasing intracellular adenosine. It has both immunomodulator and anti-inflammatory effects. Its strongest effect is on rapidly dividing cells, particularly those in the S phase of the cell cycle. Methotrexate is unique among disease-modifying antirheumatic drugs because its antirheumatic effect occurs within 4 to 6 weeks. Oral, subcutaneous, and intramuscular and/or intravenous routes are equally effective for low dosages.

- Methotrexate is used extensively in rheumatoid arthritis and has a place in the treatment of psoriatic arthritis, peripheral arthritis of seronegative spondyloarthropathies, and the arthritis in systemic lupus erythematosus and scleroderma.
- The antirheumatic effect occurs within 4-6 weeks.

Of rheumatoid arthritis patients receiving treatment with methotrexate, 80% have significant improvement within the first year of therapy. At 5 years, it is estimated that at least 35% of patients treated with methotrexate still take it. No other disease-modifying antirheumatic drug has this combination of efficacy and tolerability. Most patients with rheumatoid arthritis have a severe flare of their disease within 3 weeks after discontinuation of methotrexate therapy. This drug should not be used in patients with significant renal dysfunction (creatinine >2.0 mg/dL). Coadministration of trimethoprim sulfa antibiotics and methotrexate increases the risk of hematologic toxicity.

- 80% of rheumatoid arthritis patients taking methotrexate have significant improvement within the first year of treatment.
- Most rheumatoid arthritis patients have a severe flare of their disease within 3 weeks after discontinuation of methotrexate therapy.

Gastrointestinal toxic reactions are common side effects of methotrexate. Nausea and vomiting may persist for 24 to 48 hours after ingestion. Stomatitis and diarrhea are insurmountable problems for some patients. Methotrexate treatment should be withheld from patients with significant gastric ulceration until their ulcers have healed. Increased liver enzyme levels suggest a subclinical hepatic toxic effect due to methotrexate. Persistent increase in aspartate aminotransferase levels or decreasing albumin levels are markers for developing hepatic fibrosis and, potentially, cirrhosis. Cryptic cirrhosis may develop without liver enzyme abnormalities being detected. Stomatitis and the less common hematologic abnormalities such as leukopenia, thrombocytopenia, and pancytopenia may respond to folic acid supplementation. Pulmonary toxic side effects include chemical pneumonitis and insidious pulmonary fibrosis, beginning with a dry cough. Acute pneumonitis due to methotrexate may be associated with eosinophilia. Neurologic features such as headache and seizure are uncommon. Methotrexate is teratogenic and should be withheld for 3 months before the patient attempts to conceive.

● Gastrointestinal toxic reactions are the common side effects of methotrexate.
● Methotrexate should not be used in patients with significant renal dysfunction.
● Stomatitis and diarrhea are insurmountable problems for some patients.

Leflunomide

Leflunomide (Arava) is an immunoregulatory agent that interferes with pyrimidine synthesis and is approved for the treatment of rheumatoid arthritis. Its efficacy may be comparable to that of methotrextate and is noted within 12 weeks after initiating therapy. Toxicity is also comparable to that of methotrexate, although no pulmonary complications or cirrhosis has been reported. The most common side effects include gastrointestinal distress, rashes, and alopecia. The toxic-side-effect monitoring that is recommended currently is the same as that recommended for methotrexate.

Azathioprine

Azathioprine and its metabolites are purine analogues. It is considered a cytotoxic agent. Azathioprine is metabolized by xanthine oxidase and thiopurine methyltransferase (TPMT). Allopurinol, an inhibitor of xanthine oxidase, delays the metabolism of azathioprine and can lead to toxic reactions if the dose of azathioprine is not decreased by 50% to 66%. Thiopurine methyltransferase can be assayed; low levels of this enzyme predict the 1 in 300 patients in whom a severe hematologic reaction to azathioprine will develop. Controlled studies have documented the efficacy of azathioprine in the treatment of rheumatoid arthritis and systemic lupus erythematosus.

The most common problem with azathioprine is gastrointestinal toxic effects. An idiosyncratic, acute pancreatitis-like attack is an absolute contraindication to further treatment with this drug. Cholestatic hepatitis is rare, but if it occurs, it generally does so within the first several weeks after drug administration. If tolerated initially, hematologic toxic effects become the most significant concern. In patients who have undergone organ transplant, azathioprine treatment increases the risk of neoplasia, particularly lymphomas, leukemias, and skin and cervical malignancies. Azathioprine does not alter fertility, but it may have some teratogenic potential. For pregnant women, azathioprine should be reserved for those with severe or life-threatening rheumatic diseases.

● Azathioprine is a cytotoxic agent.
● The most common problems with azathioprine are gastrointestinal toxic effects and cytopenias.
● Allopurinol should be avoided in patients taking azathioprine.

Cyclophosphamide

Cyclophosphamide is a potent alkylating agent. It acts on dividing and nondividing cells, interfering with cellular DNA function. It depletes T cells and B cells, causing considerable immunosuppression. Oral cyclophosphamide is well absorbed and completely metabolized within 24 hours, and most of its metabolites are excreted in the urine. Allopurinol increases the risk of leukopenia in patients taking cyclophosphamide. Short-term studies document significant efficacy of this drug in the treatment of rheumatoid arthritis at doses of 1 to 2 mg/kg per day. Unequivocal healing and arresting of erosive change occur. The considerable toxicity associated with chronic administration of cyclophosphamide has raised questions about whether it should be used in rheumatoid arthritis. It is the drug of choice in the treatment of generalized Wegener granulomatosis. Intravenous administration of cyclophosphamide is efficacious in managing systemic necrotizing vasculitis and severe systemic lupus erythematosus, including proliferative glomerulonephritis. Short-term advantages of intravenous pulse cyclophosphamide may include fewer toxic effects on the bladder and perhaps a lower risk of infection.

● Cyclophosphamide depletes T cells and B cells, causing considerable immunosuppression.
● Allopurinol increases the risk of leukopenia in patients taking cyclophosphamide.
● Cyclophosphamide is efficacious in managing systemic necrotizing vasculitis and severe systemic lupus erythematosus.

Dose-related bone marrow suppression is common in patients receiving cyclophosphamide and requires close laboratory monitoring. Immune suppression from treatment with cyclophosphamide increases the risk of infection. Herpes zoster infection occurs in most patients receiving the drug orally. Cyclophosphamide directly affects ovarian and testicular function. Premature ovarian failure frequently occurs in premenopausal lupus patients taking the drug. Spermatogenesis can also be affected by this drug, which causes atrophy of seminiferous tubules. Cyclophosphamide has teratogenic potential. Alopecia, stomatitis, cardiomyopathy (with drug doses used to treat cancer), and pulmonary fibrosis may complicate cyclophosphamide therapy. The metabolites of this drug, including acrolein, accumulate in the bladder. Acrolein has direct mucosal toxic effects and causes hemorrhagic cystitis. This complication is potentially life-threatening. The chronic use of cyclophosphamide taken orally is associated with increased risk of neoplasia, including hematologic and bladder malignancies. The risk of malignancy with intravenous pulse therapy has not been established. All patients who have had cyclophosphamide therapy should have urinalysis and urine cytology performed at regular intervals for life.

- Cyclophosphamide: dose-related bone marrow suppression is common.
- Cyclophosphamide directly affects ovarian and testicular function.
- The chronic use of cyclophosphamide is associated with increased risk of neoplasia.

Glucocorticosteroids

Glucocorticosteroids modify the inflammatory response dramatically. They are potent inhibitors of neutrophil function. Glucocorticosteroids suppress cellular immune activity and, to a lesser extent, inhibit the humoral response. Low doses of glucocorticosteroids (<10 mg of prednisone per day) are frequently used in the day-to-day management of the articular manifestations of rheumatoid arthritis. At least one-third of all patients with rheumatoid arthritis take glucocorticosteroids chronically. High doses of glucocorticosteroids (1-2 mg of prednisone per kilogram of patient body weight) may be required for life-threatening or serious inflammatory disorders, including systemic vasculitis and complications of systemic lupus erythematosus. Prednisone doses greater than 30 mg/day are associated with higher risk of infection, including *Pneumocystis carinii*. This is particularly the case if prednisone is given in addition to cyclophosphamide, azathioprine, or methotrexate. Many clinicans add one double-strength trimethoprim-sulfa tablet twice a week to these immunosuppressive regimens as porphylaxis against *Pneumocystis* infection.

- Glucocorticosteroids are potent inhibitors of neutrophil function.
- They suppress cellular immune activity and, to a lesser extent, inhibit the humoral response.
- One-third of all patients with rheumatoid arthritis take glucocorticosteroids chronically.

These drugs have many side effects, which are not idiosyncratic but actually unwanted effects of the medication. The longer patients receive them and the higher the dose used, determine how fast an unwanted effect appears. Many patients with rheumatoid arthritis tolerate prednisone doses in the 1 to 5 mg/day range for years without having serious side effects. Patient concerns about glucocorticosteroids include weight gain from increased appetite, water retention, and hirsutism. Longer-term concerns include thinning of the skin, bruising easily, progressive osteoporosis (unclear if this happens with physiologic doses of prednisone) and compression fractures, high blood pressure, glucose intolerance, cataract formation, and aggravation of glaucoma. The psychoactive potential of high doses of glucocorticosteroids is an additional factor in treating older patients. Glucocorticosteroid psychosis can complicate the diagnosis of neuropsychiatric lupus.

- Many patients with rheumatoid arthritis tolerate prednisone doses in the 1-5 mg/day range for years without having serious side effects.
- Long-term concerns: thinning of the skin, progressive osteoporosis and compression fractures, high blood pressure, glucose intolerance, cataract formation, and aggravation of glaucoma.
- Glucocorticosteroid psychosis can complicate the diagnosis of neuropsychiatric lupus.
- Glucocorticosteroids interfere with wound healing and increase risk of opportunistic infection.

PART II
Marc D. Cohen, M.D.

CRYSTALLINE ARTHROPATHIES

Hyperuricemia and Gout

Hyperuricemia has been described in 2% to 18% of normal populations. Hyperuricemia is associated with hypertension, renal insufficiency, obesity, and arteriosclerotic heart disease. The prevalence of clinical gouty arthritis ranges from 0.1% to 0.4%. There is a family history of gout in 6% to 18% of patients with gouty arthritis. Genetic studies suggest a multifactorial inheritance pattern. Of patients with hyperuricemia whose uric acid level is more than 9 mg/dL, gout develops in 5 years in approximately 20%.

- Hyperuricemia is associated with hypertension, renal insufficiency, obesity, and arteriosclerotic heart disease.
- The prevalence of gouty arthritis is 0.1%-0.4%.
- 6%-18% of patients with gouty arthritis have a family history of gout.
- In patients with uric acid level more than 9 mg/dL, gout develops in 20% in 5 years.

Overproduction of uric acid is the cause of hyperuricemia in 10% or less of patients with primary gout. Of these 10%, about 15% have one of the two X-linked inborn errors of purine metabolism: 1) hypoxanthine-guanine phosphoribosyltransferase deficiency (Lesch-Nyhan syndrome) and 2) 5-phosphoribosyl-1-pyrophosphate synthetase overactivity. Of the remaining 85% of patients who have overproduction, most are obese, but the cause of overproduction and the relationship between obesity and overproduction of uric acid remain unknown.

- 90% of patients with gout have underexcretion of uric acid. They have reduced filtration of uric acid, enhanced tubular reabsorption, or decreased tubular secretion.
- 10% or less of patients with gout have overproduction of uric acid.

Events leading to initial crystallization of monosodium urate in a joint after many years of asymptomatic hyperuricemia are unknown. Trauma with disruption of microtophi in cartilage may lead to release of urate crystals into synovial fluid. The urate crystals become coated with immunoglobulin and then complement. They are then phagocytosed by leukocytes with subsequent release of chemotactic protein, activation of the kallikrein system, and disruption of the leukocytes, which release lysosomal enzymes into synovial fluid.

Important Enzyme Abnormalities in Uric Acid Pathway (Fig. 22-8)

Lesch-Nyhan syndrome is a complete deficiency of hypoxanthine-guanine phosphoribosyltransferase. It is characterized by X-linked disorder in young boys, hyperuricemia, self-mutilation, choreoathetosis, spasticity, growth retardation, and severe gouty arthritis.

Overactivity of 5-phosphoribosyl-1-pyrophosphate synthetase is associated with hyperuricemia, X-linked genetic inheritence, and gouty arthritis.

Adenosine deaminase deficiency is inherited in an autosomal recessive pattern. It causes a combined immunodeficiency state with severe T-cell and mild B-cell dysfunction. There is a buildup of deoxyadenosine triphosphate in lymphocytes, which is toxic to immature lymphocytes. Features of the disorder are hypouricemia, recurrent infection, chondro-osseous dysplasia, and an increased deoxyadenosine level in plasma and urine. Treatment for the disorder is with irradiated frozen red blood cells or marrow transplantation.

Xanthine oxidase deficiency is also inherited in an autosomal recessive pattern. It is characterized by hypouricemia, xanthinuria with xanthine stones, and myopathy associated with deposits of xanthine and hypoxanthine.

Causes of Secondary Hyperuricemia

Secondary hyperuricemia can be attributed to overproduction or underexcretion of uric acid (Table 22-21).

- Important causes of overproduction of uric acid include cancers, psoriasis, and sickle cell anemia.
- Important causes of underexcretion of uric acid include many causes of chronic renal insufficiency, lead nephropathy, alcohol, diabetic ketoacidosis, and drugs, notably thiazide diuretics, nicotinic acid, and cyclosporine.

Causes of Hypouricemia

Increased urinary excretion of uric acid contributes to hypouricemia. It can develop in healthy persons with an isolated defect in tubular reabsorption of uric acid. It also can be related to diminished reabsorption of urate, such as in Fanconi syndrome, Fanconi syndrome associated with Wilson disease, carcinoma of the lung, acute myelogenous leukemia,

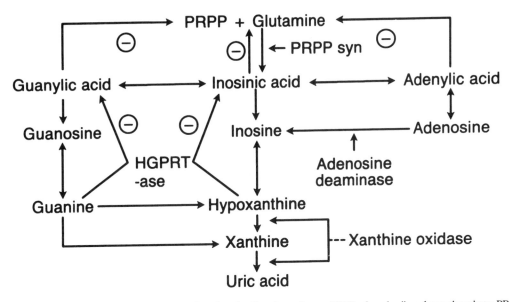

Fig. 22-8. Purine metabolism. HGPRTase, hypoxanthine-guanine phosphoribosyltransferase; PRPP, phosphoribosylpyrophosphate; PRPP syn, phosphoribosylpyrophosphate synthetase; ⊖, feedback inhibition.

light-chain diseases, and use of outdated tetracycline. Malignant neoplasms, such as carcinoma, Hodgkin disease, and sarcoma, also are associated with increased excretion of uric acid. Hypervolemia caused by inappropriate secretion of antidiuretic hormone also can be a factor. Drugs involved in increased excretion of uric acid are high-dose aspirin, probenecid and other uricosuric agents, and glyceryl guaiacolate. Radiographic contrast agents that can cause hypouricemia are iopanoic acid (Telopaque), iodipamide meglumine (Cholografin), and diatrizoate sodium (Hypaque). It also can occur in severe liver disease.

Decreased synthesis of uric acid also can cause hypouricemia. The drug allopurinol inhibits the enzyme xanthine oxidase, causing hypouricemia. The decrease also can be caused by congenital deficiencies in enzymes involved in purine biosynthesis: 5-phosphoribosyl-1-pyrophosphate synthetase deficiency, adenosine deaminase deficiency, purine nucleoside phosphorylase deficiency, and xanthine oxidase deficiency (xanthinuria). Acquired deficiency in xanthine oxidase activity (metastatic adenocarcinoma of lung) also can cause decreased synthesis of uric acid, as can acute intermittent porphyria.

Predisposing Factors to Gout and Pseudogout

The following can predispose to an attack of gout or pseudogout: trauma, surgery (3 days after), major medical illness (myocardial infarction, cerebrovascular accident, pulmonary embolus), fasting, alcohol use, infection, and acidosis. The attacks are precipitated by changes in the urate equilibrium between the blood and joints.

● Factors that precipitate gout and pseudogout include trauma, surgery, alcohol use, and acidosis.

Clinical Manifestations of Acute Gout

In 50% of patients with gout, the metatarsophalangeal joint of the great toe is involved initially (podagra), and this joint is eventually involved in more than 75% of patients. Rapid joint swelling is associated with extreme tenderness. Uric acid crystals, which are needle-like and strongly negatively birefringent under polarized light, are always found in the joint during an acute attack. The diagnosis of gout is established by the demonstration of uric acid crystals in the joint aspirate. The joint fluid is usually inflammatory with between 5,000 and 75,000 polymorphonuclear neutrophils.

Gout occurs most commonly in middle-aged men, but, after menopause, the incidence of gout in women approaches that in men. Although gout is usually monarticular and usually involves the joints in the lower extremity, attacks may become polyarticular over time in some patients.

● Podagra is the initial presentation of gout in 50% of cases.
● Uric acid crystals are negatively birefringent under polarized light microscopy.
● Gout is usually monarticular and most often involves the joints in the lower extremities.

Treatment of Acute Gouty Arthritis

Indomethacin or other nonsteroidal anti-inflammatory drugs (NSAIDs) are the drugs of choice for the treatment of acute gouty arthritis and should be used for a 7- to 10-day course.

Table 22-21. —Causes of Secondary Hyperuricemia

Overproduction
  Myeloproliferative disorders
    Polycythemia, primary or secondary
    Myeloid metaplasia
    Chronic myelocytic leukemia
  Lymphoproliferative disorders
    Chronic lymphatic leukemia
  Plasma cell proliferative disorders
    Multiple myeloma
  Disseminated carcinoma and sarcoma
  Sickle cell anemia, thalassemia, and other forms of chronic
    hemolytic anemia
  Psoriasis
  Cytotoxic drugs
  Infectious mononucleosis
  Obesity
  Increased purine ingestion
Underexcretion
  Intrinsic renal disease
    Chronic renal insufficiency of diverse cause
    Saturine gout (lead nephropathy)
  Drug-induced
    Thiazide diuretics, furosemide, ethacrynic acid,
      ethambutol, pyrazinamide, low-dose aspirin,
      cyclosporine, nicotinic acid, laxative abuse, levodopa
  Endocrine conditions
    Adrenal insufficiency, nephrogenic diabetes insipidus,
      hyperparathyroidism, hypoparathyroidism,
      pseudohypoparathyroidism, hypothyroidism
  Metabolic conditions
    Diabetic ketoacidosis, lactic acidosis, starvation,
      ethanolism, glycogen storage disease type I, Bartter
      syndrome
  Other
    Sarcoidosis
    Down syndrome
    Beryllium disease

These drugs are relatively contraindicated in patients with congestive heart failure, peptic ulcer disease, or renal insufficiency. NSAIDs should not be used in patients with nasal polyps and aspirin sensitivity because they may cause bronchospasm.

- NSAIDs are the initial drug of choice for an acute attack of gouty arthritis.
- Avoid NSAIDs in patients with congestive heart failure, peptic ulcer disease, and renal insufficiency.

Intra-articular or oral corticosteroids and subcutaneous adrenocorticotropic hormone are other treatments, especially in patients who have contraindications to colchicine and NSAIDs. Oral corticosteroids may need to be given for 10 days to avoid relapses. Do not administer allopurinol or probenecid until the acute attack completely subsides. Because of severe gastrointestinal side effects, high-dose oral colchicine is rarely used for an acute attack. Intravenously administered colchicine in a single dose (1 to 2 mg) has no gastrointestinal side effects. It has increased toxicity in patients with renal insufficiency, bone marrow depression, sepsis, and immediate prior use of oral colchicine. Repeat dosages should be avoided. It can cause severe extravasation if it infiltrates into subcutaneous tissues.

- Colchicine: there is potential for gastrointestinal side effects with the oral form, but there are no gastrointestinal side effects with single-dose intravenous administration.
- Avoid intravenous colchicine in patients with renal insufficiency, bone marrow depression, sepsis, or immediate prior use of oral colchicine.

Treatment During Intercritical Period
Oral colchicine, 0.6 mg twice a day, may be given prophylactically with probenecid or allopurinol for 6 to 12 months to prevent exacerbation of acute gout.

Probenecid is uricosuric. It inhibits tubular reabsorption of filtered and secreted urate, thereby increasing urinary excretion of uric acid. It should not be used if the patient has a history of kidney stones or if the 24-hour urine uric acid value is more than 1,000 mg (normal, less than 600 mg/day). Probenecid delays the renal excretion of indomethacin and thereby increases its blood level. Probenecid delays the renal excretion of acetylsalicylic acid (ASA), and ASA completely blocks the uricosuric effect of probenecid. ASA also blocks tubular secretion of urates. Do not use probenecid with methotrexate because probenecid increases methotrexate blood levels, increasing toxicity.

- Probenecid inhibits tubular reabsorption of filtered and secreted urate.
- Probenecid should not be used if patient has a history of kidney stones or if 24-hour uric acid value is more than 1,000 mg.
- Probenecid delays renal excretion of indomethacin and ASA.

Allopurinol is a xanthine oxidase inhibitor. It is the drug of choice to prevent gouty attacks if the patient has a history of renal stones or renal insufficiency. Allopurinol and probenecid usually are not used simultaneously unless the patient has extensive tophaceous gout with good renal function.

Allopurinol can cause a rash and a severe toxicity syndrome consisting of eosinophilia, fever, hepatitis, decreased renal function, and an erythematous desquamative rash. This syndrome usually occurs in patients with decreased renal function. Allopurinol should be given in the lowest dose possible to keep the uric acid value less than 6 mg/dL. If allopurinol is used, the dose of 6-mercaptopurine or azathioprine needs to be reduced by 25%.

- Allopurinol is a xanthine oxidase inhibitor.
- It can precipitate gout.
- It is the drug of choice if patient has a history of renal stones or renal insufficiency.
- It can cause severe toxicity syndrome: eosinophilia, fever, hepatitis, decreased renal function, erythematous desquamative rash.

The indications for use of allopurinol rather than probenecid for lowering the uric acid level are tophaceous gout, gout complicated by renal insufficiency, uric acid excretion more than 1,000 mg/day, history of uric acid calculi, use of cytotoxic drugs, and allergy to uricosuric agents. Allopurinol should be used before treatment of rapidly proliferating tumors. The nucleic acid liberated with cytolysis is converted to uric acid and can cause renal failure secondary to precipitation of uric acid in collecting ducts and ureters (acute tumor lysis syndrome). Patients also should have adequate hydration and alkalinization of the urine before chemotherapy.

- Indications for allopurinol include tophaceous gout, gout complicated by renal insufficiency, history of uric acid calculi, and use of cytotoxic drugs.

Renal Disease and Uric Acid

Renal function is not necessarily adversely affected by an increased serum urate concentration. The incidence of interstitial renal disease and renal insufficiency is no greater than that in patients of comparable age with similar degrees of hypertension, arteriosclerotic heart disease, diabetes, and primary renal disease. Correction of hyperuricemia (to 10 mg/dL or less) has no apparent effect on renal function.

Most rheumatologists do not treat asymptomatic hyperuricemia if the uric acid level is less than 10.0 mg/dL (normal to 8.0). When hyperuricemia is associated with a urinary uric acid of more than 1,000 mg/24 hours, which increases the risk of uric acid stones, renal function should be monitored closely. Excessive exposure to lead may contribute to the renal disease found in some patients with gout.

- Renal function is not adversely affected by an increased serum urate concentration.

- Correction of hyperuricemia (to 10 mg/dL or less) has no apparent effect on renal function.

Miscellaneous Points of Importance

- Positive diagnosis of a crystalline arthritis requires identification of crystal by polarization microscopy.
- Do not start allopurinol therapy during an acute attack of gout.
- 30% of patients with chronic tophaceous gout are positive for rheumatoid factor (usually weakly positive).
- 10% of patients with acute gout will be positive for rheumatoid factor (usually weakly positive).
- 5%-10% of patients will have gout and pseudogout attack simultaneously.
- 50% of synovial fluids aspirated from first metatarsophalangeal joints of asymptomatic patients with gout have crystals of monosodium urate.
- Up to 20% of patients with acute gout have a normal level of serum uric acid at the time of the acute attack.
- Gout in a premenopausal female is very unusual.
- Sulfinpyrazone is also uricosuric and potentially therapeutic.
- There have been many recent reports of superimposed gout occurring in Heberden and Bouchard nodes in older women taking thiazide diuretics.
- A septic joint can trigger a gout or pseudogout attack in a predisposed person. Always obtain synovial fluid analysis for crystals, Gram stain, and culture.
- The frequency of gout in patients who have had cardiac transplantation is high (25%). (Both cyclosporine and diuretics cause hyperuricemia.)

Calcium Pyrophosphate Deposition Disease

Etiologic Classification

Calcium pyrophosphate deposition disease (CPPD) is classified as idiopathic, hereditary, or associated with metabolic disease. The associated diseases include hyperparathyroidism, hemochromatosis-hemosiderosis, hypothyroidism, gout, hypomagnesemia, hypophosphatasia, Wilson disease, and ochronosis. CPPD also is associated with amyloidosis, Bartter syndrome, osteoarthritis, and Paget disease.

- CPPD disease associations include hyperparathyroidism, hemochromatosis-hemosiderosis, hypothyroidism, and hypomagnesemia.

Pseudogout

When CPPD causes an acute inflammatory arthritis, the term "pseudogout" is applied. CPPD crystals are weakly positively birefringent and are rhomboid-shaped. Pseudogout rarely involves the first metatarsophalangeal joint. It most commonly affects the knees, but the wrists, elbows, ankles, and intervertebral disks may be involved. It usually occurs in older individuals. Most patients with pseudogout have chondrocalcinosis on radiography. The presence of chondrocalcinosis does not necessarily mean that a patient will have pseudogout or even CPPD.

- Pseudogout is an acute inflammatory arthritis caused by CPPD.
- CPPD crystals are weakly positively birefringent under polarized light microscopy.
- Pseudogout most commonly affects the knees, but the wrists, elbows, ankles, and intervertebral disks can be affected.
- Chondrocalcinosis is found on radiographs in most patients with pseudogout.
- Chondrocalcinosis does not mean that patients will have pseudogout or even CPPD.

Treatment of Pseudogout

For treatment of acute attacks, NSAIDs or injection of a steroid preparation can be used. Intravenously administered colchicine is effective for acute attacks, but oral administration is not consistently effective. Prophylactic oral colchicine (0.6 mg twice to three times daily) can lead to a decrease in the frequency and severity of pseudogout attacks. In patients with underlying metabolic disease, the frequency of acute attacks of pseudogout does not decrease with treatment of the underlying disease (such as hypothyroidism or hyperparathyroidism).

- Treatment of acute attacks of pseudogout: NSAIDs, injection of steroid preparation, or colchicine given intravenously.
- Prophylactic oral colchicine can lead to a decrease in the frequency and severity of attacks.

Hydroxyapatite Deposition Disease (Basic Calcium Phosphate Disease)

Presentation

Clinical presentations include 1) acute inflammation, including calcific tendinitis, osteoarthritis with inflammatory episodes, periarthritis/arthritis dialysis syndrome, calcinotic deposits in scleroderma and 2) chronic inflammation, including osteoarthritis and Milwaukee shoulder: glenohumeral osteoarthritis, rotator cuff tear, noninflammatory paste-like joint fluid containing hydroxyapatite.

- Hydroxyapatite deposition disease can present as acute or chronic inflammation.

Diagnosis and Treatment

Individual crystals cannot be seen on routine polarization microscopy (Table 22-22). Small, round (shiny coin) bodies 0.5 to 100 µm are seen. On electron microscopy, these represent lumps of needle-shaped crystals. Positive identification requires transmission electron microscopy or elemental analysis. Alizarin red stain showing calcium staining provides a presumptive diagnosis (if CPPD is excluded). Treatment involves NSAIDs and intra-articular steroids.

- Individual crystals are not seen on polarization microscopy.
- Positive identification requires transmission electron microscopy.

Calcium Oxalate Arthropathy

This disorder occurs in patients with primary oxalosis and in patients undergoing chronic hemodialysis. It can cause acute inflammatory arthritis. Crystals are large, bipyramidal, and birefringent. Calcium oxalate can cause chondrocalcinosis or large soft tissue calcifications.

Table 22-22.—Differential Diagnosis According to Results of Synovial Fluid Analysis

Diagnosis	Leukocyte count, per mm^3	Differential	Polarization microscopy
Degenerative joint disease	<1,000	Mononuclear cells	Negative
Rheumatoid arthritis	5,000-50,000	PMNs	Negative
Gout	5,000-100,000	PMNs	Monosodium urate
Pseudogout	5,000-100,000	PMNs	CPPD
Hydroxyapatite	5,000-100,000	PMNs	Negative
Septic arthritis	≥100,000	PMNs	Negative

CPPD, calcium pyrophosphate deposition disease; PMN, polymorphonuclear leukocytes.

● Calcium oxalate arthropathy occurs in patients with primary oxalosis and patients undergoing chronic hemodialysis.

Other Crystals Implicated in Joint Disease

Cholesterol crystals are a nonspecific finding and have been found in the synovial fluid of patients with various types of chronic inflammatory arthritis. Cryoglobulin crystals are found in essential cryoglobulinemia and paraproteinemia. Corticosteroid crystals are found in an arthritis flare after a corticosteroid injection, and Charcot-Leyden crystals have been found in hypereosinophilic syndromes. In patients undergoing hemodialysis, aluminum phosphate crystals can develop.

SPONDYLOARTHROPATHIES

Conditions that form the spondyloarthropathies include ankylosing spondylitis, Reiter syndrome, reactive arthritis, enteropathic spondylitis, and psoriatic arthritis.

Spondyloarthropathies are characterized by involvement of the sacroiliac joints (uncommon in rheumatoid arthritis), peripheral arthritis (usually asymmetric oligoarticular), absence of rheumatoid factor, and an association with HLA-B27. They are enthesopathic disorders.

The HLA region of chromosome 6 contains genes of the human histocompatibility complex. Every person has two 6th chromosomes, one inherited from each parent. On each of these there is an HLA-A and HLA-B allele. Therefore, everyone has two HLA-A types and two HLA-B types. With regard to inheritance, an offspring has a 50% chance of acquiring a specific HLA-A or HLA-B antigen from a parent (Fig. 22-9). Siblings have a 25% chance of being identical for all four HLA-A and HLA-B alleles.

The frequency of HLA-B27 in control populations is as follows: whites (United States), 8%; African blacks, 0%; Asians, 1%; Haida (North American Indian), 50%.

The rheumatic diseases associated with HLA-B27 are ankylosing spondylitis (HLA-B27 in more than 90%), Reiter syndrome or reactive arthritis (more than 80%), enteropathic spondylitis (approximately 75%), and psoriatic spondylitis (approximately 50%).

● Ankylosing spondylitis is associated with HLA-B27 in more than 90% of cases.

Many theories have been proposed to explain the association between HLA-B27 and the spondyloarthropathies: B27 may act as a receptor site for an infective agent; B27 is a marker for an immune response gene that determines susceptibility to an environmental trigger; and B27 may induce tolerance to foreign antigens with which it cross-reacts.

An offspring of a person with HLA-B27 has a 50% chance of carrying the antigen. In randomly selected persons with HLA-B27, the chance of the disease developing is 2%. In B27-positive relatives of B27-positive patients with ankylosing spondylitis, the risk of the disease developing is 20%.

Ankylosing Spondylitis

Ankylosing spondylitis is a chronic systemic inflammatory disease that affects the sacroiliac joints, the spine, and the peripheral joints. Sacroiliac joint involvement defines this disease, and back pain, decreased spinal motion, and reduced chest expansion also are often found

● Sacroiliac joint involvement defines ankylosing spondylitis, and back pain, decreased spinal motion, and reduced chest expansion also are often found.

Features

Characteristic features of low back pain in ankylosing spondylitis are age at onset usually between 15 and 40 years, insidious onset, duration of more than 3 months, morning stiffness, improvement with exercise, family history, involvement of other systems, and diffuse radiation of back pain.

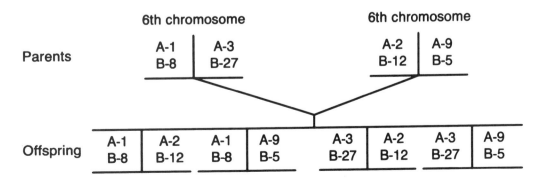

Fig. 22-9. Inheritance of HLA antigens.

- Features of low back pain in ankylosing spondylitis include age at onset between 15 and 40 years, insidious onset, and improvement with exercise.

Findings of ankylosing spondylitis on physical examination are listed in Table 22-23. Other physical findings in ankylosing spondylitis are listed in Table 22-24.

The radiographic findings in ankylosing spondylitis are 1) sacroiliac involvement with erosions, "pseudowidening" of joint space, sclerosis (both sides of sacroiliac joint; this finding is needed for diagnosis), and fusion and 2) spine involvement with squaring of superior and inferior margins of vertebral body, syndesmophytes, and bamboo spine.

- Radiographic findings in ankylosing spondylitis include erosions, syndesmophytes, bamboo spine.

Laboratory Findings

The erythrocyte sedimentation rate may be increased, there may be an anemia of chronic disease, rheumatoid factor is absent, and 95% of white patients are positive for HLA-B27.

Extraspinal Involvement

Enthesopathic involvement distinguishes spondyloarthropathies from rheumatoid arthritis and consists of plantar fasciitis, Achilles tendinitis, and costochondritis. Hip and shoulder involvement are common (up to 50%), but peripheral joints can be affected, usually with asymmetric involvement of the lower extremities. Some patients diagnosed with juvenile rheumatoid arthritis, especially male adolescents, may have juvenile ankylosing spondylitis in which peripheral arthritis preceded the low back pain.

- Enthesopathic involvement is characteristic of ankylosing spondylitis and the other spondyloarthopathies: plantar fasciitis, Achilles tendinitis, costochondritis.
- Hip and shoulder involvement are common (up to 50%).

Table 22-23.--Findings in Ankylosing Spondylitis

Characteristic	
Scoliosis	Absent
Decreased range of movement	Symmetric
Tenderness	Diffuse
Hip flexion with straight-leg raising	Normal
Pain with sciatic nerve stretch	Absent
Hip involvement	Frequently present
Neurodeficit	Absent

Extraskeletal Involvement

Other findings in active disease include 1) fatigue, 2) weight loss, 3) low-grade fever, and 4) iritis (25% of patients). Iritis is an important clinical clue in the diagnosis of spondyloarthropathies. It is not found in adults with rheumatoid arthritis.

- Iritis is an important clue to the diagnosis of spondyloarthropathies and is not found in adults with rheumatoid arthritis.

Late complications can include 1) cord compression due to traumatic spinal fracture, 2) cauda equina syndrome (symptoms include neurogenic bladder, fecal incontinence, leg pain), 3) fibrotic changes in upper lung fields (cavities can develop and aspergillomas have been reported), 4) aortic insufficiency in 3% to 5% of patients, 5) complete heart block, and 6) amyloidosis.

- Late complications of ankylosing spondylitis include cord compression due to traumatic spinal fractures, cauda equina syndrome, fibrotic changes in upper lung fields, and aortic insufficiency.

Ankylosing Spondylitis in Men and Women

Ankylosing spondylitis has been thought to be a disease primarily of men, but it is now recognized that the incidence in women is higher than originally thought, although women have less tendency for spinal ankylosis. The ratio of men to women is approximately 3:1. Women more frequently have osteitis pubis and peripheral joint involvement.

Differential Diagnosis

The differential diagnosis includes diffuse hypertrophic skeletal hyperostosis (DISH), osteitis condensans ilii, fusion of sacroiliac joint in paraplegia, osteitis pubis, and degenerative joint disease. The clinical symptoms of DISH are "stiffness" of spine and relatively good preservation of spine motion. It generally affects middle-aged and elderly men. Patients with DISH can have dysphagia related to cervical osteophytes. Criteria for DISH are "flowing" ossification along the anterolateral aspect of at least four contiguous vertebral bodies, preservation of disk height, absence of apophyseal joint involvement, absence of sacroiliac joint involvement, and extraspinal ossifications, including ligamentous calcifications.

Osteitis condensans ilii usually affects young to middle-aged females with normal sacroiliac joints. Radiography shows sclerosis on the iliac side of the sacroiliac joint only.

The sacroiliac joint also can be involved with 1) tuberculosis, 2) metastatic disease, 3) gout, 4) Paget disease, or 5) infection (*Brucella, Serratia, Staphylococcus*).

Table 22-24.—Results of Testing in Ankylosing Spondylitis

Test	Method	Results
Schober	Make a mark on the spine at level of L-5 and one at 10 cm directly above with the patient standing erect. Patient then bends forward maximally and the distance between the two marks is measured	An increase of <5 cm indicates early lumbar involvement
Chest expansion	Measure maximal chest expansion at nipple line	Chest expansion of <5 cm is clue to early costovertebral involvement
Sacroiliac compression	Exert direct compression over sacroiliac joints	Tenderness or pain suggests sacroiliac involvement

- Osteitis condensans ilii usually affects young to middle-aged females; radiography shows sclerosis on the iliac side of the sacroiliac joint only.
- The sacroiliac joint can be involved with metastatic disease, gout, Paget disease, or infection (*Brucella, Serratia, Staphylococcus*).

Treatment

Treatment involves physical therapy (upright posture is very important), exercise (swimming), cessation of smoking, genetic counseling, and drug therapy with NSAIDs such as indomethacin; aspirin is not as effective. Sulfasalazine and methotrexate therapy also may provide benefit, especially in patients with peripheral joint involvement.

Reiter Syndrome

This is a seronegative, asymmetric arthropathy predominantly affecting the lower extremities. One or more of the following conditions also may occur: 1) urethritis, 2) dysentery, 3) inflammatory eye disease (conjunctivitis or iritis), and 4) mucocutaneous disease (balanitis, oral ulcerations, or keratoderma). In addition, approximately 80% of patients are HLA-B27-positive. Keratoderma blennorrhagicum is a characteristic skin finding that is indistinguishable clinically and histologically from psoriasis. Joint predilection is for the toes and asymmetric large joints in the lower extremities. It can cause "sausage" toe, as can psoriatic arthritis. The distal interphalangeal joints in the hands can be affected also. Cardiac conduction disturbances and aortitis can develop. Sacroiliitis (sometimes unilateral) and iritis can occur. Long-term studies indicate that the disease remains episodically active in 75% of patients and that disability is a frequent outcome.

- Reiter syndrome is characterized by a seronegative, asymmetric arthropathy with urethritis, dysentery, inflammatory eye disease, or mucocutaneous disease.

- 80% of patients are HLA-B27-positive.
- Cardiac conduction disturbances and aortitis can develop.

Treatment is with NSAIDs (indomethacin), sulfasalazine, and methotrexate. Treatment with tetracycline or erythromycin-type antibiotics may decrease the duration and severity of illness in some cases of *Chlamydia*-triggered Reiter syndrome.

Reactive Arthritis

This is an aseptic arthritis induced by a host response to an infectious agent rather than direct infection. HLA-B27 is associated in 80% of cases. The condition develops after infections with *Salmonella* organisms, *Shigella flexneri, Yersinia enterocolitica,* and *Campylobacter jejuni,* which cause diarrhea, and *Chlamydia* and *Ureaplasma urealyticum,* which cause nonspecific urethritis. In addition to polyarthritis, clinical features of Reiter syndrome, including sacroiliitis, may develop. Patients usually have self-limited disease. Joint destruction is *not* common. The condition is usually managed with NSAIDs. Treatment with tetracycline antibiotics may decrease the duration and severity of the illness.

- Reactive arthritis: aseptic arthritis induced by a host response to an infectious agent rather than direct infection.
- HLA-B27 is associated in 80% of cases.
- Develops after infections with *Salmonella, Shigella flexneri, Yersinia enterocolitica, Campylobacter jejuni, Chlamydia, Ureaplasma urealyticum.*
- Clinical features of Reiter syndrome may develop.

Arthritis Associated With Inflammatory Bowel Disease

Two distinct types of arthritis are associated with chronic inflammatory bowel disease: 1) a *non*destructive oligoarthritis of the peripheral joints tending to correlate with the activity of the bowel disease and 2) ankylosing spondylitis (enteropathic spondylitis). The spondylitis is not a complication of the bowel disease. It may be diagnosed many years before the onset of bowel symptoms, and its subsequent progress bears little relationship to the bowel disease. Approximately 75% of patients with ankylosing spondylitis and inflammatory bowel disease are HLA-B27-positive. Patients with inflammatory bowel disease alone do not have an increased frequency of HLA-B27 and are not at increased risk for development of spondylitis.

- Patients with inflammatory bowel disease may have a non-destructive oligoarthritis of the peripheral joints which tends to correlate with the activity of the bowel disease.

Psoriatic Arthritis

Psoriatic arthritis develops in 7% or less of patients with psoriasis. Pitting of nails is strongly associated with joint disease. Patients with more severe skin disease are at higher risk for the development of arthritis. Hyperuricemia is present in 15% of all patients with psoriasis whether or not they have arthritis. A "sausage" finger or toe is characteristic of psoriatic arthritis and is very uncommon in rheumatoid arthritis. Radiographic evidence of involvement of the distal interphalangeal joint with erosions is common in psoriasis and uncommon in rheumatoid arthritis. Psoriatic arthritis also can cause a characteristic "pencil-in-cup" deformity of the distal interphalangeal and proximal interphalangeal joints on radiography.

- Psoriatic arthritis develops in 7% or less of patients with psoriasis.
- Pitting of nails is strongly associated with joint disease.
- Hyperuricemia is present in 15% of all patients with psoriasis.
- "Sausage" finger or toe is characteristic.
- "Pencil-in-cup" deformity of the distal and proximal interphalangeal joints is radiographic finding.

There are five clinical groups of psoriatic arthritis: 1) predominant distal interphalangeal joint involvement, 2) arthritis mutilans, 3) symmetrical polyarthritis-like rheumatoid arthritis but negative for rheumatoid factor, 4) asymmetrical oligoarthritis, and 5) psoriatic spondylitis (HLA-B27-positive in 50%-75% of cases). Treatment is with NSAIDs, methotrexate, and azathioprine.

IRITIS AND RHEUMATOLOGIC DISEASES

Various rheumatologic diseases are associated with iritis, particularly the seronegative spondyloarthopathies. Iritis is uncommon in rheumatoid arthritis and systemic lupus erythematosus. Nongranulomatous iritis without any other associated symptoms may be associated with HLA-B27 in almost 50% of patients.

BEHÇET SYNDROME

Behçet syndrome is most common in Middle Eastern countries and Japan. In addition to oral and genital ulcerations, uveitis, synovitis, cutaneous vasculitis, and meningoencephalitis may be present. The pathergy reaction (hyperreactivity of the skin in response to superficial trauma) is also seen. Migratory, superficial thrombophlebitis and erythema nodosum also have been associated with this syndrome. The combination of recurrent aphthous dermatitis, similar ulcerations in the genital area, and uveitis is most common. Treatment is with corticosteroids, although more aggressive immunosuppression is often required.

OSTEOID OSTEOMA

Osteoid osteoma is a benign bone tumor. It usually occurs between the ages of 5 and 30 years in males and females with equal frequency. The classic symptom is bone pain at night, which is relieved completely with aspirin or another NSAID. The diagnosis is made with routine radiography, but often this is negative and a bone scan may be helpful in localizing the tumor. Tomography or computed tomography then can be done for better visualization. Radiography shows a small nidus, usually less than 1 cm, varying from radiolucent to radiopaque, depending on the age of the lesion. There is usually a lucent ring around the nidus and adjacent bone sclerosis. Definitive treatment includes excision, which is curative.

- Osteoid osteoma is a benign bone tumor.
- Bone pain at night is relieved by aspirin or other NSAID.
- Treatment includes excision, which is curative.

BYPASS ARTHRITIS

This occurs in patients who have undergone intestinal bypass operations, including jejunocolic or jejunoileal. The arthritis may be acute or subacute, is usually intermittent, and can last occasionally for short periods only to recur. The most commonly affected joints are the metacarpophalangeal, proximal interphalangeal, wrists, knees, and ankles. It is commonly associated with a dermatitis, which can be pustular in nature. Circulating immune complexes composed of bacterial antigens have been found in both the circulation and the synovial fluid and are thought to be the cause of this disorder. Treatment consists of NSAIDs and antibiotics such as tetracycline, but many times reanastomosis may be necessary for resolution of symptoms.

- Bypass arthritis occurs in patients who have had intestinal bypass operations.
- Most commonly affected joints: metacarpophalangeal, proximal interphalangeal, wrists, knees, ankles.
- Bypass arthritis is commonly associated with a dermatitis.

SYSTEMIC LUPUS ERYTHEMATOSUS

Systemic lupus erythematosus (SLE) is a chronic inflammatory disease of unknown cause with a wide spectrum of clinical manifestations and variable course. Antibodies that react with nuclear antigens commonly are found in patients with the disease. Genetic, hormonal, and environmental factors seem to be important in the cause. Multiple organs may be affected, and the disease course is variable and characterized by exacerbations and remission.

- Genetic, hormonal, and environmental factors seem important in the cause of SLE.
- SLE is characterized by exacerbations and remissions.

Diagnosis

At least *four* of the following findings are needed for the diagnosis of SLE: malar rash; discoid lupus; photosensitivity; oral ulcers; nonerosive arthritis; proteinuria (protein >0.5 g/day) or cellular casts; seizures or psychosis; pleuritis or pericarditis; hemolytic anemia, leukopenia, lymphopenia, or thrombocytopenia; antibody to nDNA, antibody to Sm (Smith), IgG or IgM anticardiolipin antibodies, positive test for lupus anticoagulant, or false-positive results of VDRL test; and positive results of fluorescent antinuclear antibody test.

Epidemiology

The female:male ratio is 8:1 during the reproductive years. The first symptoms usually occur between the second and fourth decades of life. The disease seems to be less severe in the elderly. In SLE with onset at an older age, the female:male ratio is equal. The frequency of SLE is increased in American blacks, Native Americans, and Asians.

- Female:male ratio in SLE is 8:1 during the reproductive years.
- Increased frequency of SLE in American blacks, Native Americans, Asians.

Etiology

Type C oncornavirus is present in NZB/W mice developing a lupus-like illness, and both viral protein and antibody to protein are found in affected mouse glomeruli. A direct causal relationship has *not* been established. In human disease, viral-like particles in glomeruli of patients with SLE also are seen in other kinds of kidney damage. Attempts to isolate viruses have been unsuccessful. Patients with SLE have increased antibody titers to a wide range of antigens without much sign of specificity for a particular viral agent.

- In SLE, increased antibody titers to a wide range of antigens without much sign of specificity for a particular viral agent.

Genetics

Among relatives of patients with SLE, 20% have an immunologic disease. Another 25% have antinuclear antibodies, circulating immune complexes, antilymphocyte antibodies, or a false-positive result on VDRL test without clinical disease. Concordance for SLE among monozygotic twins is much greater than among dizygotic twins. Multiple genetic and environmental factors are important in the development of SLE. Immune complex levels are much higher in persons with close contact to the SLE patients than in unexposed consanguineous relatives. The frequency of HLA-B8, HLA-DR2, and HLA-DR3 is increased.

- 20% of relatives of patients with SLE have an immunologic disease.
- In SLE, the frequency of HLA-B8, HLA-DR2, and HLA-DR3 is increased.

Immune System

There is a change in the activity of the cellular immune system with an absolute decrease in T-suppressor cells. There is an increase in the activity of the humoral immune system with B-cell hyperactivity resulting in polyclonal activation.

- In SLE, there is an absolute decrease in T-suppressor cells with an increase in the humoral immune system with B-cell hyperactivity.

Pathogenesis

Circulating immune complexes (anti-nDNA) may contribute to glomerulonephritis and skin disease, among other manifestations. Immune complexes bind complement, which initiates the inflammatory process. Organ-specific autoantibodies also contribute to the pathophysiology of the disease and include antibodies that are 1) antierythrocyte, 2) antiplatelet, 3) antileukocyte, 4) antineuronal, and 5) antithyroid.

- Circulating immune complexes (anti-nDNA) are responsible for glomerulonephritis and certain skin manifestations.
- Organ-specific autoantibodies also may contribute to the pathophysiology.

Late complications of SLE are related to vascular damage, sometimes in the relative absence of active immunologic disease. Damage to the intima during active disease may result in premature deterioration of vasculature and various thrombotic, ischemic, and hypertensive manifestations.

Clinical Manifestations

Fever in SLE usually is caused by the disease, but infection *must* be ruled out. Shaking chills and leukocytosis strongly suggest infection.

Articular

Arthritis is characteristically nondeforming and nonerosive. Avascular necrosis of bone occurs, and not only in patients taking steroids. The femoral head, navicular bone, and tibial plateau are most commonly affected.

Dermatologic

Discoid lupus involves the face, scalp, and extremities. There is follicular plugging with atrophy leading to scarring. Subacute cutaneous LE is a subset of SLE that primarily has skin involvement with psoriasiform or annular erythematous lesions. Patients may be negative for antinuclear antibodies but frequently are positive for antibodies to the extractable nuclear antigen SS-A (Ro).

Cardiopulmonary

Cardiac involvement in SLE is manifested by pericarditis, myocarditis, valvular involvement, accelerated coronary atherosclerosis, and coronary vasculitis.

Pulmonary involvement in SLE is manifested by any of the following: pleurisy, pleural effusions, pneumonitis, pulmonary hypertension, hemorrhage, and diaphragmatic dysfunction.

Neuropsychiatric

Central nervous system lupus is a most variable and unpredictable phenomenon. Manifestations such as impaired cognitive function, seizures, long tract signs, cranial neuropathies, psychosis, and migraine-like attacks occur with little apparent relationship to each other or to other systemic manifestations. Immune complexes in the choroid plexus are *not* specific for central nervous system disease. They also occur in patients without central nervous system disease. There is no specific laboratory abnormality. Patients may have increased cerebrospinal fluid protein (IgG), pleocytosis, and anti-neuronal antibodies.

Results of electroencephalography can be abnormal. Brain scanning is of no help. Magnetic resonance imaging usually shows areas of increased signal in the periventricular white matter, similar to that found in multiple sclerosis. Magnetic resonance imaging findings are often nonspecific and some-

times can be seen in patients who have SLE without central nervous system manifestations. Pathologic examinations of autopsy specimens usually reveal microinfarcts, nerve cell loss, vasculitis, or no detectable abnormalities.

Proposed pathogenetic mechanisms causing neuropsychiatric manifestations include autoneuronal antibodies, vasculitis, leukoagglutination, antiphospholipid-associated hypercoagulability, and cytokine effect.

Psychosis caused by steroid therapy is probably rarer than previously thought. When in doubt about the cause of the psychosis, the steroid dose can be increased and the patient observed. Patients rarely can have isolated central nervous system involvement and normal results of cerebrospinal fluid examination and no other organ involvement.

Particularly with neuropsychiatric symptoms or respiratory symptoms, secondary causes must be considered, particularly infection, hypertension, anemia, hypoxia, and fever. Fever should be considered due to infection until proved otherwise.

- Central nervous system lupus is a most variable and unpredictable phenomenon.
- Immune complexes in choroid plexus are *not* specific for central nervous system disease.
- Electroencephalography can be abnormal in SLE.
- Magnetic resonance imaging findings are nonspecific.
- Particularly with neuropsychiatric symptoms or respiratory symptoms, secondary causes must be considered, particularly infection, hypertension, anemia, hypoxia, and fever.
- Fever should be considered due to infection until proved otherwise.

Pregnancy and SLE

Women with SLE who become pregnant have a high prevalence of spontaneous abortion. Because abortion itself may lead to a flare of the disease, therapeutic abortion ordinarily is not recommended after the first trimester. Flares of disease should be treated with steroids, particularly during the postpartum period.

In infants of mothers with SLE, thrombocytopenia and leukopenia can develop from passive transfer of antibodies. They also can have transient cutaneous lesions and transient complete heart block. Mothers usually have anti-SS-A (Ro), which crosses the placenta and is transiently present in the infant. Mothers usually are HLA-B8/DR3-positive, but there is no HLA association in the child. In some affected infants, no clinical disease is present in the mother, although antibodies are present.

Renal Involvement

The types of renal disease in SLE are 1) mesangial, 2) focal glomerulonephritis, 3) membranous glomerulonephritis, 4) diffuse proliferative glomerulonephritis, 5) interstitial nephritis with defects in the renal tubular handling of K^+, and 6) renal vein thrombosis with nephrotic syndrome.

Treatment of renal disease depends in part on the results of renal biopsy. Patients with mesangial changes alone do not require aggressive therapy. Patients with active diffuse proliferative glomerulonephritis are treated with high-dose steroids and immunosuppressive agents. Immunosuppressive agents lower the incidence of renal failure in patients with diffuse proliferative glomerulonephritis and may improve overall survival. Appropriate treatment for focal proliferative glomerulonephritis and membranous glomerulonephritis is controversial because the prognosis is more favorable. Renal biopsies can be helpful in directing therapy. Patients with high activity indices such as active inflammation, proliferation, necrosis, and crescent formation are considered for aggressive therapy. Patients with high chronicity indices such as tubular atrophy, scarring, and glomerulosclerosis are less likely to respond to aggressive therapy.

- Renal biopsies are helpful for directing therapy.
- Active diffuse proliferative glomerulonephritis is treated with high-dose steroids and immunosuppressive agents.
- Patients with mesangial changes alone do not require aggressive therapy.

Laboratory Findings

Anemia of chronic disease and hemolytic anemia (Coombs positive) can occur. Leukopenia usually does not predispose to infection. Antilymphocyte antibodies cause lymphopenia in SLE. Idiopathic thrombocytopenic purpura with the presence of platelet antibodies can be the initial manifestation of SLE. Polyclonal gammapathy due to hyperactivity of the humoral immune system is common. The erythrocyte sedimentation rate usually correlates with disease activity.

Hypocomplementemia (CH_{50}, C3, C4) usually correlates with active disease. Hypocomplementemia with increased anti-nDNA antibodies usually implies renal disease (or skin disease). Complement split products (such as C3a, C5a, Ba/BB) are increased in active disease. A total complement value too low to measure with normal C3 and C4 values suggests a hereditary complement deficiency. Familial C2 deficiency is the most common complement deficiency in SLE, but C1r, C1s, C1q, C4, C5, C7, and C8 deficiencies also have been reported.

Patients with SLE may have false-positive results of the VDRL test as a result of antibody to phospholipid, which cross-reacts with VDRL. Patients with SLE also can have false-positive results of the fluorescent treponemal antibody test, but this is usually of the "beaded pattern" of fluorescence. LE cells are present in approximately 70% of patients with SLE and are caused by antibody to deoxyribonucleoprotein (DNP). This test is not specific and is not performed in many centers. Anti-DNP also is detected by the fluorescent antinuclear antibody test in a homogeneous pattern.

Anti-nDNA levels fluctuate with disease activity, whereas levels of other autoantibodies (ribonucleoprotein, Sm, antinuclear antibody) show *no* consistent relationship to levels of anti-nDNA or disease activity. Methods used to measure anti-nDNA are 1) an immunofluorescent method using *Crithidia lucilia*, an organism with a kinetoplast that contains helical native DNA free of other nuclear antigens—therefore, there is no single-stranded DNA contamination; and 2) radioimmunoassay and other techniques, which suffer from the difficulty of maintaining DNA in its native double-stranded state and so are contaminated with single-stranded DNA.

Although all patients with lupus should have positive results of antinuclear antibody tests, a positive result is by no means specific for lupus. Antinuclear antibody patterns are outlined in Table 22-25. Other autoantibodies and disease associations are outlined in Table 22-26.

- Hemolytic anemia (Coombs positive) can occur in SLE.
- Idiopathic thrombocytopenic purpura can be the initial manifestation of SLE.
- Hypocomplementemia (CH_{50}, C3, C4) usually correlates with active disease.
- Hypocomplementemia with increased anti-nDNA antibodies usually implies renal disease (or skin disease).
- Anti-nDNA levels fluctuate with disease activity.

Table 22-25.—Antinuclear Antibody Patterns

Fluorescent pattern	Antigen	Disease association
Rim, peripheral, shaggy	nDNA	SLE
Homogeneous	DNP	SLE, others
Speckled	ENA	MCTD, SLE, others
Nucleolar	RNA	Scleroderma

DNP, deoxyribonucleoprotein; ENA, extractable nuclear antigens; MCTD, mixed connective tissue disease; RNA, ribonucleic acid; SLE, systemic lupus erythematosus.

Table 22-26.—Autoantibodies in Rheumatic Diseases

Antibody	Disease association
Anti-ssDNA	SLE, 100%
	High frequency in other CTD; also chronic infection, CAH, interstitial lung disease
Anti-nDNA	SLE, 50%-60%
Anti-Sm (Smith)	SLE, 30%
Anti-RNP (ribonuclear protein)	MCTD, 100% high titer
	SLE, 30% titer
	Scleroderma, low frequency, low titer
Anti-SS-A	Sjögren, 70%
	SLE, 35%
	Scleroderma + MCTD, low frequency, low titer
Anti-SS-B	Sjögren, 60%
	SLE, 15%
Antihistone	Drug-induced SLE, 95%
	SLE, 70%
	RA, 20%
Anti-Sc1-70 (antitopoisomerase I)	Scleroderma, 25%
Anticentromere	CREST, 70%-90%
	Scleroderma, 10%-15%
Anti-PM1	PM, 50%
Anti-Jo1 (histidyl-tRNA synthetase)	PM/interstitial lung disease, 30%

CAH, chronic active hepatitis; CREST, syndrome of *c*alcinosis cutis, *R*aynaud phenomenon, *e*sophageal dysmotility, *s*clerodactyly, *t*elangiectasia; CTD, connective tissue disease; MCTD, mixed connective tissue disease; PM, polymyositis; RA, rheumatoid arthritis; SLE, systemic lupus erythematosus.

● A positive result of an antinuclear antibody test is by no means specific for lupus.

Treatment

Treatment should match the activity of SLE in the individual patient. Serial monitoring of organ function and appropriate immunologic evaluation (anti-nDNA, C3, erythrocyte sedimentation rate) allow rapid recognition and treatment of flares and appropriate tapering of steroid dose during periods of disease quiescence. Table 22-27 provides guidelines for treatment, and Table 22-28 outlines the complications of treatment.

Outcome

The 10-year survival rate is 90% in newly diagnosed SLE. Prognosis is worse in blacks and Hispanics than in whites. Prognosis is worse in patients with creatinine values more than 3.0 mg/dL. The major causes of death are 1) renal disease, 2) infection, 3) central nervous system involvement, and 4) vascular disease (such as myocardial infarction).

● The 10-year survival rate is 90% in newly diagnosed SLE.
● The prognosis is worse in blacks and Hispanics.

DRUG-INDUCED LUPUS

Many drugs have been implicated in drug-induced lupus. The most common drugs are listed in Table 22-29. One must differentiate between the clinical syndrome of drug-induced lupus and only a positive antinuclear antibody result without clinical symptoms. Many drugs can cause a positive antinuclear antibody result without ever causing the clinical syndrome of drug-induced lupus. Only hydralazine and procainamide have been strongly implicated in drug-induced lupus. A drug-induced lupus syndrome develops in approximately 5% of persons taking hydralazine, and approximately 15% to 25% of those who take procainamide for 1 year will have a positive result of the antinuclear antibody test.

● Only hydralazine and procainamide are strongly implicated in drug-induced lupus.
● Virtually all patients taking procainamide for 1 year have a positive result of the antinuclear antibody test.

Clinical Features

The clinical manifestations of drug-induced lupus are arthralgias and polyarthritis, which occur in approximately

Table 22-27.—Treatment of Manifestations of Systemic Lupus Erythematosus

Manifestation	Treatment
Arthritis, fever, mild systemic symptoms	ASA, NSAID
Photosensitivity, rash	Avoidance of sun, use of sunscreens
Rash, arthritis	Hydroxychloroquine (Plaquenil)
Significant thrombocytopenia, hemolytic anemia	Steroids
Renal disease, CNS disease, pericarditis, other significant organ involvement	Steroids
Rapidly deteriorating renal function	Cytotoxic agents

ASA, acetylsalicylic acid; CNS, central nervous system; NSAID, nonsteroidal anti-inflammatory drug.

Table 22-28.—Complications of Treatment for Systemic Lupus Erythematosus

Treatment	Complication
Ibuprofen	Aseptic meningitis (headache, fever, stiff neck, CSF pleocytosis)
NSAID	Decreased renal blood flow
ASA	Salicylate hepatitis (common), benign
Cyclophosphamide	Hemorrhagic cystitis, alopecia, opportunistic lymphomas, infection, increased incidence of lymphomas (CNS)
Hydroxychloroquine (Plaquenil)	Retinal toxicity

ASA, acetylsalicylic acid; CNS, central nervous system; CSF, cerebrospinal fluid; NSAID, nonsteroidal anti-inflammatory drug.

Table 22-29.—Implicated Agents in Drug-Induced Lupus

Definite	Probable
Common	Phenytoin
Procainamide	Carbamazepine
Hydralazine	Ethosuximide
Uncommon	Propylthiouracil
Isoniazid	Penicillamine
Methyldopa	Sulfasalazine
Chlorpromazine	Lithium carbonate
Quinidine	Acebutolol
	Lovastatin

80% of cases. Malaise is common, and fever has been reported in up to 40% of cases. Cardiopulmonary involvement is common, and approximately 30% of patients have pleural-pulmonary manifestations as their presenting symptoms. Pericarditis has been reported in approximately 20% of cases. Diffuse interstitial pneumonitis has been noted. Asymptomatic pleural effusions may be found on routine chest radiography. A few cases of pericardial tamponade have been reported. In contrast to SLE, the incidence of renal and central nervous system involvement is low in drug-induced lupus. Therefore, it is regarded as more benign than SLE. Clinical differences include a lower incidence of skin manifestations, lymphadenopathy, and myalgias in drug-induced disease.

- In drug-induced lupus, arthralgias and polyarthritis occur in about 80% of cases.
- Malaise is common, and fever occurs in up to 40% of cases.
- About 30% of patients have pleural-pulmonary manifestations.
- Pericarditis is reported in about 20% of cases.
- The incidence of renal and central nervous system involvement is low.

Other differences between drug-induced lupus and SLE include age and sex distribution. SLE is predominantly a disease of premenopausal females, whereas drug-induced disease has an almost equal sex distribution and occurs in an older population. This disparity in age reflects the use of hydralazine and procainamide in primarily an older population.

Laboratory Abnormalities

Virtually all patients with SLE and drug-induced lupus have antinuclear antibodies. Although patients with SLE and drug-induced lupus are serologically similar in many respects, there are notable differences. Antibodies to native DNA are found in only a small percentage of cases of drug-induced lupus but in approximately 60% of cases of SLE. Serum total hemolytic complement, C3, and C4 are usually normal in drug-induced disease, in contrast to SLE. Antibodies such as anti-SM, SS-A, SS-B, and RNP are also unusual in drug-induced lupus. The frequency of antihistone antibodies in drug-induced lupus is high (>95% of cases), but these also occur in approximately 60% of cases of SLE. Other, less frequent laboratory abnormalities in drug-induced lupus can include a positive LE preparation, positive Coombs test, positive rheumatoid factor, false-positive result of serologic test for syphilis, circulating anticoagulants, and cryoglobulins.

Metabolism

Drugs involved in drug-induced lupus have different chemical structures, but three of them—isoniazid, procainamide, and hydralazine—contain a primary amine or hydralazine that is acetylated by the hepatic N-acetyltransferase system. Persons who are taking one of these drugs and who are *slow* acetylators have a much higher incidence of serologic abnormalities and clinical disease than rapid acetylators. These manifestations also occur over a shorter period in slow acetylators than in rapid acetylators.

- Slow acetylators have a much higher incidence of serologic abnormalities and clinical disease.

Treatment

When possible, patients with drug-induced lupus should stop using the offending drug. Symptoms usually subside within several weeks, although the duration for complete resolution varies depending on the drug. Serologic abnormalities can remain for years after resolution of clinical symptoms. Patients taking procainamide are most likely to have a rapid remission once use of the drug is stopped, but patients taking hydralazine might have prolonged clinical manifestations. Treatment depends on the clinical manifestations and could include aspirin or other NSAIDs or possibly prednisone if needed.

OVERLAP SYNDROMES

An overlap syndrome is a disease characterized by features of more than one connective tissue disease. Secondary Sjögren syndrome accompanying another connective disease is not classified as an overlap syndrome.

Mixed Connective Tissue Disease

This is described as a distinct disease with variable features of SLE, polymyositis, systemic sclerosis, and rheumatoid arthritis. The incidence of renal disease is low. It is serologically characterized by a positive antinuclear antibody and by a high titer of the autoantibody anti-RNP. Anti-nDNA antibodies usually are not present. Raynaud phenomenon is common.

Undifferentiated Connective Tissue Disease

This category includes patients with symptoms that do not fulfill the diagnostic criteria for a definite or specific connective tissue disease. Common symptoms include Raynaud phenomenon, arthralgias, fatigue, and variable joint or soft tissue swelling. The antinuclear antibody may be positive, but other autoantibodies are not present. Patients need to be observed to determine whether progression to a distinct connective tissue disease occurs.

ANTIPHOSPHOLIPID SYNDROME

The lupus anticoagulant and various phospholipid antibodies have been associated with recurrent arterial and venous thromboses. Antiphospholipid antibodies may be either the IgG or the IgM immunoglobulin class and are routinely measured as anticardiolipin antibodies. The hallmark of the antiphospholipid antibody syndrome is prolongation of all phospholipid-dependent coagulation tests. The antibodies prolong the partial thromboplastin time at the level of the prothrombin activator complex of the clotting cascade. The antiphospholipid antibodies are thought to interact with the β_2-glycoprotein-1 that binds to phospholipid or the phospholipid itself, interfering with the calcium-ion-dependent binding of prothrombin factor Xa to the phospholipid. The failure of normal plasma to correct the prolonged clotting time distinguishes the lupus anticoagulant and antiphospholipid antibodies from antibodies directed against specific clotting factors and from clotting factor deficiencies. In the usual coagulation screening tests, the lupus anticoagulant results in prolongation of the activated partial thromboplastin time with or without slight prolongation of the prothrombin time (Table 22-30).

- Antiphospholipid antibodies are of either the IgG or the IgM immunoglobulin class.
- Prolongation of all phospholipid-dependent coagulation tests is the laboratory hallmark of the antiphospholipid antibody syndrome.
- Activated partial thromboplastin time is prolonged and not corrected by adding normal plasma.

Various other tests are reported to be sensitive for detection of lupus anticoagulants, including the plasma clot time, kaolin

Table 22-30.—Coagulation Tests Characterizing the Lupus
Anticoagulant

Screening tests
    Prothrombin time (PT) normal or prolonged
    Partial thromboplastin time (PTT) prolonged
    Plasma clot time prolonged
Tests identifying the lupus anticoagulant
    Prolonged PTT not corrected by adding normal plasma

clotting time, a platelet neutralization procedure, and modified Russell viper venom time.

Many, but not all, patients with lupus anticoagulant have increased IgG or IgM antiphospholipid antibody levels.

The lupus anticoagulant and antiphospholipid antibodies are commonly associated with SLE, but they also have been reported in various other autoimmune, malignant, infectious, and drug-induced diseases. Other diseases include Sjögren syndrome, rheumatoid arthritis, idiopathic thrombocytopenic purpura, Behçet syndrome, myasthenia gravis, and mixed connective tissue disease. The antibodies also can be found in persons who have no apparent disease but in whom recurrent thrombosis develops.

- Lupus anticoagulant and antiphospholipid antibodies also have been reported in various other autoimmune, malignant, infectious, and drug-induced diseases.

Clinical Features

There is an association between the presence of the lupus anticoagulant and antiphospholipid antibodies and recurrent venous or arterial thrombosis. Thrombotic events described have included stroke, transient ischemic attacks, myocardial infarctions, brachial artery thrombosis, deep venous thrombophlebitis, retinal vein thrombosis, hepatic vein thrombosis resulting in Budd-Chiari syndrome, and pulmonary hypertension. Other manifestations include recurrent fetal loss, thrombocytopenia, positive results of Coombs test, migraines, chorea, epilepsy, chronic leg ulcers, livedo reticularis, and progressive dementia resulting from cerebrovascular accidents. Recently, acquired valvular heart disease, especially aortic insufficiency, has been described. The mechanism or mechanisms by which antiphospholipid antibodies are associated with thromboembolic manifestations remain unclear. Blocking the production of prostacyclin from vascular endothelial cells, inhibition of the prekallikrein activity protein C pathway and fibrinolysis, and decreased plasminogen activator release have all been described.

Although many patients with lupus and other diseases can have a lupus anticoagulant or antiphospholipid antibodies, of either the IgG or the IgM class, thrombosis will not necessarily develop. In general, patients with the highest levels of antiphospholipid antibodies are more prone to thrombosis than those with lower levels. Also, the IgG antiphospholipid antibody is much more strongly associated with recurrent thrombosis than is the IgM antiphospholipid antibody. If there is no history of thrombosis, most physicians are reluctant to treat the patient for a lupus anticoagulant or increased antiphospholipid antibodies alone without clinical manifestations.

- There is association between the presence of the lupus anticoagulant and antiphospholipid antibodies and recurrent venous or arterial thrombosis.
- Other manifestations: recurrent fetal loss, thrombocytopenia, positive Coombs test, migraines, chorea, epilepsy, chronic leg ulcers, livedo reticularis, and progressive dementia from cerebrovascular accidents.
- Acquired valvular heart disease, especially aortic insufficiency, has been described.
- Patients with the highest levels of antiphospholipid antibodies are more prone to thrombosis.
- IgG antiphospholipid antibody is more strongly associated with recurrent thrombosis.

Treatment

For most patients who have recurrent thrombosis and high-titer anticardiolipin antibody, warfarin (Coumadin) is prescribed in doses sufficient to yield INR values close to 3 and will need to be taken for life. Low-dose aspirin and subcutaneous heparin have been used in pregnant women to prevent fetal loss. Corticosteroids have not been clearly demonstrated to be efficacious in preventing thrombosis.

RAYNAUD PHENOMENON

This is biphasic or triphasic color changes (pallor, cyanosis, erythema) accompanied by pain and numbness in the hands or feet. Cold is a common precipitating agent. Associated factors are listed in Table 22-31.

- Cold is a common precipitating agent for Raynaud phenomenon.

Raynaud phenomenon is related to an abnormality of the microvasculature associated with intimal fibrosis. In male patients with Raynaud phenomenon, a rare occurrence, a connective tissue disease may develop. Although Raynaud phenomenon is common in females, it usually is not associated with a connective tissue disease unless the patient has positive results for antinuclear antibody, which suggest that a connective tissue disease may develop in the future.

Table 22-31.—Causes of Secondary Raynaud Phenomenon

Chemotherapeutic agents
   Bleomycin
   Vinblastine
Toxins
   Vinyl chloride
Vibration-induced injuries
   Jackhammer use
Vascular occlusive disorders
   Thoracic outlet obstruction
   Atherosclerosis
   Vasculitis
Connective tissue diseases
   Scleroderma, 90%-100%
   Mixed connective tissue disease, 90%-100%
   Systemic lupus erythematosus, 15%
   Rheumatoid arthritis, <10%
   Polymyositis
Miscellaneous
   Cryoglobulinemia
   Cold agglutinins
   Increased blood viscosity

Skin capillary microscopy reveals tortuous, dilated capillary loops in systemic sclerosis, mixed connective tissue disease, and polymyositis. They also may be present in patients with Raynaud phenomenon who will go on to develop systemic sclerosis, polymyositis, or mixed connective tissue disease.

Treatment involves smoking cessation, wearing gloves, biofeedback, 2% nitrol paste, and antihypertensive agents (methyldopa, prazosin, dibenzyline, nifedipine). A stellate ganglion block or digital nerve block is used if ischemia is severe. β-Adrenergic blockers increase spasm and so are not used.

To differentiate primary Raynaud phenomenon from the secondary form (resulting from a connective tissue disease), clinical features are considered. In primary Raynaud disease, females are usually affected, the onset is at menarche, usually all digits are involved, and attacks are very frequent. The severity of symptoms is mild to moderate, and they can be precipitated by emotional stress. Digital ulceration and finger edema are rare, as is periungual erythema. Livedo reticularis is frequent. In persons with Raynaud phenomenon due to a connective tissue disease, both males and females are affected. The onset of Raynaud phenomenon is in the mid-20s or later. It often begins in a single digit, and attacks are usually infrequent (zero to five a day). The severity is moderate to severe, and the disorder is not precipitated by emotional stress. Digital ulceration occurs in 30% to 50% of cases, and finger edema and periungual erythema are frequent. Livedo reticularis is uncommon.

SYSTEMIC SCLEROSIS (SCLERODERMA)

For the diagnosis of systemic sclerosis, one major criterion or two or more minor criteria need to be present. The major criterion is symmetrical induration of the skin of the fingers and skin proximal to metacarpophalangeal or metatarsophalangeal joints. The minor criteria are sclerodactyly, digital pitting scars or loss of substance from the finger pad, and bibasilar pulmonary fibrosis.

- Systemic sclerosis is characterized by symmetrical induration of the skin of the fingers and skin proximal to metacarpophalangeal or metatarsophalangeal joints, sclerodactyly, fingertip pitting or scarring, and bibasilar pulmonary fibrosis.

Clinical Manifestations

Skin

Patients are at risk for the development of rapidly progressive acral and trunk skin thickening and early visceral abnormalities. Skin and visceral changes tend to parallel each other in severity, but not always. Some patients have rapid progression for 2 to 3 years and then arrest of the disorder, allowing for some improvement of the disorder.

Raynaud Phenomenon

Raynaud phenomenon occurs in almost *all* patients. It usually occurs more than 2 years before skin changes. The vasospasm in the hands can be associated with reduced perfusion to the heart, lungs, kidneys, and gastrointestinal tract. If Raynaud phenomenon is not present but skin findings are suggestive of scleroderma, another disease such as eosinophilic fasciitis should be considered.

Articular

Nondeforming symmetrical polyarthritis similar to rheumatoid arthritis may precede cutaneous manifestations by 12 months. Patients can have both articular erosions and nonarticular bony resorptive changes of ribs, mandible, radius, ulna, and distal phalangeal tufts which are unique to systemic sclerosis. Up to 60% of patients have "leathery" crepitation of the tendons of the wrist.

Pulmonary

A significant decrease in CO diffusion can be present with a normal chest radiograph. Diffuse interstitial fibrosis occurs in approximately 70% of patients and is the most common pulmonary abnormality. Pleuritis (with effusion) is very rare. Pulmonary hypertension is more common in patients with CREST variant.

- A significant decrease in CO diffusion can be present with a normal chest radiograph.
- Diffuse interstitial fibrosis occurs in approximately 70% of patients and is the most common pulmonary abnormality.
- Pleuritis is very rare.
- Pulmonary hypertension is more common in patients with CREST variant.

Cardiac

Cardiac abnormalities occur in up to 70% of patients. Conduction defects and supraventricular arrhythmias are most common. Pulmonary hypertension with cor pulmonale is the most serious problem.

- Cardiac abnormalities occur in up to 70% of patients.
- Pulmonary hypertension with cor pulmonale is a serious potential problem.

Gastrointestinal

Esophageal dysfunction is the most frequent gastrointestinal abnormality. It occurs in 90% of patients and often is asymptomatic. Lower esophageal sphincter incompetence with acid reflux may produce esophageal strictures or ulcers. Medications to reduce acid production are important. Reduced esophageal motility may respond to therapy with metoclopramide, cisapride, or erythromycin. Small bowel hypomotility may be associated with pseudo-obstruction, bowel dilatation, bacterial overgrowth, and malabsorption. Treatment with tetracycline may be helpful, but pro-motility agents are less effective. Colonic dysmotility also occurs.

Renal

Renal involvement may result in fulminant hypertension, renal failure, and death if not treated aggressively. Proteinuria, newly diagnosed *mild* hypertension, microangiopathic hemolytic anemia, vascular changes on renal biopsy, and rapid progression of skin thickening may precede overt clinical findings of renal crisis. Renal involvement with hyper-reninemia requires the use of angiotensin-converting enzyme inhibitors. Aggressive early antihypertensive therapy can extend life expectancy.

Laboratory Findings

Antitopoisomerase I antibody (anti-Scl-70) is found in approximately 25% of patients with scleroderma, and anti-centromere antibody occurs in 10% to 20%.

Treatment

No remissive or curative therapy is available. Retrospective studies suggest that D-penicillamine (750 mg daily) may decrease skin thickness, prevent or delay internal organ involvement, and prolong life expectancy. Aggressive nutritional support, including hyperalimentation, may be required for extensive gastrointestinal disease.

- No remissive or curative therapy is available for systemic sclerosis.

CREST SYNDROME

This is characterized by *c*alcinosis cutis, *R*aynaud phenomenon, *e*sophageal dysmotility, *s*clerodactyly, and *t*elangiectasias. Skin involvement progresses slowly and is limited to the extremities. Development of internal organ involvement occurs but is delayed. Lung involvement occurs in 70% of patients. Diffusing capacity is low, and pulmonary hypertension can develop. The latter is more common in CREST than in diffuse scleroderma. Onset of Raynaud phenomenon occurs before skin changes (less than 2 years before skin changes). Anticentromere antibody is found in 70% to 90% of patients and antiscleroderma-70 antibody in 10%. The incidence of primary biliary cirrhosis is increased.

- In CREST syndrome, 70% of patients have lung involvement.
- The diffusing capacity is low, and pulmonary hypertension can develop.
- Anticentromere antibody is present in 70%-90% of patients.
- There is an increased incidence of primary biliary cirrhosis.

The clinical manifestations of limited and systemic scleroderma are listed in Table 22-32.

SCLERODERMA-LIKE SYNDROMES

Disorders Associated With Occupation or Environment

This group includes polyvinyl chloride disease, organic solvents, jackhammer disease, silicosis, silicone implants (still a controversial association), and toxic oil syndrome.

Eosinophilic Fasciitis

Clinical features of this disorder include tight bound-down skin of the extremities, characteristically sparing the hands and feet. Peau d'orange skin changes can develop. Onset after vigorous exercise is common. Raynaud phenomenon does not occur, and there is no visceral

Table 22-32.—Clinical Findings in Limited and Diffuse Scleroderma

Clinical finding	Cutaneous disease	
	Limited	Diffuse
Raynaud phenomenon	Precedes other symptoms by years	Onset associated with other symptoms within 1 year
Nailfold capillaries	Dilated	Dilated with dropout
Skin changes	Distal to elbow	Proximal to elbow with involvement of trunk
Telangiectases, digital ulcers, calcinosis	Frequent	Rare early, but frequent later in the course
Joint and tendon involvement	Uncommon	Frequent (tendon rubs)
Visceral disease	Pulmonary hypertension	Renal, intestinal, and cardiac disease; pulmonary interstitial fibrosis
Autoantibodies	Anticentromere (40%-70%)	Antitopoisomerase 1 (Scl-70) (25%-40%)
10-year survival	>70%	<70%

involvement. Flexion contractures and carpal tunnel syndrome can develop.

Laboratory findings are peripheral eosinophilia, increased sedimentation rate, and hypergammaglobulinemia. The diagnosis is based on the findings of inflammation and thickening of the fascia on deep fascial biopsy. Treatment is with prednisone (40 mg daily). The response is usually good. Associated conditions are aplastic anemia and thrombocytopenia (both antibody-mediated) as well as leukemia and myeloproliferative diseases.

- Eosinophilic fasciitis is characterized by tight bound-down skin of the extremities, usually sparing the hands and feet.
- There is no visceral involvement.
- Laboratory findings include peripheral eosinophilia.
- Treatment with prednisone provides good response.

Metabolic Causes of Scleroderma-Like Syndrome

This group includes porphyria, amyloidosis, carcinoid, and diabetes mellitus (flexion contractures of the tendons in the hands can develop).

Other Causes

As a manifestation of *graft-versus-host disease*, skin induration develops in up to 30% of patients who receive bone marrow transplant. *Drug-induced disorders* are caused by carbidopa, bleomycin, and bromocriptine. *Eosinophilic myalgia syndrome* is associated with ingestion of contaminated L-tryptophan. Eosinophilia, myositis, skin induration, fasciitis, and peripheral neuropathy develop. Skin changes are similar to those of eosinophilic fasciitis. There is a poor response to steroids. *Scleredema* frequently occurs after streptococcal upper respiratory tract infection in children. It is usually self-limiting. Swelling of the head and neck is common. In adults, diabetes mellitus often is associated. *Scleromyxedema* is associated with IgG monoclonal protein. Cocaine use and appetite suppressants also cause scleroderma-like illness.

THE INFLAMMATORY MYOPATHIES

Inflammatory myopathies can be classified into several categories, including polymyositis, dermatomyositis, myositis associated with malignancy, childhood-type, and overlap connective tissue disease. Polymyositis is an inflammatory myopathy characterized by proximal muscle weakness. Patients with dermatomyositis can have an associated rash that includes a heliotrope hue of the eyelids, a rash on the metacarpophalangeal and proximal interphalangeal joints (Gottron papules), and photosensitivity dermatitis of the face. Most patients have an increased creatine kinase level, a characteristic electromyogram, and a characteristic muscle biopsy.

The electromyogram is characteristic but not diagnostic of inflammatory myopathies. It shows decreased amplitude and increased spike frequency, it is polyphasic, and conduction speed is normal. Fibrillation is not specific for inflammatory myopathies, but when present it indicates active disease. Loss of fibrillation usually means the inflammatory myopathy is under control, but if the electromyogram is still myopathic, it suggests an associated steroid myopathy caused by treatment. The muscle biopsy, which is mandatory in all patients with inflammatory myopathy, shows degeneration, necrosis, and regeneration of myofibrils and lymphocytic plus monocytic infiltrate in a perivascular or interstitial distribution.

In patients older than 40 years, perhaps 10% of those with dermatomyositis have an associated malignancy. The antibody anti-Jo1 is associated with polymyositis and dermatomyositis in approximately 25% of cases. This antibody is associated with inflammatory arthritis, progressive interstitial lung disease, Raynaud phenomenon, and increased mortality primarily due to respiratory failure. The autoantibody anti-Mi-2 is associated with dermatomyositis in 2% to 20% of patients.

- Polymyositis is an inflammatory myopathy characterized by proximal muscle weakness.
- Dermatomyositis is an inflammatory myopathy plus a rash that includes heliotrope hue of eyelids.
- Electromyogram is characteristic but not diagnostic of polymyositis.
- Perhaps 10% of patients older than 40 years with dermatomyositis have associated malignancy.
- Anti-Jo1 is associated with polymyositis and dermatomyositis in about 25% of cases.

Treatment of polymyositis includes prednisone (60 mg daily), usually for 1 to 2 months, until the muscle enzyme values normalize. The dosage is slowly reduced thereafter, and the clinical course and creatine kinase values are monitored. In steroid-resistant cases, either azathioprine (1-2 mg/kg per day) or methotrexate can be used.

Aspiration pneumonia can occur as a result of pharyngeal weakness. If so, a liquid diet, feeding tube, or feeding gastrostomy is needed until there is clinical improvement.

Inclusion Body Myositis

With regard to the differential diagnosis of inflammatory myopathies, inclusion body myositis needs to be considered. This usually occurs in the older age group. The onset of weakness is more insidious, occurring over many years. The creatine kinase value often is only minimally to several times increased, and distal weakness and proximal weakness occur. The electromyogram, besides showing a myopathic picture, also can have an associated neuropathic picture. The diagnosis of inclusion body myositis is made from biopsy. Histopathologic findings are indistinguishable from those of polymyositis except for the presence of eosinophilic inclusions and rimmed vacuoles with basophilic enhancement. Inclusion body myositis responds poorly to prednisone and immunosuppressive therapy, and the course is one of slow, progressive weakness.

- Inclusion body myositis usually occurs in older age group.
- Diagnosis is made from biopsy.
- It responds poorly to prednisone.

DRUG-INDUCED MYOPATHIES

Muscle Disease

Drugs may cause an inflammatory myopathy. The myopathy associated with colchicine mimics polymyositis, and patients have muscle weakness and an increased creatine kinase level. This often occurs in the setting of a patient with gout and renal insufficiency taking long-term colchicine. Lipid-lowering drugs such as lovastatin, zidovudine, D-penicillamine, and addictive drugs such as heroine or cocaine have all been associated with myopathy.

INFECTIOUS ARTHRITIS

An infectious cause should be ruled out immediately in a patient with acute monarticular arthritis. Approximately 5% to 10% of patients with septic arthritis present with multiple joint involvement.

Bacterial Arthritis

Nongonococcal bacterial arthritis is caused by hematogenous spread of bacteria, direct inoculation (which is usually traumatic), or extension of soft tissue infection with osteomyelitis into the joint space. Large joints are more commonly affected. Patients who are elderly or immunosuppressed are predisposed to septic arthropathy, including patients with cancer, diabetes mellitus, chronic renal failure, liver disease, or sickle cell anemia. Patients with chronic inflammatory and degenerative arthritis are also at increased risk for septic arthritis, and the possibility of septic arthritis should be considered in patients with a preexisting polyarthritis who have a single joint flare that is out of proportion to the rest of their joint symptoms. In any patient with a septic joint, the possibility of infectious endocarditis, other septic joints, or a disk space infection should be considered.

Septic arthritis is a medical emergency. A thorough search for a source of an infection is important. Joint aspiration is required. Gram staining of centrifuged synovial fluid and appropriate cultures should be performed. Typically, patients with nongonococcal septic arthritis have a leukocyte value of more than 50,000/μL in the synovial fluid. Low glucose levels in synovial fluid and high levels of lactic acid are common but not specific for septic arthritis. Blood cultures should be performed when septic arthritis is considered. Radiographs of an involved joint may demonstrate an associated osteomyelitis or previous local trauma, but radiographic findings of infection usually lag considerably behind clinical symptoms.

Staphylococcus aureus is the most common pathogen in adult patients with nongonococcal bacterial arthritis. In sickle cell anemia, *Salmonella* is the organism commonly causing septic arthritis. *Pseudomonas* should be considered in the context of cat or dog bites, and an aerobic infection should be considered in cases of human bites. Intravenous drug users may have bacteremia with unusual organisms, such as *Pseudomonas* or *Serratia*, and this may present with septic arthritis in unusual locations, such as the sternoclavicular or sacroiliac joints. The portal of entry may help predict the infecting organism; for example, gram-negative bacilli, such as *E. coli* and *Klebsiella*, may cause septic arthritis in older patients with gastrointestinal or genitourinary infections or instrumentation.

Broad-spectrum antibiotics should be used until culture results are available. Daily aspiration of the affected joint should be performed until clinical improvement is obvious. Synovial fluid leukocytes and volume should decrease, or orthopedic arthroscopic or open drainage should be considered. Such drainage usually is indicated in joints such as the hip, which are not readily accessible. The duration of treatment depends on the virulence of the organisms, but antibiotics usually are given intravenously for at least 2 weeks.

- Nongonococcal bacterial arthritis usually is caused by hematogenous spread of bacteria, direct inoculation (which is usually traumatic), or extension of soft tissue infection or osteomyelitis.
- Synovial fluid Gram stain and culture are essential.
- The portal of entry may predict the organism causing septic arthritis.
- Antibiotics should be initiated even before culture results are available.
- If repeated aspiration and antibiotics do not lead to clinical improvement as well as a decrease in synovial fluid volume and leukocytosis, then arthroscopic or open drainage and debridement may be necessary.

Gonococcal Arthritis

Disseminated gonococcal infection develops in approximately 0.2% of patients with gonorrhea. The male-to-female ratio is 3:1. This is the most common form of septic arthritis in younger, sexually active persons who may be asymptomatic carriers of gonococci. When gonococcal infection is suspected, specimens from the pharynx, joints, rectum, blood, and genitourinary tract should be cultured. Females present with gonococcal arthritis commonly during pregnancy or within 1 week after onset of menses, possibly related to the pH of vaginal secretions. The most common form of gonococcal arthritis is the disseminated gonococcal arthritis syndrome with fever, dermatitis, and an inflammatory tenosynovitis. Approximately 50% of these patients present with an inflammatory arthritis, commonly of the knee, wrist, or ankle. Tenosynovitis is more common than large joint effusions. Rash, sometimes with pustules or hemorrhagic vesicles, is common. The second form

of gonococcal arthritis commonly begins as a migratory polyarthralgia, which subsequently localizes to one or more joints.

Synovial fluid cultures are positive in only 30% of patients with known disseminated gonococcal infection. Culture of the skin lesion is positive for gonococcus in 40% to 60% of patients with disseminated gonococcal infection. The leukocyte count in the joint fluid may be lower than in the other types of septic arthritis. Joint effusions in patients with disseminated gonococcal infection may be related to a *reactive* postinfectious response rather than to bacterial invasion. Patients who have recurrent disseminated gonococcal infection may have an associated terminal complement component deficiency (C5-C9).

Most patients with disseminated gonococcal arthritis are treated as outpatients. Current treatment recommendations suggest a later third-generation cephalosporin, such as ceftriaxone, 1.0 g per day. Treatment involves a minimum of a 7-day course. Treatment should include an anti-chlamydial antibiotic.

- Gonococcal arthritis develops in 0.2% of patients with gonorrhea.
- In the disseminated gonococcal arthritis syndrome, fever, dermatitis, and tenosynovitis are common.
- In the nonbacteremic form of gonococcal arthritis, migratory polyarthralgias are followed by inflammation localizing to one or more joints.
- Synovial fluid cultures are positive in 30% of patients with known disseminated gonococcal infection.
- Joint fluid leukocyte counts may be lower than in other types of septic arthritis.
- Joint effusions may be related to a reactive or postinfectious arthritis.
- Treatment recommendations are the use of a later third-generation cephalosporin (e.g., ceftriaxone).
- Treatment should include an anti-chlamydial antibiotic.

Mycobacterial and Fungal Joint Infections

These types of organisms usually cause chronic bone and joint infections. Months are required for radiographic changes to be obvious. A synovial biopsy and culture may be required to document these infections. Tuberculous arthritis is often otherwise asymptomatic and usually is caused by direct extension from adjacent bony infection. Atypical mycobacterial infection may cause an inflammatory arthritis and tenosynovitis. Surgical excision and prolonged treatment with multiple drug regimens are often required. Sporotrichosis and blastomycosis are the fungi most likely to have osteoarticular manifestations.

- Tuberculous arthritis is often otherwise asymptomatic and is caused by direct extension from adjacent bony infection.

- Atypical mycobacteria may cause an inflammatory arthritis and tenosynovitis.
- Sporotrichosis and blastomycosis are the fungi most likely to have osteoarticular manifestations.

Spinal Septic Arthritis

This condition should be suspected in patients with acute or chronic, unrelenting back pain associated with fever and marked local tenderness. The thoracolumbar region is most commonly affected. An antecendent infection or procedure predisposing to bacteremia may help suggest this diagnosis. Imaging studies usually have evidence for infection crossing the disc space. In tuberculous spinal septic arthritis (Pott disease), the site of involvement is most commonly T10-L2, and there is usually an associated paraspinal abscess.

Intravertebral disc infection is often a difficult diagnosis to establish because pain patterns may be unusual and localizing signs may be absent. Bone scanning may be helpful, but magnetic resonance imaging may be very helpful, particularly because of the ability to show extension of infection into surrounding tissues.

Infected Joint Prostheses

Infection in joint prostheses occurs in approximately 1% to 5% of all joint replacements. Symptoms and signs of infection may be difficult to detect during the postoperative period. Fever may not be present, and laboratory findings are often unhelpful. There may or may not be evidence of loosening of the cement holding the new joint in place, and radiographs may reveal lytic changes around the prosthesis. A negative bone scan is reassuring. Aspiration of fluid from the prosthetic joint is necessary to confirm infection. Prosthetic joint arthritis usually is caused by gram-positive organisms, particularly *Staphylococcus aureus* and *Staphylococcus epidermidis* in the first 6 months after the replacement surgery and by gram-negative and fungal organisms after 6 months. In long-standing prosthetic joints, return of pain and evidence of prosthetic loosening may be the only signs and symptoms. Patients with prosthetic joints require antibiotic prophylaxis before invasive dental, gastrointestinal, or genitourinary procedures.

- Prosthetic joint arthritis usually is caused by a gram-positive organism within the first 6 months after joint replacement.
- Prosthetic joint infections usually are caused by gram-negative or fungal organisms beyond the initial 6 months after joint replacement.

LYME DISEASE

Lyme disease is a tick-borne spirochetal illness with acute and chronic manifestations affecting the skin, heart, joints, and nervous system primarily. Diagnosis is important because treatment with appropriate antibiotics at an early stage of disease can prevent chronic sequelae. Even some chronic symptoms are treatable. Endemic areas in the United States include Connecticut, Delaware, Maryland, Massachusetts, New Jersey, New York, Pennsylvania, Rhode Island, Minnesota, Wisconsin, California, Nevada, Oregon, and Utah.

- Lyme disease is a tick-borne spirochetal illness.
- Acute and chronic manifestations affect skin, heart, joints, and nervous system.

The Tick

Ticks that transmit Lyme disease include *Ixodes dammini* in the northeastern and midwestern United States and *Ixodes pacificus* in the western United States. *Amblyomma americanum* ("lone star" tick) is a possible vector in the eastern, southern, and western United States. *Ixodes scapularis* is the common deer tick. It has a wide distribution. Humans are accidental hosts.

The Spirochete

Borrelia burgdorferi was an unknown organism until isolated initially from ticks by Burgdorfer in 1983. It is similar to an organism causing relapsing fever. It apparently exists only in the digestive tract of tick vectors.

Clinical Stages

Signs and symptoms occur in stages that may overlap. Later stages may occur *without* evidence of previous disease.

Stage I

About 50% of patients experience erythema chronicum migrans. Flu-like symptoms, including fever, headache, malaise, and adenopathy, can occur. They usually occur several days to a month after the tick bite.

- In stage I Lyme disease, about 50% of patients experience erythema chronicum migrans.

Stage II

Symptoms begin weeks to months after the initial symptoms in stage I. Disseminated infection develops and can include symptoms of the skin, musculoskeletal system, heart, and nervous system. In approximately 15% of patients, neurologic symptoms develop, including Bell palsy, meningoencephalitis, and sensory and motor radiculoneuritis. Approximately 5% of patients have cardiac abnormalities, including heart block. About 30% to 50% of patients have arthritis. This usually affects large joints, primarily the knees, and joint fluid analysis shows a leukocytosis similar to that in rheumatoid arthritis. Baker cysts may form early and are prone to rupture in patients who have arthritis of the knees.

- In stage II Lyme disease, symptoms begin weeks to months after initial symptoms of stage I.
- Disseminated infection develops.
- 15% of patients have neurologic symptoms.
- 5% of patients have cardiac abnormalities.
- 30%-50% of patients have arthritis.

Stage III

This usually occurs several years after the initial onset of illness. Episodes of arthritis can develop and become chronic. Histologically, the synovium resembles that in rheumatoid arthritis, although a unique feature of Lyme arthritis is the finding of an obliterative endarteritis. Spirochetes occasionally are seen in and around the blood vessels. Patients in whom chronic joint disease develops have increased frequency of HLA-DR4, often in combination with HLA-DR2. Patients with chronic arthritis have a poor response to antibiotics.

- Stage III Lyme disease occurs several years after initial onset of illness.
- Episodes of arthritis can be chronic.
- Synovium resembles that in rheumatoid arthritis.
- A unique feature of Lyme arthritis is obliterative endarteritis in the synovium.
- Patients with chronic joint disease have increased frequency of HLA-DR4, often in combination with HLA-DR2.

Diagnosis

Culturing the organism is difficult and of low yield. Antibody to spirochete can be measured by several techniques. The enzyme-linked immunosorbent assay (ELISA) is most commonly performed, but this is not standardized and there is a significant frequency of false-positive results. Patients with other autoimmune disease can have false-positive results. Also, such results may occur in syphilis, relapsing fever, and Rocky Mountain spotted fever. Although patients with syphilis have false-positive Lyme serologic results by ELISA, patients with Lyme disease have negative results of the VDRL test. Up to 25% of patients with lupus and rheumatoid arthritis have false-positive results of Lyme test by ELISA. It is important to remember that test results remain negative for up to 4 to 6 weeks after infection. Also, if patients are treated early with tetracycline or another antibiotic, the results might never be positive, although symptoms of chronic Lyme disease can result. The Western blot assay for Lyme disease is now being used as a confirmatory test if the ELISA test result is positive.

- In Lyme disease, culturing the organism is difficult and of low yield.
- The ELISA assay is commonly performed but is not standardized.
- There is a significant frequency of false-positive results with ELISA.
- False-positive ELISA results may occur in syphilis, relapsing fever, and Rocky Mountain spotted fever.
- Up to 25% of patients with lupus and rheumatoid arthritis have false-positive results of Lyme test by ELISA.
- Patients treated early with tetracycline or other antibiotic may never have positive results.

Treatment

For early treatment of Lyme disease, either oral tetracycline or doxycycline, or amoxicillin in children, can prevent later complications. The optimal treatment for patients with chronic symptoms is unclear but can include the use of penicillin G (20 million units intravenously daily for 14 days) or ceftriaxone (2 g intravenously daily for 14 days). Patients with Lyme disease can experience worsening of symptoms analogous to the Jarisch-Herxheimer reaction and can be treated with acetaminophen.

- Early treatment of Lyme disease is either oral tetracycline or doxycycline (amoxicillin in children).

RHEUMATIC FEVER AND POSTSTREPTOCOCCAL REACTIVE ARTHRITIS

Arthritis affects two-thirds of all patients with rheumatic fever. One-third of patients with acute rheumatic fever have no obvious antecedent pharyngitis. In adults, arthritis may be the only clinical feature of acute rheumatic fever and often occurs early. The arthritis usually involves the large joints, particularly the knees, ankles, elbows, and wrists. The arthritis may be migratory with each joint remaining inflamed for approximately 1 week. The arthritis of rheumatic fever is nonerosive; however, repeated attacks may result in a "Jaccoud deformity," in which the metacarpophalangeal joints are in ulnar deviation as a result of tendon laxity rather than bony damage.

Patients with joint symptoms without carditis may be treated with high-dose salicylates (3-6 g per day). Corticosteroids may be required if patients do not respond to salicylates. Joint symptoms may rebound when anti-inflammatory therapy is discontinued.

- The arthritis in rheumatic fever may be migratory and usually involves the large joints, particularly the knees, ankles, elbows, and wrists.

- Repeated attacks of rheumatic fever may result in "Jaccoud deformity."
- The mainstay treatment for the arthritis of rheumatic fever is high-dose salicylates (3 to 6 g per day).

VIRAL ARTHRITIS

Viruses associated with arthralgia and arthritis include human immunodeficiency virus (HIV), hepatitis B, rubella, parvovirus, and, less commonly, mumps, adenovirus, herpesvirus, and enterovirus. Most viral-related arthritides have joint symptoms with a semiacute onset, but fortunately they are usually of brief duration. The arthritis is nondestructive.

Although *parvovirus* infection in children is usually mild, in adults associated arthralgias and arthritis are common, and the distribution of involved joints is symmetrical and may mimic rheumatoid arthritis. Joint symptoms in adults are usually self-limited, but chronic disease develops in a small number of patients. The diagnosis of parvovirus infection is made by demonstrating the presence of anti-B19 IgM antibodies, but these may be increased in patients for only 2 months after acute infection. Because the joint symptoms usually occur approximately 1 to 3 weeks after the initial infection, the antibodies are usually present at the time of onset of rash or joint symptoms. Treatment is usually conservative and includes anti-inflammatory medications, but in more chronic infections more aggressive treatment such as low-dose corticosteroids may be warranted. Parvovirus infection also has been associated rarely with significant hematologic abnormalities.

Hepatitis B virus infection has been associated with an immune complex-mediated arthritis, which can be dramatic. The arthritis is usually limited to the pre-icteric prodrome, although patients with chronic types of hepatitis may have recurrent arthralgias or arthritis. Polyarteritis nodosa and mixed essential cryoglobulinemia have been associated with chronic hepatitis. Recently, *hepatitis B* and *C* also have been associated with cryoglobulinemia. *Rubella* virus infection is frequently associated with joint complaints in adults. In a few patients, the symptoms have persisted for months to years. Joint symptoms may occur just before or after the appearance of the characteristic rash.

- Parvovirus infection in adults may cause a symmetrical polyarthritis mimicking rheumatoid arthritis.
- Parvovirus infection can be documented by demonstrating the presence of anti-B19 IgM antibodies. Parvovirus infection may cause a chronic arthritis.
- Hepatitis B virus infection has been associated with an arthritis limited to the pre-icteral prodrome.
- Hepatitis B and C viremia have been associated with cryoglobulinemia and vasculitis.

- Rubella virus infection frequently is associated with joint complaints in young adults.

RHEUMATOLOGIC MANIFESTATIONS OF HIV INFECTION (TABLE 22-33)

Musculoskeletal complaints can be some of the first manifestations of HIV infection. Articular manifestations can be extremely debilitating. Epidemiologic studies have not concluded whether HIV infection predisposes to arthritis or whether other viral or new mechanisms associated with HIV infection have a role in the pathogenesis of arthritis.

Reiter Syndrome and Undifferentiated Spondyloarthropathy

Signs and symptoms of Reiter syndrome, psoriatic arthritis, or a nonspecific enthesopathy and related destructive arthritis may occur before or simultaneously with the onset of HIV infection. The prevalence of these conditions in HIV-infected patients varies from 0.5% to 10% in reports. These HIV-associated spondyloarthropathies have a predisposition for HLA-B27 and frequently are associated with severe enthesopathy and dactylitis. Except for several cases of mild sacroiliitis, progressive axial involvement may be less common in HIV-associated arthritides. The foot and ankle are common sites of enthesopathy in Reiter syndrome and may be severe. Symptoms may be episodic. Most HIV-infected patients with Reiter syndrome have skin and mucocutaneous manifestations, including urethritis, keratoderma blennorrhagicum, circinate balanitis, or painless oral ulcers, but conjunctivitis is unusual. In approximately one-third of patients, the onset of

Table 22-33.—Rheumatologic Manifestations of Human Immunodeficiency Virus (HIV)

Arthralgia
Painful articular syndrome
HIV arthropathy
Reiter syndrome
Psoriatic arthritis
Undifferentiated spongyloarthropathy
Myositis
Vasculitis
Raynaud phenomenon
Sjögren-like syndrome (diffuse infiltrative lymphocytosis syndrome)
Septic arthritis
Fibromyalgia
Serologic abnormalities

HIV-associated Reiter syndrome has been linked to a documented infection with specific enteric organisms known to precipitate reactive arthritis. Genitourinary tract infection with *Ureaplasma* or *Chlamydia* is less common.

- Enthesopathy and dactylitis may be severe in HIV-infected patients.
- Mucocutaneous features are common, but conjunctivitis is unusual.

Lupus-Like Illnesses in HIV Infection

Some of the features of systemic lupus erythematosus are similar to those in patients with HIV infection. Fever, lymphadenopathy, mucous membrane lesions, rashes, arthritis, and hematologic abnormalities are common to both lupus and HIV infection. HIV infection also may be associated with polyclonal B-cell activation resulting in autoantibody production, including antinuclear and antiphospholipid antibodies. HIV infection should be considered in the differential diagnosis of systemic lupus erythematosus in any patient who is at risk for HIV. Antinuclear antibodies in high titer have not been observed in HIV infection, and antibodies to double-stranded DNA are absent.

- Although some features of HIV infection may resemble lupus, antinuclear antibodies are present in low titer only and antibodies to double-stranded DNA are absent.

HIV-Associated Vasculitis

Different types of vasculitic syndromes have been described in association with HIV infection. Primary angiitis of the central nervous system, angiocentric lymphoproliferative lesions related to lymphomatoid granulomatosis, and polyarteritis nodosa have been reported. It has not been established whether the association of vasculitis and HIV infection is coincidental, related to comorbidities such as drugs or other infections, or represents a direct pathogenetic role for the HIV virus. All patients with primary angiitis of the central nervous system and lymphoproliferative angiocentric vasculopathies should be tested for HIV. Any person with known HIV infection who presents with new mononeuritis should be evaluated for vasculitis.

Other HIV-Associated Rheumatic Syndromes

The diffuse, infiltrative lymphocytosis syndrome (DILS) is manifested by xerostomia, xerophthalmia, and salivary gland swelling mimicking Sjögren syndrome. The glands are infiltrated with CD8 lymphocytes. In contrast to Sjögren syndrome, these HIV-positive patients usually do not have antibodies to SS-A or SS-B and are usually rheumatoid factor-negative.

There is an inflammatory articular syndrome associated with HIV infection which is distinct from any resemblance to spondyloarthropathy. This is usually an oligoarthritis affecting joints of the lower extremities and is usually short-lived.

There is an acquired immunodeficiency syndrome (AIDS)-associated myopathy that may be viral as well as a myopathy due to zidovudine therapy. Fibromyalgia also has been reported in up to 25% of HIV-infected patients.

OTHER TYPES OF INFECTIOUS ARTHRITIS

Whipple disease is a rare cause of arthropathy and usually is associated with constitutional symptoms, fever, neurologic symptoms, malabsorption, lymphadenopathy, and hyperpigmentation. There may be a slow progressive dementia. The infectious agent is *Tropheryma whippeli*. Small bowel or synovial biopsy may be necessary to establish the diagnosis. Treatment is usually with doxycycline or trimethoprim-sulfamethoxazole, often for several months.

QUESTIONS

Multiple Choice (choose the one best answer)

1. A 32-year-old working, single mother with 3 children with a 3-month history of progressively severe rheumatoid factor-negative inflammatory polyarthritis is referred by a family practitioner. She has not responded well to trials of two different NSAIDs, each for 3 weeks. She has been unable to work outside of the home for the last 2 weeks. She cannot make a complete fist with either hand. The most reasonable next step in her treatment is:
   a. A trial of a third NSAID
   b. Hydroxychloroquine
   c. Low-dose oral methotrexate
   d. Inject carpal tunnels and send to physical therapy
   e. Low-dose oral daily prednisone

2. A contraindication to the use of nonacetylated salicylates in a 57-year-old woman with asthma and symptomatic osteoarthritis of the knees includes:
   a. Nasal polyps
   b. Peptic ulcer disease
   c. Severe hypertension
   d. Renal failure
   e. Warfarin anticoagulation

3. A 31-year-old woman developed seropositive destructive rheumatoid arthritis. Which of the following correctly describes the risk of her daughter developing rheumatoid arthritis?
   a. About half that of the normal population
   b. About 3 times that of the normal population
   c. About 6 times that of the normal population
   d. About 30 times that of the normal population
   e. About 60 times that of the normal population

4. A 41-year-old male physician has a 6-week history of persistent painful, swollen, and stiff proximal interphalangeal joints, wrists, and ankles. The most reasonable next diagnostic step is:
   a. Radiography of hand and wrist
   b. Check for HLA-B27
   c. Hepatitis B serology testing
   d. Rheumatoid factor and anti-nuclear antibody
   e. Joint aspirate for microcrystals

5. A 3-week trial of which of the following rheumatoid arthritis treatments would be considered an adequate trial to test the efficacy of the drug?
   a. Methotrexate
   b. IM gold
   c. Sulfasalazine
   d. Hydroxychloroquine
   e. Naproxen

6. A 52-year-old man referred to you with recurrent pneumonia and neutropenia has a 13-year history of nodular, destructive, inflammatory polyarthritis. He complains of dry eyes and mouth and has, in addition to joint swelling and deformity, splenomegaly and petechial rash on his legs. Laboratory findings include a positive rheumatoid factor, ANA, SS-A, and normal complement. The most likely diagnosis is:
   a. Sjögren syndrome
   b. Adult Still disease
   c. Rheumatoid arthritis with secondary Sjögren syndrome
   d. Felty syndrome
   e. Systemic lupus erythematosus

7. Joan, a 45-year-old new car salesperson with newly diagnosed seropositive rheumatoid arthritis, wants to know her chances of working to age 60. A good estimate of her risk of complete disability within the first 15 years of her disease is:
   a. With good medical care, she has no increased risk of disability
   b. There is little chance that she will still be working in 15 years
   c. There is a 1 in 7 chance of total disability within the first 15 years of her disease
   d. About half of all seropositive rheumatoid arthritis patients are disabled in 15 years
   e. It all depends on whether she has disability insurance

8. A diagnosis of primary osteoarthritis is suggested by which of the following radiographic appearances and histories:
   a. Flowing osteophytes linking six thoracic vertebrae and osteoarthritis of the left hip in a 56-year-old male carpenter
   b. Chondrocalcinosis and left knee asymmetric joint-space narrowing of the lateral compartment in a 62-year-old obese diabetic female
   c. Large osteophytes at the metacarpophalangeal joints of a farmer from Missouri
   d. Hypertrophic changes, joint-space narrowing, and superior humeral head subluxation of the right shoulder of a 48-year-old accountant and high school tennis star
   e. Left ankle and subtalar osteoarthritis in a 52-year-old farmer with diabetes mellitus for the past 31 years

9. COX-2 enzyme inhibition
   a. Does not occur at clinically significant levels with

currently available NSAIDs
b. Causes interference with prostaglandin-dependent renal function
c. Causes interference with gastric mucous barrier
d. Inhibits platelet thromboxane inhibition
e. Is safe in asthmatics with aspirin allergy and nasal polyps

10. A patient with systemic lupus taking allopurinol for recurrent gout requires more aggressive anti-inflammatory treatment. Which drug requires significant dosage reduction in this setting?
a. Methotrexate
b. Indomethacin
c. Prednisone
d. Hydroxychloroquine
e. Azathioprine

11. A 48-year-old woman has a 10-year history of progressive fatigue and widespread musculoskeletal aches and pains. She is finding it harder and harder to work full time. You suspect fibromyalgia. The next step in her diagnosis is:
a. ANA, rheumatoid factor, erythrocyte sedimentation rate
b. Neurology consultation
c. Psychiatry consultation
d. Muscle biopsy
e. Physical examination

12. Treatment that has shown to influence the symptoms of fibromyalgia includes:
a. Magnesium supplements
b. Complete rest with permanent disability
c. Management of coexisting depression when present
d. High dose of NSAIDs
e. Gammaglobulin given intravenously

13. A 31-year-old male lumberyard foreman reports a 2-week history of low back pain. The pain has kept him from working for the last 3 work days. The pain is localized to the low back, about the lumbosacral junction, but does not radiate below the level of the knees. The pain worsens with cough. There is no compromise of bowel or bladder function, and he has no difficulty getting an erection. He denies leg or foot numbness or weakness. Physical examination is remarkable only for tenderness at the lumbosacral junction and a decreased left ankle reflex compared with the right. Which of the following is true?
a. He needs MRI to rule out a disk lesion
b. A week of bedrest is essential before sending him for

neurologic review
c. Plain radiographs if normal would be very reassuring and should be obtained if there is a history of lifting that precipitated the pain
d. He needs formal physical therapy, including pelvic traction or a trial of a transcutaneous electrical nerve stimulator unit
e. Reassure the patient, prescribe simple analgesics, and leave him to his own devices

14. A 71-year-old man has a one-week history of low grade fever, anorexia, stiffness and pain in his neck, shoulders, and thighs. He is so stiff he can barely roll out of bed in the morning. He denies any other new symptoms. His examination, including heart, lungs, abdomen, and joints, is normal with the exception of reduced shoulder motion. The most likely diagnosis is:
a. Myositis
b. Shoulder bursitis and viral infection
c. Fibromyalgia
d. Polymyalgia rheumatica
e. Widespread bony metastases

15. Following a sore throat, a healthy 18-year-old man taking no medication gets severe abdominal cramps, hematochezia, diarrhea, nonblanching tiny red spots on his legs and buttocks, pain, and swelling of his ankles. Urinalysis documented moderate proteinuria. Normal or negative studies include ANA, rheumatoid factor, ANCA, complement, and cryoglobulins. The most likely diagnosis is:
a. ANA-negative systemic lupus erythematosus
b. Wegener granulomatosis
c. Hypersensitivity vasculitis
d. Schönlein-Henoch purpura
e. Ulcerative colitis and associated rash/arthritis

16. A 62-year-old man has a 3-month history of anorexia, weight loss, night sweats, and arthralgias of the knees and ankles. One week ago, he suddenly developed left foot drop with associated pain, then numbness over the dorsum of the left foot. Physical examination confirmed foot drop. Screening laboratory studies suggested a systemic inflammatory process. You suspect systemic vasculitis. The confirmatory test of choice is:
a. ANCA
b. Chest radiography and lung biopsy if abnormal
c. Electromyography, nerve conduction studies, and sural nerve biopsy if abnormal
d. Visceral angiography
e. Testicular biopsy

17. A 71-year-old woman has had good health her entire life. Three weeks before presentation she has a flu-like illness, and her symptoms do not go away. In addition to widespread muscle aches and stiffness, she continues to have low grade fever and a dry cough. In the past week, her scalp has been sore to touch and at breakfast her jaw aches after every mouthful of cold cereal she eats. Screening laboratory tests document a normocytic anemia and an elevated erythrocyte sedimentation rate. The most critical diagnosis to consider at this time is:
    a. Giant cell arteritis
    b. Occult cancer
    c. Multiple myeloma with bony metastasis
    d. Atypical pneumonia (*Legionella*)
    e. Asthma with Churg-Strauss syndrome

18. An 18-year-old woman with a previous diagnosis of fibromyalgia describes feeling ill for several months, with fatigue, low-grade fevers, light-headed spells, and aches and swelling of her ankles and knees. Over the last 2 weeks, she has had a cramping discomfort in her left buttock and thigh when she walks for more than a few minutes. Her blood pressure cannot be determined in the left arm, and it is 170/95 mm Hg in the right arm. Which of the following is true?
    a. A temporal artery biopsy should be diagnostic
    b. An ANCA blood test should be diagnostic
    c. Her fibromyalgia is flaring, but she needs MRI of the lumbar spine to rule out disk rupture
    d. No further evaluation is necessary if erythrocyte sedimentation rate is normal
    e. Aortic angiography should be diagnostic

19. A 69-year-old man has epistaxis, nasal crusting, thick-walled cavitary nodules on chest radiography, and creatinine of 1.5 mg/dL, with a nephritic-appearing urinalysis. His c-ANCA is positive. The best treatment plan for this man is:
    a. Trimethoprim-sulfa
    b. Prednisone
    c. Cyclophosphamide
    d. Immunoglobulin given intravenously
    e. Referral to a rheumatologist

20. A 22-year-old white man has recurrent episodes of iritis and an 8-month history of low back pain with morning stiffness. Which of the following is the most useful test for establishing a diagnosis?
    a. Rheumatoid factor
    b. Antinuclear antibody
    c. HLA-B27

d. Antineutrophilic cytoplasmic antibodies
e. Radiograph of pelvis

21. A 61-year-old white man has had recurrent episodes of gout. The uric acid value is 8.4 mg/dL (normal, <8.0). Radiographs of his feet reveal erosive changes of the first metatarsophalangeal joints, and tophi are apparent on physical examination. He is asymptomatic at examination. A 24-hour urinary uric acid value is 300 mg (normal, <1,000). Which of the following would be most appropriate in the treatment of this patient?
    a. Continued observation and treatment of the acute attacks when they occur
    b. Indomethacin, 50 mg 4 times a day with food
    c. Begin allopurinol therapy
    d. Begin probenecid therapy
    e. Begin allopurinol in conjunction with colchicine therapy

22. A 34-year-old white man presents with an acutely swollen right ankle. He had severe, self-limiting diarrhea on a recent foreign trip. What is the most likely diagnosis?
    a. Reactive arthritis
    b. Gout
    c. Ankylosing spondylitis
    d. Arthritis of inflammatory bowel disease
    e. Rheumatoid arthritis

23. A 26-year-old man presents because of a 2-week history of pain and swelling of his right knee and left ankle. Five weeks before his visit, he presented with a purulent urethral discharge. Urethritis was diagnosed and treated with an antibiotic. After treatment, the patient had significant improvement but experienced residual dysuria, which cleared after 1 week. Physical examination now demonstrated bilateral conjunctivitis and synovitis of the right knee and left ankle. Joint aspiration shows cloudy, yellow fluid containing 41,000 leukocytes/μL. What is the most likely joint fluid culture result?
    a. Culture positive for *Neisseria gonorrhoeae*
    b. Culture positive for *Campylobacter jejuni*
    c. Culture positive for *Ureaplasma urealyticum*
    d. Culture sterile
    e. Culture positive for *Chlamydia trachomatis*

24. A 48-year-old man presents with severe right shoulder pain and loss of abduction of the right arm. There is no history of trauma or overuse. A radiograph of the affected shoulder demonstrates periarticular calcification. The patient is treated with a nonsteroidal anti-inflammatory agent and 1 week later is asymptomatic. Also, at that time

a chest radiograph obtained before an elective herniorrhaphy demonstrates that the right shoulder is normal. What is the probable cause of the patient's shoulder pain?

a. Gout
b. Pseudogout
c. Bicipital tendinitis
d. Rotator cuff tear
e. Hydroxyapatite periarthritis

25. A 66-year-old man with mild knee aching for more than a year presents with a 3-day history of pain and swelling in his left knee. There is no history of trauma. A radiograph shows tibial spurring and medial compartmental narrowing bilaterally with chondrocalcinosis. Which of the following is the most likely cause of the acute left knee pain?

a. Avascular necrosis
b. Anserine bursitis
c. Tear of the medial meniscus
d. Pseudogout
e. Gout

26. Which of the following is considered a late complication of ankylosing spondylitis?

a. Scleromalacia perforans
b. Dactylitis
c. Cauda equina syndrome
d. Pulmonary hemorrhage
e. Small vessel vasculitis

27. A 46-year-old man presents with a 10-week history of pain and swelling in the right second metacarpophalangeal joint, the left knee, the right ankle, and the proximal interphalangeal joint of the third toe. He has a history of an erythematous scaling rash on the scalp, which recently improved with topical application of an over-the-counter corticosteroid ointment. There is no history of gastrointestinal, urinary tract, or ophthalmologic symptoms. Examination confirms swelling and local pain in the affected joints, but the remainder of the examination is completely normal. Laboratory studies demonstrate a normal complete blood cell count, a normal erythrocyte sedimentation rate, normal liver function test, and a negative determination for rheumatoid factor. You prescribed indomethacin, 150 mg daily, and a week later the patient reports impressive symptomatic improvement. Which of the following is the most appropriate diagnostic step?

a. HLA-B27 testing
b. Evaluation of the scalp rash if it occurs
c. Antinuclear antibody testing

d. Radiography of the affected joints as soon as possible
e. Colonoscopy

28. A 35-year-old woman presents with a sudden onset of severe pain in the right ankle which began 12 hours ago. There were no similar previous episodes. One year ago she received a renal transplant because of chronic glomerulonephritis. Daily medications include cyclosporine (300 mg daily), azathioprine (100 mg daily), and prednisone (10 mg daily). On physical examination the patient is afebrile and has a blood pressure of 142/98 mm Hg. The right ankle is swollen and tender with limited motion. She has no rash, nodules, or tophi. Her cardiovascular examination is normal. Laboratory evaluation demonstrates a stable creatinine value of 2.2 mg/dL and a serum uric acid level of 9.8 mg/dL. A radiograph of the right ankle shows soft tissue swelling without narrowing of the joint space or bony abnormalities. The ankle joint is aspirated, and synovial fluid analysis demonstrates numerous granulocytes with intracellular negatively birefringent crystals. A Gram stain of the fluid shows no organisms. Which of the following is the most appropriate treatment for this patient's current joint problem?

a. Allopurinol, 100 mg twice daily
b. Colchicine, 0.6 mg orally twice daily
c. Indomethacin, 50 mg orally every 6 hours
d. Colchicine, 1 mg intravenously followed by 0.5 mg every 12 hours for 48 hours
e. Triamcinolone, 20 mg by intra-articular injection into the right ankle

29. A 43-year-old white woman has a 10-year history of systemic lupus erythematosus. Multiple flares of her disease during the past several years have necessitated courses of high-dose prednisone. She now presents with a 2-week history of pain in the left groin with ambulation. She denies fever, chills, or other symptoms that she has equated with a flare in the past. Routine radiography of her pelvis, including hips, is normal. Which one of the following would be most helpful for determining the cause of her symptoms?

a. Electromyography
b. Sedimentation rate and anti-nDNA determinations
c. Magnetic resonance imaging of the hips
d. Empiric trial of a corticosteroid injection into the hip under fluoroscopy
e. Bone scanning

30. A 65-year-old man has been taking procainamide for 1 year for a cardiac arrhythmia. He is feeling well. His

cardiac rhythm is now normal. Antinuclear antibody testing is positive at 1:640. Which of the following is an appropriate course of action?
a. Stop the procainamide treatment
b. Obtain other serologic evidence for SLE systemic lupus erythematosus, including anti-nDNA and complement determinations
c. Prescribe prednisone, 10 mg daily
d. Prescribe prednisone, 60 mg daily, and stop the procainamide treatment
e. Continue with current medication and observe

31. Proximal muscle weakness and dysphagia develop in a 53-year-old woman. The creatine kinase value is 10,000 U/L (normal, 50-250). The patient is Jo-1 antibody-negative. Which of the following would be the most likely cause of death during the first 3 months of illness?
a. Pericardial tamponade
b. Renal disease
c. Aspiration pneumonia
d. Progressive pulmonary interstitial disease
e. Myoglobinuria

32. A 42-year-old woman presents with a 2-month history of a facial rash, arthritis, and pleurisy. Urinalysis reveals 40 to 50 erythrocytes per high-power field with erythrocyte casts and +2 protein. Testing for which of the following best corresponds with the renal involvement?
a. Anti-SS-A antibodies
b. Antihistone antibodies
c. Anti-ssDNA antibodies
d. Anti-nDNA antibodies
e. Anticardiolipin antibodies

33. Which of the following laboratory findings is consistent with the antiphospholipid antibody syndrome?
a. Microangiopathic hemolytic anemia
b. Thrombocytopenia
c. Prolonged prothrombin time
d. Normal Russell viper venom time
e. Prolonged bleeding time

34. A 50-year-old man with hypertension, hypothyroidism, and hypercholesterolemia is treated with a thiazide diuretic, levothyroxine, and lovastatin. The patient presents for follow-up examination with arthralgias, muscle cramping, and fatigue for the past week. Laboratory results are as follows:

Serum potassium	4.1 mEq/L (normal)
Serum calcium	9.6 mg/dL (normal)
Serum phosphorus	3.1 mg/dL (normal)
Serum creatine kinase	642 U/L (3 times increased)
Serum uric acid	10.4 mg/dL (increased)
Thyroid-stimulating hormone	3.2 mU/L (normal)

Which is the best course of action?
a. Give supplemental potassium
b. Increase the levothyroxine dose
c. Add allopurinol
d. Discontinue use of the thiazide diuretic
e. Discontinue use of lovastatin

35. A 32-year-old man presents with fever and swollen painful upper arms. He played basketball for several hours 3 days ago at a family reunion, but previously he had been inactive. The arm symptoms began the day after this vigorous exercise and have been progressive. On examination, the skin over both upper arms is tender, edematous, and described as indurated or woody. The fingers and hands are normal. Needle aspiration is attempted but yields no fluid. Blood cultures are negative. A complete blood cell count is normal except for 11% eosinophils. The erythrocyte sedimentation rate is 42 mm/hour. A biopsy of the affected skin and muscle is likely to be consistent with which of the following?
a. Necrotizing fasciitis
b. Edematous phase of systemic sclerosis
c. Polymyositis
d. Eosinophilic fasciitis
e. Axillary vein thrombosis

36. A 24-year-old woman presents with the onset of pain overlying the left ankle. The ankle is slightly swollen, but passive extension and flexion cause severe pain. She also has difficulty fully extending the left elbow which is also slightly swollen and mildly tender. She has a hemorrhagic vesicle on the right palm but no other evidence of rash. Aspiration of synovial fluid from the left ankle demonstrates a slight leukocytosis, but no organisms are seen on Gram stain. Which of the following is the most appropriate treatment?
a. Intra-articular injection of corticosteroid into the left ankle
b. Amoxicillin, 500 mg orally 3 times daily
c. Indomethacin, 25 mg orally 3 times daily
d. Ceftriaxone, 1 g intravenously daily
e. Doxycycline, 100 mg orally twice daily

37. A 37-year-old woman presents with a 2-year history of skin tightening over the fingers. She also has a long-standing history of Raynaud phenomenon with some

symptomatic worsening during the past 8 months. She reports increasing difficulty with swallowing of solid foods. Physical examination shows a slightly reduced oral opening and scattered telangiectasias on the face and fingers. There is moderate sclerodactyly. Dilated capillaries are noted in the periungual areas. Which of the following antibodies is most likely to be present in this patient?

a. Antitopoisomerase I (Scl-70)
b. Anti-Jo1
c. Anticentromere
d. Anti-Sm
e. Antihistone

38. A 31-year-old woman is referred with a 1-week history of stiffness and swelling in the hands, wrists, knees, and feet. She has a low-grade fever and a faint rash over the trunk and extremities. Her 4-year-old son recently was sent home from school because of a facial rash. Four weeks ago she took amoxicillin for 10 days for treatment of the pharyngitis, which resolved. Examination demonstrates a faint erythematous rash over the arms and trunk. There is mild swelling in the wrists, metacarpophalangeal joints, proximal interphalangeal joints, knees, and metatarsophalangeal joints. The remainder of her examination is completely normal. Laboratory studies show a normal complete blood cell count, a normal erythrocyte sedimentation rate, and a negative determination for rheumatoid factor and antinuclear antibodies. The total hemolytic complement level is normal. Which of the following is the most likely diagnosis?

a. Arthritis due to rubella
b. Rheumatic fever
c. Prodromal hepatitis B
d. Reaction to amoxicillin
e. Arthritis due to parvovirus infection

39. A 26-year-old homosexual man presents with bilateral swelling of the parotid glands. He also describes a gritty sensation in the eyes and dramatic mouth dryness. He has no symptoms of arthritis. Physical examination demonstrates bilateral parotid swelling, diffuse cervical lymphadenopathy, and a Schirmer test result showing lack of normal tear production. The most appropriate diagnostic laboratory test at this time includes:

a. Anti-SSA
b. Anti-SSB
c. Antinuclear antibody determination
d. Rheumatoid factor determination
e. HIV antibody determination

ANSWERS

1. Answer e.

The person needs to be able to care for herself and others. She does not have the 6 weeks to wait for methotrexate to start to work, although this should be considered soon in her case. None of the other choices provide a good chance that she will be able to provide for her family, except for the use of low-dose prednisone daily. Once she is functional, discussion about methotrexate treatment should begin.

2. Answer d.

Nonacetylated salicylates do not inhibit COX-1. They do not significantly influence the housekeeping prostaglandin maintenence of the gastric mucous barrier, platelet thromboxane synthesis, or renal blood flow. They would not aggravate hypertension or influence asthma/nasal polyps in most patients. They, like all salicylates, are contraindicated in renal insufficiency/renal failure because they do not follow classic first-order kinetics.

3. Answer b.

The genetics of rheumatoid arthritis are complex and incompletely understood. More than one gene contributes to the risk of rheumatoid arthritis. If one parent has rheumatoid arthritis, the child has no more than 2.5 to 3.5 times the risk of the normal population of getting rheumatoid arthritis. If one fraternal twin has rheumatoid arthritis, the other has a 6-fold increase in the risk of getting rheumatoid arthritis.

4. Answer d.

This is early polyarticular synovitis. That it is has been present for 6 weeks implies a chronic process. Symmetric small joint inflammation is not the usual presentation of an

HLA-B27-associated arthropathy. It is best to consider both rheumatoid arthritis and systemic lupus erythematosus, which should be the clinical models of this sort of presentation.

5. Answer e.

The first four answers are slow-acting antirheumatic agents. Even the fastest acting of the group, methotrexate, takes 6 weeks for clinical effects to appear; the others require 3 to 4 months. Naproxen, however, is in a different class, the NSAIDs. Most of the time, a 3-week trial is more than enough to assess the efficacy of any given NSAID.

6. Answer d.

The keys to the right answer here are the long duration of the nodular, destructive inflammatory arthritis, which could only be rheumatoid arthritis. Also, the patient has neutropenia, cutaneous vasculitis, splenomegaly, and, of course, secondary Sjögren syndrome. The combination of seropositive rheumatoid arthritis (particularly severe, nodular rheumatoid arthritis of long duration), neutropenia, and splenomegaly is called "Felty syndrome" and affects about 1% of all seropositive rheumatoid arthritis patients.

7. Answer c.

Rheumatoid arthritis is a disabling condition for many. The severity (number of joints involved, nodularity) of the disease and the type of work all influence the disability risk. Overall, however, about 15% of patients who perform light tasks are disabled after 15 years (1 in 7). Patients need an accurate assessment of this sort of risk to plan for the future.

8. Answer a.

Secondary osteoarthritis is suggested by involvement of the shoulder or metacarpophalangeal joints. Secondary osteoarthritis is also suggested with chondrocalcinosis or when one knee or ankle is affected out of proportion to other joints (trauma or neuropathic arthritis). The only one of the conditions that does not meet this definition of secondary, and is therefore primary, osteoarthritis is the patient with diffuse idiopathic skeletal hyperostosis of the spine (flowing osteophytes) and osteoarthritis of the hip.

9. Answer e.

COX-2 inhibition occurs at clinically significant levels with all currently available NSAIDs, which are otherwise not COX-2 specific. Only answer e is true. The rest deal with COX-1 inhibition.

10. Answer e.

Of these drugs, only azathioprine metabolism is influenced by allopurinol.

11. Answer e.

The correct response is physical examination. A history and physical exam will make all the other answers unnecessary, except for a psychiatry consultation. This is not a good move initially. I introduce the topic of cryptic depression or emotional decompensation slowly and try to keep the patient's confidence.

12. Answer c.

Only psychiatric treatment of depression, when it exists, has been shown to make a difference in the long-term outcome of fibromyalgia.

13. Answer e.

Simple back pain (the absent left ankle reflex by itself does not correlate with a root lesion, but if it did, the initial management would be the same) should be managed with a good examination, simple analgesics, and modifications to lifestyle, including frequent changes in position, best left to the patient.

14. Answer d.

Polymyalgia rheumatica is the best bet. Myositis rarely hurts and is not associated with muscle stiffness. Shoulder bursitis would uncommonly, suddenly affect both shoulders simultaneously. Think of alternatives to fibromyalgia if the first sign of it occurs after age 60. Also, metastases do not present acutely in so many places.

15. Answer d.

ANA-negative lupus is extremely rare. Wegener granulomatosis would most likely be ANCA-positive and have a nephritic sediment. Hypersensitivity vasculitis is much more common, over age 21, and is associated with new drug ingestion or recent infection. The association of gut involvement is very uncommon in hypersensitivity vasculitis. The description is classic for late onset Schönlein-Henoch purpura. Ulcerative colitis may present with necrotizing vasculitis of the lower extremity, or erythema nodosum, but not widespread petechiae. Colonoscopy could settle the diagnosis. The biopsy of inflamed mucosa would show the same pathologic features (leukocytoclastic vasculitis with IgA deposition) that one would see with biopsy of a skin lesion.

16. Answer c.

Confirmatory testing is usually angiography or biopsy of affected tissue. In this case, the leading diagnosis is polyarteritis, with the biopsy-accessible organ system, the peripheral nerve.

17. Answer a.

Giant cell arteritis is the best bet in this age group and with these symptoms. The other diagnoses are possible (except for

Legionella pneumonia), but none of them has the critical nature of diagnosis and treatment to avoid the 15% risk of blindness that the diagnosis of giant cell arteritis carries with it.

18. Answer e.

Aortic angiography will demonstrate Takayasu arteritis, which is the only arteritis in this age group that would affect the large elastic arteries needed to give these symptoms.

19. Answer e.

Refer to a rheumatologist. Answers a, b, and c, otherwise come closest to the answer, but still are incomplete.

20. Answer e.

The patient has ankylosing spondylitis manifested by inflammatory eye disease and sacroiliitis. The sacroiliac joints are likely to show some early radiographic evidence of disease, either marginal erosions or perhaps sclerosis. Although rheumatoid arthritis can affect the eye, it usually causes episcleritis or scleritis. In patients with seronegative spondyloarthropathy tests for rheumatoid factor, antinuclear antibody and antineutrophil cytoplasmic antibodies are usually negative. Although this patient may be HLA-B27 positive, it does not establish the active diagnosis because approximately 8% of the population is HLA-B27–positive without an active spondyloarthropathy.

21. Answer e.

This man has erosive changes on radiographs and tophi with a relatively low urinary uric acid value. Indications for the initiation of allopurinol therapy include tophi, high urinary uric acid values (more than 1,000 mg), uric acid stone disease, and impaired renal function. Allopurinol should initially be given with colchicine prophylaxis to prevent exacerbating an attack of gout. The patient is currently asymptomatic, therefore indomethacin is not appropriate. The presence of tophi eliminates the usefulness of probenecid. The presence of tophi and the erosive changes make continued observation without treatment untenable.

22. Answer a.

The patient's history is compatible with a gastrointestinal infection, possibly with *Yersinia, Campylobacter,* or *Salmonella.* Although the diarrhea has resolved, this patient seems to have developed a reactive arthritis, probably triggered by the previous infection. There is insufficient history to support a diagnosis of inflammatory bowel disease, although this remains a possibility. The diagnoses of gout, ankylosing spondylitis, and rheumatoid arthritis would not explain the previous gastrointestinal problems and are therefore less likely.

23. Answer d.

The patient's history is compatible with a urethritis that may be related to any of the infective organisms listed. The joint manifestations in this patient, however, represent a reactive arthritis, and synovial fluid cultures are most often negative. The arthritis is inflammatory but aseptic.

24. Answer e.

The clinical presentation and radiographs suggest a calcific periarthritis, which is usually self-limited and related to pain and swelling around the tendon sheath adjacent to the affected joint. After the acute attack the calcific densities may disappear. When analyzed, the calcium deposits are most consistent with basic calcium phosphate and hydroxyapatite. Gout would be an unusual cause of shoulder pain and is not calcified. The calcification of pseudogout tends to be a linear, intra-articular deposition in cartilage. Bicipital tendinitis does not usually restrict abduction. A rotator cuff tear usually does not respond so completely or quickly to conservative therapy.

25. Answer d.

The chondrocalcinosis is associated with pseudogout rather than gout. This man has osteoarthritis, explaining his more chronic symptoms, but the acute pain and swelling involving the left knee are most likely pseudogout because there is no history to suggest trauma. Avascular necrosis does not usually cause significant effusion and there are no obvious risk factors mentioned. Similarly, anserine bursitis does not cause acute swelling of the knee.

26. Answer c.

There are many late complications of ankylosing spondylitis. Cauda equina syndrome with symptoms, including leg pain, a neurogenic bladder, and fecal incontinence, may occur in patients with long-standing ankylosing spondylitis. This results in characteristic changes on magnetic resonance imaging and myelography. Other later complications include cord compression due to traumatic spinal fracture, fibrotic changes in the upper lung fields, aortic insufficiency, complete heart block, and amyloidosis. None of the other answers are common in early or long-standing ankylosing spondylitis.

27. Answer b.

The asymmetric oligoarthritis associated with the erythematous scaling rash is typical of psoriatic arthritis. Laboratory tests are often normal in these patients, in particular a rheumatoid factor determination should be negative. HLA-B27 testing will not confirm the diagnosis and is not usually of any help in the diagnosis of psoriatic arthritis. The duration of the joint findings is probably not sufficient to result in characteristic radiographic findings. Although patients with inflammatory bowel disease may manifest an inflammatory polyarthritis, the lack of gastrointestinal symptoms and the presence of a rash suggesting psoriasis probably do not warrant colonoscopy at this time. Similarly, although the rash of systemic lupus erythematosus may resemble psoriasis, this patient had no other criteria to suggest lupus at this time. If the rash recurs, evaluation to confirm psoriasis would be most reasonable with a more aggressive topical treatment if the symptoms warrant.

28. Answer e.

Although gout occurs extremely rarely in premenopausal female patients, this patient is taking cyclosporine, which is one of the drugs that predisposes patients to gout. The presence of intracellular negatively birefringent crystals confirms this diagnosis, with no evidence of concurrent infection. With regard to treatment options, allopurinol should not be used in acute gout. Colchicine twice daily usually is not adequate. Indomethacin should be avoided in a patient with renal insufficiency. The dosage of intravenous colchicine is initially correct, but the multiple doses should be avoided, particularly in patients with chronic renal insufficiency. Intra-articular steroid injection should be adequate to treat the acute symptoms in this patient.

29. Answer c.

Both systemic lupus erythematosus and corticosteroid exposure are risk factors for avascular necrosis. Early in the course, routine radiographs may be interpreted as normal. Magnetic resonance imaging is the diagnostic study of choice at this time. The patient has no symptoms to suggest active lupus. A bone scan might be positive but would not differentiate avascular necrosis from other causes of increased uptake, including infection. Further attempts at establishing a diagnosis should be undertaken before attempting an empiric trial of corticosteroid injections.

30. Answer e.

Many patients exposed to procainamide for longer than a year will test positive for antinuclear antibodies. This patient has nothing to suggest a clinically active drug-induced lupus syndrome. Further evaluation, new drug treatment, or even stopping the procainamide treatment should not be necessary at this time.

31. Answer c.

Aspiration pneumonia is a complication of polymyositis which can occur in patients with weak pharyngeal muscles. This is a potential problem early in the course of patients with aggressive disease. Although progressive pulmonary interstitial disease also can be a complication, it tends to be later

and associated with Jo-1 antibodies. Renal disease and pericardial tamponade are uncommon in polymyositis. Myoglobinuria is not characteristic of polymyositis and not related to cause of death in this disease.

32. Answer d.

Only antibodies to "native" or double-stranded DNA correlate with disease activity in systemic lupus erythematosus. Antibodies to double-stranded DNA may correspond with renal involvement, whereas none of the other antibodies tend to correlate with disease activity in patients with lupus and specifically do not correlate with renal involvement.

33. Answer b.

Thrombocytopenia is associated with the antiphospholipid antibody syndrome. The antiphospholipid antibody has not been associated with a microangiopathic hemolytic anemia. Patients with the antiphospholipid antibody syndrome have prolonged activated partial thromboplastin times but usually normal prothrombin times and normal bleeding times. The Russell viper venom time is usually prolonged and may be a relatively helpful finding in patients with the syndrome.

34. Answer e.

Several drugs may cause a low-grade inflammatory myopathy. Lovastatin is one of these medications. The laboratory values and clinical symptoms suggest a myopathy. Giving potassium would not help this patient, and his increased uric acid level is not contributing to his current symptoms, although it may warrant treatment and justify discontinuing use of the thiazide diuretic. His thyroid-stimulating hormone level is normal, suggesting that increasing his exogenous thyroid dose is not necessary and would not be helpful. Other lipid-lowering agents and zidovudine also have been associated with myopathy.

35. Answer d.

This patient has eosinophilic fasciitis of the upper extremities characterized by a woody-like swelling of the affected extremities associated with hypereosinophilia. This disease often has its onset after unusual physical exertion. Necrotizing fasciitis is not often bilateral, and there is no obvious site of infection. Polymyositis often presents with weakness but without the skin and fascia involvement implied in this patient. Axillary vein thrombosis is not often bilateral and probably would cause peripheral swelling also. The edematous phase of systemic sclerosis usually is a distal event, initially most often involving the hands, which are spared in this patient. To establish the diagnosis of eosinophilic fasciitis, a deep skin-to-muscle biopsy, which includes fascia, is important.

36. Answer c.

Young patients with an inflammatory monarthritis should be considered to have gonococcal arthritis until proved otherwise. This may be associated with tenosynovitis and dermatologic lesions such as pustules or hemorrhagic vesicles. Synovial fluid cultures are positive in less than half of patients with gonococcal arthritis. Indomethacin may be used for symptoms, but it is not the primary treatment for septic arthritis. Similarly, corticosteroids should be avoided. Although some strains of *Gonococcus* are sensitive to penicillin, current initial treatment recommendations suggest a parenteral, later-generation cephalosporin, such as ceftriaxone.

37. Answer c.

This patient has criteria suggesting a CREST syndrome. Anticentromere antibodies are present in a significant percentage of cases of this syndrome. Antitopoisomerase I antibodies are more characteristic of diffuse or systemic sclerosis. Anti-Jo1 antibodies are associated with polymyositis, often in association with progressive interstitial lung disease. Anti-Sm antibodies are relatively specific, although not very sensitive, for systemic lupus erythematosus. Antihistone antibodies are present in patients with drug-induced lupus and in some patients with systemic lupus erythematosus.

38. Answer e.

Parvovirus may cause manifestations in infected adults which may be indistinguishable from early rheumatoid arthritis. This patient's symptoms are characteristic of parvovirus, and presumably her child also was infected, the manifestations in children usually being milder than those in adults. Rubella infection is less likely and often is not associated with synovitis. Hepatitis B viral infection has been associated with inflammatory polyarthritis, but this is usually limited to the pre-icteric, prodromal phase. The manifestations of rheumatic fever are more likely to be migratory and usually involve larger joints. A reaction to amoxicillin usually does not result in synovitis.

39. Answer e.

This patient has the HIV-associated rheumatic syndrome of diffuse, infiltrating lymphocytosis manifested by xerostomia, xerophthalmia, and salivary gland swelling, which may mimic Sjögren syndrome. The glands are usually infiltrated with CD8 lymphocytes. These HIV-positive patients usually do not have antibodies to SSA or SSB and are also often negative for rheumatoid factor.

CHAPTER 23
VASCULAR DISEASES

Thom Rooke, M.D.

ANEURYSMS

Abdominal Aortic Aneurysms

Although congenital or acquired aneurysms can affect any blood vessel in the body, abdominal aortic aneurysms are the ones most commonly encountered by the general medical practitioner. In autopsy series or studies in which unselected adult patients are screened with ultrasonography, the frequency of abdominal aortic aneurysms (usually defined as a vessel diameter ≥3 cm) ranges from 1.5% to 3.2%. In high-risk patients, such as those with coronary or peripheral vascular disease, the rate may be as high as 5% to 10%. The growth rate of these aneurysms is typically 0.3 to 0.5 cm per year, and 95% are located below the origin of the renal arteries. Five percent of all aneurysms are the so-called inflammatory type. For a patient with an abdominal aortic aneurysm, the chance that a first-degree relative also has one is approximately 20%.

- Abdominal aortic aneurysms (vessel diameter ≥3 cm) are the most common aneurysm encountered by the general practitioner.

- Frequency is 1.5%-3.2%.
- In high-risk patients, frequency is as high as 5%-10%.
- Growth rate is 0.3-0.5 cm per year.
- 95% are below origin of renal arteries.
- Chance that first-degree relative has aneurysm is about 20%.

Cause

Most aneurysms are associated with atherosclerosis and hypertension, but predisposing factors such as connective tissue disease (the Marfan syndrome, Ehlers-Danlos syndrome), infection, trauma, vasculitis, and others may also be involved.

- Most abdominal aortic aneurysms are associated with atherosclerosis and hypertension.
- Other predisposing factors: connective tissue disease (Marfan syndrome, Ehlers-Danlos syndrome), infection.

Diagnosis

Various imaging methods are used to diagnose aneurysms (Fig. 23-1).

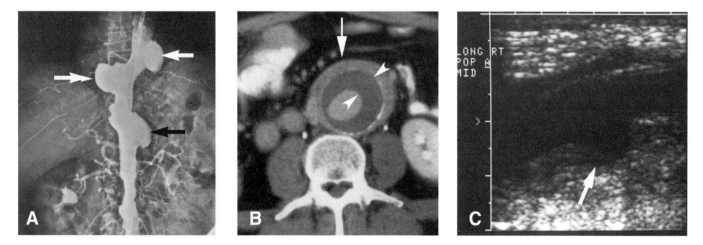

Fig. 23-1. Aneurysms can be diagnosed and evaluated with many imaging methods. *A*, Aortogram shows multiple saccular aneurysms (*arrows*) protruding from abdominal aorta. *B*, Computed tomogram cuts through a large, inflamed abdominal aortic aneurysm (*arrow*). Eccentric layer of laminated thrombus (*arrowheads*) surrounds lumen. *C*, Ultrasound scan shows a saccular aneurysm protruding from popliteal artery (*arrow*).

935

Rupture

The overall mortality rate with ruptured abdominal aortic aneurysm is 80%, and 50% of patients die before they reach the hospital. Of those who survive to reach the hospital, 25% die before operation can be performed, and 40% die during or after operation. The risk of rupture is directly related to aneurysm size. For aneurysms of 5.0, 6.0, or 7.0 cm in diameter, the yearly rate of rupture is less than 5%, 5% to 10%, and 20%, respectively.

- Overall mortality rate with ruptured abdominal aortic aneurysm is 80%.
- 50% of patients die before they reach the hospital.
- Of those who survive to reach the hospital, 25% die before operation.
- 40% of patients die during or after operation.
- Risk of rupture is related to aneurysm size.

Treatment

In the series with the best results, the surgical mortality rate for elective aneurysm resection is 3% to 5%. If the operation is performed on high-risk patients, on elderly patients (>80 years), or in hospitals not specializing in vascular surgery, the mortality rate doubles to 7% to 10%. A reasonable approach to management is based on the size of the aneurysm: less than 4.5 cm in diameter, observe; 4.5 to 6.0 cm, operate electively if the patient is a good surgical risk; and more than 6.0 cm, consider operation even when the patient is a less-than-optimal surgical risk.

- Surgical mortality rate for elective resection of abdominal aortic aneurysm is 3%-5%.
- Rate in high-risk patients is 7%-10%.
- Management based on aneurysm size: <4.5 cm, observe; 4.5-6 cm, operate electively; >6.0 cm, consider operation even if patient is not a good surgical risk.

Other Aneurysms

Other aneurysms that are occasionally encountered by the internist include popliteal aneurysms (these typically thrombose rather than rupture, and when they do so they may cause limb-threatening embolizations or acute ischemia); splenic aneurysms (these often appear in the left upper quadrant as calcified masses on radiographs of the chest or abdomen); iliac aneurysms (almost always seen in conjunction with abdominal aortic aneurysm); and thoracic aortic aneurysms (ascending or descending). Whenever an aneurysm is detected, it is essential that the clinician screen for the presence of other occult aneurysms.

- Popliteal aneurysms typically thrombose rather than rupture.
- When an aneurysm is detected, clinician must screen for occult aneurysms.

ACUTE ARTERIAL OCCLUSION

Cause

Most cases of acute arterial occlusion can be attributed to one of three causes: thrombosis, emboli, and dissection.

Thrombosis

Thrombosis in situ usually occurs at the site of an underlying vascular abnormality such as an atherosclerotic lesion (plaque rupture) or within an aneurysm. Clotting disorders are only rarely the cause of spontaneous arterial thrombosis. Both antiplatelet and anticoagulant agents may be useful in preventing arterial thrombosis.

- Thrombosis that causes acute arterial occlusion often occurs at the site of atherosclerotic lesion or within aneurysm.
- Antiplatelet and anticoagulant agents may prevent arterial thrombosis.

Emboli

Emboli large enough to occlude relatively large arteries usually (in >95% of cases) have a cardiac source. The most common abnormalities producing cardiac-derived emboli include ventricular mural thrombus (typically caused by an infarct or cardiomyopathy), valvular disease (native or prosthetic), and atrial disorders such as chronic or paroxysmal atrial fibrillation. Mural tumors such as atrial myxoma rarely embolize. Other unusual causes of large arterial emboli include paradoxic emboli, in which a thrombus originating in the deep venous system passes through an atrial septal defect or patent foramen ovale and enters the arterial system. Antiplatelet drugs or anticoagulants may prevent some types of emboli.

- Emboli large enough to occlude large arteries usually have a cardiac source.
- Cardiac-derived emboli result from ventricular mural thrombus, valvular disease, paroxysmal atrial fibrillation.
- An unusual cause of emboli is paradoxic emboli: thrombus passes through atrial septal defect or patent foramen ovale and enters arterial system.

Dissection

Dissections are usually associated with hypertension, atherosclerosis, aneurysms, or certain degenerative or connective tissue disorders. As invasive diagnostic and therapeutic cardiovascular interventions have become more popular, iatrogenic dissection has markedly increased in frequency. Trauma (blunt or penetrating) also accounts for a significant number of dissections.

- Dissections are usually associated with hypertension, atherosclerosis, aneurysms, or certain degenerative or connective tissue disorders.
- Iatrogenic dissection has increased in frequency.

Clinical Manifestations

Remember the six P's: 1) pulseless, 2) polar (cool), 3) pallor, 4) pain, 5) paresthesias, and 6) paralysis. It is essential to remember that when acute arterial occlusion occurs, the first abnormalities noted include pulselessness, limb coolness, and limb pallor; although these are important findings, they do not necessarily imply critical ischemia, and the limb can generally be watched as long as necessary. When pain and paresthesia occur, revascularization is necessary and should be performed at the earliest convenient opportunity. However, when motor weakness or paralysis begins to develop in a patient with acute arterial occlusion, the potential for limb loss is high, and revascularization should be performed immediately (within 2 or 3 hours if possible).

- Six P's of acute arterial occlusion: 1) pulseless, 2) polar (cool), 3) pallor, 4) pain, 5) paresthesias, and 6) paralysis.
- When motor weakness or paralysis begins to develop, potential for limb loss is high; immediate revascularization is needed.

Treatment

Specific forms of treatment depend on the cause of the occlusion and are largely beyond the scope of this chapter. Thrombosis may be treated surgically or with lytic agents. Emboli may be treated surgically, including percutaneous removal with a Fogarty balloon catheter. Dissection typically requires operation or percutaneous stenting, although in some situations a dissection may heal with conservative therapy. In most cases, anticoagulation, control of hypertension, and limb protection are indicated.

VASCULITIS (SMALL AND MEDIUM-SIZED VESSELS)

Cause

Several processes may produce vasculitis of small and medium-sized vessels; although none of these are individually common, as a group they are encountered by the internist on a regular basis. In general, immunologic or autoimmune phenomena are thought to be involved in the production of most vasculitides, although the exact mechanism(s) by which this occurs is poorly understood.

Specific Vasculitides

The most commonly encountered types of vasculitis include polyarteritis nodosa, Wegener granulomatosis, and rheumatoid vasculitis.

Polyarteritis Nodosa

This is an acute, necrotizing vasculitis (Fig. 23-2) that affects primarily medium-sized and small arteries. It is a systemic disorder that may involve the kidneys, joints, skin, nerves, and various other tissues. The diagnosis is usually made with biopsy (the affected tissues generally show necrotizing changes and disruption of the blood vessels) or angiography (focal stenoses and microaneurysms are typical). Corticosteroids and cytotoxic agents (such as cyclophosphamide and azathioprine) are frequently effective for treatment.

- Polyarteritis nodosa: acute, necrotizing vasculitis that affects medium-sized and small arteries.
- It is a systemic disorder.
- Diagnosis is made with biopsy or angiography.
- Corticosteroids and cytotoxic agents are effective therapy.

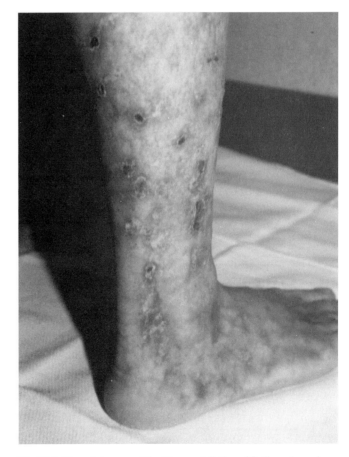

Fig. 23-2. Necrotizing vasculitis. The constellation of findings shown here (ulcerations, livedo, petechial skin lesions) are typical of many vasculitic processes that affect small or medium-sized vessels.

Wegener Granulomatosis

This granulomatous, necrotizing process can affect blood vessels in the respiratory tract and kidneys. In severe cases, surrounding structures, including the skin, may be involved. The syndrome is typically fatal without treatment. The diagnosis has been aided in recent years by the ability to test for antineutrophil cytoplasmic antibodies; although they are present in many vasculitides, a typical granular pattern is seen in Wegener granulomatosis. Treatment consists of prednisone, cyclophosphamide, and, in some cases, trimethoprim-sulfamethoxazole.

- Wegener granulomatosis can affect blood vessels in respiratory tract and kidneys.
- Syndrome is typically fatal without treatment.
- Diagnosis is aided by testing for antineutrophil cytoplasmic antibodies.
- Treatment consists of prednisone and cyclophosphamide.

Rheumatoid Vasculitis

Blood vessels are frequently involved in rheumatoid and other collagen vascular diseases. The findings frequently resemble those of polyarteritis nodosa, although the skin is affected more often. In the United States, rheumatoid vasculitis is one of the most common causes of chronic leg ulcers, after neuropathy, atherosclerosis, and venous disorders. Prednisone is usually effective, with or without other immunosuppressive agents.

- Rheumatoid vasculitis is similar to polyarteritis nodosa, except skin is affected more often.
- It is a common cause of chronic leg ulcers in United States.
- Prednisone is usually effective treatment.

Other Vasculitides

A wide variety of other vasculitides may affect small and medium-sized vessels. These include allergic angiitis (Churg-Strauss syndrome), cryoglobulinemia, Schönlein-Henoch purpura, various forms of hypersensitivity vasculitis, serum sickness, and numerous nonspecific necrotizing and non-necrotizing vasculitides. In general, most of these can be treated with corticosteroids or a steroid-sparing immunosuppressant.

BUERGER DISEASE

Cause

The cause of Buerger disease (thromboangiitis obliterans) remains unknown, but its association with smoking is powerful and well known. Few, if any, cases occur in the absence of tobacco use. Pathologically, the disease resembles a vasculitis; the vessel is typically thrombosed and infiltrated with inflammatory cells. Granuloma formation and microabscesses are common.

- Cause of Buerger disease is unknown.
- Association with smoking is powerful and well known.
- Granuloma and microabscesses are common.

Clinical Manifestations

The disease usually affects the small distal arteries first and progresses proximally if smoking is continued. Veins are also often involved; the first manifestation of Buerger disease may be superficial phlebitis. If smoking is discontinued, the process is frequently arrested; if smoking continues, the disease almost always progresses. Interestingly, whereas other vasculitides typically demonstrate an elevated erythrocyte sedimentation rate, in Buerger disease it is often minimally elevated or normal.

- Buerger disease affects small distal arteries first.
- Veins are also involved.
- First manifestation may be superficial phlebitis.
- Erythrocyte sedimentation rate is minimally elevated or normal.

Diagnosis

The diagnosis is usually made on the basis of the history. The patient is typically younger than 40 years, has distal disease (Fig. 23-3), and has a history of cigarette use. Men were once thought to be primarily affected, but as women have started to smoke in greater numbers, the frequency with which they develop this disease has increased. Angiography shows typical findings that can aid in the diagnosis, and definitive pathologic findings can often be obtained on appropriate biopsy.

- Typical patient with Buerger disease: <40 years old, has distal disease, has history of cigarette use.

Treatment

Cessation of smoking is an absolute necessity. Other treatments (such as pentoxifylline and sympathectomy) are of variable benefit.

- Cessation of smoking is a necessity in Buerger disease.

ERGOTISM

Mechanism of Action

Ergotamine and ergot derivatives are potent arterial vasoconstrictors. They are thought to produce vasoconstriction by cross-reacting with α-adrenergic (and to a lesser extent, serotonergic) receptors in the blood vessel wall. These compounds are typically given either orally or by suppository. Their major indication is for the treatment of vasomotor (migraine) headache.

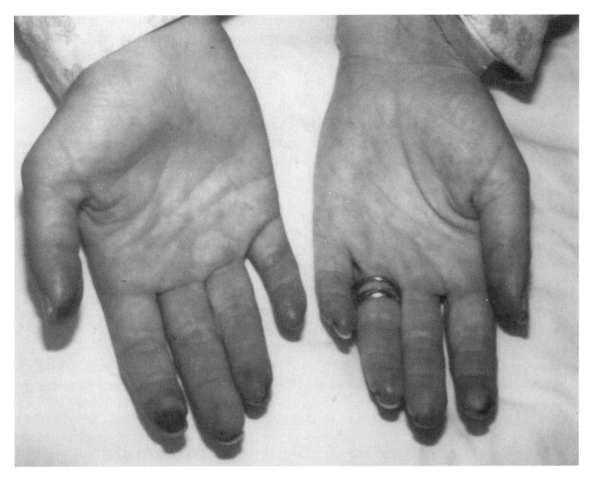

Fig. 23-3. Buerger disease. Distal portions of digits are severely ischemic. Bilateral ischemia affecting multiple digits is suggestive of Buerger disease, thromboembolic disease, or a connective tissue disorder.

- Ergotamine and ergot derivatives are potent arterial vasoconstrictors.
- They cross-react with α-adrenergic receptors in the blood vessel wall.

Clinical Manifestations

The typical patient with ergotism is a young female with a history of headaches. The patient may complain of vasospastic phenomena such as Raynaud disease or Prinzmetal angina. However, the vasospasm may be so persistent and severe that it mimics or leads to arterial occlusion. Myocardial infarction, mesenteric insufficiency or infarction, limb ischemia, neurologic findings, cutaneous infarctions, and other ischemic syndromes may result from its use.

- Typical patient with ergotism: young female with history of headaches.
- Vasospastic phenomena may be present, such as Raynaud disease or Prinzmetal angina.

Diagnosis

The diagnosis of ergot toxicity is almost always made from the history and by exclusion. It is often difficult to elicit a history of ergot use from patients, many of whom use the compound unknowingly, fail to recognize the significance of its use, or use it in an intentionally abusive way.

- Diagnosis of ergot toxicity is almost always made from history and by exclusion.

Treatment

Discontinuing the use of ergot usually leads to relief of symptoms. Occasionally, vasodilator therapy is indicated. Sodium nitroprusside is generally effective in this regard, although calcium or α-adrenergic blockers may also be useful.

- Discontinuing use of ergot leads to relief of symptoms.
- Sodium nitroprusside is generally effective.

THORACIC OUTLET SYNDROME

Cause

Thoracic outlet syndrome occurs when the brachial plexus, subclavian artery, or subclavian vein becomes compressed in the region of the thoracic outlet (Fig. 23-4). Symptoms are thought to result from nerve compression in 90% to 95% of cases; only a small number are clearly due to venous or arterial compression. Thoracic outlet syndrome is the most common cause of acute arterial occlusion in the upper extremity of adults younger than 40 years. Repetitive trauma to the artery can lead to intimal damage, embolization, aneurysm formation, or acute thrombosis. Thoracic outlet syndrome is also the most common cause of upper extremity acute venous occlusion in the young adult. "Stress" thrombosis, which occurs during periods of intense upper extremity activity such as lifting heavy weights, is typically the consequence of intermittent venous occlusion.

- Symptoms of thoracic outlet syndrome are thought to result from nerve compression in 90%-95% of cases.
- Thoracic outlet syndrome is most common cause of acute arterial occlusion in upper extremity of adults <40 years old.
- Thoracic outlet syndrome is the most common cause of upper extremity acute venous occlusion in young adults.

Diagnosis

Arterial involvement is suggested by radial or brachial pulse obliteration during provocative maneuvering of the arms, although this finding may also be a normal variant. Nerve involvement is much more difficult to determine; electromyography and nerve conduction studies have not proved consistently useful for diagnosis. Intermittent venous compression is also difficult to document, and when it is found (on ultrasound duplex scanning or magnetic resonance imaging) its significance is uncertain. One of the most useful clinical tests is the elevated arm stress test (EAST), in which the patient raises his or her hands above the head and clenches and unclenches the fist for 1 or 2 minutes. The appearance of typical symptoms, with or without signs of vascular involvement such as delayed capillary refilling, is suggestive of the syndrome.

- Indicator of possible thoracic outlet syndrome: positional obliteration of radial pulse.
- Nerve involvement is more difficult to determine.
- Useful test is elevated arm stress test.

Treatment

Conservative measures should be tried first. These include exercise, stretching activities, and avoidance of aggravating factors. When conservative measures fail and symptoms warrant, surgical resection of the first rib is curative in 80% to 85% of patients. In those with significant arterial involvement (such as intimal damage or aneurysm formation), the involved section of artery should be replaced with a graft. Patients with recent venous thrombosis can have the clot cleared with thrombolytic therapy before rib resection.

- For thoracic outlet syndrome, conservative measures should be tried first.
- Surgical resection of first rib is curative in 80%-85% of cases.

MICROEMBOLI

Cause (Fig. 23-5)

Whereas macroemboli most frequently originate in the heart, microemboli more commonly originate from the peripheral vessels, although cardiac sources can occur. The most common variety are atheroemboli, which are small thrombi or cholesterol particles given off by fragmenting atherosclerotic plaques. Malfunctioning cardiac valves (native or prosthetic), dissection flaps, intracardiac tumors, and a host of other lesions can also spawn microemboli. Plaque rupture may occur spontaneously, but it is increasingly found as a complication of invasive (catheter) procedures.

- Microemboli commonly originate from peripheral vessels.
- Most common variety are atheroemboli.
- Plaque rupture may occur spontaneously or as a complication of invasive procedure.

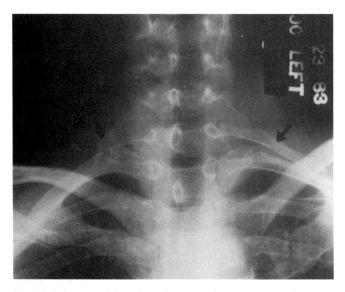

Fig. 23-4. Positional thoracic outlet obstruction is frequently due to the presence of a cervical rib (*arrow*).

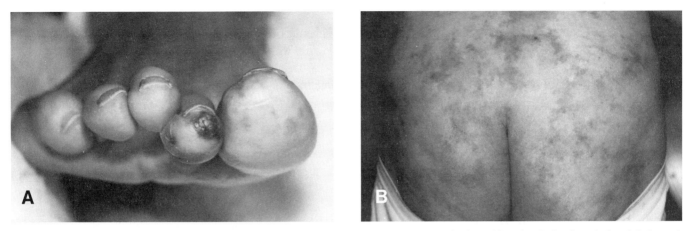

Fig. 23-5. Embolic disease. *A,* Distal infarcts and petechia. *B,* Emboli to buttocks after aortic catheterization. This patient had catheter-induced cholesterol microemboli that caused small infarctions and petechiae over back and buttocks.

Clinical Manifestations

Microemboli may produce livedo, rubor, petechia, focal cutaneous necrosis, and organ ischemia or infarction. These findings depend on the distribution and extent of embolization. Diffuse microembolization from a source proximal to the renal or mesenteric vessels is a catastrophic occurrence that can lead to visceral and renal infarction and severe peripheral ischemia.

● Microemboli may produce livedo, rubor, petechia, focal cutaneous necrosis, and organ ischemia or infarction.

Treatment

The only reliable treatment of persistent microemboli is identification and removal of the embolic source. Because atherosclerosis is a diffuse process, the search for an embolic source often demonstrates widespread disease for which no simple surgical repair is readily apparent. Medical therapy, such as aspirin or anticoagulation, may help but often does not. Indeed, there is a well-recognized syndrome in which warfarin triggers or exacerbates atheroemboli. The exact mechanism of this phenomenon remains uncertain. Dipyridamole has been advocated by some, but it remains of unproven value.

● Only reliable treatment for microemboli is identification and removal of embolic source.
● There is a syndrome in which warfarin triggers or exacerbates atheroemboli.

DISSECTION

Cause

Dissection, like aneurysm formation, is a degenerative condition that can affect most large or medium-sized arteries.

Dissection occurs when the intima or media separates from the remainder of the artery, creating a flap that can obstruct the lumen of the vessel (Fig. 23-6). Aneurysm formation or rupture of the weakened wall may occur. Marfan syndrome, Ehlers-Danlos syndrome, cystic medial necrosis, and a host of other conditions can predispose to dissection. Hypertension is frequently present. The aorta is the artery most frequently affected by dissection. Iatrogenic dissection may occur because of invasive diagnostic or therapeutic intravascular procedures, blunt trauma, or deceleration injuries.

● Dissection is a degenerative condition affecting most large or medium-sized arteries.
● Marfan syndrome, Ehlers-Danlos syndrome, and cystic medial necrosis predispose to dissection.
● Hypertension is frequently present.
● Aorta is the artery most frequently affected by dissection.

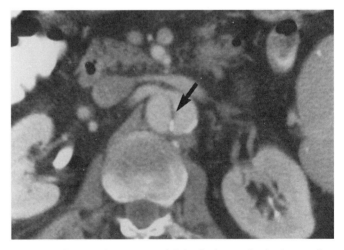

Fig. 23-6. Computed tomogram of abdominal aorta clearly shows a flap (*arrow*) resulting from a dissection. Dissections can also be studied with angiography or ultrasonography.

Classification

The two most common systems for classifying aortic dissection are the Stanford and the DeBakey systems, defined as follows:

Stanford A: any dissection involving the ascending aorta regardless of the site of primary intimal tear or distal extent of propagation

Stanford B: any dissection confined entirely to the distal aorta (i.e., distal to the aortic arch)

DeBakey type 1: equivalent to Stanford A

DeBakey type 2: a dissection limited to the ascending portion of the aorta

DeBakey type 3: equivalent to Stanford B.

Diagnosis

The sudden onset of "tearing" chest, scapular, or abdominal pain should alert the clinician to the possibility of aortic dissection. The pain commonly migrates as the dissection extends. Evidence of arterial occlusion may be present if the dissection flap causes vascular obstruction. Care must be taken to avoid misdiagnosing dissection as myocardial infarction because the administration of thrombolytics in this setting is potentially lethal. Several tests may be used to screen for, or confirm the diagnosis of, dissection. Aortography is the historical standard, although computed tomography (conventional and ultrafast) and transesophageal echocardiography are rapidly emerging as equivalent or possibly superior technologies. Magnetic resonance imaging, digital subtraction angiography, transthoracic or abdominal duplex ultrasonography, and other similar tests are less desirable because of their limited ability to visualize the flap and their increased expense.

- Symptoms of aortic dissection: "tearing" chest, scapular, or abdominal pain.
- Pain commonly migrates as dissection extends.
- Misdiagnosis as myocardial infarction needs to be avoided.
- Aortography is the standard test.

Treatment

Dissections involving the ascending aorta (Stanford A, DeBakey type 1 or 2) should be treated with an emergency operation. The mortality rate for patients in this group who are treated medically is more than 90%. The perioperative mortality rate is 20% or less. When the dissection involves the aortic valve, replacement or repair of the valve is necessary. Dissections involving the descending aorta (Stanford B or DeBakey type 3) may be treated either medically or surgically. Generally, medical therapy can be attempted first (β-adrenergic blockade, reduction of blood pressure as much as tolerated), and if the pain resolves promptly the patient can be followed. Operation should be performed if pain persists or

recurs, aneurysms develop or enlarge, or limb or abdominal ischemia occurs. Regardless of the treatment used, serial follow-up with computed tomography should be performed to look for enlargement or resolution of the dissection and the integrity of the graft anastomosis.

- Dissections of ascending aorta should be treated with emergency operation.
- Mortality rate with medical treatment of dissection of ascending aorta is >90%.
- Dissection of descending aorta may be treated medically or surgically.
- Operation for dissection of descending aorta is needed if pain persists or recurs, aneurysms develop, or limb or abdominal ischemia occurs.

Other Dissections

Dissections of the coronary artery can result from diagnostic catheterization or interventional therapeutic procedures such as percutaneous transluminal coronary angioplasty. Spontaneous carotid dissection can occur and is manifested by a constellation of symptoms that include unilateral headache, focal cerebral ischemic symptoms, and pulsatile tinnitus. Although there is no surgical option for this condition, spontaneous resolution is the rule. In contrast, spontaneous renal dissection is usually treated surgically. Iliofemoral dissections are usually the result of diagnostic or therapeutic catheter procedures performed through groin puncture sites.

- Carotid dissection resolves spontaneously.
- Renal dissection is usually treated surgically.

FIBROMUSCULAR DYSPLASIA

Background

Fibromuscular dysplasia (FMD) is a dysplastic disease affecting medium-sized and small arteries. Women are affected much more frequently than men. Most patients with FMD have renovascular involvement (60%-70%), and about 30% have cerebrovascular involvement. FMD can affect any layer of the arterial wall (intima, media, adventitia); the pathologic classification of this disease is usually based on the site of involvement. The most common form of FMD is medial (medial fibroplasia), which represents 70% to 95% of all forms of FMD.

- FMD is a dysplastic disease of medium-sized and small arteries.
- Renovascular involvement occurs in 60%-70% of cases.
- Cerebrovascular involvement occurs in about 30% of cases.

Diagnosis

In patients with renovascular hypertension or arterial occlusive disease, an FMD-related cause can be determined by angiography. In the most common forms of dysplasia the artery has a "string-of-beads" appearance (Fig. 23-7). These beads typically represent alternating stenotic and aneurysmal regions of blood vessels. Examination of biopsy specimens, when available, can aid in the diagnosis of FMD. Pathogenically, FMD can produce stenotic lesions that may limit or occlude blood flow. It can also predispose to aneurysm formation or dissection.

- FMD is diagnosed with angiography.
- Artery has "string-of-beads" appearance.
- FMD can produce stenotic lesions or predispose to aneurysm formation or dissection.

Treatment

FMD is best treated, when possible, by percutaneous transluminal angioplasty (PTA). Nearly two-thirds of patients with renovascular FMD will be "cured" by PTA alone. Operation should be reserved for patients in whom PTA fails, or in whom aneurysm or dissection is present. In certain patients, particularly those in whom PTA has failed and who are poor surgical risks, drug therapy alone may be adequate.

- FMD is best treated by percutaneous transluminal angioplasty.
- Almost two-thirds of patients are "cured" by angioplasty alone.
- Operation is used when angioplasty fails or when aneurysm or dissection is present.

GIANT CELL ARTERITIS

Background

Giant cell arteritis is a granulomatous vasculitic process of unknown cause. The large arteries are primarily affected. The two major syndromes of giant cell arteritis are Takayasu arteritis and temporal arteritis.

- Giant cell arteritis is a granulomatous vasculitic process.
- Two major syndromes: Takayasu arteritis and temporal arteritis.

Takayasu Arteritis

Takayasu arteritis (Fig. 23-8) affects primarily the aorta and its major branches, particularly those of the aortic arch. It is more common in females than in males. Also known as pulseless disease, it frequently leads to complete occlusion of the

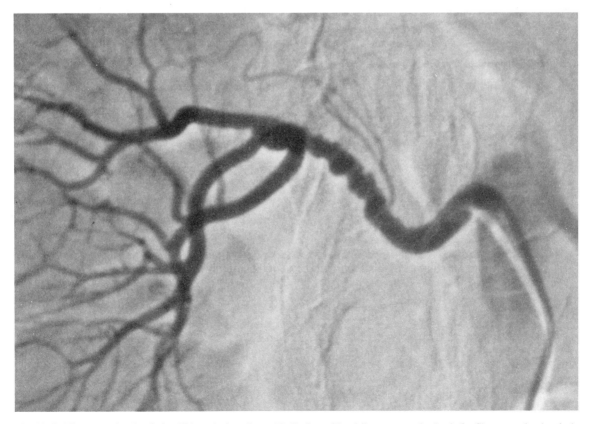

Fig. 23-7. Fibromuscular dysplasia. This typical angiographic "string-of-beads" appearance is classic for fibromuscular dysplasia.

brachiocephalic vessels. Patients are almost always younger than 50 years. Affected arteries may occasionally form aneurysms. The diagnosis is usually made from the history, examination, and arteriography. Angiographic findings include tapered narrowings (such as the "string" sign) of the brachiocephalic vessels; these occasionally go on to produce occlusion. When necessary, or when tissue is available, the diagnosis can be made from biopsy. The erythrocyte sedimentation rate is almost always increased in patients with active Takayasu arteritis, and it can serve as an index of disease activity. Other acute-phase reactants, such as C-reactive protein, are occasionally useful.

- Takayasu arteritis is more common in females.
- Patients are almost always <50 years old.
- Diagnosis is made from the history, examination, and arteriography.

Therapy primarily involves the use of prednisone. High-dose prednisone (50-100 mg daily in single dose or divided doses) is usually instituted for 3 to 6 weeks, or until the sedimentation rate has stabilized in the normal range. Slow taper (2.5-5.0 mg every 2-4 weeks) is the rule, with the taper slowing to as little as 1 mg per month once the daily dose reaches 10 mg. The rate of taper should be modified according to the sedimentation rate and the clinical picture. In some cases, low-dose prednisone may be needed for prolonged periods or even indefinitely. Occasionally, vessels that were stenotic during the active phase of the disease will "reopen" during treat-

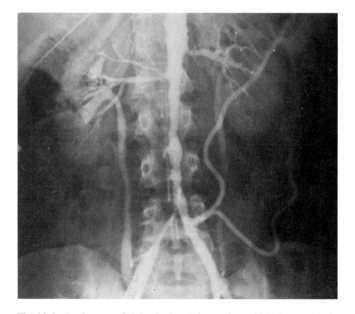

Fig. 23-8. Angiogram of abdominal aorta in a patient with Takayasu arteritis shows multiple areas of stenosis involving distal aorta, iliac arteries, and renal arteries. Narrowed regions represent areas of the artery which have undergone inflammation or scarring.

ment. When surgical correction is necessary, efforts should be made to hold off until the disease has been adequately treated, or preferably until it is "burned out."

- Treatment of Takayasu arteritis is with high-dose prednisone that is slowly tapered.

Temporal Arteritis

Temporal arteritis primarily affects people older than 50 years. It predominantly affects secondary or tertiary branches from the aorta. Like Takayasu arteritis, its systemic manifestations may include fatigue, malaise, fever, and myalgias. It is pathologically indistinguishable from Takayasu arteritis. Temporal arteritis should be suspected in any patient with systemic symptoms and pain or tenderness localized to the temporal arteries. As with Takayasu arteritis the erythrocyte sedimentation rate is typically increased, and the degree of increase can be used to monitor the activity of the disease. Although angiography can be used to make the diagnosis, biopsy is much more commonly used because of the accessibility of the temporal artery. Biopsy should include as long a piece of the temporal artery as possible, and it may need to be performed bilaterally before the disease can be excluded.

- Temporal arteritis primarily affects people >50 years old.
- Systemic manifestations: fatigue, malaise, fever, myalgias.
- Temporal arteritis is pathologically indistinguishable from Takayasu arteritis.
- Diagnosis should be suspected in any patient with pain or tenderness localized to the temporal arteries.

Like Takayasu arteritis, the treatment of temporal arteritis involves the use of corticosteroids. A typical program is 50 to 100 mg of prednisone per day, and treatment is usually maintained for 3 to 6 weeks or until the erythrocyte sedimentation rate has stabilized in the normal range. The relapse rate during taper is higher than that for Takayasu arteritis, and in some series it approaches 50%. Longer-term, higher-dose corticosteroid programs may be necessary.

If the diagnosis of temporal arteritis is being seriously considered, treatment with prednisone should begin immediately. This approach prevents the sudden, unexpected complication of blindness due to occlusion of the central retinal artery. Biopsy results remain accurate if biopsy is performed within several days after starting treatment with corticosteroids.

- For temporal arteritis, treatment with prednisone should begin immediately to prevent sudden, unexpected blindness due to occlusion of the central retinal artery.

RAYNAUD PHENOMENON

Background

Raynaud phenomenon refers to any inappropriate or excessively intense episode of cutaneous, digital, or limb vasoconstriction. It most commonly affects the upper limb. Females are affected far more commonly than males. Attacks are usually triggered by exposure to the cold or by emotional stress. The disease can be divided into two categories, primary and secondary, depending on cause.

● Raynaud phenomenon is inappropriate or excessively intense episode of cutaneous, digital, or limb vasoconstriction.

Primary Raynaud Phenomenon

The cause of primary Raynaud phenomenon is unknown. Episodes are usually bilateral. Digital ulcerations are rare but may occur occasionally. The symptoms are usually stable and may be related to abnormalities in adrenergic function, blood viscosity, or endothelial disorders.

● Episodes of primary Raynaud phenomenon are usually bilateral.
● Digital ulcerations are rare.

Secondary Raynaud Phenomenon

This refers to Raynaud phenomenon occurring as the result of some other underlying abnormality. Predisposing factors include atherosclerosis, arteritis, cancer, collagen vascular disease, thoracic outlet syndrome, embolic occlusions, occupational disease, certain drugs (β-adrenergic blocker, nicotine, ergotamine), and various other conditions. Secondary Raynaud phenomenon is occasionally unilateral (perhaps affecting a single digit) and may produce skin breakdown.

● Secondary Raynaud phenomenon is the result of some other underlying abnormality.

Diagnosis

The diagnosis of Raynaud phenomenon is made primarily on clinical grounds. Provocative testing to document and assess normal vasoconstriction is often of limited value because of the difficulty in reliably reproducing symptoms in the laboratory setting.

● Diagnosis of Raynaud phenomenon is made on clinical grounds.

Treatment

The treatment of Raynaud phenomenon is often difficult. In cases of secondary Raynaud phenomenon, treatment of the underlying condition should be attempted whenever possible. Simple conservative measures such as dressing warmly, avoiding unnecessary exposure to the cold, and intermittent hand warming may improve the condition substantially. Biofeedback is effective in certain cases. Drugs with a potential for causing vasoconstriction should be avoided. Occasionally it is necessary to move to a warmer climate to achieve complete relief. Certain vasodilators, especially nifedipine, prazosin, and other calcium or α-adrenergic blockers, may help in selected cases. Interruption of the sympathetic nerves, either through ganglionic injection or surgical sympathectomy, is often useful in patients with severe symptoms.

● Simple treatment for Raynaud phenomenon: dressing warmly, avoiding exposure to cold, intermittent hand warming.
● Certain vasodilators may help in selected cases.

ACUTE DEEP VENOUS THROMBOSIS

Cause

The factors predisposing to deep venous thrombosis (DVT) include those of the Virchow triad: stasis, trauma, and hypercoagulability. Underlying conditions or factors that can predispose to DVT include cancer, inflammatory bowel disease, pregnancy or estrogen use, obesity, age, tobacco use, surgery or trauma, congestive heart failure, previous DVT, and a host of others.

● Factors in DVT include the Virchow triad: stasis, trauma, hypercoagulability.

Clinical Manifestations

Acute DVT is notoriously difficult to diagnose on clinical grounds only. Swelling, pain, discoloration, positive Homans sign, cord palpation, and other typical features can suggest the diagnosis but are frequently misleading. In many cases extensive DVT may be minimally symptomatic or even asymptomatic, whereas in others the proximal DVT is so massive that the leg becomes mottled, cyanotic, markedly tender, and ischemic; this condition is referred to as phlegmasia cerulea dolens.

● DVT is notoriously difficult to diagnose on clinical grounds only.

Diagnosis

Venography has long been the standard method for definitively diagnosing DVT, but duplex scanning (with or without color flow) is rapidly emerging as an equivalent method for the diagnosis of proximal DVT. Nonimaging (functional) methods such as impedance plethysmography and continuous-wave Doppler remain reliable, cost-efficient methods for detecting proximal DVT. They are unreliable for excluding below-knee thrombus. Fortunately, the embolic potential of below-knee thrombus is extremely low, and in many clinical situations it is safe to follow patients who have negative results of functional studies such as impedance plethysmography.

- Venography is standard method to diagnose DVT.
- Duplex scanning is an equivalent method for diagnosis of proximal DVT.

Treatment

Patients with acute, proximal DVT are traditionally hospitalized and treated with intravenously administered heparin, although in selected cases therapy may be performed in the outpatient setting with subcutaneously administered heparin. When unfractionated heparin is used, the activated partial thromboplastin time should be kept at 2.0 to 2.5 times the control value. The dose of low-molecular-weight heparin must be adjusted according to body weight. Treatment with oral warfarin is started as soon as possible and is overlapped with heparin therapy for at least 5 days; use of heparin is discontinued when the prothrombin time is therapeutic and stable. If hospitalization is required, the patient should remain hospitalized until the prothrombin time is therapeutic (1.5-2.0 times control value, or INR of 2-3) and the patient is able to ambulate without pain. Use of warfarin should be maintained for at least 3 months. In most cases of DVT, an elastic compression stocking should be prescribed and worn during treatment with warfarin.

- Treatment for DVT: hospitalization, intravenously administered heparin.
- Patient is hospitalized until prothrombin time, while receiving warfarin, is therapeutic.
- Warfarin is used for at least 3 months.

Unprecipitated DVT

In patients with unprecipitated DVT, be sure to search for an underlying, occult disorder that may be predisposing the patient to clot formation.

- For unprecipitated DVT, search for underlying disorder.

PULMONARY EMBOLISM

Background

Pulmonary embolism is a major cause of death in the United States and may cause as many as 250,000 fatalities per year. It is estimated that up to 80% of significant pulmonary emboli escape detection and that 50% of patients suspected of having pulmonary emboli on clinical grounds actually do not. The mortality rate is between 20% and 35% for untreated pulmonary emboli, and it is 8% when the condition is properly diagnosed and treated.

- Mortality rate with untreated pulmonary emboli: 20%-35%.

Pathophysiology

The risk factors for pulmonary emboli are the same as those for deep venous thrombosis (see page 901). Emboli are most likely to originate in the large, deep veins of the lower extremity (iliofemoral system), although 10% of pulmonary emboli come from the upper extremity. Thrombi in the superficial veins or deep venous system distal to the knee do not commonly give rise to clinically significant emboli.

- Emboli are most likely to originate in large, deep veins of the lower extremity.
- 10% of emboli come from the upper extremity.

Signs and Symptoms

There is generally poor correlation among symptoms, clinical findings, and the presence or absence of pulmonary emboli. Most pulmonary emboli occur silently. When signs and symptoms occur, they are highly variable. In the Urokinase Pulmonary Embolism Trial, the most common signs and symptoms included tachypnea (respiration rate >16 per minute), 92%; dyspnea, 85%; pleuritic chest pain, 74%; apprehension, 59%; rales, 58%; and cough, 53%. Phlebitis was clinically apparent in only 32%. Other common findings included an accentuated second heart sound, tachycardia, fever, hemoptysis, diaphoresis, and syncope. Massive pulmonary embolism may cause syncope, cor pulmonale, cardiogenic shock, and cardiac arrest with electromechanical dissociation. Chronic pulmonary emboli may lead to pulmonary hypertension and the development of cor pulmonale.

- Correlation is poor among symptoms, clinical findings, and the presence or absence of pulmonary emboli.
- Most pulmonary emboli occur silently.
- Chronic pulmonary emboli may lead to pulmonary hypertension.

Screening Tests

The most common electrocardiographic abnormality noted in pulmonary embolism is sinus tachycardia. Classic electrocardiographic findings such as an S_1, Q_3, T_3 pattern, right bundle branch block, right-axis deviation, and increased P wave are present in only one-fourth of patients. Chest radiography is likewise nonspecific; findings include pleural effusion in 50%, right-sided cardiomegaly, pulmonary infarction, elevation of the hemidiaphragm, and atelectasis. The arterial blood gas may show decreased PO_2 and PCO_2.

Specific Tests

Ventilation-perfusion scanning is one of the most widely used tests to screen for pulmonary embolism. It should be viewed as a useful test when the findings suggest either a high probability or normal results. Intermediate- or low-probability results should be viewed as nondiagnostic. Pulmonary angiography remains the standard diagnostic method. Computed tomography, especially ultrafast, is also a useful diagnostic tool.

- Ventilation-perfusion scanning is widely used to screen for pulmonary embolism.
- Pulmonary angiography is standard diagnostic method.

Treatment

Anticoagulation is the mainstay of treatment for acute pulmonary embolism. It should be started immediately with heparin, which is usually given for 5 to 10 days. The regimen is then switched to warfarin, which should be maintained for 3 to 6 months. In cases of massive pulmonary embolism, thrombolytic therapy should be considered. Streptokinase, urokinase, and tissue-plasminogen activator are all potentially useful agents. In patients with massive, life-threatening pulmonary embolism who have contraindications to thrombolytic therapy or who have not responded to an attempt at lysis, or in whom severe, chronic pulmonary embolism is present, surgical embolectomy can be considered. Patients who cannot tolerate anticoagulation should be considered for a caval filter to prevent recurrent, possibly lethal, pulmonary embolism.

CHRONIC DEEP VENOUS INSUFFICIENCY (POSTPHLEBITIC SYNDROME)

Background

Chronic deep venous insufficiency (DVI) is among the most common causes of leg ulcer in the United States (Fig. 23-9). The condition develops when veins become chronically obstructed, or when venous valvular incompetence develops. These recurrences are often caused by deep venous thrombosis. Although the exact mechanism by which venous insufficiency produces chronic changes is unknown, it appears that chronically increased venous pressure is the culprit.

- DVI is one of the most common causes of leg ulcer in the United States.
- Recurrences are usually caused by deep venous thrombosis.

Clinical Manifestations

DVI may lead to limb swelling, pigmentation (from hemosiderin deposition in the perivascular tissues), induration and cellulitis, dermatitis, and ulceration. The most commonly affected area of the leg is the region around the medial malleolus, although any portion of the lower part of the leg may be involved.

- DVI most often affects the medial malleolar region.

Diagnosis

The diagnosis is made from the clinical history, physical findings, and objective testing. Specific tests for DVI include continuous-wave Doppler (with or without duplex imaging), various types of plethysmographic studies, and descending venography.

Treatment

DVI is treated primarily with measures to control swelling. The leg should be elevated whenever possible, and long periods of standing or sitting should be avoided. Elastic compression, either in the form of stockings or wrap, is essential. The compression must be graduated and of sufficient magnitude to prevent swelling. If stockings are to be used, the swelling should be maximally reduced before fitting. Additional compression can be supplied by the use of elastic pads. Dermatitis and other forms of inflammation are often improved by the use of corticosteroid cream. Antibiotics should be reserved for situations in which infection is apparent. Anticoagulation is not necessary unless recurrent clotting has developed or is likely. Venous stripping or perforator ligation may be useful in a limited number of cases with refractory ulcers. The stripping of superficial veins should be avoided if deep venous obstruction is present, because the superficial veins may be acting as collaterals. Occasionally a chronic

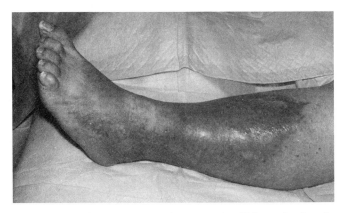

Fig. 23-9. Leg of a man with severe deep venous insufficiency. Persistently elevated venous pressure produces changes including swelling, inflammation, and hemosiderin deposition. The extensive region of discoloration is due to hemosiderin that has been deposited in the skin.

arteriovenous fistula may mimic DVI. This possibility should be considered when penetrating trauma, surgical procedures, or other causes of fistula are present.

- Elastic compression is essential for DVI.
- Venous stripping or perforator ligation is useful in a limited number of cases.
- Chronic arteriovenous fistula may mimic DVI.

LYMPHEDEMA

Background

Lymphedema is the result of hypoplasia, dysfunction, or obstruction of the lymphatic vessels (Fig. 23-10). As a result, lymphatic fluid accumulates in the interstitial space and the extremity becomes swollen. Pitting edema is present early in the disease, but in chronic cases the subcutaneous tissues become fibrotic and hyperplastic, producing woody nonpitting edema.

- Lymphedema results from hypoplasia, dysfunction, or obstruction of lymphatic vessels.
- Pitting edema occurs early in disease.

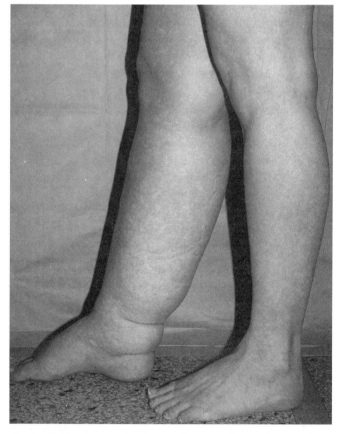

Fig. 23-10. Right leg is swollen because of obstructed lymphatic vessels. Note that the dorsum of the foot is involved in this process.

Cause

Lymphedema may be primary (due to a congenital abnormality or predisposition) or secondary (due to trauma, infection, cancer, and other disorders). Primary lymphedema most commonly becomes manifest at puberty (lymphedema praecox) and may be familial in about 15% of cases. Secondary lymphedema is a worldwide problem of major proportion. In tropical countries, the most common cause of lymphedema is filarial infection, and the lymphedema produced can be severe (elephantiasis). In Western or industrialized countries, tumors (such as breast, prostate, gynecologic) and recurrent infections are the most common causes. The treatment of breast cancer may produce edema of the upper extremity. The likelihood and severity of lymphedema depend on the type and extent of operation and the use of adjuvant therapy such as radiation or chemotherapy.

- Primary lymphedema manifests at puberty (lymphedema praecox) and may be familial.
- In tropical countries, the most common cause of lymphedema is filarial infection.
- In Western countries, tumor and recurrent infections are commonly associated with lymphedema.

Diagnosis

The diagnosis of lymphedema can usually be made from the history and physical examination. When a confirmatory study is necessary, the best technique is lymphoscintigraphy. In this test, a small amount of radiolabeled colloid is injected in the web space between the digits, where its progress through the lymphatics is followed with nuclear scanning. The patency of lymphatics can thus be determined. Lymphangiography has been considered the standard, but it should be avoided whenever possible because of its invasive nature and tendency to cause lymphangitis, which may worsen lymphedema.

- Lymphoscintigraphy is best diagnostic technique for lymphedema.
- Lymphangiography should be avoided because of its invasive nature.

Treatment

In most cases, lymphedema is incurable but treatable. Good hygiene and protection from trauma are among the most important elements of care. The limb should be elevated as often as possible to drain the tissue and keep swelling to a minimum. Elastic compression stockings (often with pressures as high as 50 or 60 mm Hg) are the mainstay of treatment. Sequential compression pumps capable of generating pressures of 80 to 100 mm Hg can be used to "milk" lymphatic fluid out of the legs. Massage therapy also may be useful in selected patients for reducing edema and maintaining limb size. Antibiotics should be used liberally to treat or provide prophylaxis against bacterial infection. In some cases, surgical techniques to reduce the size of the limb or bypass blocked lymphatics are possible.

- Elastic compression stockings are mainstay of treatment for lymphedema.
- Pumps or massage may be used to reduce or maintain limb size.

ARTERIOVENOUS MALFORMATION OR FISTULA

Background

Arteriovenous malformation or fistula (Fig. 23-11) may be acquired or congenital. Acquired cases are generally due to penetrating trauma, iatrogenic processes such as surgery or catheterization, or spontaneous degeneration of blood vessels. Congenital malformation or fistula may involve primarily arterial, venous, capillary, or lymphatic tissues; at times the lesions are mixed and involve elements of all four.

- Arteriovenous malformations may be acquired or congenital.

Consequences

Arteriovenous malformations may be of cosmetic significance only, or they can produce pain, tissue destruction, or limb hypertrophy, especially when the flow is high. In some patients, congestive heart failure has occurred as a result of the high demand for blood flow associated with these lesions.

Treatment

The treatment of many arteriovenous malformations is difficult because the malformation may involve deep or vital structures and make resection impossible; vessels feeding or draining the lesion may be difficult to identify, reach, and ligate; the lesion has a propensity to redevelop after resection; and successful treatment may produce ischemia in regions distal to the malformation. Thus, conservative measures are frequently used. When pain, swelling, congestive heart failure, the possibility of malignancy, or other problems force a consideration of interventional therapy, surgery or embolization is usually attempted. Catheter-directed embolization is showing increasing utility in this regard.

- Treatment of arteriovenous malformation is difficult.

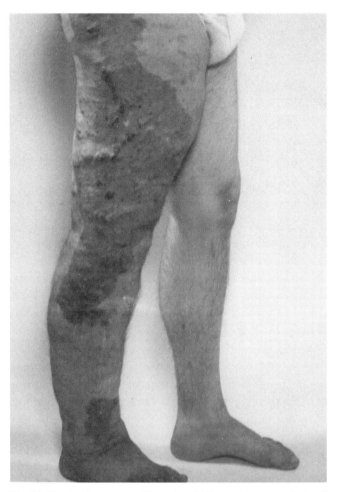

Fig. 23-11. Arteriovenous malformation. This extensive congenital malformation has led to venous volume and pressure overload. As a result, many of the clinical findings are similar to those of chronic venous insufficiency. If blood flow is high enough, heart failure may develop.

ULCERS

Types

Vascular ulcers can be divided into four categories: ischemic, venous, arteriolar, and neurotrophic.

Ischemic

Ischemic ulcers (Fig. 23-12) result from arterial occlusive disease (large or small vessels) that reduces blood flow below the level necessary for maintaining skin viability. The ulcers tend to be distal (digits or foot) and may be triggered by trauma, including mild abrasion from shoes. They often become infected. Ischemic ulcers are usually painful unless associated neuropathy is present.

- Ischemic ulcers result from arterial occlusive disease.
- Ischemic ulcers tend to be distal (digits or foot).
- Ulcers are usually painful.

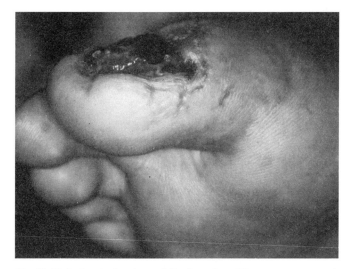

Fig. 23-12. Ischemic ulcer located distally on foot. There was poor wound granulation, and the ulcer was very painful.

Venous

Venous ulcers (Fig. 23-13) were discussed on page 947. They result from skin breakdown associated with chronic venous insufficiency. Other signs or symptoms of venous stasis are usually present around the ulcer, including swelling, pigmentation, and indurated cellulitis. Trauma is often a precipitating factor. The ulcers are usually located over the medial malleolus, but they may occur on any part of the leg. They are typically painful, but not as painful as ulcers caused by ischemia.

● Venous ulcers are associated with chronic venous insufficiency.
● Venous ulcers are not as painful as ischemic ulcers.

Arteriolar

Also known as "hypertensive" ulcers, arteriolar ulcers (Fig. 23-14) result from small-vessel occlusion. They tend to have punched-out or irregular (serpiginous) borders and are usually extremely painful. A wide variety of processes can lead to the small-vessel occlusion producing arteriolar ulcers; these include hypertension, vasculitis, and collagen vascular diseases.

● Arteriolar ulcers result from small-vessel occlusion.
● They have punched-out or irregular (serpiginous) borders.
● They are extremely painful.

Neurotrophic

Patients with neuropathy, particularly those who are diabetic, frequently develop neurotrophic ulcers (Fig. 23-15) as a result of chronic trauma. The ulcers are painless and pale and typically have associated thick edges and callous formation. They are almost always present over pressure points or sites of repetitive trauma.

● Neurotrophic ulcers often develop in patients with neuropathy (diabetes).
● Ulcers are painless and pale and have thick edges and callous formation.

LOOK-ALIKES

Several processes can produce leg ulcers that may mimic vascular disease. These include pyoderma gangrenosum, Kaposi sarcoma, various infections, cutaneous tumors, lipedema (mimicking lymphedema), myxedema, trauma, and various other problems.

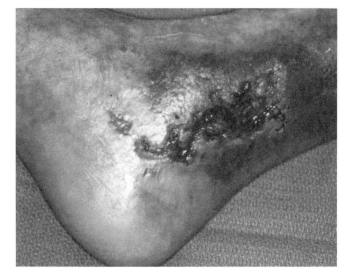

Fig. 23-13. Venous ulcer. Note location over medial malleolus and surrounding hyperpigmentation and cellulitis.

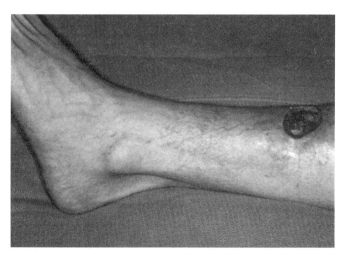

Fig. 23-14. Arteriolar (vasculitis) ulcer. This case has a clean, punched-out appearance.

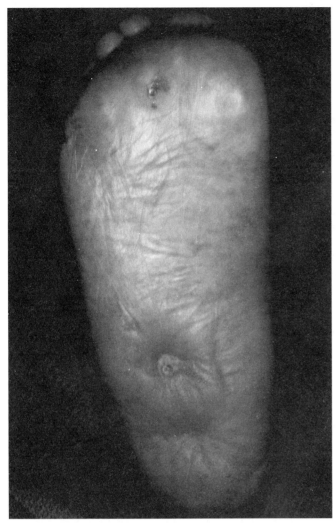

Fig. 23-15. Neurotrophic ulcers over pressure points on insensitive foot.

WARFARIN NECROSIS

This rare entity occurs in less than 1% of patients receiving the medication. It usually develops 3 to 6 days after initiation of therapy (more often in women) and is characterized by the sudden development of erythematous or hemorrhagic skin lesions. These eventually become gangrenous, and the overlying skin sloughs. Areas of skin with underlying fatty deposits (e.g., breasts and buttocks) are most commonly affected. The exact cause of this reaction is unknown, but a decreased level of protein C may be involved. When it occurs, the use of warfarin should be discontinued immediately.

- Warfarin necrosis occurs in <1% of patients receiving the medication.
- It develops 3-6 days after therapy.
- It is characterized by erythematous or hemorrhagic skin lesions that become gangrenous.
- Use of warfarin should be discontinued immediately.

HEPARIN-INDUCED THROMBOCYTOPENIA

The frequency of heparin-induced thrombocytopenia is probably 1% or 2%, but estimates as high as 30% have been reported. It typically begins 5 to 10 days after the initiation of heparin therapy. Patients with this condition are frequently asymptomatic but may develop hemorrhagic or thrombotic complications. The cause probably involves an antigen/antibody interaction, but the exact mechanism is poorly understood. Treatment consists of discontinuing use of heparin when the problem is identified.

- Heparin-induced thrombocytopenia occurs in 1% or 2% of patients receiving the medication.
- It begins 5-10 days after initiation of therapy.
- Cause involves antigen/antibody interaction.

IATROGENIC VASCULAR DISEASE AND TRAUMA

Vascular trauma is an increasingly common occurrence. Interventional procedures such as catheterization can produce occlusion, dissection, or bleeding. Other common sources of trauma include penetrating injuries, acceleration injuries, and blunt trauma.

QUESTIONS

Multiple Choice (choose the one best answer)

1. Which of the following is *not* associated with arterial aneurysm formation?
   a. Vasculitis
   b. Atherosclerosis
   c. Marfan syndrome
   d. Cytotoxic drugs
   e. Fibromuscular dysplasia

2. Which of the following is usually *not* directly associated with smoking?
   a. Lymphedema
   b. Raynaud phenomenon
   c. Atherosclerosis
   d. Buerger disease
   e. Venous thromboembolic disease

3. Which of the following statements about fibromuscular dysplasia is *false*?
   a. Most types have a "string-of-beads" appearance on angiography
   b. The most commonly affected vessel is the renal artery
   c. Fibromuscular dysplasia may cause stenosis but rarely causes aneurysms or dissection
   d. Renal artery fibromuscular dysplasia can often be treated with balloon angioplasty
   e. Hypertension is common when renal fibromuscular dysplasia is severe

4. Which statement about Takayasu arteritis and temporal arteritis is *false*?
   a. Both are associated with sudden blindness if steroids are not given
   b. Both show giant cells on pathologic specimen
   c. Both affect primarily the large arteries
   d. Both may be associated with an increased sedimentation rate
   e. Both may "burn out" and become inactive over time

5. Which of the following is *not* associated with lymphedema?
   a. Filariasis
   b. Cancer
   c. Infection
   d. Radiation therapy
   e. Steroids

6. Which of the following is *not* a sign of acute arterial occlusion involving a digit or limb?
   a. Pain
   b. Pitting edema
   c. Pallor
   d. Paresthesias
   e. Paralysis

7. In thoracic outlet syndrome, most symptoms are caused by which of the following?
   a. Intermittent compression of the nerve
   b. Intermittent compression of the artery
   c. Intermittent compression of the veins
   d. Continuous compression of the artery
   e. Continuous compression of the vein

8. Which statement about vascular ulcers is *false*?
   a. Venous ulcers usually occur on the medial malleolus
   b. Diabetic ulcers are usually painful
   c. Ischemic ulcers are usually associated with atherosclerosis
   d. Arteriolar ulcers may be produced by hypertension, vasculitis, or collagen vascular diseases
   e. Certain tumors or infections can mimic vascular ulcers

9. Which statement is *false*?
   a. Microemboli commonly originate from peripheral vessels
   b. Microemboli are often cholesterol particles from arterial plaques
   c. Plaque rupture may occur spontaneously or as the result of trauma
   d. Microemboli can usually be treated effectively with lytic agents or anticoagulants
   e. Microemboli cannot be removed surgically

10. Which one of the following statements about Buerger disease (thromboangiitis obliterans) is false?
    a. Thromboangiitis obliterans usually affects small distal arteries before affecting larger, proximal arteries
    b. The disease can affect upper or lower extremities
    c. An initial manifestation of Buerger disease may be superficial thrombophlebitis
    d. Buerger disease is often associated with aortic dissection
    e. Buerger disease is usually associated with smoking but not with excessive alcohol use

ANSWERS

1. Answer d.

Vasculitis, atherosclerosis, Marfan syndrome, and fibromuscular dysplasia are all examples of processes that damage or weaken the arterial wall and lead to the formation of aneurysms. Cytotoxic drugs do not classically do this.

2. Answer a.

Smoking can predispose to atherosclerosis, clotting, vasospasm, and Buerger disease. It does not directly cause lymphedema.

3. Answer c.

Fibromuscular dysplasia both causes stenosis and may predispose to aneurysm formation or dissection.

4. Answer a.

Temporal arteritis is associated with sudden-onset blindness, but Takayasu arteritis is not. Steroids can prevent the blindness.

5. Answer e.

Steroids can cause edema, but they do not cause lymphatic blockage (lymphedema) the way the other processes can.

6. Answer b.

Pitting edema is not a sign of acute arterial occlusion. Pitting edema may occur in limbs (usually the lower extremity) with *chronic* edema because the patient keeps the limb in a dependent position in order to assist arterial inflow.

7. Answer a.

All of these can occur, but most symptoms (more than 90%) are caused by intermittent compression of the nerves of the shoulder.

8. Answer b.

Diabetic ulcers are classically painless.

9. Answer d.

Microemboli often contain cholesterol or fragments of atherosclerotic plaque. These agents do not dissolve with the use of lytics or anticoagulants. Surgery can be used to treat microembolic disease by removing the source of emboli, but it is not useful for opening the occluded small vessels.

10. Answer d.

Buerger disease usually affects distal arteries and small vessels, and it is not a classic cause of dissection.

NOTES

INDEX

Note: Page numbers in italics refer to figures; page numbers followed by "t" refer to tables.

A

Abdominal aortic aneurysms, 935–936
ABIM. *See* American Board of Internal Medicine
Absorption, toxic, prevention of, 139–140
  activated charcoal, 140
  gastric lavage, 140
  induced emesis, 139–140
Acanthosis nigricans, 181
ACE. *See* Angiotensin-converting enzyme
  hypertension and, 501
Acetaminophen, 143, *144*
  poisoning, antidote, 141
Acetylcholine receptor antibodies, 682
Acid-base balance
  arterial blood gases, 155–157
  Henderson-Hasselbalch equation, 155
  patterns, 156–157
    metabolic acidosis, 156
    metabolic alkalosis, 156–157
    mixed acid-base disorders, 157
    respiratory acidosis, 156
    respiratory alkalosis, 156
Acid-base disorders, 630–632, 632t
Acitretin, 176
Acquired immunodeficiency syndrome
  dementia with, 415
  gastrointestinal manifestations of, 311–312
    adenovirus, 311
    bacteria, 311–312
      Campylobacter jejuni, 312
      Mycobacterium avium, 311–312
      Salmonella, 312
      Shigella flexneri, 312
    fungi, 312
      Candida albicans, 312
      Histoplasma capsulatum, 312
    protozoa, 312
      Blastocystis hominis, 312
      Cryptosporidium, 312
      Entamoeba histolytica, 312
      Giardia lamblia, 312
      Isospora belli, 312
      microsporidia, 312
    viral, 311
      cytomegalovirus, 311
      herpes simplex virus, 311
  heart and, 55
  hematology, 479
  malignancies with, 574

neurologic complications, 689
  psychologic aspects of, 742–743
Acrodermatitis enteropathica, 184
Acromegaly, 209–210
  clinical features, 209
  endocrine diagnosis, 209
  etiology, 209
  pituitary tumor, 209–210
  radiologic diagnosis, 209
  therapy, 209–210
ACTH-producing tumors, 210
Actinomycosis, 530, 853
Activities of daily living, ability to perform, 408
Acyclovir, 587–588
Addison disease, 235–236
  mood disorder with, 738
Adenocarcinoma, 805
Adenocorticotropic hormone, function of, 203
Adenoma, toxic, 217
Adenovirus, with AIDS, 311
Adjustment disorder
  with anxious mood, 739
  with depressed mood, 735–736
ADL. *See* Activities of daily living
Adolescents, male hypogonadism, 246
Adrenal mass, incidentally discovered, 244–245
  diagnosis, 244
  etiology, 244
  therapy, 244–245
Adrenergic agonists, 777
Adrenergic inhibitors, hypertension, 498–500
Adrenocortical failure, 235–238
  adrenal crisis, 236
    management of, 237–238
  clinical features, 236
  diagnosis, 236–237
    endocrine, 236–237
    etiologic, 237
  etiology, 235
    Addison disease, 235–236
    secondary, 236
  therapy, 237–238
    acute illness coverage, 237
    primary adrenocortical failure, 237
Adrenocorticotropic hormone. *See* ACTH
Adult respiratory distress syndrome, 160t, 160–162, 161t
Advance directives, 167, 608–609, 609–610

Aging. *See* Geriatrics
Agoraphobia, 739
AIDS. *See* Acquired immunodeficiency syndrome
Air travel, 802
Airway management, 158, 163
Akathisia, 746
Alcohol, 148–149
  cardiovascular system, 88
  ethanol, 148
  ethylene glycol, 148–149
  hypertension, 496
  isopropyl alcohol, 148
  liver disease, 333–334
    cirrhosis, 334
    hepatitis, 333–334
  methanol, 148
Alcoholic myopathy, 671
Alcoholism, 744–745
Aldosteronism, primary, 240–242, 506
  clinical features, 240, 506
  diagnosis, 240–241, 506–507
  differential diagnosis, 241–242
  endocrine diagnosis, 240–241
  etiologic diagnosis, 241
  etiology, 240
  laboratory features, 506
  therapy, 242
Alkaline phosphatase liver test, 325
Alkaptonuria, 874
Allergic bronchopulmonary aspergillosis, 791. *See also* Pulmonary disease
Allergic contact dermatitis, 175–176
Allergic granulomatosis syndrome, 183
Allergy, 9–34
  asthma, 10–18
    acute, management of, 15–18, *17*
    allergic bronchopulmonary aspergillosis, 18, *18,* 18t
    angiotensin-converting enzyme, 12
    aspirin ingestion, 12
    atenolol, as allergen, 12
    beta agonists, 14, 15
    beta blockers, as allergens, 12
    chronic, management of, 15, *16*
    cigarette smoking and, 13
    corticosteroids, 14–15
      bronchial hyperresponsiveness, 13
    cromolyn, 10
    cytokines, characteristics of, 11t